Collins
Alternative
Health Guide

The A-to-Z, Everything-You-Need-to-Know Guide
to Conditions, Natural Remedies, Herbs, and Supplements

STEVEN BRATMAN, M.D.

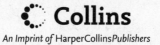 Collins

An Imprint of HarperCollinsPublishers

This book will educate the reader about medical conditions, natural herbs and supplements, alternative therapies and treatments, drug interactions, and diet and nutrition. It is designed to be informational and to help the reader be a more informed consumer of medical and health services. It should by no means be considered a substitute for advice from a medical or naturopathic professional, who should be consulted by the reader in specific matters relating to his or her health and particularly in respect to any symptoms which may require medical attention. While every effort has been made to ensure that selections of natural drugs, remedies, treatments, medicines, cures, and applicable dosages are in accordance with current recommendations and practices, because of ongoing research and other factors, the reader is cautioned to check with his or her health professional about specific recommendations for the reader's condition and needs. The author and publisher expressly disclaim responsibility for any adverse effects arising from the use or application of the information contained in this book.

COLLINS ALTERNATIVE HEALTH GUIDE. Copyright © 2007 by EBSCO PUBLISHING, INC. All rights reserved. Printed in the United States of America. No part of this book may be used or reproduced in any manner whatsoever without written permission except in the case of brief quotations embodied in critical articles and reviews. For information, address HarperCollins Publishers, 10 East 53rd Street, New York, NY 10022.

HarperCollins books may be purchased for educational, business, or sales promotional use. For information, please write: Special Markets Department, HarperCollins Publishers, 10 East 53rd Street, New York, NY 10022.

FIRST EDITION

Library of Congress Cataloging-in-Publication Data is available upon request.

ISBN: 978-0-06-112018-3
ISBN-10: 0-06-112018-9

07 08 09 10 11   WBC/RRD   10 9 8 7 6 5 4 3 2 1

CONTENTS

Herbs and Supplements

Alternative Therapies

Drug Interactions

WHAT MAKES THIS BOOK DIFFERENT?

The interest in natural medicine has never been greater. According to surveys, the majority of people in America use alternative therapies and yet it is hard for the consumer to find trustworthy sources of information about this field. Why? Frankly, natural medicine has had a checkered history. From snake oil potions sold at the turn of the century to those books, magazines, and product catalogs that hype miracle cures today, this is a field where exaggerated claims are too often standard practice.

Proponents of natural medicine have tended to abuse science, treating it more as a marketing tool than a means of discovering the truth. However, proponents of mainstream medicine too often exhibit prejudices in the opposite direction, requiring higher standards of evidence for alternative therapies than for unproven treatments that are a familiar part of conventional practice. What is needed is a level playing field where science rather than prejudice determines opinion.

In medicine, the only reliable source of truth is the double-blind, placebo-controlled study. In the last decade, there has been an exponential increase in such studies involving herbs, supplements, and other alternative therapies. At present, for a number of natural treatments, it is possible to give reasonably scientific answers to the questions: How well does this work? How safe is it? What types of conditions is it best used for?

The Collins Alternative Health Guide is designed to cut through the hype and tell you what we know and what we don't know about popular natural treatments. This book is more scientifically objective than most others available, more honest about the weaknesses and strengths of alternative medicine approaches, and more fair in its comparisons of natural and conventional treatments. You won't find any miracle cures here, but you will discover useful options that can help you become healthier.

Why Choose Natural Treatments?

Although the science behind natural medicine continues to grow, this is still a much less scientifically validated field than conventional medicine. One might ask, "Why should I resort to an herb that is only partly proven, when I could take a drug with solid science behind it?" There are at least three good reasons to consider natural alternatives.

First, a few alternative therapies may offer benefits that are not matched by any conventional drug. For example, evidence suggests that certain types of zinc lozenges may actually shorten the duration of the common cold. About no conventional treatment can this claim be made.

A second reason to consider natural therapies is that some may offer benefits comparable to those of drugs with fewer side effects. The herb St. John's wort is a good example. Very strong scientific evidence suggests that this herb is an effective treatment for major depression of mild to moderate severity, while producing fewer side effects on average than conventional medications. Saw palmetto for benign enlargement of the prostate, ginkgo for relieving symptoms of Alzheimer's disease, and acupuncture for the pain of tendinitis are other examples. This is not to say that alternative therapies are completely harmless—they're not—but for most the level of risk is quite low.

Finally, there is a philosophical point to consider. For many people, it "feels" better to use a treatment that comes from nature instead of from a laboratory. Just as you might rather wear all-cotton clothing than polyester or look at a mountain landscape rather than the skyscrapers of a downtown city, natural treatments may simply feel more compatible with your view of life. We can quibble endlessly about just what "natural" means and whether a certain treatment is "actually" natural or not, but such arguments are beside the point. The difference is in the feeling, and feelings matter. In fact, having a good feeling about taking an herb may lead you to use it more consistently than you would a prescription drug.

Of course, at times synthetic drugs may be necessary and even lifesaving. But on many other occasions it may be quite reasonable to turn to an herb, supplement, or alternative therapy instead of a drug.

To make good decisions you need good information. Unfortunately, while hundreds of books on alternative medicine are published every year, many are highly misleading. The phrase "studies prove" is often used when the studies in question are so small or so badly conducted that they prove nothing at all. You may even find that the "data" from other books comes from studies with petri dishes and not real people!

You can't even assume that books written by well-known authors are scientifically sound. Many of these authors rely on secondary writers, leading to a game of "telephone" where misconceptions are passed around from book to book. And there's a strong tendency to exaggerate the power of natural remedies, whitewashing them with selective reporting.

The Collins Alternative Health Guide gives you the balanced information you need to make informed decisions about your health needs. Setting a high standard of accuracy and objectivity, this book takes a realistic look at the alternative therapies you read about in the news. You will encounter both favorable and unfavorable studies in these pages and will learn about both the benefits and the risks of natural treatments.

The Collins Alternative Health Guide is the source you can trust.

                                    STEVEN BRATMAN, M.D.

INTRODUCTION

So that you can easily access the information you need, the Collins Alternative Health Guide is divided into four parts. *Part One: Conditions* contains information about hundreds of illnesses and health problems, from acne to warts. In each entry, you will find a description of the condition, as well as the various conventional treatments, herbs, supplements, and lifestyle changes that might help. Treatments that have fairly good evidence behind them or are widely used are called *Principal Proposed Natural Treatments*; the remainder are called *Other Proposed Natural Treatments*.

If you're interested primarily in herbs, vitamins, minerals, and other supplements, then turn to *Part Two: Herbs and Supplements*. For each herb or supplement, we discuss its various uses, the scientific evidence behind those uses, and dosage information, as well as safety issues of which you should be aware. If there is considerable evidence for a substance's effectiveness for a given condition, or if it is widely used for that purpose, that condition is listed under *Principal Proposed Uses*. Otherwise, it falls into the category of *Other Proposed Uses*.

Part Three: Alternative Therapies takes the same approach to other therapies such as acupuncture, chiropractic, and massage.

In some cases, use of natural therapies can interfere with the actions of medications, while in other cases, supplementation may be beneficial. In *Part Four: Drug Interactions*, we discuss possible harmful and helpful interactions between drugs and herbs or supplements.

Throughout the book, you will see terms in boldface. This means that there is a section about this subject in one of the other parts. For example, if you're reading about a condition and a treatment for it is listed in boldface, you can turn to the page mentioned in parentheses to learn more about that treatment in general, including its history, current uses, the scientific studies performed, and dosage and safety information.

Resources Used

The Collins Alternative Health Guide is based on science, not opinion, anecdote, or folk wisdom. It relies fundamentally on the double-blind, placebo-controlled study. More than 10,000 such studies make up the foundation of this book. To print them in the book itself, however, would increase the book's size to an impractical extent and for this reason they cannot appear. We hope to mount them on the Internet in the future.

Why Does This Book Rely on Double-blind Studies?

At first glance, it might seem that you can discover whether a treatment is successful quite simply: just try it and see. However, a close analysis of the subject reveals that it's much harder to identify effective treatments than one might think. Decades of investigation have led scientists gradually to the conclusion that there's only one truly trustworthy source of information on whether a medical therapy really works: the double-blind, placebo-controlled study. The reasons behind this conclusion are complicated and run counter to almost everybody's intuition. Here, we explore this crucial topic in depth.

For a hint why double-blind studies are so important, consider the following examples: in medical trials of drugs used to treat the symptoms of menopause, many of the participants were given a fake treatment (placebo) without being informed that it was fake. The combined results of multiple studies showed that women given placebo experienced a 51% reduction in hot flashes! Similarly, in a large study of men with prostate enlargement, participants given placebo therapy showed significantly improved symptoms and maintained at least some improvement for a full two years.

Effects like these can be highly misleading to both physicians and patients. Suppose, for example, a physician prescribes a new drug for menopausal symptoms or prostate enlargement and his or her patients report wonderful improvements. Does this indicate that the drug is effective? Not at all. As we know from the results described in the previous paragraph, many patients will report improvement no matter what they are taking. Thus, a drug can seem to be effective even if it doesn't possess any healing powers beyond the power of suggestion.

For a particularly dramatic example of this phenomenon, consider what happened when orthopedic surgeon Bruce Moseley, team physician for the Houston Rockets, decided he needed to properly evaluate the efficacy of an operation commonly used to treat the pain caused by arthritic knees. This surgery involves scraping away rough areas in the knee's cartilage. It is widely believed to be effective and as many as 400,000 such surgeries are performed each year.

Moseley decided to see if the surgery really worked. He conducted a study in which five patients were given the real surgery and five were given fake surgery consisting of little incisions over the knee. He then followed his patients for two years.

The results were amazing. Interviews showed that pain and swelling were reduced just as much in the placebo group as in the group that received the real surgery. Four out of the five participants who experienced the fake surgery said it was so helpful they'd gladly recommend it to a friend. Glowing testimonials, in other words, mean nothing.

A follow-up trial of 180 individuals confirmed these results, and this surgical approach is on its way to well-deserved oblivion. However, if these properly designed trials had not been undertaken, surgeons might have continued to scrape arthritic knees. No doubt, there are other ineffective surgeries that pass for effective, as well as ineffective herbs, supplements, and alternative therapies.

The double-blind, placebo-controlled trial is the best way to eliminate such misleading results. Such trials are the foundation of modern evidence-based medicine, and they are the foundation of the information in the Collins Alternative Health Guide as well.

In the following discussion, we'll begin by exploring the many factors that can deceive medical researchers. We'll continue with an explanation of how the double-blind study design solves these problems. After that, we'll analyze the many difficulties involved in performing a meaningful double-blind study and properly interpreting the results. Finally, we'll look at other forms of scientific evidence, and explain their limitations.

Confounding Effects: Why Treatments Can Appear Effective Even When They Are Not

At least twelve factors tend to confound (confuse) the results of studies.

➣ Observer Bias

First, researchers tend to observe what they expect to observe, a confounding factor known as *observer bias*. One placebo-controlled study evaluated a new treatment for multiple sclerosis. The researchers behind this study added an interesting twist: while most of the physicians assigned to evaluate the participants for improvement were blinded, a few were not blinded and they knew which participants were receiving placebo. As it happened, the treatment proved to be no more effective than placebo. However, the unblinded physicians managed to "observe" a significant difference in outcome between patients on placebo and those getting the treatment under study. In other words, they imagined they saw improvement where they expected to see it. No doubt this happens frequently in the daily life of a practicing physician, who is never blinded. For this reason the professional opinions of practicing doctors are far less reliable than the outcomes of double-blind, placebo-controlled studies.

➣ Rosenthal Effect

Not only do observers' expectations influence their own observations, they can also cause study participants to behave in the way the observers expect. This is the *Rosenthal effect*, and it is startlingly powerful. In one famous set of experiments, graduate students were given several photographs and told to show them to their subjects. The subjects were supposed to rate their impression of the people in the photos on a scale whose extremes were "big success in life" and "utter failure in life." (The photos were selected from magazines and were intended to show rather normal people.)

Next, half the graduate student experimenters were informed by their professors that their subjects would rate most of the people in the photos as failures. The rest of the graduate students were led to expect their subjects to rate the photos as showing only successful people.

Almost invariably, subjects gave precisely the ratings experimenters expected. This is particularly amazing because the graduate students were only allowed to read a set speech to their subjects. They were not allowed to change a single word and did not do so. Apparently, they managed to communicate their expectations through small changes in inflection of voice.

➣ Reinterpretation Effect

One of the reasons study participants respond to observer expectation in medical studies is a desire to please their physician. Patients tend to stress improvements and downplay problems if that's what they sense the doctor wants to hear. This does not necessarily involve lying. Participants may simply reinterpret their own experience to show improvement. A good example of this reinterpretation effect occurs when you take vitamin C over the winter and then decide, no matter how many colds you had, you would have gotten more if you didn't use the vitamin C. You don't really know this, but you may tell yourself it is true nonetheless.

➣ *Placebo Effect*

An entirely different possibility is that the power of suggestion may actually improve your health. This is the concept of the placebo effect. It may be, for example, that if you expect your knee arthritis to improve, it really will improve, through the power of the mind. (The concept of the placebo effect has recently undergone serious challenge, but it probably does occur at least to some extent.)

➣ *Memory Distortion*

Memory distortion effects also influence the apparent outcome of treatments. Physicians (like everyone else) have a tendency to remember their greatest successes and most extreme failures and drop from their memory everything in between. This can lead to a very skewed recall of the effectiveness of a treatment. Suppose a surgery works dramatically 15 times, fails absolutely 5 times, and yields mediocre results in the great majority of patients. The surgeon will most likely recall the surgery as highly effective.

➣ *Cognitive Dissonance*

Cognitive dissonance is another influence that makes physician impression unreliable. It is a well-established principle of experimental psychology that if you state out loud that something is true (for example, that a treatment is effective), your mind will jump through hoops to make you experience the results as consistent with your beliefs. If you make your living doing something, you will similarly experience a strong tendency to believe that what you are doing really works.

➣ *Natural Course of the Disease: Illusion of Agency*

Another major confusing influence is the natural course of the disease. Many diseases eventually run their course and symptoms improve on their own. This can give a false impression that a treatment has worked. However, due to a very powerful psychological tendency called the *illusion of agency*, a doctor will tend to feel that his or her efforts caused this improvement.

➣ *Regression Toward the Mean*

A related effect is called *regression toward the mean*. This term refers to a statistical principle. Simply put, most objective measurements of the state of the body fluctuate over time. Cholesterol level is a good example. People who are admitted to a study because their cholesterol levels are high may simply have high cholesterol at the moment they were tested for the study. During the subsequent several months, their cholesterol level will naturally move up and down. Suppose they happened to have been caught at a time of particularly high levels at the beginning of the study. By the end of that study, odds are they will show a lower reading. You might object that the effect should be symmetrical, and they just as well could have been caught at a low cholesterol moment at the beginning of the study. However, if that had been the case, they wouldn't have been allowed to participate in the study, because they wouldn't appear to have high cholesterol. Thus, this effect tends to produce an impression of improvement when in fact what is being observed is simply the workings of chance.

➣ *Study Effect*

Another influence is called the *study effect*. Individuals in scientific studies (or under the care of a physician generally) often feel motivated to take better care of themselves overall. If you have diabetes, for example, and you enroll in a study of a new diabetes treatment, you may subconsciously begin to take your insulin shots more religiously, control your diet more enthusiastically, and make sure that you don't miss any doctors' appointments. The net result may be an improvement in symptoms that has nothing to do with a specific therapy under study.

➣ *Study Dropouts*

Finally, participants with bad results may drop out of a study (or stop going to a physician), while those with good results remain. This will tend to bias the apparent outcome toward more positive results.

All of these factors combine to make it immensely tricky to informally discover whether a treatment is effective. Neither a physician's clinical experience nor a patient's personal experience is particularly trustworthy. By the 1960s, researchers had begun to settle on an effective solution to this problem.

Enter the Double-blind Study

Medical researchers now agree that a treatment cannot really be said to be proven effective unless it has been examined in properly designed and sufficiently large double-blind studies.

In such experiments, half the participants are randomly assigned to receive the "real thing"—the treatment being tested. The other half receives a fake treatment designed to appear as much as possible like the real thing (the placebo control). Both participants and researchers are kept in the dark regarding which is which. Hence, they are both "blind"—resulting in the term *double-blind*.

If performed correctly, a double-blind study can eliminate all the confounding effects described above. If the people in the real treatment group fare significantly better than those in the placebo group, it is a strong indication that the treatment really works on its own merits.

Problems in Performing Double-blind Trials

However, conducting a proper double-blind, placebo-controlled study isn't easy.

One problem is that participants may be able to discern whether they are getting a real treatment or placebo. For example, the smell and taste of a liquid preparation of some herbs is distinctive. Creating a substance that looks and tastes similar but lacks any active ingredients is difficult. This means that it's possible for those in the treatment group to know they are taking the real thing and for those in the control group to know they are taking placebo. Technically, this is described as *breaking the blind* and it can invalidate the results of a study. Similar difficulties occur in studies of conventional medications. If a treatment causes side effects, participants and physicians may be able to tell whether they are part of the treated group rather than the untreated (placebo) group. A top quality study will report on the success researchers had in efforts to keep the participants "blind." Surprisingly, many studies of medications reported in prestigious medical journals fail to do so.

In addition, some treatments are difficult or impossible to fit into the double-blind format, and others may be impossible. Studies on therapies such as acupuncture, physical therapy, diet, surgery, chiropractic, and massage are quite challenging to design in a double-blind manner. How do you keep the acupuncturist or surgeon in the dark as to whether he or she is performing real or fake treatment? How do you make study participants unaware of what they are eating?

Even properly designed double-blind studies aren't perfect. For example, individuals willing to participate in studies may not be representative of the general population. This could skew the results. It's not clear what can be done to eliminate this issue.

☙ Statistical Significance

Another important issue regards a subject called *statistical significance*. Sometimes you will read that people in the treatment group did better than those in the placebo group but that the results were not statistically meaningful. This means you cannot assume that the results proved the treatment was effective.

Evaluation of statistical significance is a mathematical analysis used to ensure that the apparent improvement seen in the treated group represents a genuine difference, rather than just chance. Consider the following analogy: Suppose you flip one coin 20 times and end up with 9 heads. Then, you flip a second coin 20 times and count 12 heads. Does this mean that the first coin is less likely to fall with the head side up than the second coin? Or was the difference just due to chance? A special mathematical technique can help answer this question. The bottom line is that when study results look good but aren't statistically significant, they can't be taken any more seriously than the apparent "bias" of the coin that happens to fall heads more often when you flip it a few times.

A related issue is called *statistical power*. If a study enrolls too few people, the chance of discovering a true treatment effect diminishes. The number of enrollees necessary to identify a benefit depends on the strength of the treatment—a powerful treatment can be identified as effective in a relatively small study, but a modestly effective treatment may require hundreds of study participants to identify an effect. This effect is compounded when it is tricky to measure the benefits of a treatment.

Antidepressant drugs and herbs are a good example of a form of treatment requiring very large studies to demonstrate benefit. There are two reasons for this. First, in antidepressant studies, people given placebo typically show about 75% as much improvement as those in the treated group. Additionally, the method of rating depression severity—a questionnaire—is relatively coarse and subject to wide variations in interpretation. The net result is a great deal of statistical "noise." In consequence, numerous studies of antidepressants have failed to identify any difference between treatment and placebo. This doesn't mean that the drugs don't work—only that very large studies are necessary to show that they do work. Similarly, when small trials fail to find an herb effective, one shouldn't think they have proven it ineffective. They simply have failed to find it effective. Only relatively large negative trials truly prove that a treatment doesn't work. Small trials may simply lack sufficient statistical power to show benefit.

☙ Data Dredging

Another statistical problem involves what is called data dredging. Before performing an experiment, researchers are supposed to pick one or two hypotheses that their study will test. This is called the *primary outcome measure(s)*. For example, in a study of a treatment for Alzheimer's disease, the primary outcome measure may be the score on a given memory test. The researchers hypothesize that scores on this test will improve and then conduct the study to determine whether their hypothesis is correct.

Once a study has begun, however, there's a temptation to gather more information by applying numerous tests to the participants. These are called *secondary outcome measures*. In the Alzheimer's example, these may involve such ratings as questionnaire assessments of ability to perform a daily task, physician opinion of overall progress, caregiver assessment of overall progress, and other perfectly reasonable ways of evaluating the success of therapy. There is a problem, however, with using a multitude of secondary outcomes: by the laws of statistics, if you measure enough things, some will indicate improvement just by chance. Researchers who look at dozens of factors in hopes of finding evidence of improvement in a few of them are said to be engaged in *data dredging*. Only the results on the primary outcome measure are trustworthy. There is simply too much leeway to find favorable data by digging deep in the mass of other data recorded.

This is not a complete list of the challenges involved in designing a proper double-blind trial. There are numerous other tricky considerations, including ethical issues that interfere with an accurate determination of outcome. Nonetheless, when properly designed, the double-blind, placebo-controlled trial is the best method we have of objectively determining the effectiveness of a treatment.

Other Types of Studies

There are many other types of studies besides double-blind, placebo-controlled trials; however, none can be considered as reliable.

➢ *Double-blind, Comparative Trials*

Some double-blind studies compare a new treatment against an accepted treatment. If the comparative treatment is known to be effective beyond a shadow of a doubt and the new treatment proves equally effective, such a study can provide evidence of effectiveness. However, it is preferable that such studies should also include a placebo group to enhance their meaningfulness.

➢ *Single-blind Studies*

In a single-blind trial, even though participants are not informed of who is receiving real treatment and who is not, researchers know the difference. Studies of acupuncture are typically single-blind, because it is difficult to design a study in which acupuncturists can deliver fake acupuncture without knowing it. Similar problems apply in studies of modalities such as physical therapy, surgery, chiropractic, and massage.

The problem with single-blind trials is that they can't eliminate all the confounding factors described above. Some can be prevented by using blinded evaluators; in other words, the acupuncturists know who is receiving real treatment, but a separate researcher evaluates how well participants have improved and that researcher has no idea who received real treatment. Nonetheless, a single-blind study can't eliminate all confounding factors. The Rosenthal effect described above, for example, still has full sway to bias the results.

➢ *Controlled Studies Using an Untreated Group*

In some studies, a portion of the participants simply receives no treatment at all. Their outcome is compared to those who do receive treatment. Unfortunately, this form of study proves little. Every one of the confounding factors described above comes into play and the results almost universally indicate that the tested treatment is successful, regardless of what it is.

➢ *Observational Studies*

Double-blind studies involve giving participants a treatment; in other words, "intervening" in their lives. They all fall into the category of an *intervention trial*.

Observational studies (also called *epidemiologic* or *population studies*), on the other hand, simply follow large groups of people for years and keep track of a great deal of information about them, including diet. Researchers do not do anything to them; they just examine the collected data closely and try to identify which dietary and lifestyle factors are associated with better health and longer life. Researchers in these studies don't change anything; they simply observe what is already going on. Such studies have most often tried to find connections between what people eat and the development of different diseases. A few have looked at the effect of taking nutrition supplements.

Observational studies are often the only practical way to gain information about the long-term health effects of nutrition and lifestyle. As noted above, how would you set up a study with placebo diet in which neither participants nor researchers knew who was eating what? It's basically impossible.

Furthermore, when looking for changes in events like heart attacks, you need to enroll enormous numbers of people and you have to follow them for decades. It is simply very expensive and difficult to conduct double-blind studies that meet such requirements.

Thus, for many treatments, such as low fat diets, observational studies are the primary source of information on their effects. Unfortunately, the results of observational studies can be misleading. Consider, for example, an observational study that discovers the following piece of data: people who consume high levels of saturated fat develop more heart disease. Does this mean that reducing saturated fat in the diet will reduce heart disease risk? Not necessarily. It is quite possible that the saturated fat in the diet was an innocent bystander, not the cause of the heart disease. Perhaps people who eat a great deal of saturated fat also tend to exercise less and smoke more cigarettes than other people. Those habits, and not the fat, might play the most important role.

Researchers try to look closely at the data and eliminate such factors, but it can never be done perfectly. Knowing this, scientists reporting the results of observational studies tend to make very cautious statements, such as "high saturated fat intake is associated with increased heart disease," rather than "high saturated fat intake causes heart disease." However, the media will frequently rephrase the results to make them more impressive. This leads to the all-too-frequent situation in which scientists appear to change their minds from year to year. In many cases, it's not that the scientists have revised their opinion; just that those who report the studies (including physicians, who should know better) have drawn unwarranted, firm conclusions from them.

In the Collins Alternative Health Guide, when we report the results of observational studies, we add the caveat that they can't be taken as definitive proof.

Even Less Reliable Studies

An *in vitro* study is a trial that tests a substance in a test tube. Such studies are really only spurs for further research, as they don't prove that a treatment is effective in real life. An herb or supplement taken by mouth must be absorbed into the bloodstream, survive processing by the liver, and still manage to be effective when diluted by the fluids of the body. It's a long leap from a test tube result to a treatment that actually works.

Evidence from studies enrolling animals means more than evidence from *in vitro* studies. However, because animals may process nutrients and herbs differently than we do, the results can't be taken as completely reliable.

Sometimes a group of people are given a treatment and simply followed for a period of time to see if they improve. The results of such *open studies* mean practically nothing at all. Due to all the influences described above, one can expect even before conducting the trial that improvements will be reported. Such studies are mostly worthwhile for discovering harmful effects of new treatments.

The Limitations of this Book

Remember that no book can substitute for individualized medical care from a physician. Every person is different and has specific health needs only a doctor can assess. Furthermore, in many cases it is possible to use combinations of treatments—both natural and pharmaceutical—in sophisticated ways that cannot be described in a book of this type. The information contained in the following text should be regarded as an introduction, a suggestion for where to start.

CONDITIONS

Acne

RELATED TERMS: *Pimples*

PRINCIPAL PROPOSED NATURAL TREATMENTS: *Niacinamide Gel, Zinc*

OTHER PROPOSED NATURAL TREATMENTS: *Ayurvedic Medicine, Burdock, Chromium, Gugulipid, Red Clover, Selenium, Tea Tree Oil, Vitamin E*

The blackheads and sometimes painful pimples that we know as acne occur most commonly during adolescence, but they may persist into later life as well. There is much we still don't understand about what causes acne. We do know that during adolescence and other times of hormonal imbalance, such as around menopause, glands in the skin increase their levels of oil secretions. A combination of naturally occurring yeast and bacteria then breaks down these secretions, causing the skin to become inflamed and the pimples to eventually rupture. In severe cases, acne can lead to permanent scars.

Conventional treatment, which usually is quite successful, consists primarily of oral or topical antibiotics, cleansing agents, and chemically modified versions of **vitamin A**.

Note: Do not rely on any of the natural treatments discussed in this article to treat severe acne in which scarring is a possibility.

Principal Proposed Treatments for Acne

Zinc

Studies suggest that people with acne have lower-than-normal levels of zinc in their bodies. This fact alone does not indicate that taking zinc supplements will help acne.

Several double-blind, placebo-controlled studies have found zinc more effective than placebo but less effective than antibiotic therapy.

In one of these studies, 54 people were given either placebo or 135 mg of zinc as zinc sulfate daily. Zinc produced slight but measurable benefits. Similar results have been seen in other studies using 90 to 135 mg of zinc daily, although others failed to find that zinc helped.

Relatively weak evidence suggests that a lower and safer dose, 30 mg daily, may also be helpful.

A large double-blind trial (332 participants) compared 30 mg daily of zinc against a **tetracycline-family medication** often used for acne (minocycline at 100 mg daily). The results showed minocycline is more effective than zinc. Tetracycline taken at a dose of 250 mg daily, appears to be no more effective than zinc, but when taken at 500 mg daily it seems to be considerably more effective.

Keep in mind that the dosages of zinc used in most of these studies are much higher than daily requirements and have the potential for causing toxicity. Indeed, case reports indicate that people have made themselves extremely ill by taking zinc in hopes of treating their acne symptoms.

For more information, see the full **zinc** article.

Niacinamide

In a double-blind trial, 76 individuals with moderately severe acne were treated with either 4% **niacinamide** gel or 1% clindamycin gel (a standard antibiotic treatment). Niacinamide proved to be just as effective as the antibiotic over an 8-week trial period. However, because this study lacked a placebo group, its results are unreliable.

Other Proposed Treatments for Acne

Ayurvedic medicine has shown some promise for acne. One study evaluated the potential benefits of an herbal combination containing the following constituents: *Aloe barbadensis, Azardirachta indica,* **Curcuma longa,** *Hemidesmus indicus, Terminalia chebula,* **Terminalia arjuna,** and **Withania somnifera.** In this 4-week, double-blind, placebo-controlled study of 53 people with acne, combined topical and oral use of the herbal preparation significantly improved acne symptoms. Oral treatment alone was not effective.

Another controlled trial compared an extract of the Ayurvedic herb **guggul** against tetracycline for the treatment of acne and found them equally effective. Unfortunately, the study report does not state whether this trial was double-blind and, for this reason, the results are not reliable. (For information on why double-blinding matters, see **Why Does This Book Rely on Double-blind Studies?**)

Tea tree oil has antiseptic properties and has been suggested as an alternative to benzoyl peroxide for direct application to the skin. One study that compared the two treatments found benzoyl peroxide significantly more effective; tea tree oil also improved symptoms but, due to the absence of a placebo group, this trial cannot be taken as evidence that tea tree oil is effective.

Other commonly mentioned natural treatments for acne include **chromium**, **vitamin E**, **selenium**, **burdock**, and **red clover**. There haven't been any well-designed studies examining these treatments, however.

Herbs and Supplements to Use Only with Caution

Various herbs and supplements may interact adversely with drugs used to treat acne. For more information on this potential risk, see the individual drug article in the Drug Interactions section of this book.

Acute Bronchitis

RELATED TERMS: *Bronchitis (Acute), Chest Cold*
PRINCIPAL PROPOSED NATURAL TREATMENTS: *Essential Oil Monoterpenes (Oral), Pelargonium sidoides*
OTHER PROPOSED NATURAL TREATMENTS: *All Treatments Used for Colds or Asthma, Elecampane, Essential Oils (Inhaled), Ivy Leaf, Licorice, Marshmallow, Milk Avoidance, Mullein, Primrose-root and Thyme, Slippery Elm, Vitamin C, Yerba Santa*

The term *bronchitis* refers to inflammation of the major air passageways in the lungs, the bronchi. There are two principal types of bronchitis: acute bronchitis and chronic bronchitis. The latter is closely related to emphysema and is discussed in the article on **chronic obstructive pulmonary disease** (COPD). Acute bronchitis, the subject of this article, is a condition that frequently develops during the course of a common cold. Symptoms may include cough (dry or productive), sensation of heaviness in the chest, and difficulty breathing.

In recent years, it has become clear that, in many cases, symptoms of bronchitis represent temporary asthma brought on by a respiratory infection. For this reason, anti-asthma drugs are now commonly a major component of treatment. Antibiotics may be used as well.

Principal Proposed Natural Treatments

Essential Oil Monoterpenes

A fixed combination of essential oils has been extensively evaluated as a treatment for respiratory problems. This mixture, called *essential oil monoterpenes*, consists of cineole from **eucalyptus**, d-limonene from citrus fruit, and alpha-pinene from pine. Numerous double-blind, placebo-controlled trials, many of substantial size, indicate that essential oil monoterpenes can aid recovery from sinusitis, bronchitis, and other respiratory conditions.

One large study evaluated the effectiveness of essential oil monoterpenes for acute bronchitis. In this 2-week, double-blind, placebo-controlled trial of 676 people with acute bronchitis, participants received either placebo, essential oil monoterpenes, or one of two antibiotics. The results indicate that the essential oil mixture was significantly more effective than placebo and at least as effective as antibiotic therapy.

For more information, including dosage and safety issues, see the full **Essential Oil Monoterpene** article.

Pelargonium sidoides

An extract made from the herb *Pelargonium sidoides*, has undergone meaningful study as a treatment for a variety of respiratory problems. In one double-blind, placebo-controlled trial, 468 adults with recent onset of acute bronchitis were given either placebo or a standard alcohol extract of *Pelargonium sidoides* 3 times daily for a week. The results showed significantly greater improvement in symptoms in the treatment group as compared to the placebo group. On average, participants who received the real treatment were able to return to work 2 days earlier than those given placebo. A high dropout rate, however, somewhat diminishes the meaningfulness of these results.

For more information, including dosage and safety issues, see the full *Pelargonium* article.

Other Proposed Treatments for Acute Bronchitis

In a double-blind, placebo-controlled study of 150 people with acute bronchitis, a combination primrose-root and thyme extract significantly decreased the severity and duration of symptoms.

One double-blind, placebo-controlled study found that use of 200 mg per day of **vitamin C** enhanced recovery among 57 elderly patients hospitalized for respiratory conditions, including bronchitis.

Inhaled essential oils have a long, traditional use for respiratory infections. However, there is no more than scant preliminary scientific support for such treatments.

Numerous herbs have a reputation for helping bronchitis. These include **elecampane**, **ivy leaf**, **licorice**, **marshmallow**, **mullein**, **slippery elm**, and **yerba santa**.

It is widely believed by many proponents of alternative medicine that cow's milk and related dairy products increase mucus in the lungs and sinuses and should, therefore, be avoided by people with bronchitis problems. However, there has not been sufficient scientific investigation into this belief to either confirm or deny it.

Because acute bronchitis tends to develop during the course of a common cold, all of the natural treatments used to prevent or treat colds are worth considering. See the **Common Cold** article for detailed information on these options. In addition, because bronchitis is often a form of temporary asthma, the treatments discussed in the entry on **asthma** are worth considering as well.

Acute Mountain Sickness

RELATED TERMS: *Altitude Sickness, High-Altitude Sickness, Mountain Sickness*

PRINCIPAL PROPOSED NATURAL TREATMENTS: *None*

OTHER PROPOSED NATURAL TREATMENTS: *Antioxidants (Vitamin C, Vitamin E, Lipoic Acid), Glutamine, High-Carbohydrate Diet, Magnesium, Milk Thistle, Rhodiola rosea*

PROBABLY NOT EFFECTIVE TREATMENTS: *Ginkgo Biloba, Arginine*

Acute mountain sickness is a set of symptoms caused by the lower pressure and reduced amount of oxygen at high altitudes (above 7,000 feet). The symptoms are headache, dizziness, shortness of breath, fatigue, and nausea, or, in serious cases, extreme fatigue, impaired motor control, and fluid accumulation in the brain and lungs. In general, the greater the altitude and the more rapid the ascent, the greater the likelihood of severe symptoms. Many deaths on Mt. Everest and other high mountains can be attributed to the effects of altitude sickness. However, in most cases, altitude sickness is a benign condition that afflicts people from sea level when they go on a ski vacation or hiking in the mountains.

The best treatment for altitude sickness is prevention. Individuals planning an ascent of high mountains such as Mt. Everest should take as much time as possible to acclimate to the starting elevation. Keep in mind that full adjustment to the reduced oxygen content of the air may take several weeks. In general, ascents should be gradual: one recommendation suggests 2 days for an 8,000-foot elevation gain plus 1 day for each 1,000 to 2,000 feet afterwards.

However, such recommendations are not practical for people who fly to a vacation destination such as a ski resort and must deal with the effects of reduced oxygen all at once. To prevent or treat mild cases of altitude sickness, you should drink plenty of water and avoid alcohol, caffeine, and salty foods. If severe symptoms develop, the best response is to descend as rapidly as possible.

Conventional treatments include acetazolamide or dexamethasone for prevention or treatment of mild altitude sickness and nifedipine for people prone to pulmonary edema. Ibuprofen and related drugs may help with headache.

Proposed Natural Treatments for Altitude Sickness

A double-blind trial of 18 mountaineers climbing to the Mt. Everest base camp found that use of an antioxidant vitamin supplement (providing 1,000 mg of **vitamin C**, 400 IU of **vitamin E**, and 600 mg of **lipoic acid** daily) significantly improved symptoms of altitude sickness as compared to placebo. Treatment was begun 3 weeks prior to ascent and continued during the 10 days of climbing. However, this was a very small study and its results cannot be taken as reliable.

Two small double-blind trials found preliminary evidence that the herb *Ginkgo biloba* can help prevent altitude sickness. Based on these encouraging results, researchers conducted a large-scale, double-blind study enrolling 10 times more people than the total number enrolled in the other two trials combined. In this definitive trial, ginkgo failed to prove more effective than placebo. (The drug acetazolamide, however, did provide significant benefits.)

High-carbohydrate meals are sometimes recommended for preventing altitude sickness. The reasoning is that carbohydrate ingestion increases carbon dioxide production, which in turn stimulates an increased rate of breathing. However, studies on this treatment have resulted in contradictory results.

Magnesium, **glutamine**, and **milk thistle**, alone or in combination, have been suggested for altitude sickness, but there is no meaningful evidence that they work. The herb *Rhodiola rosea* has also been proposed as an altitude sickness treatment, but current evidence is more negative than positive. One study of the supplement **arginine** found that it *increased* elevation-related headaches.

Adolescent Health

RELATED TERMS: *Teenage Health*

Fortunately, the human body is strong during the teenage years. If it weren't, many of us wouldn't survive! Poor diet, lack of sleep, and, often, experimentation with alcohol and other drugs mark the teenage years of many people in our culture.

Many teenagers show marginal malnutrition in a number of vitamins and minerals. For this reason, taking a general multivitamin/multimineral supplement is perhaps the easiest important health-promoting step that any teenager should consider. For treatment of particular health problems especially relevant to teenagers, see the following articles:

Young Women:

- Acne
- Athlete's Foot
- Bladder Infections
- Canker Sores
- Cervical Dysplasia
- Cigarette Addiction

- Colds and Flus
- Depression
- Dysmennorhea
- Eating Disorders
- Endometriosis
- Fatigue
- Herpes
- Immune Function
- Insomnia
- Migraine Headaches
- Minor Injuries
- Premenstrual Syndrome (PMS)
- Rosacea
- Sports Performance
- Strep Throat
- Stress
- Sunburn
- Vaginal Infections
- Weight Control
- Yoga

Aging Skin

Young Men:

- Acne
- Athlete's Foot
- Canker Sores
- Cigarette Addiction
- Colds and Flus
- Fatigue

- Herpes
- Immune Function
- Insomnia
- Minor Injuries
- Sports Performance
- Strep Throat
- Stress
- Sunburn

Aging Skin

RELATED TERMS: *Photoaging, Sun-damaged Skin*

PRINCIPAL PROPOSED NATURAL TREATMENTS: *Alpha-hydroxy acids (AHAs), Antioxidants (Carotenoids, Green Tea, Milk Thistle, Oligomeric Proanthocyanidin Complexes [OPCs], Selenium, Soy Isoflavones, Vitamin C, Vitamin E)*

OTHER PROPOSED NATURAL TREATMENTS: *Acupuncture, Aloe, Arnica, Beta-carotene, Calendula, Chamomile, Dead Sea Minerals, Glucosamine, Gotu Kola, Niacinamide, PABA, Silicon, Thuja, Vitamin A, IGF-1, IGF-2, TGF-A, and other growth factors, "Growth Hormone Enhancers"*

HERBS AND SUPPLEMENTS TO USE ONLY WITH CAUTION: *St. John's Wort, Vitamin A (Among People Using Tretinoin)*

The substances collagen and elastin give skin its firmness and elasticity. With age, though, the collagen and elastin content of the skin gradually decreases. As a result, the skin becomes looser, weaker, less elastic, and drier. In addition, the fat pads under the skin begin to disappear. Wrinkles form and the skin begins to sag.

This gradual loss of structure has several causes: genetic programming (a built-in "clock" that causes aging), cumulative sun damage (photoaging), and direct chemical effects from **cigarette smoking** and/or abrasive chemicals. Sun damage additionally causes fine wrinkles that disappear when stretching the skin, surface roughness, mottled pigmentation, "liver" spots, and skin cancer.

In people who already have signs of aging skin and wish to reverse it, a number of treatments are available.

The drug tretinoin (retinoic acid, or Retin-A), a substance related to **vitamin A**, has been shown effective for reversing the fine wrinkles, splotchy pigmentation, and rough skin of sun damage.

The hormone estrogen is thought to help restore normal skin tone in menopausal women, but the evidence for this widely held belief remains weak.

More aggressive treatments for aging skin include injections of botulin toxin, dermabrasion, chemical peels, soft tissue augmentation, laser resurfacing, and GORE-TEX® threads. For detailed information on the relative merits and demerits of these methods, consult a dermatologist or plastic surgeon.

Principal Proposed Natural Treatments

Two classes of natural treatments have shown promise in the treatment of aging skin: alpha-hydroxy acids (AHAs) and **antioxidants**. However, the evidence that they work remains incomplete and AHAs can cause significant side effects.

Alpha-hydroxy Acids

Alpha-hydroxy acids, such as glycolic acid and lactic acid, are substances derived from fruit and dairy products. These are milder relatives of the substances used by dermatologists in chemical peels, which are designed to remove damaged layers of the skin. In recent years, cosmetic manufacturers have begun to add AHAs to numerous skin-care products.

Meaningful evidence in support of AHAs comes from one double-blind, placebo-controlled study reported in 1996. This 22-week study enrolled 74 women with sun-damaged skin. Participants received either 8% glycolic acid, 8% L-lactic acid, or placebo cream, and applied it to the face and forearm. Although participants showed improvements in each of the three groups, superior results were achieved with each of the AHA creams than with the placebo cream.

Another double-blind study compared estrogen cream, glycolic acid cream, and their combination against placebo. Both estrogen and glycolic acid improved skin aging.

AHAs are not always harmless. Possible side effects include burning, blistering, severe redness, swelling (especially in the area of the eyes), bleeding, rash, and increased sensitivity to the sun. There are also concerns that AHAs may increase risk of skin cancer. For all these reasons, the FDA is currently investigating the use of AHAs in cosmetic products to determine whether they should be reclassified as drugs.

Antioxidants

The ultraviolet light from the sun creates free radicals, naturally occurring substances that can harm many tissues of the body, including the skin. Antioxidants are substances that neutralize free radicals. On this basis, various antioxidants have been investigated for their potential usefulness in treating or preventing photoaging.

A small 3-month, double-blind, placebo-controlled study found benefit with a cream containing 5% alpha-lipoic acid. Use of this antioxidant substance improved several measures of aging skin as compared to placebo, especially skin roughness.

Preliminary studies, including one small double-blind, placebo-controlled study, have found that cream containing **vitamin C** produces positive changes in sun-damaged skin.

Oligomeric proanthocyanidin complexes (OPCs) made from grape seed or pine bark are also marketed for the treatment of aging skin. These substances, closely related to **bioflavonoids**, have strong antioxidant properties. They also appear to protect and strengthen collagen and elastin. These effects provide theoretical reasons to believe that OPCs might be helpful for the treatment of aging skin. Again, unfortunately, there are no reliable double-blind, placebo-controlled trials to consult.

In an 8-week, double-blind, placebo-controlled study

of 40 women who already had sun-damaged skin, combined use of oral **green tea** and a topical green tea cream failed to prove more effective than placebo in improving the condition of sun-damaged skin. Some possible benefits were seen in microscopic evaluation of skin condition.

Antioxidant substances have also been studied as aids to *preventing* sun damage.

Studies on laboratory animals found that topical vitamin C and **vitamin E** helped prevent burning on exposure to ultraviolet light.

One small, double-blind study found that 2 g of vitamin C and 1,000 IU of vitamin E taken orally for 8 days resulted in a modest decrease of "sunburn" induced by ultraviolet light. In addition, a 50-day, placebo-controlled study of 40 people found that higher doses of these vitamins provided a sun protection factor of about 2. (Compare this to the sun protection factor of 15 or higher in many sunscreens.) It appears that these vitamins must be taken together for best effect; when used alone they do not appear to work.

Oral use of **beta-carotene**, **lycopene**, and other **carotenoids** has shown preventive effects in some but not all studies. Benefits have also been seen with mixtures of various antioxidants taken together (vitamin E, carotenoids, and others).

Oral vitamin A has shown some promise for preventing skin cancer in people at risk for it, but the doses used in studies were quite high, considerably above current recommendations for the maximum safe dose. (**Note:** Do not use vitamin A along with the drug tretinoin (see Herbs and Supplements to Use Only with Caution below).

Because these antioxidants work in an entirely different manner from standard sunscreen, it appears reasonable to believe that they might offer a synergistic effect if taken with sunscreen. However, this hypothesis has not been studied.

Other substances with antioxidant actions that have shown some promise for treating or preventing aging skin include **milk thistle**, **selenium**, **soy isoflavones**, and **zinc**. However, the supporting evidence that use of these substances (taken either orally or topically) offers any benefit for the skin remains far too preliminary to be relied upon at all.

Other Proposed Natural Treatments

In a double-blind study of 50 women with signs of aging skin, use of topical **niacinamide** cream significantly improved skin appearance and elasticity as compared to placebo cream.

The substance **glucosamine** is widely used for osteoarthritis in part because it seems to help collagen regenerate. For this reason, it has been advocated as a treatment for aging skin. However, the only evidence that it works comes from one poorly designed study. In this single-blind trial, 72 women with symptoms of aging skin were divided into two unequal groups: a small group that received no treatment and a much larger one that received a proprietary mixture of glucosamine, amino acids, and minerals. The results indicated greater improvement in the treated group as compared to the untreated group. However, because this was not a double-blind, placebo-controlled study, the results cannot be taken as reliable.

The mineral **silicon** has also been proposed as a treatment for aging skin. In the one potentially meaningful published study, 50 women with sun-damaged skin were given either 10 mg silicon daily (as orthosilicic acid) or placebo for 20 weeks. Measurements of skin roughness and elasticity showed improvement in the silicon group as compared to the placebo group. However, this study, performed by the manufacturer of a silicon product, leaves much to be desired in design and reporting.

Numerous herbs and other natural products have been advocated for the treatment of aging skin, including **aloe**, arnica, **calendula**, **chamomile**, dead sea minerals, **gotu kola**, **PABA**, thuja, and **vitamin A**. Other products claim to contain biological substances called *growth factors*—with names such as IGF-1, IGF-2, TGF-A, TGF-B, EGF, and FGF—and go on to claim that these growth factors improve skin condition. Still others supposedly raise levels of human growth hormone in the body and, therefore, help produce youthful skin. However, there is no meaningful evidence that any of these treatments actually work.

So-called *acupuncture face lifts* are widely available for treating facial wrinkles. They involve a series of treatments in which fine needles are inserted into the face. However, there is no evidence to indicate this method produces any benefit.

Herbs and Supplements to Use Only with Caution

The herb **St. John's wort** contains a substance, hypericin, that increases the skin's sensitivity to the sun. For this reason, it is possible that use of St. John's wort could accelerate sun damage of skin.

People using the drug tretinoin (Retin-A) should not take high doses of vitamin A, as each might increase the toxicity of the other.

Alcoholic Hepatitis

RELATED TERMS: *Alcoholic Liver Disease, Hepatitis, Alcoholic; Liver Disease, Alcoholic*

PRINCIPAL PROPOSED NATURAL TREATMENTS: *Reduce alcohol consumption*

OTHER PROPOSED NATURAL TREATMENTS: *General Nutritional, Support, Magnesium, Milk Thistle, Omega-3 Essential Fatty Acids, Omega-6 Essential Fatty Acids, S-Adenosylmethionine (SAMe), Trimethylglycine (TMG)*

HERBS AND SUPPLEMENTS TO AVOID: *Beta-carotene (Excessive Dose), Coltsfoot, Comfrey, Germander, Greater Celandine, Kava, Kombucha, Pennyroyal, Prepackaged Chinese Herbal Remedies, Vitamin A (Excessive Dose)*

The liver is a marvelously sophisticated chemical laboratory, capable of carrying out thousands of chemical transformations on which the body depends. The liver produces some important chemicals from scratch and modifies others to allow the body to use them better. In addition, the liver neutralizes an enormous range of toxins. Without a functioning liver, you cannot live for long.

Unfortunately, a number of influences can severely damage the liver, of which alcohol is the most common. This powerful liver toxin harms the liver in three stages: alcoholic fatty liver, alcoholic hepatitis, then cirrhosis.

Although the first two stages of injury are usually reversible, cirrhosis is not. Generally, liver cirrhosis is a result of more than 10 years of heavy alcohol abuse.

Usually, alcoholic hepatitis is discovered through blood tests that detect levels of enzymes released from the liver. The blood levels of these enzymes—known by acronyms such as SGOT, SGPT, ALT, AST, and GGT—rise as damage to the liver (by any cause) progresses.

If blood tests show that you have alcoholic hepatitis (or any other form of liver disease), it is essential that you stop drinking. There is little in the way of specific treatment beyond this.

Principal Proposed Natural Treatments

Several herbs and supplements have shown promise for protecting the liver from alcohol-induced damage. However, none of these has been conclusively proven effective and cutting down (or eliminating) alcohol consumption is undoubtedly more effective than any other treatment. For information regarding natural treatments that can help people stop drinking, see the article on **alcoholism**. The alcoholism article also discusses the depletion of certain nutrients, which may affect people who consume enough alcohol to damage the liver.

Below, we concentrate on treatments used specifically to treat early liver damage caused by alcohol. Treatments for more advanced alcohol-induced liver damage are discussed in the liver cirrhosis article.

Numerous double-blind, placebo-controlled studies enrolling a total of several hundred people have evaluated whether the herb milk thistle can successfully counter alcohol-induced liver damage. However, these studies have yielded inconsistent results.

For example, a double-blind, placebo-controlled study performed in 1981 followed 106 Finnish soldiers with alcoholic liver disease over a period of 4 weeks. The treated group showed a significant decrease in elevated liver enzymes and improvement in liver structure as evaluated by biopsy in 29 subjects.

Two similar studies enrolling a total of approximately 60 people also found benefits. However, a 3-month, double-blind, placebo-controlled study of 116 people showed little to no additional benefit, perhaps because most participants reduced their alcohol consumption and almost half of them stopped drinking entirely. Another study found no benefit in 72 patients who were followed for 15 months. For more information, including dosage and safety issues, see the full **Milk Thistle** article.

Other Proposed Natural Treatments

The supplement **SAMe** has also shown some promise for preventing or treating alcoholic hepatitis, but as yet there is no reliable evidence to support its use for this purpose.

The supplement **TMG** helps the body create its own SAMe and has also shown promise in very preliminary studies.

Herbs and Supplements to Avoid

High doses of the supplements beta-carotene and vitamin A might cause alcoholic liver disease to develop more rapidly in people who abuse alcohol. Nutritional supplementation at the standard daily requirement level should not cause a problem. See the articles on **vitamin A** and **beta-carotene** for more information.

Although one animal study suggests that the herb **kava** might aid in alcohol withdrawal, the herb can cause liver damage; therefore, it should not be used by people with alcoholic liver disease (and probably not by anyone at all). Numerous other herbs possess known or suspected liver-toxic properties, including **coltsfoot, comfrey, germander, greater celandine, kombucha, pennyroyal,** and various prepackaged **Chinese herbal remedies.** For this reason, people with alcoholic liver disease should use caution before taking any medicinal herbs.

Alcoholism

RELATED TERMS: *Addiction, Alcohol; Chemical Dependency, Alcohol; Nutritional Support, Alcohol*

PRINCIPAL PROPOSED NATURAL TREATMENTS: *General Nutritional Support, Milk Thistle, SAMe*

OTHER PROPOSED NATURAL TREATMENTS: *Acupuncture, Kudzu, Passionflower, Phosphatidylcholine, Prickly Pear Cactus* (Opuntia ficus indica), *TMG*

HERBS AND SUPPLEMENTS TO AVOID: *Arginine, Beta-carotene (Excessive Dose), Kava, Kombucha, Prepackaged Chinese Herbal Combinations, Vitamin A (Excessive Dose), White Willow*

Alcoholic beverages present a perfect example of the ancient virtue of moderation. While small amounts of alcohol (the equivalent of one to two drinks daily) may actually enhance health, excessive consumption of alcohol wreaks gradual havoc throughout the entire body. The liver is often the first organ to show injury, followed by (in no set order) the brain, circulatory system, pancreas, stomach, and throat.

Conventional treatment of alcoholism involves nutritional support and various means to induce and maintain abstinence. Alcoholics Anonymous is the most effective known abstinence-promoting method, but other programs and techniques are also in use. The drugs acamprosate (Campral) and naltrexone (ReVia) have shown considerable promise. It is not clear whether disulfiram (Antabuse) actually offers any benefit.

Principal Proposed Natural Treatments

The herb milk thistle and the supplement SAMe have shown promise for protecting the liver from alcohol-induced damage. However, keep in mind that neither of these has been conclusively proven effective and that abstinence is undoubtedly more effective than any treatment. For additional information, see the articles on **alcoholic hepatitis** and **cirrhosis**.

In addition to damaging the liver, alcoholism causes a general depletion of nutrients. People who drink to excess (either because they have not quit drinking or because they are in the process of quitting), may benefit from supplementation.

Milk Thistle

Numerous double-blind, placebo-controlled studies enrolling a total of several hundred participants have evaluated whether milk thistle can successfully counter alcohol-induced liver damage. Unfortunately, most of the studies were flawed in design and reporting, and their results were less than consistent. At present, therefore, it is not possible to draw firm conclusions about milk thistle's usefulness for people who over-consume alcohol. For more information, see the full **milk thistle** article.

SAMe

The supplement S-adenosylmethionine (SAMe) has been proposed for the treatment of alcoholic liver disease, but there is as yet no meaningful evidence that it is effective. A 2-year, double-blind, placebo-controlled study of 117 people with alcoholic liver cirrhosis found that treatment with SAMe reduced mortality and/or the need for a liver transplant in those with less advanced disease, but not in the group as a whole. For more information, see the full **SAMe** article.

Nutritional Support

Chronic over-consumption of alcohol may lead to improper metabolism or outright deficiencies of numerous vitamins and minerals. For this reason, use of a **general nutritional supplement** may be advisable. (See, however, the warning regarding beta-carotene and vitamin A in Herbs and Supplements to Avoid below.)

Other Proposed Natural Treatments

In a double-blind study of 64 people, use of an extract made from the skin of the fruit of the prickly pear cactus *Opuntia ficus indica* significantly reduced hangover symptoms as compared to placebo. The greatest improvements were seen in symptoms of nausea, loss of appetite, and dry mouth. Overall, the rate of severe hangover symptoms was 50% lower in the treatment group as compared to the placebo. The researchers involved in this study hypothesized that hangovers are caused by inflammation and that the herb reduced inflammation.

Artichoke leaf is much better known than prickly pear cactus as a means of preventing hangover symptoms. However, the one double-blind study on the subject failed to find artichoke any more effective than placebo.

The supplement **trimethylglycine** (TMG) stimulates the formation of SAMe and might be helpful for alcoholic liver disease. However, no meaningful double-blind, placebo-controlled clinical trials have been reported.

The supplement **phosphatidylcholine** has been advocated as a treatment for early alcohol-related liver damage (especially fatty liver), but the results of highly preliminary studies have been inconsistent. One study in baboons even found evidence of *increased* liver toxicity.

Other herbs and supplements that have been proposed for protecting the liver, but only on the basis of extremely weak evidence, include **andrographis**, **barberry**, beet leaf, **boldo, dandelion, inositol, licorice, lipoic acid**, liver extracts, **N-acetylcysteine**, *Picrorhiza kurroa*, **schisandra, taurine, thymus extract**, and **turmeric**.

The herb **kudzu** has been widely advocated as an aid for quitting alcohol, based on studies using hamsters or rats. However, small double-blind studies in humans have yielded inconsistent results at best.

Acupuncture has also been proposed as an aid to alcohol withdrawal. However, study results have been contradictory and the largest trial failed to find any benefit. This 3-week, single-blind trial study of 503 alcoholics failed to find any difference between real ear acupuncture and placebo ear acupuncture. In addition, a 10-week, single-blind, placebo-controlled study of 72 alcoholics found no difference in drinking patterns or cravings between sham acupuncture and real acupuncture groups. Negative results were also seen in a similar trial of 56 participants, and in one of 48 people. However, a single-blind trial of 54 people did find benefit, as did a single-blind trial of 80 people.

The herb **passionflower** has been proposed as an aid to alcohol withdrawal, primarily on the basis of the study of people addicted to opiates.

Herbs and Supplements to Avoid

High doses of the supplements beta-carotene and vitamin A might cause alcoholic liver disease to develop more rapidly in people who abuse alcohol. Nutritional supplementation at the standard daily requirement level should not cause a problem. See the articles on **vitamin A** and **beta-carotene** for more information.

All forms of **vitamin B₃**, including niacin, niacinamide (nicotinamide), and inositol hexaniacinate, may damage the liver when taken in high doses. (Again, nutritional supplementation at the standard daily requirement level should not cause a problem.)

One animal study suggests that the herb **kava** may have value as an aid to alcohol withdrawal. However, people who abuse alcohol should probably not take kava at all; even in healthy people, the herb has caused severe liver damage.

Numerous herbs and supplements have known or suspected liver-toxic properties, including, but not limited to, **barberry**, borage, chaparral, **coltsfoot, comfrey, germander**, germanium (a mineral), **greater celandine, kombucha, mistletoe, noni, pennyroyal, pokeroot, sassafras**, and various herbs and minerals used in **traditional Chinese herbal medicine**. In addition, herbs that are not liver-toxic in themselves are sometimes adulterated with other herbs of similar appearance accidentally harvested in a misapprehension of their identity (for example, germander found in **skullcap** products). Other forms of contamination are possible as well. Blue-green algae species such as **spirulina** may at times be contaminated with liver-toxic substances called *microcystins* (for which no highest safe level is known).

Some articles claim that the herb **echinacea** is potentially liver-toxic, but this concern appears to have been based on a misunderstanding of its constituents. (Echinacea contains substances in the pyrrolizidine alkaloid family. However, while many pyrrolizidine alkaloids are liver-toxic, those found in echinacea are not believed to have that property.)

Whole **valerian** contains liver-toxic substances called *valepotriates*. However, valepotriates are thought to be absent from most commercial valerian products and case reports suggest that even very high doses of valerian do not harm the liver.

Herbs and supplements with the potential to irritate the stomach, such as **white willow** and **arginine**, should be used only with caution by people who consume excessive alcohol.

Allergies, Respiratory

Allergies, Respiratory

RELATED TERMS: *Hay Fever, Pollen Allergy, Seasonal Allergy*

PROPOSED NATURAL TREATMENTS: *None*

OTHER PROPOSED NATURAL TREATMENTS: *Acupuncture, Adrenal Extract, Ayurvedic Medicine, Bacopa Monniera (Brahmi), Barberry, Bee Pollen, Betaine Hydrochloride, Butterbur, Cat's Claw, Coleus forskohlii, Enzyme Potentiated Desensitization (EPD), Fish Oil, GLA (Gamma-Linolenic Acid), Hypnosis, MSM, Nettle Leaf, OPCs, Other Flavonoids, Quercetin, Rosmarinic Acid/Perilla Frutescens, Spirulina, Sublingual Immunotherapy (SLI), Tinospora Cordifolia, Topical Capsaicin, Traditional Chinese Medicine, Vitamin B$_6$, Vitamin B$_{12}$, Vitamin C, Vitamin E*

For other types of allergies, see Asthma and Eczema.

About 7% of all Americans suffer from hay fever, an allergic condition that can cause runny nose, sneezing, and teary eyes. It is known officially as *allergic rhinitis*, *allergic sinusitis*, or *allergic conjunctivitis*, depending on whether symptoms manifest mainly in the nose, sinuses, or eyes, respectively. Hay fever usually peaks when particular plants are pollinating or when molds are flourishing. People who suffer from year-round hay fever (*perennial rhinitis*) may be allergic to persistent allergens in the environment coming from such sources as dust mites, mice, and cockroaches.

Here's how hay fever works. In response to the triggers noted above, an individual prone to allergies develops an exaggerated immune response. Substances known as *IgEs* flood the nasal passages, white blood cells called *eosinophils* arrive by the millions and billions, and inflammatory substances such as histamine, prostaglandins, and leukotrienes are released in massive amounts. The overall effect is the familiar one of swelling, dripping, itching, and aching.

The mechanism of allergic response is fairly well understood. Why allergic people react so excessively to innocent bits of pollen, however, remains a complete mystery.

Conventional treatment for hay fever primarily involves non-sedating antihistamines and nasal steroids, and is usually quite effective.

Principal Proposed Natural Treatments

The herb butterbur is best known as a promising new treatment for migraine headaches. However, butterbur may also be helpful for allergic rhinitis.

In a 2-week, double-blind, placebo-controlled study of 186 people with intermittent allergic rhinitis, use of butterbur at a dose of three standardized tablets daily, or one tablet daily, reduced allergy symptoms as compared to placebo. Significantly greater benefits were seen in the higher dose group. Such "dose dependency" is taken as a confirming sign that a treatment really works.

In another double-blind study, 330 people were given either butterbur extract (one tablet three times daily), the antihistamine fexofenadine (Allegra), or placebo. The results showed that butterbur and fexofenadine were equally effective and both were more effective than placebo.

A previous 2-week, double-blind study of 125 individuals with hay fever (technically, seasonal allergic rhinitis) compared a standardized butterbur extract against the antihistamine drug certizine. According to ratings by both doctors and patients, the two treatments proved about equally effective. Unfortunately, this study did not use a placebo group.

Two much smaller studies produced inconsistent results. For more information, including dosage and safety issues, see the full **butterbur** article.

Other Proposed Natural Treatments

Several natural products have shown potential benefit for allergic rhinitis in one or more preliminary controlled trials. These include a freeze-dried extract of stinging **nettle**, probiotics, an extract of soy sauce (Shoyu polysaccharides), the herb *Tinospora cordifolia*, rosmarinic acid, a substance found in the herb **rosemary** and many other herbs, including **Perilla frutescens**, and an **Ayurvedic** herbal formula containing *Commiphora mukul, Tinospora cordifolia, Rubia cordifolia, Emblica officinalis, Moringa pterygosperma,* and *Glycyrrhiza glabra*.

Traditional Chinese herbal medicine has also shown some promise for allergies. Another traditional Chinese treatment, **acupuncture**, is commonly recommended for allergies, but a controlled trial of 40 people failed to find significantly more benefit with real acupuncture than with fake acupuncture.

One rather unusual study tested a nasal spray containing capsaicin, the "hot" in cayenne and other hot peppers. It's not clear how practical this is—researchers had to use local anesthetic in the nose prior to using the spray!

Highly preliminary evidence suggests **spirulina** may counter allergic reactions of the type involved in hay fever.

A sizable (112-participant) double-blind study of **vitamin E** at a dose of 800 mg daily for hay fever found modest benefits at best. A smaller study failed to find any benefits.

Vitamin C is often suggested as a treatment for allergies, but the research results are preliminary and somewhat contradictory.

Test-tube studies suggest that flavonoids—biologically active compounds found in many plants—may help reduce allergy symptoms. A particular flavonoid, **quercetin**, seems to be one of the most active. Many texts on natural medicine claim that quercetin works like the drug cromolyn (Intal) by stopping the release of allergenic substances in the body. However, while we have direct evidence that cromolyn is effective, there have not been any published studies in which people were given quercetin and their allergic symptoms decreased. It is a long way from test-tube studies to real people.

OPCs from grape seed or pine bark are also often said to be effective. However, an 8-week, double-blind trial of 49 individuals found no benefit from grape seed extract (dose not stated).

Adrenal extracts, **bee pollen**, *Bacopa monniera* (brahmi), **barberry**, vitamin B_6, vitamin B_{12}, **cat's claw**, *Coleus forskohlii*, **GLA**, **fish oil**, **MSM**, and **betaine hydrochloride** are sometimes recommended for hay fever, but there is as yet no significant evidence that they are effective.

An alternative to allergy shots known as *sublingual immunotherapy* (SLI) involves using allergenic substances placed under the tongue. Several double-blind, placebo-controlled studies indicate that SLI can improve symptoms of allergic rhinitis when the offending allergens are known. Treatment, however, may take 2 years to show significant benefit.

While SLI is fairly well accepted in conventional medicine, another form of "alternative" allergy shots remains firmly in the alternative medicine field: Enzyme Potentiated Desensitization (EPD). This method involves injections of allergens combined with certain enzymes. In one double-blind, placebo-controlled study, EPD failed to prove more helpful than placebo for seasonal allergic rhinitis.

In one study, self-hypnosis appeared to provide some benefits.

Alzheimer's Disease and Non-Alzheimer's Dementia

PRINCIPAL PROPOSED NATURAL TREATMENTS: *Acetyl-L-carnitine, Ginkgo, Huperzine A, Phosphatidylserine, Vinpocetine*

OTHER PROPOSED NATURAL TREATMENTS: *Aromatherapy, Carnosine, Citrulline, Choline or Phosphatidylcholine, Treating High Homocysteine, DHEA, Lemon Balm, N-Acetylcysteine (NAC), Sage*

Alzheimer's disease is the most common cause of severe mental deterioration (dementia) in the elderly. It has been estimated that 30% to 50% of people over 85 years old suffer from this condition. It's cause is not known. However, microscopic examination of the brains of people who have died of Alzheimer's shows loss of cells in the thinking part of the brain, particularly cells that release a chemical called *acetylcholine*.

Alzheimer's begins with subtle symptoms, such as loss of memory for names and recent events. It progresses from difficulty learning new information to a few eccentric behaviors to depression, loss of spontaneity, and anxiety. Over the course of the disease, the person gradually loses the ability to carry out the activities of everyday life. Disorientation, asking questions repeatedly, and an inability to recognize friends are characteristics of moderately severe Alzheimer's. Eventually, virtually all mental functions fail.

Similar symptoms may be caused by conditions other than Alzheimer's disease, such as multiple small strokes (called *multi-infarct* or *vascular dementia*), severe alcoholism, and certain more rare causes. It is very important to begin with an examination to discover what is causing the symptoms of mental decline. Various easily treatable conditions, such as depression, can mimic the symptoms of dementia.

Four drugs have shown at least modest benefit for Alzheimer's disease or non-Alzheimer's dementia: Reminyl, Exelon, Aricept, and Cognex. These medications usually produce a modest improvement in mild to moderate Alzheimer's disease by increasing the duration of action of acetylcholine. However, they can cause sometimes severe side effects due to the exaggeration of acetylcholine's action in other parts of the body.

Principal Proposed Natural Treatments

There are two natural treatments for Alzheimer's disease with significant scientific evidence behind them: ginkgo and phosphatidylserine. Huperzine A and vinpocetine, while more like drugs than natural remedies, may also improve mental function in people with dementia. Acetyl-L-carnitine was once considered a promising option for this condition as well, but current evidence suggests that it does not work.

Ginkgo

The most well-established herbal treatment for Alzheimer's disease is the herb *Ginkgo biloba*. Numerous double-blind, placebo-controlled studies indicate that ginkgo is effective for treating various forms of dementia. One of the largest was a U.S. trial that enrolled more than 300 participants with Alzheimer's disease or non-Alzheimer's dementia. Participants were given either 40 mg of *Ginkgo biloba* extract or placebo 3 times daily. The results showed significant (but far from dramatic) improvements in the treated group.

On the other hand, one fairly large study of ginkgo extract found no benefit. This 24-week, double-blind, placebo-controlled study of 214 participants with either mild to moderate dementia or ordinary age-associated memory loss found no effect with ginkgo extract at a dose

of 240 or 160 mg daily. However, this study has been sharply criticized for a number of serious flaws in its design.

For more information, including dosage and safety issues, see the full **Ginkgo** article.

Phosphatidylserine

Phosphatidylserine (PS) is one of the many substances involved in the structure and maintenance of cell membranes. Double-blind studies involving a total of more than 1,000 people suggest that phosphatidylserine is an effective treatment for Alzheimer's disease and other forms of dementia.

The largest of these studies followed 494 elderly subjects in northeastern Italy over a course of 6 months. All suffered from moderate to severe mental decline, as measured by standard tests. Treatment consisted of 300 mg daily of either PS or placebo. The group that took PS did significantly better in both behavior and mental function than the placebo group. Symptoms of depression also improved.

These results agree with those of numerous smaller double-blind studies involving a total of more than 500 people with Alzheimer's and other types of age-related dementia.

However, the form of phosphatidylserine available as a supplement has altered since the studies described above were performed and the currently available form may not be equivalent. For more information, including dosage and safety issues, see the full **Phosphatidylserine** article.

Huperzine A

Huperzine A is a chemical derived from a particular type of club moss (*Huperzia serrata*). Like caffeine and cocaine, huperzine A is a medicinally active, plant-derived chemical that belongs to the class known as alkaloids. This substance is really more a drug than an herb, but it is sold over the counter as a dietary supplement for memory loss and mental impairment.

According to three Chinese double-blind trials enrolling a total of more than 450 people, use of huperzine A can significantly improve symptoms of Alzheimer's disease and other forms of dementia. One double-blind trial failed to find evidence of benefit, but it was relatively small.

For more information, including dosage and safety issues, see the full **Huperzine A** article.

Vinpocetine

Vinpocetine is a chemical derived from vincamine, a constituent found in the leaves of common periwinkle

(*Vinca minor*) as well as the seeds of various African plants. It is used as a treatment for memory loss and mental impairment.

Developed in Hungary more than 20 years ago, vinpocetine is sold in Europe as a drug under the name Cavinton. In the U.S. it is available as a so-called dietary supplement, although the substance probably doesn't fit that category by any rational definition. Vinpocetine doesn't exist to any significant extent in nature. Producing it requires significant chemical work performed in the laboratory.

Several double-blind studies have evaluated vinpocetine for the treatment of Alzheimer's disease and related conditions. Unfortunately, most of these suffered from significant flaws in design and reporting. A review of the literature found three studies of acceptable quality, enrolling a total of 583 people. Perhaps the best of these was a 16-week, double-blind, placebo-controlled trial of 203 people with mild to moderate dementia which found significant benefit in the treated group. However, even this trial suffered from several technical limitations and the authors of the review concluded that vinpocetine cannot yet be regarded as a proven treatment. Currently, several better quality trials are under way.

For more information, including dosage and safety issues, see the full **Vinpocetine** article.

Acetyl-L-carnitine

Carnitine is a vitamin-like substance that is often used for angina, congestive heart failure, and other heart conditions. A special form of carnitine, acetyl-L-carnitine, has been extensively tested for the treatment of dementia: double- or single-blind studies involving a total of more than 1,400 people have been reported.

However, while early studies found evidence of modest benefit, two large and well-designed studies failed to find acetyl-L-carnitine effective at all. The first of these was a double-blind, placebo-controlled trial that enrolled 431 participants for 1 year. Overall, acetyl-L-carnitine proved no better than placebo. However, because a close look at the data indicated that the supplement might help people who develop Alzheimer's disease at an unusually young age, researchers performed a follow-up trial. This 1-year, double-blind, placebo-controlled trial evaluated acetyl-L-carnitine in 229 patients with early-onset Alzheimer's. Unfortunately, no benefits were seen here either.

One review of literature interpreted the cumulative results to mean that acetyl-L-carnitine may be mildly helpful for mild Alzheimer's disease. However, another

review concluded that if acetyl-L-carnitine does offer benefits for any form of Alzheimer's disease, they are too minor to make much of a practical difference.

For more information, including dosage and safety issues, see the full **Carnitine** article.

Other Proposed Natural Treatments

Two small double-blind studies performed by a single research group found evidence that the herbs **sage** and **lemon balm** can improve cognitive function in people with mild to moderate Alzheimer's disease.

One study found that **vitamin E** (dl-alpha-tocopherol) at the high dosage of 2,000 IU daily may slow the progression of Alzheimer's disease, but another did not. A physician's supervision is essential when taking this much vitamin E because of potential risks of bleeding complications.

Very preliminary evidence suggests that **N-acetyl-cysteine** (NAC) might also be helpful for slowing the progression of Alzheimer's disease.

Lavender oil used purely as **aromatherapy** (treatment involving inhaling essential oils) has been advocated for reducing agitation in people with dementia; however, people with dementia tend to lose their sense of smell, making this approach seem somewhat unlikely to work. Topical use of essential oil of the herb lemon balm has also shown promise for reducing agitation in people with Alzheimer's disease; the researchers who tested it considered their method aromatherapy because the fragrance wafts up from the skin, but essential oils are also *absorbed* through the skin and this mechanism of action seems more plausible. Oral use of lemon balm extract has also shown promise.

As we explained at the beginning of this article, drugs used for Alzheimer's disease affect levels of acetylcholine in the body. The body makes acetylcholine out of the nutrient choline. On this basis, supplements containing choline or the related substance **phosphatidylcholine** have been proposed for the treatment of Alzheimer's disease, but the results of studies have not been positive. One special form of choline, however, has shown more promise. In a 6-month, double-blind study of 261 people with Alzheimer's disease, use of choline alfoscerate at a dose of 400 mg 3 times daily significantly improved cognitive function as compared to placebo.

Elevated blood levels of the substance **homocysteine** have been suggested as a contributor to Alzheimer's disease and multi-infarct dementia. However, a double-blind, placebo-controlled study failed to find that homocysteine-lowering treatment using B-vitamins was helpful for multi-infarct dementia.

Bee pollen, carnosine, citrulline, DMAE, inositol, magnesium, pregnenolone, vitamin B$_1$, and **zinc** have also been suggested as treatments for Alzheimer's disease. However, as yet there is no reliable scientific evidence to support their use.

Early reports suggested that declining levels of the hormone **DHEA** cause impaired mental function in the elderly. On this basis, DHEA has been promoted as a cognition-enhancing supplement. However, the one double-blind study that tested DHEA for Alzheimer's disease found little to no benefit.

Colistrinin, a substance derived from **colostrum,** has shown some promise for treatment of Alzheimer's.

Amenorrhea

RELATED TERMS: *Menstruation, Absence*

PRINCIPAL PROPOSED NATURAL TREATMENTS: *None*

OTHER PROPOSED NATURAL TREATMENTS: *Progesterone, Chasteberry, Alfalfa Seed, Angelica, Asafetida, Blue Cohosh, Bugleweed, Motherwort, Parsley, Rue, Vitamin B$_6$, Zinc*

HERBS AND SUPPLEMENTS TO AVOID: *Flaxseed, Lignans*

The term *amenorrhea* literally means "an absence of menstrual bleeding." In medicine, it is used to indicate one of two conditions: the cessation of menstrual cycle in a woman of menstrual age or the failure to develop a menstrual cycle at all in a young woman who has reached the age of 16 years old. This article only addresses the first of these conditions, technically called *secondary amenorrhea.* To avoid using this lengthy term, we will simply refer to the condition here as *amenorrhea.*

There are many causes of amenorrhea. Severe weight loss, such as may occur in a woman with anorexia nervosa, can cause the menstrual period to stop. So can extreme exercise, such as marathon running, bodybuilding, or professional-caliber ballet dancing.

Young women who go to college may develop amenorrhea too, possibly from stress or perhaps as a reflex reaction to what the body considers a "migration." Pregnancy and nursing stop the menstrual cycle by design. Finally, women who have used oral contraceptives may find that it takes a while for a normal menstrual cycle to return after discontinuing them.

More rarely, amenorrhea may indicate a serious medical condition, such as a disorder of the pituitary gland, the hypothalamus, or the ovaries. For this reason, it's a good idea to check with your doctor if you miss more than one menstrual period to see if more evaluation is needed. Medical treatment for amenorrhea depends on the cause. If examination reveals no underlying cause, physicians may recommend a period of oral contraceptive use to start up the cycle.

Proposed Natural Treatments

The hormone **progesterone,** available (probably inappropriately) as an ingredient in some "natural" creams, may help restore the menstrual cycle. In one double-blind, placebo-controlled trial, oral use of a micronized form of progesterone restored a normal menstrual cycle in women with secondary amenorrhea. However, although progesterone is marketed as a "natural hormone," it is as much a drug as estrogen and should never be used without medical supervision.

In some women, the pituitary gland produces excess levels of prolactin. Prolactin is a hormone that naturally rises during pregnancy to stimulate milk production; it can also cause amenorrhea. Excessive pituitary prolactin release is a condition that must be investigated medically because it may indicate the presence of a tumor. However, it is possible that slight abnormalities in prolactin level without a dangerous medical cause may trigger amenorrhea in some women. The herb **chasteberry** is thought to reduce prolactin levels and, for this reason, it has been tried for amenorrhea. However, as yet no double-blind, placebo-controlled trials on this potential use of chasteberry have been reported. The herb **bugleweed** is also thought to reduce prolactin levels, but it too has not been tested for amenorrhea.

Other commonly proposed natural treatments for amenorrhea include the supplements **vitamin B$_6$** and **zinc** and the herbs **blue cohosh**, angelica, asafetida, alfalfa seed, motherwort, **parsley**, and rue. However, there is no meaningful scientific evidence to indicate whether they are effective.

For reasons that are not entirely clear, women with amenorrhea often have an accelerated rate of bone loss, potentially leading to osteoporosis. Women who have developed amenorrhea due to heavy exercise tend to experience an accelerated rate of bone loss, which may lead to osteoporosis. Unfortunately, calcium and vitamin D supplements are not sufficient to protect bone mass under these circumstances. Stronger measures, such as reducing exercise or using medications, may be necessary.

Herbs and Supplements to Avoid

Substances called *lignans*, found in many foods but most especially in flax seeds, may increase levels of prolactin. As noted above, this could tend to cause amenorrhea.

Finally, certain herbs and supplements may interact with oral contraceptive drugs used to treat amenorrhea. For more information, see the **Oral Contraceptive** article in the Drug Interactions section of this book.

Amyotrophic Lateral Sclerosis

RELATED TERMS: *Lou Gehrig's Disease, ALS*

PRINCIPAL PROPOSED NATURAL TREATMENTS: *None*

OTHER PROPOSED NATURAL TREATMENTS: *BCAAs, CoenzymeQ$_{10}$, Genistein, Guanidine, Multivitamins, L-Threonine, Vitamin B$_{12}$*

PROBABLY NOT EFFECTIVE: *Creatine, Vitamin E*

Amyotrophic lateral sclerosis (ALS) is a nerve disorder that causes progressive muscle weakness. It usually begins with weakness in the hands or feet, which then spreads to the rest of the body. Affected muscles become spastic (tight and prone to spasm) and ineffective. As the weakness spreads, speaking, breathing, and swallowing become difficult. Most people die within 3 years of being diagnosed. However, for reasons that are unclear, some individuals (such as the physicist Stephen Hawking) live much longer.

The cause of ALS is unknown and there is no cure for the disorder. Physical therapy can help the muscles maintain strength and flexibility for a time. Drugs such as baclofen may reduce muscle spasms and cramping. Eventually, individuals with ALS must be fed through a tube and sustained on a ventilator.

Proposed Natural Treatments

Vitamin E

Vitamin E is a potent antioxidant, capable of fighting dangerous natural substances known as *free radicals*. It has been hypothesized that free radicals might play a role in ALS and that, therefore, antioxidants might slow the progression of the disease.

Based on this theory, a 1-year, double-blind, placebo-controlled trial of 289 people with ALS was conducted in which participants were given the drug riluzole plus either vitamin E (alpha-tocopherol, 500 mg twice daily) or placebo. However, to the disappointment of researchers, use of vitamin E failed to improve survival time or measurably improve movement ability.

By looking closely at the data, the researchers did manage to find one benefit: according to one measurement of disease severity, vitamin E did appear to delay the progression of mild ALS to its more severe form. Unfortunately, this finding is quite likely a statistical fluke: when researchers look at enough measures of a disease, benefit will tend to be seen in one or two simply as the result of chance.

Some vitamin E proponents felt that the dose of vitamin E used in this study might have been too low. Researchers therefore conducted another study using *10 times* the dose, this one lasting 18 months and enrolling 160 people. Once again, vitamin E failed to prove significantly more effective than placebo.

One study supposedly found that vitamin E along with high consumption of polyunsaturated fats reduced the risk of developing ALS, but the study was in fact too low in quality to provide any meaningful evidence at all.

Branched-chain Amino Acids

Branched-chain amino acids (BCAAs) are most well-known as a **sports supplement**, but have also been tried as a treatment for ALS. The theory behind this treatment is that people with ALS might not metabolize the substance glutamate properly. Glutamate plays a major role in nerve function. Since BCAAs help the body to metabolize glutamate, they could be useful for ALS. However, at best, BCAAs have been found only modestly effective in ALS and study results have been mixed.

One very small double-blind, placebo-controlled study found that people treated with BCAAs for 1 year maintained muscle strength and the ability to walk longer than those on placebo. However, other studies found no effect and one actually found a slight increase in deaths during the study period among those treated with BCAAs compared to placebo.

L-Threonine

L-Threonine, an essential amino acid, has been tried for ALS because, like BCAAs, it affects glutamate metabolism. Open trials and one double-blind study have shown some short-term improvement in symptoms, but in other research the results have not been impressive.

Creatine

Another sports supplement, **creatine**, has been tried for ALS based on studies showing that it can improve muscle performance in certain situations. Evidence from animal and open human trials had suggested that creatine improved strength and slowed the progression of the disease and for these reasons many people with ALS have tried it. However, hopes raised by these findings were dashed in 2003 when the results of a 10-month, double-blind, placebo-controlled trial of 175 people with ALS were announced. Use of creatine at a dose of 10 g daily failed to provide any benefit at all in terms of symptoms or disease progression.

Creatine also failed to prove effective in another study, this one enrolling 104 people and using a dose of 5 g daily for 6 months.

Other Natural Treatments

Other nutrients that have been tried for ALS with some promising results in extremely preliminary research include **vitamin B$_{12}$**, **CoenzymeQ$_{10}$**, **genistein**, and guanidine. However, there is no solid evidence as yet that they are effective.

Non-nutrient nutritional supplements have been tried for ALS but have failed to prove effective in studies. These include **multivitamins**, AMP, and **policosanol**.

One very small trial tested a combination pill containing amino acids, antioxidants, and the calcium-channel blocker nimodipine, finding some evidence that it might slow the progression of the disease.

Angina

PRINCIPAL PROPOSED NATURAL TREATMENTS: *L-Carnitine and L-Propionyl-Carnitine, Magnesium*

OTHER PROPOSED NATURAL TREATMENTS: *Arginine, Coenzyme Q$_{10}$ (CoQ$_{10}$),* Coleus forskohlii, *Fish Oil, Glutamine, Hawthorn, Khella, Vitamin E,* Terminalia arjuna

PROBABLY NOT EFFECTIVE TREATMENTS: *Chelation Therapy*

Essentially, angina is a muscle cramp in the heart—the one muscle that cannot take a rest. It develops when the heart muscle does not receive enough oxygen for its needs from the arteries that supply it: the coronary arteries. Angina is, therefore, a symptom of coronary artery disease. Atherosclerosis is the most common cause

of coronary artery disease; it causes thickened arterial walls and impaired blood flow.

People usually experience angina as a squeezing chest pain, as if a heavy weight rested on the chest or a tight band wrapped around it. This is often accompanied by sweating, shortness of breath, and possibly pain radiating into the left arm or neck. Usually, angina is brought on by exercise—the more rapidly the heart pumps, the more oxygen it needs. Atherosclerosis (hardening of the arteries) is the most common cause of angina.

People with angina are at high risk for a **heart attack** and treatment must take that into account. Drugs that expand (dilate) the heart's arteries, such as nitroglycerin, can give immediate relief. Other drugs help over the long term by making the heart's work easier. It is also important to slow or reverse the progression of atherosclerosis by treating high blood pressure and high cholesterol, and by reducing other risk factors. Surgical treatments (such as angioplasty and coronary artery bypass grafting) physically widen the blood vessels that feed the heart.

Principal Proposed Natural Treatments

Angina is a serious disease that absolutely requires conventional medical evaluation and supervision. No one should self-treat for angina. However, alternative treatments may provide a useful adjunct to standard medical care when monitored by an appropriate health-care professional. We intentionally do not give dosages in this section as they should be individualized by your physician; however, you can find general guidelines in the separate articles on each substance.

Note: Because angina is usually caused by atherosclerosis, other relevant information may be found in the **Atherosclerosis** article.

L-Carnitine

The vitamin-like substance L-carnitine might be a good addition to standard therapy for angina. Carnitine plays a role in the cellular production of energy. Although carnitine does not address the cause of angina, it appears to help the heart produce energy more efficiently, thereby enabling it to get by with less oxygen.

In one controlled study, 200 individuals with angina (the exercise-induced variety) received either a daily dose of L-carnitine or were left untreated. All the study participants continued to take their usual medication for angina. Those taking carnitine showed improvement in several measures of heart function, including a significantly greater ability to exercise without chest pain. They were also able to reduce the dosage of some of their heart medications (under medical supervision) as their symptoms decreased.

Unfortunately, the results of this study can't be fully trusted, because it didn't use a double-blind, placebo-

controlled design. (For information on why double studies are so important, see **Why Does This Book Rely on Double-blind Studies?**.) A smaller trial that did use a double-blind, placebo-controlled format evaluated 52 people with angina. The results showed that daily use of L-carnitine significantly improved symptoms as compared to placebo.

Other studies (both single- and double-blind) used a special form of L-carnitine called *L-propionyl-carnitine* and found evidence of benefit. Consult with your physician regarding dosage and specific safety issues.

For more information, including dosage and safety issues, see the full **L-carnitine** article.

Magnesium

Magnesium has actions in the body that resemble those of drugs in the **calcium channel blocker family**, although much weaker. Since these drugs are useful for angina, magnesium has been tried as well.

In a 6-month, double-blind, placebo-controlled study, 187 individuals with angina were given either daily oral magnesium or placebo. The results showed that use of magnesium significantly improved exercise capacity, lessened exercise-induced chest pain, and improved general quality of life.

Similarly, a double-blind, placebo-controlled trial of 50 individuals with coronary artery disease found that supplementation with magnesium significantly improved exercise tolerance.

For more information, including dosage and safety issues, see the full **magnesium** article.

Other Proposed Treatments for Angina

A 1-week, double-blind, placebo-controlled crossover trial of 58 people evaluated the effectiveness of the herb *Terminalia arjuna* for angina by comparing it against placebo and the standard drug isosorbide mononitrate. The results indicated that the herb reduced anginal episodes and increased exercise capacity. It was more effective than placebo and approximately as effective as the medication. A subsequent 3-month study compared the effectiveness of *Terminalia arjuna* against placebo in 40 people with a recent heart attack. All participants in this study suffered from a particular complication of a heart attack called *ischaemic mitral regurgitation*. The results showed that use of the herb improved heart function and reduced angina symptoms. Another study found benefits with an **Ayurvedic** herbal combination containing *Terminalia arjuna*.

Preliminary evidence suggests that the amino acids **arginine** and glutamine might improve exercise tolerance in angina. **Coenzyme Q$_{10}$** (CoQ$_{10}$) is best known as a treatment for congestive heart failure, but it may offer benefits in angina as well.

N-acetyl cysteine may be helpful when taken along with the drug nitroglycerin, but severe headaches may develop.

Results are conflicting on whether fatty fish or **fish oil** are helpful for people with angina.

The herbs **hawthorn**, khella, and *Coleus forskohlii* are often recommended for angina by herbalists, but as yet there is no meaningful evidence that they work. **Vitamin E** has been found only slightly effective at best

for angina, and **beta-carotene** may actually increase angina.

Chelation therapy is widely promoted for the treatment of angina, but there is no meaningful evidence that it is effective and some evidence that it is not.

Herbs and Supplements to Use Only with Caution

Various herbs and supplements may interact adversely with drugs used to treat angina. For more information on this potential risk, see the individual drug article in the Drug Interactions section of this book.

Anxiety and Panic Attacks

RELATED TERMS: *Nervousness*

PRINCIPAL PROPOSED NATURAL TREATMENTS: *None*

OTHER PROPOSED NATURAL TREATMENTS: *5-HTP (5-Hydroxytryptophan), Acupuncture, Aromatherapy, Bach Flower Remedies, Biofeedback, Chamomile, Chinese Skullcap, Flaxseed Oil, GABA, Gamma Oryzanol, Gotu Kola, Hops, Inositol (for Panic Disorder), Kava, Lemon Balm, Linden, Magnesium, Hawthorn and* Eschscholtzia californica *(California poppy) Combination, Massage, Melatonin, Multivitamin/Mineral Supplements, Passionflower, Relaxation Therapies (Meditation and Guided Imagery), Selenium, European Skullcap, Suma, Valerian*

As W. H. Auden pointed out, we live in the age of anxiety. Most of us suffer from a certain level of chronic anxiety because modern life is jagged, fast-paced, and divorced from the natural rhythms that tend to create a harmonious inner life. For some, this existential unease goes further and becomes a psychological disorder.

Typical symptoms of anxiety disorder include feelings of tension, irritability, worry, frustration, turmoil, and hopelessness, along with insomnia, restless sleep, grinding of teeth, jaw pain, an inability to sit still, and an incapacity to cope. Physical sensations frequently arise as well, including a characteristic feeling of being unable to take a full, satisfying breath; dry mouth; rapid heartbeat; heart palpitations; a lump in the throat; tightness in the chest; and cramping in the bowels. Anxiety can also give rise to panic attacks. These may be so severe that they are mistaken for heart attacks. The heart

pounds and palpitates, the chest feels tight and painful, and the whole body tenses with unreasonable fear. Such attacks can be triggered by anxiety-provoking situations, but they may also come out of nowhere, perhaps even awakening you from sleep. When a person tends to suffer more from panic attacks than generalized anxiety, physicians call the illness *panic disorder*.

The medical treatment of anxiety involves antianxiety drugs in the benzodiazepine family, the unique drug BuSpar (buspirone), and antidepressants. Panic attacks are generally more difficult to treat than other forms of anxiety.

Proposed Natural Treatments

There are no natural treatments for anxiety that have been shown to be safe and effective. However, some treatments have shown promise for generalized anxiety disorder and related conditions. No natural treatment is likely to be effective for panic disorder.

Valerian: May Provide Calming Effects

The herb valerian is best known as a remedy for insomnia. However, because many drugs useful for insomnia also reduce anxiety, valerian has been proposed as an anxiety treatment as well.

In a double-blind, placebo-controlled study, 36 people with generalized anxiety disorder were given either valerian extract, valium, or placebo for a period of 4 weeks. The study failed to find statistically significant differences among the groups, presumably due to its small size. However, a careful analysis of the results hints, at least, that valerian was helpful.

In addition, a preliminary double-blind study found that valerian may produce calming effects in stressful situations. Again, though, this study was too small to provide definitive results.

For more information, including dosage and safety issues, see the full **Valerian** article.

Kava

Up until 2002, the herb kava was widely used in Europe as a medical treatment for anxiety, based on the evidence of a substantial body of double-blind, placebo-controlled studies. However, because of recent concerns involving its potential effects on the liver, it has been withdrawn from the market in many countries and we do not recommend its use. For more information, see the full **Kava** article.

Other Herbs and Supplements

A large (264-participant) 3-month, double-blind, placebo-controlled study tested the possible antianxiety benefits of a combination therapy containing the mineral **magnesium** (150 mg twice daily), the herb **hawthorn** (150 mg twice daily of a standardized extract), and the seldom-studied herb *Eschscholtzia californica* (California poppy, 40 mg twice daily). Study participants all suffered from generalized anxiety disorder of mild-to-moderate intensity. The results indicated that the combination treatment was more effective than placebo. No significant side effects were seen. This particular combination therapy is currently used in France.

A double-blind, placebo-controlled trial of 80 healthy male volunteers found that 28 days of treatment with a **multivitamin and mineral supplement** (containing calcium, magnesium, and zinc) significantly reduced anxiety and the sensation of stress.

The supplement **5-HTP** is best known as a proposed treatment for depression. An 8-week, double-blind, placebo-controlled study compared 5-HTP and the drug clomipramine in 45 individuals suffering from anxiety disorders. The results indicated that 5-HTP was effective, but clomipramine was more effective.

Based on its ability to promote sleep, **melatonin** has been tried as a treatment for reducing anxiety while waiting for surgery to begin. A double-blind, placebo-controlled study of 75 women waiting for surgery compared melatonin against the standard drug midazolam and found it effective. Benefits were also seen in a subsequent double-blind trial of 84 women about to receive anesthesia, conducted by the same researcher. Whether melatonin is effective for other forms of anxiety has not been determined.

A 4-week, double-blind study of 36 individuals with anxiety (specifically, generalized anxiety disorder) compared the herb **passionflower** to the standard drug oxazepam. Oxazepam worked more quickly, but by the end of the 4-week trial, both treatments proved equally effective. Furthermore, passionflower showed a comparative advantage in terms of side-effects: use of oxazepam was associated with more impairment of job performance. However, because this study lacked a placebo group, it would be premature to conclude from it that passionflower has been shown to be an effective treatment for anxiety. The only other supporting evidence for passionflower comes from animal studies.

Several small double-blind studies by a single research group have found preliminary evidence that oral use of **lemon balm** (*Melissa officinalis*) may reduce anxiety levels. Like other antianxiety agents, it may also impair mental function to some degree. A combination of lemon balm and valerian has also been tested, with generally positive results.

A double-blind, placebo-controlled trial of 40 individuals found that **gotu kola** reduced the "startle" response to sudden loud noises. This suggests, but doesn't prove, that gotu kola may be helpful for anxiety.

A very small double-blind, placebo-controlled crossover study found that use of the herb **European skullcap** reduced general anxiety levels.

Two exceedingly preliminary studies that evaluated **linden** flower for potential sedative or antianxiety effects returned contradictory results.

One study found weak evidence that **sage** might reduce anxiety.

Other herbs or supplements that are frequently recommended for anxiety attacks include **Chinese skullcap**, **flaxseed oil**, **chamomile**, **gamma pryzanol**, **hops**, **selenium**, and **suma**, as well as **inositol** for panic disorder. However, there is no reliable supporting evidence to indicate that they work.

The substance GABA (gamma-aminobutyric acid) is a neurotransmitter that, in the brain, acts to reduce anxiety. However, it is unlikely that GABA taken orally gets to where it can do any good.

Alternative Therapies

Various alternative therapies have shown some promise for the treatment of anxiety, including **acupuncture**, **aromatherapy** (either alone or combined with massage), **biofeedback**, **massage** (either alone or combined with aromatherapy), and **relaxation therapies** (such as meditation and guided imagery). However, the supporting evidence to indicate that these treatments actually work remains weak.

Two studies suggest that **Bach flower remedies** are *not* helpful for situational anxiety.

Herbs and Supplements to Use Only with Caution

Various herbs and supplements may interact adversely with drugs used to treat anxiety. For more information on this potential risk, see the individual drug article in the Drug Interactions section of this book.

Arthritis

RELATED TERMS: *Rheumatism, Joint Pain*

The term arthritis (or, archaically, rheumatism) refers to any condition that involves pain in the joints. There are many possible causes of joint pain, of which three are discussed in the Collins Alternative Health Guide:

➤ **Osteoarthritis**
➤ **Rheumatoid arthritis**
➤ **Gout**

Asthma

PRINCIPAL PROPOSED NATURAL TREATMENTS: *Boswellia*, Coleus forskohlii, *Tylophora*, *Vitamin C*, *Ephedra (Unsafe)*

OTHER PROPOSED NATURAL TREATMENTS: *Acupuncture, Adrenal Extract, Aloe, Antioxidants, Astha-15 (an Ayurvedic Herbal Combination), Brahmi (Bacopa monniera), Beta-carotene, Betaine Hydrochloride, Butterbur, Chamomile, Damiana, Elecampane, Elimination Diet, Essential Fatty Acids (Omega-3 and Omega-6 Fatty Acids), Essential Oil of Eucalyptus, Fish Oil, Flaxseed Oil, Food Allergen Elimination Diet, Garlic, GLA from Evening Primrose Oil, Green-lipped Mussel, Grindelia, Horehound, Hyssop, Hypnosis, Ivy Leaf, Licorice,* Lobelia Inflata, *Magnesium, Marshmallow, Massage, Melatonin, Mullein, Onion, OPCs (Oligomeric Proanthocyanidins), Osteopathic Manipulation, Quercetin, Reishi, Relaxation Therapy, Selenium, Vitamin B$_6$, Vitamin B$_{12}$, Vitamin E, Yerba Santa, Yoga*

People who are having an asthma attack have real trouble taking a breath. Many people with stuffy noses from hay fever or colds say, "I can't breathe," but they retain the option of breathing through the mouth. Asthmatics, however, know what "I can't breathe" really means. Instead of their nasal passages, it is the bronchial tubes in their lungs that become swollen and clogged. Breathing can become frighteningly difficult.

Asthma involves two conditions: (1) contraction of the small muscles surrounding the bronchial tubes and (2) inflammation of the lining of those tubes. Traditionally, treatment primarily addressed the first aspect of asthma; but in the two decades, it has become clear that tissue swelling is the underlying cause.

The conventional treatment of asthma is highly effective for most people. Treatments include both short- and long-acting bronchodilators, which relax the bronchial muscles, and anti-inflammatory medication, which helps relieve the swelling of tissue. Bronchodilators alone may be sufficient treatment for mild asthma, or asthma that occurs only with exercise. Anti-inflammatory steroids in the cortisone family taken by inhalation are the mainstay of treatment for moderate to severe asthma. Although these are much safer than oral steroids, they may still increase risk of osteoporosis and other problems when they are taken in high doses or for a long time. Other drugs used to reduce inflammation include montelukast (Singulair), nedocromil (Tilade), and cromolyn (Intal). (Interestingly, Intal is derived from a Mediterranean herb named khella.) The newest drug treatment for asthma, omalizumab (Xolair), appears to be very safe and effective, but it is cur-

rently extremely expensive and, for this reason, it is seldom used.

Principal Proposed Natural Treatments

Warning: None of these treatments have been shown to be effective for severe asthma. Do not stop your standard asthma medication except on the advice of a physician.

The herb *Tylophora indica* (also called *Tylophora asthmatica*) appears to offer some promise as a treatment for asthma. It has a long history of use in the traditional Ayurvedic medicine of India. However, all of the studies on this herb were performed in India decades ago and fail to reach modern standards of design and reporting.

In a double-blind, placebo-controlled study of 195 individuals with asthma, the participants who were given 40 mg of a tylophora alcohol extract daily for 6 days showed significant improvement as compared to placebo. Similar results were seen in two double-blind, placebo-controlled studies involving more than 200 individuals with asthma. However, the design of these studies was a bit convoluted and various pieces of information are missing from the reports, causing some difficulty in evaluating the validity of these trials.

Another double-blind study that enrolled 135 individuals and followed a more straightforward design found no benefit from tylophora.

The bottom line: Although tylophora is promising, larger and better studies are necessary to discover whether tylophora is truly effective.

For more information, including dosage and safety issues, see the full **Tylophora** article.

Asthma

Boswellia: Possibly Helpful

The herb boswellia has shown promise as a treatment for **rheumatoid arthritis**. It is thought to work by inhibiting inflammation. Since asthma involves inflammation as well and can be treated by some of the same drugs that treat rheumatoid arthritis, boswellia has been tried for this purpose too.

One 6-week, double-blind, placebo-controlled study of 80 individuals with relatively mild asthma found that treatment with boswellia at a dose of 300 mg 3 times daily reduced the frequency of asthma attacks and improved objective measurements of breathing capacity. However, further research needs to be performed to follow up this pilot study before boswellia can be described as a proven treatment for asthma.

For more information, including dosage and safety issues, see the full **Boswellia** article.

Coleus forskohlii: May Be Effective, but More Like a Drug Than an Herb

Another herb sometimes recommended for asthma also comes from India, *Coleus forskohlii*. While there is some preliminary evidence that it might have value, this evidence is currently far too weak to be relied on. Furthermore, as presently sold, the herb is more like a drug than an herb. Natural *Coleus forskohlii* contains small amounts of a potent chemical called *forskolin*. Manufacturers deliberately modify the herb to dramatically increase its forskolin content; therefore, when using such products, one is essentially using an unlicensed drug. Forskolin appears to be safe, but more studies need to be undertaken before it can be recommended for self-treatment.

Vitamin C: Appears to Provide Some Benefits

Many studies have been conducted on the effects of vitamin C in treating asthma. When you put all the results together, it appears that the regular use of high-dose vitamin C provides some modest benefits.

For more information, including dosage and safety issues, see the full **Vitamin C** article.

Ma Huang: Effective, but Not Safe

The Chinese herb ma huang, also called *ephedra*, is definitely effective for mild asthma, because it contains the drug ephedrine. However, we cannot recommend using it because of safety concerns. This Chinese herb is a member of a primitive family of plants that look like thin, branching, connected straws. A related species,

Ephedra nevadensis, grows wild in the American Southwest and is widely called *Mormon tea*. However, only the Asian species of ephedra contains the active compounds ephedrine and pseudoephedrine.

Ma huang was traditionally used by Chinese herbalists in the early stages of respiratory infections and for the short-term treatment of certain kinds of asthma, eczema, hay fever, narcolepsy, and edema.

Japanese chemists isolated ephedrine from ma huang at the turn of the twentieth century and it soon became a primary treatment for asthma in the United States and abroad. Ephedra's other major ingredient, pseudoephedrine, became the decongestant Sudafed.

Although ephedrine can still be found in a few over-the-counter asthma drugs, physicians seldom prescribe it today. The problem is that ephedrine mimics the effects of adrenaline and causes symptoms such as rapid heartbeat, high blood pressure, agitation, insomnia, nausea, and loss of appetite. The newer asthma drugs are much safer and easier to tolerate. This is a situation in which synthetic drugs are less dangerous than a natural one. We recommend against using ma huang for asthma.

Other Herbs and Supplements

In a double-blind trial, 32 people with steroid-dependent asthma were given either placebo or **essential oil** of eucalyptus for 12 weeks. The results showed that people using eucalyptus were more able to gradually reduce their steroid dosage than those taking placebo.

Two double-blind, placebo-controlled studies enrolling a total of over 80 people with asthma suggests that **OPCs** from pine bark might reduce symptoms.

An extract made from **ivy leaf** has been advocated for the treatment of childhood asthma, but at present the meaningful supporting evidence is again limited to one placebo-controlled trial.

Another small double-blind, placebo-controlled study evaluated the effects of 4 weeks of treatment with a Japanese herbal mixture traditionally called *Saiboku-To*. Researchers tested the tendency of the bronchial tubes to contract in response to an asthma-producing substance called *methacholine*. The results indicated that use of Saiboku-To helped prevent such contractions and also reduced lung inflammation. Another study reportedly found benefit with a combination named *Mai-Men-Dong-Tang*.

There is only weak and/or inconsistent evidence regarding whether two antioxidants in the **carotenoid** family, **lycopene** and **beta-carotene**, might help prevent exercise-induced asthma.

One double-blind comparative study provides weak evidence that the **Ayurvedic herbal combination** called *Astha 15* might be helpful for mild asthma.

Vitamin B$_6$ is often mentioned as a treatment for asthma, but the evidence that it works is weak and contradictory at best. A double-blind study of 76 children with asthma found significant benefit from vitamin B$_6$ after the second month of usage. Children in the treated group were able to reduce their doses of bronchodilators and steroids. However, a recent double-blind study of 31 adults who also used either inhaled or oral steroids did not show any benefit.

Supplementation with **vitamin B$_{12}$** is also often said to be effective for asthma. However, the scientific evidence in its favor consists almost entirely of open studies that did not attempt to eliminate the placebo effect.

Magnesium is frequently mentioned as a treatment for asthma, but no good studies have shown that oral magnesium is helpful. A 4-month, double-blind, placebo-controlled study of 300 people with asthma failed to find benefit with either **vitamin C** (1 g daily) or magnesium (450 mg daily). However, some evidence exists that intravenous or inhaled magnesium may be beneficial.

The flavonoid **quercetin** is often recommended as a treatment for asthma on the basis of test-tube studies that show it can inhibit the release of inflammatory substances from special cells called *mast cells*. Because the asthma drugs Intal (cromolyn sodium) and Tilade are believed to work in the same way, many natural medicine authorities have often recommended quercetin as an equivalent treatment. However, even though significant direct evidence exists that Tilade and Intal actually work, no such evidence yet exists for quercetin.

Very preliminary evidence hints that the herb **butterbur** may be helpful for asthma.

Essential fatty acids, such as **GLA** and those found in **fish oil** and **flaxseed oil**, may inhibit inflammatory responses such as those that occur in asthma. However, of the studies that tried fish oil as a treatment for asthma, most failed to find significant benefit. One study found that fish oil can actually worsen aspirin-related asthma. However, there is some evidence from one research group that fish oil might be helpful for exercise-induced asthma.

A preliminary double-blind, placebo-controlled trial suggests that **green-lipped mussel** extract might be helpful for allergic asthma.

One study suggests that the natural substance hyaluronic acid might be helpful for asthma when taken by inhalation.

Other natural products commonly recommended for asthma include the herbs **aloe**, **Brahmi** (*Bacopa monniera*), **chamomile**, **damiana**, **elecampane**, **garlic**, grindelia, **horehound**, **hyssop**, **licorice**, **marshmallow**, **mullein**, onion, **reishi**, and **yerba santa**, as well as the supplements **adrenal extract** and **betaine hydrochloride**. *Lobelia inflata* is sometimes recommended as an herbal treatment for asthma; but according to traditional directions, it should be taken to the point of vomiting, a process we can hardly recommend. None of these treatments have any meaningful supporting evidence.

Antioxidants, such as **vitamin E**, **beta-carotene**, and **selenium**, are frequently recommended for asthma on the grounds that they may protect inflamed lung tissue. However, there is no direct scientific evidence at this time that they work. A rather theoretical study found evidence that use of vitamin E might decrease the inflammatory response in children with asthma exposed to ozone. However, a far more meaningful double-blind, placebo-controlled study found vitamin E (as 500 mg of natural vitamin E) *ineffective* for asthma.

Children with asthma may have reduced growth, possibly due to use of inhaled steroids. One study failed to find protective benefits with a **multivitamin** that contained **vitamin D**. The tested supplement did not contain calcium. Other studies have found that combination treatment with both **calcium** and vitamin D may protect bone density in people taking oral corticosteroids (for various reasons, including asthma).

Two exceedingly preliminary studies reported by one research group has led to publicized concerns that use of the insomnia supplement **melatonin** may worsen nighttime asthma. However, one double-blind study of melatonin in people with asthma found evidence of improved sleep without worsening of asthma symptoms.

Acupuncture

Although there have been numerous reports on **acupuncture** treatment for asthma, the results have been contradictory.

A team of three researchers analyzed 13 trials on acupuncture in the treatment of asthma. These studies were scored on the basis of design quality, with a maximum possible score of 100 points. Criteria for assigning points included size of the study population, randomization procedure, description of treatment, measurement of effects, follow-up, and the like. Eight studies earned more than 50 points and the highest score was 72 points. However, the overall quality of studies was judged to be mediocre and, in any case, the results were contradictory. The conclusion was that "claims that acupuncture is effective in the treatment of asthma are not based on the results of well-performed clinical trials."

A more recent review of acupuncture for asthma came to identical conclusions.

Other Alternative Therapies

Some people with asthma may also have **food allergies**. If this is the case, eliminating the offending food from the diet might reduce asthma symptoms. The only reliable way to discover if you are allergic to a certain food is through eliminating potentially allergenic foods from the diet then systematically reintroducing them to see if a reaction occurs.

A special breathing technique called *Buteyko breathing* may reduce medication use and subjective symptoms, though it does not appear to actually improve lung function. One of the studies of Buteyko failed to find Ayurvedic-style breathing (pranayama) helpful for asthma.

Hypnosis, **massage**, **yoga**, and some forms of **relaxation therapy** appear to offer no more than slight benefits at best for asthma.

In two controlled studies, **chiropractic spinal manipulation** has failed to prove more effective than fake manipulation for treatment of asthma. One study of **osteopathic manipulation** reportedly found benefits, but the study design was flawed.

Atherosclerosis and Heart Disease Prevention

PRINCIPAL PROPOSED NATURAL TREATMENTS: *Omega-3 Fatty Acids, Lifestyle Changes*

OTHER PROPOSED NATURAL TREATMENTS: *Antioxidants, Astragalus, Bilberry Fruit and Leaf, Chromium, Coenzyme Q_{10}, Copper, Flaxseed, Garlic, Genistein, Ginger, Ginkgo, GLA (Gamma-linolenic Acid), Grass Pollen, Green Tea or Black Tea, Hawthorn, Lipoic Acid, Lutein, Magnesium, Mesoglycan, OPCs (Oligomeric Proanthocyanidins), Resveratrol, Selenium, Turmeric, Vitamin C, TMG (Trimethylglycine)*

PROBABLY NOT EFFECTIVE TREATMENTS: *Beta-carotene, Vitamin E*

Atherosclerosis, often known as hardening of the arteries, leads to cardiovascular disease and is the leading cause of death in men over age 35 and all people over 45. Most heart attacks and strokes are due to atherosclerosis. Although the origin of this condition is not completely understood, we know that it is accelerated by factors such as **hypertension** (high blood pressure), **high cholesterol**, **diabetes** and milder forms of impaired glucose tolerance, **smoking**, physical inactivity, and **obesity**. Chronic inflammation in the body (of various types) is also hypothesized to play a role.

Current theories suggest that atherosclerosis begins with injury to the lining of the arteries. High blood pressure physically stresses this lining, while circulating substances such as low-density lipoprotein (LDL) cholesterol, homocysteine, free radicals, and nicotine chemically damage it. White blood cells then attach to the damaged wall and take up residence. Then, for reasons that are not entirely clear, the artery lining begins to accumulate cholesterol and other fats. Platelets also latch on, releasing substances that cause the formation of fibrous tissue. The overall effect is a thickening of the artery wall called a *fibrous plaque*.

Over time, the thickening increases, narrowing the bore of the artery. When blockage of the *coronary arteries* (the arteries supplying the heart) reaches 75 to 90%, symptoms of angina develop. In the lower legs, blockage of the blood flow leads to leg pain with exercise, a condition called *intermittent claudication*.

Blood clots can develop on the irregular surfaces of arteries and may become detached and block downstream blood flow. Fragments of plaque can also detach. Heart attacks are generally caused by such blood clots, whereas strokes are more often caused by plaque fragments or gradual obstruction. Furthermore, atherosclerotic blood vessels are weak and can burst.

With a disease as serious and progressive as atherosclerosis, the best treatment is prevention. Conventional medical approaches focus on lifestyle changes, such as increasing aerobic exercise, reducing the consumption of saturated fats, and quitting smoking. The regular use of **aspirin** also appears to be quite helpful by preventing platelet attachment and blood clot formation. If necessary, drugs may be used to lower cholesterol levels or blood pressure.

Principal Proposed Natural Treatments

This section presents some promising and not-so-promising natural approaches for preventing cardiovascular disease by fighting atherosclerosis. Note that we have left out two classes of treatments: those that reduce elevated **cholesterol** or **blood pressure**. These are discussed in their own articles. It has also been suggested that reducing levels of **homocysteine** might reduce cardiovascular disease risk, a subject also discussed in a separate article. In addition, other sections of this book contain articles on several conditions caused by atherosclerosis, such as **angina**, **heart attacks**, **intermittent claudication**, and **stroke**.

Omega-3 Fatty Acids

Omega-3 fatty acids are healthy fats, found in certain foods such as cold-water fish. Inconsistent evidence suggests fish or fish oil might help fight atherosclerosis.

Study results on fish or fish oil for cardiovascular disease have yielded contradictory results. One review (technically a meta-analysis) of many studies on the subject concluded that when all the evidence is put together, it appears that fish or fish oil can slightly reduce overall mortality, heart disease mortality, and sudden cardiac death (heart stoppage due to arrhythmia). However, a subsequent comprehensive review that included additional studies came to a more pessimistic conclusion. According to the authors working for the prestigious Cochrane Collaboration, "it is not clear that dietary or supplemental omega-3 fats alter total mortality, combined cardiovascular events or cancers in people with, or at high risk of, cardiovascular disease or in the general population."

If it does provide benefit, fish oil is thought to do so primarily by reducing serum **triglycerides**. Like cholesterol, triglycerides are a type of fat in the blood that tends to damage the arteries, leading to heart disease. According to most, but not all studies, fish oil can modestly reduce triglyceride levels. However, the standard drug, gemfibrozil, appears to be more effective than fish oil for this purpose. The most important omega-3 fatty acids found in fish oil are called *eicosapentaenoic acid* (EPA) and *docosahexaenoic acid* (DHA). DHA and EPA may have different effects on triglycerides, but as typical for studies involving marginally effective treatments, study results are not consistent; some found EPA more effective than DHA, while others did not find a difference.

Similarly, some but not all studies also suggest that fish, fish oil, or EPA or DHA separately can modestly raise levels of HDL ("good") cholesterol.

Additionally, fish oil may help the heart by "thinning" the blood and by reducing blood levels of homocysteine. Blood clots play a major role in heart attacks and homocysteine is an amino acid that appears to raise the risk of heart disease. One study directly indicates that fish oil may be able to help prevent blood clots from blocking the synthetic grafts inserted in people undergoing kidney dialysis.

Studies contradict one another on whether fish oil can lower blood pressure. A 6-week, double-blind, placebo-controlled study of 59 overweight men suggests that the DHA in fish oil, but not the EPA, can reduce blood pressure.

For more information, including dosage and safety issues, see the full **Fish Oil** article.

Flaxseed oil (another source of omega-3 fatty acids) has been suggested as an alternative to fish oil. While fish oil is much better studied, there is some evidence, including two double-blind studies, that flaxseed oil or **whole flaxseed** may reduce LDL ("bad") cholesterol, perhaps slightly reduce hypertension, and slow down atherosclerosis.

Lifestyle Approaches

There is no doubt that quitting smoking will significantly reduce heart disease risk. Increasing exercise and losing weight (if you are overweight) will most likely help as well. Although for years there has been an emphasis on reducing fat in the diet, the balance of current evidence indicates that it's more useful to substitute healthy fats for saturated fats than to try to reduce total fat intake. Evidence suggests that any low-calorie diet, whether low-carb, low-fat, or in-between, will result in weight loss and reduced cardiac risk—provided you stick to it.

However, while it may not be important to cut down on total fat, accumulating evidence hints that trans-fatty acids, a type of fatty acid found in margarine and other hydrogenated oils, increase risk of cardiovascular disease. In July 2002, the U.S. Institute of Medicine concluded that there is no safe intake level of trans-fatty acids and recommended that overall consumption should be kept as low as possible.

The moderate use of alcohol, and specifically wine, appears to help prevent atherosclerosis, although this is controversial. Contrary to some reports, coffee drinking does not appear to increase risk of heart disease, although unfiltered coffee may be harmful.

Other Proposed Natural Treatments

Several natural products have shown some promise for helping to prevent atherosclerosis.

Garlic

Garlic is generally said to produce several effects that together reduce atherosclerosis risk. Although garlic is no longer believed to strongly reduce cholesterol levels, it may improve cholesterol profiles to a modest extent; in addition, it may mildly lower blood pressure levels, as well as protect against free radicals and reduce the tendency of the blood to coagulate. However, the actual evidence for benefit is quite incomplete.

Garlic preparations have been shown to slow the development of atherosclerosis in rats, rabbits, and human blood vessels, reducing the size of plaque deposits by nearly 50%. Furthermore, in a double-blind, placebo-controlled study that followed 152 individuals for 4 years, standardized garlic powder at a dosage of 900 mg per day significantly slowed the development of atherosclerosis as measured by ultrasound. Unfortunately, this study suffered from some significant statistical problems.

An observational study of 200 people suggests that garlic protects the arteries in other ways as well. The study measured the flexibility of the aorta, the main artery exiting the heart. Participants who took garlic showed less evidence of damage to their arteries. However, observational studies are notoriously unreliable.

Finally, in another study, 432 people who had suffered a heart attack were given either garlic oil extract or no treatment over a period of 3 years. The results showed a significant reduction of second heart attacks and an approximately 50% reduction in death rate among those taking garlic. Unfortunately, the researcher's failure to use a placebo in this trial greatly decreases the meaningfulness of the results.

For more information, including dosage and safety issues, see the full **Garlic** article.

Other Potentially Beneficial Treatments

Mesoglycan is a substance obtained from the intestines of pigs. In one study, 200 mg per day of mesoglycan significantly slowed the rate of thickening of arteries. After 18 months of treatment, the additional layering of the inside vessel lining was 7.5 times less in the group receiving mesoglycan than in the group that did not receive any treatment. However, because this was not a double-blind, placebo-controlled trial, the results can't be taken as truly reliable. Preliminary evidence suggests that this supplement may work in several ways: supplying material for repair of arteries, "thinning" the blood, and improving cholesterol levels.

Magnesium also appears to be helpful. In a 6-month, double-blind, placebo-controlled study, 187 individuals with angina were given either 365 mg of magnesium daily or placebo. The results showed that use of magnesium significantly improved exercise capacity, lessened exercise-induced chest pain, and improved general quality of life. Additionally, magnesium may reduce the atherosclerosis risk caused by hydrogenated oils, margarine-like fats found in many "junk" foods.

Mildly impaired responsiveness to insulin (short of outright diabetes) is a fairly common condition that appears to increase the risk of heart disease. **Chromium** supplementation might restore normal insulin responsiveness, as well as aid in weight loss and possibly improve cholesterol levels. The net result might be decreased risk of heart disease. In support of this theory, an observational trial found associations between higher chromium intake and reduced risk of heart attack.

Some but not all observational studies suggest that **green tea** might help prevent heart disease. **Black tea** has shown inconsistent promise as well.

Many herbs and supplements appear to decrease platelet stickiness, including **bilberry, feverfew, ginger, ginkgo, policosanol,** and **hawthorn.** Whether this translates into an actual benefit for preventing atherosclerosis remains unknown.

Indirect evidence suggests that **DHEA** might help prevent heart disease, especially in men.

Frequent consumption of nuts may reduce the risk of heart disease, probably because the monounsaturated fats in nuts reduce cholesterol levels.

For other natural substances that may help prevent atherosclerosis by lowering its major risk factors, see the articles on **cholesterol** and **hypertension**. For natural substances that may be helpful for *consequences* of atherosclerosis, see the articles on **angina**, **congestive heart failure**, **heart attack**, **intermittent claudication**, and **stroke**.

Chelation therapy, a technique that involves intravenous administration of the substance EDTA, is widely promoted in some alternative medicine circles as a treatment for atherosclerosis. However, there is no meaningful evidence that it works and growing evidence that it does not work.

Antioxidants: Probably Not Effective

The body is engaged in a constant battle against damaging chemicals called *free radicals* or *pro-oxidants*. These highly reactive substances are believed to play a major role in atherosclerosis, cancer, and aging in general.

To counter the harmful effects of free radicals, the body manufactures **antioxidants** to chemically neutralize them. However, the natural antioxidant system may not always be equal to the task. Sources of free radicals, such as cigarette smoke and smoked meat, may overwhelm this defense mechanism.

Certain dietary nutrients augment the body's natural antioxidants and may be able to help out when the primary system is under stress. Vitamins E and C and beta-carotene are the best known, but many other substances found in fruits and vegetables are also strong antioxidants. For years we've been thinking that antioxidant supplements might offer considerable protection against heart disease, especially vitamin E. However, current evidence appears to dampen these high expectations.

Before presenting this disappointing information, it is necessary to explain the weaknesses of the observational studies that raised our hopes. Observational studies are relatively inexpensive and are often used to evaluate the potential health benefits of nutrients such as antioxidants. This type of study follows large groups of people for years and keeps track of a great deal of information about them, including diet. Researchers then examine the data closely and try to identify which dietary factors are associated with better health and longer life.

However, the results can be misleading. For example, if an observational study finds that people who take vitamin supplements live longer, it is not necessarily the vitamins that deserve the credit. Vitamin users also tend to exercise more and to eat more healthful foods, habits that may play a more important role than the vitamins. It is impossible to know for sure simply by evaluating the results of such a study.

Similarly, several observational studies have found that men who consume more foods that are rich in lycopene are less likely to develop prostate cancer. But does this mean that taking lycopene supplements will reduce prostate cancer risk? Not necessarily. Such foods contain many other nutrients as well and they may be more important than lycopene.

A more reliable kind of study is the intervention trial. In these studies, some people are given a specific substance, such as a vitamin, and then compared to others who are given a placebo (or sometimes no treatment at all). The best intervention trials use a double-blind, placebo-controlled design. The results of intervention trials are far more conclusive than those of observational studies. In the field of antioxidant therapy for preventing atherosclerosis, observational studies raised hopes, but intervention trials dashed them. (For more information on why double-blind trials are essential, see **Why Does This Book Rely on Double-Blind Studies.**)

Vitamin E

Most but not all observational studies have found associations between high intake of vitamin E and reduced risk of cardiovascular disease. However, as noted above, observational studies alone cannot be relied upon to identify useful treatments. Intervention trials, which provide much more convincing evidence of effectiveness, have generally failed to find vitamin E supplements effective.

The Heart Outcomes Prevention Evaluation (HOPE) trial found that natural vitamin E (d-alpha-tocopherol) at a dose of 400 IU daily did not reduce the number of heart attacks, strokes, or deaths from heart disease any more than placebo. The details of this well-designed, double-blind trial were published in the January 20, 2000, issue of *The New England Journal of Medicine*. The trial followed more than 9,000 men and women who had existing heart disease or were at high risk for it.

In addition, a large open trial compared the effectiveness of aspirin and vitamin E for the prevention of heart attacks, strokes, and other diseases related to atherosclerosis. While aspirin treatment proved somewhat helpful, vitamin E produced little to no benefit.

Negative results have been seen in other large trials as well. A few have even found weak indications that use of vitamin E may worsen certain outcomes.

When the results of these studies began to come in, some antioxidant proponents suggested that the individuals enrolled in these trials already had too advanced disease for vitamin E to help. However, a large trial found vitamin E ineffective for slowing the progression of heart disease in healthy people as well.

On balance, the evidence strongly suggests that vitamin E in the form used in these studies (alpha-tocopherol) is *not* helpful for preventing heart disease. It has been suggested that another form of vitamin E, gamma-tocopherol might be more helpful than alpha-tocopherol. Gamma-tocopherol is present in the diet much more abundantly than alpha-tocopherol and it could be that the studies showing benefits with dietary vitamin E actually tracked the influence of gamma-tocopherol. However, an observational study specifically looking to see if gamma-tocopherol levels were associated with risk of heart attack found no relationship between the two. Nonetheless, intervention trials of gamma-tocopherol are currently under way.

For more information, including dosage and safety issues, see the full **Vitamin E** article.

Beta-Carotene

The study results involving **beta-carotene** are interesting. Beta-carotene is one member of a large category of substances in foods known as *carotenoids*, which are found in high levels in yellow, orange, and dark green vegetables.

Many studies suggest that eating foods high in carotenoids can prevent atherosclerosis. However, isolated beta-carotene in supplement form may not help and could actually increase your risk, especially if you consume too much alcohol.

A huge, double-blind intervention trial involving 29,133 Finnish male smokers found 11% *more* deaths from heart disease and 15 to 20% *more* strokes in those participants taking beta-carotene supplements. This certainly does not encourage one to take it.

Similar poor results with beta-carotene were seen in another large, double-blind study in smokers. Furthermore, beta-carotene supplementation was also found to increase the incidence of angina in smokers.

What is happening here? Clearly, smoking presents a challenge to antioxidants. However, the question remains: Why should beta-carotene not only fail to help but actually worsen the situation?

One possible explanation is that beta-carotene in the diet always comes along with other naturally occurring carotenes. It is quite likely that other carotenoids in the diet are equally or more important than beta-carotene

alone. Taking beta-carotene supplements may actually promote deficiencies of other natural carotenes and overall that may hurt more than it helps.

The moral of the story is that you should eat your vegetables but maybe not take beta-carotene supplements.

Other Antioxidants

A high intake of **vitamin C** from fruits and vegetables appears to reduce the risk of heart disease. However, there is little evidence that vitamin C supplements provide the same benefits. Foods containing vitamin C also contain many other healthful ingredients (such as bioflavonoids and carotenes), so it's not clear that pills containing only vitamin C are helpful.

One double-blind study suggests that the antioxidant **coenzyme Q_{10}** may help prevent the progression of atherosclerosis after a heart attack. Many other antioxidant vitamins, supplements, and herbs have been suggested as preventive treatments for atherosclerosis, including **selenium**, **OPCs** from grape seed or pine bark, **lipoic acid**, **turmeric**, and **resveratrol** from red wine and grape skins. However, although a number of interesting studies have suggested that these substances may be beneficial, the state of the evidence is still too preliminary to draw any conclusions.

Combined Antioxidants

It has been suggested that the best approach is to use a *combination* of antioxidants. This makes sense theoretically because, for example, vitamin E fights free radicals that dissolve in fats while vitamin C fights those that dissolve in water. However, evidence for benefit with such combinations comes only from observational studies. A 3-year, double-blind, placebo-controlled study of 160 individuals found no benefit with combined antioxidant treatment providing vitamin E (800 IU), vitamin C (1,000 mg), beta-carotene (25 mg), and selenium (100 mcg). Similarly, a 3-year, double-blind, placebo-controlled study of 423 menopausal women with **coronary artery disease** found no benefit with combined vitamin E (800 IU daily) and vitamin C (1,000 mg daily). Furthermore, a 7-year, double-blind, placebo-controlled study of more than 13,000 French men and women failed to find any significant reduction of cardiovascular disease rates through use of a daily supplement containing 120 mg of vitamin C, 30 mg of vitamin E, 6 mg of beta-carotene, 100 mcg of selenium, and 20 mg of zinc.

Herbs and Supplements to Use Only with Caution

Various herbs and supplements may interact adversely with drugs used to treat atherosclerosis. For more information on this potential risk, see the individual drug article in the Drug Interactions section of this book.

Athlete's Foot

RELATED TERMS: *Fungal Infection (Foot), Onychomycosis, Ringworm, Tinea Pedis*

PRINCIPAL PROPOSED NATURAL TREATMENTS: *Tea Tree Oil*

OTHER PROPOSED NATURAL TREATMENTS: *Essential Oils, Garlic, Ozonized Vegetable Oil,* Solanum chrysotrichum *(sosa), Various Tropical/Traditional Medicinal Plants*

A thlete's foot is the common name for a fungal infection of the foot, often called *ringworm* (although there is no worm involved). The three fungi most commonly implicated in athlete's foot, *Trichophyton rubrum, T. mentagrophytes,* and *Epidermophyton floccosum,* favor the warm, moist areas between the toes and tend to flare up during warm weather. Similar infections can occur in the nails, scalp, groin, and beard.

Infection with these fungi generally causes mild scaling between the toes, but it can also cause more severe scaling, an itchy red rash, or blisters that cover the toes and the sides of the feet. Since the fungus may also cause the skin to crack, it can lead to bacterial infections, especially in older people or those with poor circulation in their feet. If the infection takes root under the toenails, it is called *onychomycosis* and can be very difficult, if not impossible, to eradicate.

Because the fungi that cause athlete's foot thrive in warm, moist areas, it's important to keep the feet clean and dry. Over-the-counter or prescription topical antifungal treatments containing miconazole, clotrimazole, econazole, or ketoconazole can generally cure athlete's foot, but treatment may have to be continued for a month or more for full results. In severe cases, oral antifungal medications may be necessary.

Principal Proposed Natural Treatments

Preliminary evidence suggests that tea tree oil might be helpful for athlete's foot.

Tea tree oil (*Melaleuca alternifolia*) has a long traditional use in Australia for the treatment of skin and other infections. This use is supported by evidence that tea tree oil is an effective antiseptic, active against many bacteria and fungi. Three double-blind studies suggest it may be helpful for athlete's foot.

In a double-blind, placebo-controlled trial, 158 people with athlete's foot were treated with placebo, 25% tea tree oil solution, or 50% tea tree oil solution, applied twice daily for 4 weeks. The results showed that the two tea tree oil solutions were more effective than placebo at eradicating infection. In the 50% tea tree oil group, 64% were cured; in the 25% tea tree oil group, 55% were cured; in the placebo group, 31% were cured. These differences were statistically significant. A few people developed dermatitis in response to the tea tree oil and had to drop out of the study, but most people did not experience any significant side effects.

Another double-blind, placebo-controlled trial followed 104 people given either a 10% tea tree oil cream, the standard drug tolnaftate, or placebo. The results showed that tea tree oil reduced the symptoms of athlete's foot more effectively than placebo, but less effectively than tolnaftate.

A third double-blind study followed 112 people with fungal infections of the toenails, comparing 100% tea tree oil to a standard topical antifungal treatment, clotrimazole. The results showed equivalent benefits; however, because topical clotrimazole is not regarded as a particularly effective treatment for this condition, the results mean little.

For more information, including dosage and safety issues, see the full **Tea Tree** article.

Other Proposed Natural Treatments

Vegetable oils treated with ozone have antifungal properties. A double-blind (but not placebo-controlled) study of 200 people with athlete's foot found that ozonized sunflower oil was effective as the drug ketoconazole cream.

Solanum chrysotrichum (sosa) is an herb used in Mexico for the treatment of athlete's foot and related infections. In a double-blind study of 101 people, 4- weeks' application of a special extract made from this herb produced benefits equivalent to those of the drug ketoconazole (as 2% cream). However, due to the lack of a placebo group, these results cannot be taken as fully reliable.

Garlic has known topical antifungal properties, and there is preliminary evidence suggesting that cream containing *ajoene*, a compound derived from garlic, might help treat athlete's foot.

Besides tea tree oil, other **essential oils** may be helpful as well, but the evidence remains weak. One open study hints that oil of bitter orange, a flavoring agent made from dried bitter orange peel, might have some effectiveness against athlete's foot when applied topically. Test-tube studies indicate that the aromatic constituents of other essential oils, such as peppermint and eucalyptus, also have antifungal activity, but they have yet to be tested on people.

More than 120 plants traditionally used to treat skin diseases in Mexico, Palestine, British Columbia, and Guatemala have demonstrated antifungal properties in test-tube studies. Further research is needed to determine if they are safe and effective for athlete's foot or other fungal infections.

Attention Deficit Disorder

RELATED TERMS: *AADD, ADD, ADHD, Adult Attention Deficit Disorder, Attention Deficit and Hyperactivity Disorder, Hyperkinetic Syndrome*

PRINCIPAL PROPOSED NATURAL TREATMENTS: *DMAE, Zinc*

OTHER PROPOSED NATURAL TREATMENTS: *Bach Flower Remedies, Blue-Green Algae, Calcium, Combined Amino Acids (GABA), Combined Polysaccharides (Galactose), Food Allergen Avoidance and Other Dietary Changes, Fucose, Glucose, Glycine, Inositol, Iron, L-Glutamine, L-Phenylalanine, L-Tyrosine, Magnesium, Mannose, Massage, Melatonin, N-acetylgalactosamine, N-acetylglucosamine, N-acetylneuraminic Acid, St. John's Wort, Taurine, Trace Minerals, Xylose*

PROBABLY NOT EFFECTIVE TREATMENTS: *Essential Fatty Acids (Fish Oil), Evening Primrose Oil*

Originally, the term attention deficit disorder (ADD) referred to children who were incapable of concentrating at school. *Hyperkinesia* was used somewhat synonymously as a descriptive term for children who simply couldn't sit still. Today, the definition has broadened to include many adults and has been refined into two conditions: ADD and ADHD (attention deficit and hyperactivity disorder). Characteristics include difficulty sustaining attention or completing tasks, easy distractibility, impulsive behavior, and, in the case of ADHD, an excessive inclination to fidget and move about. These problems make it difficult to succeed at work or at school.

Conventional treatment focuses on stimulants, such as amphetamine, dextroamphetamine, and methylphenidate (Ritalin, Concerta), as well as the newer drug atomoxetine (Strattera). Certain antidepressants may also be useful.

Proposed Natural Treatments

DMAE

There is some evidence that the supplement DMAE (2-Dimethylaminoethanol) may be helpful for ADD, according to studies performed in the 1970s. Two such studies were reported in a review article. Fifty children aged 6 to 12 years who had been diagnosed with hyperkinesia participated in a double-blind study comparing DMAE to placebo. The dose was increased from 300 mg daily to 500 mg daily by the third week and continued for 10 weeks. Evaluations revealed statistically significant test score improvements in the treatment group compared to the placebo group.

Another double-blind study compared DMAE with both Ritalin and placebo in 74 children with "learning disabilities" (it appears that today, the participants would have been given a diagnosis of ADD). It found significant test score improvement for both treatment groups over a 10-week period.

For more information, including dosage and safety issues, see the full **DMAE** article.

Zinc

The mineral zinc has shown some promise for treatment of ADHD. In a large double-blind, placebo-controlled study (approximately 400 participants), use of zinc at a dose of 35 mg daily produced statistically significant benefits as compared to placebo. This dose of zinc is higher than nutritional needs, but not so high as to be unsafe. However, the benefits seen were quite modest: about 28% of the participants given zinc showed improvement, but so did 20% in the placebo group.

Another, much smaller study evaluated whether zinc at 15 mg per day could enhance the effect of Ritalin. Again, modest benefits were seen. Finally, exceedingly weak evidence hints that zinc might enhance the effectiveness of evening primrose oil for ADHD (see next section).

For more information, including dosage and safety issues, see the full **Zinc** article.

Essential Fatty Acids

Essential fatty acids (EFAs) are "good fats," substances as important to your general health as vitamins. Based on evidence that essential fatty acids are necessary for the proper development of brain function in growing children, EFAs found in **fish oil** and **evening primrose oil** have been tried for the treatment of ADHD and related conditions. However, the results have been less than impressive.

In a double-blind, placebo-controlled study of 50 children with ADHD, use of essential fatty acids from fish oil and evening primrose oil failed to provide any consistent, significant benefit above and beyond the placebo effect. (The placebo effect, however, was considerable.) In a slightly smaller double-blind, placebo-controlled trial, weak evidence of benefit was seen, but

the results are difficult to interpret due to the high number of people who dropped out of the study.

In a double-blind, placebo-controlled trial of children already using stimulant therapy, the addition of the essential fatty acid docosahexaenoic acid (DHA, found in fish oil) for 4 months failed to further improve symptoms.

Evening primrose oil alone failed to prove effective for attention deficit disorder in a small double-blind, placebo-controlled trial. In a placebo-controlled, comparative trial, evening primrose oil proved less effective than standard medical treatment. However, a close look at the data in this last trial hinted that evening primrose oil might have been more effective in people with adequate zinc levels. This suggests that combination therapy with zinc and evening primrose oil should be tested, but thus far this approach has not undergone meaningful study.

Other Natural Treatments

A small double-blind, placebo-controlled crossover trial evaluated the possible efficacy of the supplement carnitine for ADD in boys 13 and younger. Approximately 50% of the participants responded to **carnitine**, a significantly higher percentage than responded to placebo. These promising results suggest that a larger trial is warranted.

A combination of **American Ginseng** and **ginkgo** has shown some promise for treatment of ADHD.

Vitamin B$_3$ (niacin), **vitamin B$_6$**, and **multivitamin/ multimineral supplements** have been recommended for the treatment of ADD. However, a review of the literature found no meaningful evidence to indicate that any of these treatments are effective.

One study is sometimes said to have proven **magnesium** helpful for ADD, but in fact the study design was inadequate to prove much of anything.

Other supplements that are sometimes recommended for ADD include **calcium**, **iron**, **inositol**, trace minerals, blue-green algae, combinations of amino acids (usually GABA, glycine, **taurine**, **L-glutamine**, **L-phenylalanine**, and **L-tyrosine**), and combinations of the polysaccharides galactose, glucose, mannose, N-acetylneuraminic acid, fucose, N-acetylgalactosamine, N-acetylglucosamine, and xylose. **St. John's wort** has also become popular recently. However, there is no reliable evidence for any of these treatments at this time. **Note:** St. John's wort interacts with many medications and could conceivably impair the effectiveness of conventional treatments for ADD.

One study hints that **massage** might be helpful for ADD.

It is commonly said that eliminating sugar, food additives, and **food allergens** improves ADD symptoms. However, the body of published evidence regarding these therapies remains incomplete and contradictory.

A double-blind study reported in 2005 failed to find benefits for ADD with a treatment known as **Bach flower remedies**.

One study found that the supplement **melatonin** may be helpful for improving sleep in children with ADHD taking stimulant medications.

Autism Spectrum Disorder

PRINCIPAL PROPOSED NATURAL TREATMENTS: *None*

OTHER PROPOSED NATURAL TREATMENTS: *Carnosine, Food Allergen Avoidance, Massage Therapy, Vitamin B$_6$ (Alone or Combined with Magnesium), Multivitamin/Multimineral Supplements, Vitamin C*

Autism spectrum disorder (ASD, previously called *autism*) is a poorly understood family of related conditions. People with ASD generally lack normal social interaction skills and engage in a variety of unusual and often characteristic behaviors, such as repetitive movements. There is no specific medical treatment for ASD and its cause remains unclear. Anecdotal evidence of remarkable cures with the use of the substance secretin had raised hopes, but these hopes faded when numerous formal research trials found secretin ineffective.

Despite public concerns that the measles, mumps, and rubella (MMR) vaccine may cause autism spectrum disorder, the balance of the evidence strongly suggests that this is not true.

Proposed Natural Treatments

Nutrients

Some physicians involved with natural medicine believe that autism spectrum disorder, as well as many other illnesses, are caused by genetic defects in the body that interfere with the metabolism of certain nutrients. For example, there is some evidence that children with autism spectrum disorder may have trouble metabolizing vitamin B$_6$. Based on this theory, various supplements have been advocated for the treatment of autism spectrum disorder. However, despite a number of favorable anecdotal reports, as yet there is no reliable supporting evidence from meaningful studies. As the secretin example shows (see above), anecdotes can easily be misleading.

One 10-week, double-blind, placebo-controlled, crossover study of 18 autistic children evaluated high doses of **vitamin C** for its effects on behavior. Participants received 8 g of vitamin C for every 70 kg of body weight. In this rather complex study, all participants received vitamin C for 10 weeks. After that, half received vitamin C and the other half received placebo for 10 weeks. During the third and final 10-week period, the vitamin C and placebo groups were switched. The results indicated that use of vitamin C caused significant improvements in behavior when compared to use of placebo. This study was small and suffered from various design problems. Nonetheless, it does suggest that further research into using vitamin C for autism spectrum disorder might be advisable. Note: At this level of vitamin C intake, many people experience diarrhea.

Another double-blind, placebo-controlled, crossover study found indications that very high doses of **vitamin B$_6$** may produce beneficial effects in the treatment of autism spectrum disorder. Again, however, this study was small and poorly designed; furthermore, it used a dose of vitamin B$_6$ so high that it could cause toxicity.

It has been suggested that combining magnesium with vitamin B$_6$ could offer additional benefits, such as reducing side effects or allowing a reduced dose of the vitamin. However, the two reasonably well-designed studies using combined vitamin B$_6$ and **magnesium** have failed to find benefits. Therefore, it isn't possible at present to recommend vitamin B$_6$ with or without magnesium as a treatment for autism spectrum disorder.

One small study found that use of a **multivitamin/**

multimineral supplement improved sleep and gastrointestinal problems in people with autistic spectrum disorder to a greater extent than placebo.

Other Natural Approaches

An 8-week, double-blind, placebo-controlled trial of 31 children found preliminary evidence that the supplement **carnosine** at a dose of 400 mg twice daily might be helpful for autism spectrum disorder.

Massage therapy might also be helpful for autism spectrum disorder, according to one small controlled study.

It has been suggested that food additives, **food allergies**, or other dietary factors may play a role in autism spectrum disorder, but meaningful supporting evidence for this theory has not been presented. One very small but well-designed study failed to find benefit through eliminating gluten and casein from the diet. The study followed a double-blind design; interestingly, parents generally thought they saw improvement, but perceived improvements were equally divided between the treatment group and the placebo group.

Back Pain

RELATED TERMS: *Backache, Back Strain, Lower Back Pain*
PRINCIPAL PROPOSED NATURAL TREATMENTS: *Acupuncture, Chiropractic, Prolotherapy, White Willow*
OTHER PROPOSED NATURAL TREATMENTS: *Boswellia, Butterbur, Chondroitin, Comfrey (Topical Cream),*
Devil's Claw, Ginger, Glucosamine, Osteopathic Manipulation, Proteolytic Enzymes, Turmeric, Yoga

Low back pain is one of the most common health conditions today. According to some estimates, each year nearly 15 to 20% of the United States population experiences low back problems and as many as 80% of all adults experience significant low back pain at some point during their lives. Back pain is the second most common reason adults under age 45 miss days from work (after the common cold). The total cost of back pain has been estimated to reach $25 billion per year in the U.S.

When back pain occurs suddenly (after lifting a heavy object, for example), it is called *acute back pain* or *sprain*. In most cases, acute back pain eventually improves by itself, but there may be weeks of discomfort, time lost from work, and impaired function at home.

When back pain persists over months or years, it is called *chronic back pain*. In the majority of cases, the cause of chronic back pain is unknown. Identifiable causes include **osteoarthritis**, fracture, or injury to the discs between the vertebrae.

Conventional treatment of acute back pain involves **anti-inflammatory drugs**, muscle relaxants, and the passage of time. Chronic back pain requires a medical workup to make sure there are no serious underlying causes, although evidence suggests that in most cases X rays are not necessary. Treatment may also include physical therapy and a graded exercise program. However, there is little reliable evidence that these treatments actually provide much benefit. Surgery may be recommended in certain cases, such as when there are severe disc problems, but most forms of back surgery also lack reliable supporting evidence.

Principal Proposed Natural Treatments

Extract of the herb white willow appears to be helpful for acute and chronic back pain, presumably because of its similarity to aspirin. The little-known injection technique known as prolotherapy may be effective for back pain as well. Lesser evidence supports the use of chiropractic and acupuncture.

White Willow

Willow bark has been used as a treatment for pain and fever in China since 500 BC. It contains the substance salicin, which is chemically related to aspirin. Another ingredient of white willow, tremulacin, may also be important.

In a 4-week, double-blind, placebo-controlled study of 210 individuals with chronic back pain, two different doses of willow bark extract were compared against placebo. The higher-dose group received extract supplying 240 mg of salicin daily; in this group, 39% were pain-free for at least the last 5 days of the study. In the lower-dose group (120 mg of salicin daily), 21% became pain-free. In contrast, only 6% of those given placebo became pain-free. Stomach distress did not occur in this study. The only significant side effect seen was an allergic reaction in one participant given willow.

Note: White willow should not be combined with standard anti-inflammatory drugs, such as ibuprofen. For more information, including dosage and safety issues, see the full **White Willow** article.

Prolotherapy

Invented in the 1950s by George Hackett, prolotherapy is based on the theory that chronic pain is often caused by laxness of the ligaments that are responsible for the joint's stability. When ligaments and associated tendons are loose, the body is said to compensate by using muscles to hold the joint stable. The net result, according to prolotherapy theory, is muscle spasms and pain.

Prolotherapy treatment involves injections of chemical irritant solutions into the area around such ligaments. These solutions cause tissue to proliferate (grow), increasing the strength and thickness of ligaments. This tightens up the joint and presumably allows the associated muscles to stop having spasms. In the case of arthritic joints, increased ligament strength may allow the joint to function more efficiently, reducing pain.

Prolotherapy has not yet been widely accepted in conventional medicine. However, highly respected institutions have studied it, and standard textbooks of orthopedics and rehabilitation medicine mention the technique. It is used by prolotherapy practitioners to treat many conditions including **fibromyalgia**, osteoarthritis, plantar fasciitis, **sciatica**, **sports injuries**, **temporomandibular joint** (TMJ) disorder, **tendinitis**, and **tension headaches**. The best evidence at present is for its use in back pain and osteoarthritis.

Animal and human studies have found that prolotherapy injections increase strength and thickness of ligaments.

In a double-blind study, 81 individuals with low back pain of many years' duration were given either prolotherapy injections or placebo treatment. Both groups

also received intense spinal manipulation with local anesthetic on the first visit, although in the treatment group this was more extensive. The injections were given 6 times on a weekly basis. The prolotherapy group received a mixture of dextrose, glycerin, and phenol (along with local anesthetic), thought to irritate tissues and cause ligament growth. The placebo group received saline (saltwater) injections.

The results were positive. Prolotherapy-treated participants showed significantly less pain and disability within a month and the relative benefit continued for the full 6 months of the study.

A subsequent double-blind study using the same prolotherapy mixture (but without manipulation) also found benefits.

However, a third study of similar size and using the same mixture failed to find benefit. Furthermore, a study of 110 people using a different prolotherapy mixture (20% glucose plus local anesthetic) also failed to find prolotherapy more effective than placebo.

What can one make of this contradictory evidence? The most likely conclusion is that prolotherapy, if it is effective at all, offers no more than modest benefits for back pain.

For more information, see the full **Prolotherapy** article.

Chiropractic

Chiropractic spinal manipulation is one of the most popular treatments for acute and chronic back pain in the U.S. and it may provide at least modest benefit; however, as yet research evidence has failed to find chiropractic manipulation convincingly more effective than standard medical care.

Chiropractic does seem to be more effective than placebo, if not by a great deal. For example, a single-blind, controlled study of 84 people suffering from low back pain compared manipulation to treatment with a diathermy machine (a physical therapy machine that uses microwaves to create heat beneath the skin) that was not actually functioning. The researchers asked the participants to assess their own pain levels within 15 minutes of the first treatment, then 3 and 7 days after treatment. The only statistically significant difference between the two groups was within 15 minutes of the manipulation. (Chiropractic had better results at that point.)

In another single-blind, placebo-controlled study, researchers assigned 209 participants to one of three groups: a high-velocity, low-amplitude (HVLA) spinal manipulation, a sham manipulation group, or a back education program. Though this has been reported as a positive study, most of the differences seen between the groups were too small to be statistically significant.

Unimpressive results were also seen in a well-designed study of 321 people with back pain, comparing chiropractic manipulation, a special form of physical therapy (the Mackenzie method), and the provision of an educational booklet in treating low back pain. All groups improved to about the same extent.

Several studies evaluated the effectiveness of chiropractic manipulation combined with a different kind of treatment called *mobilization*, but they too found little to no benefit.

On a positive note, one study of 100 people with back pain and sciatica symptoms (pain down the leg due to disc protrusion) found that chiropractic manipulation was significantly more effective at relieving symptoms than sham chiropractic manipulation.

Several studies have found that chiropractic is at least as helpful as other commonly used therapies for low back pain, such as muscle relaxants, soft-tissue **massage**, and physical therapy. Furthermore, in one well-designed study, 2 months of chiropractic spinal manipulation produced somewhat greater pain relief than exercise therapy and this relative superiority endured to the 1-year follow-up point.

For more information, see the full **Chiropractic** article.

Acupuncture

The ancient technique of acupuncture has become increasingly popular as a treatment for pain and other conditions. However, thus far, research has not produced evidence that acupuncture is effective for back pain.

For example, in a controlled trial of 113 people with back pain, some received traditional acupuncture, some sham acupuncture, and some no treatment. Twenty sessions of traditional acupuncture generally failed to produce significantly more benefit than sham acupuncture. Both sham and real acupuncture, however, were far more effective than no treatment, demonstrating the placebo power of acupuncture.

Also, in a single-blind, sham-acupuncture and no-treatment controlled study of 298 people with chronic back pain, use of real acupuncture failed to prove significantly more effective than sham-acupuncture. Other studies have failed to find benefit as well; in several controlled studies enrolling a total of about 200 people, real acupuncture also failed to prove more effective than sham-acupuncture or other placebo treatments.

One study compared the effects of acupuncture, massage, and education (such as videotapes on back care) for 262 people with chronic back pain over a 10-week period. The exact type of acupuncture and massage was left to practitioners, but only 10 visits were permitted. At the 10-week point, evaluations showed benefit with massage but not with acupuncture. One year later, massage and education were nearly equivalent, and both were superior to acupuncture.

Many other studies have compared acupuncture to such treatments as TENS, physical therapy, chiropractic care, and massage. In many of these trials, acupuncture provided benefits comparable to the other options tested. However, because TENS, physical therapy, and so forth have not been proven effective for back pain, studies of this type cannot be taken as evidence that acupuncture is effective. One study found acupressure massage more effective than standard physical therapy; however, it was performed in a Chinese population that may have had more faith in this traditional approach than in physical therapy.

For more information, see the full **Acupuncture** article.

Other Proposed Natural Treatments

In a double-blind, placebo-controlled study enrolling 215 people with back pain, use of a topical cream made from the herb **comfrey** produced statistically significant benefits as compared to placebo.

The herb **devil's claw** is used for the treatment of osteoarthritis and has been tried for back pain as well. However, the results have been less than impressive. A double-blind, placebo-controlled study of 197 individuals with chronic back pain found devil's claw only marginally effective at best. Similarly poor results were seen in an earlier 4-week, double-blind, placebo-controlled study of 118 individuals with acute back pain. However, a 4-week, double-blind, placebo-controlled study of 63 people with mild to moderate chronic muscular tension in the neck, back, and shoulders did find some benefit.

The herb **cayenne** contains capsaicin, a substance that produces an immediate burning sensation but later reduces pain. One double-blind study found a topical cayenne treatment more effective than placebo in 320 people with low back pain. However, on the face of it, one finds it difficult to believe that this study was truly double-blind. When cayenne is applied to the skin, it causes such an intense sensation that participants could hardly fail to notice it. When people in a study know whether they are getting real treatment or placebo treatment, the validity of the study's results is greatly decreased.

Osteopathic manipulation (OM) is a form of treatment related to chiropractic manipulation, but it tends to use gentle, extended movements (low velocity, high amplitude) rather than the quick, short, cracking movements of chiropractic. Although OM has shown some promise for the treatment of back pain, one of the best-designed trials failed to find it a superior alternative to conventional medical care. In this 12-week study of 178 individuals, OM proved no more effective than standard treatment for back pain. Another study failed to find osteopathic manipulation more effective than sham manipulation.

The **Alexander Technique** is a special method of postural training popular among dancers. A review of the literature found no more than weak preliminary evi-

dence that Alexander may help with back pain, but concluded that further research is warranted.

Biofeedback and also **hatha yoga** have shown some preliminary promise for back pain.

Preliminary evidence suggests that **proteolytic enzymes** might be helpful for back pain.

Other herbs and supplements sometimes recommended for back pain, but with no real supporting evidence, include **boswellia**, **butterbur**, **chondroitin**, **ginger**, **glucosamine**, and **turmeric**.

Herbs and Supplements to Use Only with Caution

Various herbs and supplements may interact adversely with drugs used to treat back pain. For more information on this potential risk, see the individual drug article in the Drug Interactions section of this book.

Bed-Wetting

RELATED TERMS: *Nocturnal Enuresis, Primary Nocturnal Enuresis, PNE*

PRINCIPAL PROPOSED NATURAL TREATMENTS: *None*

OTHER PROPOSED NATURAL TREATMENTS: *Acupuncture, Bach Flower Remedies, Chinese Herbal Medicine, Food Allergies, Hypnosis, Juniper, Lobelia, Marshmallow Root, Parsley Root, Uva Ursi*

Nocturnal enuresis, or bed-wetting, is defined as unintended nighttime urination in a child over 5 years old. In most cases, there is no underlying medical cause, in which case the condition is called *primary nocturnal enuresis* (PNE). When enuresis occurs as a result of another illness, it is called *secondary nocturnal enuresis.*

In adults, when the bladder becomes full during the night, it signals to the brain that this has occurred; in turn, the brain informs the bladder not to empty and also begins the process leading to wakefulness. The ability to carry out this process is not present at birth, but most children gradually develop this capacity and achieve it in full by age six. However, as many as 7% of 10-year-olds and 1 to 2% of 15-year-olds continue to have trouble. Nearly all children with primary nocturnal enuresis will cease bed-wetting by the time they reach puberty. However, PNE remains a problem for up to 1% of adults.

Enuresis occurs more commonly in boys than in girls. In addition, there is a strong genetic predisposition: if both parents have enuresis, there is a 75% chance that a child will; this decreases to 40% if only one parent has enuresis.

Nocturnal enuresis is not a disease, but it can lead to significant embarrassment and limitation of activities and, for this reason, treatment may be desired. The first step is a medical examination to rule out rare underlying causes, such as infection. Common sense steps follow, such as not drinking much liquid near bedtime, and voiding just before going to bed. More specific treatment can be delayed as long as desired because, in the great majority of cases, nocturnal enuresis will eventually disappear. For older children who wish to accelerate the process, nighttime alarm systems that wake the child in response to moisture in the child's underpants are often highly effective. Other methods include bladder exercises and a schedule of planned nighttime waking. If these behavioral methods fail, use of various medications may be considered.

Proposed Natural Treatments

No one wants to give a healthy child medication and, for this reason, many parents turn to alternative medicine for the treatment of nocturnal enuresis if behavioral methods don't work. However, no alternative therapies have as yet been proven effective for this condition.

Hypnosis has shown some promise for nocturnal enuresis. In one study, 50 children were given either the drug imipramine, or hypnotherapy, for 3 months. The results showed substantial and approximately equal benefits in the two groups. Subsequently, children in the hypnosis group practiced self-hypnosis for another 6 months, while those in the imipramine group did not utilize any special therapy. At the end of the 6 months, children practicing self-hypnosis had maintained their benefits to a much greater extent than those in the imipramine group. Other studies found benefits with hypnosis as well ; however, all had significant design limitations and, overall, the evidence supporting hypnosis for nocturnal enuresis is not yet strong.

It has been suggested that food allergies may play a role in nocturnal enuresis. However, there is only incomplete evidence that allergen avoidance or any other dietary approaches can help.

Herbs used for miscellaneous bladder problems are often recommended for nocturnal enuresis, on general principles. These include juniper, lobelia, marshmallow root, parsley root, and uva ursi. However, there is no evidence that these herbs help the condition and some, such as uva ursi, may have toxic properties, especially when given for the long term.

Acupuncture, Bach flower remedies, and Chinese herbal medicine are also sometimes recommended for nocturnal enuresis, but there is no reliable evidence that they are effective. One reasonably well-designed study found evidence that a special form of chiropractic (Activator technique) is *not* effective for bed-wetting.

Herbs and Supplements to Use Only with Caution

Various herbs and supplements may interact adversely with drugs used to treat nocturnal enuresis. For more information on this potential risk, see the individual drug article in the Drug Interactions section of this book.

Bell's Palsy

RELATED TERMS: *Facial Nerve Palsy; Facial Paralysis; Idiopathic Facial Paralysis; Palsy, Facial; Paralysis, Facial*

PRINCIPAL PROPOSED NATURAL TREATMENTS: *None*

OTHER PROPOSED NATURAL TREATMENTS: *Acupuncture, Biofeedback, Hyperbaric Oxygen Therapy, Vitamin B_{12} Injections*

Overview

Bell's palsy is the common name for a condition in which paralysis strikes the seventh cranial nerve, which controls much of the face. Only one side of the face is affected. Symptoms usually come on suddenly and painlessly and are first noticed as a droop in one corner of the mouth and an inability to smile properly. Other symptoms may include drooling, an inability to close the eye on the same side, tearing, impairment of taste, and occasionally

pain. While anyone can develop Bell's palsy, it occurs most often in pregnant women and people who have diabetes, hypertension, or a respiratory infection.

Conventional treatment for Bell's palsy currently involves corticosteroid drugs (such as prednisone) and sometimes the antiviral drug acyclovir. However, according to a review published in 2002, there is no reliable evidence that either treatment provides any benefit. A study published subsequent to the review did show a slight benefit with early, high-dose corticosteroid treatment.

Useful supportive measures for Bell's palsy include

patching the affected eye at night and using artificial tears. Surgery or electrical stimulation of the nerve are used rarely.

Note: Medical evaluation is essential because, in rare cases, Bell's palsy may be caused by an underlying condition that requires specific treatment, such as a tumor.

Proposed Natural Treatments for Bell's Palsy

Hyperbaric oxygen therapy involves breathing 100% oxygen at increased pressure. It is used both by conventional and alternative practitioners. A placebo-controlled study found hyperbaric oxygen more effective than prednisone. In this trial, a total of 79 people with Bell's palsy were randomly assigned to receive either hyperbaric oxygen (1 hour twice daily, 5 days a week, for 30 sessions or up to full recovery) or prednisone. Placebo pills were given along with hyperbaric therapy, and fake hyperbaric therapy was given along with prednisone. The results showed a significantly greater speed of recovery as well as a higher percentage of full recovery in the hyperbaric oxygen group compared to the prednisone group.

Many alternative practitioners recommend the use of injected **vitamin B$_{12}$** for Bell's palsy. However, the only scientific support for this approach comes from one study that was not double-blind. (For information on the importance of a double-blind design, see **Why Does The Natural Pharmacist Rely on Double-blind Studies?**)

Other treatments sometimes recommended for Bell's palsy, but with inadequate supporting evidence, include **acupuncture** and **biofeedback**.

Benign Prostatic Hyperplasia

RELATED TERMS: *Prostate Enlargement*

PRINCIPAL PROPOSED NATURAL TREATMENTS: *Beta-Sitosterol, Grass Pollen, Nettle Root, Pygeum, Saw Palmetto*

OTHER PROPOSED NATURAL TREATMENTS: *Flaxseed Oil, Green Tea, Maca, Oat Straw, Pumpkin Seeds, Zinc*

If you're a man and you live long enough, you will almost certainly develop benign prostatic hyperplasia (BPH). Ninety percent of all men show signs of such prostatic enlargement by the age of 80. Symptoms include difficulty in starting urination, a diminished force of urinary stream, a sensation of fullness in the bladder after urination, and the need to urinate many times at night. Ultimately, the obstruction can become so severe that urination is impossible.

The most common treatment for BPH is surgery that removes most of the prostate gland. Medications such as Cardura, Flomax, Hytrin, and Proscar can relieve symptoms of BPH. In addition, Proscar has been shown to shrink the prostate and reduce the need for surgery. However, all of these medications can cause significant side effects.

Principal Proposed Natural Treatments

Men who suspect they may suffer from BPH should make sure to see a physician to rule out prostate cancer. After this has been done, many natural options are available that have good scientific backing. Indeed, there are few other conditions for which so many natural therapies have good supporting evidence for efficacy. However, there is one potential advantage for standard medications: some have been shown sufficiently effective at slowing the progression of BPH to help men avoid surgery, while this has not been shown to be true of any natural options.

Saw Palmetto

The best-documented herbal treatment for BPH is the oil of the berry of the saw palmetto tree. This herb is so well accepted in Europe that synthetic pharmaceuticals are considered alternative therapy for BPH. Saw palmetto offers two potential advantages over conventional drug treatment. The most obvious is that it usually causes no side effects. Another advantage is that saw palmetto does not change protein-specific antigen (PSA) levels. Lab tests that measure PSA are used to screen for prostate cancer. The widely used drug Proscar can artificially lower PSA levels, which may have the unintended effect of masking prostate cancer.

The scientific evidence that saw palmetto is effective for prostate enlargement is quite impressive, although not perfect.

At least 10 double-blind, placebo-controlled studies involving a total of about 900 participants have compared the benefits of saw palmetto against placebo over a period of 1 to 12 months. In all but three of these studies, the herb significantly improved urinary flow rate and most other measures of prostate disease. However, in the most recent and perhaps best-designed of these studies, a 1-year trial of 225 men, saw palmetto product failed to prove more effective than placebo.

A double-blind study followed 1,098 men who received either saw palmetto or the drug Proscar over a period of 6 months. According to the results, the two treatments were about equally successful at reducing noticeable symptoms and neither produced much in the way of side effects. However, Proscar lowered PSA levels, presenting a risk of masking prostate cancer. Saw palmetto did not cause this problem. On the other hand, careful measurements showed that Proscar caused men's prostates to shrink by 18%, while saw palmetto caused only a 6% decrease in size. Although prostate size does not correlate well with severity of symptoms, such a decrease in size might indicate a reduced likelihood of need for surgery. This is a potential advantage for the drug.

A 52-week, double-blind study of 811 men compared saw palmetto to a standard drug for BPH in another class: the alpha-blocker tamsulosin. Once again, both treatments proved equally effective. However, saw palmetto caused fewer side effects than the drug. In addition, the herb caused some prostate shrinkage, while the drug allowed a slight prostate enlargement.

Although there are many theories about how saw palmetto works, none have been conclusively established. The best evidence suggests that the herb affects male hormones.

For important dosage and safety information, see the full **Saw Palmetto** article.

Pygeum

The pygeum tree is a tall evergreen native to central and southern Africa. Its bark has been used since ancient times for urinary problems.

At least 17 double-blind trials of pygeum for BPH have been performed, involving a total of almost 1,000 individuals and ranging in length from 45 to 90 days. Many of these studies were poorly reported and/or de-

signed. Nonetheless, overall, the results do suggest that pygeum can reduce symptoms such as nighttime urination, urinary frequency, and residual urine volume.

The best of these trials was conducted at 8 sites in Europe and included 263 men between 50 and 85 years of age. Participants received 50 mg of a pygeum extract or placebo twice daily. The results showed significant improvements in various measures of BPH severity.

We don't really know how pygeum works. Unlike the standard drug finasteride, it does not appear to work by affecting the conversion of testosterone to dihydrotestosterone. Rather it is thought to reduce inflammation in the prostate and to inhibit prostate growth factors, substances implicated in inappropriate prostate enlargement. We don't know whether pygeum can reduce the need for prostate surgery or whether it affects PSA levels.

For more information, including dosage and safety issues, see the full **Pygeum** article.

Nettle Root

Anyone who lives in a locale where nettle grows wild will likely discover the powers of this dark green plant. Depending on the species, the fine hairs on its leaves and stem cause burning pain that lasts from hours to weeks. Both its leaves and roots can be used as medicine. The root is a popular European treatment for BPH. However, it has not been as well studied as saw palmetto or pygeum.

In a double-blind, placebo-controlled study performed in Iran, 558 people were given either placebo or nettle root for 6 months. The results indicated that nettle root is significantly more effective than placebo on all major measures of BPH severity. Benefits were seen in three other double-blind studies as well, enrolling a total of more than 150 men.

For more information, including dosage and safety issues, see the full **Nettle** article.

Beta-Sitosterol

Numerous plants contain cholesterol-like compounds called *sitosterols* and their close relatives *sitosterolins*. A special mixture of these called *beta-sitosterol* is used for the treatment of BPH.

A review of the literature, published in 1999, found a total of four randomized double-blind, placebo-controlled studies on beta-sitosterol for BPH, enrolling a total of 519 men. All but one of these studies found significant benefits in both perceived symptoms and objective measurements, such as urine flow rate. The largest trial followed 200 men with BPH for a period of

6 months. After the study was completed, many of the participants were followed for an additional year, during which the benefits continued. Similar results were seen in a 6-month, double-blind trial of 177 individuals with BPH.

For more information, including dosage and safety issues, see the full **Beta-sitosterol** article.

Grass Pollen

Grass pollen is also used to treat BPH. The grasses used for this preparation are 92% rye, 5% timothy, and 3% corn. Related grass pollen extracts are used for allergy shots. However, the grass pollen extracts described here are different in that they have their allergenic components removed. Grass pollen is also an entirely different product than bee pollen.

Two double-blind, placebo-controlled studies found that grass pollen extract can improve symptoms of prostate enlargement. There have also been open studies that compared grass pollen to different treatments for BPH.

In the first double-blind, placebo-controlled study, 103 individuals with BPH were assigned to take either placebo or 2 capsules of a standardized grass pollen extract 3 times daily for a period of 12 weeks. At the end of the study, 69% of the participants who had been taking the grass pollen had reduced the number of trips they had to make to the bathroom at night. In the placebo group, only 37% reported improvement in this symptom. The amount of urine remaining in the bladder following urination was reduced in the treatment group by 24 ml and by 4 ml for the placebo group. Both of these were statistically significant improvements for those taking grass pollen.

The second double-blind, placebo-controlled study lasted longer but enrolled fewer participants. Fifty-seven men with prostate enlargement were enrolled in the study, with 31 taking 92 mg of the grass pollen extract daily for 6 months and the remaining 26 taking placebo. As with the previous study, statistically significant improvements in nighttime frequency of urination and emptying of the bladder were found with use of grass pollen extract. Additionally, 69% of the participants receiving treatment reported overall improvement, while only 29% of the group taking the placebo felt they had improved, another statistically significant difference.

An important finding in this study was that the prostates of the men taking grass pollen significantly decreased in size according to ultrasound measurements taken.

No one is certain how the grass pollen extract causes the beneficial results seen in the studies. One theory is that it inhibits the body's manufacturing of prostaglandins and leukotrienes, which might relieve prostate congestion by reducing inflammation.

For more information, including dosage and safety issues, see the full **Grass Pollen Extract** article.

Combination Treatment

A 48-week, double-blind trial of 543 men with early BPH compared combined saw palmetto and nettle root against Proscar and found equal benefits. The same combination proved superior to placebo in a 24-week, double-blind study of 257 men.

In a 3-month, double-blind, placebo-controlled study of 144 men with BPS, use of a combination product containing saw palmetto, grass pollen extract, beta-sitosterol, and **vitamin E** significantly reduced symptoms.

A 6-month, double-blind, placebo-controlled trial of 44 men given a saw palmetto herbal blend (containing, in addition, nettle root and pumpkin seed oil) found shrinkage in prostate tissue. No significant improvement in symptoms was seen, but the authors pointed out that the study size was too small to statistically detect such improvements if they did occur. Another small study failed to find significant benefit with a combination of pygeum and nettle root.

Other Proposed Natural Treatments

One study provides weak evidence that **green tea** extracts taken orally might reduce symptoms of BPH.

Pumpkin seeds are approved for use in BPH by Germany's Commission E. The mineral **zinc** is also commonly recommended in both Europe and the United States as a treatment for prostate disease, as are both **whole flaxseed** and **flaxseed oil**, along with the herbs **maca** (*Lepidium meyenii*) and **oat straw** (*Avena sativa*). However, there is no meaningful evidence to indicate that any of these proposed options are effective.

Bipolar Disorder

RELATED TERMS: *Manic-Depression, Manic-Depressive Disease*

PRINCIPAL PROPOSED NATURAL TREATMENTS: *None*

OTHER PROPOSED NATURAL TREATMENTS: *Choline, Fish Oil, Flaxseed Oil, Folate, Inositol, Lecithin, Vitamin B$_{12}$, Vitamin C*

HERBS AND SUPPLEMENTS TO USE ONLY WITH CAUTION FOR BIPOLAR DISORDER: *Chromium Picolinate, Ginseng, Glutamine, Inositol, S-adenosylmethionine (SAMe), St. John's Wort, Vanadium*

Previously known as manic-depressive disease, bipolar disorder is a relatively common mental health condition manifested in its classic form by alternating periods of mania—extreme high energy—and deep depression. In the "up" or *manic phase*, people may sleep little, talk fast, develop grand and unworkable plans, and sometimes behave bizarrely—for example, giving away all their money overnight. In the "down" phase, they may contemplate suicide. In many people with this disorder the "down" phase predominates and for that reason the diagnosis may be missed. Other, more subtle versions of the condition also exist.

Bipolar disorder is dangerous unless treated, leading to a high rate of suicide and injury. The mineral **lithium** has been shown to dramatically improve symptoms of mania and reduce the rate of suicide. Various antiseizure medications also appear to help against mania.

Proposed Natural Treatments for Bipolar Disorder

Note: There are no natural treatments that can substitute for medications in the treatment of bipolar disorder. However, some might help enhance the effectiveness of standard treatment.

In a double-blind study reported in 1999, 30 people with bipolar disorder took either **fish oil** capsules or placebo for 4 months, in addition to their regular medications. Those taking the fish oil had longer symptom-free periods than those taking placebo. The researchers used five different standardized tests to measure symptoms, examining levels of depression, mania, and overall progress. The people taking fish oil proved emotionally healthier than those taking placebo on all but one of these tests. Another study found that ethyl-EPA (a modified form of a constituent of fish oil) was helpful along with standard treatment for the depressed phase of bipolar disorder.

The same researchers who conducted the fish oil study have also experimented with **flaxseed oil** for bipolar disorder. Flaxseed oil contains alpha-linoleic acid (ALA), an omega-3 fatty acid related to the fatty acids in fish oil. In the researchers' informal observations of 22 people with bipolar disorder, all but four appeared to benefit from flaxseed oil. However, lacking a double-blind study, these results can't be taken as meaningful. When a double-blind study is finally performed, flaxseed oil may turn out not to be helpful at all.

One somewhat questionable study reported that an herbal combination utilized in **Traditional Chinese Medicine** ("Free and Easy Wanderer") may augment the effectiveness of carbamazepine treatment for bipolar disorder.

Very weak evidence suggests possible benefits with **choline**, **lecithin**, **vitamin C**, and **inositol**. Inositol may also reduce psoriasis symptoms caused by lithium. (However, caution is advised with inositol. See Herbs and Supplements to Use Only with Caution below.)

A special form of **magnet therapy** called *rTMS* has shown some promise for bipolar disorder.

Various supplements may help reduce side effects of antiseizure drugs. For more information, see the articles on **valproate**, **carbamazepine**, and **phenytoin** in the Drug Interaction section.

Despite promising preliminary indications, a double-blind study failed to find that **folate** enhances the effect of the drug lithium.

Note: Lithium is sometimes sold as a mineral supplement for treating bipolar disorder. However, this proposed use is based on a misunderstanding. When lithium is used medically as treatment for bipolar disorder, it is taken at doses far above any possible nutritional need. No researcher has seriously suggested that lithium *deficiency* causes bipolar symptoms and low doses of lithium are unlikely to have any effect at all.

Herbs and Supplements to Use Only with Caution

Antidepressant drugs may cause manic episodes in people with bipolar disorder. For this reason, herbs and supplements with antidepressant properties might also be risky. Case reports suggest that **SAMe**, **St. John's wort**, and **inositol** can indeed trigger manic episodes.

The supplement **L-glutamine**, while not normally considered to have antidepressant properties, has reportedly triggered episodes of mania in two people not previously known to have bipolar disorder. A **ginseng** product has also been associated with an episode of mania.

The supplement **chromium** is often sold in the form of chromium picolinate. Picolinate can alter levels of neurotransmitters. This has led to concern among some experts that chromium picolinate might be harmful to people with bipolar disorder.

It has been suggested that the drug lithium works, in part, by reducing the body's level of **vanadium**. For this reason, it might be advisable for people with bipolar disorder to avoid using supplements that contain vanadium.

Finally, numerous herbs and supplements may interact adversely with drugs used to prevent or treat bipolar disorder. For example, people who use lithium should avoid herbal diuretics. For more information on this potential risk, see the appropriate individual drug articles in the Drug Interactions section of this book.

Bladder Infection

RELATED TERMS: *Urinary Tract Infection*

PRINCIPAL PROPOSED NATURAL TREATMENTS: *Cranberry, Uva Ursi*

OTHER PROPOSED NATURAL TREATMENTS: *Buchu, Cleavers, Goldenseal, Goldenrod, Juniper, Lapacho, Low-sugar Diet, Methionine, Probiotics, Sandalwood, Vitamin C, Zinc*

Bladder infections are a common problem for women, accounting for more than 6 million office visits each year. Men, because of the greater distance between their bladder and urethral opening, only rarely develop bladder infections.

The primary symptoms of a bladder infection are burning during urination, frequency of urination, and urgency to urinate, possibly accompanied by pain in the lower abdomen and cloudy or bloody urine. Occasionally, the infection spreads upward into the kidneys, producing symptoms such as intense back pain, high fever, chills, nausea, and diarrhea.

Conventional treatment for bladder infections consists of appropriate antibiotic treatment guided by urine culture. Women with frequent bladder infections may keep on hand a prescription for antibiotics to be used when symptoms arise. Some women may choose to take antibiotics continuously to prevent infection. Certain hygiene habits, such as showering before or urinating after oral sex or intercourse are commonly said to be helpful, although this has not been proven.

Principal Proposed Natural Treatments

Women who do not want to use antibiotics may be able to find some help through the use of herbs. However, if symptoms do not improve or signs of a kidney infection develop, medical attention is essential to prevent serious complications.

Cranberry

Cranberry juice is commonly used to prevent bladder infections as well as to overcome low-level chronic infections. The cranberry plant is a close relative of the common blueberry. Native Americans used it both as food and as a treatment for bladder and kidney diseases. The Pilgrims learned about cranberry from local tribes and quickly adopted it for their own use. Subsequent physicians used it for bladder infections, for "bladder gravel," and to remove "blood toxins."

In the 1920s, researchers observed that drinking cranberry juice makes the urine more acidic. Because common urine infection bacteria such as *E. coli* dislike acidic surroundings, physicians concluded that they had discovered a scientific explanation for the traditional uses of cranberry. This discovery led to widespread medical use of cranberry juice for bladder infections. Cranberry fell out of favor after World War II, only to return in the 1960s as a self-treatment for bladder infections.

More recent research has revised the conclusions reached by scientists in the 1920s. It appears that cranberry's acidification of the urine is not likely to play an important role in the treatment of bladder infections; current research has instead focused on cranberry's apparent ability to interfere with the bacteria establishing a foothold on the bladder wall. If the bacteria can't hold on, they will be washed out with the stream of urine. Studies suggest that in women who frequently develop bladder infections, bacteria have an especially easy time holding on to the bladder wall. Thus when taken regularly, cranberry juice might fix this problem and break the cycle of repeated infection.

The best evidence for the use of cranberry juice for preventing bladder infections comes from a 1-year, double-blind, placebo-controlled study of 150 sexually active women that compared placebo against both cranberry juice (8 ounces 3 times daily) and cranberry tablets. The results showed that both forms of cranberry significantly reduced the number of episodes of bladder infections.

A double-blind study of 376 hospitalized seniors attempted to determine whether a low dose of cranberry juice cocktail would help prevent acute infections. It failed to find benefit, most likely due to the minimal dosage of cranberry: only 10 ounces daily of cranberry juice *cocktail*. Furthermore, because of the low rate of infections, it would necessarily have been more difficult for this study to produce statistically significant results.

Another double-blind study evaluated cranberry juice cocktail for treatment of chronic bladder infections. This trial followed 153 women with an average age of 78.5 years for a period of 6 months. Many women of this age group have what are called *chronic asymptomatic bladder infections*: signs of bacteria in the urine without any symptoms. Half of the participants were given 10 ounces per day of a standard commercial cranberry cocktail drink, the other a placebo drink prepared to look and taste the same. Both treatments contained the same amount of vitamin C to eliminate the possible effect of that supplement. Despite the weak preparation of cranberry used, the results showed that the treatment significantly reduced bacteria and white blood cells in the urine.

In addition, a year-long open trial of 150 women

found that regular use of a cranberry juice/lingonberry combination reduced the rate of urinary tract infection as compared to a probiotic drink or no treatment. However, because this study was not double-blind, the results are unreliable. (For more information on why double-blind studies are so important, see **Why Does This Book Rely on Double-blind Studies?**.)

On the negative side, three double-blind, placebo-controlled studies failed to find cranberry extract helpful for preventing bladder infection in people with bladder paralysis (neurogenic bladder).

For more information, including dosage and safety issues, see the full **Cranberry** article.

Uva Ursi

Uva ursi has a long history of use for urinary conditions in both America and Europe. Until the development of sulfa antibiotics, its principal active component, arbutin, was frequently prescribed by physicians as a treatment for bladder and kidney infections. It appears that the arbutin contained in uva ursi leaves is broken down in the intestine to another chemical, hydroquinone. This is altered a bit by the liver and then sent to the kidneys for excretion. Hydroquinone then acts as an antiseptic in the bladder. (It is, however, potentially quite toxic.)

The European Scientific Cooperative on Phytotherapy (ESCOP) is a scientific organization assigned the task of harmonizing herb policy among European countries. ESCOP recommends uva ursi for "uncomplicated infections of the urinary tract such as cystitis when antibiotic treatment is not considered essential."

Despite this recommendation, surprisingly little research has been done on uva ursi.

Two studies evaluated the antibacterial power of the urine of people who were taking uva ursi and found activity against most major bacteria that infect the urinary tract. While this is interesting, what is really needed is a double-blind trial to discover whether use of uva ursi helps people with actual urinary tract infections, and none have been done.

One study did evaluate uva ursi for prevention of bladder infections. This double-blind trial followed 57 women for 1 year. Half were given a standardized dose of uva ursi (in combination with dandelion leaf, intended to promote urine flow), while the others received placebo. Over the course of the study, none of the women on uva ursi developed a bladder infection, whereas five of the untreated women did. However, this study is a bit of an aberration, because most experts do not believe that continuous treatment with uva ursi is a good idea.

As noted above, hydroquinone is toxic and, for this reason, most experts recommend that uva ursi should not be used for more than a couple of weeks.

For more information, including dosage and safety issues, see the full **Uva Ursi** article.

Other Proposed Natural Treatments

Probiotics (friendly bacteria) have shown some promise for preventing bladder infections. The best results have been seen with an unusual type of probiotic consisting of a *harmless* form of *E. coli*. This double-blind trial enrolled 453 women with an ongoing bladder infection at the beginning of the study. Participants received either the *E. coli* or placebo for 90 days, then went 3 months without treatment, and then received treatment again for the first 10 days in months 7, 8, and 9. The results showed that as compared to placebo, use of the probiotic led to a 34% reduction of UTIs. However, another study failed to find benefit with a more common *lactobacillus* probiotic.

The herb **goldenseal** is widely recommended for bladder infections based on the antibiotic properties of its ingredient berberine. However, it is unlikely that goldenseal taken by mouth provides enough berberine in the bladder wall to have any effect.

Many nutritionally oriented physicians believe that regularly taking **vitamin C** and **zinc** supplements and decreasing sugar in the diet will help improve immunity against bladder infections. Herbs such as **buchu, dandelion, goldenrod, juniper, cleavers, parsley,** and **sandalwood** may increase urine flow, which could be helpful for increasing speed of recovery from an infection that has already occurred. The herb **lapacho** and the supplement **methionine** are also sometimes recommended for bladder infections, but there is no real evidence that they work.

Blepharitis

PRINCIPAL PROPOSED NATURAL TREATMENTS: *N-Acetyl Cysteine*

OTHER PROPOSED NATURAL TREATMENTS: *Barberry, Bayberry, Beta-carotene, Bilberry, Calendula, Chamomile, Citrus Bioflavonoids, Dandelion, Evening Primrose Oil, Eyebright, Fish Oil, Goldenseal, Lutein, Passionflower, Red Clover, Selenium, Vitamin A, Vitamin B Complex (a Mixture of Vitamins B_1, B_2, B_3, B_6, and B_{12}, Pantothenic Acid, Biotin, Folate, Inositol, and Choline), Vitamin C, Vitamin E, Zinc*

Blepharitis is a common eye disease that affects the edge of the eyelids and the eyelash hair follicles. Symptoms include red and swollen eyelids; crusting of the eyelashes on awakening; redness of the eye; sensitivity to light; excessive tearing; frothy tears; and an itching, burning, or foreign-body sensation in the eye.

There are two forms of blepharitis. *Anterior blepharitis* involves the portion of the eyelid where the eyelashes attach. It is caused either by a bacterial infection or as part of the same skin condition that causes dandruff (seborrheic dermatitis).

Posterior blepharitis occurs when the oil-secreting glands inside the eyelid (the *meibomian glands*) become inflamed and eventually cannot secrete properly. This leads to changes in the liquid bathing the eye (the *tear film*). Like anterior blepharitis, posterior blepharitis may occur as part of seborrheic dermatitis. Acne rosacea has also been associated with the condition.

Treatment of blepharitis primarily involves various methods to keep the eyelids clean and free of crusts. In some cases, antibiotic or steroid eyedrops are used.

Principal Proposed Natural Treatments

N-Acetyl Cysteine (NAC) is a specially modified form of the dietary amino acid *cysteine*. When taken orally, NAC is thought to help the body make the important antioxidant enzyme **glutathione**. It is also thought to help loosen secretions and, for this reason, it has been tried as a treatment for loosening the thick crusty secretions that block the oil-secreting glands in posterior blepharitis.

As noted above, in posterior blepharitis, the tear film becomes abnormal. A controlled but not blinded study evaluated the potential benefits of NAC in 50 people with chronic posterior blepharitis. All participants received standard eye care for blepharitis. In addition, about half the participants received NAC at a dose of 100 mg 3 times daily for 8 weeks. Researchers used various methods to objectively evaluate the quality of the tear film and found that use of NAC brought about significant improvements.

Further research, including double-blind, placebo-controlled trials, will be necessary to determine whether these apparent benefits translate into meaningful improvement for people with chronic blepharitis.

For more information, see the full **NAC** article.

Other Proposed Natural Treatments

For various theoretical reasons, numerous other natural treatments have been recommended for blepharitis, including **beta-carotene**, **citrus bioflavonoids**, **dandelion**, **evening primrose oil**, **fish oil**, **lutein**, **red clo-**ver, **selenium**, vitamin B complex (a mixture of **vitamins B₁, B₂, B₃, B₆, and B₁₂, pantothenic acid, biotin**, and **folate**, possibly with **inositol** and **choline**), **vitamins A, C**, and **E**, and **zinc**. However, there is no meaningful scientific evidence to indicate that they are helpful.

Certain herbs have been used, traditionally in the form of eyedrops, to treat blepharitis and related conditions, including **barberry**, bayberry, **bilberry, calendula, chamomile, eyebright, goldenseal**, and **passionflower**. However, again, there is no meaningful evidence to indicate that they are effective. Furthermore, using herbal preparations in the eye is risky and should not be attempted except under the supervision of a qualified health care provider.

Natural treatments used for seborrheic dermatitis or acne rosacea may also be worth considering, as these conditions are closely related to blepharitis.

Breast Enhancement

RELATED TERMS: *Breast Augmentation; Enlargement, Breast*

Each year, as many as a quarter of a million women in the U.S. utilize surgery to increase their breast size. Many other women purchase natural products touted to achieve the same goal without surgery. However, there is no meaningful evidence that any of these herbs and supplements actually have this effect and no theoretical evidence to suppose that they would. In this article, we discuss the information that is available on this subject.

Clinically Proven Products

Many manufacturers of breast enhancement products claim that their treatments are clinically proven. A typical website may quote a study that says something like this: "One hundred women were given this product and after 6 months their breast size increased by 10%!" However, while this may sound promising, it actually shows *nothing* at all.

The problem lies in a deeply rooted feature of human perception: when people expect to observe something, they usually do observe it, whether or not it actually occurred. In the hypothetical breast enhancement study just described, researchers would find it almost impossible *not* to "discover" an improvement. Measurement of breast size is an inexact art that allows for considerable leeway. Human nature would inevitably incline researchers to err on the side of finding improvement when they make their measurements at the end of the study. This would be the case even if the researchers were completely impartial and it is even more of a problem if they are paid by the product's manufacturer (which is usually the case). This is not to say that they're lying, it's just that they are human.

In order to get around this problem, medical researchers use a special type of study: the double-blind, placebo-controlled trial. In these trials, some participants receive real treatment, others receive fake treatment, and neither the participants nor the researchers know which is which (until the study is over). When performed correctly, double-blind, placebo-controlled studies eliminate the influence of bias (and other confounding factors) and, for this reason, they are the accepted source of reliable knowledge regarding medical treatments.

Unfortunately, there are no published double-blind, placebo-controlled studies of breast enhancement products at the time of this writing. Until breast enhancement products are subjected to this form of study, it is not possible to take any of them as evidence-based.

In lieu of clinical evidence, one might possibly be encouraged to try breast enhancement products if they had a reasonable theoretical likelihood of increasing breast size. But here, again, these products fall short.

There are three basic categories of herbs and supplements found in breast enhancement products: phytoestrogens, herbs and supplements said to raise progesterone levels, and miscellaneous herbs and supplements that have no real relationship to breast enhancement. We will discuss each one individually.

Phytoestrogens

The hormone estrogen, if taken in high enough doses, increases breast size by stimulating growth of breast tissue. However, it is not safe to use estrogen in this way because when breast cells are stimulated to grow, they are more likely to turn cancerous. A woman who took enough estrogen to enlarge her breasts would greatly increase her risk of breast cancer.

Many herbs and supplements provided in breast enhancement products are included there because they act somewhat like estrogen in the body. These substances are called *phytoestrogens*, meaning "plant-based estrogens," and include the following:

- Alfalfa
- Fennel
- Flaxseed
- Hops
- Isoflavones
- Licorice
- Lignans
- Red clover
- Sage
- Soy
- Verbena

Other herbs and supplements that are not phytoestrogens, but are widely promoted as if they were, are added to breast enhancement products. These include **black cohosh**, chasteberry, **dong quai**, **ginseng**, and Mexican yam. Black cohosh may have estrogen-like actions in some parts of the body, but probably not in breast tissue; the other herbs are probably not phytoestrogenic at all.

According to manufacturers of breast enhancement products, phytoestrogens can enlarge the breasts, like estrogen, but without incurring estrogen's risks.

However, there are several problems with this hypothesis.

Perhaps the most important is that phytoestrogens generally act to *decrease* the estrogen-related functions of the body, rather than *increase* them. Here's why: Natural human estrogen exerts its effects in the body by latching on to special sites on cells called *estrogen receptors*. Phytoestrogens also latch on to estrogen receptors. However, when they do so, they only produce a partial effect. In addition, they block the ability of real estrogen to bind to those receptors. The net effect in women of menstrual age is to *reduce* the action of estrogen. This may be a very useful effect because, in theory, it could decrease a woman's chance of developing breast cancer. However, the same line of reasoning suggests that phytoestrogens should *decrease* breast size, not increase it.

Furthermore, studies indicate that many breast enhancement products do not even contain substantial amounts of phytoestrogens.

In any case, if a breast enhancement product were to contain a powerful phytoestrogen in sufficient quantities to actually stimulate growth of breast cells (a very big if), it would also increase the risk of breast cancer! You can't get one effect without the other. Measurement of estrogenic breast cell stimulation is, in fact, one way of determining the breast cancer risk posed by a substance under study, whether it is a supplement or an environmental contaminant.

Thus, there is no particular reason to believe that phytoestrogens can enhance breast size, nor, if they did, that they would produce such an effect safely.

Raising Progesterone Levels

Other constituents of breast enhancement products are used because of their supposed effect on the hormone progesterone. This approach does have a certain logic to it. When taken as a pill, progesterone does increase breast size and is fairly safely. However, it does so by stimulating the growth and development of milk-producing cells, an effect that most non-nursing women would wish to avoid.

The herb chasteberry, added to breast enhancement products, might increase progesterone levels in some women. However, there is no evidence that it increases breast size.

Another herb widely added to breast enhancement

products as a source of progesterone, Mexican yam, does not in fact raise levels of progesterone at all. The widespread belief that it does so is based on a misconception.

For more information, see the full **chasteberry** and **Mexican yam** articles.

Other Herbs and Supplements

Numerous herbs and supplements are added to breast enhancement formulas merely on the basis that they have been used for some condition that affects women.

Some of the more commonly mentioned include **damiana** (an unproven herbal treatment for sexual dysfunction in women), **saw palmetto** (an unproven herbal treatment for problems with nursing), **fish oil** (possibly helpful for painful menstruation), and **calcium** (probably helpful for PMS), among literally hundreds of others. However, there is no reason whatsoever to believe that an herb or supplement used to treat an unrelated women's health condition will enhance breast size.

Breast-Feeding Support

RELATED TERMS: *Weaning; Nursing Support; Breast Milk, Enhancing; Breast Engorgement; Milk Production*

PRINCIPAL PROPOSED NATURAL TREATMENTS: *None*

OTHER PROPOSED NATURAL TREATMENTS:

Enhancing Milk Production: *Acupuncture, Fenugreek, Milk Thistle*

Weaning/Breast Engorgement: *Sage, Proteolytic Enzymes*

Preventing Allergies In Children: *Probiotics, Reducing Saturated Fats*

General Nutritional Support: *Calcium, Multivitamin/Multimineral Supplement, Omega-3 Fatty Acids*

PROBABLY INEFFECTIVE TREATMENTS:

Breast Engorgement/Weaning: *Cabbage Leaves*

HERBS AND SUPPLEMENTS TO USE ONLY WITH CAUTION: *Many natural treatments are potentially unsafe for use by nursing mothers. See the discussion at the end of this article.*

It was one of the more shameful chapters of conventional medicine when, for many decades, physicians actively discouraged women from breast-feeding. Fortunately, by the 1970s, the poor judgment inherent in this recommendation had become abundantly clear. Today, there is no longer any doubt regarding what should have been obvious from the beginning: that human breast milk is the ideal food for a human infant.

Not only does breast milk contain all the necessary nutrients, it contains additional substances such as **colostrum** that provide important health benefits. In addition, human breast milk lacks allergenic substances found in infant formulas based on cow or soy milk; for this reason, breast-feeding as opposed to formula feeding may reduce the risk of the infant developing allergy-related diseases, such as **eczema**.

However, nursing can also cause difficulties for the mother of a newborn. Milk flow may be insufficient, the breasts may become inflamed or infected, and when it comes time to stop nursing, there may be an interval of severe discomfort. There are medical treatments available for some of these problems, although in many cases they are more traditional and low-tech than gleamingly modern.

In addition, the constituents of human breast milk can be affected in both positive and negative ways by the mother's diet. Herbs and supplements, like drugs, should be considered risky in breast-feeding until demonstrated otherwise—but on the other hand, certain supplements for the mother might benefit the baby.

There is considerable overlap on this subject between conventional and alternative medicine, and only the more "alternative" of the relevant information is presented here.

Breast-Feeding Support

Proposed Natural Treatments

Weaning/Breast Engorgement

Sage leaf tea traditionally has been recommended to dry up milk supply and reduce breast engorgement for the purpose of weaning, but supporting scientific studies are lacking. One early double-blind, placebo-controlled trial did find some benefit for breast engorgement with the use of **proteolytic enzymes**, but considerably more evidence would be necessary before it could be considered an effective treatment.

According to traditional wisdom, the application of cabbage leaves to the breast can reduce the discomfort of breast engorgement during weaning, but controlled studies indicated that it is *not* effective for this purpose.

Promoting Milk Supply

The herbs **milk thistle** and **fenugreek** have been used historically to promote milk supply, but no studies have been performed to establish whether or not they actually provide any benefit.

The herb **chasteberry** has also been used traditionally for this purpose, but we do not recommend it. (See Herbs and Supplements to Avoid below.)

Acupuncture has also been proposed for increasing milk supply. However, no benefits were seen in a well-designed and reasonably large (almost 180-participant) trial.

Preventing Eczema and Other Allergic Conditions in Children

Double-blind, placebo-controlled trials suggest that nursing women may be able to help ward off **eczema** and other allergic conditions in their children by taking **probiotics** (friendly bacteria). Cutting down on saturated fat (animal fat) may be helpful as well.

General Nutritional Support

Because breast-feeding requires a woman to supply nutrients to another human being, use of a general **multivitamin/multimineral supplement** is advisable. However, such supplements seldom contain adequate amounts of calcium and for that reason a separate **calcium** supplement should be taken. Calcium supplements offer the additional benefit of reducing lead levels in breast milk.

Essential fatty acids in the **omega-3** family are thought to be essential for infant health, especially brain development and, for this reason, it has been suggested that nursing women should supplement their diet with this nutrient.

Finally, while human breast milk supplies nearly all essential nutrients, it does not contain an adequate amount of **iron**. This problem is exacerbated by the modern practice of rapidly cutting the umbilical cord, which has the effect of reducing the infant's iron stores. For this reason, some physicians routinely recommend that breast-fed infants should receive iron supplements. However, some evidence suggests that this practice is only warranted if the infant is anemic; otherwise, supplementation may decrease growth rate.

Herbs and Supplements to Avoid

Virtually no medicinal herb has been established as safe in nursing, and even herbs that might seem safe because of their wide use in cooking could cause problems when they are taken in the form of highly concentrated extracts. There could even be problems with herbs traditionally recommended for use by nursing mothers. For example, the herb chasteberry is traditionally used to promote milk supply. However, it inhibits prolactin, a hormone that is vital to milk production, and for this reason could very well have the reverse effect.

Supplements that are essential nutrients, such as vitamins, generally have a maximum safe intake established for them by a governmental agency. However, other supplements that are not essential nutrients are in much the same position as herbs and could conceivably cause harm. This may even be the case for apparently safe supplements. For example, one double-blind, placebo-controlled study found that if a nursing woman consumes the supplement **conjugated linoleic acid** (CLA), the fat content of her breast milk will be reduced, with potentially harmful effects.

Brittle Nails

RELATED TERMS: *Onychorrhexis, Onychoschisis, Onychoschizia*

PRINCIPAL PROPOSED NATURAL TREATMENTS: *Biotin*

OTHER PROPOSED NATURAL TREATMENTS: *Calcium, Cysteine, Gelatin, Horsetail* (Equisetum arvense), *Iron, Silicon, Vitamin A, Zinc*

Brittle fingernails are a common condition, occurring in about 20% of people; more women than men develop brittle nails. Brittle nails usually break or peel off in horizontal layers, starting at the nail's free end. The term *brittle nails* can also refer to a condition in which lengthwise splits appear in the nail. In either case, the nail's structure is faulty.

Brittleness in the nail may be caused by trauma, such as repeated wetting and drying, repeated exposure to detergents and water, and excessive exposure to harsh solvents, such as those found in nail polish remover. If your nails are regularly exposed to such stresses, it may be worth trying protective gloves when washing dishes and doing other chores. In the case of nail polish remover, gentler, less toxic brands have recently become available. Check with retailers of natural cosmetic products.

Nail brittleness may also be caused by an underlying medical condition, such as **Raynaud's disease**, low thyroid function (**hypothyroidism**), or lung conditions. Other possible causes include skin diseases (**psoriasis**, lichen planus, alopecia areata) as well as endocrine disorders, tuberculosis, **Sjogren's syndrome**, and malnutrition. **Selenium** poisoning can also cause brittle nails.

Because of all these possibilities, it is important to rule out a serious underlying problem before trying nutritional or herbal treatments for brittle nails. If a medical cause for this condition is not found, it may be worth considering some of the approaches described below.

Principal Proposed Natural Treatments

Although no herb or supplement has been proven effective for brittle nails, there is some evidence that the B vitamin biotin might help.

Animal studies suggest that biotin supplementation can be helpful for deformed hooves in horses and pigs. Since animal hooves are made of keratin, the same substance from which human nails are made, these findings have encouraged researchers to study the effects of biotin on brittle nails in humans.

Preliminary evidence from a small controlled study suggests that biotin may increase the thickness of brittle nails, reduce their tendency to split, and improve their microscopic structure. To arrive at their results, the researchers used a scanning electron microscope to examine the effects of biotin in 8 women with brittle nails who were given 2.5 mg of biotin daily over 6- to 9-month periods. (An additional 24 individuals were also studied; 10 served as controls, and the other 14 were examined in a way that makes the interpretation of their results questionable.) Because all nail clippings were examined without the researchers being aware of whose clippings they were looking at, these results have some validity. However, the study was too small to allow definitive conclusions.

Two small open studies also reported benefits with biotin supplementation. However, because there was no control group in either study, the results can't be taken as reliable.

For more information, including dosage and safety issues, see the full **Biotin** article.

Other Proposed Natural Treatments

The mineral **silicon** has been widely marketed for decades as a treatment for brittle nails, brittle hair, and aging skin. However, the first potentially meaningful clinical trial was not reported until 2004. In this double-blind, placebo-controlled study of 50 women, use of 10 mg silicon daily (as orthosilicic acid) for 20 weeks did appear to improve the condition of their nails. However, this study, performed by the manufacturer of a silicon product, leaves much to be desired in design and reporting.

The herb **horsetail** (*Equisetum arvense*), naturally high in silicon, is also sometimes mentioned as a treatment for brittle nails. A number of other nutritional therapies have been tried as well, including **calcium**, cysteine, gelatin-containing preparations, **iron**, **vitamin A**, and **zinc**. However, as of yet, there is no real evidence that any of these treatments are effective.

Burning Mouth Syndrome

PRINCIPAL PROPOSED NATURAL TREATMENTS: *Lipoic Acid*

OTHER PROPOSED NATURAL TREATMENTS: *Treatments for Yeast Hypersensitivity, Vitamin B₁, Vitamin B₂, Vitamin B₆, Zinc*

Burning mouth syndrome (BMS) is a poorly understood condition in which a person experiences ongoing moderate to severe pain in the tongue and/or mouth. Although the cause of BMS remains unclear, some patterns have become clear to researchers. The pain is generally worst in the late afternoon and early evening, but disappears at night. Most often, more than one part of the mouth is involved. Common areas of burning pain include the tongue, the hard palate (the front part of the roof of the mouth), and the lower lip. Many people recover spontaneously within 6 or 7 years. Dry mouth and altered taste sensations often, but not always, accompany the pain.

Burning mouth syndrome is thought to fall in the general category of *neuropathic pain*, meaning that it probably results from altered nerve function, possibly in the nerves carrying taste sensation. Use of drugs in the ACE inhibitor family has been implicated in some cases of BMS, but the reason for this apparent connection remains unclear.

Conventional treatment for BMS consists of drugs used to treat neuropathic pain in general, including anticonvulsants, sedatives in the benzodiazepine family, and tricyclic antidepressants. There is inadequate research at present to determine the precise efficacy of these treatments.

Principal Proposed Natural Treatments

The supplement lipoic acid has shown promise for the treatment of diabetic neuropathy, another form of neuropathic pain. Lipoic acid has also shown some promise for burning mouth syndrome.

In a double-blind trial, 60 people with burning mouth syndrome received either lipoic acid (200 mg 3 times daily) or placebo for a period of months. Researchers reported that almost all people receiving lipoic acid showed significant improvement, while none of those taking placebo improved, and relative benefits endured at 12-month follow-up.

While these are promising results, the total lack of benefit seen in the placebo group is somewhat difficult to believe, and raises concerns about the study's reliability. Nonetheless, positive findings such as these are sufficiently encouraging to warrant a larger study by an independent research group.

It is not known how lipoic acid might help burning mouth syndrome; the supplement's strong antioxidant effects might play a role. For more information, including dosage and safety issues, see the full **Lipoic Acid** article.

Other Proposed Treatments for Burning Mouth Syndrome

The yeast *Candida albicans* can infect the mouth, causing a condition called *thrush*. Thrush may cause symptoms similar to BMS. Some alternative practitioners believe that **excessive candida or hypersensitivity to it** is the cause of many illnesses. For this reason, they recommend using anti-yeast treatments to treat BMS. However, there is no direct evidence to support this approach, and it appears that people with BMS are no more likely to have detectable candida in the mouth than people without it.

Inconsistent evidence suggests that people with BMS might have deficiencies in various nutrients, such as **vitamins B₁, B₂,** and **B₆,** and **zinc.** However, there is no evidence as yet that supplementation with these nutrients will have any effect on BMS symptoms.

Herbs and Supplements to Avoid

Numerous herbs and supplements may interact adversely with drugs used to treat burning mouth syndrome. For more information on this potential risk, see the individual drug articles in the Drug Interactions section of this book.

Bursitis

PRINCIPAL PROPOSED NATURAL TREATMENTS: *None*

OTHER PROPOSED NATURAL TREATMENTS: *Boswellia, Devil's Claw, Evening Primrose Oil, Fish Oil, Movement Therapies (such as Pilates and Feldenkrais), Proteolytic Enzymes, Tai Chi, White Willow, Yoga*

The muscles and bones of the body work together like a smoothly oiled machine. Some of the "oil" is provided by fluid-filled sacs called *bursae*. Bursae are strategically located in areas where muscles, ligaments, and tendons might otherwise rub against bones. The smooth surface of a bursa allows tissues to move across each other without friction.

Bursae, however, can become inflamed, leading to a condition called *bursitis*. One of the main causes of bursitis is repetitive motion. For example, custodians who use a vacuum cleaner may develop bursitis in the elbow. Excessive pressure, such as caused by prolonged kneeling, can also injure a bursa. More rarely, gout, arthritis, and certain infections can cause bursitis.

Bursitis occurs most commonly in the hip, knee, elbow, or heel. Symptoms include tenderness, swelling, and pain with motion.

Conventional treatment involves resting the affected area and using anti-inflammatory drugs. If an attack of bursitis does not respond to this treatment, drainage of the bursa and injection of corticosteroids may be used.

Various practical steps can help prevent bursitis. Using knee pads can protect the bursa of the knee from pressure injury. Exercises that strengthen the muscle around a joint are thought to reduce stress on the bursae in the area. Finally, it is important to break up repetitive movements with alternative movement patterns as well as periods of rest.

Proposed Natural Treatments

There are no natural treatments for bursitis that have meaningful scientific support.

The herb **white willow** has effects similar to those of aspirin and on this basis it might be expected to offer some benefit in bursitis. However, white willow has not been directly studied for that purpose.

Other treatments sometimes recommended for bursitis, but that also lack reliable supporting evidence, include **boswellia**, **fish oil**, **evening primrose oil**, **proteolytic enzymes**, and **devil's claw**.

Yoga increases flexibility, and might help bursitis by stretching tendons and ligaments, and, therefore, by releasing tension in the area around the bursa. Movement therapies, such as Pilates and Feldenkrais, involve deliberate retraining of movement and could, therefore, alter the repetitive movements that can cause bursitis. **Tai Chi** might also lead to improved movement habits.

Cancer Prevention (Reducing the Risk)

PRINCIPAL PROPOSED NATURAL TREATMENTS: *Folate, Garlic, Green Tea, Isoflavones, Selenium, Soy, Tomatoes (Lycopene), Vitamin C, Vitamin E*

OTHER PROPOSED NATURAL TREATMENTS: *Betulin, Black Tea, Blue-green Algae, Boron, Bromelain, Calcium, Cartilage, Catechins (from Green Tea), Citrus Bioflavonoids, Conjugated Linoleic Acid, Cordyceps, Coriolus versicolor, Diindolylmethane (DIM), Ellagic Acid, Fiber, Fish Oil, Flaxseed (Lignans), Genistein, Ginseng, Glycine, Grapes (Resveratrol), Grass Pollen, Indole-3-Carbinol (I3C), Inositol Hexaphosphate (Phytic Acid, IP6), Isoflavones, Kelp, Licorice, Ligustrum, Melatonin, Milk Thistle, MSM (Methyl Sulfonyl Methane), N-Acetylcysteine (NAC), Nettle, OPCs (Oligomeric Proanthocyanidins), Papaw Tree Bark, Probiotics, Quercetin, Rosemary, Schisandra, Sulforaphane, Turmeric, Vitamin D*

PROBABLY NOT EFFECTIVE TREATMENTS: *Beta-carotene*

Cancer is the second major cause of death (after heart disease) in the United States. It claims the lives of more than half a million Americans each year out of the nearly 1.4 million who get the disease. The probability of getting cancer increases with age. Two-thirds of all cases are in people older than 65.

Cancer is believed to begin with a mutation in a single cell. However, a cell doesn't become cancerous overnight. Several mutations in a row are necessary to create all the characteristic features of cancer. Ordinarily, cells have a self-destruct mechanism that causes them to die when their DNA is damaged. However, in developing cancer cells, something interferes with the self-destruct sequence. It may be that the cancer-causing mutations themselves turn off the countdown.

The DNA alterations that create a cancer cell give it a certain independence from the ordinary rules of cell behavior. Normal cells are highly influenced by nearby cells, with the result that they "get along" well with their neighbors. For example, the growth of a healthy cell is ruled by special growth factors given off by surrounding tissues. However, cancer cells either grow without such growth factors or simply make their own. Many types of cancer cells can also trigger the growth of new blood vessels to feed them.

The rate of cancerous mutations is increased by exposure to carcinogenic substances. Cigarette smoke is a powerful carcinogen. Many carcinogens exist in the diet as well, even in fruits and vegetables.

Principal Proposed Natural Treatments

Before we can get into detailed discussion of natural products proposed to help prevent cancer, we must first discuss some fundamental issues regarding the nature of medical evidence.

It is rather difficult to prove that taking a certain supplement will reduce the chance of developing cancer. One really needs enormous long-term, double-blind, placebo-controlled studies in which some people are given the supplement while others are given placebo. However, relatively few studies of this type have been performed.

For most supplements, the evidence that they help prevent cancer comes from observational studies, which are much less reliable. Observational studies have found that people who happen to take in high levels of certain vitamins in their diets develop a lower incidence of specific cancers. However, in such studies it is very difficult to rule out other factors that may play a role. For example, individuals who take vitamins may also exercise more, or take better care of themselves in other ways. Such confounding factors make the results of observational studies less reliable.

Although this may sound like a theoretical issue, it has very practical consequences. For example, based primarily on observational studies, hormone replacement therapy was promoted as a heart-protective treatment for post-menopausal women. However, when placebo-controlled studies were performed, hormone replacement therapy proved to *increase* the risk of heart disease.

It is now thought that apparent benefits of hormone replacement therapy were due to the fact that women who used it belonged to a higher socioeconomic class than those who did not use it. (For a variety of reasons, some of which are obscure, higher income is associated with improved health.)

Only two supplements have any evidence from double-blind trials to support their potential usefulness for cancer prevention: vitamin E and selenium, and even that evidence is weak. For all other supplements, supporting evidence is limited to observational studies, as well as preliminary evidence from animal and test-tube studies.

Vitamin E

The results of observational trials have been mixed, but on balance, they suggest that high intake of vitamin E is associated with reduced risk of many forms of cancer, including stomach, mouth, colon, throat, laryngeal, lung, liver, and prostate cancer.

However, as noted above, the results of observational studies are unreliable as guidelines to treatment. The results of double-blind, placebo-controlled studies are far more persuasive in drawing conclusions about cause and effect. Unfortunately, these studies generally failed to find vitamin E helpful for the prevention of cancer.

The one positive note came in a double-blind study of 29,133 smokers. Those who were given 50 mg of synthetic vitamin E (dl-alpha-tocopherol) daily for 5 to 8 years showed a 32% reduction in the incidence of prostate cancer and a 41% drop in prostate cancer deaths. Surprisingly, results were seen soon after the beginning of supplementation. This was unexpected because prostate cancer grows very slowly. A cancer that shows up in the prostate today actually started to develop many years ago. The fact that vitamin E almost immediately lowered the incidence of prostate cancer suggests that it may somehow block one of the last steps in the development of detectable prostate cancer.

Nonetheless, the negative results regarding most other types of cancer have made scientists hesitant to place too much hope in these findings. Some researchers believe that better results will be seen with a form of vitamin E called *gamma-tocopherol* rather than the alpha-tocopherol used in the trials mentioned above. Others suggest that vitamin E might be more helpful for cancer prevention in low-risk people. Further research is currently under way to settle these questions.

For more information, including dosage and safety issues, see the full **Vitamin E** article.

Selenium

It has long been known that severe selenium deficiency increases the risk of cancer. One double-blind study found some evidence that selenium supplements might help prevent cancer even in the absence of severe deficiency. The study was actually designed to detect selenium's effects on skin cancer. It followed 1,312 individuals, half of whom were given 200 mcg of selenium daily. People participating in the study were not deficient in selenium. The participants were treated for an average of 2.8 years and were followed for about 6 years. Although no significant effect on skin cancer was found, the researchers were startled when the results showed that people taking selenium had a 50% reduction in overall cancer deaths and significant decreases in cancer of the lung (40%), colon (50%), and prostate (66%). The findings were so remarkable that the researchers felt obliged to break the blind and allow all the participants to take selenium.

Subsequent reevaluation of the results, including additional data from follow-up, indicated that lung cancer and colon cancer benefits were seen only in participants with somewhat low levels of selenium in the blood to begin with. (At the time of this writing, researchers had not announced whether the same was true regarding prostate cancer prevention.)

While this evidence is promising, it has one major flaw: the laws of statistics tell us that when researchers start to deviate from the question their research was designed to answer, the results may not be trustworthy. As an illustration of this, yet another after-the-fact statistical analysis of the data hints selenium supplements might actually *increase* risk of certain forms of skin cancer. This, however, may not be a real concern either, as all such statistical manipulation is suspect. Further research will be necessary before we know whether selenium supplements actually help prevent cancer.

For more information, including dosage and safety issues, see the full **Selenium** article.

Mixed Antioxidants

A large double-blind, placebo-controlled study evaluated the potential benefits of a low-dose combination **antioxidant** supplement providing 120 mg of ascorbic acid, 30 mg of vitamin E, 6 mg of beta-carotene, 100 mcg of selenium, and 20 mg of zinc taken daily for about 7.5 years. The results as a whole failed to show benefit. However, analysis by sex showed a significant reduction in cancer incidence in men but not in women. It is not clear whether these results are meaningful.

Beta-carotene

The story of beta-carotene and cancer is full of contradictions. It starts in the early 1980s when the cumulative results of many studies suggested that people who eat a lot of fruits and vegetables are significantly less likely to get cancer. A close look at the data pointed to carotenes as the active ingredients in fruits and vegetables. It appeared that a high intake of dietary carotene might significantly reduce the risk of cancers of the lung, bladder, breast, esophagus, and stomach.

However, as noted above, observational studies cannot prove cause and effect. When researchers gave beta-carotene to study participants, the results have been impressively negative.

Most studies enrolled people in high-risk groups, such as smokers, because it is easier to see results when you look at people who are more likely to develop cancer to begin with.

The anticancer bubble burst for beta-carotene in 1994 with the results of the Alpha-Tocopherol, Beta-Carotene (ATBC) study. These results showed that beta-carotene supplements did not prevent lung cancer, but actually *increased* the risk of getting it by 18%. This trial followed 29,133 male smokers in Finland who took supplements of about 50 IU of vitamin E (alpha-tocopherol), 20 mg of beta-carotene (more than 10 times the amount necessary to provide the daily requirement of vitamin A), both, or placebo daily for 5 to 8 years. (In contrast, vitamin E was found to reduce the risk of cancer, especially prostate cancer.)

In January 1996, researchers monitoring the Beta-Carotene and Retinol Efficacy Trial (CARET) confirmed the prior bad news with more of their own: the beta-carotene group had 46% more cases of lung cancer deaths. This study involved smokers, former smokers, and workers exposed to asbestos. Alarmed, the National Cancer Institute ended the $42 million CARET trial 21 months before it was planned to end.

At about the same time, the 12-year Physicians' Health Study of 22,000 male physicians was finding that 50 mg of beta-carotene (about 25 times the amount necessary to provide the daily requirement of vitamin A) taken every other day had no effect—good or bad—on the risk of cancer or heart disease. In this study, 11% of the participants were smokers and 39% were ex-smokers.

Similarly, another study of beta-carotene supplements failed to find any effect on the risk of cancer in women.

What is the explanation for these discrepancies? One possibility is that beta-carotene alone is not effective. Fruits and vegetables contain many carotenoids (carotene-like substances) that may be more important for preventing cancer than beta-carotene. One researcher has suggested that taking beta-carotene supplements actually depletes the body of other beneficial carotenoids.

It is also possible that intake of carotenes as such are unrelated to cancer and that some unrelated factor common to individuals with a high carotene diet is the cause of the benefits seen in observational trials.

For more information, including dosage and safety issues, see the full **Beta-carotene** article.

Tomatoes (Lycopene)

Lycopene, a carotenoid-like beta-carotene, is found in high levels in tomatoes and pink grapefruit. Lycopene appears to exhibit about twice the antioxidant activity of beta-carotene and may be more helpful for preventing cancer.

In one observational study, elderly Americans consuming a diet high in tomatoes showed a 50% reduced incidence of cancer. Men and women who ate at least seven servings of tomatoes weekly developed fewer stomach and colorectal cancers compared to those who ate only two servings weekly.

In another study, 47,894 men were followed for 4 years in an observational study looking for influences on prostate cancer. Their diets were evaluated on the basis of how often they ate fruits, vegetables, and foods containing fruits and vegetables. High levels of tomatoes, tomato sauce, and pizza in the diet were strongly connected to reduced incidence of prostate cancer. After an evaluation of known nutritional factors in these foods as compared to other foods, lycopene appeared to be the common denominator. Additional impetus has been given to this idea by the discovery of lycopene in reasonably high levels in the human prostate, as well as evidence that men with higher lycopene levels in the blood have a lower risk of prostate cancer.

Similar evidence suggests that foods containing lycopene might help prevent other forms of cancer as well, including lung, colon, and breast cancer.

A few poorly designed intervention trials have also been performed, and these suggest that lycopene or a standardized tomato extract containing lycopene might be helpful for the prevention or treatment of prostate or breast cancer.

For more information, including dosage and safety issues, see the full **Lycopene** article.

Vitamin C

Several observational studies have found a strong association between high dietary vitamin C intake and a reduced incidence of stomach cancer. It has been proposed that vitamin C may prevent the formation of carcinogenic substances known as *N-nitroso compounds* in the stomach.

Observational studies have also linked higher vitamin C in the diet with reduced risk of cancers of the colon, esophagus, larynx, bladder, cervix, rectum, breast, and perhaps lung. However, dietary vitamin C intake does not appear to be associated with reduced rate of prostate cancer.

One study found that vitamin C supplementation at 500 mg or more daily was associated with a lower incidence of bladder cancer. However, another study found no association. Similarly, in another observational study, 500 mg or more of vitamin C daily over a period of 6 years was not associated with reduced incidence of breast cancer. Another study found similar results.

For more information, including dosage and safety issues, see the full **Vitamin C** article.

Green Tea

Both green tea and black tea come from the plant *Camellia sinensis*, which has been cultivated in China for centuries. The key difference between the two is in preparation. For black tea, the leaves are allowed to oxidize, a process believed to lessen the potency of the presumed active ingredients in green tea, catechin polyphenols. Green tea is made by lightly steaming the freshly cut leaf, a process that prevents oxidation and possibly preserves more of the therapeutic effects.

Laboratory and animal studies suggest that tea consumption protects against cancers of the stomach, lung, esophagus, duodenum, pancreas, liver, breast, and colon. A 1994 study of skin cancer in mice found that both black and green teas, even decaffeinated versions, inhibited skin cancer in mice exposed to ultraviolet light and other carcinogens. After 31 weeks, mice given the teas brewed at the same concentration humans drink had 72 to 93% fewer skin tumors than mice given only water.

However, results from observational studies in humans have not been so clear-cut—some have found evidence of a protective effect and others have not.

One study followed 8,552 Japanese adults for 9 years. Women who drank more than 10 cups of green tea daily had a delay in the onset of cancer and also a 43% lower total rate of cancer occurrence. Males had a 32% lower cancer incidence, but this finding was not statistically significant.

A study in Shanghai, China, found that those who drank green tea had significantly less risk of developing cancers of the rectum and pancreas than those who did not. No significant association with colon cancer incidence was found. A total of 3,818 residents aged 30 to 74 were included in the population study. For men, those who drank the most tea had a 28% lower incidence of rectal cancer and a 37% lower incidence of pancreatic cancer compared to those who did not drink tea regularly. For women, the respective differences in cancer frequency were even greater: 43% and 47%.

Another study in Shanghai found similar associations for stomach cancer. Green tea drinkers were 29% less likely to get stomach cancer than nondrinkers, with those drinking the most tea having the least risk. Interestingly, the risk of stomach cancer did not depend on the person's age at which he or she started drinking green tea. Researchers suggested that green tea may disrupt the cancer process at both the intermediate and the late stage.

However, in an observational study of 26,311 Japanese individuals, no reduction in stomach cancer rates were seen. Lack of benefit was also seen in a study conducted in Hawaii. In any case, observational studies are intrinsically unreliable.

Green tea may exert an estrogen-blocking effect that is helpful in preventing breast and uterine cancer, and another study suggests that it might prevent the development of tumors by blocking the growth of new blood vessels.

The main catechin polyphenol found in green tea is epigallocatechin gallate (EGCG). Preliminary experimental studies suggest that EGCG may help prevent skin cancer if it is applied directly to the skin.

For more information, including dosage and safety issues, see the full **Green Tea** article.

Soy

In many animal studies, soybeans, soy protein, or other soy extracts decreased cancer risk, and observational studies in people have found suggestive associations between higher soy consumption and lower incidence of hormone-related cancers such as prostate, breast, and uterine cancer.

Soybeans provide estrogen-like compounds known as **isoflavones**, especially **genistein** and daidzein. These substances bind to the same sites in the body as estrogen, occupying these sites and keeping natural estrogen away. Estrogen stimulates certain forms of cancer, but soy isoflavones exert a milder estrogen-like effect that may not stimulate cancer as much as natural estrogen. This could help protect against cancer. Soy may additionally reduce levels of the body's own estrogen, which would also have a protective effect.

However, not all evidence on soy and cancer is positive. Because the isoflavones work somewhat like estrogen, there are theoretical concerns that they may not be safe for women who have *already* had breast cancer. Studies in animals have found suggestive evidence that under certain circumstances soy isoflavones might stimulate breast cancer cells. Furthermore, evidence from two preliminary studies in humans found changes suggesting that soy might slightly increase breast cancer risk. Other studies in women have found reassuring results; nonetheless, prudence suggests that women who have had breast cancer, or are at high risk for it, should consult a physician before taking any isoflavone product.

In men, estrogen is used as a treatment for prostate cancer. There is weak evidence that soy might be helpful for treating (or preventing) prostate cancer too.

For more information, including dosage and safety issues, see the full **Soy** article.

Folate

Folate deficiency may predispose individuals toward developing cancer of the cervix, colon, lung, breast, pancreas, and mouth. Large observational studies suggest that folate supplements may help prevent colon cancer, especially when taken for many years. Folate has similarly shown a bit of promise for preventing colon cancer in people with **ulcerative colitis**. Since deficiency of this essential vitamin is quite common (and quite unhealthy), you really can't go wrong taking extra folate at the recommended dose.

For more information, including dosage and safety issues, see the full **Folate** article.

Other Proposed Natural Treatments

Some, but not all, observational and intervention studies have found evidence that **calcium** supplementation may reduce the risk of colon cancer. However, calcium supplements might *increase* risk of prostate cancer (in men).

Some studies have connected higher **vitamin D** levels with a lower incidence of cancer of the breast, colon, pancreas, and prostate, as well as melanoma, but overall research has yielded mixed results.

Dietary fiber has long been thought to help prevent colon cancer. However, several recent studies have found either little evidence of benefit or none at all.

Substances known as **lignans** are found in several foods and may produce anticancer benefits. They are converted in the digestive tract to estrogen-like substances known as *enterolactone* and *enterodiol*. Like soy isoflavones (see the previous discussion under the heading Soy), these substances prevent estrogen from attaching to cells and may thereby block its cancer-promoting effects. Lignans are found most abundantly in **flaxseed**, a high-fiber grain that has been cultivated since ancient Egyptian times. Both flaxseed and **flaxseed oil** have been recommended for prevention or treatment of cancer, but the supporting evidence is still extremely preliminary. Contrary to some reports, flaxseed *oil* contains no lignans. Instead, it contains the alpha-linolenic acid, which is also hypothesized to have cancer-preventive effects.

Evidence from observational studies suggests that **garlic** taken in the diet as food may help prevent cancer, particularly cancer of the colon and stomach. In one of the best of these studies, the Iowa Women's Study, women who ate significant amounts of garlic were found to be about 30% less likely to develop colon cancer. Similar results were seen in other observational studies performed in China, Italy, and the United States. However, no meaningful intervention studies have been reported.

Resveratrol is a phytochemical found in at least 72 different plants, including mulberries and peanuts. Grapes and red wine are particularly rich in resveratrol. This substance has shown anticancer properties in test-tube studies.

One large observational study suggests that higher intake of **boron** may reduce risk of prostate cancer.

Provocative evidence suggests that a substance called *sulforaphane*, found in broccoli and related vegetables, may possess anticancer properties. Recently, broccoli sprouts have been touted for cancer prevention on the basis of their high content of sulforaphane. However, this recommendation is still highly speculative. Another constituent of broccoli-family vegetables, **indole-3-carbinol**, has also shown promise as a cancer-preventative agent; however, there is some evidence that this substance might actually increase the risk of cancer in certain circumstances. Much the same is true of the related substance dindolylmethane (DIM).

One study provides preliminary supporting evidence for the notion that **fish oil** reduces the risk of prostate cancer; however, there is no reliable evidence that fish oil has a general cancer-preventive effect.

Weak evidence hints that **N-acetylcysteine** (NAC) treatment may help to prevent colon cancer.

Several studies have experimented with using very high doses of **vitamin A** to prevent skin cancer, doses considerably above levels ordinarily considered safe. Some have found possible benefits regarding preventing some forms of skin cancer, while others have not. This approach should not be tried except under physician supervision.

Vitamin K has shown a slight bit of promise for helping to prevent liver cancer in people with chronic viral hepatitis.

Innumerable other herbs and supplements have shown promise in test tube and animal studies, including but not limited to **cordyceps**, *Coriolus versicolor*, **ligustrum, quercetin, citrus bioflavonoids, conjugated linoleic acid**, *Morina citrifolia* (**noni**), **turmeric, rosemary**, betulin (from white birch tree), **bromelain**, ellagic acid (from grapes, raspberries, strawberries, apples, walnuts, and pecans), **ginseng, glycine, grass pollen, inositol hexaphosphate** (phytic acid, IP6), **kelp, licorice, melatonin, MSM, milk thistle, nettle, OPCs** (oligomeric proanthocyanidins), papaw tree bark, **probiotics** or "friendly" bacteria, **schisandra**, and **blue-green algae**.

While it is commonly stated as a fact that high consumption of fruits and vegetables reduces cancer risk, the evidence is limited to inherently unreliable observational studies, and even among these the results are inconsistent. Similarly, meat consumption might or might not increase colon cancer risk. Current data does *not* suggest that diets high in sugar or other simple carbohydrates increase colon cancer risk or that reducing fat in the diet reduces colon or breast cancer risk.

Cancer Treatment

PRINCIPAL PROPOSED NATURAL TREATMENTS: *None*

OTHER PROPOSED NATURAL TREATMENTS:

Improving Effectiveness of Conventional Treatment: *American Ginseng;* Coriolus versicolor; *Docosahexaenoic Acid;* Eleutherococcus senticosus; Ginkgo biloba; *Lycopene; Melatonin; Mistletoe Extract, Injected; N-Acetylcysteine; Shark Cartilage; Social Support; Vitamin A; Vitamin C; Vitamin D*

Reducing Side Effects of Chemotherapy: *Acetyl-L-carnitine, Acupuncture/Acupressure, Beta-carotene, Chamomile Cream, Colostrum, CoenzymeQ*$_{10}$*, Creatine, Docosahexaenoic Acid, Ginger, Glutamine, Hypnosis, Melatonin, Milk Thistle, N-Acetylcysteine, Probiotics, Relaxation Therapy, Vitamin E*

Reducing Side Effects of Radiation Therapy: Aloe vera *Gel, Calendula Cream, Chamomile Cream, Probiotics, Proteolytic Enzymes, Zinc*

Treating lymphedema Caused By Breast Cancer Surgery: *Citrus Bioflavonoids, OPCs, Oxerutins*

Treating Weight Loss Caused By Cancer or Cancer Treatment: *See the Undesired Weight Loss article.*

Herbs and Supplements To Use Only with Caution: *Alfalfa, Androstenedione, Beta-carotene, Black Cohosh, Boron, Dong Quai, Estriol, Folate, Genistein,* Panax ginseng, *Hops, Licorice, Red Clover, Resveratrol, Soy, St. John's Wort, Vitamin C, Vitamin E*

Not only is cancer the second leading cause of death in the United States (after heart disease), its insidious nature gives it a special terror. Most diseases give warning in the form of escalating symptoms, while others strike so suddenly that there's no time to brood on it. Cancer follows a different, stealthier path. A

Cancer Treatment

person who feels perfectly well may come back from the doctor's office with a diagnosis of potentially fatal cancer and plenty of time to fear what comes next.

Conventional treatments for cancer also have frightening qualities to them: disfiguring surgery, arduous chemotherapy, and treatment with invisible radiation. In many cases, when cancer is found early enough, conventional treatment can lead to a permanent cure. But often the prognosis is given in statistics—a percentage chance of survival—or, worse, in months remaining to live.

No wonder, then, that people turn to alternative medicine. It would be wonderful if there were some powerful alternative approach that could rout cancer at its root. Unfortunately, the reality is that no alternative treatment offers a sure and simple route to recovery. Worse still, there are plenty of unscrupulous people who will take advantage of a cancer victim's desperation. Even the most scrupulous providers of alternative cancer therapy mislead in one sense: they display a conviction and enthusiasm even though they do not know, in truth, whether their approach really works. It simply isn't possible for a medical practitioner to fairly judge the effectiveness of a therapy from apparent clinical results. Only double-blind, placebo-controlled studies can do that. (For information on why this form of study is essential, see **Why Does This Book Rely on Double-blind Studies?**)

It is possible, of course, that some alternative therapies for cancer may truly work, even if they haven't yet been proven. However, we may never know which ones are real and which ones offer only false promises. Proper studies require money and patience with the scientific process, and proponents of alternative cancer therapies may lack one or both of those. In addition, ethical considerations make it difficult to study an unproven therapy for a fatal disease, when therapies that provide a chance of cure are available. For this reason, most studies of alternative therapies for cancer have involved adding a natural treatment to a standard cancer regimen; alternatively, they enrolled individuals who have already failed to respond to existing methods. These latter circumstances could potentially hide the benefits of an effective natural therapy. If a treatment only worked in the absence of chemotherapy, for example (as some alternative cancer therapy proponents claim about their methods) or could cure only early cases of cancer, these ethical obstacles would prevent researchers from finding out.

This article discusses the relatively small amount of information that is known from a scientific perspective about alternative treatments for cancer. We also discuss natural options that may reduce side effects of standard cancer therapies, as well as possible interactions between herbs and supplements and drugs.

Proposed Natural Treatments for Cancer

Various natural supplements have shown some promise for improving the effectiveness of conventional cancer therapy (specifically, surgery, chemotherapy, and radiation) or reducing its side effects. In most cases, however, the supporting evidence remains weak and the most rigorous studies have often failed to find benefit.

Note: If you are receiving cancer treatment, do not use any herbs or supplements except under the supervision of your physician.

For information on treatments to *prevent* cancer, see the full **Cancer Prevention** article.

Improving Effectiveness of Conventional Cancer Treatment

Numerous natural therapies have been proposed for enhancing the cancer-fighting effects of standard therapies. However, as noted above, most of the supporting research falls short of the necessary standard for proof: a double-blind, placebo-controlled study.

Shark Cartilage

Based on the belief that sharks don't get cancer, **shark cartilage** has been heavily marketed as a cure for cancer. While this is a myth (sharks do get cancer), shark cartilage has, in fact, shown some promise. Shark cartilage tends to inhibit the growth of new blood vessels, a process called *angiogenesis*. Since cancerous tumors must build new blood vessels to feed themselves, this effect might be beneficial.

Shark cartilage also inhibits substances called *matrix metalloproteases* (MMPs). These little-understood enzymes affect the extracellular matrix, the framework of substances that lie between cells in the body. MMPs are thought to play a role in diseases of the cornea, gums, skin, blood vessels, and joints, as well as in cancer and illnesses that involve excessive fibrous tissue.

A number of test tube experiments have found that shark cartilage extracts prevent new blood vessels from forming in chick embryos and other test systems. These findings have led to other test tube experiments, animal studies, and preliminary human trials to investigate the possible anticancer effects of shark cartilage. The results suggest that a particular liquid shark cartilage extract might be useful in the treatment of various cancers, including lung, prostate, and breast cancer. However, not all studies have been positive.

Social Support and Other Psychological Factors

Cancer treatment puts tremendous stress, both physical and emotional, on those that undergo it. Several studies have examined the potential benefits of social support for women with breast cancer. According to most, but not all, studies, such support improves survival and/or enhances quality of life. In one famous study of women with advanced breast cancer, participants who attended a support group twice weekly doubled their survival time as compared to study participants who did not attend the group.

It is also commonly said that certain psychological coping styles (for example, fighting spirit versus helpless acceptance) can lead to longer life in people with cancer. However, a review of the evidence found that in fact there is little to no evidence that psychological attitude makes much of a difference. People with cancer should not feel pressured into adopting particular coping styles to improve survival or reduce the risk of recurrence, the study's authors concluded.

One study evaluated guided imagery and **relaxation therapy** following surgery for colon cancer. The results indicated no more than a short-term mood-elevating benefit; those receiving the treatment did not recover more quickly.

Vitamin C

Cancer treatment is one of the more controversial proposed uses of **vitamin C**. An early study tested vitamin C in 1,100 terminally ill cancer patients. One hundred patients received 10,000 mg daily of vitamin C, while the other 1,000 patients (the control group) did not receive vitamin C. Those taking the vitamin C survived more than 4 times longer on average (210 days) than those in the control group (50 days). A large (1,826 subjects) follow-up study by the same researchers found a nearly doubled survival rate (343 days versus 180 days) in vitamin C–treated patients whose cancers were deemed "incurable," as compared to people not treated with vitamin C. Benefits were also seen in a similarly designed Japanese study.

However, while these results seem promising—almost miraculous—they, in fact, show next to nothing

because they lacked a placebo group. When proper double-blind, placebo-controlled studies were performed on vitamin C for cancer, they failed to find any benefit.

Vitamin C proponents have criticized these trials on various grounds, but the fact remains that there is as yet no reliable positive evidence for vitamin C in cancer.

PC-SPES for Prostate Cancer

PC-SPES is a formulation of eight natural substances: seven are plants and one is a fungus. The name is derived from the common abbreviation for prostate cancer (PC) and the Latin word *spes*, meaning "hope."

After its commercial launch in 1996, PC-SPES received increasing interest from the general public and prostate cancer researchers. Preliminary evidence suggested that it has significant effects on prostate cancer cells, perhaps due in part to its estrogen-like action.

However, chemical analysis reported in 2002 showed that PC-SPES is not truly a purely herbal product; samples of the product dating back to 1996 have been found to contain a form of pharmaceutical estrogen, diethylstilbestrol (DES), as well as indomethacin (an anti-inflammatory medication in the ibuprofen family), and warfarin (a strong blood thinner). Samples subsequent to 1999 contain less DES, but they also have shown less effectiveness in treating prostate cancer.

There is little doubt that DES is active against prostate cancer, but it presents a variety of risks, including blood clots in the legs. The other two pharmaceutical contaminants might actually reduce the risk of blood clots (which may be why they were covertly added), but present various risks all on their own. For these reasons, we strongly recommend against using PC-SPES at all.

Other Herbs and Supplements

Literally hundreds of herbs and supplements have been shown in test-tube studies to fight cancer cells. However, it is a long way from a test tube to a human body, and such findings are not at all meaningful.

In this subsection we discuss several natural supplements that have received at least preliminary study in humans. Keep in mind that none of the positive studies cited below reached the level of rigor required to truly show a treatment effective. (Most of them lacked a control group, for example.) In contrast, several properly designed studies failed to find benefit.

According to most but not all reported trials, extracts of the fungus *Coriolus versicolor* may enhance the effectiveness of various forms of standard cancer therapy.

Coriolus is thought to work by stimulating the immune system.

The supplement DHA (docosahexaenoic acid), a constituent of **fish oil**, has shown promise for enhancing the effects of the cancer chemotherapy drug doxorubicin.

The herb **ginkgo** is thought to increase blood flow. An uncontrolled study evaluated combination therapy with ginkgo extract and the chemotherapy drug 5FU for the treatment of pancreatic cancer on the theory that ginkgo might enhance blood flow to the tumor and thereby help 5FU penetrate better. The results were promising.

Scant preliminary evidence suggests that **American ginseng** may aid treatment of breast cancer and that so-called **Siberian ginseng** (properly known as *Eleutherococcus senticosus*) may be useful in the treatment of breast cancer and other forms of cancer.

A small unblinded study using a no-treatment control group found indications that use of a standardized tomato extract containing the supplement **lycopene** might slow the growth of prostate cancer. In a small double-blind, placebo-controlled study, a combination of **soy**, **isoflavones**, lycopene, silymarin (from **milk thistle**) and **antioxidants** showed some potential benefit for preventing recurrence of prostate cancer after prostate cancer surgery.

Preliminary studies, including unblinded controlled trials, suggest that the hormone **melatonin** may enhance the effectiveness of standard therapy for breast cancer, prostate cancer, brain glioblastomas, non–small-cell lung cancer, and other forms of cancer. However, no double-blind studies have been reported. Melatonin may also help decrease cancer chemotherapy side effects (see below).

Mistletoe extract taken by injection has been evaluated as a cancer treatment in a number of studies, including double-blind, placebo-controlled trials. The results, however, have not been particularly encouraging. In general, only the poor quality studies found benefit; more rigorous studies found no improvement in survival time, survival rate, or quality of life.

Note: The safety of mistletoe is not established, and one report suggests that it can damage the liver.

An uncontrolled study found that use of a special **spleen extract** (spleen peptide preparation) somewhat reduced side effects of chemotherapy for head and neck cancer.

In a double-blind, placebo-controlled trial, neither **vitamin A** nor **N-acetylcysteine** proved helpful for head and neck cancer or for lung cancer.

Vitamin D may decrease bone pain and increase muscle strength in prostate cancer.

Reducing Side Effects of Chemotherapy

Various herbs and supplements have shown promise for reducing the side effects of chemotherapy.

Many chemotherapy drugs work by interfering with rapidly dividing cells. Unfortunately, cancer cells aren't the only cells that divide rapidly. The intestinal tract constantly rebuilds its lining, and chemotherapy may interfere with that process. The result: Gastrointestinal side effects, such as mouth sores, nausea, loss of appetite, and diarrhea.

Several herbs and supplements have shown promise for alleviating these conditions, although none have been definitively proven effective.

Diarrhea and Other Gastrointestinal Side Effects

A well-designed double-blind, placebo-controlled trial of 70 participants undergoing cancer chemotherapy with the drug 5-FU evaluated the potential benefits of the supplement **glutamine** for reducing chemotherapy-induced diarrhea. The results suggest that use of glutamine at a dose of 18 g daily may reduce intestinal damage and diminish symptoms of diarrhea. These promising findings indicate a need for larger trials to accurately determine the extent of benefit.

A double-blind, placebo-controlled study of 164 people undergoing chemotherapy with 5-FU found some evidence that a special **probiotic** could reduce gastrointestinal side effects.

In highly preliminary trials, the supplement **colostrum** has also shown some potential for reducing chemotherapy-induced gastrointestinal side effects.

In one study, use of the supplement **creatine** failed to help maintain muscle mass in people undergoing chemotherapy for colon cancer.

Mouth Sores

In an uncontrolled study, use of the herb **chamomile** mouthwash appeared to help prevent mouth sores in people undergoing various forms of chemotherapy. However, uncontrolled studies prove nothing. A rigorous double-blind, placebo-controlled trial of 164 people did *not* find chamomile mouthwash effective for treating the mouth sores caused by the chemotherapy drug 5-FU.

Beta-carotene and **vitamin E** have also shown some promise for preventing mouth sores (caused by various forms of cancer treatment) in preliminary studies, but rigorous studies of adequate size have not been reported.

Nausea

A very preliminary trial hints that **ginger** may reduce nausea caused by the chemotherapy drug 8-MOP. However, another study failed to find ginger helpful for nausea in people using the drug **cisplatin**.

Psychological methods such as hypnosis and relaxation therapy may reduce nausea and other symptoms caused by cancer therapy.

Studies of **acupressure** or **acupuncture** for reducing nausea in people undergoing chemotherapy have generally found marginal benefits at best.

Various Side Effects of Certain Chemotherapy Drugs

In highly preliminary trials, the supplement N-acetyl-cysteine has shown promise for reducing various side effects of the drug ifosfamide.

An animal study suggests that a constituent of fish oil called *docosahexaenoic acid* (DHA) might decrease side effects caused by the drug irenotecan.

The hormone melatonin has shown some promise for reducing the side effects of various chemotherapy drugs.

In preliminary studies, the supplement *coenzymeQ*$_{10}$ has shown some potential for preventing the heart damage caused by the drug doxorubicin, but the results are far from conclusive. Vitamin E has been tried for this purpose as well, but one preliminary trial failed to find benefit.

One animal study hints that the herb milk thistle might protect against kidney damage caused by the drug cisplatin. A highly preliminary human study hints that acetyl-L-carnitine might reduce peripheral neuropathy symptoms caused by cisplatin or paclitaxel.

Reducing Side Effects of Radiation Therapy

Although the symptoms are generally less intense than with chemotherapy, radiation therapy can also cause problems, such as diarrhea, skin damage, and fatigue. Certain supplements may offer benefit.

A double-blind, placebo-controlled study of more than 200 people undergoing radiation therapy found that use of probiotics significantly improved diarrhea.

An unblinded controlled study of 75 people receiving radiation therapy for various forms of cancer found some evidence that soap enriched with *Aloe vera* gel can help protect the skin from radiation damage. However, researchers had to use questionable statistical methods to find evidence of benefit, making the results less than fully reliable. A double-blind, placebo-controlled study that evaluated the effects of aloe gel in 225 women undergoing radiation therapy for breast cancer failed to find benefit. Another study failed to find aloe vera beneficial for reducing side effects of radiation therapy for head and neck cancer.

One study compared cream made from **calendula** flowers with the standard treatment trolamine for protecting the skin during radiation therapy and found calendula more effective. However, it is not known whether trolamine is beneficial, neutral, or harmful when used for this purpose and, for this reason, it's not possible to draw firm conclusions from the study.

One study failed to find **OPCs** from grape seed helpful for reducing the side effects of radiation therapy for breast cancer.

Cream made from chamomile has also been tried for protecting the skin, but one controlled trial failed to find it effective.

Radiation treatment in the vicinity of the mouth may cause alterations in taste sensation. In a small double-blind, placebo controlled trial, use of **zinc** supplements tended to counter this symptom.

Radiation treatment to the pelvic area can cause nausea, vomiting, and fatigue. A double-blind, placebo-controlled trial with 56 participants evaluated the potential effectiveness of **proteolytic enzymes** for reducing these symptoms. Unfortunately, no benefits were seen.

Another large study failed to find **aromatherapy** more helpful than placebo for reducing psychological distress among people undergoing radiation therapy for cancer.

The use of antioxidants during radiation therapy is controversial. One study found that use of antioxidants decreased radiation therapy side effects, but may have decreased radiation therapy effectiveness as well.

Treating Lymphedema Caused by Breast Cancer Surgery

Many women experience lymphedema (chronic arm swelling caused by damage to the lymph drainage system) following breast cancer surgery. Natural treatments for this condition include **oxerutins**, **citrus bioflavonoids**, and OPCs. For more information see the **Surgery Support** article.

Hot Flashes After Mastectomy

Women who have had breast cancer surgery frequently experience annoying hot flashes. Estrogen treatment is not an option, as it might increase the risk of cancer recurrence.

In a 2-month, double-blind trial, 85 women who had undergone treatment for breast cancer received either the herb **black cohosh** or placebo. The results were not encouraging: black cohosh did not reduce overall hot-flash symptoms.

Four double-blind, placebo-controlled trials evaluated soy isoflavones as a treatment for hot flashes, but again failed to find benefit.

Treating Weight Loss Caused by Cancer or Cancer Treatment

Cancer can cause a condition called *tumor-induced weight loss* (TIWL), in which symptoms of starvation occur despite apparently adequate nutrition. The cause is thought to be a particular form of inflammation caused by the cancer. Cancer chemotherapy can also cause weight loss. For information on natural treatments that may be helpful, see the **Undesired Weight Loss** article.

Cancer Cures

Numerous herbs have been claimed effective for treatment of cancer, including:

- Bloodroot
- Burdock
- Cat's claw
- Flaxseed (based on lignan content)
- Lapacho
- Maitake
- Noni
- Oregon grape
- Pokeroot
- Red clover
- Reishi

However, there is no reliable evidence to indicate that they actually help, and one, pokeroot, is actively toxic.

Various herbal combinations have also been promoted for the treatment of cancer, including the Hoxsey cancer cure, Essiac, and Jason Winter's cancer-cure tea. Again, however, there is no reliable evidence that they really work.

Similarly, while various dietary approaches, such as macrobiotics and raw foods, have been claimed to be effective for treating cancer, there is no meaningful evidence that they work.

Herb and Supplement Interactions With Specific Cancer Drugs

Various herbs and supplements may interact adversely with drugs used to treat cancer. We strongly recommend that individuals under treatment for cancer do not use any herb or supplement except under a physician's supervision. A few important categories of potential interactions are described here. Follow the links to the indicated article for detailed information.

The herb **St. John's wort** interacts with many medications, including various chemotherapy drugs.

The drug **methotrexate** causes the body to become deficient in **folate**. For this reason, people who take methotrexate for **rheumatoid arthritis**, juvenile rheumatoid arthritis, or **psoriasis** are sometimes advised to take folate supplements. Studies indicate that in those conditions, use of folate does not impair the action of the drug. However, no studies have as yet established that folate supplements are safe to take with methotrexate when it is used to treat cancer.

The citrus bioflavonoid tangeretin may interact with the breast cancer drug **tamoxifen**.

One highly preliminary study found that black cohosh might interfere with the action of the chemotherapy drug **cisplatin**.

The Antioxidant Controversy

Heated disagreement exists regarding whether it is safe or appropriate to combine antioxidants (such as vitamin E, vitamin C, and beta-carotene) with standard chemotherapy drugs. The reasoning behind the concern is that some chemotherapy drugs may work in part by creating free radicals that destroy cancer cells and antioxidants might interfere with this beneficial effect. However, there is little good evidence that antioxidants actually interfere with chemotherapy drugs and growing evidence that, not only do they not cause harm, they might, in certain cases, offer benefits. However, the effects are likely to vary with the specific situation (for example, type and stage of cancer, and kind of treatment used), and there is far more that we do not know about this than we know. Therefore, we strongly recommend that you do not take antioxidants (or any other supplements) while undergoing cancer chemotherapy except on the advice of a physician.

A similar situation exists regarding radiation therapy. One study found that use of antioxidants decreased radiation therapy side effects, but may have decreased radiation therapy effectiveness as well.

Herbs that May Increase Breast Cancer Recurrence Risk

Women who have had breast cancer are at high risk for a recurrence. As noted above, use of estrogen promotes the development of breast cancer and, for this reason, it is off limits. However, certain natural products may present a similar risk. Numerous herbs and supplements have estrogen-like properties, including the following:

> Alfalfa
> Genistein
> Hops
> Licorice
> Red clover
> Resveratrol
> Soy

Contrary to popular belief, black cohosh is probably not estrogenic.

Other supplements, such as **androstenedione** and **boron**, may raise estrogen levels in the body. Finally, although the herbs **dong quai** and *Panax ginseng* do not appear to act in an estrogen-like manner, they may nonetheless stimulate growth of breast cancer cells. Women who have undergone breast cancer surgery should use these herbs and supplements only under the advice of a physician.

The weak estrogen, **estriol**, is sometimes advocated by alternative practitioners as a safer choice than standard estrogen. However, test-tube studies suggest that estriol is just as likely to cause breast cancer as any other form of estrogen.

Candida/Yeast Hypersensitivity Syndrome

PRINCIPAL PROPOSED NATURAL TREATMENTS: *None*

OTHER PROPOSED NATURAL TREATMENTS: *Barberry; Betaine Hydrochloride; Capryllic Acid; Garlic; Grapefruit Seed Extract; Lapacho; Certain Essential Oils, such as: Lavender Oil, Oregano Oil, Peppermint Oil, and Tea Tree Oil; Probiotics; Red Thyme*

Candida albicans is a naturally occurring yeast that flourishes in moist areas, such as the digestive tract, the vagina, and skin folds. Ordinarily, its population is kept in check by bacteria that live in the same areas. When normal bacteria are disturbed by antibiotics, however, yeast populations can grow to abnormally high levels.

For women, the most common form of excess candida is a **vaginal yeast infection**, as marked by itchiness, redness, burning on urination, and a yeasty odor. Candida can also overpopulate in the mouth (thrush), in the warm moist environment under a diaper (diaper rash), and in other areas.

Candida usually confines itself to the surface of mucous membranes and does not penetrate deeply into the body. However, in people whose immune systems are severely depressed, such as those with AIDS or leukemia, candida can become a dangerous, invasive organism. The medical name for this rare and dire condition is *systemic candidiasis*.

Besides this official meaning, *systemic candidiasis* has another meaning that was coined in the world of alternative medicine. As used there, it is a loose term connoting a whole syndrome of symptoms proposed as related to candida overgrowth. Equivalent terms are *chronic candida*, the *yeast syndrome*, the *yeast hypersensitivity syndrome*, or just plain *candida* for short.

Conventional medicine does not recognize this alternative use of the term *systemic candidiasis* as valid. However, for several years it was practically impossible to walk into an alternative practitioner's office and not walk out with the diagnosis of candida. Fortunately, this excess enthusiasm has cooled in recent years.

The story of "the yeast syndrome" begins in 1983, when Orion Truss published *The Missing Diagnosis*. This was followed by William Crook's much more famous *The Yeast Connection*. These books claim that a person who is chronically colonized by too much candida may develop an allergy-like hypersensitivity to it. The symptoms of this allergy are said to be similar to those of other allergies, including sinus congestion, fatigue, intestinal gas, difficulty concentrating, depression, muscle aches, and many other common complaints.

The regimen outlined by Dr. Crook consists of two parts: treatments that tend toward diminishing the total body burden of candida, and less convincing recommendations that attempt to lessen allergic reactions toward yeast in general.

To decrease the amount of yeast in the body, Dr. Crook recommended avoiding certain substances, including antibiotics, corticosteroids, birth control pills, sugar, and most sweet foods (it is his contention that dietary sugar "feeds yeast"). He also recommended the use of various supplements and even strong prescription drugs to directly kill yeast or at least interfere with its growth.

Next, Dr. Crook recommended avoiding foods containing yeast of any type, for he believed that those who are allergic to candida will also be allergic to other members of the fungus family. Thus Dr. Crook forbade fermented foods, such as beer, cheese, breads containing baker's yeast, tomato paste (which has a significant mold content), and even mushrooms.

Some evidence suggests that individuals diagnosed with this condition do not, in fact, have excessive growth of candida in the digestive tract. Nonetheless, one study suggests that antifungal treatment might provide some benefits, perhaps through effects on other yeasts. This 4-week, double-blind, placebo-controlled study of 116 individuals with symptoms believed to be characteristic of the yeast syndrome evaluated the effects of treatment with the antifungal drug nystatin. The results showed that treatment with nystatin modestly improved overall symptoms as compared to placebo. In addition, some participants voluntarily undertook a sugar- and yeast-free diet, and reported even better results; how much of this latter effect was due to the power of suggestion cannot be determined. A previous study of 42 women failed to find benefit with nystatin, but the study design was somewhat convoluted.

Proposed Natural Treatments for Candida/ Yeast Hypersensitivity Syndrome

Many treatments can reduce the amount of yeast in the body. Unfortunately, it isn't possible to eliminate *Candida albicans* permanently. No matter how successful a treatment may be, as soon as it is stopped, candida will return. It has to because it is a natural inhabitant of the body. However, we know from other conditions, such as vaginal yeast infections, that sufficient intake of *probiotics*, or "friendly" bacteria, can help keep yeast regrowth within reasonable bounds. It is probably best to use a mixture of organisms, including acidophilus, bulgaricus, and bifidus. For more information, including dosage and safety issues, see the full **probiotics** article.

Other agents that may reduce the amount of yeast in the body (especially the digestive tract) include capryllic acid, grapefruit seed extract, **betaine hydrochloride**, **barberry**, red thyme, pau d'arco (also called *lapacho*), and **garlic**. Various **essential oils** have also been proposed for this purpose, including **peppermint oil**, **oregano oil**, lavender oil, and **tea tree oil**. However, the scientific foundation for the use of any of these treatments in candida infections is weak, and some may be toxic if taken to excess or for prolonged periods.

Canker Sores

RELATED TERMS: *Aphthous Stomatitis*

PRINCIPAL PROPOSED NATURAL TREATMENTS: *None*

OTHER PROPOSED NATURAL TREATMENTS: *Acidophilus, Calendula, Caraway, Deglycyrrhizinated Licorice (DGL), Oak Bark, Rhizophora mangle (Red Mangrove), Slippery Elm, Vitamin B$_1$, Witch Hazel*

Canker sores are small ulcers in the mouth caused by an assortment of viruses. A susceptibility to canker sores tends to run in families. No successful conventional treatment is available.

Proposed Natural Treatments for Canker Sores

A highly preliminary study suggests that a chemically altered form of the herb licorice known as **deglycyrrhizinated licorice** (DGL) may be useful for speeding the resolution of canker sores. However, because this study lacked a control group, its results are not reliable. (See **Why Does This Book Rely on Double-blind Studies?**.) Besides the absence of proof of its efficacy, DGL must be sucked to coat the canker sores and some people find its taste objectionable.

A product containing vitamins and minerals as well as the herbs paprika, **rosemary**, **peppermint**, milfoil, **hawthorn**, and **pumpkin seed** has been used in Scandinavia for many years as a treatment for various mouth-related conditions. A small 6-month study reported that use of this product could reduce frequency of canker sores. However, two subsequent studies failed to find any meaningful benefit.

One small double-blind study found benefits with an extract of the bark of the red mangrove tree, *Rhizophora mangle*.

Other herbs and supplements sometimes recommended for canker sores but lacking supporting evidence include **caraway**, **oak bark**, **witch hazel**, **acidophilus**, **calendula**, **slippery elm**, and **vitamin B$_1$**.

One study failed to find that alpha-linolenic acid from perilla oil reduced incidence of canker sores.

Cardiac Arrhythmia

RELATED TERMS: *Palpitations, Heart Palpitations, Arrhythmia, Heart Arrhythmia, Atrial Fibrillation, Irregular Heartbeat, Sinus Arrhythmia*

PRINCIPAL PROPOSED NATURAL TREATMENTS: *None*

OTHER PROPOSED NATURAL TREATMENTS: *Fish Oil, Hawthorn, Magnesium*

HERBS AND SUPPLEMENTS TO AVOID: *Cola Nut, Ephedra, Guarana*

Operating under the control of a complex internal electrical system, the heart beats out a continual rhythm from a few weeks after conception until death. This rhythm is ordinarily even and regular, changing speed as necessary to adjust to the body's need for oxygen.

Sometimes, however, the heart's rhythm becomes disturbed (*arrhythmic*). The most common and benign form

of arrhythmia is the common "heart palpitation," known technically as *sinus arrhythmia*. Generally, these are felt as a short run of thumps or flutters in the chest. Sinus arrhythmia is often caused by stress and anxiety. It poses no danger, although it can be annoying.

More serious forms of heart arrhythmia may occur as well. In later life, many people develop atrial fibrillation, a condition in which part of the heart contracts at excessive speed and another part follows along irregularly. Although some people live for years in a state of atrial fibrillation, this is a potentially dangerous condition that requires medical attention.

Other forms of heart arrhythmia are more dangerous still, including ventricular tachycardia and ventricular fibrillation. These frequently occur after a heart attack. They are often heralded by ventricular premature complexes.

Conventional treatment for arrhythmia depends on the type involved. Sinus arrhythmias are often left untreated. More serious rhythm disturbances are addressed through the use of medications, defibrillation, or a pacemaker.

Note: Heart arrhythmias are far too dangerous for self-treatment. In all but the most obviously benign cases, medical supervision is mandatory.

Proposed Natural Treatments for Cardiac Arrhythmia

Evidence is conflicting on whether **fish oil** helps prevent dangerous heart arrhythmias.

The mineral **magnesium** tends to stabilize the heart and intravenous infusions of magnesium are sometimes given to people in cardiac intensive care. However, a 6-month, double-blind, placebo-controlled study of 170 people did not find oral magnesium effective for maintaining normal heart rhythm in people with a tendency to develop atrial fibrillation.

Diuretic drugs in the **thiazide** family tend to deplete the body of the minerals potassium and magnesium. People using such drugs are usually advised to take **potassium** supplements because potassium deficiency can cause arrhythmias. One small double-blind study failed to find that additional supplementation

with magnesium further stabilized the heart. Apparently, the extent of magnesium deficiency caused by thiazide diuretics is not severe enough to destabilize the heart's rhythm.

However, the drug **digoxin** appears to sensitize the heart to magnesium deficiency. People with **congestive heart failure** (CHF) are likely to use both digoxin and loop diuretics (another type of diuretic that depletes magnesium), and the net result can be cardiac arrhythmias. One small double-blind, placebo-controlled study found that magnesium supplements reduced episodes of ventricular arrhythmia in people with CHF.

The herb **hawthorn** is widely used to treat mild palpitations, but scientific evidence to show that it is effective consists only of partially relevant test-tube studies.

When palpitations are caused by **anxiety** or **stress**, herbs and supplements used for those conditions may be helpful. See the individual articles for more information.

Other herbs and supplements sometimes recommended for palpitations, but which have little supporting evidence, include **vitamin D**, **calcium**, **corydalis**, **valerian**, **skullcap**, and **lady's slipper**.

Herbs and Supplements to Avoid

Caffeine stimulates the heart and may cause minor palpitations. Herbs containing caffeine, such as **guarana** and **cola nut**, would be expected to cause similar problems. The herb **ephedra** also stimulates the heart and should be avoided by people with palpitations.

A few reports suggest that the supplement **creatine** could, at times, cause heart arrhythmias.

Numerous herbs and supplements may interact adversely with drugs used to prevent or treat arrhythmias. For more information on this potential risk, see the individual drug articles in the Drug Interactions section of this book.

Cardiomyopathy

RELATED TERMS: *Arrhythmogenic Right Ventricular Cardiomyopathy, Dilated Cardiomyopathy, Hypertrophic Cardiomyopathy, Idiopathic Dilated Cardiomyopathy, Idiopathic Hypertrophic Cardiomyopathy, Idiopathic Restrictive Cardiomyopathy, Restrictive Cardiomyopathy*

PRINCIPAL PROPOSED NATURAL TREATMENTS: *None*

OTHER PROPOSED NATURAL TREATMENTS: *Carnitine, Coenzyme Q_{10} (CoQ_{10})*

Cardiomyopathy is a little understood condition in which the muscle tissue of the heart becomes diseased. There are several distinct forms of cardiomyopathy that may or may not be similar in origin. Medical treatment consists mainly of medications that attempt to compensate for the increasing failure of the heart to function properly. A heart transplant may ultimately be necessary.

Proposed Natural Treatments

Note: Cardiomyopathy is certainly not a disease that you should treat yourself! For this reason, we deliberately do not discuss dosage or safety issues in this section, although general guidelines can be found in the articles on these substances.

Coenzyme Q_{10}

Preliminary evidence suggests that the naturally occurring substance coenzyme Q_{10} (CoQ_{10}) might offer benefit in some forms of cardiomyopathy.

In a 6-year trial, 143 people with moderately severe cardiomyopathy were given CoQ_{10} daily in addition to standard medical care. The results showed a significant improvement in cardiac function (technically, *ejection fraction*) in 84% of the study participants. Most of them improved by several stages on a scale that measures the severity of heart failure (technically, *NYHA class*). Furthermore, a comparison with individuals on conventional therapy alone appeared to show a reduction in mortality.

This study was an open trial, meaning that participants knew that they were being treated, and such studies are not fully reliable. There have been a few double-blind, placebo-controlled trials of CoQ_{10} in cardiomyopathy as well. One such trial followed 80 people with various forms of cardiomyopathy over a period of 3 years. Of those treated with CoQ_{10}, 89% improved significantly, but when the treatment was stopped, their heart function deteriorated.

No benefit was seen in another double-blind study, but it was a smaller and shorter trial and enrolled only people who had one particular type of cardiomyopathy (idiopathic dilated cardiomyopathy).

For more information on coenzyme Q_{10}, including dosage and safety issues, see the full **Coenzyme Q_{10}** article.

Carnitine

A small amount of evidence indicates that the vitamin-like supplement carnitine may be useful in cardiomyopathy. For more information on carnitine, including dosage and safety issues, see the full **Carnitine** article.

Herbs and Supplements to Use Only with Caution

Various herbs and supplements may interact adversely with drugs used to treat cardiomyopathy. For more information on these potential risks, see the individual drug article in the Drug Interactions section of this book.

Carpal Tunnel Syndrome

PRINCIPAL PROPOSED NATURAL TREATMENTS: *None*

OTHER PROPOSED NATURAL TREATMENTS: *Arnica, Bromelain, Laser Therapy, Magnet Therapy, Proteolytic Enzymes, Vitamin B$_6$, Vitamin B$_{12}$, Yoga*

Carpal tunnel syndrome (CTS) is a common and often disabling condition most often associated with data entry and general computer use, but it can affect anyone who performs repetitive hand motions. CTS occurs in women more often than men and is a relatively common temporary complication of pregnancy (due to fluid retention). It also occurs frequently among people with **rheumatoid arthritis** or **diabetes**.

CTS is caused by compression of the median nerve. On its way to the hand, the median nerve passes through an opening in the wrist called the *carpal tunnel*. Constant, repetitive hand motion may aggravate the ligaments and tendons encased in the tunnel, causing them to swell. As the tunnel walls close in, they compress the median nerve. This causes tingling and numbness in the thumb, index finger, middle finger, and half of the ring finger. The discomfort of CTS often wakes people during the night and eventually makes it difficult to grasp small objects.

Most instances of CTS are job-related. Paying attention to proper ergonomics is essential for preventing CTS. This might involve repositioning a computer keyboard or taking breaks more often. Conventional medical treatment for more stubborn CTS cases is variable in its success. Splinting the affected hand, especially at night, may help reduce symptoms. **Nonsteroidal anti-inflammatory medications**, such as ibuprofen or naproxen, may help slightly. Surgery is considered the ultimate treatment, but corticosteroid injections may be equally or slightly more effective. In some cases, a person with work-related CTS may have no choice but to change vocation.

Proposed Natural Treatments

There are no natural treatments for carpal tunnel syndrome that have any meaningful supporting evidence. Those that have been scientifically evaluated to any extent at all include vitamin B$_6$, yoga, and magnet therapy.

Vitamin B$_6$

More than 25 years ago, researchers noted that people with CTS seemed to be deficient in vitamin B$_6$. This led to widespread use of B$_6$ as a CTS remedy. However, a recent study found no association between CTS and B$_6$ deficiency. In any case, even if B$_6$ deficiency were common in CTS, that by itself wouldn't prove that taking B$_6$ *supplements* can reduce symptoms.

A few studies have investigated the effectiveness of vitamin B$_6$ for CTS. Most were poorly designed and involved few people. The two (albeit small) randomized, double-blind, placebo-controlled studies that do exist found no evidence that vitamin B$_6$ effectively treats CTS. The first study, which enrolled only 15 people, found no significant difference after 10 weeks among those taking vitamin B$_6$, placebo, or nothing at all. The second, involving 32 people, did find some benefits, but these were fairly minor. There was no improvement in nighttime pain, numbness, or tingling, nor in objective measurements of median nerve function. Some benefit, however, was seen in the relatively less important symptoms of finger swelling and discomfort after repetitive motion.

The bottom line: Because vitamin B$_6$ has not been proven effective and may be harmful in high doses, we do not recommend it for carpal tunnel syndrome.

For more information, including dosage and safety issues, see the full **Vitamin B$_6$** article.

Yoga

Hatha yoga, a system of stretching and balancing exercises, has been tried for carpal tunnel syndrome. In one study, 42 individuals with carpal tunnel syndrome were randomly assigned to receive either yoga instruction or a wrist splint for a period of 8 weeks. The results indicated that yoga was more effective than the wrist splint.

However, this study has a serious flaw: participants in the control group were simply offered the wrist splint and given the choice of using it or not; it would have been preferable for them to have received an option with more "glamour," such as fake laser acupuncture or, even better, phony yoga postures. Experience from numerous studies shows that when people believe they are receiving an effective treatment, they report improvement, regardless of the nature of the treatment. (See, for example, the magnet therapy study described below.)

For more information on hatha yoga, see the full **Yoga** article.

Magnet Therapy

In the one reported double, placebo-controlled study of magnet therapy for carpal tunnel syndrome, 30 people with CTS received treatment with either a real or a fake static magnet. Dramatic, long-lasting benefits were seen with the magnet treatment; however, identical, dramatic long-lasting benefits were seen with placebo treatment as well! This study underscores the need for a placebo group in studies—had there not been one in this trial, magnet therapy would have seemed to show itself quite effective for CTS. For more information on magnet therapy, see the full **Magnet Therapy** article.

Other Treatments

Bromelain and other **proteolytic enzymes** are sometimes recommended for the treatment of carpal tunnel syndrome, but there is no evidence as yet that they are effective.

In a double-blind, placebo-controlled study of 37 people undergoing surgery for CTS, an ointment made from the herb arnica (combined with homeopathic arnica tablets) proved slightly more effective than placebo for relieving pain after surgery.

People who have a stroke that renders one hand paralyzed may develop CTS due to overuse of the remaining functional hand. One poorly designed study found preliminary evidence that mecobalamin, a form of **vitamin B_{12}**, might provide some benefit.

One study failed to find low-level laser therapy helpful for CTS.

Cataracts

PRINCIPAL PROPOSED NATURAL TREATMENTS: *Antioxidants, Beta-carotene, Lutein, Lycopene, Vitamin C, Vitamin E*

OTHER PROPOSED NATURAL TREATMENTS: *Bilberry, Carnosine, Ginkgo, Lipoic Acid, OPCs (Oligomeric Proanthocyanidins), Selenium, Taurine, Turmeric, Vitamin B_2 (Riboflavin), Vitamin B_3 (Niacin), Whey Protein, Zinc*

Cataracts—an opaque buildup of damaged proteins in the lens of the eye—are the leading cause of visual decline in those over 65. In fact, most people in that age group have at least the beginnings of cataract formation. Many factors contribute to the development of cataracts but damage by free radicals is believed to play a major role. (See the article on **atherosclerosis** for a description of free radicals.)

Cataracts can be removed surgically. Although this has become a relatively quick, safe, easy, and painless surgery, it does not result in completely normal vision. Clearly, preventing cataracts, if possible, would be preferable.

Principal Proposed Natural Treatments

Numerous observational studies suggest that high intake of **antioxidants**, such as **vitamin C**, **vitamin E**, and ca-

rotenoids (beta-carotene, **lutein**, and **lycopene**) are associated with a reduced incidence of cataracts. However, this by itself does not prove that the use of antioxidant supplements can prevent cataracts. Only double-blind, placebo-controlled studies can do that. (For information on why the double-blind design is so important, see **Why Does This Book Rely on Double-blind Studies?**.) Unfortunately, the results of two large studies of this type were not encouraging.

One double-blind, placebo-controlled trial studied the effects of antioxidant supplements in 4,629 older individuals. Participants received either placebo or an antioxidant supplement containing 500 mg of vitamin C, 400 IU of vitamin E, and 15 mg of beta-carotene. The results over more than 6 years showed no effect on the risk of development of cataracts nor the rate at which existing cataracts progressed to greater severity.

Similarly, a 5-year double-blind, placebo-controlled study of 798 people in Southern India failed to find benefit with supplemental antioxidants, despite the fact that dietary antioxidant deficiency was common among the people studied.

A previous double-blind, placebo-controlled study examined the use of beta-carotene or vitamin E alone and failed to find them effective. On a more positive note, though, one large study found that beta-carotene supplements helped prevent cataracts in the subgroup of study participants who smoked. However, no benefits were seen in the group as a whole and, in any case, people who smoke are generally not advised to take extra beta-carotene. (For the reasons behind this concern, see the **beta-carotene** article.)

A very small, 2-year study found some evidence that lutein may improve visual function in people who already have cataracts.

Other Proposed Natural Treatments

Herbs high in antioxidant flavonoids are frequently suggested for preventing cataracts. These include **bilberry**, **ginkgo**, **OPCs**, and **turmeric**. For various theoretical reasons, the supplements **carnosine**, **lipoic acid**, **niacin** (vitamin B₃), **riboflavin** (vitamin B₂), **selenium**, **taurine**, **whey protein**, and **zinc** have also been proposed. However, there is little real evidence that any of these treatments actually help.

Cervical Dysplasia

RELATED TERMS: *Abnormal Pap Smear*

PRINCIPAL PROPOSED NATURAL TREATMENTS: *None*

OTHER PROPOSED NATURAL TREATMENTS: *Black Cohosh, Blessed Thistle, DHEA, Diindolylmethane, "Emmenagogue" Herb, False Unicorn, Folate, Indole-3-Carbinol, Motherwort, Multivitamin and Mineral Supplement, Selenium, Squaw Vine, True Unicorn*

Very few cancers can be identified so far ahead of the danger point as cancer of the cervix. A decade or more before invasive cancer develops, the cells lining the surface of the cervix begin to show changes visible under a microscope—in plenty of time for definitive treatment. For this reason, a regular, properly performed and interpreted Pap smear is one of medicine's most effective preventive methods.

The stages of progression from a healthy cervix to cancer begin with what is called *mild dysplasia*: precancerous alterations in structure and activity. Prolonged infection with human papillomavirus (HPV) is thought to be the primary cause of these changes. Subsequently, altered cells spread from the surface of the cervix down toward the underlying tissue. In the early stages, cancerous changes may disappear on their own, but once these cells fully penetrate the lining, progression to true cancer usually occurs within 5 to 10 years.

Medical treatment consists of watchful waiting for spontaneous regression during the early stages of dysplasia and, if no regression occurs, more aggressive removal

of the cervical lining by laser, freezing, or other techniques. These options are usually successful; however, they are invasive and frequently uncomfortable.

The newly invented vaccine for preventing HPV infection is expected to markedly reduce cervical cancer risk.

Proposed Natural Treatments

It has been claimed that various natural herbs and supplements can improve the odds of early stages of dysplasia changing back to normal cells. If your physician suggests watchful waiting and a repeat examination, it should be safe to try some of these methods during the waiting period. However, there is no reliable scientific evidence that these treatments are effective and, in all circumstances, close medical supervision is necessary to verify good results or identify failure. Alternative treatment is definitely not advisable for advanced cervical dysplasia.

Folate deficiency is thought to increase the ease with which cervical cancer can develop. However, taking extra folate does not appear to reverse cervical dysplasia once it has occurred.

Indole-3-carbinol (I3C) is a substance found in broccoli-family vegetables. One small double-blind, placebo-controlled trial found evidence that I3C at a dose of 200 or 400 mg per day can improve the chances of cervical dysplasia returning to normal by itself. The related substance, **diindolylmethane**, might also offer benefit.

Observational studies have found that women with cervical dysplasia tend to show a high frequency of general nutritional deficiencies, as high as 67% in one survey. Particular vitamin deficiencies most closely associated with cervical dysplasia include **beta-carotene**, **vitamin C**, **vitamin B₆**, **selenium**, and, as previously mentioned, folate. However, observational studies are notoriously unreliable; it is quite possible, for example, that people who do not eat healthily also have other risk factors for cervical dysplasia. Only double-blind, placebo-controlled studies can actually show a treatment effective, and these have so far not been promising. For example, a double-blind placebo-controlled study of 141 women found that neither vitamin C nor beta-carotene supplements taken daily in doses of 500 mg and 30 mg, respectively, could reverse cervical dysplasia. Negative results were also seen in studies that investigated beta-carotene by itself.

Some practitioners of herbal medicine feel that a class of herbs known as *emmenagogues* can be helpful in cervical dysplasia. These include squaw vine, **motherwort**, true unicorn, **false unicorn**, **black cohosh**, and **blessed thistle**. However, there is no meaningful scientific evidence to indicate that any of these herbs are effective for cervical dysplasia.

Vaginal use of the hormone **DHEA** (dehydroepiandrosterone) has also been suggested for the treatment of early cervical dysplasia, but as yet no controlled studies have been reported.

Chemical Dependency (Narcotic)

RELATED TERMS: *Addiction, Drug; Addiction, Methamphetamine; Chemical Dependency, Cocaine; Chemical Dependency, Heroin; Cocaine Addiction; Drug Addiction; Heroin Addiction; Methamphetamine Addiction; Narcotic Addiction*

PRINCIPAL PROPOSED NATURAL TREATMENTS: *None*

OTHER PROPOSED NATURAL TREATMENTS: *Acupuncture,* Bacopa monniera *(Brahmi), Velvet Antler, Ginkgo, Lobelia, Passionflower, Rosemary, Yoga*

The family of drugs loosely known as *narcotics* includes chemicals in the opiate family, such as heroin, along with cocaine and variations of methamphetamine ("speed"). All of these drugs produce intense psychological symptoms during withdrawal and most cause physical symptoms as well, making them some of the most addictive substances known.

The process of overcoming narcotic addiction involves short-term assistance to ease the immediate withdrawal period, long-term psychological work to induce behavior change, and, in some cases, maintenance treatment with long-acting narcotics, such as methadone. New classes of medications are under investigation for aiding withdrawal as well.

Proposed Natural Treatments

There are no well established natural treatments to aid the treatment of drug addiction, but some have shown a bit of promise.

Passionflower

The herb **passionflower** is thought to have mild sedative properties and has been suggested as an aid to drug withdrawal. A 14-day, double-blind trial enrolled 65 men addicted to opiate drugs and compared the effectiveness of passionflower combined with the drug clonidine to clonidine alone. Clonidine is used widely to assist in narcotic withdrawal. It effectively reduces physical symptoms, such as increased blood pressure. However, it does not help emotional symptoms, such as drug-craving, anxiety, irritability, agitation, and depression. These symptoms can be quite severe and they often cause enrollees in drug treatment programs to end participation.

In this 14-day study, the use of passionflower along with clonidine significantly eased the emotional aspects of withdrawal compared to use of clonidine alone. However, more research will be necessary to prove this treatment effective.

Acupuncture

Although some animal studies suggest that various forms of **acupuncture** may have some benefits for chemical dependency, study results in humans have been mixed at best, with the largest studies reporting no benefits.

For example, a single-blind, placebo-controlled trial that evaluated 620 cocaine-dependent adults found acupuncture no more effective than sham acupuncture or relaxation training. Similarly, a single-blind, placebo-

controlled study enrolling 236 residential clients found no benefit from ear acupuncture for cocaine addiction. However, benefits *were* seen in a much smaller single-blind trial.

Finally, a single-blind, controlled trial of 100 participants with heroin addiction evaluated the potential benefits of ear acupuncture. However, a high dropout rate makes the results difficult to interpret.

Other Natural Approaches

A 10-week, double-blind trial failed to find **ginkgo** helpful for cocaine addiction.

Another study failed to find **hatha yoga** helpful for enhancing the effectiveness of a methadone maintenance treatment for heroin addiction.

Weak evidence hints that the substance lobeline from the herb **lobelia** might offer benefit for methamphetamine addiction.

Even weaker evidence hints at potential benefits for opiate addiction with the herbs **brahmi** (*Bacopa monniera*), **rosemary**, and **velvet antler**.

Children's Health

Because young people are more sensitive and delicate than adults, many parents wish to spare their children treatment with potentially harsh medications, so they turn to natural medicine. However, this desire meets an opposing impulse: the fact that parents are worried about their children's health and are less willing to experiment with treatments that may or may not help. The net effect for the parents is often increased anxiety about which course to take.

Other complications arise as well. For example, some treatments favored by natural medicine are particularly difficult for children to tolerate (such as restrictive diets) and use of them runs the risk of causing emotional harm. Furthermore, many alternative practitioners believe that immunizations are harmful for children and actively crusade against them, while conventional practitioners present vaccines as a matter of necessity.

Common sense, fortunately, suggests a way through this confusing situation: alternative medicine (especially in its gentler, more child-friendly forms) may be appropriate for relatively mild conditions, where there is not

much risk of serious harm. Whenever there is risk of serious illness, however, medical diagnosis and treatment is preferable to the more speculative approaches of alternative medicine.

For a discussion of specific natural medicine issues of particular relevance to children, see the following articles in the *Collins Alternative Health Guide*:

> **Attention Deficit Disorder**
> **Autism Spectrum Disorder**
> **Bed-wetting**
> **Colic**
> **Ear Infections**
> **Eczema**
> **Insect Bites**
> **Strep Throat**
> **Warts**

For information on natural treatments of particular relevance to older children, see the full article on **adolescent health**.

Chronic Fatigue Syndrome

RELATED TERMS: *Myalgic Encephalomyelitis, Post-viral Fatigue Syndrome*

PRINCIPAL PROPOSED NATURAL TREATMENTS: *None*

OTHER PROPOSED NATURAL TREATMENTS: *Beta-carotene, Carnitine, DHEA, Echinacea, Essential Fatty Acids (GLA and Fish Oil), Eleutherococcus, Licorice, Melatonin, Multivitamin and Mineral Supplementation, NADH, Panax ginseng, Traditional Chinese Herbal Medicine*

Chronic fatigue syndrome (CFS) has been a subject of controversy for many years. Medical authorities were once quite skeptical regarding whether it even existed. However, in 1988, the Centers for Disease Control officially recognized CFS. Today, CFS is defined essentially as follows: Unexplained, persistent, or relapsing fatigue with a definite beginning; it is not the result of exertion; it is not relieved by rest; and it results in significant reduction of activities.

In addition, at least four of the following symptoms persist or recur for 6 or more consecutive months of the illness:

➤ **Impairment in short-term memory or concentration**
➤ **Sore throat**
➤ **Tender lymph nodes in the neck or armpits**
➤ **Muscle pain**
➤ **Pain in many joints, without redness or swelling**
➤ **Headache of new pattern or severity**
➤ **Unrefreshing sleep**
➤ **Malaise following exercise, that lasts for more than 24 hours**

Frequently, symptoms of CFS follow a viral infection; some individuals with CFS describe their symptoms as a flu that never goes away.

The cause (or causes) of CFS remains unknown. Because its symptoms somewhat resemble those of mononucleosis (caused by the Epstein-Barr virus), for a time the disease was called *chronic Epstein-Barr syndrome*. However, further investigation disclosed that evidence of past or current Epstein-Barr infection is no more common in individuals with CFS than in the general population. Nonetheless, this erroneous and misleading term still crops up in literature on CFS.

Other syndromes with a similar pattern of symptoms to CFS include fibromyalgia, multiple chemical sensitivities (MCS), and food allergies; some consider these conditions to be closely related to each other, but there is no real evidence to support this hypothesis.

There is no dramatically effective treatment for CFS. Antidepressants (such as Prozac and Zoloft) may improve energy and mood; older antidepressants (such as amitriptyline) may improve sleep; antihistamines and decongestants can help allergic symptoms that frequently occur in CFS; and nonsteroidal anti-inflammatory drugs (such as ibuprofen and naproxen) may help pain. Careful attention to lifestyle issues, such as exercise level and use of caffeine, may also offer benefit.

Other approaches to CFS that have been tried include magnesium injections, corticosteroid treatment, and the antidepressant fluoxetine combined with graded exercise.

For a time, researchers expressed some excitement over initial findings that deliberately raising blood pressure might help individuals with CFS. However, a double-blind, placebo-controlled study of 25 people given a 6-week course of fludrocortisone and increased dietary sodium to raise blood pressure found no improvement in CFS symptoms.

Proposed Natural Treatments

There are some promising natural treatments for CFS, but the scientific evidence for them is not yet strong.

Essential Fatty Acids

In a double-blind, placebo-controlled study, 63 people were given either a combination of essential fatty acids containing evening primrose oil (a source of **GLA**) and **fish oil**, or liquid paraffin placebo over a 3-month period. At 1 and 3 months, participants in the treatment group reported significant improvement in CFS symptoms as compared to the placebo group. The researchers also found that at the beginning of the study many participants had abnormal essential fatty acid levels and these improved with treatment.

However, in 1999, researchers tried to replicate this study with 50 other people, using more precise means of measuring CFS symptoms. The results showed no difference between individuals given essential fatty acids and those given placebo (sunflower oil). These researchers also found no difference in fatty acid levels between individuals with CFS and individuals without CFS who served as controls.

NADH (Nicotinamide Adenine Dinucleotide)

Nicotinamide adenine dinucleotide (NADH) is a naturally occurring chemical that plays a significant role in cellular energy production. NADH supplements have been tried in hopes they might improve energy levels in athletes and in individuals with chronic fatigue.

A double-blind, placebo-controlled crossover trial that followed 26 people given 10 mg of NADH for a 4-week period showed some improvement in symptoms during NADH treatment as compared to the period of placebo treatment (31% versus 8%). However, larger studies will have to be performed to actually prove a benefit with this supplement.

Carnitine

Carnitine is a substance the body uses to convert fatty acids to energy. Early studies reported decreased carnitine levels in people with CFS. Based on these, an unblinded crossover trial (8 weeks with each treatment, and a 2-week "washout" period in between) enrolled 30 individuals with CFS to evaluate the potential benefits of carnitine supplements. The results suggest potential benefit with this supplement.

However, this study was severely flawed. One problem was that, rather than using a placebo group for comparison purposes, researchers chose to investigate the antiviral drug amantadine. This drug has no proven efficacy in CFS and it caused so many side effects that more than half of the participants dropped out during the period they were taking amantadine. This high dropout rate makes statistical interpretation of the results unreliable. In addition, the lack of blinding in the study also impairs the trustworthiness of the results.

Other Herbs and Supplements

Traditional Chinese herbal medicine is part of a comprehensive and unique approach to healing developed over many centuries in Asia. A double-blind, placebo-controlled study of 29 people suggests that the use of an herbal formula originating in this system may be helpful for CFS.

A test tube study of echinacea and *Panax ginseng* found that both increased cellular immune function in cells taken from people with CFS. However, many herbs and supplements can cause measurable changes in immune function and such observations do not prove that there will be an actual benefit in people with the disease.

Both beta-carotene and DHEA have been suggested as treatments for CFS, but the evidence that they work remains extremely preliminary at best.

Based on the theory mentioned above that CFS might be related to low blood pressure, the herb licorice has been recommended for CFS by some herbalists. Licorice raises blood pressure (and causes other potentially harmful effects) when taken in high doses for a long time. However, there is no evidence that it works for CFS, and other treatments to raise blood pressure have proven ineffective for CFS.

Although some authorities have suggested that CFS might be caused by deficiencies of multiple vitamins and minerals, a double-blind, placebo-controlled study of 42 people found no significant improvement in CFS symptoms when a vitamin-mineral supplement was given four times daily after meals for 3 months. Another trial failed to find benefit with a multivitamin/multimineral supplement as well.

A fairly substantial (96-participant) double-blind, placebo-controlled study failed to find *Eleutherococcus senticosus* ("Siberian ginseng") helpful for people with CFS. Over the 2-month study period, both eleutherococcus and placebo reduced fatigue symptoms, but there was no statistically significant difference. (The researchers managed to find some benefit by resorting to statistically questionable after-the-fact procedures.)

Another study failed to find melatonin helpful for CFS.

People with CFS may at times attribute their symptoms to chemical exposures, thereby relating chronic fatigue syndrome to another loosely defined condition known as multiple chemical sensitivities, or MCS. One study evaluated people with chronic fatigue syndrome who believed that certain chemical triggers affected their mental function, causing mental sluggishness and confusion. The results showed decreased mental function on testing following exposure to supposed chemical triggers; however, the decrease was the same whether the actual chemical or a substitute placebo was used. In other words, it was the *belief* that a substance causes harm, rather than actual harm caused by the substance, that produced the symptoms.

Chronic Obstructive Pulmonary Disease

RELATED TERMS: *Chronic Bronchitis, COPD, Emphysema*

PRINCIPAL PROPOSED NATURAL TREATMENTS: *N-Acetyl Cysteine (NAC)*

OTHER PROPOSED NATURAL TREATMENTS: *Antioxidant-rich Diet, Ayurvedic Herbal Medicine, L-Carnitine, Coenzyme Q$_{10}$, Creatine, Echinacea (in Combination with Wild Indigo and White Pine), Essential Oil Monoterpenes, Fish Oil, High-fat, Low-carbohydrate Diet, Ivy Leaf, Plantain*

Chronic obstructive pulmonary disease (COPD) is a permanent lung condition caused, most often, by cigarette smoking. It starts with a wheezing cough and gradually progresses to a shortness of breath that accompanies even the slightest exertion, such as dressing or eating. COPD encompasses both emphysema and chronic bronchitis.

Emphysema consists of the destruction of the tiny air sacs (alveoli) in the lungs and the weakening of the support structure around them. This leads to a collapse of the small airways in the lungs, especially on inhalation, and reduces the body's ability to take in oxygen and expel carbon dioxide.

Chronic bronchitis consists of chronic inflammation of the airways, causing a persistent productive cough. This inflammation also impairs the body's ability to exchange new air for old. COPD also involves spasm of the airways similar to what occurs in asthma. Finally, occasional flare-ups occur when bacteria grow in the lungs, leading to acute exacerbation of symptoms.

Because cigarette smoking contributes to both emphysema and chronic bronchitis, anyone who has COPD should stop smoking. Quitting smoking won't reverse the condition, but it might stop COPD from getting worse. Airborne irritants such as chemical fumes exacerbate symptoms and should also be avoided. Standard treatment for COPD includes using bronchodilators such as ipratropium and albuterol to reduce muscle spasms, and corticosteroids to control inflammation in the airways. Acute flare-ups are treated with antibiotics. Severe COPD may require continuous oxygen therapy.

Malnutrition is common among people with COPD and seems to correspond to the severity of the condition. It's been suggested that the caloric needs of people with COPD increase as the disease progresses. Because malnutrition in turn can worsen lung function and make people more prone to infection, many researchers now recommend that individuals with COPD receive supplemental nutrition as part of their treatment.

Principal Proposed Natural Treatments

N-acetyl cysteine (NAC) may improve breathing in people with COPD.

N-acetyl cysteine is a specially modified form of the dietary amino acid cysteine. Regular use of NAC may diminish the number of severe bronchitis attacks. A review and meta-analysis of available research focused on eight reasonably well-designed double-blind, placebo-controlled trials of NAC in COPD. The results of these studies, involving a total of about 1,400 individuals, suggest that NAC taken daily at a dose of 400 to 1,200 mg can reduce the number of acute attacks of severe bronchitis. However, a subsequent 3-year, double-blind, placebo-controlled study of 523 people with COPD failed to find benefit with 600 mg of NAC daily.

N-acetyl cysteine was once thought to aid lung conditions by helping to break up mucus. However, continuing research has tended to cast doubt on this explanation of its action.

For more information, including dosage and safety issues, see the full **NAC** article.

Other Proposed Natural Treatments

Evidence from three double-blind placebo-controlled studies enrolling a total of 49 individuals suggests that the supplement **L-carnitine** can improve exercise tolerance in COPD, presumably by improving muscular efficiency in the lungs and other muscles.

Eucalyptus is a standard ingredient in cough drops and in oils sometimes added to humidifiers. A combination **essential oil** therapy containing cineole from eucalyptus, d-limonene from citrus fruit, and alpha-pinene from pine has been studied for a variety of respiratory conditions. Because these oils are all in a chemical family called *monoterpenes*, the treatment is called *essential oil monoterpenes*. A 3-month, double-blind trial of 246 individuals with chronic bronchitis found that oral treatment with essential oil monoterpenes helped prevent acute flare-ups of chronic bronchitis. A previous double-blind study, too small to provide reliable results, hints that oral use of essential oil monoterpenes can enhance the effects of antibiotics for acute flare-ups once they do occur. It is thought that essential oil monoterpenes work by improving the lungs' ability to clear secretions.

A mixture of extracts from **echinacea**, **wild indigo**, and white cedar has shown promise for treating a variety of respiratory infections. A well-designed double-blind, placebo-controlled trial of 53 people tested its benefits in acute exacerbations of chronic bronchitis. All participants in this trial received standard antibiotic therapy. The results showed that people receiving the herbal medication experienced more rapid improvements in lung function than those given placebo.

In one poorly designed and reported study, use of an **Ayurvedic herbal combination** appeared to offer some benefit.

It has been suggested that the sports supplement **creatine** might improve muscle strength in people with COPD, but results from small double-blind studies have been inconsistent.

Slight evidence from a small open trial suggests that **coenzyme Q_{10}** improves lung function in individuals with COPD.

The herbs **ivy leaf** and **plantain** have been suggested for chronic bronchitis, but there is no meaningful evidence that they actually help. One study failed to find pomegranate juice helpful for COPD.

Observational studies suggest a correlation between respiratory problems and diets low in **antioxidants** from food, such as **vitamin A**, **vitamin E**, **vitamin C**, and **beta-carotene**. However, such studies don't prove that taking supplements of such nutrients will help—only double-blind, placebo-controlled studies can do that. (For information on the reasons why, see **Why Does This Book Rely on Double-blind Studies?**.) Indeed, a double-blind study of vitamin E and beta-carotene supplementation found no effect on COPD symptoms.

The effects of other antioxidant supplements on COPD haven't yet been studied.

Evidence from several studies suggests that the standard approved diet, low in fat and high in carbohydrates, worsens exercise performance and lung function in people with COPD, whereas a **low-carbohydrate diet** may improve COPD symptoms. Carbohydrates cause the body to produce increased amounts of carbon dioxide and people with COPD have trouble getting rid of carbon dioxide.

Herbs and Supplements to Use Only With Caution

Various herbs and supplements may interact adversely with drugs used to treat chronic obstructive pulmonary disease. For more information on these potential risks, see the individual drug article in the Drug Interactions section of this book.

Cigarette Addiction

RELATED TERMS: *Chemical Dependency, Nicotine; Chemical Dependency, Tobacco; Chemical Dependency, Cigarettes; Smoking Addiction; Nicotine Withdrawal; Addiction, Cigarettes; Stop Smoking*

PRINCIPAL PROPOSED NATURAL TREATMENTS: *None*

OTHER PROPOSED NATURAL TREATMENTS: *Acupuncture; Alfalfa; Eucalyptus; Gotu Kola; Hops; Licorice; Lobelia; Melatonin; Passionflower; Skullcap; Wild Oats (Avena sativa)*

Nicotine is one of the most addictive drugs known. When you combine this chemical with the flavor of tobacco smoke and the oral satisfaction of a cigarette, you get an addiction that is very difficult to break.

Conventional treatment for smoking addiction focuses primarily on methods to separate nicotine addiction from the other habit-forming features of cigarettes. These include the nicotine patch and the nicotine inhaler. In addition, the drug bupropion (Zyban) may help decrease the addictive urge.

Proposed Natural Treatments

There are no proven natural aids for treating cigarette addiction.

The herb **lobelia** has been widely promoted for stopping smoking. The origin of this idea appears to be a misconception that has been passed along for some years: that a constituent of lobelia—lobeline—closely resembles the drug nicotine. In fact, lobeline and nicotine are not biochemically similar and they are not believed to have generally similar actions in the nervous system. Nonetheless, intriguing research suggests that lobeline might have some unusual effects on the nervous system that could make it helpful for treating addiction, especially to amphetamines. But keep in mind that it's a long way from theoretical findings of this type to practical usage.

The herb **wild oats** (*Avena sativa*) has also been suggested as a treatment for cigarette addiction, but on balance the evidence indicates that it is not effective.

Weak evidence supports a role for **melatonin** in reducing nicotine withdrawal symptoms.

Numerous other herbs are promoted for stopping smoking, including **alfalfa**, **eucalyptus**, **gotu kola**, **hops**, **licorice**, **passionflower**, and **skullcap**, but they have not been evaluated scientifically.

Acupuncture, especially in the form of ear acupuncture (auriculopuncture) is widely used as a treatment for cigarette addiction. However, a 1999 meta-analysis of 12 placebo-controlled trials did not find acupuncture more effective than sham-acupuncture for smoking cessation. A subsequent double-blind, placebo-controlled study in 2000 of 330 adolescent smokers also found no benefit. On a more positive note, one study found that while acupuncture may not be effective for treating cigarette addiction on its own, it might (in some unknown manner) increase the effectiveness of smoking cessation education. In this placebo-controlled study of 141 adults, acupuncture plus education was twice as effective as sham acupuncture plus education, and four times as effective as acupuncture alone. Nonetheless, these benefits were seen only in the short term; at long-term follow-up, acupuncture's advantage disappeared.

Smoking is believed to cause increased need for a variety of nutrients, including **beta-carotene**, **folate**, **vitamin B$_{12}$**, **vitamin C**, and **vitamin E**. For this reason, people who smoke might benefit by taking a supplement that provides these nutrients at a little more than standard nutritional doses. (For more information, see the **Nutrition for Cigarette Smokers** article.) However, there is no reason to think that use of these supplements will help you *quit* smoking.

Cluster Headaches

RELATED TERM: *Headaches, Cluster*

PRINCIPAL PROPOSED NATURAL TREATMENTS: *None*

OTHER PROPOSED NATURAL TREATMENTS: *Melatonin, Hyperbaric Oxygen Therapy, Magnesium*

First recognized in 1867, cluster headaches remain one of the most painful and frustrating headache syndromes. Their cause is unclear, and no treatment is fully effective. People with cluster headaches may go for more than a year without any attacks and then suddenly the headaches appear and strike several times a day. Each headache lasts from 30 minutes to 2 hours and consists of very severe pain on one side of the head, generally in the region of the eye. These daily headaches continue for 4 to 8 weeks, and then disappear for another year or more. A more chronic, continuous form of cluster headaches can also occur.

Cluster headaches are different from migraine headaches (although they may possess some underlying similarities) and much more difficult to treat. During cluster headache episodes, rapid-acting treatments are used, including aerosolized ergotamine, pure oxygen, lidocaine nasal spray, and anesthetic inhalation. For prevention, drugs such as ergotamine, prednisone, methysergide, and lithium may reduce the severity and frequency of attacks.

Proposed Natural Treatments

Some evidence suggests that people with cluster headaches have lower than average levels of the hormone **melatonin**. In a double-blind, placebo-controlled study of 20 people with cluster headaches, use of melatonin (10 mg daily) for 14 days significantly reduced headache severity and/or frequency compared to placebo. About half the participants given melatonin responded well.

As noted above, inhalation of 100% oxygen is sometimes used to treat cluster headache attacks. In preliminary controlled trials, use of hyperbaric oxygen (oxygen under pressure) not only treated the headaches, but also helped prevent further attacks.

Intravenous use of **magnesium** has shown promise for cluster headache relief. However, use of *oral* magnesium has not been evaluated.

Colds and Flus

PRINCIPAL PROPOSED NATURAL TREATMENTS: *Andrographis (Often Combined with* Eleutherococcus*), Echinacea (Sometimes Combined with Wild Indigo and White Pine), Essential Oil Monoterpenes, Garlic,* Panax ginseng, *Probiotics, Vitamin C, Zinc*

OTHER PROPOSED NATURAL TREATMENTS: *Arginine, Ashwagandha, Astragalus, Chlorella, Colostrum, Elderberry, Ginger, Glutamine, Hyssop, Ivy Leaf, Kelp, Kudzu, Linden, Maitake, Marshmallow, Mistletoe, Mullein, Multivitamin/Multimineral Supplement, Oregano, Osha,* Pelargonium sidoides, *Peppermint, Propolis, Reishi, Thymus Extract, Sage, Suma, Yarrow*

A cold is a respiratory infection caused by one of hundreds of possible viruses. However, because these viruses are so widespread, it is perhaps more accurate to say that colds are caused by a decrease in immunity that allows one of these viruses to take hold.

Colds occur more frequently in winter, but no one knows exactly why. Nearly everyone catches colds occasionally, but some people catch colds quite frequently, and others tend to stay sick an unusually long time.

Influenza B, commonly called the *flu*, occurs in the form of a worldwide epidemic every winter. The predominant symptoms of flu are fever, malaise, and muscle aches. Cold-like respiratory symptoms are usually fairly minor with the flu. However, a dangerous type of pneumonia can develop as a complication of influenza, especially in seniors.

Conventional medicine can neither cure nor prevent the common cold. Furthermore, none of the over-the-counter treatments have been found to shorten the duration of a cold or even provide significant temporary relief. Cough syrup, in fact, seems to be no better than placebo. Some of the natural treatments described in this section may be able to do better.

People often want to take antibiotics for colds and many physicians will prescribe them—even though antibiotics have no effect on viruses. Many believe that when the mucus turns yellow, it means that a bacterial infection has occurred for which antibiotic treatment is indicated. However, viruses can also produce yellow mucus and even if bacteria have made a home in the excess mucus, they may be only innocent bystanders and produce no symptoms.

Colds, however, can be complicated by bacterial infections. In such cases, antibiotic treatment may be indicated.

The situation is somewhat better for influenza. The "flu shot" provides protection against several strains of influenza. There are also prescription antiviral medications that can help prevent flu and also reduce its length and severity if you do come down with it.

Principal Proposed Natural Treatments

Various natural treatments have shown promise for treating or preventing colds, and they are described below. See also the treatments discussed in the **Acute Bronchitis** article.

Zinc

One famous alternative treatment for colds is the use of zinc in nasal gel or lozenges. When you take zinc this way, you are not using it as a nutrient. Rather, certain forms of zinc release ions that are thought to directly inhibit viruses in the nose and throat.

Taking zinc orally as a nutrient might also be useful in some cases. The immune system does not function properly if you don't have enough zinc in your body. Because zinc is commonly deficient in the diet, especially among senior citizens, nutritional zinc supple-

mentation may certainly be useful for those who get sick easily. Indeed, a 2-year, double-blind study suggests that zinc and selenium taken together in nutritional doses can reduce the number of infections in nursing home residents. Ten other studies performed in Third World countries have found that zinc supplements at nutritional doses can increase resistance to infection. However, more isn't better; once you do have enough zinc, getting extra won't help and might even hurt.

➤ *What Is the Scientific Evidence for Zinc Nasal Gel and Lozenges?*

Use of lozenges containing zinc gluconate or zinc acetate have shown somewhat inconsistent but generally positive results for reducing the severity and duration of the common cold. For example, in a double-blind trial, 100 people who were experiencing the early symptoms of a cold were given a lozenge that either contained 13.3 mg of zinc from zinc gluconate or was a placebo. Participants took the lozenges several times daily until their cold symptoms subsided. The results were impressive. Coughing disappeared within 2.2 days in the treated group versus 4 days in the placebo group. Sore throat disappeared after 1 day versus 3 days in the placebo group, nasal drainage in 4 days (versus 7 days), and headache in 2 days (versus 3 days). Positive results have also been seen in double-blind studies of zinc acetate. Not all studies have shown such positive results. However, the overall results appear to be favorable.

It has been suggested that the exact formulation of the zinc lozenge plays a significant role. Flavoring agents, such as citric acid and tartaric acid, appear to prevent zinc from inhibiting viruses, and chemical forms of zinc other than zinc gluconate or zinc acetate may not work; in particular, zinc sulfate may be ineffective. Sweeteners such as sorbitol, sucrose, dextrose, and mannitol are fine, but the information on glycine as a flavoring agent is equivocal.

Use of zinc in the nose is somewhat more controversial. In addition to showing inconsistent results in studies, use of zinc nasal gel can cause pain and possibly loss of sense of smell.

In one double-blind, placebo-controlled trial, 213 people with a newly starting cold used one squirt of zinc gluconate gel or placebo gel in each nostril every 4 hours while awake. The results were significant: treated participants stayed sick an average of 2.3 days, while those receiving placebo were sick for an average of 9 days, a 75% reduction in the duration of symptoms. Somewhat more modest but still significant relative benefits were seen

Colds and Flus

with zinc nasal gel in a double-blind, placebo-controlled study of 80 people with colds. However, a slightly larger study of a similar zinc gluconate nasal gel found no benefit. Another study—this one involving 77 people—failed to find benefit, even with near constant saturation of the nasal passages with zinc gluconate nasal spray.

For more information, including dosage and safety issues, see the full **Zinc** article.

Echinacea

Until the 1930s, echinacea was the number one cold and flu remedy in the United States. It lost its popularity with the arrival of sulfa antibiotics. Ironically, sulfa antibiotics are as ineffective against colds as any other antibiotic, while echinacea does seem to be at least somewhat helpful. In Germany, echinacea remains the main remedy for minor respiratory infections.

Echinacea is generally thought to work by temporarily stimulating the immune system, although most (but not all) recent evidence has tended to cast doubt on this belief. Contrary to popular belief, however, there is little reason to believe that echinacea strengthens or "nourishes" the immune system when taken over the long term.

There are three main species of echinacea: *Echinacea purpurea*, *Echinacea angustifolia*, and *Echinacea pallida*. A mixture containing all the parts of *E purpurea* above the ground (flowers, leaves, stems) has the best supporting evidence for effectiveness in treating colds and flus; the root of *E. purpurea* is probably not effective, while the root of *E. pallida* may be the active part of that species.

Echinacea has shown promise for reducing the symptoms and duration of colds and aborting a cold once it has started. However, echinacea does not appear to be helpful for preventing colds. It may also not be effective in children.

➣ Reducing the Symptoms and Duration of Colds

Double-blind, placebo-controlled studies enrolling a total of more than 1,000 people have found that various forms and species of echinacea can reduce the symptoms and duration of a common cold, at least in adults.

For example, in one double-blind, placebo-controlled trial, 80 individuals with early cold symptoms were given either *E. purpurea* extract or placebo. The results showed that individuals who were given echinacea recovered significantly more quickly: in just 6 days among the echinacea group versus 9 days among the placebo group.

Another double-blind, placebo-controlled trial looked at reduction of the severity of cold symptoms. The results in 246 participants showed that treatment with *E. purpurea* significantly improved cold symptoms, such as runny nose, sore throat, sneezing, and fatigue. Symptom reduction with *E. purpurea* was also seen in a double-blind, placebo-controlled study of 282 people.

In addition, three double-blind, placebo-controlled studies enrolling a total of about 600 participants found similar benefits with a combination product containing *E. purpurea* and *E. pallida* root, along with **wild indigo** and white pine.

While the above evidence tends to suggest that the above-ground portion of *E. purpurea* is active against the common cold, two studies have failed to find benefit. One of these was a double-blind, placebo-controlled study enrolling 120 adults, the other an even larger trial (407 participants) involving children. The reason for these negative outcomes is not clear. *E. angustifolia* root has also failed to prove effective in a large study.

➣ Aborting a Cold

A double-blind study suggests that echinacea can not only make colds shorter and less severe, it might also be able to stop a cold that is just starting. In this study, 120 people were given *E. purpurea* or a placebo as soon as they started showing signs of getting a cold.

➣ Preventing Colds

Several studies have attempted to discover whether the daily use of echinacea can prevent colds from even starting, but the results have not been promising.

In one double-blind, placebo-controlled trial, 302 healthy volunteers were given an alcohol tincture containing either *E. purpurea* root, *E. angustifolia* root, or placebo for 12 weeks. The results showed that *E. purpurea* was associated with perhaps a 20% decrease in the number of people who got sick, and *E. angustifolia* with a 10% decrease. However, the difference was not statistically significant. This means that the benefit, if any, was so small that it could have been due to chance alone.

Another double-blind, placebo-controlled study enrolled 109 individuals with a history of four or more colds during the previous year and gave them either *E. purpurea* juice or placebo for a period of 8 weeks. No benefits were seen in the frequency, duration, or severity of colds. (Note: this paper is actually a more detailed look at a 1992 study widely misreported as providing evidence of benefit.)

Three other studies also failed to find statistically significant preventive effects.

A study often cited as evidence that echinacea can prevent colds actually found no benefit in the 609 participants taken as a whole. Only by looking at subgroups of participants (a statistically questionable procedure) could researchers find any evidence of benefit, and it was still slight.

However, a recent study using a combination product containing echinacea, **propolis**, and vitamin C did find preventive benefits. In this double-blind, placebo-controlled study, 430 children age 1 to 5 years were given either the combination or placebo for 3 months during the winter. The results showed a statistically significant reduction in frequency of respiratory infections. It is not clear which of the components of this mixture was responsible for the apparent benefits seen.

For more information, including dosage and safety issues, see the full **Echinacea** article.

Andrographis

Andrographis is a shrub found throughout India and other Asian countries, sometimes called *Indian echinacea* because it is believed to provide much the same benefits. It has been used historically in epidemics, including the Indian flu epidemic in 1919, during which andrographis was credited with stopping the spread of the disease. Recently, it has become popular in Scandinavia as a treatment for colds.

Although we don't know how andrographis might work for colds, some evidence suggests that it might stimulate immunity. Interestingly, the ingredient of andrographis used for standardization purposes, andrographolide, does not appear to affect the immune system as much as the whole plant extract.

According to a few well-designed studies, andrographis can reduce the symptoms of colds. It may offer the additional useful benefit of helping to prevent colds.

☞ *Reducing Cold Symptoms*

A total of seven double-blind, placebo-controlled studies enrolling a total of about 900 people have found that andrographis (or a combination containing it as the presumed primary ingredient) significantly reduces the duration and severity of cold symptoms.

For example, a 4-day, double-blind, placebo-controlled trial of 158 adults with colds found that treatment with andrographis significantly reduced cold symptoms. Participants were given either placebo or 1,200 mg daily of an andrographis extract standardized

to contain 5% andrographolide. The results showed that by day 2 of treatment, and even more by day 4, individuals given the actual treatment experienced significant improvements in symptoms as compared to participants in the placebo group. The greatest response was seen in earache, sleeplessness, nasal drainage, and sore throat, but other cold symptoms improved as well.

Three other double-blind, placebo-controlled studies, enrolling a total of about 400 people, evaluated an herbal combination treatment containing both andrographis and *Eleutherococcus senticosus* (so-called Russian Ginseng). One study suggests that this combination may be more effective than echinacea.

The same combination has also shown promise in two double-blind studies for reducing the duration, severity, and rate of complications of influenza.

Andrographis has also been compared to **acetaminophen** (Tylenol). In a double-blind study of 152 adults with sore throat and fever, participants received andrographis (in doses of 3 or 6 g per day for 7 days) or acetaminophen. The higher dose of andrographis (6 g) decreased symptoms of fever and throat pain to about the same extent as acetaminophen, but the lower dose of andrographis (3 g) was not as effective. There were no significant side effects in either group.

☞ *Preventing Colds*

According to one double-blind, placebo-controlled study, andrographis may increase resistance to colds. A total of 107 students, all 18 years old, participated in this 3-month trial that used a dried extract of andrographis. Fifty-four of the participants took two 100-mg tablets standardized to 5.6% andrographolide daily—considerably less than the 1,200 to 6,000 mg per day that has been used in studies on treatment of colds. The other 53 students were given placebo tablets with a coating identical to the treatment. Then, once a week throughout the study, a clinician evaluated all the participants for cold symptoms.

By the end of the trial, only 16 people in the group using andrographis had experienced colds, compared to 33 of the placebo-group participants. This difference was statistically significant, indicating that andrographis reduces the risk of catching a cold by a factor of two as compared to placebo.

For more information, including dosage and safety issues, see the full **Andrographis** article.

Vitamin C

Vitamin C may mildly reduce symptoms of colds when they occur, but it probably does help prevent colds.

➤ *Treating Colds*

Numerous studies have found that vitamin C supplements taken at a dose of 1,000 mg or more daily can modestly reduce symptoms of colds and help you get over a cold faster. In addition, one study suggests that vitamin C can enhance the effect of standard cold treatments, such as acetaminophen.

Note: In most of these studies, participants used vitamin C throughout the cold season and found that when they developed colds, the colds were less severe. (This method of using vitamin C does not, however, appear to help *prevent* colds. See below.) Many people use vitamin C for colds in a different way: they only begin taking it when cold symptoms start. Relatively few studies have evaluated this approach.

➤ *Preventing Colds*

Although two relatively recent studies suggest that regular use of vitamin C throughout the cold season can help prevent colds, most other studies have found little to no benefit along these lines. Vitamin C has shown a bit more promise for prevention of one type of cold, the *post-marathon sniffle*. These are colds that develop after endurance exercise; use of vitamin C before and during competition may help keep you cold-free afterwards. In addition, vitamin C seems to help prevent respiratory infections among individuals who are actually deficient in the vitamin.

For more information, including dosage and safety issues, see the full **Vitamin C** article.

Essential Oils

Eucalyptus is a standard ingredient in cough drops and in oils meant to be added to humidifiers. A standardized combination of three essential oils has been tested for its usefulness in respiratory conditions. The studied combination, called *essential oil monoterpenes*, includes cineole from eucalyptus, d-limonene from citrus fruit, and alpha-pinene from pine. Numerous double-blind trials have found them effective when taken orally for acute bronchitis, **chronic bronchitis**, sinus infections, and other respiratory conditions, in both adults and children. Cineole alone at a dose of 200 mg three times daily showed benefit in a double-blind, placebo-controlled study of 152 people with cold symptoms. For more information, including dosage and safety issues, see the full **eucalyptus** and **essential oil monoterpenes** articles.

Ginseng

Although most people in the West think of ginseng as a stimulant, in Eastern Europe ginseng is widely believed to improve overall immunity to illness. As we have seen, echinacea does not seem to prevent respiratory infections. But it appears that regular use of ginseng might be able to provide this important benefit.

There are three different herbs commonly called *ginseng*: Asian or Korean ginseng (*Panax ginseng*), American ginseng (*Panax quinquefolius*), and Siberian "ginseng" (*Eleutherococcus senticosus*). The latter herb is actually not ginseng at all, and is not discussed here.

A double-blind, placebo-controlled study of 323 people found meaningful evidence that an extract of American ginseng taken at 400 mg daily may help prevent the common cold. Participants who used the extract over 4 months experienced a reduced number of colds as compared to those taking the placebo. Comparative benefits were also seen regarding the percentage of participants who developed two or more colds and the severity and duration of cold symptoms that did develop. Similar benefits were also seen in a study of 43 people.

Two double-blind, placebo-controlled studies enrolling a total of about 100 people indicate that American ginseng may also help prevent flu-like illness in seniors.

A double-blind, placebo-controlled study suggests that *Panax ginseng* can also help prevent flu-like illnesses as well as improve response to influenza vaccination. This trial enrolled 227 participants at three medical offices in Milan, Italy. Half were given ginseng at a dosage of 100 mg daily, the other half placebo. Four weeks into the study, all participants received influenza vaccine. The results showed a significant decline in the frequency of colds and flus in the treated group compared to the placebo group (15 versus 42 cases). Also, antibody measurements in response to the vaccination rose higher in the treated group than in the placebo group.

For more information, including dosage and safety issues, see the full **Ginseng** article.

Garlic

The herb garlic has a long history of use for treating or preventing colds. However, up until 2001, there was no scientific evidence that it actually works for this purpose. In fact, many people joked that garlic merely makes you smell so bad people stay away from you, so you don't catch their cold.

However, there is now some evidence that garlic may really work.

In one 12-week, double-blind, placebo-controlled trial, 146 individuals received either placebo or a garlic extract between November and February.

The results showed that participants receiving garlic were almost two-thirds less likely to catch cold than those receiving placebo. Furthermore, participants who did catch cold recovered about one day faster in the garlic group as compared to the placebo group.

Benefits were also seen in a smaller double-blind study.

Note that these studies do not indicate that taking garlic will help once you already have a cold.

For more information, including dosage and safety issues, see the full **Garlic** article.

Probiotics

Probiotics are healthy organisms that colonize the digestive tract. Not only can they help preventive intestinal infections, they appear to help prevent colds as well.

A 7-month, double-blind, placebo-controlled study of 571 children in day-care centers in Finland found that use of milk fortified with the probiotic bacteria *Lactobacillus* GG modestly reduced the number and severity of respiratory infections. Benefits were also seen in three other large studies, in which probiotics alone or combined with multivitamins and minerals helped prevent colds and/or reduce their duration and severity in adults.

For more information, see the full **Probiotic** article.

Other Proposed Natural Treatments

Various other natural treatments have shown some promise for preventing or treating colds and flus.

Preventing Respiratory Infections

Use of multivitamin/multimineral supplements, or supplements containing zinc and **selenium** alone, may help prevent respiratory infections in elderly individuals, according to some but not all studies. However, serious concerns have been raised that one of the researchers involved in studying this topic might have engaged in questionable scientific practices.

One small double-blind study suggests that the supplement **arginine** might be helpful for preventing colds in children.

There is some evidence that the supplement **glutamine** may, like vitamin C, help prevent post-exercise infections. For example, a double-blind, placebo-controlled study evaluated the benefits of supplemental glutamine (5 g) taken at the end of exercise in 151 endurance athletes. The result showed a significant decrease in infections among treated athletes. Only 19% of the athletes taking glutamine got sick, as compared to 51% of those on placebo.

In contrast, some evidence suggests that a combination of **vitamin E** and **beta-carotene** treatment might *increase* risk of exercise-associated colds.

The evidence regarding whether vitamin E alone can *prevent* respiratory infections is conflicting.

The thymus gland plays a role in immunity. A 1-year, double-blind, placebo-controlled trial of 16 children with frequent respiratory infections found that treatment with **thymus extract** could reduce the rate of infection. However, a double-blind, placebo-controlled trial of 60 athletes failed to find any significant evidence of benefit with thymus extract for preventing post-exercise infections.

An extract of rice bran has shown some promise for preventing or treating colds in seniors.

A throat spray made from **sage** has shown considerable promise for reducing sore throat pain.

A study widely reported as showing that the supplement **colostrum** can help prevent colds was actually far too preliminary to prove anything at all.

There is some evidence that elements in **kelp** might help to prevent infection with several kinds of viruses, including influenza. However, the evidence thus far is more theoretical than practical.

Various herbs are said to enhance immunity over the long term, including **ashwagandha**, **astragalus**, **garlic**, **maitake**, **reishi**, and **suma**. However, there is as yet no meaningful evidence that they really work. In addition, several herbs, including **ginger**, **kudzu**, **osha**, and **yarrow**, are said to help avert colds when taken at the first sign of infection; but again, there is no scientific evidence that they are effective.

Products containing colloidal **silver** are sometimes used in the belief that they will prevent colds and otherwise **strengthen the immune system**; however, because colloidal silver can cause permanent color changes in the skin, we recommend that you do not use it.

Some seniors do not respond fully to the influenza vaccine. There is some evidence that vitamin E supplements may strengthen the immune response to vaccinations. Similarly, evidence from two double-blind trials, but not a third, suggests that combined **multivitamin/multimineral** supplements may improve their response. However, in another trial, a multivitamin tablet without minerals actually worsened participants' response to the vaccine. The reason for these discrepancies is unclear; however, serious concerns have been raised that one of the scientists who reported benefits in some of these trials engaged in questionable scientific practices.

In a double-blind, placebo-controlled study of 124 people, the supplement **chlorella** at a dose of 200 mg or 400 mg daily failed to enhance response to influenza vaccine. Another study failed to find benefit with a remedy from **traditional Chinese herbal medicine**, Hochu-ekki-to.

Treatment of Respiratory Infections

A standardized product containing **elderberry** combined with small amounts of echinacea and bee propolis has been widely marketed as a cold and flu remedy. Weak evidence suggests that this mixture may stimulate the immune system and also inhibit viral growth. In a preliminary double-blind study, the combination significantly reduced the recovery time from epidemic influenza B (a relatively mild form of influenza). Another small double-blind study found similar benefits in both influenza A and B.

One small study found that the popular Throat Coat brand of medicinal beverage teas actually does reduce sore throat discomfort, as compared to placebo tea.

Inhaled **essential oils** have shown a slight bit of promise for the treatment of colds.

The herb *Pelargonium sidoides* is used in Europe for the treatment of colds, but the only relevant double-blind support for its effectiveness involved people with acute bronchitis rather than the common cold.

In double-blind, placebo-controlled studies enrolling a total of more than 300 people, a combination of herbs (primrose, **gentian root**, elderberry, common sorrel, and **vervain**) has shown promise for treatment of sinusitis.

Other herbs sometimes recommended to reduce cold symptoms, but that lack meaningful supporting scientific evidence, include **hyssop**, **ivy leaf**, **linden**, **marshmallow**, **mistletoe**, **mullein**, **oregano**, and **peppermint**.

In a double-blind, placebo-controlled trial, **colostrum** was not helpful for people with sore throat. (The researchers made sure to exclude people with **strep throat**, but some participants may have had sore throat caused by bacteria rather than cold viruses.)

Colic

RELATED TERMS: *Infantile Colic*

PRINCIPAL PROPOSED NATURAL TREATMENTS: *Fennel Seed Oil, Dietary Changes, Behavioral Methods*

OTHER PROPOSED NATURAL TREATMENTS: *Chiropractic Spinal Manipulation, Herbal Combinations*

The mere thought of a colicky baby is often enough to strike fear in the heart of the parents of a newborn child. A baby with colic may cry for hours despite the parents' attempts at consolation; although the colicky phase will eventually end, it may seem like an eternity while it continues.

Colic is generally defined as excessive (frequently inconsolable) crying that lasts for more than three hours at least three days per week, continuing for at least three weeks; additionally, there must be no medical problem causing the crying.

Other symptoms frequently associated with colic include pulling the knees up towards the stomach, a hard and/or swollen stomach, and excessive gas. Crying occurs most often in the evening. Colic typically ends by the age of 4 to 5 months.

Colicky babies may be at an increased risk of abuse at the hands of exhausted and frustrated parents. Additionally, the parent may not properly bond with the child because of feelings of inadequacy and anger, leading to developing behavioral problems as the child grows.

No one knows for sure what causes colic, although there are many theories. One view attributes it to painful digestive cramps and/or excessive gas caused by allergic reaction to foods (such as milk). Another theory suggests that some babies may simply have a sensitive temperament, possibly compounded by a parental inability to respond to the infant's needs. Finally, what we call colic may just be an extreme version of normal infant crying or an increased perception of normal crying by parents with less tolerance for it.

The antispasmodic and sedating drugs dicyclomine and dicycloverine appear to be effective for colic, but they can have dangerous side effects in infants and are not recommended. The gas-relieving drug dimethicone is also sometimes recommended, but evidence suggests that it does not work.

Principal Proposed Natural Treatments

A number of natural approaches to colic have preliminary supporting evidence.

Fennel Seed Oil

In a double-blind, placebo-controlled study, 125 infants with colic were given either placebo or fennel seed oil at a dose of 12 mg daily per kg of body weight. The results were promising. About 40% of the infants receiving fennel showed relief of colic symptoms, as compared to only 14% in the placebo group, a significant difference. Another way to look at the results involves hours of inconsolable crying. In the treated group, infants cried about 9 hours per week, compared to 12 hours in the placebo group.

While these are encouraging results, confirmation by an independent research group is necessary before the treatment can be accepted as effective. Furthermore, the safety of fennel seed oil for infants has not been conclusively established.

For more information, see the full **Fennel** article.

Dietary Changes

Cow's milk can cause **allergic reactions**. Most infant formula contains cow's milk and can cause reactions in allergic babies. There is also some evidence that breast-fed infants may have allergic responses to cow's milk proteins in the mother's diet.

Numerous small, open and double-blind studies have evaluated the effects of cow's milk or cow's milk protein in the diet of infants with colic. Most (but not all) of these found an improvement in crying when cow's milk protein was removed from the diet of formula-fed infants or from the diet of the mothers in breast-fed infants.

As an alternative to standard cow's milk–based formula, researchers primarily used hypoallergenic formula made from hydrolyzed (processed) whey or casein. Formula based on these sources of protein may be superior to those based on soy because soy itself can cause allergic reactions in sensitive children.

If no improvement is seen through eliminating cow's milk, some experts recommend searching in the breastfeeding mother's diet for other potential food allergens, such as wheat, soy, or eggs. However, it is important to keep nutritional needs in mind: the nursing mother who eliminates certain foods needs to maintain an adequate intake of calcium, protein, and other nutrients.

It should be noted that most infants with colic are able to tolerate cow's milk protein as they get older, so neither the mother nor the baby are doomed to life without milk. Researchers propose that this might be the result of an immature digestive system; according to this theory, maturation of the digestive tract is the reason that colic usually disappears on its own in time.

Milk also contains lactose, a form of sugar that many adults can't digest (see the **Lactose Intolerance** article for more information). However, reducing the lactose content of infant formula has *not* been found helpful in treating colic.

Behavioral Methods

Many doctors believe that the cause of colic is not physical; rather, that it results from a child's oversensitivity to stimuli in the environment. Overanxious parents might contribute to the problem by adding more stimulation in an attempt to calm their child. Other parents might underreact in the belief that paying too much attention to the infant's cries will "spoil" him. Either response could set up a vicious cycle leading to long periods of inconsolable crying.

Based on these theories, some authorities recommend counseling the parents of a colicky infant on appropriate coping strategies, including building a personal support system and occasionally leaving the child with a different caregiver to provide a respite.

Studies evaluating the effects of carrying a colicky child more or using a motion-simulation device have not found benefit.

Colic

Other Proposed Natural Treatments

A 1-week, double-blind, placebo-controlled study of 93 breast-fed, colicky infants found benefits with a standardized extract of **fennel**, **lemon balm**, and **chamomile**. Another double-blind, placebo-controlled study found benefits with a combination of chamomile, **vervain**, **licorice**, fennel, and lemon balm. However, the safety of these herbal combinations in infants have not been established.

Chiropractic spinal manipulation has also been tried for colic. One controlled study compared chiropractic treatments with the drug dimethicone. Fifty infants were randomly assigned one of the treatments for 2 weeks. By the sixth day of treatment, the spinal manipulation group cried significantly less than those on dimethicone. Whether this was a specific effect of the manipulation or a general response to attention and touch is difficult to determine.

In Britain, a preparation called *gripe water* is widely sold for the treatment of colic. Varying formulations exist; however, all include aromatic oils, such as dill, spearmint, or **caraway**, combined with alcohol, sucrose (sugar), and sodium bicarbonate. There is no scientific evidence to show whether or not gripe water works. It should be noted that at the recommended dosage, the infant would receive the equivalent of five shots of whiskey. That would be enough to calm anyone.

Other herbs sometimes recommended for colic include cardamom, angelica, peppermint, **yarrow**. However, no scientific evidence as yet supports their use.

The use of salt substitutes containing potassium have also been recommended, but they can be dangerous.

Congestive Heart Failure

PRINCIPAL PROPOSED NATURAL TREATMENTS: *Coenzyme Q_{10} (CoQ_{10}), Hawthorn, Vitamin B_1*

OTHER PROPOSED NATURAL TREATMENTS: *Arginine, Creatine, L-Carnitine, Magnesium, Ribose, Taurine*

When the heart sustains injury that weakens its pumping ability, a complicated physiological state called *congestive heart failure* (CHF) can develop. Fluid builds up in the lungs and lower extremities, the heart enlarges, and many symptoms develop, including severe fatigue, difficulty breathing while lying down, and altered brain function.

Medical treatment for this condition is quite effective and sophisticated and consists of several drugs used in combination.

Principal Proposed Natural Treatments

Note: CHF is too serious a condition for self-treatment. The supervision of a qualified health-care professional is essential. However, given medical supervision, some of the following treatments may be quite useful. The herb hawthorn appears to be effective for mild CHF, and may be helpful for more severe CHF, as well. However, while standard drugs have been shown to help reduce hospitalizations and mortality associated with CHF, there is no similar evidence as yet for hawthorn.

Also, adding the supplement coenzyme Q_{10} to standard treatment may improve results. Finally, the supplement vitamin B_1 (thiamin) may be helpful for individuals who take loop diuretics (such as furosemide) for CHF.

Hawthorn

At least nine double-blind, placebo-controlled trials, involving a total of about 750 participants have found hawthorn helpful for the treatment of mild to moderate congestive heart failure.

In one of the best of these studies, 209 people with relatively advanced congestive heart failure (technically, New York Heart Association [NYHA] class III) were given either 1,800 mg or 900 mg of standardized hawthorn extract or matching placebo. The results after 16 weeks of therapy showed significant improvements in the hawthorn groups as compared to the placebo groups. Benefits in the high-dose hawthorn group included a reduction in subjective symptoms, as well as an increase in exercise capacity. Subjective symptoms improved to about the same extent in the lower-dose hawthorn group, but there was no improvement in exercise capacity.

A comparative study suggests that hawthorn extract (900 mg) is about as effective as a low dose of the conventional drug captopril. However, while captopril and other standard drugs in the same family have been shown to help reduce hospitalizations and mortality associated with CHF, there is no similar evidence for hawthorn.

Like other treatments used for CHF, hawthorn improves the heart's pumping ability. However, it may offer some important advantages over certain conventional drugs used for this condition.

Digoxin, as well as other medications that increase the power of the heart, also make the heart more susceptible to dangerous irregularities of rhythm. In contrast, preliminary evidence indicates that hawthorn may have the unusual property of both strengthening the heart and stabilizing it against arrhythmias. It is thought to do so by lengthening what is called the *refractory period*. This term refers to the short period following a heartbeat during which the heart cannot beat again. Many irregularities of heart rhythm begin with an early beat. Digoxin shortens the refractory period, making such a premature beat more likely, while hawthorn seems to protect against such potentially dangerous breaks in the heart's even rhythm.

Another advantage of hawthorn involves toxicity. With digoxin, the difference between the proper dosage and the toxic dosage is dangerously small. Hawthorn has an enormous range of safe dosing.

However, keep in mind that digoxin is itself an outdated drug. There are many newer drugs for CHF (such as ACE inhibitors) that are much more effective and have been proven to save lives. Hawthorn has not been shown to provide the same benefit. Furthermore, it is not clear whether one can safely combine hawthorn with other drugs that affect the heart.

For more information, including dosage and safety issues, see the full **Hawthorn** article.

Coenzyme Q_{10}

People with CHF have significantly lower levels of coenzyme Q_{10} (CoQ_{10}) in heart muscle cells than healthy people. This fact alone does not prove that CoQ_{10} supplements will help CHF; however, it prompted medical researchers to try using CoQ_{10} as a treatment for heart failure.

In the largest study, 641 individuals with moderate to severe CHF were monitored for 1 year. Half were given 2 mg/kg of body weight of CoQ_{10} daily; the rest were given placebo. Standard therapy was continued in both groups. The participants treated with CoQ_{10} experienced a significant reduction in the severity of their symptoms. No such improvement was seen in the placebo group. The people who took CoQ_{10} also had significantly fewer hospitalizations for heart failure.

Similarly positive results were also seen in other double-blind studies involving a total of more than 250 participants.

However, two recent and very well-designed double-blind studies enrolling a total of about 85 individuals with CHF failed to find any evidence of benefit. The reason for this discrepancy is not clear.

For more information, including dosage and safety issues, see the full **CoenzymeQ_{10}** article.

Vitamin B_1

Evidence suggests that the strong diuretics (technically, loop diuretics, such as furosemide) commonly used to treat CHF may interfere with the body's metabolism of vitamin B_1 (thiamin).

Since the heart depends on vitamin B_1 for proper function, this finding suggests that taking a supplement may be advisable; and, in fact, preliminary evidence suggests that thiamin supplementation may indeed improve heart function in individuals with CHF.

For more information, including dosage and safety issues, see the full **Vitamin B_1** article.

Other Proposed Natural Treatments

Several studies (primarily by one research group) suggest that the amino acid **taurine** may be useful in CHF and could be more effective than CoQ_{10}.

Another treatment for CHF that has some evidence is the expensive supplement **L-carnitine**, especially when given in the special form called *propionyl-L-carnitine*. Carnitine is frequently combined with CoQ_{10}.

Three small, double-blind studies enrolling a total of about 70 individuals with CHF found that the supplement **arginine** significantly improved symptoms of CHF, as well as objective measurements of heart function.

Evidence suggests that the sports supplement **creatine** may offer some help for the sensation of fatigue that often accompanies CHF.

One small double-blind study found preliminary evidence that the supplement **ribose** may improve CHF symptoms.

Combination therapy with several of the supplements mentioned above may also be helpful. A double-blind trial of 41 individuals found that use of a supplement containing taurine, CoQ$_{10}$, creatine, and carnitine, as well as other nutrients, improved objective measures of heart function.

A study performed in China reported that berberine (a constituent of various herbs, including goldenseal and Oregon grape) can decrease mortality and increase quality of life in CHF.

There is some evidence that supplementing with **magnesium** may be helpful for individuals taking both digoxin and diuretics; diuretics can deplete the body of magnesium and this, in turn, may increase risk of digoxin

side effects. One study found that use of magnesium (as magnesium orotate) may improve exercise capacity and reduce heart arrhythmias in people with CHF who have just undergone bypass graft surgery.

In addition, it is important to pay attention to all the general considerations that bring health to the heart, such as those described in the article on atherosclerosis.

Vitamin E has been proposed as a treatment for CHF, but a small, double-blind study did not find it effective.

Herbs and Supplements to Use Only with Caution

Various herbs and supplements may interact adversely with drugs used to treat congestive heart failure. For more information on this potential risk, see the individual drug article in the Drug Interactions section of this book.

Conjunctivitis

PRINCIPAL PROPOSED NATURAL TREATMENTS: *None*

OTHER PROPOSED NATURAL TREATMENTS: *Barberry, Bee Propolis, Calendula, Chamomile, Eyebright, Goldenseal, Oregon Grape, Vitamin A*

Also called *pinkeye*, conjunctivitis is an inflammation of the conjunctiva, which is the clear membrane that covers the eyeball. Symptoms in the affected eye include a bloodshot appearance, crusty discharge, and discomfort that may feel like something has gotten in the eye. Conjunctivitis is frequently caused by a viral infection, sometimes of the same viruses that cause colds. In such cases, conjunctivitis could be called "a cold in the eye" and is really no more serious than any other cold. Other causes of conjunctivitis include bacterial infections, allergies, environmental irritants, such as smoke or pollution, exposure to chemicals such as chlorine or contact lens solution, or injuries to the eye.

Medical treatment varies depending on the cause of the inflammation. Common viral conjunctivitis does not require treatment—but if conjunctivitis is due to the *Herpes* virus, urgent treatment is necessary. For

bacterial eye infections, antibiotic ointment or oral antibiotics are usually prescribed; for allergic conjunctivitis, prescription eyedrops and/or antihistamines may be used.

Proposed Natural Treatments

Herbal Teas

Traditionally, herbal teas have been applied to the eyes directly, in compress or poultice form. **Note**: We do not recommend this method because, if absolute sterility is not assured, further serious infection may occur. Furthermore, allergic reactions to herbal products are relatively common and may themselves cause eye irritation.

As the name indicates, eyebright is a traditional herbal treatment for eye conditions; however, this recommendation may be based more on the bloodshot appearance of its petals rather than any actual medicinal effect.

The herbs **barberry**, **Oregon grape**, and **goldenseal** contain berberine, a substance with antimicrobial and antibacterial properties. A special berberine preparation is used as a pharmaceutical treatment for conjunctivitis in Germany, but is not used widely elsewhere.

The herb **calendula** is thought to possess anti-inflammatory and antiseptic properties, and has been used traditionally as an eye compress.

Chamomile tea has also traditionally been used to soothe conjunctivitis symptoms.

Vitamin A

There is some evidence that individuals with chronic conjunctivitis may have a **vitamin A** deficiency. However, this does not prove that taking vitamin A supplements would be helpful in treating or preventing conjunctivitis.

Bee Propolis

Preliminary studies suggest **bee propolis** may be helpful for treating conjunctivitis. However, because it was applied topically to the eye in these trials, we do not recommend this treatment out of concerns regarding sterility.

Constipation

PRINCIPAL PROPOSED NATURAL TREATMENTS: *Cascara Sagrada, Dandelion, He Shou Wu, Increased Dietary Fiber (Debittered Fenugreek Seeds, Flaxseed, Glucomannan, Psyllium Husks), Increased Water Intake, Methyl Sulfonyl Methane (MSM), Probiotics (Alone or with Prebiotics), Senna, Traditional Chinese Herbal Medicine*

OTHER PROPOSED NATURAL TREATMENTS: *Acupuncture, Aloe, Ayurvedic Herbal Combinations, Basil, Barberry, Bladderwrack, Biofeedback, Buckthorn, Cayenne, Dandelion, Goldenseal, He Shou Wu, Red Raspberry, Slippery Elm*

In the nineteenth century, a naturopathic concept came into being whose influence persists today: namely, that regular, frequent, and complete bowel movements are necessary for optimum health. William Harvey Kellogg, of Kellogg's cereal fame, wrote extensively of the dangers of "autointoxication" purportedly caused by inadequate elimination. He and others claimed that a concrete-like sludge builds up on the wall of the colon, increasing in thickness over time and destroying the health of the body.

However, in modern times physicians have performed millions of direct examinations of the colon, using the procedure known as colonoscopy, without finding any evidence of such a coating. Caked colons are a myth.

Furthermore, conventional medicine has never observed any connection between elimination and overall health. Many people eliminate only once a week or so and their health appears to be no worse than that of the population at large.

In addition, one study found that there is no connection between constipation and colon cancer.

Nonetheless, most people find occasional constipation unpleasant and for some it becomes a severe chronic problem.

Conventional treatment for constipation involves mainly increasing exercise and intake of dietary fiber and water while reserving laxatives, suppositories, and enemas for emergencies.

Principal Proposed Natural Treatments

Occasional constipation can be safely self-treated. However, if constipation becomes a chronic problem, it should be evaluated by a physician.

Increasing dietary fiber and water intake is the first treatment to try for chronic constipation. Whole grains and fruits and vegetables add fiber in the diet. In addition, fiber supplements may be taken in the form of psyllium husks, debittered **fenugreek** seeds, **glucommannan**, and **flaxseed**. A typical dosage of fiber is 5 to 10 g 1 to 3 times daily with at least 16 ounces of liquid. Start with the lower doses and work up gradually, as too much fiber all at once can actually worsen constipation.

The herbs cascara sagrada and **senna** are stimulant laxatives approved as over-the-counter treatments for constipation. They work by virtue of chemical constituents called *anthraquinones* that irritate the colon wall. When taken to excess, these laxatives can cause dependence. In addition, if overused, they can cause depletion of potassium. This is especially dangerous for people taking drugs in the **digoxin** family.

Traditional Chinese herbal medicine offers numerous herbal combinations for the treatment of constipation. One such combination has undergone study: a combination of the herbs rhubarb and licorice called *Daio-kanzo-to*. In this 2-week, double-blind, placebo-controlled trial, 132 people complaining of constipation were randomly assigned to one of three groups: placebo, low-dose Daio-kanzo-to, or high-dose Daio-kanzo-to.

The results indicate that the higher-dose group, but not the lower-dose group, experienced statistically significant improvements in constipation compared to placebo. These findings are not surprising because rhubarb, like cascara and senna, contains anthraquinones. The licorice constituent of this formula is said to reduce side effects by protecting mucous membranes. However, there is no meaningful evidence for any such protective effect, nor indication that such a protective effect is needed. Furthermore, licorice presents significant safety risks if taken for more than a short time. See the full **Licorice** article for more information.

Some evidence indicates that **probiotics** ("friendly bacteria") alone, or taken in combination with **prebiotics** (nutrients that encourage the growth of probiotics) may improve constipation.

The psychological aspect of constipation should be considered as well. Like sleep, elimination is inhibited by thinking too much about it. Part of the key to solving chronic constipation problems is to decrease the sense of worry and anxiety that surrounds the issue. Although constipation is certainly unpleasant, its evils have been greatly exaggerated. Thinking less about it will often go a long way toward solving the problem.

Other Proposed Natural Treatments

Numerous herbs are used alone or in combination formulas for the treatment of constipation, including **aloe**, **Ayurvedic herbal combinations**, **barberry**, **bladderwrack**, basil, buckthorn, **cayenne**, **dandelion**, **goldenseal**, **He shou wu**, **red raspberry**, and **slippery elm**. However, the effectiveness of these therapies has not been scientifically evaluated.

Besides herbs, other alternative medicine therapies have been proposed for use in the treatment of constipation. **Biofeedback** has shown promise in preliminary trials. However, one small study failed to find **acupuncture** helpful for constipation.

Cough

PRINCIPAL PROPOSED NATURAL TREATMENTS: *None*

OTHER PROPOSED NATURAL TREATMENTS: *Marshmallow; Elecampane; Garlic; Horehound; Hyssop; Ivy Leaf; Lobelia; Licorice; Mullein; Plantain; Primula Root; Slippery Elm; Soap Bark; Essential Oils of Anise, Eucalyptus, Fennel, Peppermint, and Thyme*

The cough reflex is intended to expel mucus and other unwanted material from the breathing passages. However, sometimes it takes on a life of its own and causes an unproductive cough that seems to serve no purpose except to keep you awake.

The most common cause of coughing is a viral infection. Sometimes a chronic cough may indicate **asthma**, either caused by allergies or created temporarily by a respiratory infection. Other causes of cough include sinus drainage tickling the throat and chronic bronchitis.

First and foremost, medical treatment for cough involves treating the underlying condition, if possible. When appropriate, cough suppressants may be prescribed as well to hold coughing to manageable levels. Most cough remedies contain codeine or the codeine-like drug dextromethorphan to suppress the cough reflex, as well as guaifenesin, which is thought to loosen mucus. Other common ingredients, such as decongestants and antihistamines, do not directly affect coughs. Unfortunately, there is no reliable evidence that any over-the-counter cough suppressant actually works. Furthermore, while it is often said that prescription codeine cough syrups are more effective than dextromethorphan, one study found that neither codeine nor dextromethorphan reduced night-time coughing in children to any greater extent than placebo. In another study, prescription codeine cough syrup failed to prove more effective than dextromethorphan.

Proposed Natural Treatments

Although many herbs have been used historically to treat coughs, none has been shown effective in a double-blind, placebo-controlled trial. Without such trials it is impossible to know whether a treatment really works, regardless of its reputation. (For a discussion of the many ways in which people can be fooled into thinking that an ineffective treatment is effective, see **Why Does This Book Rely on Double-blind Studies?**.) A few studies that lack a placebo group are sometimes cited in support of traditional cough remedies, but these are almost as unreliable as completely unscientific anecdotes.

Weak evidence indicates that the herb **marshmallow** may help soothe coughs. The herb **coltsfoot** has been used since ancient times to relieve cough; its scientific name, *Tusillago farfara*, means "cough dispeller" in Latin. However, there is no scientific evidence to indicate that coltsfoot actually works. Furthermore, the root of the plant contains high levels of liver-toxic pyrrolizidine alkaloids. The leaves and flowers are safer, but they also may contain these toxins.

Many herbs are categorized as mucilaginous (gluey) and are said to coat the throat. These include marshmallow, **mullein**, **plantain**, and **slippery elm**. The herbs **ivy leaf**, primula root, and soap bark contain chemicals called *saponins*, which are said to loosen mucus. Other herbs used for coughs include **elecampane**, **garlic**, **horehound**, **hyssop**, **lobelia**, and **licorice**. Essential oils such as anise, **eucalyptus**, **fennel**, **peppermint**, and thyme are often included in cough preparations or added to a vaporizer. As noted above, there is no meaningful scientific evidence that any of these treatments are effective. However, since much the same situation exists for standard cough suppressants, they may be worth trying.

The most common cause of a cough is a respiratory infection; for this reason, herbs and supplements used to treat **colds** may be worth considering as well.

Crohn's Disease

RELATED TERMS: *Granulomatous Ileitis, Ileocolitis, Inflammatory Bowel Disease, Regional Enteritis*

PRINCIPAL PROPOSED NATURAL TREATMENTS: *Nutritional Support*

OTHER PROPOSED NATURAL TREATMENTS: *Acupuncture, Avoidance of Allergenic Foods, Boswellia, Fish Oil, Glutamine, Probiotics*

Crohn's disease is a disease of the bowel that is closely related to **ulcerative colitis**. The two are grouped in a category called *inflammatory bowel disease* (IBD) because they both involve inflammation of the digestive tract.

The major symptoms of Crohn's disease include fever, non-bloody or bloody diarrhea, abdominal pain, and fatigue. The rectum may be severely affected, leading to fissures, abscesses, and fistulas (hollow passages). Intestinal obstruction can occur and over time fistulas may develop in the small bowel. Other complications include gallstones, increased risk of cancer in the small bowel and colon, and pain in or just below the stomach that mimics the pain of an ulcer. Arthritis, skin sores, and liver problems may develop as well.

Crohn's disease tends to wax and wane, with periods

of remission punctuated by severe flare-ups. Medical treatment aims at reducing symptoms and inducing and maintaining remission.

Sulfasalazine is one of the most commonly used medications for Crohn's disease. Given either orally or as an enema, it can both decrease symptoms and prevent recurrences. Corticosteroids such as prednisone are used similarly, sometimes combined with immunosuppressive drugs such as azathioprine. In severe cases, partial removal of the bowel may be necessary.

Another approach involves putting people with Crohn's disease on an *elemental* diet. This involves special formulas consisting of required nutrients but no whole foods. Sometimes, after a period on such a diet, whole foods can be restarted one at a time.

Principal Proposed Natural Treatments

People with Crohn's disease can easily develop deficiencies in numerous nutrients. Malabsorption, decreased appetite, drug side effects, and increased nutrient loss through the stool may lead to mild or profound deficiencies of protein, **vitamins A, B$_{12}$, C, D, E, and K, folate, calcium, copper, magnesium, selenium**, and **zinc**. Supplementation to restore adequate body supplies of these nutrients is highly advisable and may improve specific symptoms as well as overall health. We recommend working closely with your physician to identify any nutrient deficiencies and to evaluate the success of supplementation to correct them.

Other Proposed Natural Treatments

Several natural treatments have shown promise for Crohn's disease, but none have been proven effective.

The herb **boswellia** is thought to have some anti-inflammatory effects. An 8-week, double-blind, placebo-controlled trial of 102 people with Crohn's disease compared a standardized extract of boswellia against the drug mesalazine. Participants taking boswellia fared at least as well as those taking mesalazine, according to a standard method of scoring Crohn's disease severity.

Fish oil also has anti-inflammatory effects. However, the evidence regarding whether it is helpful for Crohn's disease remains contradictory. A 1-year, double-blind trial involving 78 participants with Crohn's disease in remission who were at high risk for relapse found that fish oil supplements helped keep the disease from flaring up. In contrast, a 1-year, double-blind, placebo-controlled trial that followed 120 people with Crohn's disease did not find any reduction of relapse rates. A smaller study did find benefit. These opposing results suggest that fish oil is at best modestly effective.

One preliminary double-blind study found indications that the **probiotic** yeast *Saccharomyces boulardii* may be helpful for reducing Crohn's symptoms. However, two studies failed to find benefit with *Lactobacillus* probiotics. On a positive note, some evidence hints that probiotics might reduce the joint pain that commonly occurs in people with inflammatory bowel disease.

Glutamine has been suggested as a treatment for Crohn's disease, but the most meaningful of the reported studies on its potential benefits failed to find it helpful.

A bit of evidence hints that **acupuncture** might be helpful for Crohn's.

Preliminary investigations hint that **food allergies** might play a role in Crohn's disease. However, there is as yet no meaningful evidence that avoiding allergenic foods can improve Crohn's symptoms.

Herbs and Supplements to Use Only with Caution

Various herbs and supplements may interact adversely with drugs used to treat Crohn's disease. For more information on this potential risk, see the individual drug articles in the Drug Interactions section of this book.

Cyclic Mastalgia

RELATED TERMS: *Breast Pain, Cyclic; Breast Tenderness, Cyclic; Cyclic Mastitis; Fibrocystic Breast Disease*
PRINCIPAL PROPOSED NATURAL TREATMENTS: *Chasteberry, Ginkgo*
OTHER PROPOSED NATURAL TREATMENTS: *Diindolylmethane, Evening Primrose Oil/GLA, Iodine, Red Clover Isoflavones, Soy*

Some women's breasts are unusually tender and lumpy, with symptoms of pain and dull heaviness that vary with the menstrual cycle. This condition is called *cyclic mastalgia* or *cyclic mastitis* and is often associated with premenstrual syndrome (PMS). When the lumps become significant enough to be called *cysts*, the condition is called *fibrocystic breast disease.*

Besides discomfort, perhaps the worst problem of this condition is that it can mimic the appearance of breast cancer on mammograms, leading to false alarms. To make matters worse, fibrocystic changes can also hide true cancers and some evidence hints that women with fibrocystic breast disease may also have a greater tendency toward breast cancer.

The cause of cyclic breast pain is unclear. One theory, popular in Europe, suggests that higher than normal levels of the hormone prolactin may be involved. Another theory attributes the condition to an imbalance of essential fatty acids.

Conventional treatment for cyclic mastalgia involves anti-inflammatory medications and, sometimes, hormonal treatments.

Principal Proposed Natural Treatments

Cyclic mastalgia often occurs in connection with PMS. (See the **Premenstrual Syndrome** article for information on related treatments.)

Chasteberry

In Germany, the herb chasteberry is frequently used to treat cyclic mastalgia and other symptoms of PMS because of its effect on the pituitary gland to suppress the release of prolactin.

Some evidence suggests that it is in fact effective for this purpose. For example, a double-blind trial of 104 women compared placebo against two forms of chasteberry (liquid and tablet) for at least three menstrual cycles. The results showed statistically significant and comparable improvements in the treated groups as compared to placebo.

Another double-blind, placebo-controlled study, enrolling 178 women, evaluated chasteberry for PMS in general. The results over three menstrual cycles indicated that chasteberry reduced breast tenderness and other PMS symptoms. Benefits were also seen in two other double-blind trials enrolling a total of more than 250 women.

For more information, including dosage and safety issues, see the full **Chasteberry** article.

Ginkgo

Although the herb ginkgo is primarily used to enhance memory and mental function (see the article on **Alzheimer's disease**), it may be helpful for breast tenderness as well. A double-blind, placebo-controlled study evaluated 143 women with PMS symptoms, 18 to 45 years of age, and followed them for two menstrual cycles. Each woman received either the ginkgo extract (80 mg twice daily) or placebo on day 16 of the first cycle. Treatment was continued until day 5 of the next cycle and resumed again on day 16 of that cycle.

As compared to placebo, ginkgo significantly relieved major symptoms of PMS, especially breast pain.

For more information, including dosage and safety issues, see the full **Ginkgo** article.

Other Proposed Natural Treatments

Evening primrose oil contains relatively high concentrations of the essential omega-6 fatty acid named **gamma-linolenic acid** (GLA). On the theory that essential fatty acid imbalances play a role in cyclic mastalgia, evening primrose oil became a popular treatment for this condition. However, despite numerous positive anecdotes, there are considerable doubts regarding whether it is actually effective. The main supporting evidence for GLA comes from three small double-blind studies. Unfortunately, all of these suffered from significant limitations in study design and reporting. A very large (555-participant) and well-designed study failed to find GLA, with or without antioxidants, any more effective than placebo. (The placebo by itself, however, was found to be quite effective, possibly explaining why so many doctors and patients believe that evening primrose oil is helpful.) Another well-designed study found that evening primrose oil, by itself or with **fish oil**, is not more effective than placebo for cyclic breast pain. Other studies found evening primrose oil ineffective for established breast cysts.

Fish oil taken alone has thus far failed to prove effective for cyclic breast pain.

According to one small double-blind trial, the substance **diindolylmethane** (DIM) might be helpful for cyclic mastalgia.

A small and poorly reported double-blind, placebo-controlled trial provides weak evidence that **red clover isoflavones** might reduce symptoms of cyclic mastalgia. Another small study suggests possible benefit with **soy** protein.

Very weak evidence suggests the supplement **iodine** may also be helpful for cyclic mastalgia.

Like chasteberry, the herb **bugleweed** appears to reduce prolactin levels and, for this reason, has also been tried for the treatment of cyclic mastalgia. However, this herb affects the thyroid gland, and we do not recommend it.

Finally, many conventional and alternative practitioners suggest avoiding caffeine. However, despite the popularity of this intervention, there is no consistent evidence that caffeine really causes a problem. Physicians of all types are often overly willing to speak ill of foods that people enjoy, in accordance with an impulse that some call "health Puritanism."

Depression (Mild to Moderate)

PRINCIPAL PROPOSED NATURAL TREATMENTS: *St. John's Wort*

OTHER PROPOSED NATURAL TREATMENTS: *5-Hydroxytryptophan (5-HTP), Acetyl-L-Carnitine, Acupuncture, Ayurveda, Beta-carotene, Chromium, Damiana, Dehydroepiandrosterone (DHEA), Exercise, Fish Oil, Folate, Ginkgo, Hatha Yoga, Inositol, Lavender, Massage, NADH, Phenylalanine, Phosphatidylserine, Pregnenolone, S-Adenosylmethionine (SAMe), Repetitive Transcranial Magnetic Stimulation (rTMS), Saffron* (Crocus sativus), *Tyrosine, Vitamin B$_6$, Vitamin B$_{12}$, Zinc*

Depression is a common emotional illness that varies widely in its intensity. Many of the natural treatments described in this section have been evaluated in people with major depression of mild to moderate intensity. This apparently contradictory language indicates a level of clinical depression that is significantly more intense than simply feeling "blue," but not as disabling as major depression of severe intensity, which usually requires hospitalization.

Typical symptoms of major depression of mild to moderate severity include depressed mood, lack of energy, sleep problems, anxiety, appetite disturbance, difficulty concentrating, and poor stress tolerance. Irritability can also be a sign of depression.

More severe depression includes markedly depressed mood complicated by symptoms such as slowed speech, slowed (or agitated) responses, markedly impaired memory and concentration, excessive (or diminished) sleep, significant weight loss (or weight gain), intense feelings of worthlessness and guilt, recurrent thoughts of suicide, and lack of interest in pleasurable activities. This form of clinical depression is a dangerous and excruciating illness. The emotional structure of the brain has frozen into a pattern of misery that cannot be altered by willpower, a change of scenery, or the most earnest efforts of friends. In a sense, the brain has locked up like a crashed computer.

One of the earliest successful treatments for major depression was shock therapy. This technique is in some ways analogous to rebooting a computer and, in cases of major depression, its effects were revolutionary. For the first time, a reliable way was available to bring people out of the depths of severe major depression.

However, shock treatment was overused at first and became unpopular as a result. The accidental discovery of antidepressant drugs provided a route with fewer interventions. The original antidepressants, known as MAO inhibitors, could bring people out from the depths of major depression as successfully as shock treatment. However, MAO inhibitors can cause serious and even fatal side effects. No one would ever think of using MAO inhibitors to treat mild to moderate depression.

Subsequently, antidepressants with progressively fewer side effects came on the market, but most of them still caused significant fatigue. Since fatigue is one of the most characteristic symptoms of mild to moderate depression, such medications were seldom found useful for anything other than severe depression. With the appearance of the selective serotonin reuptake inhibitor (SSRI) class of antidepressants, however, suddenly there was a practical option for depression that was less than catastrophic. Practically overnight, enormous numbers of people began taking Prozac and similar drugs for mild to moderate depression, as well as for the related but more mild condition known as *dysthymia*.

The big advantage of the SSRIs is that they usually don't cause severe fatigue. Many people find them to be entirely side effect–free. However, side effects are not uncommon and include sexual disturbances (such as impotence in men and the loss of the ability to experience an orgasm in women), insomnia, and nervousness. The antidepressant drug Wellbutrin is an option for people who have sexual side effects from SSRIs.

Principal Proposed Natural Treatments

Alternative medicine offers numerous options for treating depression, but only one has strong scientific evidence behind it: the herb St. John's wort.

What Is the Scientific Evidence for St. John's Wort?

Numerous double-blind, placebo-controlled studies have examined the effectiveness of St. John's wort for the treatment of mild to moderate major depression and most have found the herb more effective than placebo. In addition, at least eight studies have found that St. John's wort is at least as effective as standard antidepressants, including fluoxetine (Prozac), sertraline (Zoloft), citalopram (Celexa), and paroxetine (Paxil). The total number of patients in these trials runs into the several thousands and compares favorably to the evidence-base for approved drugs.

Much has been made of two double-blind, placebo-controlled trials performed in the United States that failed to find St. John's wort more effective than placebo. However, two studies cannot overturn a body of positive research. Approximately 35% of double-blind studies involving pharmaceutical antidepressants have also failed to find the active agent significantly more effective than placebo. As if to illustrate this, in the more recent of the two trials in which St. John's wort failed to prove effective, the drug sertraline (Zoloft) also failed to prove effective. The reason for these negative outcomes is not that Zoloft (or Prozac, or any other drug) does not work. Rather, statistical effects can easily hide the benefits of a drug, especially in a condition like depression where there is a high placebo effect and no truly precise method for measuring symptoms.

St. John's wort seldom causes immediate side effects. However, it interacts adversely with a large number of critical medications and may present other safety issues as well. For more information, see the full **St. John's Wort** article.

Other Proposed Natural Treatments

There are a number of other herbs and supplements that may be helpful in depression, although the evidence for them is nowhere near as strong as that for St. John's wort.

Folate

In the body, the vitamin folate works in tandem with SAMe. Studies have suggested that depressed people have reduced folate levels and that folate supplements may help alleviate depression. In addition, people with particularly low folate levels may respond poorly to antidepressants. Based on these findings, a study examined the effects of combining folate with antidepressant treatment.

This 10-week, double-blind, placebo-controlled trial of 127 people with severe major depression found that folate supplements at a dose of 500 mcg daily significantly improved the effectiveness of fluoxetine (Prozac) in female participants. Improvement in male participants was not significant, but blood tests conducted during the study suggest that higher intake of folate might be necessary for men.

For more information, including dosage and safety issues, see the full **Folate** article.

S-adenosylmethionine

The supplement S-adenosylmethionine (SAMe) has been widely marketed for the treatment of depression, but the evidence to indicate that it works remains incomplete.

Several double-blind, placebo-controlled studies have found SAMe effective in relieving depression; however, most were small and poorly reported. In addition, many used injected SAMe rather than the oral supplement. Furthermore, the most recent and best-designed of these, a double-blind, placebo-controlled study of 133 depressed people, actually failed to find intravenous SAMe more effective than placebo. (Researchers managed to find some benefit to report by resorting to questionable statistical manipulation of the data.)

In addition to placebo-controlled studies, several trials have compared SAMe against antidepressant drugs in the **tricyclic** family. Again, many of these studies were poorly reported and designed, or used injected SAMe rather than the oral supplement. Of the studies using oral SAMe, the best was a 6-week, double-blind trial of 281 people with mild depression. The results showed that SAMe was about as effective as the drug imipramine. However, the lack of a placebo group in this trial makes the results less than fully reliable.

Other small studies have also compared the benefits of oral or intravenous SAMe to those of tricyclic antidepressants and have found generally equivalent results, although, again, poor reporting and inadequacies of study design (such as too limited a treatment interval) mar the meaningfulness of the outcomes.

For more information, including dosage and safety issues, see the full **S-adenosylmethionine** article.

Ginkgo

Ginkgo is used mainly for age-related mental decline such as that from **Alzheimer's disease**. However, during the studies on impaired mental function, researchers frequently observed improvements in mood and relief from symptoms of depression. This incidental discovery led scientists to investigate whether ginkgo might be useful as an antidepressant treatment.

One double-blind study, published in 1990, evaluated this effect in 60 people who suffered from depressive symptoms along with other signs of dementia. The results showed significant improvement among participants given ginkgo extract instead of placebo.

Another study followed 40 depressed people over the age of 50 who had not responded successfully to antidepressant treatment. Those who were given ginkgo showed an average drop of 50% in scores on the Hamilton Depression scale, whereas the placebo group showed only a 10% improvement.

In 1994 an interesting piece of research was reported that may shed light on the mechanism by which ginkgo may reduce depression. This study examined levels of serotonin receptors in rats of various ages. When older rats were given ginkgo, the level of serotonin-binding sites increased. However, the same effect was not observed in younger rats. The researchers theorized that ginkgo may block an age-related loss of serotonin receptors. Reduced receptors for serotonin may mean that the body needs more serotonin to produce a normal effect. Thus, ginkgo might improve the brain's ability to respond to serotonin (at least in older people). However, this is still highly speculative.

For more information, including dosage and safety issues, see the full **Ginkgo** article.

Phenylalanine

Phenylalanine is a naturally occurring amino acid that we all consume in our daily diets. There is some evidence that phenylalanine supplements may help reduce symptoms of depression.

Phenylalanine occurs in a right-hand and a left-hand form, known as *D*- and *L-phenylalanine*, respectively. Some studies have evaluated the D form and others have evaluated a mixture of the D and L forms. Both formulations may provide some measure of relief for symptoms of depression. The mixed form (DLPA) is the one most commonly available in stores.

A 1978 study compared the effectiveness of D-phenylalanine against the antidepressant drug imipramine (taken in daily doses of 100 mg) and found them to be equally effective. A total of 60 people were randomly assigned to either one group or the other and followed for 30 days. D-phenylalanine worked more rapidly, producing significant improvement in only 15 days.

Another double-blind study followed 27 people, half of whom received DL-phenylalanine and the other half imipramine in higher doses of 150 to 200 mg daily. When the participants were reevaluated in 30 days, the two groups had improved by the same amount.

Unfortunately, there do not seem to have been any properly designed studies that compared phenylalanine to placebo. Until these are performed, phenylalanine cannot be considered a proven treatment for depression, but it is certainly promising.

For more information, including dosage and safety issues, see the full **Phenylalanine** article.

5-hydroxytryptophan

When the body sets about manufacturing serotonin, it first makes 5-hydroxytryptophan (5-HTP). The theory behind taking 5-HTP as a supplement is that providing the one-step-removed raw ingredient might raise serotonin levels.

There have been several preliminary studies of 5-HTP. The best of these trials was a 6-week study of 63 people given either 5-HTP (100 mg 3 times daily) or an antidepressant in the Prozac family (fluvoxamine, 50 mg 3 times daily). The results showed equal benefit between the supplement and the drug. Actually, 5-HTP worked a little better, but from a mathematical perspective, the difference was not statistically significant.

5-HTP caused fewer and less severe side effects than fluvoxamine. The only real complaint was occasional mild digestive distress.

For more information, including dosage and safety issues, see the full **5-hydroxytryptophan** article.

Fish Oil

According to most but not all studies, **fish oil** or the related substance ethyl-EPA may be helpful for depression when taken along with standard antidepressant treatment.

For example, a 4-week, double-blind, placebo-controlled trial evaluated the potential benefits of fish oil in 20 individuals with depression. All but one of the participants were also taking standard antidepressants and had been for at least 3 months. By week 3 of the trial, the level of depression had improved to a significantly greater extent in the fish oil group than in placebo group. Six of 10 participants given fish oil, but only 1 of 10 given placebo, showed at least a 50% reduction in depression scores by the end of the trial. (A reduction of this magnitude is considered a cure.) In addition, a double-blind, placebo-controlled study of 70 people with depression that did not respond well to drug treatment found that the addition of ethyl-EPA (a modified form of a primary ingredient of fish oil) improved the response.

However, the largest (77 participants) study unexpectedly failed to find fish oil more effective than placebo. The reason for this discrepancy is unclear.

Exercise

Exercise may be helpful for depression. In a review published in the journal *Sports Medicine*, researchers analyzed the published research on this subject. Their conclusion: A very qualified "yes."

In seven out of eight studies reviewed, various forms of exercise proved beneficial for depression. Aerobic exercise, weight training, dancing, and racquetball all produced improvements in mood as compared to no exercise.

However, the findings of the one negative study reported in this review cast doubt on the others. In this trial, some participants exercised, while others took a course at school and didn't exercise at all. The results: Equal benefits in both groups. This suggests that it may not be the exercise itself that is helping, but rather the general effects of participation in an organized activity.

Another feature of the positive studies also tends to cast doubt on the value of exercise per se in depression. You'd think that if it were exercise itself improving mood, the more effectively the participants exercised the greater the effect. However, no correlation was seen between how much participants increased their physical fitness and how significantly their depression improved.

Other Herbs and Supplements

Like ginkgo, the supplement **phosphatidylserine** is used mainly for mental decline in the elderly, but it may also offer antidepressant benefits for seniors. Limited evidence hints that **acetyl-L-carnitine** may also offer benefits for seniors, as well as, potentially, for younger people.

Diets low in **vitamin B$_6$** or **vitamin B$_{12}$** have been associated with symptoms of depression. While there is little direct evidence that taking these supplements can help depression, deficiencies of B$_6$ are common and B$_{12}$ deficiencies occur more often with advancing age, so it may be a good idea to take these vitamins on general principles.

In a small double-blind, placebo-controlled study, tincture of **lavender** enhanced the antidepressant effectiveness of the drug imipramine. The hormone **DHEA** has shown some promise for depression.

When depression is characterized by rapid mood changes, excessive sleeping and eating, a sense of leaden paralysis, and extreme sensitivity to negative life events, the condition is called *atypical depression*. A very small (15 participants) double-blind, placebo-controlled study found that **chromium picolinate** might be helpful for this form of depression; however, a much larger study failed to find convincing benefits.

One study found weak evidence that **zinc** supplements may enhance the effectiveness of standard antidepressants.

According to three preliminary double-blind studies, use of the herb **saffron** (*Crocus sativus*) at 30 mg daily is more effective than placebo and equally effective as standard treatment for major depression. However, all these studies were small and were performed by a single research group (in Iran). Larger studies and independent confirmation will be necessary to determine whether saffron truly is effective for depression.

Beta-carotene, damiana, NADH, pregnenolone, and **tyrosine** are also sometimes recommended for depression, but there is little evidence as yet that they really work.

A double-blind study of 42 people with severe depression found no improvement with the supplement **inositol**.

Alternative Therapies

Various alternative therapies have shown some promise for the treatment of depression. These include **acupuncture, Ayurveda, hatha yoga,** and **massage**.

In addition, a growing body of evidence suggests, on balance, that **repetitive transcranial magnetic stimulation** (rTMS), may be helpful for depression.

Herbs and Supplements to Use Only with Caution

Various herbs and supplements may interact adversely with drugs used to treat depression. For more information on this potential risk, see the individual drug article in the Drug Interactions section of this book.

Diabetes, Complications of

RELATED TERMS: *Autonomic Neuropathy, Diabetic; Cardiac Autonomic Neuropathy, Diabetic; Cataracts; Cataracts, Diabetic; Diabetes, Complications of; Diabetic Neuropathy; Diabetic Retinopathy; Peripheral Neuropathy, Diabetic; Retinopathy, Diabetic*

PRINCIPAL PROPOSED NATURAL TREATMENTS:

Peripheral Neuropathy: *Acetyl-L-Carnitine, Lipoic Acid, Evening Primrose Oil (GLA)*

Cardiac Autonomic Neuropathy: *Lipoic Acid*

OTHER PROPOSED NATURAL TREATMENTS:

Peripheral Neuropathy: *Fish Oil, Magnet Therapy, Selenium, Vitamin E*

Cardiac Autonomic Neuropathy: *Vitamin E*

Lower Leg Swelling (Microangiopathy): *Oxerutins*

Retinopathy: *Bilberry, OPCs (Oligomeric Proanthocyanidins)*

Cataracts: *Bilberry*

Immunity and Infections: *Multivitamin/Multimineral Supplements*

For more information on natural treatments for diabetes in general, see the full **Diabetes** article. This entry discusses natural treatments for the *complications* of diabetes.

Diabetes is an illness that damages many organs in the body, including the heart and blood vessels, nerves, kidneys, and eyes. Most of this damage is believed to be caused by the toxic effects of abnormally high blood sugar, although other factors may play a role as well.

So-called tight control of blood sugar greatly reduces all complications of diabetes. Some of the natural treatments described here may help as well.

Principal Proposed Natural Treatments

Several supplements may help prevent or treat some of the common complications of diabetes. However, because diabetes is a dangerous disease, alternative treatment should not be attempted as a substitute for conventional medical care.

Atherosclerosis is one of the worst problems associated with diabetes and all the suggestions discussed in the article on that topic may be useful. Similarly, natural treatments helpful in general for improving cholesterol and triglyceride profiles may be useful to people with diabetes.

Note: Contrary to some early concerns, both **fish oil** and **niacin** (treatments used for improving triglyceride and cholesterol levels, respectively) appear to be safe for people with diabetes.

High levels of blood sugar can damage the nerves leading to the extremities, causing pain and numbness. This condition is called *diabetic peripheral neuropathy*. Nerve damage may also develop in the heart, a condition named *cardiac autonomic neuropathy*. Below, we discuss three natural supplements—acetyl-L-carnitine, lipoic acid, and gamma-linolenic acid (GLA)—that have shown promise for the treatment of diabetic nerve damage.

Acetyl-L-Carnitine

The supplement acetyl-L-carnitine (ALC) has shown promise for diabetic peripheral neuropathy. Two 52-week, double-blind, placebo-controlled studies involving a total of 1,257 people with diabetic peripheral neuropathy evaluated the potential benefits of ALC taken at 500 mg or 1000 mg daily. The results showed that use of ALC, especially at the higher dose, improved sensory perception and decreased pain levels. In addition, the supplement appeared to promote nerve fiber regeneration.

ALC has also shown some promise for cardiac autonomic neuropathy.

For more information, including full dosage and safety issues, see the **Carnitine** article.

Lipoic Acid

The DEKAN (Deutsche Kardiale Autonome Neuropathie) study followed 73 people with cardiac autonomic neuropathy for 4 months. Treatment with 800 mg of oral lipoic acid daily showed significant improvement compared to placebo and no important side effects.

Lipoic acid has been widely proposed as a treatment for diabetic peripheral neuropathy as well. However, a review of the evidence shows that while *intravenous* lipoic acid has shown promise for treating this condition, there is no real evidence to indicate that *oral* lipoic acid can help. For example, a double-blind, placebo-controlled study that enrolled 503 people with diabetic peripheral neuropathy found that intravenous lipoic acid helped reduce symptoms over a 3-week period. However, subsequent long-term supplementation with oral lipoic acid was *not* effective.

Other double-blind, placebo-controlled trials also found benefit in the short term with intravenous lipoic acid, but they did not evaluate oral lipoic acid at all.

The positive evidence for oral lipoic acid in diabetic peripheral neuropathy is limited to open studies or double-blind trials that were too small to be conclusive.

Preliminary evidence hints that lipoic acid may be more effective for neuropathy if it is combined with GLA (gamma-linolenic acid, described in the next section).

For more information, including dosage and safety issues, see the full **Lipoic Acid** article.

Gamma-linolenic Acid (from Evening Primrose Oil)

Gamma-linolenic acid, GLA, is an essential fatty acid in the omega-6 category. The most common sources of GLA are evening primrose oil, borage oil, and black currant oil.

Many studies in animals have shown that evening primrose oil can protect nerves from diabetes-induced injury. Human trials have also found benefits. A double-blind study followed 111 people with diabetes for a period of 1 year. The results showed an improvement in subjective symptoms of peripheral neuropathy, such as pain and numbness, as well as objective signs of nerve injury. People with good blood sugar control improved the most. A much smaller double-blind study also reported positive results.

For more information, including dosage and safety issues, see the full **GLA** article.

Other Proposed Natural Treatments

A 4-month, double-blind, placebo-controlled trial found that **vitamin E** at a dose of 600 mg daily might improve symptoms of cardiac autonomic neuropathy. Vitamin E as well as **selenium** have also shown promise for diabetic peripheral neuropathy. Intriguing evidence from a small study suggests that vitamin E may also help protect people with diabetes from developing damage to their eyes and kidneys. However, a large, long-term study failed to find vitamin E effective for preventing kidney damage. (Vitamin E also did not help prevent coronary artery disease.)

The supplement inositol has been tried as a treatment for diabetic neuropathy, but the results have been mixed.

In highly preliminary studies, fish oil has shown some promise for diabetic neuropathy, but human trials have not been performed.

Diabetes can cause swelling of the ankles and feet by

damaging small blood vessels (microangiopathy). A preliminary, double-blind, placebo-controlled trial suggests that **oxerutins** might be helpful for this condition.

Weak evidence suggests that the herb **bilberry** may help prevent eye damage (**cataracts** and retinopathy) caused by diabetes. Pycnogenol, a source of OPCs, has also shown promise for diabetic retinopathy.

It has been suggested that vitamin C may also help prevent cataracts in diabetes, based on its relationship to sorbitol. Sorbitol, a sugar-like substance that tends to accumulate in the cells of people with diabetes, may play a role in the development of diabetic cataracts. Vitamin C appears to help reduce sorbitol buildup. However, the evidence that vitamin C provides significant benefits by this route is at present indirect and far from conclusive.

Another study suggests that vitamin C might be helpful for reducing blood pressure in people with diabetes.

Magnetic insoles, a form of **magnet therapy**, have shown some promise for the treatment of diabetic peripheral neuropathy. A 4-month, double-blind, placebo-controlled, crossover study of 19 people with peripheral neuropathy found a significant reduction in symptoms in people using the insoles as compared to those using placebo insoles. This study enrolled people with peripheral neuropathy of various causes; however, reduction in the symptoms of burning, numbness, and tingling were especially marked in those cases of neuropathy associated with diabetes.

One small double-blind, placebo-controlled study suggests that regular use of **multivitamin/multimineral supplements** may reduce incidence of infectious illness in people with diabetes. Another study *failed* to find that general nutritional supplementation accelerated healing of diabetic foot ulcers.

Diabetes, General

RELATED TERMS: *Diabetes, Prevention; Diabetes, Nutritional Depletion*

PRINCIPAL PROPOSED NATURAL TREATMENTS:

Blood Sugar Control: *Aloe, Chromium, Ginseng*

To Correct Nutritional Deficiencies: *Calcium, Magnesium, Manganese, Taurine, Vitamin B_{12}, Vitamin C, Zinc*

Complications of Diabetes: *See associated article.*

OTHER PROPOSED NATURAL TREATMENTS:

Blood Sugar Control: *Arginine, Ayurvedic Combination Herbal Therapies, Bilberry Leaf, Biotin, Bitter Melon, Caiapo, Carnitine, Cinnamon, Coenzyme Q_{10} (CoQ_{10}), Coccinia indica, DHEA, Fenugreek, Garlic, Glucomannan, Guggul, Gymnema, Holy Basil, Lipoic Acid, Magnesium, Niacinamide, Nopal Cactus, Onion, Ooolong Tea, OPCs, Pterocarpus, Salt Bush, Traditional Chinese Herbal Medicine, Vanadium, Vitamin E*

TREATMENTS TO USE ONLY WITH CAUTION: *Conjugated Linoleic Acid (CLA), Ginkgo, Rosemary*

Diabetes has two forms. In the type that develops early in childhood (type 1), the insulin-secreting cells of the pancreas are destroyed (probably by a viral infection) and blood levels of insulin drop nearly to zero. However, in type 2 diabetes (usually developing in adults) insulin remains plentiful, but the body does not respond normally to it. (This is only an approximate description of the difference between the two types.) In both forms of diabetes, blood sugar reaches toxic levels, causing injury to many organs and tissues.

Conventional treatment for type 1 diabetes includes insulin injections and careful dietary monitoring. Type 2 diabetes may respond to lifestyle changes alone, such as increasing exercise, losing weight, and improving diet. Various oral medications are also often effective for type 2 diabetes, although insulin injections may be necessary in some cases.

Principal Proposed Natural Treatments

Several alternative methods may be helpful when used under medical supervision as an addition to standard treatment. They may help stabilize, reduce, or eliminate medication requirements, or correct nutritional deficiencies associated with diabetes. However, because diabetes is a dangerous disease with many potential complications, alternative treatment for diabetes should not be attempted as a substitute for conventional medical care.

Other natural treatments may be helpful for preventing and treating complications of diabetes, such as peripheral neuropathy, cardiac autonomic neuropathy, retinopathy, and cataracts. See the article on **Complications of Diabetes** article for more information.

Treatments for Improving Blood Sugar Control

The following treatments might be able to improve blood sugar control in type 1 and/or type 2 diabetes.

Note: Keep in mind that if these treatments work, you will need to reduce your medications to avoid hypoglycemia. For this reason, medical supervision is essential.

⇒ *Chromium*

Chromium is an essential trace mineral that plays a significant role in sugar metabolism. Some evidence suggests that chromium supplementation may help bring blood sugar levels under control in type 2 diabetes, but it is far from definitive.

A 4-month study reported in 1997 followed 180 Chinese men and women with type 2 diabetes, comparing the effects of 1,000 mcg chromium, 200 mcg chromium, and placebo. The results showed that HbA1c values (a measure of long-term blood sugar control) improved significantly after 2 months in the group receiving 1,000 mcg, and in both chromium groups after 4 months. Fasting glucose (a measure of short-term blood sugar control) was also lower in the group taking the higher dose of chromium.

A double-blind, placebo-controlled trial of 78 people with type 2 diabetes compared two forms of chromium (brewer's yeast and chromium chloride) against placebo.

This rather complex crossover study consisted of four 8-week intervals of treatment in random order. The results in the 67 participants who completed the study showed that both forms of chromium significantly improved blood sugar control. Positive results were also seen in other small double-blind, placebo-controlled studies of people with type 2 diabetes. However, several other studies have failed to find chromium helpful for improving blood sugar control in type 2 diabetes. These contradictory findings suggest that the benefit, if any, is small.

One placebo-controlled study of 30 women with gestational diabetes (diabetes during pregnancy) found that supplementation with chromium (at a dosage of 4 or 8 mcg chromium picolinate for each kilogram of body weight) significantly improved blood sugar control.

Chromium has also shown a bit of promise for helping diabetes caused by **corticosteroid** treatment.

For more information, including dosage and safety issues, see the full **Chromium** article.

⇒ *Ginseng*

In double-blind studies performed by a single research group, use of American ginseng (*Panax quinquefolius*) appeared to improve blood sugar control. The same researchers subsequently reported possible benefit with Korean red ginseng, a specially prepared form of *Panax ginseng*.

A different research group found benefits with ordinary *Panax ginseng*. However, in other studies (conducted by the research group mentioned in the previous paragraph), ordinary *Panax ginseng* seemed to *worsen* blood sugar control rather than improve it. It seems possible that certain ginsensosides (found in high concentrations in some American ginseng products) may lower blood sugar while others (found in high concentrations in some *Panax ginseng* products) may raise it. It has been suggested that since the actions of these various ginseng constituents are not well defined at this time, ginseng should *not* be used to treat diabetes until more is known.

For more information, including dosage and safety issues, see the full **Ginseng** article.

⇒ *Aloe*

The succulent aloe plant has been valued since prehistoric times as a topical treatment for burns, wound infections, and other skin problems. However, recent evidence suggests that oral aloe might be useful for type 2 diabetes.

Evidence from two human trials suggests that aloe gel can improve blood sugar control.

A single-blind, placebo-controlled trial evaluated the potential benefits of aloe in either 72 or 40 people with diabetes (the study report appears to contradict itself). The results showed significantly greater improvements in blood sugar levels among those given aloe over the 2-week treatment period.

Another single-blind, placebo-controlled trial evaluated the benefits of aloe in people who had failed to respond to the oral diabetes drug glibenclamide. Of the 36 people who completed the study, those taking glibenclamide and aloe showed definite improvements in blood sugar levels over 42 days as compared to those taking glibenclamide and placebo.

While these are promising results, large studies that are double- rather than single-blind will be needed to establish aloe as an effective treatment for improving blood sugar control.

Note that in the above we are referring to the *gel* of the aloe vera plant, and not the *leaf skin* (the latter is drug aloe, not aloe gel). However, some confusion has been introduced by the fact that some leaf skin may find its way into gel products and that could be the actual active ingredient in aloe gel regarding diabetes. It is possible, therefore, that completely pure aloe gel might not work.

For more information, including dosage and safety issues, see the full **Aloe** article.

☞ Other Treatments That May Help Control Blood Sugar

The food spice **fenugreek** might also help control blood sugar, but the supporting evidence is weak. In a 2-month, double-blind study of 25 people with type 2 diabetes, use of fenugreek (1 g daily of a standardized extract) significantly improved some measures of blood sugar control and insulin response as compared to placebo. Triglyceride levels decreased and HDL ("good") cholesterol levels increased, presumably due to the enhanced insulin sensitivity. Similar benefits have been seen in animal studies and open human trials as well. However, it is possible that the effects of fenugreek are simply due to its dietary fiber content.

A few preliminary studies suggest that the Ayurvedic (Indian) herb **gymnema** may help improve blood sugar control. It might be helpful for mild cases of type 2 diabetes when taken alone or in combination with standard treatment (under a doctor's supervision in either case).

Cinnamon has been widely advertised as an effective treatment for type 2 diabetes as well as **high cholesterol**. The primary basis for this claim is a single study performed in Pakistan. In this 40-day study, 60 people with type 2 diabetes were given cinnamon at a dose of 1, 3, or 6 g daily. The results reportedly indicated that use of cinnamon improved blood sugar levels by 18 to 29%, total cholesterol by 12 to 26%, LDL ("bad") cholesterol by 7 to 27%, and triglycerides by 23 to 30%. These results were said to be statistically significant as compared to the beginning of the study and to the placebo group. However, this study has some odd features. The most important is that it found no significant difference in benefit between the various doses of cinnamon. This is called lack of a *dose-related effect* and it generally casts doubt on the results of a study.

In an attempt to replicate these results, a group of Dutch researchers performed a carefully designed 6-week double-blind, placebo-controlled study of 25 people with diabetes. All participants were given 1.5 g of cinnamon daily. The results failed to show *any* detectible effect on blood sugar, insulin sensitivity or cholesterol profile. Although this second study was smaller than the first, because it had fewer groups (arms), overall its statistical power is similar. Another study, this one involving 79 people given 3 g of cinnamon daily for 4 months, found marginal benefits at most. At present, therefore, it would be premature to consider cinnamon an evidence-based treatment for diabetes or high cholesterol.

Studies in rats with and without diabetes suggest that high doses of the mineral **vanadium** may have an insulin-like effect, reducing blood sugar levels. Based on these findings, preliminary studies involving human subjects have been conducted, with mostly promising results. However, this evidence is too limited to be taken as definitive proof. Furthermore, the doses of vanadium used are vastly higher than nutritional needs, and therefore present concerns of toxicity.

Preliminary (in some cases, highly preliminary and/or inconsistent) evidence suggests that the herbs **bilberry leaf**, **bitter melon** (*Momordica charantia*), Caiapo, *Coccinia indica*, **garlic**, **guggul**, holy basil (*Ocimum sanctum*), **maitake**, **nopal cactus** (*Opuntia stredptacantha*), onion, oolong tea, **OPCs**, pterocarpus, and **salt bush**, and the supplements **arginine**, **carnitine**, **coenzyme Q$_{10}$** (CoQ$_{10}$), **DHEA**, **glucomannan**, **lipoic acid**, **magnesium**, and **vitamin E** might also help control blood sugar levels, at least slightly.

Conjugated linoleic acid (CLA) has also shown promise in preliminary trials. However, other studies have found that CLA might worsen blood sugar control. (See Supplements to Use Only with Caution below for more information.)

Other herbs traditionally used for diabetes that might possibly offer some benefit include *Anemarrhena asphodeloides, Azadirachta indica* (**neem**), *Catharanthus roseus, Cucurbita ficifolia, Cucumis sativus, Cuminum cyminum* (cumin), *Euphorbia prostrata, Guaiacum coulteri, Guazuma ulmifolia, Lepechinia caulescens, Medicago sativa* (**alfalfa**), *Musa sapientum L.* (banana), **Phaseolus vulgaris**, *Psacalium peltatum, Rhizophora mangle, Spinacea oleracea, Tournefortia hirsutissima,* and *Turnera diffusa.*

Combination herbal therapies used in **Ayurvedic medicine** have also shown some promise for improving blood sugar control.

A double-blind study of more than 200 people evaluated the effectiveness of a combination herbal formula used in **traditional Chinese herbal medicine** (Coptis Formula). This study evaluated Coptis Formula with and without the drug glibenclamide. The results hint that Coptis Formula may enhance the effectiveness of the drug, but that it is not powerful enough to treat diabetes on its own.

In one study the herb *Tinospora crispa* did not work and showed the potential to cause liver injury.

If your child has just developed diabetes, the supplement niacinamide—a form of niacin, also called *vitamin B₃*—might slightly prolong what is called the *honeymoon period*. This is the interval during which the pancreas can still make some insulin and the body's need for insulin injections is low. However, the benefits (if any) appear to be minor. A cocktail of niacinamide plus **antioxidant** vitamins and minerals has also been tried, but the results were disappointing. (See also Preventing Diabetes below.)

Massage therapy has shown some promise for enhancing blood sugar control in children with diabetes.

According to most studies, **fructo-oligosaccharides** (FOS, also known as *prebiotics*) do *not* improve blood sugar control in people with type 2 diabetes.

Treating Nutritional Deficiencies in Diabetes

Both diabetes and the medications used to treat it can cause people to fall short of various nutrients. Making up for these deficiencies (either through diet or the use of supplements) may or may not help your diabetes specifically, but it should make you a healthier person overall.

One double-blind study found that people with type 2 diabetes who took a **multivitamin/multimineral supplement** were less likely to develop an infectious illness than those who took placebo.

People with diabetes are often deficient in **magnesium** and one double-blind study suggests that magnesium supplementation may enhance blood sugar control. People with either type 1 or type 2 diabetes may also be deficient in the mineral **zinc**. **Vitamin C** levels have been found to be low in many people on insulin, even though they were consuming seemingly adequate amounts of the vitamin in their diets. Deficiencies of **taurine** and **manganese** have also been reported.

The drug **metformin** can cause **vitamin B₁₂** deficiency. Interestingly, taking extra **calcium** may prevent this.

Preventing Diabetes
➢ *Niacinamide*

Evidence from a large study conducted in New Zealand suggests that the supplement niacinamide—a form of niacin, also known as *vitamin B₃*—might be able to reduce the risk of diabetes in children at high risk. In this study, more than 20,000 children were screened for diabetes risk by measuring certain antibodies in the blood (ICA antibodies, believed to indicate risk of developing diabetes), it turned out that 185 of these children had detectable levels. About 170 of these children were then given niacinamide for 7 years (not all parents agreed to give their children niacinamide or have them stay in the study for that long). About 10,000 other children were not screened, but they were followed to see if they developed diabetes.

The results were positive. In the group in which children were screened and given niacinamide if they were positive for ICA antibodies, the incidence of diabetes was reduced by almost 60%.

These findings suggest that niacinamide is an effective treatment for preventing diabetes. (The study also indicates that tests for ICA antibodies can very accurately identify children at risk for diabetes.)

At present, a long-term trial of enormous scale called the European Nicotinamide Diabetes Intervention Trial is being conducted to definitively determine whether regular use of niacinamide can prevent diabetes. Results from the German portion of the study have been released and they were not positive; however, until the entire study is complete, it is not possible to draw conclusions.

As noted above, a small trial evaluated the effects of niacinamide plus antioxidant vitamins and minerals for children who had just started to show signs of diabetes and failed to find any benefits in terms of preventing the disease from worsening.

Warning: Medical supervision is essential before giving your child long-term niacinamide treatment.

➢ *Dietary Changes*

The related terms *glycemic index* and *glycemic load* indicate the tendency of certain foods to stimulate insulin release. It has been suggested that foods that rank high on these scales, such as white flour and sweets, might tend to exhaust the pancreas, and therefore lead to type 2 diabetes. For this reason, **low-carbohydrate** and **low glycemic-index** diets have been promoted for the prevention of type 2 diabetes. However, the results from studies on this question have been contradictory and far from definitive.

There is no question, however, that people who are obese have a far greater tendency to develop type 2 diabetes than those who are relatively slim; therefore, **weight loss** (especially when accompanied by increase in exercise) is clearly an effective step for prevention.

➢ *Other Natural Treatments*

Several observational studies suggest that **vitamin D** may also help prevent diabetes. However, studies of this type are far less reliable than double-blind trials.

One observational study failed to find that high consumption of **lycopene** reduced risk of developing type 2 diabetes.

Supplements to Use Only with Caution

In a double-blind, placebo-controlled study of 60 overweight men, use of **conjugated linoleic acid** (CLA) unexpectedly worsened blood sugar control. These findings surprised researchers, who were looking for potential diabetes-related benefits with this supplement. Other studies corroborate this as a potential risk for people with type 2 diabetes and for overweight people without diabetes. At present, therefore, people with type 2 diabetes or at risk for it should not use CLA except under physician supervision.

There are some indications that the herb **ginkgo** might alter insulin release in people with diabetes. The effect appears to be rather complex; the herb may cause some increase in insulin output, and yet might actually lower insulin levels overall through its effects on the liver and perhaps on oral medications used for diabetes. Until this situation is clarified, people with diabetes should use ginkgo only under the supervision of a physician. There is another worry with ginkgo as well: it may impair the action of some oral drugs used for diabetes.

For information on other herbs and supplements that may interact adversely with drugs used by people with diabetes, see the individual drug articles in the Drug Interactions section of this book.

One study hints that the herb **rosemary** might worsen blood sugar control in people with diabetes.

Despite earlier concerns, vitamin B$_3$ (niacin) and fish oil appear to be safe for people with diabetes.

A few early case reports and animal studies had raised concerns that glucosamine might be harmful for individuals with diabetes, but subsequent studies have tended to allay these worries. There are still slight concerns that glucosamine might increase risk of **cataracts** in people with diabetes.

Finally, as noted above, if any herb does help decrease blood sugar levels, this could potentially lead to dangerous hypoglycemia. A doctor's supervision is strongly suggested.

Diarrhea

RELATED TERMS: *Stools (Loose)*

PRINCIPAL PROPOSED NATURAL TREATMENTS: *Probiotics*

OTHER PROPOSED NATURAL TREATMENTS: *Acupuncture, Bilberry, Carob, Chamomile, Colostrum,* Eleutherococcus, *Fiber, Fructo-oligosaccharides, Folate, Food Allergen Identification and Avoidance, Goldenseal, Green Banana, Lactase, Marshmallow, Pectin, Red Raspberry, Sangre de Drago, Slippery Elm, Tormentil Root* (Potentilla tormentilla), *Witch Hazel, Wood Creosote*

SUPPLEMENTS TO AVOID: *Magnesium, Vitamin C*

Diarrhea, or loose bowel movements, can occur for many reasons. Food poisoning and infections are the most common causes of acute (short-lived) diarrhea. Chronic diarrhea may be caused by ongoing illnesses of the digestive tract, such as **inflammatory bowel disease** and **irritable bowel syndrome**.

Conventional treatment for diarrhea involves addressing the cause, if possible, and, in some cases, treating symptoms with medications that slow down the action of the digestive tract.

Principal Proposed Natural Treatments

Supplements called *probiotics* have shown considerable promise for safely preventing or treating various kinds of diarrhea. The following section summarizes much of the evidence regarding this treatment. For more information, see the full **Probiotics** article.

Probiotics

Certain bacteria and fungi play a helpful role in the body. For this reason, they are known collectively as *probiotics* (literally, "pro life"). Some of the most common include the yeast *Saccharomyces boulardii* and the following bacteria:

> *Lactobacillus acidophilus*
> *L. bulgaricus*
> *L. reuteri* (often studied in the proprietary form Lactobacillus G.G.)
> *L. plantarum*
> *L. casei*
> *B. bifidus*
> *Saccharomyces salivarius*
> *Streptococcus thermophilus*

The digestive tract is like a rain forest ecosystem, with billions of bacteria and yeasts instead of trees and frogs. Some of these internal inhabitants are more helpful to your body than others.

Probiotics not only help digestive tract function, they also reduce the presence of less healthful organisms by competing with them for the limited available space. For this reason, use of probiotics can help prevent infectious diarrhea.

Antibiotics being taken to treat an infection can disturb the balance of the "inner ecosystem" by killing friendly bacteria. When this occurs, harmful bacteria and yeasts can move in and flourish, which can lead to diarrhea. Probiotic therapy may help prevent this problem. Probiotics also appear to be helpful for preventing or treating forms of diarrhea with different causes.

➣ Traveler's Diarrhea

According to several studies, it appears that regular use of various probiotics can help prevent traveler's diarrhea, an illness caused by eating contaminated food, usually in developing countries. One double-blind, placebo-controlled study followed 820 people traveling to southern Turkey and found that use of a probiotic called *Lactobacillus* GG significantly protected against intestinal infection.

An even larger double-blind, placebo-controlled study found benefits from using the yeast product *S. boulardii*. This trial enrolled 3,000 Austrians traveling to a variety of countries. The greatest benefits were seen in travelers who visited North Africa and Turkey. The researchers noted that the benefit depended on consistent use of the product and that a dosage of 1,000 mg daily was more effective than 250 mg daily.

Diarrhea

Substances called *prebiotics* are thought to enhance the growth of probiotics. On this basis, a prebiotic called *fructo-oligosaccharides* (FOS) has been suggested for preventing traveler's diarrhea. However, in a 244-participant, double-blind study, FOS at a dose of 10 g daily offered only minimal benefits.

⋙ Infectious Diarrhea

Children frequently develop diarrhea caused by infectious viruses. Probiotics may help prevent or treat this condition and may also be useful for viral diarrhea in adults.

A review of the literature published in 2001 found 13 double-blind, placebo-controlled trials on the use of probiotics for acute infectious diarrhea in infants and children. Ten of these trials involved treatment, and three involved prevention. Benefits have been seen in subsequent studies as well, including one that included almost 1,000 infants. Overall, the evidence strongly suggests that use of probiotics can significantly reduce the severity and duration of diarrhea, and perhaps help prevent it.

One double-blind, placebo-controlled trial of 269 children (ages 1 month to 3 years) with acute diarrhea found that those treated with *Lactobacillus* GG recovered more quickly than those given placebo. The best results were seen among children with rotavirus infection. (Rotavirus can cause severe diarrhea in children.) In another double-blind, placebo-controlled study, *Lactobacillus* GG helped prevent diarrhea in 204 undernourished children. The probiotics B. *bifidum*, S. *thermophilus*, L. *casei*, L. *reuteri*, and S. *boulardii* have also shown promise for preventing or treating diarrhea in infants and children. However, probiotic therapy is probably not helpful for acute, severe, dehydrating diarrhea. Keep in mind that diarrhea in young children can be serious. If it persists for more than a couple of days or is extremely severe, it would be wise to contact the child's physician.

In addition, a large (211-participant), double-blind, placebo-controlled study found that adults with infectious diarrhea can also benefit from probiotic treatment.

⋙ Antibiotic-related Diarrhea

The results of most (but not all) double-blind and open trials suggest that probiotics, especially S. *boulardii* and *Lactobacillus* GG, may help prevent or treat antibiotic-related diarrhea (including the most severe form, *Clostridium difficile* diarrhea). It is sometimes said that it is useless to begin probiotic treatment until after the antibiotics are finished, but evidence appears to indicate that it is better to begin treatment with probiotics along with the initial use of antibiotics, then continue it for a week or two afterwards.

Note: Diarrhea that occurs in the context of antibiotics may be dangerous; for this reason, physician consultation is essential.

⋙ Inflammatory Bowel Disease

Crohn's disease and **ulcerative colitis** fall into the family of conditions known as *inflammatory bowel disease*. Chronic diarrhea is a common feature of these conditions.

A double-blind trial of 116 people with ulcerative colitis compared a special probiotic treatment using *E. coli* to a relatively low dose of the standard drug mesalazine. The results suggest that this probiotic treatment might be as effective as low-dose mesalazine for controlling symptoms and maintaining remission. Evidence of benefit was seen in other trials as well.

Another study found S. *boulardii* helpful for treating diarrhea resulting from Crohn's disease. However, two studies failed to find benefit with *Lactobacillus* probiotics.

⋙ Other Forms of Diarrhea

Preliminary evidence suggests that probiotics may be helpful for reducing diarrhea and other gastrointestinal side effects caused by cancer treatment (radiation or chemotherapy).

One study found that S. *boulardii* can increase the effectiveness of standard treatment for amoebic infections.

Small, double-blind studies suggest S. *boulardii* might be helpful for treating chronic diarrhea in people with **HIV** and hospitalized patients who are being tube-fed.

⋙ Irritable Bowel Syndrome (Spastic Colon)

People suffering from irritable bowel syndrome (IBS) experience crampy digestive pain, alternating diarrhea and constipation, and other symptoms. Although the cause of IBS is not known, one possibility is a disturbance in healthy intestinal bacteria. Based on this theory, probiotics have been tried as a treatment for IBS, but the results have been inconsistent.

Other Proposed Natural Treatments

One double-blind study found that an extract of **tormentil root** (*Potentilla tormentilla*) can reduce the severity and duration of rotavirus infection in children. Another study found it approximately equally effective as the drug loperamide for the treatment of non-specific diarrhea in adults. The herbal extract was particularly effective for reducing symptoms of abdominal cramping. Wood creosote is the principal ingredient in the widely used traditional herbal treatment Seirogan. It has undergone a certain amount of safety testing, and appears to be relatively safe, at least for short-term use.

A preliminary, double-blind study found that an extract of the Amazonian herb **sangre de drago** might be helpful for diarrhea associated with HIV infection. The supplement **medium-chain triglycerides** (MCTs) has also shown promise for this condition.

Wheat germ might enhance the effects of standard treatments for giardiasis.

A double-blind clinical trial of 41 infants with diarrhea found that **carob** powder (at a dose of 1 g per kilogram per day) significantly speeded resolution of diarrhea as compared to placebo.

The herb *Eleutherococcus* might be useful in the treatment of antibiotic-associated diarrhea. Brewer's yeast, a bitter-tasting product recovered from the beer-making process, might be helpful as well.

The herb **goldenseal** contains berberine, a substance with antimicrobial properties. One study suggests that berberine can help in diarrhea caused by *E. coli* bacteria. However, it is not clear that goldenseal itself would have the same effect. The herbs **barberry** and **Oregon grape** also contain berberine.

Allergy to milk and other foods may trigger diarrhea. Milk can also cause diarrhea in a completely different way—through **lactose intolerance**. This condition is the inability to digest milk sugar and it occurs in many adults. Use of the enzyme lactase should help.

Weak (and in some cases inconsistent) evidence partially supports the use of the following as treatments for various forms of diarrhea: **colostrum**, fiber, **folate**, and green banana or pectin.

Other herbs that are suggested for diarrhea but have no meaningful supporting evidence include agrimony, **bilberry**, blackberry leaf, **chamomile**, **marshmallow**, **oak bark**, **red raspberry**, **slippery elm**, and **witch hazel**. The supplement **glutamine** has been advocated for chronic diarrhea, but again there is no meaningful supporting evidence.

Acupuncture has been studied for its beneficial effects on diarrhea, but to date there is no compelling evidence for its effectiveness.

Supplements to Avoid

Excessive intake of **vitamin C** or **magnesium** can cause diarrhea.

Diverticular Disease

PRINCIPAL PROPOSED NATURAL TREATMENTS: *None*

OTHER PROPOSED NATURAL TREATMENTS: *Fiber Supplements: Psyllium, Glucomannan, and Methylcellulose*

Almost half of all Americans over the age of 60 develop diverticulosis: small, bulging pouches (diverticula) in the colon. In most cases, these diverticula do not cause any discomfort. However, in perhaps 15% of people with diverticulosis, diverticula may become inflamed or infected. The result is a condition called *diverticulitis*. Symptoms of diverticulitis include pain, nausea, and sometimes fever.

It is thought that the main cause of diverticulosis is the relatively low-fiber diet consumed in developed countries. Treatment of diverticulitis includes dietary changes, antibiotics, and, sometimes, surgery.

Proposed Natural Treatments

Fiber supplements have shown promise for both preventing and treating diverticulosis and diverticulitis.

Studies suggest (but do not prove) that diets high in fiber and low in total fat and red meat may help prevent diverticular disease.

Furthermore, high fiber consumption may help prevent diverticulitis from developing in people with diverticulosis. However, this has not been proven and the results of the scant published controlled trials on the topic have been inconsistent.

Common fiber supplements include psyllium, **glucomannan**, and methylcellulose.

Note: Use of fiber supplements during an active bout of diverticulitis is not advisable because the colon needs to rest.

Contrary to some reports, there is no evidence that obesity or consumption of caffeine or alcohol increases risk of diverticular disease. However, high levels of physical activity may reduce the risk of developing the condition.

Dupuytren's Contracture

PRINCIPAL PROPOSED NATURAL TREATMENTS: *None*

OTHER PROPOSED NATURAL TREATMENTS: *Vitamin E*

Named after a nineteenth-century French baron, Dupuytren's contracture is a thickening of tissue in the palm that causes an inability to straighten one or more fingers, usually the ring finger or little finger. The involved tissue hardens and shrinks forming a small lump or "cord" in the palm. Discomfort is unusual. The condition can involve both hands or even the toes and tends to progress slowly.

If you have Dupuytren's contracture, you may wonder if you injured your hand in some way, but if injury plays any role it is probably not a major one. Although the exact cause of the condition is unknown, the disorder appears to be at least partially inherited.

If the contracture becomes very troublesome, surgery may be useful.

Proposed Natural Treatments

There are no well-documented natural treatments for Dupuytren's contracture. However, in the 1940s, a number of physicians reported attempts to treat the condition with vitamin E. Most reported some success; however, their reports were incomplete and highly subjective, leading others to question their findings.

In 1952, two different researchers added an objective measure to their investigations by examining plaster casts of patients' hands before and after treatment, but their results were conflicting.

One researcher treated a group of 19 people with 300 mg daily of oral vitamin E for 300 days and reported moderate improvement in the amount of contraction. In contrast, the other researcher found no improvement among 46 people receiving 200 mg of vitamin E daily for 3 months.

However, since neither of these studies used a control group, the results are not particularly meaningful. Only double-blind, placebo-controlled studies can prove a treatment effective, and none have been reported for vitamin E in the treatment of Dupuytren's.

For more information, including dosage and safety issues, see the full **Vitamin E** article.

Dysmenorrhea

RELATED TERMS: *Menstrual Cramps*

PRINCIPAL PROPOSED NATURAL TREATMENTS: *Fish Oil, Magnesium, Vitamin E*

OTHER PROPOSED NATURAL TREATMENTS: *Acupuncture, Black Cohosh, Boswellia, Bromelain, Calcium, Chiropractic,* Coleus forskohlii, *Cramp Bark, Dong Quai, Fennel, Krill Oil, Manganese, Magnet Therapy, Turmeric, White Willow*

Medicine does not know why menstruation is uncomfortable or why it is much more uncomfortable for some women than for others, or from month to month.

Occasionally, severe menstrual pain indicates the presence of **endometriosis** (a condition in which uterine tissue is growing in places other than the uterus) or uterine fibroids (benign tumors in the uterus), but in most cases no such identifiable abnormality can be found. Natural substances known as *prostaglandins* seem to play a central role in menstrual pain, but their detailed actions are not fully understood. **Anti-inflammatory drugs**, such as ibuprofen and naproxen, relieve pain and reduce levels of some prostaglandins; these drugs are the mainstay of conventional treatment for menstrual pain. Oral contraceptive treatment may also help.

Principal Proposed Natural Treatments

There is some evidence that the supplements fish oil, magnesium, and vitamin E may help reduce menstrual pain.

Fish Oil

The omega-3 fatty acids in fish oil are thought to have anti-inflammatory effects and may relieve dysmenorrhea by affecting the metabolism of prostaglandins and other factors involved in pain and inflammation.

In a 4-month study of 42 young women ages 15 to 18, half the participants received a daily dose of 6 g of fish oil, providing 1,080 mg of EPA (eicosapentaenoic acid) and 720 mg of DHA (docosahexaenoic acid) daily. After 2 months, they were switched to placebo for another 2 months. The other group received the same treatments in reverse order. The results showed that these young women experienced significantly less menstrual pain while they were taking fish oil.

Another double-blind study followed 78 women, who received either fish oil, seal oil, fish oil with vitamin B_{12} (7.5 mcg daily), or placebo for three full menstrual periods. Significant improvements were seen in all treatment groups, but the fish oil plus B_{12} proved most effective and its benefits continued for the longest time after treatment was stopped (3 months). The researchers offered no explanation why B_{12} should be helpful.

Krill oil, another source of omega-3 fatty acids, might be helpful as well.

For more information, including dosage and safety issues, see the full **Fish Oil** article.

Vitamin E

In a double-blind, placebo-controlled trial, 100 young women complaining of significant menstrual pain were given either 500 IU vitamin E or placebo for 5 days. Treatment began 2 days before and continued for 3 days after the expected onset of menstruation. While both groups showed significant improvement in pain over the 2 months of the study (due to the power of placebo), pain reduction was greater in the treatment group than the placebo group.

In another study performed in Iran, 278 adolescents with dysmenorrhea were given either placebo or 200 IU of vitamin E twice daily on the same schedule as above. Again, vitamin E proved more effective than placebo.

It is not clear how vitamin E could affect menstrual pain.

For more information, including dosage and safety issues, see the full **Vitamin E** article.

Magnesium

Preliminary studies suggest that magnesium supplementation may be helpful for dysmenorrhea. A 6-month, double-blind, placebo-controlled study of 50 women with menstrual pain found that treatment with magnesium significantly improved symptoms. The researchers reported evidence of reduced levels of prostaglandin F_2 alpha, one of the prostaglandins involved in menstrual pain.

Similarly positive results were seen in a double-blind, placebo-controlled study of 21 women.

For more information, including dosage and safety issues, see the full **Magnesium** article.

Other Proposed Natural Treatments

One small double-blind trial suggests that making sure to get enough **calcium** and **manganese** may help control symptoms of menstrual pain.

The herb cramp bark has traditionally been used to relieve menstrual pain. Unfortunately, it has not received any significant scientific attention. Numerous other herbs and supplements have been suggested for menstrual pain relief, including **boswellia, bromelain,** *Coleus forskohlii,* **dong quai, turmeric,** and **white willow.** However, there is no reliable scientific support for these treatments.

One study has been reported as finding the herb **fennel** helpful for menstrual pain; however, a close look at the study shows that it merely found fennel *less* effective than the drug mefenamic acid. The study did not have a placebo control group and, for this reason, it is quite possible that the relatively mild benefits seen in the fennel group simply reflect the placebo effect.

A double-blind study of 43 women found some evidence that **acupuncture** can be effective for control of menstrual pain. In addition, a controlled study of 61 women evaluated the effects of a special garment designed to stimulate acupuncture points related to menstrual pain. Unfortunately, researchers chose to compare treatment to no treatment, rather than to placebo treatment. For this reason, the results (which were positive) mean little.

According to one small double-blind study, use of **magnet therapy** (applying the magnets to the pelvic area) might improve menstrual pain.

A controlled study failed to find **chiropractic spinal manipulation** helpful for menstrual pain.

Herbs and Supplements to Use Only With Caution

Various herbs and supplements may interact adversely with drugs used to treat dysmenorrhea. For more information on this potential risk, see the individual drug article in the Drug Interactions section of this book.

Dyspepsia

RELATED TERMS: *Gas, Indigestion, Poor Digestion, Stomach Upset*

PRINCIPAL PROPOSED NATURAL TREATMENTS: *Artichoke Leaf, Turmeric*

OTHER PROPOSED NATURAL TREATMENTS: *Banana Powder, Betaine Hydrochloride, Boldo, Cayenne, Chamomile, Essential Oils of Carminative Herbs, Herbal Combinations Containing Candytuft (Iberis amara), Lemon Balm, Pancreatic Enzymes*

Dyspepsia is a catchall term that includes a variety of digestive problems, such as stomach discomfort, gas, bloating, belching, appetite loss, and nausea. Although many serious medical conditions can cause digestive distress, the term *dyspepsia* is used when no identifiable medical cause can be detected. In this way, dyspepsia is like a stomach version of the symptoms in the intestines called **irritable bowel syndrome**.

The standard medical approach to dyspepsia begins by looking for an identifiable medical condition, such as **gallstones, ulcers,** or **esophageal reflux.** If none is found, various treatments are often suggested on a trial-and-error basis, including medications that reduce stomach acid as well as those that decrease spasm in the digestive tract. The drugs cisapride (Propulsid) and metoclopramide (Reglan) increase stomach emptying and have also been tried for dyspepsia. However, cisapride has been taken off the market and metoclopramide causes many side effects.

It's thought that stress plays a role in dyspepsia, as it

does with irritable bowel syndrome. Interestingly, one study of 30 people with dyspepsia found that after 8 weeks of treatment with placebo, 80% reported their symptoms had improved. This unusually high placebo response emphasizes the emotional contribution to this condition.

In Europe, it is widely believed, though without much supporting evidence, that dyspepsia is commonly caused by inadequate function of the gallbladder.

Principal Proposed Natural Treatments

Artichoke Leaf

An extract of artichoke leaf has undergone considerable study in the last few years as a treatment for a variety of conditions, most prominently **high cholesterol**. Artichoke leaf is one of many herbs thought to stimulate gallbladder function. In 2003, a large (247-participant) study evaluated artichoke leaf as a treatment for dyspepsia. In this carefully conducted study, artichoke leaf extract proved significantly more effective than placebo for alleviating symptoms of functional dyspepsia. A study of an herbal combination containing artichoke leaf is described below.

For more information, including dosage and safety issues, see the full **Artichoke** article.

Turmeric

The spice turmeric contains a substance, curcumin, that may stimulate gallbladder contractions. A double-blind, placebo-controlled study including 106 people compared the effects of 500 mg of curcumin 4 times daily against placebo (as well as against a locally popular over-the-counter treatment). After 7 days, 87% of the curcumin group experienced full or partial symptom relief from dyspepsia as compared to 53% of the placebo group.

For more information, including dosage and safety issues, see the full **Turmeric** article.

Other Proposed Natural Treatments

Combination Herbal Treatments

Several studies, enrolling a total of hundreds of participants, have found benefits with an herbal combination therapy containing bitter **candytuft** (*Iberis amara*), **matricaria flower**, **peppermint** leaves, **caraway**, **licorice** root, and **lemon balm** (and, in some studies, angelica root, **celandine**, and **milk thistle** as well).

A double-blind trial of 60 people given either placebo or a combination of artichoke leaf, celandine and **boldo** found improvements in symptoms of indigestion after 14 days of treatment. Similarly positive effects were seen in a double-blind trial of 76 individuals given a combination treatment containing turmeric and celandine.

Note: Reports have raised concerns that celandine can damage the liver. In addition, boldo is dangerous for use by pregnant women, or individuals with liver or kidney disease.

Essential Oils of Carminative Herbs

Herbs believed to assist in the passing of gas are traditionally called *carminatives*. Classic carminatives include caraway, **chamomile**, dill, **fennel**, peppermint, spearmint, and turmeric. Essential oils made from some of these herbs have been studied for the treatment of dyspepsia.

For example, a double-blind, placebo-controlled study including 39 individuals found that an enteric-coated peppermint-caraway oil combination taken 3 times daily for 4 weeks significantly reduced dyspepsia pain as compared to placebo. Of the treatment group, 63.2% was pain-free after 4 weeks, compared to 25% of the placebo group.

Results from a double-blind comparative study including 118 people suggest that the combination of peppermint and caraway oil is comparably effective to the no-longer-available standard drug cisapride. After 4 weeks, the herbal combination reduced dyspepsia pain by 69.7%, whereas the conventional treatment reduced pain by 70.2%.

A preparation of peppermint, caraway, fennel, and **wormwood** oils was compared to metoclopramide in another double-blind study enrolling 60 individuals. After 7 days, 43.3% of the treatment group was pain-free compared to 13.3% of the metoclopramide group.

Note: Essential oils of herbs can present health risks. In particular, wormwood (the herb in absinthe) is dangerous when taken long term. Physician supervision is strongly recommended. See the **Essential Oil** article for more information.

Cayenne

Preliminary evidence suggests that oral use of the herb **cayenne** can reduce the pain of dyspepsia. This may seem like an odd use of the herb; intuitively, it seems that hot peppers should be hard on the stomach. However, contrary to popular belief, hot peppers don't actually inflame the tissues they contact; in fact, hot peppers aren't even harmful for ulcers! Rather, they merely produce sensations similar to those caused by actual damage.

Here's how it works: All hot peppers contain a substance called *capsaicin*. When applied to tissues, capsaicin causes release of a chemical called *substance P*. Substance P is ordinarily released when tissues are damaged; it is part of the system the body uses to detect injury. When hot peppers artificially release substance P, they trick the nervous system into thinking that an injury has occurred. The result: A sensation of burning pain. When capsaicin is applied regularly to a part of the body, substance P becomes depleted in that location. This is why individuals who consume a lot of hot peppers gradually build up a tolerance. It's also the basis for a number of medical uses of capsaicin. When levels of substance P are reduced in an area, all pain in that area is somewhat reduced. Because of this effect, capsaicin cream is widely used for the treatment of painful conditions such as shingles, arthritis, and diabetic neuropathy.

Oral use of capsaicin may also reduce discomfort in the stomach. In a double-blind study, 30 individuals with dyspepsia were given either 2.5 g daily of red pepper powder (divided up and taken prior to meals) or placebo for 5 weeks. By the third week of treatment, individuals taking red pepper were experiencing significant improvements in pain, bloating, and nausea as compared to placebo, and these relative improvements lasted through the end of the study.

Other Herbs and Supplements

A controlled (but not blinded) study of 46 people suggests that banana powder, a traditional Indian food, may help treat dyspepsia. After 8 weeks of treatment, 75% of the people taking banana powder reported complete or partial symptom relief compared to 20% of those who received no treatment.

Herbs with a reputation for relaxing a nervous stomach, such as chamomile, **valerian**, and lemon balm, are also sometimes recommended for dyspepsia. Numerous other herbs that have been recommended for dyspepsia include angelica root, anise seed, **barberry**, **bitter orange** peel, **blessed thistle**, cardamom, centaury, chicory, **dandelion** root, **cinnamon**, cloves, coriander, **devil's claw**, dill, **gentian**, **ginger**, **horehound**, **juniper**, **linden**, milk thistle, radish, **rosemary**, **sage**, St. John's **wort**, star anise, and **yarrow**.

A tea made from the "fruits" or seeds of **parsley** is a traditional remedy for colic, indigestion, and intestinal gas.

Reduced levels of digestive enzymes may play a role in dyspepsia. One double-blind study found that use of pancreatic enzyme supplements improved symptoms following consumption of a high-fat meal. However, another placebo-controlled study failed to find pancreatic enzymes helpful for dyspepsia symptoms in general.

Betaine hydrochloride increases the acidity of the stomach and on that basis it has been proposed as a digestive aid for people with inadequate stomach acid. However, there is no evidence that reduced stomach acid levels causes symptoms of indigestion.

Herbs and Supplements to Use Only with Caution

Various herbs and supplements may interact adversely with drugs used to treat dyspepsia. For more information on this potential risk, see the individual drug article in the Drug Interactions section of this book.

Ear Infections

RELATED TERMS: *Middle Ear Infection, Otitis Media*

PRINCIPAL PROPOSED NATURAL TREATMENTS: *Avoiding Passive Smoke Inhalation; Breastfeeding; Herbal Eardrop Combinations Containing Mullein and Garlic; Xylitol*

OTHER PROPOSED NATURAL TREATMENTS: *Andrographis, Cranial Sacral Osteopathy, Echinacea, Food Allergen Elimination, Ginseng, Oral Garlic, Vitamin C, Zinc*

Acute otitis media (AOM) is a painful infection of the middle ear, the portion of the ear behind the eardrum. (Another form of ear infection, otitis externa or swimmer's ear, is entirely different and is not covered here.)

AOM often follows a cold, sore throat, or other respiratory illness. Although it can affect adults, this occurs primarily in infants and young children. It's estimated that by age 7, up to 95% of all children in the U.S. will have experienced at least one bout of AOM—it's the most common reason parents take a child to the doctor.

When the Eustachian tube connecting the upper part of the throat to the middle ear is blocked by a cold's mucus and swelling, fluids pool behind the eardrum, providing an ideal place for bacteria to grow; an infection may set in, generating even more fluid. The pressure this exerts on the eardrum can be intensely painful. The eardrum turns red and bulges. Children too young to explain their discomfort cry, fuss, and pull at their ears. They might also appear unresponsive because they can't hear well—fluid buildup in the middle ear prevents the eardrum and small bones in the ear from moving, causing temporary hearing loss.

In addition, a complication called *secretory otitis media* (fluid buildup in the middle ear) may develop and cause continuous hearing loss for months. Other possible, though rare, complications of AOM include mastoiditis (an infection of the bone behind the ear) and spinal meningitis.

Without treatment, most middle ear infections resolve on their own, often through a harmless rupture of the eardrum. In the Netherlands, pediatricians take a conservative approach, generally waiting 24 to 72 hours until they are certain an ear infection warrants antibiotics.

U.S. doctors, however, tend to initiate treatment early. This practice has been criticized on several grounds.

First, aggressive antibiotic treatment has not been found effective in preventing complications, such as serous otitis, pneumococcal meningitis, or hearing loss.

In addition, antibiotic treatment does not even appear to help AOM itself very much. For example, a double-blind, placebo-controlled trial of 240 children ages 6 months to 2 years found so little benefit with antibiotic treatment that the authors recommended physician-supervised watchful waiting rather than immediate treatment.

In other published reviews, the benefits of antibiotics for AOM have also been found less than impressive. A review of 33 randomized trials involving 5,400 children concluded that antibiotics modestly improved the rate of recovery. An evaluation of six randomized, controlled studies concluded that early antibiotic use had only slight benefit, reducing pain and fever in a small percentage of children and helping to prevent the development of infection in the other ear, but not significantly speeding up recovery of hearing. Modest benefits were also seen in a more recent trial of 315 children. Finally, children with recurrent ear infections do not appear to benefit from preventive antibiotic treatment.

However, the claim (often made in alternative medicine circles) that early antibiotic treatment causes an increased rate of ear infection recurrence does not appear to be correct.

Note: Despite the issues raised above, simply withholding antibiotic treatment can be dangerous. Any child who appears to have an ear infection should be seen by a physician.

When ear infections do reoccur frequently, a physician may insert a tube into the infected ear to drain fluids and relieve pressure, a procedure called *tympanostomy*. Nearly one million American children undergo this procedure each year; however, its usefulness is somewhat controversial.

Principal Proposed Natural Treatments

Although there is as yet no natural treatment for AOM, there are several promising approaches parents can take that may help prevent children from developing ear infections or reduce symptoms.

Xylitol

A natural sugar found in plums, strawberries, and raspberries, xylitol is used as a sweetener in some "sugarless" gum and candies. One of its advantages is that it inhibits the growth of *Streptococcus mutans*, a type of bacteria that causes dental cavities. Xylitol also inhibits the growth of a related bacteria species, *Streptococcus pneumoniae*, implicated in ear infections. Additionally, xylitol acts against *Haemophilus influenza*, another bacteria that frequently causes ear infections.

Based on this evidence, xylitol has been tried as a preventive treatment for middle ear infections with some success. Two well-designed studies enrolling a total of 1,163 children found that chewing gum and syrup sweetened with xylitol helped prevent middle ear infections and decreased the need for antibiotics. Although xylitol clearly did not absolutely prevent ear infections, it significantly decreased the rate at which they occurred.

One of these studies, a large double-blind, placebo-controlled trial of 857 children investigated how well xylitol (in chewing gum, syrup, and lozenges) could prevent AOM. The gum was most effective, reducing the risk of developing AOM by a full 40%. Xylitol syrup was also effective, but less so. The lozenges weren't effective: researchers speculated that children got tired of sucking on the large candies and didn't get the proper dose of xylitol. (In addition, the children were able to distinguish between the xylitol and placebo lozenges by taste, making that portion of the study single-blind.)

Similarly positive results had been seen in an earlier double-blind study by the same researchers, evaluating about 300 children.

For more information, including dosage and safety issues, see the full **Xylitol** article.

Breast-feeding

Breast-feeding may help prevent AOM. Numerous studies tracking ear infection frequency in large groups of infants found that the infants who were breast-fed exclusively had significantly fewer middle ear infections than those fed formula. Such observational studies aren't as reliable as placebo-controlled or double-blind designs, but the results do suggest that breast-feeding is a good preventive measure.

Researchers aren't sure how breast milk might protect infants from ear infections. Studies attempting to determine if breast milk inhibits bacteria associated with AOM have yielded mixed results.

Avoidance of Cigarette Smoke

Environmental conditions may predispose a child to middle ear infections. A study of 132 daycare students found that the 45 children exposed to cigarette smoke at home had a 38% higher risk of middle ear infections than the 87 children whose parents didn't smoke.

Herbal Eardrops

The herbs mullein and garlic are traditionally combined with other herbs in oily eardrops designed to reduce the pain of ear infections. One study supports this use. Two double-blind trials enrolling a total of more than 250 children with eardrum pain caused by middle ear infection compared the effectiveness of an herbal preparation containing mullein, garlic, St. John's wort, and calendula against a standard anesthetic eardrop product (ametocaine and phenazone). The results indicated that the two treatments were equally effective. In addition, one of the studies found that use of the antibiotic amoxicillin did not add additional benefit.

However, due to the strong placebo response in pain conditions, this study would have needed a placebo group to provide truly dependable evidence that the herbs were effective.

Keep in mind that while herbal eardrop products may relieve pain, the actual infection is on the other side of the eardrum, and it is not immediately clear how the herbs can get to where they could do any good. There is some evidence, however, that **essential oils** of herbs may be able to penetrate the eardrum and reach the other side. However, essential oils can be toxic as well as irritating to tissues.

Note: Garlic and its oil are too harsh to instill into the ear. Herbal drops that contain garlic use much milder extracts of the herb.

Other Proposed Natural Treatments

Allergies

Allergies may contribute to ear infections, possibly by increasing the amount of fluid in the middle ear. There is some evidence that children allergic to pollens, dust, molds, and foods may be more likely to develop AOM. Weak evidence suggests that a **food allergen elimination diet** might help prevent middle ear infections.

Other Herbs and Supplements

Numerous natural products have been proposed for preventing or treating ear infections. These include all herbs and supplements used for **colds**, including **echinacea**, **zinc**, **vitamin C**, **andrographis**, oral **garlic**, and **ginseng**. However, there is no direct evidence that any of these treatments are helpful for AOM. The only product in the list that has been tested, echinacea, failed to prove effective in the one reported study. This placebo-controlled trial tested an echinacea extract made from *Echinacea purpurea* roots and seeds. Participants, children ages 1 to 5 years old with a history of recurrent infections, were given either echinacea or placebo for 10 days during upper respiratory infections. No benefits were seen.

The study just mentioned also failed to find **cranial-sacral osteopathy** helpful for preventing ear infections.

Easy Bruising

RELATED TERMS: *Bruising, Contusions, Ecchymoses, Hematomas*
PRINCIPAL PROPOSED NATURAL TREATMENTS: *Bilberry, Citrus Bioflavonoids, Escin (Topical), Oligomeric Proanthocyanidins (OPCs), Trypsin and Chymotrypsin, Vitamin C*
OTHER PROPOSED NATURAL TREATMENTS: *Arnica (Topical), Bromelain, Comfrey (Topical), Sweet Clover (Topical)*

Bruising and bleeding both occur because of damage to blood vessels. When a vein, artery, or capillary is torn or cut, blood flows out into the vessel's surroundings; if the escaped blood is contained within the tissues directly under the skin, we see a bruise.

While all of us bruise from time to time, some people bruise particularly easily. A number of factors, besides being accident-prone, can make this occur.

One factor contributing to easy bruising is thinning skin, caused by aging or by medications such as corticosteroids. Easy bruising can also be due to fragile blood vessel walls. Finally, difficulties with blood clotting, including problems with platelets or clotting factors, can also increase bruising. For this reason, strong blood-thinning drugs, such as heparin and warfarin (Coumadin), can lead to excessive bruising. **Warning**: if you're taking these or other anticoagulant drugs and notice increased bruising, contact your doctor, as this situation could be dangerous.

Aspirin or natural remedies, such as policosanol, ginkgo, garlic, and high-dose **vitamin E**, may also thin the blood, possibly raising the risk of bruising and other bleeding problems; and if you combine two blood-thinning substances, these effects might multiply.

Rarely, severe bruising from minor or unnoticed injuries can be a sign of leukemia or another serious health problem. Especially if this is a new development, discuss your symptoms with a doctor.

However, in most cases, there is no identifiable medical cause for easy bruising and no conventional treatment. Furthermore, once you have a bruise, there is no conventional therapy to help speed its resolution.

Principal Proposed Natural Treatments

A number of natural substances might be helpful for easy bruising, including citrus bioflavonoids, the related substances OPCs and bilberry, and vitamin C. In addition, if you already are bruised, you may find some help with a combination of two proteolytic enzymes, trypsin and chymotrypsin, or a topical preparation of escin (an extract of horse chestnut).

Citrus Bioflavonoids and Related Substances

Bioflavonoids (or flavonoids) are plant substances that bring color to many fruits and vegetables. Citrus fruits are a rich source of bioflavonoids, including diosmin, hesperidin, rutin, and naringen; studies have found these bioflavonoids may help decrease bruising. Two types of natural compounds related to bioflavonoids—OPCs (oligomeric proanthocyanidins) and anthocyanosides—have also shown promise for decreasing the tendency to bruise.

For example, a double-blind, placebo-controlled study of 96 people with fragile capillaries found that a combination of the bioflavonoids diosmin and hesperidin decreased the tendency to bruise. Participants took 2 tablets daily of these bioflavonoids or placebo for 6 weeks, while researchers used a suction cup to measure their capillaries' tendency to rupture and also looked for spontaneous bruising and other symptoms of fragile capillaries. Those individuals who received bioflavonoids had significantly greater improvements in both capillary strength and symptoms compared to those taking placebo.

Two rather poorly designed studies from the 1960s found benefits with a combination of **vitamin C** and citrus bioflavonoids for decreasing bruising in collegiate athletes. In a single-blind study of 27 wrestlers, 71% of those taking placebo were injured, with bruises making up more than half their injuries; in contrast, only 38% of those taking the supplement were injured, none of whom sustained bruises. In a follow-up double-blind study of 40 football players, the treated group received fewer severe bruises than the group taking placebo.

Test-tube studies have found that OPCs protect collagen, partly by inhibiting an enzyme that breaks it down. One rather poorly designed double-blind study of 37 people—most of whom had fragile capillaries—found that OPCs were more effective than placebo in decreasing capillary fragility; however, the authors of this study left many questions unanswered in their report, making it hard to determine how seriously to take their results.

Anthocyanosides, which are present in high concentrations in bilberry, may also strengthen capillaries through their effects on collagen. Some European physicians believe that these vessel-stabilizing properties make bilberry us ¹ as a treatment for easy bruising, but the evidence a   t is only suggestive.

For more information, including dosage and safety issues, see the full articles on **citrus bioflavonoids**, **OPCs**, and **bilberry**.

Vitamin C

Vitamin C is essential for healthy collagen; severe vitamin C deficiency, called *scurvy*, can lead to easy bruis-

ing. Fortunately, scurvy is extremely rare in Western countries today—but marginal vitamin C deficiency is not rare, and might lead to increased risk of bruising.

A 2-month, double-blind study of 94 elderly people with marginal vitamin C deficiency found that vitamin C supplements decreased their tendency to bruise.

If your diet is low in fresh fruits and vegetables, you may wish to supplement it with vitamin C. In the study mentioned above, bruising in elderly people decreased significantly with 1 g of oral vitamin C given daily for 2 months.

For more information, including dosage and safety issues, see the full **Vitamin C** article.

Trypsin and Chymotrypsin

Trypsin and chymotrypsin, naturally produced in the body to help digest protein, are often called *proteolytic enzymes*. (Bromelain, discussed below, is a proteolytic enzyme from a plant source.) It is theorized that trypsin and chymotrypsin reduce swelling by breaking down protein fibers that trap fluids in the tissues after an injury, thereby restoring normal circulation in the area. Three small double-blind studies, involving a total of about 80 athletes, found that treatment with proteolytic enzymes significantly speeded healing of bruises and other mild athletic injuries as compared to placebo.

For more information, including dosage and safety issues, see the full **Proteolytic Enzymes** article.

Escin

An extract of horse chestnut called *escin* may also help with bruising. Horse chestnut has been traditionally used to treat varicose veins and other problems involving blood vessels and swelling. One double-blind study of 70 people found that about 10 g of 2% escin gel, applied externally to bruises in a single dose 5 minutes after they were induced, reduced bruise tenderness.

For more information, including dosage and safety issues, see the full **Horse Chestnut** article.

Other Proposed Natural Treatments

Bromelain

Like trypsin and chymotrypsin, bromelain is thought to decrease bruising by breaking down proteins that trap fluids in the tissues after an injury, and it is sometimes used in Europe to speed recovery from injuries. However, better-quality studies are needed before bromelain can be said to be effective.

In one controlled study, 74 boxers with bruises on their faces and upper bodies were given bromelain until all signs of bruising had disappeared; another 72 boxers were given placebo. Fifty-eight of the group taking bromelain had lost all signs of bruising within 4 days, compared to only 10 taking placebo. Unfortunately, this study was apparently not double-blind, meaning that some of its results may have been due to the power of suggestion.

Another study—this one without any type of control group—found that bromelain reduced swelling, pain at rest, and tenderness among 59 patients with blunt injuries, including bruising.

For more information, including dosage and safety issues, see the full **Bromelain** article.

Other Herbs Used for Bruising

The herbs **comfrey**, arnica, and sweet clover are widely used externally on bruises and other minor injuries, but despite this traditional use, there is no real scientific evidence that they work.

Note: There are various safety concerns involved in using comfrey, arnica, and sweet clover internally. For the treatment of bruising, they are used as topical ointments and salves.

Eating Disorders

RELATED TERMS: *Anorexia Nervosa, Binge Eating Disorder, Bulimia Nervosa*

PRINCIPAL PROPOSED NATURAL TREATMENTS: *None*

OTHER PROPOSED NATURAL TREATMENTS: *5-Hydroxytryptophan, Dehidroepiandrosterone (DHEA),
St. John's Wort, Zinc*

There are three major types of eating disorders: anorexia nervosa, bulimia nervosa, and binge eating disorder. Anorexia nervosa involves compulsive dieting and exercise to reduce weight, leading to dangerous weight loss and, in women, the absence of menstrual periods. Bulimia nervosa is characterized by binge eating followed by purging. The recently identified binge eating disorder is marked by binge eating that isn't followed by purging.

Nearly all the people affected by eating disorders are teenage girls and young adult women from the middle and upper socioeconomic classes. The causes of the various disorders aren't known, but it seems indisputable that the current Western emphasis on slimness as a mark of feminine attractiveness contributes greatly.

Because severe anorexia can be life threatening, treatment generally combines a weight-gain program with psychotherapy and, sometimes, antidepressant drugs. Bulimia nervosa and binge eating disorder are both treated with psychotherapy, antidepressants, or appetite suppressants to help control binge eating.

Proposed Natural Treatments

While there are no well-established natural treatments for eating disorders, there is some evidence that zinc supplements, when used in conjunction with conventional medical treatments, may help people with anorexia to gain weight. Preliminary attempts to treat bulimia by altering serotonin levels are also promising. In addition, the supplement DHEA might be helpful for protecting bone mass.

Zinc

The relationship between anorexia nervosa and zinc deficiency is controversial and the subject of many studies.

Symptoms of zinc deficiency (weight loss, appetite loss, and behavior changes) resemble those of anorexia nervosa to some extent. This has led some researchers to theorize that low zinc levels may be related to the onset of the eating disorder.

Preliminary evidence including one small, double-blind trial suggests that zinc supplements might indeed be helpful in treating anorexia nervosa, possibly enhancing weight gain and helping to stabilize mood. One frequently quoted study often used to discredit the use of zinc in anorexia appears to be relatively meaningless when inspected closely.

For more information, including dosage and safety issues, see the full **Zinc** article.

Tryptophan

Animal and human studies suggest that when levels of the brain chemical serotonin rise, hunger decreases. People who engage in binge eating may have a different response to changes in serotonin levels. In an attempt to change binge eating behavior, some researchers have tried to alter serotonin levels.

Standard antidepressant drugs are most often used for this purpose. However, it might be possible to achieve similar results with tryptophan and related supplements.

The body uses the amino acid L-tryptophan to make serotonin. Preliminary evidence from a small double-blind, placebo-controlled study suggests that a combination of L-tryptophan and vitamin B_6 significantly reduced binge eating among people with bulimia. This evidence, however, is contradicted by results of another small study that found no significant difference between the effects of L-tryptophan and placebo on binge eating.

Note: L-tryptophan is no longer sold as a supplement due to safety concerns. 5-Hydroxytryptophan (5-HTP) might be a safer option; however, it has not been studied in eating disorders.

The antidepressant herb St. John's wort might also raise serotonin levels.

For more information, including dosage and safety issues, see the full **5-HTP** and **St. John's wort** articles.

Dehidroepiandrosterone (DHEA)

Women with anorexia often experience bone loss, at least in part due to decreases in estrogen levels. In a 1-year long, double-blind study, women with anorexia received either DHEA at a dose of 50 mg per day, or standard hormone replacement therapy. The results showed equivalent bone preservation in both groups. However, because there is considerable doubt that hormone replacement therapy is truly helpful for preventing bone loss caused by anorexia, these results mean little.

For more information, including dosage and safety issues, see the full **DHEA** article.

Eczema

PRINCIPAL PROPOSED NATURAL TREATMENTS:

  Oral: *Breast-feeding (Prevention), Chinese Herbal Medicine (Treatment), Probiotics (Prevention and Treatment)*

  Topical: *Calendula, Chamomile, Licorice, St. John's Wort, Vitamin B$_{12}$*

OTHER PROPOSED NATURAL TREATMENTS: *Burdock*, Coleus forskohlii, *Quercetin, Red Clover, Red Vine Leaf and Licorice, Sea Buckthorn* (Hippophae rhamnoides), *Zinc*

PROBABLY NOT EFFECTIVE TREATMENTS: *Evening Primrose Oil/GLA*

Eczema is an allergic reaction that occurs in the skin. It consists mainly of itchy, inflamed patches on the face, elbows, knees, and wrists. Eczema is most commonly found in infants and young children. Eczema is closely associated with asthma and hay fever. All together, they are called *atopy*. Atopy tends to run in families.

Medical treatment for eczema consists mainly of antihistamines and topical steroid creams.

Principal Proposed Natural Treatments

Probiotics

Probiotics are health-promoting bacteria. The most famous probiotic is *Lactobacillus acidophilus*, used to make yogurt. Probiotics are thought to have immune-regulating actions. Use of probiotics during pregnancy and after childbirth may reduce risk of childhood eczema, presumably by, in some unknown fashion, normalizing immune response.

In a double-blind, placebo-controlled trial that enrolled 159 women, participants received either placebo or *Lactobacillus GG* capsules beginning 2 to 4 weeks before expected delivery. After delivery, breast-feeding mothers continued to take placebo or the probiotic for 6 months; formula-fed infants were given placebo or probiotic directly for the same period of time. The results showed that use of *Lactobacillus GG* reduced children's risk of developing eczema by approximately 50%. A follow-up study found that these benefits were maintained for several years.

In addition, most but not all double-blind trials have found evidence that infants and children who already have eczema may benefit from the use of probiotics.

For more information, including dosage and safety issues, see the full **Probiotics** article.

Breast-feeding

Early exposure of the infant to allergenic substances found in infant formula may play a role in the development of eczema. **Breast-feeding** might, therefore, help prevent this condition.

A large study lends credence to this theory. More than 17,000 women in the Republic of Belarus were enrolled. About half were entered in a program that encouraged them to breastfeed (the "intervention group"), while the other half were enrolled in a different program that did not instigate any particular method of infant feeding (the "control group").

The results showed that women encouraged to breast-feed were much more likely to do so than other women. Furthermore, children of women in the intervention group showed almost a 50% reduction in the incidence of eczema.

Interpreting this study is trickier than it might appear. Technically, it does not prove that breast-feeding reduces risk of eczema. Rather, it shows that counseling to breast-feed reduces risk of eczema. However, the implication is fairly compelling: if you breast-feed your child, he or she is less likely to develop eczema.

Another option might be to use special infant formulas that are less allergenic.

Chinese Herbal Medicine

A combination of traditional Chinese herbs has shown promise as a treatment for eczema. This proprietary formula contains *Ledebouriella seseloides, Potentilla chinensis, Akebia clematidis, Rehmannia glutinosa, Paeonia lactiflora, Lophatherum gracile, Dictamnus dasycarpus, Tribulus terrestris, Glycyrrhiza uralensis,* and *Schizonepeta tenuifolia.* In paired double-blind, placebo-controlled trials carried out by one research group, the mixture produced significantly better effects than placebo for both adults and children. Each study enrolled approximately 40 people and used a cross-over design in which all participants received the real treatment and placebo for 8 weeks each. Use of the herbal combination significantly reduced eczema symptoms compared to placebo. However, a subsequent study of similar design performed by a different research group failed to find significant benefit. The reason for this discrepancy is not clear. However, Asian herbal creams marketed for eczema have often been found to contain (illegally) high potency corticosteroids that are not listed on the label.

For more information, including safety issues, see the **Traditional Chinese Herbal Medicine** article.

Topical Treatments

Topical creams made from **chamomile, licorice,** or **calendula,** alone or in combination, are widely used in Europe to treat eczema. One study of 161 individuals found chamomile cream equally effective as 0.25% hydrocortisone cream for the treatment of eczema. However, the report didn't state whether doctors or patients were blinded as to which treatment was which, so it isn't clear how reliable the results may be. (For information on why blinding is essential, see **Why Does This Book Rely on Double-Blind Studies?**)

A study by the same authors (also not double-blind), involving 72 individuals with eczema, found somewhat odd results: In this trial, chamomile was not significantly more effective than placebo, but both were better than 0.5% hydrocortisone cream. It is difficult to interpret what these results actually mean, but they certainly cannot be taken as proof that chamomile cream is effective.

A double-blind study of 30 people compared 1% and 2% licorice cream against placebo cream for eczema. Both proved more effective than placebo, and the 2% preparation was more effective than the 1%. A cream containing **red vine leaf** and licorice extract has shown some promise for the treatment of eczema.

The herb **St. John's wort** is most often used for the treatment of depression. St. John's wort contains a substance, hypericin, that is thought to have anti-inflammatory properties, making it potentially useful in eczema as well. In a double-blind study, a cream containing St. John's wort extract was compared against placebo cream in 21 people with mild to moderate eczema symptoms. Study participants used real cream on one arm and the placebo cream on the other. The results indicated that use of St. John's wort cream significantly reduced symptoms.

Another placebo-controlled, double-blind study, enrolling 49 people with eczema, found benefit with a cream containing **vitamin B$_{12}$** at a concentration of 0.07%. Topical B$_{12}$ is thought to work in eczema by affecting local levels of a substance called *nitric oxide* (NO).

Evening Primrose Oil/GLA

Evening primrose oil, a source of the essential fatty acid gamma-linolenic acid (GLA), is widely used in Europe for the treatment of eczema; however, the most recent and best-designed studies have generally failed to find it effective.

A review of all studies reported up to 1989 found that evening primrose oil reduced the symptoms of eczema after several months of use, with the greatest improvement noticeable in the level of itching. However, this review has been sharply criticized: it included studies of very poor design, and also, apparently, misinterpreted the results of some of the studies it evaluated.

Better designed studies published subsequent to this review have not had promising results. A double-blind, placebo-controlled study that followed 58 children with eczema for 16 weeks found no difference in effectiveness between evening primrose oil and placebo. A 24-week, double-blind study of 160 adults with eczema failed to find benefit with GLA from borage oil, as did a 12-week study of 151 adults and children. In addition, GLA from evening primrose either alone or in combination with fish oil failed to provide benefits in a 16-week, double-blind, placebo-controlled study of 102 people with eczema. A fourth double-blind trial followed 39 people with hand dermatitis for 24 weeks. Evening primrose oil at a dosage of 6 g daily produced no significant improvement as compared to the placebo.

Only one double-blind trial performed subsequent to the 1989 review found therapeutic benefit with evening primrose oil, but it used very high doses of the supplement and found only marginal benefits.

The bottom line: At the present time, the balance of the evidence suggests that evening primrose oil is probably not very effective for treating eczema.

For more information, including dosage and safety issues, see the full **GLA** article.

Other Proposed Natural Treatments

One study found that 4 weeks of **massage therapy** performed by the parents (after a one-time training session with a massage professional) significantly decreased eczema symptoms in children.

The herbs **burdock**, **red clover**, and *Coleus forskohlii* and the supplements **quercetin** and **zinc** have also been recommended for eczema, but there is as yet no meaningful evidence that they really work.

A small 30-day, double-blind trial failed to find **vitamin B$_6$** at a dose of 50 mg daily helpful for eczema.

Similarly, an 8-week, double-blind trial of zinc at the high dose of 67 mg daily failed to find any benefit for eczema symptoms. Another that tested a combination of *Eleutherococcus*, **yarrow**, and *Lamium album* also came up with negative results.

A widely publicized study supposedly found oral use of the plant sea buckthorn (*Hippophae rhamnoides*) helpful for eczema, but in fact placebo treatment proved equally or more effective.

Although it is widely believed that food allergies are a major contributor to eczema, this assumption may be incorrect.

Edema

RELATED TERMS: *Fluid Retention, Lymphedema, Swelling, Water Retention*

Many medical conditions can cause edema (swelling). The following forms of edema are discussed in their own articles.

➤ A condition related to varicose veins called *chronic venous insufficiency* can cause swelling in the legs. Numerous natural treatments have substantial supporting evidence of effectiveness for this condition.

➤ Women who have undergone a mastectomy for breast cancer may experience swelling in the arm near the affected breast. This condition is called lymphedema and natural treatments that may help are discussed in the *Surgery Support* article.

➤ *Minor injuries* as well as surgery may cause swelling as part of the healing process.

➤ *Congestive heart failure* can also cause leg swelling.

➤ Women with *premenstrual syndrome* (PMS) often experience fluid retention prior to the onset of menstruation.

➤ Edema frequently occurs during *pregnancy.*

Many of the treatments used for these conditions fall into one of two categories: bioflavonoids and diuretics.

Bioflavonoids have shown promise for conditions in which edema is caused by leaky blood vessels, including the first three items in the above list. The following relevant bioflavonoids or bioflavonoid sources have full articles in this book:

➤ Bilberry
➤ Citrus Bioflavonoids
➤ Oligomeric Proanthocyanidin Complexes (OPCs)
➤ Oxerutins

Many herbs are thought to have a diuretic effect, causing the body to increase its water excretion. This could reduce edema in the remaining items on the above list. Herbs with apparent diuretic effects include:

➤ Buchu
➤ Cleavers
➤ Rosemary
➤ Goldenrod
➤ Juniper
➤ Dandelion Leaf
➤ Parsley
➤ Horsetail

Endometriosis

PRINCIPAL PROPOSED NATURAL TREATMENTS: *None*

OTHER PROPOSED NATURAL TREATMENTS: *Acupuncture, Chasteberry, Crampbark, Dandelion Root, Fish Oil, Magnet Therapy, Traditional Chinese Herbal Medicine*

Endometriosis is a painful, chronic disease that occurs when uterine tissue (technically, endometrial tissue) grows outside the uterus. The misplaced fragments of tissue develop and bleed in response to the hormones of the menstrual cycle. In turn, this causes inflammation and damage in nearby tissues. Symptoms of endometriosis include fatigue, infertility, and cyclic pelvic pain made worse by urination, bowel movements, or sexual intercourse.

Conventional treatment may involve anti-inflammatory medications, hormone therapies, and surgery. Unfortunately, such treatment is often not fully satisfactory.

Proposed Natural Treatments

Due to the limitations of conventional treatment for endometriosis, many women with this condition turn to alternative therapies. However, there is no reliable scientific evidence to indicate that any natural treatment can relieve or heal endometriosis.

Traditional Chinese herbal medicine is one of the more commonly used alternative approaches to endometriosis. **Chinese medical theory** has its own unique way of interpreting the condition, using such concepts as "blood stasis" and "obstructed Qi." It employs herbal combinations along with **acupuncture** in the hopes of restoring normal health. Commonly used herbs include **corydalis**, cnidium, bupleurum, **dong quai**, and **perilla**. Unfortunately, no double-blind, placebo-controlled trials of Chinese herbs for endometriosis have been conducted. A trial comparing Chinese herbal therapy to standard therapy is currently under way.

Magnet therapy has been proposed for the treatment of many chronic pain conditions. However, a double-blind, placebo-controlled study of 14 women with chronic pelvic pain (due to endometriosis or other causes) found no significant benefit with 2 weeks of treatment. A larger study did find some evidence of benefit after 4 weeks of treatment, but a high dropout rate and other design problems compromised the meaningfulness of the results.

Studies in animals suggest that **fish oil**, a source of omega-3 fatty acids, may be helpful for endometriosis. However, human trials have not been reported.

Western herbs such as crampbark, **chasteberry, dandelion root**, and **prickly ash** are sometimes suggested for the treatment of endometriosis, but there is no reliable evidence that they are helpful.

Finally, some alternative practitioners associate endometriosis with **chronic candida, food allergies**, or **immune weakness**, but there is no meaningful scientific evidence to indicate that approaches based on these supposed connections provide any benefit.

Enhancing Memory and Mental Function

RELATED TERMS: *Memory Enhancement, Mental Function Enhancement, Brain Boosters, Cognitive Enhancement*

PRINCIPAL PROPOSED NATURAL TREATMENTS: Bacopa monniera *(Brahmi), Ginkgo, Ginseng, Phosphatidylserine*

OTHER PROPOSED NATURAL TREATMENTS: *Cranberry, Creatine, Dehydroepiandrosterone (DHEA), Huperzine A, Lobelia, Muira Puama, NADH, Rhodiola rosea, Rosemary, Saffron, Spanish Sage, Tyrosine, Vinpocetine, Whey protein, Vitamin B$_1$, Vitamin B$_{12}$*

Which of us wouldn't want a boost in mental function if we could get it? Whether it's remembering names, numbers, computer passwords, or why we walked into a room (so-called destinesia), we've all been frustrated by the occasional limitations of our ability to remember.

Mental function often declines particularly under conditions of stress or fatigue. In addition, most people over the age of 40 experience some memory loss, technically known as *Age-related Cognitive Decline* (ARCD) or *Age-associated Memory Impairment* (AAMI). We don't know what causes this normal experience and there is

no conventional treatment available for it. As you shall see in this section, there are a few natural treatments that might be helpful for these problems.

Certain conditions can cause a far more serious loss of mental function. These are discussed in the article on **Alzheimer's disease and related conditions**.

Principal Proposed Natural Treatments

Statistically speaking, it's easier to demonstrate a big improvement than a small one and for that reason it's more difficult to prove the effectiveness of a treatment in a mild condition than in a severe one. Because of this, there is far more evidence supporting the use of natural supplements for treating Alzheimer's disease than for improving mental function in healthy people. Nonetheless, there is some evidence for the latter and we present it here.

Ginkgo

An extract made from the herb *Ginkgo biloba* is a well-established herbal treatment for Alzheimer's disease. Ginkgo may also be helpful for improving normal age-related memory loss and even for enhancing mental function in younger people.

➤ Age-related Mental Decline

In six out of nine double-blind studies, use of *Ginkgo biloba* extract significantly improved age-related mental decline compared to placebo.

For example, in a double-blind, placebo-controlled trial, 241 seniors complaining of mildly impaired memory were given either placebo or ginkgo for 24 weeks. The results showed that ginkgo produced modest improvements in certain types of memory.

Another double-blind, placebo-controlled trial examined the effects of ginkgo extract in 40 men and women (ages 55 to 86) who did not suffer from any mental impairment. Over a 6-week period, the results showed improvements in measurements of mental function. Benefits were seen in four other trials as well, involving a total of about 135 participants.

Set against these positive findings is a large (214 people) 24-week study that found no benefit in ordinary age-related memory loss. It has been suggested that flaws in the trial's design led to this negative outcome. However, three other studies enrolling a total of about 400 seniors also failed to find significant benefit with daily use of ginkgo. Another double-blind, placebo-controlled study used a one-time dose of ginkgo and again found no benefits.

A small, double-blind, placebo-controlled study looking for immediate mind-stimulating effects did not find them.

Besides these negative trials, there is another weakness in the evidence. Those studies that did find benefits with ginkgo reported improvements in certain aspects of memory, but not in others, and the pattern was not consistent between trials. This tends to decrease the confidence one can place in these apparently positive outcomes; if ginkgo is really working, its effects on memory should theoretically be more reproducible.

The bottom line: Ginkgo may help normal age-related memory loss, but more research is necessary before we will know for sure.

➤ Improving Memory and Mental Function in Younger People

Several studies enrolling a total of about 250 people have examined the effects of ginkgo on memory and mental function in younger people. Inconsistent benefits were seen in some of these trials, but the largest study failed to find any effect. According to one study, benefits may be present early on, and then decline after several weeks.

Besides ginkgo alone, several double-blind, placebo-controlled studies evaluated combined treatment with ginseng and ginkgo or **vinpocetine** and ginkgo for enhancing mental function in young people and most found some evidence of benefit. In two studies, ginkgo combined with the Ayurvedic herb brahmi failed to improve mental function. (See the further discussion of brahmi below.)

For more information, including dosage and safety issues, see the full **Ginkgo** article.

Phosphatidylserine

Like ginkgo, the supplement phosphatidylserine (PS) is widely used in Europe to treat various forms of dementia. There is some evidence that PS can also help people with ordinary age-related memory loss.

In one double-blind study that enrolled 149 people with memory loss (but not dementia), PS provided significant benefits compared to placebo. People with the most severe memory loss showed the most improvement.

However, another double-blind trial of 120 older people with memory complaints (but not dementia) found no benefits. This discrepancy may have to do with the type of PS used—the second trial used the more modern soy-derived form of the supplement.

For more information, including dosage and safety issues, see the full **Phosphatidylserine** article.

Ginseng

Several studies have found indications that the herb ginseng might enhance mental function. However, the specific benefits seen have varied considerably from trial to trial, tending to make the actual cognitive effects of ginseng (if there are any) difficult to discern.

For example, in a 2-month, double-blind, placebo-controlled study of 112 healthy, middle-aged adults given either ginseng or placebo, results showed that ginseng improved abstract thinking ability. However, there was no significant change in reaction time, memory, concentration, or overall subjective experience between the two groups.

Another double-blind, placebo-controlled study of 50 men found that 8-week treatment with a ginseng extract improved ability to complete a detail-oriented editing task. A double-blind trial of 16 healthy males found favorable changes in ability to perform mental arithmetic in those given ginseng for 12 weeks.

More comprehensive benefits were seen in a double-blind, placebo-controlled trial of 60 seniors given 50 or 100 days of treatment. The results showed that *Panax ginseng* produced improvements in numerous measures of mental function, including memory, attention, concentration, and ability to cope. Benefits were still evident at the 50-day follow-up. However, virtually no improvement was seen in the placebo group, a result that is highly unusual and raises doubts about the accuracy of the study.

Finally, four double-blind, placebo-controlled studies evaluated combined treatment with ginseng and ginkgo and found inconsistent evidence of improved mental function.

For more information, including dosage and safety issues, see the full **Ginseng** article.

Bacopa monniera (Brahmi)

The **Ayurvedic** herb *Bacopa monniera* (brahmi) has a traditional reputation for improving memory. However, a 12-week, double-blind, placebo-controlled trial of 76 individuals that tested the potential memory-enhancing benefits of brahmi generally failed to find much evidence of benefit. The only significant improvement seen among all the many measures used was one that evaluated retention of new information. While this may sound at least somewhat promising, in fact, it means almost nothing. Here's why: When a study uses many different techniques to assess improvement, mere chance ensures that at least one of them will come up with results. Properly designed studies should focus on one test of benefit alone (the primary outcome measure) that is selected prior to running the trial. The use of multiple tests is sometimes called *fishing for results* and is frowned upon by researchers.

However, if several independent studies use multiple tests of improvement and the pattern of response is reliably maintained, then the results begin to appear

more significant. Unfortunately, this does not seem to be the case concerning brahmi. In another double-blind, placebo-controlled study of 38 individuals, short-term use of brahmi failed to produce any measurable improvements in memory, while in a third double-blind, placebo-controlled study, use of brahmi over a 2-week period did produce some benefits, but in quite a different pattern. Finally, a study found that one-time combined treatment with *Ginkgo biloba* (120 mg) and brahmi (300 mg) failed to improve mental function.

Slightly more promising results have been seen in studies of a proprietary Ayurvedic mixture containing brahmi and about 30 other ingredients. However, these studies were generally not up to modern scientific standards.

For more information, including dosage and safety issues, see the full *Bacopa monniera* article.

Other Proposed Natural Treatments

A single study suggests that the supplement **NADH** might help improve temporary mental impairment caused by jet lag.

Evidence conflicts on whether **multivitamin/multimineral tablets** may improve cognitive function in people of various age groups. **Note:** Serious allegations of fraud have been raised regarding the work of one of the scientists involved in this research.

Isoflavones in **soy** or **red clover** have inconsistently shown beneficial effects on mental function in women.

Huperzine A is a potent chemical derived from a particular type of club moss (*Huperzia serrata*). This substance is really more a drug than an herb, but it is sold over the counter as a dietary supplement for memory loss and mental impairment. Some evidence indicates that it may be helpful for Alzheimer's disease and related conditions; very weak evidence suggests benefit for healthy people. Much the same can also be said about the substance **vinpocetine**.

Other treatments proposed for enhancing mental function in healthy people and having at least slight supporting evidence from preliminary double-blind trials include **creatine** (particularly after sleep deprivation), **sage**, and **vitamin B$_1$**.

Mild **vitamin B$_{12}$** deficiency may impair mental function. Because such deficiency is relatively common in the elderly, it has been suggested that vitamin B$_{12}$ supplements may be appropriate in this age group. However, in the one study that tried it, no benefits were seen.

Seniors are also commonly deficient in vitamin B_6, but a review of the literature failed to find meaningful evidence that B_6 offers any benefits.

Preliminary double-blind trials suggest that the amino acid **tyrosine** may improve memory and mental function under conditions of sleep deprivation or other forms of stress. Other double-blind trials suggest that the herb *Rhodiola rosacea* may offer a similar benefit.

Whey protein contains alpha-lactalbumin, a protein that in turn contains high levels of the amino acid tryptophan. Tryptophan is the body's precursor for serotonin and is thought to affect mental function. In a small double-blind study, use of alpha-lactalbumin in the evening improved morning alertness perhaps by enhancing sleep quality. Another small double-blind study found weak evidence that alpha-lactalbumin improved mental function in people sensitive to stress. A third study failed to find that alpha-lactalbumin significantly improved

memory in women experiencing **premenstrual symptoms**.

Herbs that contain caffeine would be expected to enhance mental function in healthy people, at least temporarily. These include **green tea**, **black tea**, **maté**, and **guarana**.

Some reports suggested that declining levels of the hormone **DHEA** cause impaired mental function in the elderly. On this basis, DHEA has been promoted as a brain-boosting supplement. However, large studies have failed to find any correlation between DHEA levels and mental function and there is no direct evidence that DHEA supplements provide any benefit in seniors. One study did find potential benefits in younger people.

Other herbs and supplements proposed for enhancing memory and mental function, but that lack meaningful supporting evidence, include **rosemary**, **saffron**, **muira puama**, **sage**, and **lobelia**.

One study failed to find **folate** helpful for enhancing mental function in seniors.

Epilepsy

RELATED TERMS: *Generalized Seizures, Partial Complex Seizures, Seizure Disorder, Temporal Lobe Epilepsy*

PRINCIPAL PROPOSED NATURAL TREATMENTS: *Ketogenic Diet, Nutritional Support*

OTHER PROPOSED NATURAL TREATMENTS: *Acupuncture, Electromagnetic Therapy (rTMS), Fish Oil, Food Allergen Identification and Avoidance, Manganese, Melatonin, Taurine, Traditional Chinese Herbal Remedies (Saiko-Keishi-To and Sho-Saiko-To)*

HERBS AND SUPPLEMENTS TO AVOID: *5-HTP, DMAE (2-Dimethylaminoethanol), Ginkgo, Glutamine, Hyssop Essential Oil, Ipriflavone, Japanese Star Anise, Nicotinamide, White Willow*

Epilepsy is a disorder of the brain that causes recurrent episodes called *seizures*. A seizure is sometimes described as an electrical storm in the brain leading to abnormal movements, sensations, and states of consciousness. In reality, however, it is more orderly than a storm; during a seizure, nerves function in an abnormally synchronized manner, a kind of lockstep that can continue for seconds or minutes. The results range from mild changes in awareness to violent convulsions.

Isolated seizures can occur for many reasons. The term *epilepsy* is applied when a person has recurrent seizures with no known treatable cause. If the seizure occurs in a localized part of the brain, it is called a *partial seizure*. If it affects much of the brain, it is called a *generalized seizure*.

The most common forms of generalized seizures are absence seizures (*petit mal*) and tonic-clonic seizures (*grand mal*). Petit mal seizures involve a brief lapse of consciousness that occurs suddenly and lasts for a brief time before disappearing; there are usually no symptoms afterward. A grand mal seizure involves loss of consciousness, convulsions of the body, tongue biting, and often urination; a state of confusion follows the seizure.

Partial seizures come in three main varieties. They can be *simple* (involving just an arm, for example) or *complex* (involving more complicated movements and loss of consciousness). Finally, some may turn into *generalized* seizures. There are several medications used to treat epilepsy, generally with considerable success. Most of these drugs can cause significant side effects, though. Fortunately, some of these side effects may be partially correctable through nutrient supplementation (see the Nutritional Support section below).

Principal Proposed Natural Treatments

There are no well-established herbs or supplements for the treatment of epilepsy. However, a number of supplements may be useful for treating nutritional deficiencies caused by anticonvulsant drugs. Besides herbs and supplements, the ketogenic diet might be helpful for controlling seizures in children.

Note: Epilepsy is far too serious a condition for self-treatment. For this reason, none of the treatments listed below should be used without the advice and supervision of a physician.

Ketogenic Diet

Before drug treatments for epilepsy were invented, scientists noticed that fasting tends to reduce seizure frequency. Subsequent investigation pinned down a metabolic state called *ketosis* as the causative factor. Ketosis occurs during fasting and also while consuming a diet high in fat and very low in carbohydrates (the ketogenic diet).

When effective anticonvulsant drugs were developed the ketogenic diet fell into disfavor, but in recent years medical interest has returned. Today, the diet is seeing increased use in the treatment of people who do not respond fully to standard medications. Most studies have involved children because they tend to be more agreeable than adults to the diet.

Evidence suggests that the ketogenic diet may almost completely stop seizures in about half of all children with epilepsy and reduce seizure frequency less dramatically in another third. Unfortunately, the keto-

genic diet can cause side effects, such as fatigue, nausea, reduced immunity, mental confusion, dehydration, constipation, and increased tendency to bruise. Major side effects seen occasionally with certain forms of the ketogenic diet include kidney stones, gallstones, impaired liver function, severe hypoproteinemia (dangerously low levels of protein in the blood), and kidney injury. Vitamin and mineral deficiency may also occur with some ketogenic diets, but the use of a **multivitamin/multimineral supplement** can easily prevent this.

Nutritional Support

Many drugs can impair the body's ability to absorb or metabolize certain nutrients; however, anticonvulsants are particular offenders. Meaningful evidence indicates that common anticonvulsants interfere with the body's handling of folate, biotin, calcium, vitamin D, and vitamin K. In addition, one anticonvulsant, valproic acid, affects the nutrient-like substance carnitine. For these reasons, it is often recommended that people using anticonvulsants take supplements that provide these nutrients.

However, there's a potential catch to correcting such "nutrient depletions." In some cases, taking the nutrient can impair the absorption or alter the metabolism of anticonvulsant drugs. In other cases, it is possible that nutrient depletion is part of how the anticonvulsant operates. For this reason, physician supervision is essential when taking any supplements.

The following is a brief account of the interactions between nutrients and anticonvulsant medications; for more information, see the full articles on **carbamazepine** (Tegretol), **phenobarbital**, **phenytoin** (Dilantin), **primidone** (Mysoline), and **valproic acid** (Depakene).

➯ *Folate*

Folate (also known as folic acid) is a B vitamin that plays an important role in many vital aspects of health. Unfortunately, most drugs used for preventing seizures can reduce levels of folate in the body. In turn, low serum folate levels can cause elevated levels of homocysteine, possibly increasing the risk of heart disease.

Low folate levels are also linked to increased risk of a variety of birth defects. Because anticonvulsant drugs deplete folate, babies born to women taking anticonvulsants are at increased risk for such birth defects.

However, the case for taking extra folate is complicated by the fact that high folate levels may speed up the normal breakdown of phenytoin and possibly other anticonvulsants. This could lead to breakthrough seizures. For this reason, folate supplementation during anticonvulsant therapy should always be supervised by a physician.

≽ *Biotin*

Numerous anticonvulsants can reduce body levels of the essential vitamin **biotin**, probably by interfering with its absorption. Valproic acid may affect biotin to a lesser extent than other anticonvulsants.

It is not clear whether this biotin deficiency actually causes any problems. Nonetheless, it is not good to be short on any essential nutrient and, for this reason, biotin supplementation has been recommended during long-term anticonvulsant therapy. Keep in mind, though, that the action of anticonvulsant drugs may be at least partly related to their effect on biotin levels. For this reason, physician supervision is strongly advised before adding biotin to an anticonvulsant regimen.

≽ *Calcium*

Many anticonvulsant drugs increase the risk of **osteoporosis** and other bone disorders. This is believed to be due in part to the fact that they impair calcium metabolism (see also the sections on vitamin D and vitamin K below). Effects on calcium may also *increase* the tendency toward seizures by lowering blood levels of calcium.

Calcium supplementation may thus be beneficial for people taking anticonvulsant drugs. However, some studies indicate that antacids containing calcium carbonate interfere with the absorption of phenytoin and perhaps other anticonvulsants. For this reason, calcium supplements and anticonvulsant drugs should be taken several hours apart.

≽ *Vitamin D*

Anticonvulsant drugs may interfere with the activity of **vitamin D**; this may be another contributing factor to anticonvulsant-induced bone problems.

Adequate sunlight exposure may help overcome the effects of anticonvulsants on vitamin D by stimulating the skin to manufacture the vitamin. People regularly taking anticonvulsants, especially those taking combination therapy and those with limited exposure to sunlight, may additionally benefit from vitamin D supplementation.

≽ *Vitamin K*

Phenytoin, carbamazepine, phenobarbital, and primidone speed up the normal breakdown of **vitamin K** into inactive byproducts, thus depriving the body of active vitamin K. Use of these anticonvulsants by pregnant mothers can lead to vitamin K deficiencies in their unborn babies, resulting in bleeding disorders or facial-bone abnormalities in the newborns. For this reason, mothers who take these anticonvulsants may need vitamin K supplementation during pregnancy.

In other circumstances, anticonvulsants seldom deplete vitamin K enough to cause bleeding problems. However, vitamin K deficiency may contribute to anticonvulsant-induced osteoporosis.

≽ *Carnitine*

Valproic acid (Depakene) and possibly other anticonvulsants may reduce the body's levels of the substance **carnitine**. For this reason it has been suggested that people using these drugs should take supplemental carnitine. However, there is no evidence as yet that *taking* carnitine will provide any noticeable benefit; the one study that did attempt to evaluate this possibility failed to discern any meaningful effect.

Other Proposed Treatments for Epilepsy

Herbs and Supplements

The **traditional Chinese herbal remedies** known by the Japanese names *saiko-keishi-to* and *sho-saiko-to* have also been suggested for epilepsy, but the supporting evidence for their use remains highly preliminary. Both of these combination treatments consist of bupleurum, peony root, pinellia root, cassia bark, **ginger root**, jujube fruit, **Asian ginseng root**, Asian skullcap root, and **licorice root**, but the proportions vary.

Weak evidence suggests that the amino acid **taurine** might offer modest, short-term benefits in epilepsy.

A preliminary double-blind study also found no more than short term benefits with **fish oil**.

Several studies by a single research group hint that the supplement **melatonin** may improve quality of life in children with epilepsy.

People with epilepsy have lower-than-normal levels of the mineral **manganese** in their blood. This suggests (but doesn't prove) that manganese supplements might be helpful for epilepsy

Other supplements sometimes suggested for epilepsy

(but with no meaningful supporting evidence) include **vitamin B₁**, **vitamin B₆**, **beta-carotene**, and **glycine**. Herbs traditionally regarded as "nervines" or nerve-relaxants are also sometimes proposed, such as the following:

- Skullcap
- Lobelia
- Lady's slipper
- Valerian
- Kava
- Passionflower
- Lemon balm

However, there is no meaningful evidence that they can help, and some of these herbs present significant safety concerns.

Note: Most herbs used for epilepsy are sedatives, as are many anticonvulsant drugs. Combination treatment could lead to dangerous over-sedation. People with epilepsy should, therefore, seek medical supervision before using any herbs or supplements.

Alternative Therapies

A special form of **electromagnetic therapy** called *rTMS* has shown promise for epilepsy. In a double-blind, placebo-controlled trial, 24 participants with epilepsy localized to a specific part of the brain (technically, partial complex seizures or secondarily generalized seizures) and not fully responsive to drug treatment were given twice daily treatment with rTMS or sham rTMS for a week. The results showed a mild reduction in seizures among the participants given real rTMS. However, the benefits rapidly disappeared when treatment was stopped.

Weak evidence hints that **food allergen identification and avoidance** may be helpful for people with both **migraine headaches** and epilepsy.

Acupuncture has been proposed for the treatment of epilepsy. However, a single-blind, controlled trial of individualized acupuncture for 34 people with severe epilepsy found no benefit.

Herbs and Supplements to Avoid in Epilepsy

Numerous herbs and supplements have been associated with unexpected or unexpectedly severe seizures. In most cases, however, the evidence linking any particular natural product to increased seizure activity remains circumstantial. Some of the more worrisome potential "pro-seizure" agents are discussed here. In addition, we discuss herbs and supplements that may interact with medications used for seizures. See also the discussion of folate and biotin above.

Ginkgo seeds contain a seizure-promoting substance called *4-methoxypyridoxine* (MPN). Although ginkgo *seeds* are seldom used today, seizures have also been reported with the use of the more normal form of the herb: ginkgo leaf extract. One possible explanation is that ginkgo-leaf products may have been contaminated ginkgo seeds. Another possibility has been proposed as well: ginkgo may affect the brain in ways similar to tacrine, a drug also used to improve memory and which has been associated with seizures. Finally, it has been suggested that ginkgo might impair the effectiveness of dilantin and depakote. Regardless of the explanation, people with epilepsy should probably avoid ginkgo.

Many anti-epilepsy drugs work by blocking the effects of a substance called *glutamate*; for this reason, high dosages of the closely-related amino acid **glutamine** could conceivably overwhelm these drugs and pose a risk to people with epilepsy.

Manufacturers of the supplement **DMAE** warn that it might increase seizure risk.

Tea made from the herb **hyssop** is thought to be safe, but hyssop essential oil, like most **essential oils**, is toxic in excessive doses. Some of the constituents of hyssop oil are thought to increase risk of seizures. For this reason, hyssop essential oil should not be used by people with epilepsy.

Japanese star-anise contains substances that can trigger seizure activity.

Some evidence hints that the supplement **5-HTP** could potentially exacerbate or initiate a seizure-related illness called *myoclonic seizure disorder*.

Grapefruit juice slows the body's normal breakdown of several drugs, including the anticonvulsant **carbamazepine**, allowing it to build up to potentially dangerous levels in the blood; this effect can last for 3 days or more following the last glass of juice.

The supplement **ipriflavone** might increase levels of carbamazepine and phenytoin, potentially raising the risk of side effects.

The herb **white willow**, also known as willow bark, is used to treat pain and fever. White willow contains a substance closely related to aspirin known as salicin. Aspirin is known to increase phenytoin levels and toxicity during long-term use of both drugs. This raises the concern that white willow might have similar effects on phenytoin, though this has not been proven.

Nicotinamide appears to increase blood levels of carbamazepine and primidone, possibly requiring a reduction in drug dosage to prevent toxic effects.

Early reports suggested the possibility that the supplement **gamma-linolenic acid** (GLA) might worsen temporal lobe epilepsy. However, there has been no later confirmation of this.

Fatigue

RELATED TERMS: *Energy, Low; Low Energy*

Do you feel that you don't have as much energy as you would like? If so, you have company. Fatigue is one of the most common complaints that people bring to their physicians. It seems that almost everyone today feels low-energy, stressed, and worn out much of the time.

Unfortunately, there are no easy solutions to this common problem. While many medical conditions can cause fatigue, the overwhelming majority of people who experience fatigue do not have any illness that can be diagnosed. It seems most likely that the true cause of this widespread problem is modern life itself.

The body was not designed for a sedentary life. While today most of us might consider one hour of exercise daily to be ideal, in the past, eight hours of daily exercise was not uncommon. Our ancestors lived much of their lives outdoors and walked many miles every day. Today, we live indoors, sit in chairs, and seldom walk more than a mile. Not only that, instead of peaceful outdoor surroundings, we live in a fast-paced, noisy world that interrupts us constantly with its demands, and requires that we multitask our way through nerve-frazzling challenges. This way of life simply violates the body's design principles.

Furthermore, with the invention of the electric light, the body's normal sleep habits were replaced by progressively longer periods of wakefulness. Few people today get eight hours of sleep regularly, much less the 10 to 12 hours that some experts believe our ancestors ordinarily enjoyed (at least in winter).

Tiredness, in other words, is a consequence of numerous factors that confront us all and for that reason it isn't easy to fix.

Low Energy: A Common Sense Approach

If you frequently feel tired, you should begin with a medical exam to rule out identifiable medical conditions such as **hypothyroidism, depression, fibromyalgia, chronic fatigue syndrome, chronic viral hepatitis**, and anemia. Problems such as these need to be addressed specifically in order to make any headway.

If you do not prove to have any identifiable illness, the next steps to take involve common sense principles. People with inadequate energy should increase the time they give themselves to sleep, exercise daily (as much as possible), and reduce bad habits, such as **cigarette smoking** and excessive consumption of alcohol. Cutting down on coffee consumption may help, too, by improving sleep and decreasing stress. In addition, it is important not to neglect such fundamentals as enjoyable work, healthy relationships, and adequate recreation. Even very unhealthy people tend to have more energy when they love what they're doing with their lives.

Nutrient deficiencies can also cause fatigue and, for this reason, it may be useful to take supplements. For more information on this topic, see the article on **general nutritional support**.

One nutrient requires a bit of special attention: **iron**. Iron deficiency can cause anemia, which in turn can cause fatigue. Certain manufacturers of iron supplements made a leap from this fact to the conclusion (unsupported at the time) that iron supplements were useful treatments for general fatigue. This recommendation worried many experts, because there is at least some evidence that taking too much iron can be harmful. On this basis, many physicians recommended that their patients avoid iron supplements if they were not anemic. More recent evidence, however, suggests that the iron promoters may have been at least partially right. Several studies indicate that marginal deficiency of iron, too slight to cause anemia, may decrease physical performance capacity. In addition, a double-blind, placebo-controlled study of 144 women with unexplained fatigue who also had low or borderline-low levels of ferritin (a measure of stored iron) found that use of an iron supplement enhanced energy and well-being. Nonetheless, it is not advisable to take iron just because you feel tired. Make sure to get tested to see whether you are indeed deficient. With iron, more is definitely *not* better.

Other Alternative Approaches

Many alternative practitioners recommend reducing intake of sugar and other simple carbohydrates or going on a **low-carbohydrate diet**, but there is no scientific evidence as yet to show that this will increase your energy. Similarly, it is unclear whether eating organic or pesticide-free foods or becoming a vegetarian (or its opposite, going on a so-called caveman diet) will make a difference. Still, there is nothing wrong with trying these methods and some people feel that they help.

Despite widespread claims, there are no herbs or supplements proven to enhance overall energy and **well-being**. Some of the natural products claimed to have this effect include:

- Adrenal Extract
- Ashwagandha
- Bee propolis
- Carnitine
- Chromium
- L-citrulline
- Coenzyme Q_{10}
- Cordyceps
- DHEA
- *Eleutherococcus*
- Ginseng
- Guarana
- Maca
- Maitake
- NADH
- Pregnenolone
- Pyruvate
- Reishi
- *Rhodiola rosea*
- Royal jelly
- Schisandra
- Suma
- Vitamin B_{12}
- Vitamin C

The supplements **tyrosine** and **NADH** have shown promise for enhancing wakefulness under conditions of sleep deprivation, but they have not been investigated for treating ongoing fatigue.

Most systems of alternative medicine claim to be able to improve overall health and enhance energy, including **Chinese medicine**, **chiropractic**, **Ayurveda**, **homeopathy**, and **naturopathy**. Therapies such as **massage**, **Reiki**, and **Therapeutic Touch**, and exercise systems such as **yoga** and **Tai Chi** make the same claim. Furthermore, based on the theory that toxins in the environment are a major cause of illness, some alternative practitioners recommend **detoxification** methods. However, there is as yet no meaningful supporting evidence to indicate that these approaches actually improve overall energy.

People who are tired because they don't sleep well might find benefit by trying natural therapies for **insomnia**. Similarly, people who feel overwhelmed by life may benefit from natural treatments for **stress**.

In addition, many people with low energy report that they feel better when they use natural treatments for **food allergies**, **candida**, or **low immunity**; whether this is merely due to a placebo effect, however, remains unclear.

The Bottom Line

In most cases, fatigue is a complex problem that doesn't respond to simple treatment approaches. However, don't be discouraged. Simply making it a priority to feel better may eventually lead to improvement.

Female Infertility

PRINCIPAL PROPOSED NATURAL TREATMENTS: *None*

OTHER PROPOSED NATURAL TREATMENTS: *Acupuncture, Ashwagandha, Bee Propolis, Beta-carotene, Calcium, Chasteberry, False Unicorn, Maca, Multivitamins, N-Acetylcysteine, Reducing Stress, Traditional Chinese Herbal Medicine, Vitamin C, Vitamin D*

There are many possible causes of female infertility. Tubal disease and endometriosis (a condition in which uterine tissue begins to grow where it shouldn't) account for 50% of female infertility; failure of ovulation is the cause of about 30% and cervical factors cause another 10%.

An immense industry has sprung up around correcting female infertility, using techniques that range from hormone therapy to *in vitro* (test tube) babies. Although these methods have their occasional stunning successes, there is considerable controversy about the high cost and low rate of effectiveness of fertility treatments in general. The good news is that apparently infertile women often become pregnant eventually with no medical intervention at all.

Proposed Natural Treatments

Because of its effects on the hormone prolactin, the herb **chasteberry** has been tried as a fertility treatment. However, the only properly designed study of this potential use was too small to return conclusive results.

Women with a condition known as *polycystic ovary syndrome* may suffer from infertility and may not respond to the fertility drug clomiphene. One substantial (150-participant) double-blind study found some evidence that the supplement **N-acetylcysteine** may improve the effectiveness of clomiphene in women with polycystic ovary syndrome. Far weaker evidence hints that **vitamin D** and **calcium** may also be helpful in this condition.

Another small study found some evidence that supplements containing **isoflavones** may increase the effectiveness of in vitro fertilization.

In a small double-blind, placebo-controlled trial, use of **bee propolis** at a dose of 500 mg twice daily resulted in a pregnancy rate of 60%, as compared to 20% in the placebo group. This difference was statistically significant.

Another study reported that **vitamin C** supplements slightly improved pregnancy rates in women with a condition called *luteal phase defect*, but because researchers failed to give the control group a placebo and instead merely left them untreated, the results are not very meaningful. (For information on why the use of a placebo is essential, see **Why Does this Book Rely on Double-blind Studies?**.) Yet another study that had severe defects in design found that **multivitamin supplements** may slightly increase fertility.

Stress may lead to infertility, and treatments for reducing **stress** might help increase fertility.

The herb **maca** (Lepidium) is widely advocated as a fertility-enhancing herb. However, the only basis for this claim are a few animal studies.

Caffeine avoidance has also been recommended for improving fertility, but there is no evidence as yet that it really helps.

Acupuncture has a long history of traditional use for infertility, but the supporting evidence for its use is exceedingly weak. A few open trials appeared to show that acupuncture can enhance the success rate of *in vitro* fertilization. The one properly designed study failed to find acupuncture more effective than placebo.

Traditional Chinese herbal medicine also has a long history of use for infertility, but there is no meaningful evidence to indicate that it is effective. **Note:** One case report has linked use of a Chinese herbal product with reversible ovarian failure.

Other treatments sometimes recommended for female infertility include **ashwagandha**, **false unicorn**, and **beta-carotene**, but there is as yet no evidence that they work.

Fibromyalgia

RELATED TERMS: *Fibrositis, Fibromyositis, Myofascial Pain Syndrome, Myofibrositis, Primary Fibromyalgia Syndrome*

PRINCIPAL PROPOSED NATURAL TREATMENTS: *5-Hydroxytryptophan (5-HTP); Capsaicin; S-Adenosylmethionine (SAMe)*

OTHER PROPOSED NATURAL TREATMENTS: *Acupuncture, DHEA, Guided Imagery, Hypnotherapy, Magnet Therapy, Malic Acid Plus Magnesium, Massage, Melatonin, Osteopathic Manipulation, Selenium, Vitamin B$_1$, Vitamin E*

Fibromyalgia is a common chronic condition whose main symptoms are specific tender points on various parts of the body, widespread musculoskeletal discomfort, morning stiffness, fatigue, and disturbed sleep. The cause of the condition is unknown, but it occurs most often in women aged 30 to 50. Other symptoms commonly believed to be associated with fibromyalgia are irritable bowel syndrome, urinary frequency, anxiety, headache, and numbness or tingling.

Apart from tender points on the body, physical exams and lab tests for people with fibromyalgia are usually normal. Because of this, some physicians are inclined to believe that the condition is "all in the patient's head." One researcher has noted that many of the symptoms of fibromyalgia, including certain tender points, are common in the general population and goes so far as to question whether it is a real condition.

However, the current consensus is that fibromyalgia is real and the American College of Rheumatologists has given it an official medical definition. It involves the presence of widespread chronic pain and the existence of pain in at least 11 of 18 specific points on the body when pressure is applied. Although the cause of fibromyalgia is not known, it may be related to poor sleeping with incomplete muscular relaxation.

Antidepressants have been shown to help chronic pain from many causes, and have been found to be effective in reducing fibromyalgia symptoms, even when given in doses too low to treat depression. Other conventional treatment for fibromyalgia may include antidepressants, anti-inflammatory drugs, muscle relaxants, sleeping pills, and antianxiety medications.

Aerobic exercise may also be helpful for individuals with fibromyalgia, although not all studies agree.

Principal Proposed Natural Treatments

There are three natural treatments that might be helpful for fibromyalgia, although the evidence is not yet strong: SAMe, 5-HTP, and capsaicin.

SAMe

SAMe, short for S-adenosylmethionine, is a chemical derived from a combination of methionine, an amino acid, and adenosine triphosphate (ATP), the main molecule for energy in the body. More well known as a treatment for depression and also osteoarthritis, preliminary research suggests that SAMe may be helpful for fibromyalgia as well.

Four double-blind trials have studied the use of SAMe for fibromyalgia, three of them finding it to be helpful. Unfortunately, most of these studies gave SAMe either intravenously or as an injection into the muscles, sometimes in combination with oral doses. When you inject a medication, the effects can be quite different than when you take it orally. For that reason, these studies are of questionable relevance.

However, the one double-blind study that used only oral SAMe did find positive results. In this trial, 44 people with fibromyalgia took 800 mg of SAMe or placebo for 6 weeks. Compared to the group taking placebo, those taking SAMe had improvements in disease activity, pain at rest, fatigue, and morning stiffness, and in one, measurement of mood. In other respects, such as the amount of tenderness in their tender points, the group taking SAMe did no better than those taking the placebo.

It isn't clear whether SAMe is helping fibromyalgia through antidepressant effects or some other mechanism.

For more information, including dosage and safety issues, see the full **SAMe** article.

5-HTP

5-HTP, short for 5-hydroxytryptophan, is most commonly used as a treatment for depression. It is thought to work by increasing the amount of serotonin in the brain. However, evidence that it helps fibromyalgia is still preliminary.

One double-blind study of 50 people with fibromyalgia found that those taking 300 mg of 5-HTP for 30 days reported significant decreases in the number of tender points and the amount of pain they experienced, compared to those taking placebo. They also noted improvements in sleep patterns, morning stiffness, anxiety, and fatigue. Interestingly, the people taking placebo also noted significant improvements in pain and sleep, although less marked than those experienced with 5-HTP. More studies are needed to determine how much 5-HTP really helps.

For more information, including dosage and safety issues, see the full **5-HTP** article.

Capsaicin

Capsaicin, the "hot" in cayenne peppers, is widely used as a treatment for various painful conditions, such as shingles and arthritis. One double-blind study of 45 people found that it may be beneficial for fibromyalgia as well. In this study, participants used either the capsaicin cream or a placebo 4 times a day for 4 weeks, rubbing it into the tender points on one side of their body. Those who used the real treatment reported less tenderness in their tender points than those using the placebo. Interestingly, the points on their untreated sides were also less tender. There was no difference between those using capsaicin or placebo in the amount of overall pain or sleep quality. It must be noted, however, that it's hard to believe the study was really double-blind, since it's impossible to hide the burning sensation caused by capsaicin!

For more information, including dosage and safety issues, see the full **Cayenne Pepper** article.

Other Proposed Treatments for Fibromyalgia

The blue-green algae *Chlorella pyrenoidosa* might be helpful for fibromyalgia. In a double-blind, placebo-controlled trial, 37 people with fibromyalgia were given either placebo or chlorella supplements at a dose of 10 g daily. At the end of 3 months, people were switched to the opposite group and then treated for an additional 3 months. The results showed significant improvements in symptoms when participants used chlorella as compared to placebo. **Note**: There are serious safety concerns about blue-green algae. For more information, see the full **Blue-green Algae** article.

A mixture of **malic acid** and **magnesium** has been widely marketed as a treatment for fibromyalgia. However, in a double-blind study of 24 people, this treatment proved no more effective than placebo. Good results were seen in open trials, but such studies cannot eliminate the placebo effect and for that reason are not reliable. (For more information on this complicated issue, see **Why Does This Book Rely on Double-blind Studies?**)

Other proposed natural supplements for fibromyalgia include **vitamin B$_1$**, **vitamin E**, and **selenium**, but there is no real evidence that they work. A study that purportedly found **melatonin** helpful was, in fact, too poorly designed to provide meaningful evidence.

One study failed to find **DHEA** at a dose of 50 mg per day helpful for fibromyalgia.

Acupuncture appears to reduce fibromyalgia symptoms; however, the best-designed studies failed to find real acupuncture more effective than fake acupuncture. Other alternative treatments with minimal supporting evidence include **hypnotherapy**, **guided imagery**, **massage**, **magnet therapy**, **relaxation therapies**, and **osteopathic manipulation**.

One study purportedly found that use of cosmetics increases fibromyalgia symptoms, but it was too poorly designed to show anything at all.

Food Allergies and Sensitivities

RELATED TERMS: *Allergies, Food*

PRINCIPAL PROPOSED NATURAL TREATMENTS: *Elimination Diet, Hypoallergenic Infant Formula*

OTHER PROPOSED NATURAL TREATMENTS: *Bromelain, Proteolytic Enzymes, Thymus Extract*

A food allergy is defined as an abnormal immune reaction caused by the ingestion of a food or food additive. The most dramatic form of food allergy reaction occurs within minutes, usually in response to certain foods such as shellfish, peanuts, or strawberries. The effects are similar to those of a bee sting allergy, involving hives, itching, swelling in the throat, and difficulty breathing; this immediate type of allergic reaction can be life-threatening.

Other food allergy reactions are more delayed, causing relatively subtle symptoms over days or weeks. These include gastrointestinal problems (constipation, diarrhea, gas, cramping, and bloating), rashes, and headaches. However, because such delayed reactions are relatively vague and can have other causes, it has remained a controversial subject in medicine.

Some food allergy–like reactions do not actually involve the immune system. These are termed *food sensitivities* (or *food intolerance*). In most cases, the cause of such sensitivities is unknown.

Delayed-type food allergies and sensitivities might play a role in many diseases, including asthma, attention deficit disorder, rheumatoid arthritis, vaginal yeast infections, canker sores, colic, ear infections, eczema, irritable bowel syndrome, migraine headaches, psoriasis, chronic sinus infections, ulcerative colitis, Crohn's disease, and celiac disease. However, not all experts agree; practitioners of natural medicine tend to be more enthusiastic about the food allergy theory of disease than conventional practitioners.

Conventional treatment for immediate-type food allergy reactions includes desensitization (allergy shots), emergency epinephrine (adrenaline) kits for self-injection, and the antihistamine diphenhydramine (Benadryl).

Delayed-type food allergies are much more difficult to identify and treat. Although skin and blood tests are sometimes used, their reliability is questionable. A particular blood test called *ALCAT* has shown some promise, but much more study is necessary to establish its accuracy. The double-blind food challenge is the only truly reliable way to identify delayed-type food allergies. This method uses some means of disguising the possibly allergenic food, usually by mixing it with other, non-allergenic foods. Individuals are randomly given either the possibly allergenic food or placebo on a number of occasions separated by 1 or more days. Neither the physician nor the participant knows which is the possibly allergenic food and which is not. Evaluation of the response can then determine whether an allergic response is really present or not. Studies suggest that perhaps only one-third of people who believe they are allergic to a given food actually experience an allergic reaction when they are given it in a double-blind fashion; in addition, reactions are often milder than individuals believe.

Although it is the most accurate way of determining food allergies, the double-blind food challenge is still mostly used in research. The elimination diet with food challenges (described below) is the most common technique in use.

Another conventional approach for delayed-type food allergies is oral cromolyn (a drug sometimes used in an inhaled form for treating asthma and other allergic illnesses). A double-blind, placebo-controlled study of 14 children with milk and other food allergies found that cromolyn was effective in preventing allergic reactions in 11 of 13 cases, whereas placebo was effective in only 3 of 9 cases. In another study, 32 individuals were given cromolyn one half hour before meals and at bedtime. If their food allergy symptoms were prevented, the participants were entered into a double-blind, placebo-controlled crossover study using cromoglycate. Of the 31 people who completed the study, 24 experienced relief of gastrointestinal symptoms when taking cromolyn as compared to 2 when taking placebo. In addition, systemic allergic reactions were also blocked with the cromolyn. Unfortunately, the drug also had many side effects.

Principal Proposed Natural Treatments

There are no well-documented natural treatments for food allergies. The most obvious approach would be to remove known allergenic foods from the diet. Some alternative practitioners offer lab tests to identify such allergens. However, as described above, no lab tests have been proven accurate for this purpose.

The elimination diet is another approach for identifying allergenic foods. This method involves starting with a highly restricted diet consisting only of foods that are seldom allergenic, such as rice, yams, and turkey. If dietary restriction leads to resolution or improvement of symptoms, foods are then reintroduced one by one to see which, if any, will trigger reactions. There is some evidence that the elimination diet may be effective for chronic or recurrent hives; it has been tried for many other conditions as well, including irritable bowel syndrome, asthma, chronic ear infections, reflux esophagitis, and Crohn's disease.

Still another method involves simply eliminating the most common allergens. Cow's milk protein intolerance is thought to be the most common childhood allergy, followed by allergies to eggs, peanuts, nuts, and fish. Some evidence indicates that use of special hypoallergenic infant formulas rather than cow's milk formula may help prevent eczema, urticaria, and food-induced digestive distress. In addition, eliminating cow's milk from the diets of breastfeeding infants and their nursing mothers might reduce symptoms of infantile colic, although not all studies have found benefit.

In hopes of *preventing* food allergies and diseases re-lated to them, some authorities recommend that pregnant and breastfeeding mothers as well as their children should avoid allergenic foods.

However, it is not clear if this method actually provides any benefit. For example, one study evaluated 165 children at high risk of developing allergic symptoms. Careful avoidance of allergenic foods in the diets of the mothers and infants did not reduce the later development of eczema, asthma, hay fever, or food allergy symptoms.

Other Proposed Treatments for Food Allergies and Sensitivities

Digestive enzymes such as **bromelain** and other **proteolytic enzymes** have been proposed as a treatment for food allergies, based on the reasonable idea that digesting offending proteins will reduce allergic reactions to them. However, there is no real evidence as yet that they are effective against food allergies.

Thymus extract is a supplement derived from the thymus gland of cows. Highly preliminary evidence suggests that by normalizing immune function, thymus extracts may be helpful for food allergies. However, there are significant safety issues with thymus extract (see the full article for details), and this study did not prove thymus extract to be effective.

Gallstones

RELATED TERMS: *Gallbladder Pain*

PRINCIPAL PROPOSED NATURAL TREATMENTS: *None*

OTHER PROPOSED NATURAL TREATMENTS: *Artichoke Leaf, Betaine Hydrochloride, Boldo, Dandelion Root, Fumitory, Greater Celandine, Milk Thistle, Peppermint, Turmeric, Vitamin C*

The job of the gallbladder is to store the bile produced by the liver and to release it on an as-needed basis for digestive purposes. However, it isn't easy to keep this complex mixture of chemicals in liquid form. The various elements of bile have a natural tendency to form sludge, lumps, and hard deposits called *gallstones*. The body uses several biochemical methods to prevent such condensation from occurring, but this natural chemistry does not always succeed. More than 20% of women and 8% of men develop gallstones at some time in their lives.

You could have gallstones in your body for many years without experiencing any problems. However, sooner or later, a gallstone will likely plug the duct that leads out of the gallbladder, causing pain.

Generally, gallbladder pain starts in the form of occasional minor attacks that subside rapidly, separated by weeks without discomfort. During this phase, the stones block the duct temporarily and then move out of the way. Eventually, continuous obstruction may develop, causing the gallbladder to become inflamed and perhaps infected. This condition is called *cholecystitis*. Cholecystitis is a potentially life-threatening situation because an inflamed, blocked gallbladder can rupture. Another risk is that a stone may escape the gallbladder's own duct and move along to the duct that carries away secretions from both the liver and the gallbladder (the common bile duct). When this happens, the liver cannot unload the bile it produces, putting it at risk of permanent injury and creating a true surgical emergency.

The most reliable symptom of cholecystitis is intense pain beneath the right lower rib cage, often occurring from midnight to 3 a.m. Typically, pain radiates to the right shoulder and is accompanied by a loss of appetite and sometimes nausea. Removal of the gallbladder immediately solves the problem. Gallbladder surgery can usually be carried out laparoscopically, resulting in a quick and easy procedure that requires little recovery time.

Living without a gallbladder does not seem to bring any long-term consequences. However, many people are opposed on general principle to removing an organ that nature has placed there. Medications that dissolve gallstones may be another option.

Proposed Natural Treatments

The only time it is appropriate to use alternative treatments for gallstones is during the interval before cholecystitis develops. Once the gallbladder has become completely blocked, surgical treatment is urgent.

However, during the initial period in which pain is only occasional or intermittent, the risks incurred by postponing surgery are slight. If your doctor feels that a trial of stone-dissolving medications might be appropriate, some of the agents described here could present alternate possibilities. Unfortunately, none are well established as effective. Medical supervision is definitely essential.

Preliminary clinical trials suggest that formulas containing peppermint and related terpenes (fragrant substances found in plants) can dissolve gallstones.

The herb **milk thistle**, standardized to its silymarin content, has been shown to improve the liquidity of bile, although its actual effects on gallstones in real life are unknown.

Several herbs are prescribed in Germany for gallbladder pain, including **artichoke leaf**, **boldo**, **dandelion root**, fumitory, **greater celandine**, and **turmeric**. These herbs are thought to work by causing the gallbladder to contract and thereby expel its stones. However, such an effect is a mixed blessing: expelled stones might become lodged in the duct of the gallbladder, or, worse, the common bile duct. Furthermore, if the duct is already blocked, gallbladder contraction will lead to increased pain and perhaps rupture. Finally, some of these herbs are potentially toxic to the liver. The bottom line: Consult a qualified physician before trying these treatments.

There is some evidence that regular coffee drinking can reduce the risk of developing gallstones, at least in men aged 40 to 75. In an observational study that tracked about 46,000 male physicians for a period of 10 years, those who drank 2 to 3 cups of caffeinated coffee daily had a 40% reduced risk of developing gallstone disease. Those who drank more coffee had an even greater reduction of risk.

It may be the caffeine in coffee that helps, as other sources of caffeine were also associated with reduced risk of gallstones, while decaffeinated coffee didn't seem to help. Caffeine is known to increase the flow of bile, so this connection makes sense. However, it is also possible that people who drink more coffee have other unknown characteristics that make them more likely to have gallstones and that caffeine itself is an innocent bystander. Observational studies, in other words, do not show cause and effect.

Similarly weak evidence suggests that regular use of **vitamin C** supplements might help prevent gallstones in women.

Gastritis

PRINCIPAL PROPOSED NATURAL TREATMENTS: *None*

OTHER PROPOSED NATURAL TREATMENTS: Aloe vera, *Beeswax Extract, Betaine Hydrochloride, Bioflavonoids, Butterbur, Cat's Claw, Cayenne, Cinnamon, Colostrum, Cranberry, Cysteine, Fish Oil, Gamma Oryzanol, Garlic, Glutamine, Licorice, Marshmallow, Methyl Sulfonyl Methane (MSM), Probiotics, Reishi, Selenium, Slippery Elm, Suma, Vitamin A, Vitamin C, Wood Betony, Zinc*

HERBS AND SUPPLEMENTS TO USE ONLY WITH CAUTION: *Arginine, Cola Nut, Feverfew, Turmeric, White Willow*

Gastritis is a condition in which the lining of the stomach becomes inflamed, leading to discomfort. If the inflammation is prolonged, either atrophic gastritis (a condition in which the glands of the stomach lining disappear) or an ulcer may develop. Underlying causes of gastritis include infection with the organism *Helicobacter pylori*; excessive stomach acid secretion; autoimmune processes (conditions in which the body attacks itself); and damage to the stomach lining caused by alcohol, non-steroidal anti-inflammatory drugs (NSAIDs), corticosteroids, or severe stress.

Gastritis typically causes pain in the upper abdomen (just below the sternum), but it may also occur without pain. A burning sensation higher up in the chest (heartburn) generally indicates esophageal reflux. Stomach distress may also occur without inflammation of the stomach wall; in that case, it is called *dyspepsia*.

Conventional treatment for gastritis includes antibiotics to eliminate *H. pylori*; reducing stomach acidity with medications in the antacid, H$_2$ blocker, or proton pump inhibitor families; and possibly using medications to protect the stomach lining. In addition, it is important to reduce alcohol consumption and change (or, if possible, stop taking) medications that damage the stomach. Vitamin B$_{12}$ supplementation may be necessary in some cases of atrophic gastritis.

Newer anti-inflammatory drugs in the COX-2 inhibitor family, such as Celebrex (celecoxib) and Vioxx (rofecoxib), were designed to cause less harm to the stomach than the older drugs in that category (such as aspirin and ibuprofen). However, current evidence remains mixed on how much safer these drugs really are compared to the old ones. More sophisticated forms of inhibitors that are currently moving toward the market may better fulfill the promise of these medications.

Proposed Natural Treatments

No herbs or supplements have been proven effective for gastritis. The treatments mentioned here have merely shown some promise in preliminary studies.

Natural Therapies That May Affect *H. Pylori*

As discussed above, *H. pylori* is thought to contribute to many cases of gastritis. A number of treatments have been evaluated to see whether they inhibit *H. pylori*'s growth. For example, evidence suggests that various **probiotics** (friendly bacteria) in the *Lactobacillus* family can inhibit the growth of *H. pylori*. While this effect does not appear to be strong enough for probiotic treatment to eradicate *H. pylori* on its own, preliminary studies (one of which was double-blind) suggest that probiotics may help standard antibiotic therapy work better, improving the rate of eradication and reducing side effects.

Highly preliminary studies suggest that various **bioflavonoids** can inhibit the growth of *H. pylori* as well. All fruits and vegetables provide bioflavonoids, but these substances can also be taken as supplements.

Vitamin C has also shown some ability to act against *H. pylori*.

Despite early reports that **garlic** inhibits or kills *H. pylori*, studies in people have not been promising.

Fish oil in combination with antibiotic therapy has been tried as a treatment for eradicating *H. pylori*, but it did not prove particularly helpful.

The herb **cranberry** is thought to help prevent bladder infections by preventing adhesion of bacteria to the bladder. Preliminary evidence suggests that it might also help prevent the adhesion of *H. pylori* to the stomach wall. Theoretically, this could help treat gastritis, but as

Gastritis

yet there is no direct evidence regarding this potential benefit.

Cayenne does not appear to be helpful against *H. pylori*. However, some evidence suggests that cayenne can protect the stomach against damage caused by anti-inflammatory drugs. Other natural supplements that have shown promise for protecting against the side effects of these drugs include the amino acid cysteine, a special form of **licorice** known as *deglycyrrhizinated licorice* (DGL), and the breast milk constituent known as **colostrum**.

Other Natural Therapies That May Protect the Stomach Lining

A collection of substances extracted from beeswax has been studied as a treatment for preventing and treating ulcers of various kinds, with promising results. Known as *D-002*, this product is chemically related to policosanol; however, policosanol itself is not thought to have this effect. (To make matters more confusing, a similar beeswax extract is sold in the U.S. *as* policosanol.)

Very weak evidence also suggests that **butterbur** and **cinnamon** might help protect the stomach lining.

Other substances have also been suggested as aids to stomach health, but as yet there is little to no scientific evidence that they are effective for gastritis. These include the following:

- *Aloe vera*
- Cat's claw
- Gamma oryzanol
- Glutamine
- Marshmallow
- MSM
- Reishi
- Selenium
- Slippery elm
- Suma
- Vitamin A
- Vitamin C
- Wood betony
- Zinc

Many naturopathic physicians believe that the supplement **betaine hydrochloride** can aid gastritis by *increasing* stomach acid. This sounds paradoxical, since conventional treatment for this condition involves *reducing* stomach acid. However, according to one theory, lack of stomach acid leads to incomplete digestion of proteins and these proteins cause allergic reactions and other responses that lead to an increase in ulcer pain. Again, scientific evidence is lacking.

Note: Symptoms of gastritis are similar to those of non-specific dyspepsia (stomach pain with no known cause). If you suffer from stomach discomfort but your doctor does not think you have gastritis, ulcer disease, esophageal reflux, or any other specific illness, you might benefit from the natural treatments discussed in the dyspepsia article.

Herbs and Supplements to Use Only with Caution

A number of herbs and supplements might tend to increase stomach inflammation, including **arginine, cola nut, feverfew, turmeric,** and **white willow**.

In addition, various supplements may interact with drugs used to treat gastritis. For more information, see the specific drug article in the Drug Interactions section of this book.

Gastroesophageal Reflux Disease

RELATED TERMS: *Esophageal Reflux, GERD, Heartburn*

PRINCIPAL PROPOSED NATURAL TREATMENTS: *None*

OTHER PROPOSED NATURAL TREATMENTS: Aloe vera, *Betaine Hydrochloride, Bladderwrack, Carob, Folate, Licorice, Marshmallow, Multivitamin/Multimineral Supplements, Vitamin B*$_{12}$

In gastroesophageal reflux disease (GERD), acid from the stomach splashes upward, or "refluxes," and burns the esophagus (the tube connecting the mouth to the stomach). Normally, a type of sphincter muscle keeps the upper part of the stomach closed, but various factors may loosen it, allowing acid to rise more easily. The result is pain in the chest (heartburn). GERD is generally made worse by lying down because gravity no longer restrains the upward movement of stomach contents. In infants, the major issue with GERD is spitting up of food or milk rather than pain.

Certain foods may worsen GERD, including alcohol, carbonated beverages, caffeine, chocolate, citrus juices, milk, and peppermint. Cigarette smoking may also increase symptoms. Contrary to earlier beliefs, it does not appear that people with GERD need to cut down on fat intake to help control the disease.

Pregnant women frequently develop GERD due to changes in muscle tone. The connection between obesity and GERD remains unclear.

Treatment for GERD involves elevating the head of the bed and using medications that reduce the acidity of the stomach. In general, more powerful antacid medications are required for GERD than for **ulcers** or **gastritis**. Drugs in the **proton pump** category are most effective. Surgery may be recommended in certain cases.

If left untreated, GERD causes precancerous alterations in the lower part of the esophagus (a condition called *Barrett's esophagus*), which can develop into **esophageal cancer**. For this reason, people with GERD are often given a test to evaluate the condition of the esophagus.

Proposed Natural Treatments

Drugs used to treat GERD may tend to deplete the body of certain nutrients—especially **vitamin B**$_{12}$, but also **folate** and various minerals. Use of a **multivitamin/multimineral supplement** should correct this problem. For more information, see the articles on specific medications in the Drug Interactions section of this book.

Deglycyrrhizinated licorice (DGL), a special form of the herb **licorice**, has shown some promise for the treatment of ulcers. A drug (carbenoxolone) that is similar to ingredients in licorice has been studied for the treatment of GERD, with good results.

However, in these studies carbenoxolone was combined with other ingredients, including antacids and alginic acid (see next paragraph). It is not clear that carbenoxolone alone will help GERD, and it's even less clear that licorice itself offers any benefit.

A popular over-the-counter drug for GERD, Gaviscon, contains a substance called *alginic acid*. Alginic acid is thought to form a kind of protective seal at the top of the stomach, reducing reflux. The seaweed **bladderwrack** is high in alginic acid. However, there is no evidence that whole bladderwrack can reduce heartburn symptoms.

Several other natural supplements are often recommended for the treatment of GERD, including *Aloe vera*, antioxidants, artemesia, fresh **garlic**, **marshmallow**, and **slippery elm**, but there is no scientific evidence to support their use.

Milk allergy is thought to contribute to GERD in infants. Whether **food allergies** play a significant role in adult GERD remains unclear.

The herb **carob** may be helpful for infant GERD.

Many **naturopathic** physicians believe that the supplement **betaine hydrochloride** can aid GERD by *increasing* stomach acid. This sounds paradoxical, since conventional treatment involves *reducing* stomach acid. However, according to one theory, lack of stomach acid leads to incomplete digestion of proteins; these proteins cause allergic reactions and other responses that lead to an increase in reflux. Again, scientific evidence is lacking.

General Wellness

RELATED TERMS: *General Well-being*

PRINCIPAL PROPOSED NATURAL TREATMENTS: *Multivitamin/Multimineral Supplements, Ginseng*

OTHER PROPOSED NATURAL TREATMENTS: *Ashwagandha, Astragalus,* Eleutherococcus, *Garlic, Maitake, "Natural" Thyroid Hormone (T3), Reishi,* Rhodiola rosacea, *Schisandra, Shiitake, Spirulina, Suma, Various Alternative Therapies,* Vitamin B$_{12}$

PROBABLY NOT EFFECTIVE TREATMENTS: *DHEA, Selenium*

It's one of the cardinal principles of natural medicine that treatment should aim not only to treat illness but also to enhance wellness. According to this ideal, a proper course of treatment should improve your sense of general well-being, enhance your immunity to illness, raise your physical stamina, and increase mental alertness, as well as resolve the specific condition you took it for.

Unfortunately, while there can be little doubt that this is a laudable goal, it is easier to laud it than to achieve it. Conventional medicine tends to focus on treating diseases rather than increasing wellness, not as a matter of philosophical principle, but because it is easier to accomplish.

Probably the strongest force affecting wellness is genetics. Beyond that, common sense steps endorsed by all physicians include increasing exercise, reducing stress, improving diet, getting enough sleep, and living a life of moderation without bad habits, such as smoking or overeating.

Beyond this, however, it is difficult to make strong affirmations and the optimum forms of diet and exercise and other aspects of lifestyle remain unclear. In fact, they may always remain unclear, as it is impossible to perform double-blind, placebo-controlled studies on most lifestyle habits. (For information on why such studies are irreplaceable see **Why Does This Book Depend on Double-blind Studies?**.)

Principal Proposed Natural Treatments

Although no natural treatments have been proven effective for enhancing overall wellness, two have shown promise: multivitamin/multimineral tablets and the herb *Panax ginseng*.

Multivitamin/Multimineral Supplements

In order to function at our best, we need good nutrition. However, the modern diet often fails to provide people with sufficient amounts of all the necessary nutrients. For this reason, use of a multivitamin/multimineral supplement might be expected to enhance overall health and well-being, and preliminary double-blind trials generally support this view.

For example, in one double-blind study, 80 healthy men between the ages of 18 and 42 were given either a multivitamin/multimineral supplement or placebo and followed for 28 days. The results showed that use of the nutritional supplement improved several measures of well-being.

Similarly, an 8-week, double-blind, placebo-controlled study of 95 people with careers in middle management also found improvements in well-being.

Furthermore, several, although not all, studies have found that multivitamin/multimineral supplements can improve immunity in older people. General nutritional supplements may also help improve response to stress.

For more information, see the article on **general nutritional support**.

Panax ginseng

The herb *Panax ginseng* has an ancient reputation as a healthful "tonic." According to a more modern concept developed in the former USSR, ginseng functions as an *adaptogen*.

This term is defined as follows: An adaptogen helps the body adapt to stresses of various kinds, whether heat, cold, exertion, trauma, sleep deprivation, toxic exposure, radiation, infection, or psychologic stress. In addition, an adaptogen causes no side effects, is effective in treating a wide variety of illnesses, and helps return an organism toward balance no matter what may have gone wrong.

From a modern scientific perspective, it is not truly clear that such things as adaptogens actually exist. However, there is some evidence that ginseng may satisfy some of the definition's requirements.

Several studies have found that ginseng can improve the overall sense of well-being. For example, such benefits were seen in a 12-week, double-blind trial that evaluated the effects of *Panax ginseng* extract in 625 people. The average age of participants was just under 40 years old. Each participant received a multivitamin supplement daily, but for one set of participants, the multivitamin also contained ginseng. Level of well-being was measured by a set of 11 questions. The results showed that people taking the ginseng-containing supplement reported significant improvement compared to those taking the supplement without ginseng.

Similarly positive findings were reported in a double-blind, placebo-controlled study of 36 people newly diagnosed with diabetes. After 8 weeks, participants who had been taking 200 mg of ginseng daily reported improvements in mood, well-being, vigor, and psychophysical performance that were significant compared to the reports of control participants.

A 12-week, double-blind, placebo-controlled study of 120 people found that ginseng improved general well-being among women ages 30 to 60 years old and men ages 40 to 60 years old, but not among men ages 30 to 39 years old. This finding is possibly consistent with the traditional theory that ginseng is more effective for older people.

Other results suggest this as well: a double-blind, placebo-controlled trial of 30 young people found marginal benefits at most, and a 60-day, double-blind, placebo-controlled trial of 83 adults in their mid-20s found no effect.

In addition, ginseng has also shown some potential for enhancing **immunity**, **mental function**, and **sports performance**, all effects consistent with the adaptogen concept. For more information on these possibilities, as well as dosage and safety issues, see the full **Ginseng** article.

Other Proposed Natural Treatments

Besides *Panax ginseng* (discussed above), certain other herbs are regarded as adaptogens, including ***Eleutherococcus senticosus*** ("Siberian" ginseng), ***Rhodiola rosacea***, **ashwagandha**, **astragalus**, **suma**, **schisandra**, and the Asian mushrooms **maitake**, shiitake, and **reishi**. Meaningful supporting evidence for their benefits, however, is scant. In one of the better studies, a small double-blind, placebo-controlled trial of *Rhodiola rosacea*, the herb seemed to improve physical and mental performance and sense of well-being in students under stress.

Although **garlic** is not generally regarded as an adaptogen, one study found that garlic *powder* (but not garlic *oil*) enhanced well-being. However, another study failed to find such benefits with garlic powder.

"Green juices" made from such substances as **spirulina** and wheat grass are widely marketed for enhancing well-being. A double-blind study found that use of one such product improved general vitality, but so did placebo and the differences between the outcomes in the two groups were marginal.

Levels of the hormone **DHEA** naturally decrease with age and for that reason DHEA supplements have been widely hyped as a kind of fountain of youth. However, at least eight studies have found that DHEA supplementation does not improve mood or increase the general sense of well-being in older people.

A relatively large (about 500 participants) double-blind study also failed to find **selenium** helpful in seniors.

A smaller study failed to find evidence that **vitamin B_{12}** improved general sense of well-being among seniors with signs of mild B_{12} deficiency.

In some branches of alternative medicine, low levels of **thyroid hormone** are believed to be a common cause of impaired well-being. As part of this theory, it is said that the most commonly used medical form of thyroid replacement therapy (thyroxine, also called T4) is inadequate. Supposedly, better results are obtained when T4 is taken in combination with the thyroid hormone known as T3, often in the form of so-called natural thyroid extracted from animal thyroid glands. However, a double-blind study of 110 people designed to test this theory failed to find combined T3/T4 more effective than T4 alone.

Numerous other alternative therapies are claimed by their proponents to improve overall wellness, including **acupuncture, Ayurveda, chiropractic, detoxification, homeopathy, massage, naturopathy, osteopathic manipulation, Reiki, Tai Chi, Therapeutic Touch, traditional Chinese herbal medicine,** and **yoga**. However, there is as yet little meaningful evidence to support these claims.

Additional information relevant to wellness may be found in articles on **food allergies, immune support, preventive medicine, sports supplements,** and **stress**.

Glaucoma

PRINCIPAL PROPOSED NATURAL TREATMENTS: *None*

OTHER PROPOSED NATURAL TREATMENTS: *Forskolin (from* Coleus Forskohlii*), Ginkgo, Lipoic Acid, Magnesium, Melatonin, Omega-3 Fatty Acids, Vitamin C*

G laucoma is a group of related diseases that cause damage to the eye's optic nerve and result in visual impairment or blindness. Most often, glaucoma occurs in the presence of increased intraocular pressure (pressure inside the eye). However, glaucoma can also occur when intraocular pressure is normal (although treatment that reduces the pressure appears to benefit this kind of glaucoma too).

Glaucoma is the second leading cause of legal blindness in the U.S. and the first leading cause of blindness in African-Americans. Unfortunately, most of the time glaucoma presents no symptoms until permanent damage has been done. It is estimated that 2.5 million Americans have glaucoma—and half of these people do not know they have it. For this reason, regular checkups are advisable for people at high risk for glaucoma. Risk factors include:

> African-American descent
> Age over 60
> Family history of glaucoma
> Use of corticosteroid drugs (including steroid inhalers for asthma)

Physicians diagnose glaucoma by measuring intraocular pressure as well as by examining the optic nerve and using special vision tests. Eyedrops that reduce intraocular pressure are safe and highly effective for most cases of glaucoma.

Proposed Natural Treatments

A small double-blind, placebo-controlled trial found that use of **ginkgo** extract at a dose of 120 mg daily for 8 weeks significantly improved vision in people with glaucoma. Ginkgo is thought to work by enhancing circulation.

Small double-blind, placebo-controlled trials suggest that eyedrops containing the chemical forskolin, a constituent of the herb *Coleus forskohlii*, reduces intraocular pressure in people without glaucoma. However there is no evidence as yet that forskolin is an effective treatment for people with glaucoma. In any case, forskolin is not available except for research and using ordinary preparations of the herb directly in the eye is not recommended. (There is no reason to believe that oral use of *Coleus forskohlii* will benefit glaucoma.)

Highly preliminary evidence suggests that certain dietary supplements may also reduce intraocular pressure, including high-dose **vitamin C**, **melatonin**, and **omega-3 fatty acids**. However, there is as yet no reliable evidence that any of these supplements enhances the effect of standard treatment and they definitely cannot be used as substitutes for it. Weak evidence suggests that the supplement **lipoic acid** could improve vision in people with glaucoma. **Magnesium** has been suggested for the same purpose, but in one preliminary study, use of magnesium failed to produce statistically significant benefits. The herbs bilberry, **oregano**, and pilocarpus, and the supplements citrus bioflavonoids and OPCs (oligomeric proanthocyanidin complexes) are sometimes recommended for preventing or treating glaucoma, but there is no meaningful evidence to indicate that they work.

Gout

PRINCIPAL PROPOSED NATURAL TREATMENTS: *None*

OTHER PROPOSED NATURAL TREATMENTS: *Aspartic Acid, Bromelain, Celery Juice, Cherry Juice, Devil's Claw, Fish Oil, Folate, Olive Leaf, Selenium, Vitamin A, Vitamin C, Vitamin E*

Gout is an inflammatory condition that is caused by the deposit of uric acid crystals in joints (most famously the big toe) as well as other tissues. Typically, attacks of fierce pain, redness, swelling, and heat punctuate pain-free intervals.

Medical treatment consists of anti-inflammatory drugs for acute attacks and of uric acid–lowering drugs for prevention.

Proposed Treatments for Gout

The following herbs and supplements are widely recommended for gout, but as yet they have no reliable scientific support.

Vitamin C

In a double-blind, placebo-controlled study of 184 people without gout, use of vitamin C at a daily dose of 500 mg significantly reduced uric acid levels. This suggests, but falls far short of proving, that vitamin C might be helpful for preventing or treating gout.

Folate

Folate has been recommended as a preventive treatment for gout for at least 20 years. Some clinicians report that it can be highly effective. However, what little scientific evidence we have on the method is contradictory. It has been suggested that a contaminant found in folate, pterin-6-aldehyde, may actually be responsible for the positive effects observed by some clinicians.

For more information, including dosage and safety issues, see the full **Folate** article.

Devil's Claw

The herb devil's claw is sometimes recommended as a pain-relieving treatment for gout based on evidence for its effectiveness in various forms of arthritis. However, it has not been tested in gout.

For more information, including dosage and safety issues, see the full **Devil's Claw** article.

Other Supplements

On the basis of interesting reasoning but no concrete evidence of effectiveness, **fish oil**, **olive leaf**, **vitamin E**, **selenium**, **bromelain**, **vitamin A**, and aspartic acid have also been recommended for both prevention and treatment of gout.

Folk Remedies

A traditional remedy for gout (with negligible scientific evidence) calls for 1/2 to 1 pound of cherries a day. You can also buy tablets containing concentrated cherry juice.

Celery juice is another folk remedy for gout that is said to be widely used in Australia.

Herbs and Supplements to Use Only With Caution

Various herbs and supplements may interact adversely with drugs used to treat gout. For more information on these potential risks, see the individual drug article in the Drug Interactions section of this book.

Hearing Loss

RELATED TERMS: *Age-related Hearing Loss, Idiopathic Sudden Hearing Loss, Noise-induced Hearing Loss, Sudden Hearing Loss, Unilateral Idiopathic Sudden Hearing Loss*

PRINCIPAL PROPOSED NATURAL TREATMENTS:

Prevention of Noise-induced Hearing Loss: *Magnesium*

Treatment of Sudden Hearing Loss: *Ginkgo*

OTHER PROPOSED NATURAL TREATMENTS: *Lipoic Acid*

There are many possible causes of hearing loss, ranging from wax in the ear canal to problems with the nerves that receive sound and transmit it to the brain. Two of the most common causes are age-related hearing loss (presbycusis) and noise-induced hearing loss. The treatment for hearing loss depends on its cause and for that reason medical consultation is essential.

In this article, we discuss a few herbs and supplements that have shown promise for various forms of hearing loss. See also the article on **tinnitus** for hearing problems that involve ringing in the ears.

Principal Proposed Natural Treatments

Two natural treatments have been evaluated in double-blind, placebo-controlled trials for the prevention or treatment of hearing loss: magnesium and ginkgo.

Magnesium for Preventing Noise-induced Hearing Loss

Long-term exposure to loud sounds, such as gunfire or rock music, can cause permanent hearing loss. A 2-month, double-blind, placebo-controlled study of 300 military recruits found daily supplementation with magnesium helped protect the ear from noise-induced damage. The dosage used in this study was quite small—only 167 mg of magnesium daily—but tests showed that even this amount was sufficient to raise magnesium levels inside cells and apparently protect the ear from damage. Soldiers who received the magnesium were less likely to experience permanent hearing damage than those in the placebo group and when they did experience hearing damage, it was less severe.

It is not clear how magnesium might protect hearing. Studies in animals suggest that magnesium deficiency can increase the stress on cells involved with hearing and thereby make them more susceptible to

damage caused by intense noise. However, human magnesium deficiency is believed to be rare, so it is possible that supplemental magnesium acts in some entirely different way.

At present, only the use of noise-reduction devices (for example, headsets that block sound) have been proven effective for preventing noise-induced hearing loss and this study does not indicate that magnesium supplements can replace this tried-and-true approach. However, this study suggests that a safe, low dose of magnesium may add an additional level of protection.

For more information, including dosage and safety issues, see the full **Magnesium** article.

Ginkgo for Treating Sudden Hearing Loss

Some people develop hearing loss suddenly, usually in one ear. This condition is called *unilateral idiopathic sudden hearing loss*. Its cause is unknown, but problems with circulation may play a role in some cases. The herb *Ginkgo biloba* is thought to increase circulation and for that reason it has been tried as a treatment for this condition.

In a double-blind, placebo-controlled trial, 106 participants with a carefully defined form of sudden hearing loss were given either a full dose of ginkgo extract (120 mg twice daily) or a low dose of the herb (12 mg twice daily). The lower dose was chosen in the belief that it couldn't possibly offer any benefit and would therefore serve as placebo. However, researchers were surprised to find that most participants in each group recovered by the end of the 8-week trial. There are two possibilities to explain this: low-dose ginkgo is effective or many people with sudden hearing loss recover on their own anyway.

Because both groups improved to such a great extent, the overall results of the trial did not prove ginkgo effective. An exploratory look at the data provided some tantalizing hints that high-dose ginkgo may have helped ensure full recovery, but for statistical reasons these tantalizing hints can't be taken as proof.

Another double-blind study compared ginkgo to pentoxifylline, a circulation-enhancing drug used in Germany for the treatment of sudden hearing loss. The results indicate that ginkgo was at least as effective as the medication. However, because pentoxifylline is not a proven treatment for this condition, the results prove little.

Additional research will be necessary to discover whether ginkgo is actually effective for sudden hearing loss. For more information on this herb, including dosage and safety issues, see the full **Ginkgo** article.

Other Proposed Natural Treatments

A study in animals suggests that the supplement lipoic acid might help prevent age-related hearing loss. Another animal study suggests that melatonin may help prevent hearing loss induced by noise.

Free radicals are naturally-occurring substances that cause damage to many parts of the body, including the ear. Antioxidants are substances that fight free radicals. Antioxidant supplements have shown promise for preventing various forms of hearing loss, including age-related hearing loss and hearing damage caused by medications. Commonly used antioxidants include the following:

- **Citrus bioflavonoids**
- **Coenzyme Q_{10}**
- **Lipoic acid**
- **Lutein**
- **Lycopene**
- **Oligomeric Proanthocyanidins (OPCs)**
- **Vitamin C**
- **Vitamin E**

Other natural treatments sometimes used for various forms of hearing loss, but which lack meaningful scientific support, include **folate**, **manganese**, myrrh, **potassium**, **vitamin B_1**, **vitamin B_2**, **vitamin B_6**, **vitamin B_{12}**, and **zinc**.

Heart Attack

RELATED TERMS: *Myocardial Infarction*

PRINCIPAL PROPOSED NATURAL TREATMENTS: *Natural Treatments for Atherosclerosis, High Cholesterol, High Blood Pressure, and High Homocysteine*

OTHER PROPOSED NATURAL TREATMENTS: *Antioxidants (such as Vitamin A, Vitamin C, Vitamin E, and Beta-carotene), Arginine, Coenzyme Q_{10}, Fish Oil, Garlic Oil, Glycine, Hawthorn, Inosine, L-carnitine, Lifestyle Modification, Lipoic Acid, Selenium*

PROBABLY INEFFECTIVE TREATMENTS: *Chelation Therapy, Magnesium*

As an active muscle, the heart needs a continuous supply of oxygen. The coronary arteries have the job of carrying oxygen to the heart. These arteries have a difficult job to do because they undergo intense compression every time the heart beats. This job becomes even more difficult when the arteries are damaged by **atherosclerosis** (commonly, though not quite accurately, called *hardening of the arteries*) in a condition called *coronary artery disease*.

In coronary artery disease the passages inside the coronary arteries become narrowed by plaque deposits, which decreases blood flow. When the blood flow is decreased to a sufficient extent, pain caused by oxygen deprivation occurs. This pain is known as *angina pectoris*. Angina tends to wax and wane, generally worsening with exercise.

A heart attack may occur after years of angina or with no warning at all. Most heart attacks occur when a blood clot (thrombus) forms on the roughened wall of an atherosclerotic coronary artery. Such a blood clot may lead to a sudden and complete blockage of the artery. More rarely, a spasm of a coronary artery may cut off blood flow. In either case, the cells of the heart fed by that artery begin to die. The region of dead cells is called an *infarct*, leading to the technical name for a heart attack: a myocardial infarction (MI).

The classic symptom of a heart attack is intense, central chest pressure. Other common symptoms include: Pain or heaviness in the left arm, nausea, shortness of breath, increased perspiration, and a feeling of impending doom. But many people who have had an MI describe chest "discomfort," or pain in the jaw, teeth, arm, or abdomen. Women are more likely than men to feel pain in their backs. Often, symptoms come on gradually and are intermittent or vague. A quarter of patients—more often women and people with diabetes—experience no symptoms at all.

When a heart attack occurs, emergency treatment at a hospital can minimize the extent of permanent damage to the heart. "Clot busting" drugs, if given soon enough, can open the coronary arteries, allowing blood to flow again. Other methods of restoring blood flow include procedures known as *angioplasty, stenting,* and *bypass surgery.* The aim is to save those heart cells that are in danger of dying but are still hanging on to life. Recovery after a heart attack depends on the extent of heart damage. If only a small portion of the heart has died, or if it is in a relatively less important region, symptoms may be slight. More severe damage can cause the heart to pump improperly, leading to **congestive heart failure**.

During the first several days following a heart attack, the heart has a tendency to lose its normal rhythm and fall into a dysfunctional pattern of beating that does not properly circulate blood. Treatment aimed to prevent or treat this condition, called an ***arrhythmia***, is conducted in a cardiac intensive care unit.

Long-term treatment to reduce the risk of heart attacks generally involves aspirin to prevent blood clots, as well as treatments to slow, stop, or reverse atherosclerosis. The latter is accomplished through the use of medications that keep cholesterol and blood pressure within normal limits, as well as by increasing exercise and improving other aspects of lifestyle.

Principal Proposed Natural Treatments

The most important contribution natural medicine has to make to heart attacks lies in prevention, not treatment. Because heart attacks are, in almost all cases, caused by atherosclerosis, the natural treatments discussed in the atherosclerosis article are relevant to reducing heart attack risk.

In turn, atherosclerosis is accelerated by **high blood pressure** and **high cholesterol**, and possibly by **high levels of homocysteine** in the blood. Natural treatments used for these conditions may very well be worth considering.

Note: Natural therapies for high blood pressure and high cholesterol are generally less effective than the conventional approaches. If you have one or both of these conditions and you wish to treat them with natural therapies, first consult with a physician to determine how long it is safe to experiment. If natural therapies have not controlled your condition within that time, it may be the better part of valor to use conventional therapies.

Other Proposed Natural Treatments

Several natural treatments have shown promise for use along with conventional treatment in the period following a heart attack. Note, however, that people who have recently had a heart attack should not use any herbs or supplements except under the supervision of a physician.

Furthermore, none of these treatments can *substitute* for standard care; at most, they might be helpful if used in addition to it.

Coenzyme Q_{10}

The supplement **coenzyme Q_{10}** (CoQ_{10}) is thought to improve heart function. In a double-blind trial, 145 people who had recently experienced a heart attack were given either placebo or 120 mg of CoQ_{10} daily for 28 days. The results showed that participants receiving CoQ_{10} experienced significantly fewer heart-related problems, such as episodes of angina pectoris or arrhythmia, or recurrent heart attacks.

CoQ_{10} taken in combination with the mineral **selenium** has also shown promise for people who have survived a heart attack.

L-carnitine

The amino acid **L-carnitine** has shown potential value during the first few weeks after an MI. A double-blind, placebo-controlled study that followed 101 people for 1 month after a heart attack found that use of L-carnitine, in addition to standard care, reduced the size of the infarct (area of dead heart tissue). Other complications of heart attack were reduced as well. Similar benefits were also seen in a 1-year, controlled study of 160 people who had just experienced a heart attack; however, because this study was not double-blind, its results are not reliable. (For information on why double-blind studies are so important, see **Why Does This Book Rely on Double-blind Studies?**.)

In the months following a severe heart attack, the heart often enlarges and loses function. L-carnitine has shown some potential for helping the first of these complications, but not the second. In a 12-month, double-blind, placebo-controlled study of 472 people who had just experienced a heart attack, use of carnitine at a dose of 6 g per day significantly decreased the rate of heart enlargement. However, heart function was not improved. A 3-month, double-blind, placebo-controlled study of 60 people who had just undergone a heart attack also failed to find improvements in heart function with L-carnitine. (Heart enlargement was not studied.)

Results consistent with those of the studies above were seen in a 6-month, double blind, placebo-controlled study of 2,330 people who had just had a heart attack. Carnitine failed to produce significant reductions in mortality or heart failure (serious decline in heart function) over the 6-month period. However, it did find reductions in early death. (Unfortunately, for statistical reasons, the meaningfulness of this last finding is questionable: it was a secondary endpoint rather than a primary one.)

Fish Oil

Fish oil contains healthy fats in the omega-3 fatty acid category. Fish oil supplements have shown promise for helping to prevent sudden death after a heart attack. However, evidence is conflicting on whether fish oil does so by reducing risk of dangerous heart arrhythmias or simply by reducing heart rate.

Garlic

In one study, 432 people who had suffered a heart attack were given either garlic oil extract or no treatment over a period of 3 years. The results showed a significant reduction of second heart attacks and about a 50% reduction in death rate among those taking garlic.

Note: People who take aspirin to prevent heart attacks should not take garlic supplements as the combination could lead to excessive bleeding. (See the full article on **garlic** for more information.)

Antioxidants

Antioxidant supplements help neutralize free radicals, which are dangerous, naturally-occurring chemicals that may accelerate heart cell death following a heart attack (among their many other harmful effects). In a double-blind trial, people who had just experienced a heart attack were given either placebo or a mixture of antioxidants (**vitamin A**, **vitamin C**, **vitamin E**, and **beta-carotene**) for 28 days. The results indicated that use of antioxidants minimized the extent of heart cell damage.

Magnesium

The mineral **magnesium** is sometimes suggested for stabilizing the heart after a heart attack, but one study actually found a negative effect. In this 1-year, double-blind, placebo-controlled trial of 468 people who had just experienced a heart attack, use of a magnesium supplement at a dose of 360 mg daily failed to prevent heart-related events (defined as heart attack, sudden cardiac death, or need for cardiac bypass) and actually may have increased the risk slightly.

Arginine

The supplement **arginine** has been proposed for aiding recovery from a heart attack. In one double-blind study, arginine did not cause harm and showed potential modest benefit. However, in another study, arginine failed to prove helpful and possibly increased post–heart attack death rate.

Other Herbs and Supplements

Other herbs and supplements sometimes said to be useful after a heart attack, but that lack reliable substantiation, include the following:

- **Glycine**
- **Hawthorn**
- **Inosine**
- **Lipoic acid**

Lifestyle Modifications

Evidence suggests that a program of intensive lifestyle modification, involving an extremely low-fat diet along with exercise and stress reduction, can actually reverse coronary artery disease in people who have had heart attacks or are at high risk for it. It is not clear whether less ascetic approaches can achieve similar effects.

Chelation Therapy

Some alternative medicine physicians recommend use of intravenous infusions of a chemical called *ethylenediaminetetraacetic acid* (EDTA) in order to clear out the arteries of the heart, a method called **chelation therapy**. This method is based on an outmoded understanding of atherosclerosis and is most likely ineffective.

Hemorrhoids

Herbs and Supplements to Use Only with Caution

Numerous herbs and supplements may interact adversely with drugs used to prevent or treat heart attacks. For more information on these potential risks see the individual drug articles in the Drug Interactions section of this book.

Hemorrhoids

PRINCIPAL PROPOSED NATURAL TREATMENTS: *Bioflavonoids: Citrus Bioflavonoids, Oxerutins, and Bilberry*

OTHER PROPOSED NATURAL TREATMENTS: *Butcher's Broom, Calendula, Collinsonia, Gotu Kola, Horse Chestnut, Mesoglycan, Oak Bark, Oligomeric Proanthocyanidins (OPCs), Slippery Elm, Witch Hazel*

Hemorrhoids are swollen, inflamed veins in the rectum that can ache and bleed. They are very common and are usually caused by **constipation**, a low-fiber diet, a sedentary lifestyle, **pregnancy**, or **liver cirrhosis**.

The most important interventions for hemorrhoids aim at reversing their causes. Adopting a high-fiber diet, sitting down less, getting plenty of exercise, and maintaining regular bowel habits can make a significant difference.

Medical treatment consists mainly of stool softeners and moist heat. In more severe cases, surgical procedures may be used.

Contrary to popular belief, it does not appear that consumption of foods spiced with hot chile peppers causes any discomfort or harm to people with hemorrhoids; a double-blind study found no difference in symptoms following consumption of hot peppers or placebo.

Principal Proposed Natural Treatments

Bioflavonoids are colorful substances that occur widely in the plant kingdom. Reasonably good evidence suggests that the citrus bioflavonoids diosmin and hesperidin (in a special micronized combination preparation) may be helpful for hemorrhoids.

A 2-month, double-blind, placebo-controlled trial of 120 individuals with recurrent hemorrhoid flare-ups found that treatment with combined diosmin and hesperidin significantly reduced the frequency and severity of hemorrhoid attacks. Another double-blind, placebo-controlled trial of 100 individuals had positive results with the same bioflavonoids in relieving symptoms once a flare-up of hemorrhoid pain had begun. A 90-day, double-blind trial of 100 individuals with bleeding hemorrhoids also found significant benefits for both treatment of acute attacks and prevention of new ones. Finally, this bioflavonoid combination was found to compare favorably with surgical treatment of hemorrhoids. However, less impressive results were seen in a double-blind, placebo-controlled study in which all participants were given a fiber laxative with either combined diosmin and hesperidin or placebo.

Other sources of bioflavonoids have been studied as well. For example, in a 4-week, double-blind, placebo-controlled trial of 40 people with hemorrhoids, use of an extract made from the bioflavonoid-rich herb bilberry significantly reduced hemorrhoid symptoms as compared to placebo. In addition, according to some but not all double-blind studies, the semi-synthetic bioflavonoids known as oxerutins may also be helpful for hemorrhoids, including the hemorrhoids that occur during pregnancy.

Although it is not known precisely how flavonoids work, it is thought that they stabilize the walls of blood vessels, making them less susceptible to injury.

For more information, including dosage and safety issues, see the full articles on **citrus bioflavonoids, bilberry,** and **oxerutins.**

Other Proposed Natural Treatments

Preliminary evidence suggests that an extract made from pig intestines called *mesoglycan* can improve the symptoms of hemorrhoids.

The natural treatments used for **varicose veins** are also often recommended for hemorrhoids because a hemorrhoid is actually a special kind of varicose vein. Some of the most commonly mentioned include **horse chestnut, oligomeric proanthocyanidins** (OPCs), **gotu kola**, and **butcher's broom**.

Traditional herbal remedies for hemorrhoids include **calendula** (applied topically), *Collinsonia* root (oral or topical), **oak bark** (topical), **slippery elm** (oral or topical), and **witch hazel** (topical). However, there has been little to no scientific evaluation of these treatments.

Herpes

RELATED TERMS: *Cold Sores, Genital Herpes,* Herpes simplex

PRINCIPAL PROPOSED NATURAL TREATMENTS:

Prevention: *L-Lysine, Melissa*

Treatment: Aloe vera, *Melissa,* Topical Zinc

OTHER PROPOSED NATURAL TREATMENTS: *Adenosine Monophosphate, Astragalus, Bee Propolis, Cat's Claw, Elderberry,* Eleutherococcus, *Kelp, Sage/Rhubarb Cream, Sandalwood, Tea Tree Oil, Vitamin C, Witch Hazel*

PROBABLY NOT EFFECTIVE TREATMENTS: *Echinacea*

The common virus *Herpes simplex,* known simply as herpes, can cause painful blister-like lesions around the mouth and in the genitalia. Slightly different strains of herpes predominate in each of these two locations, but the infections are essentially identical. In both areas, the herpes virus has the devious habit of hiding out deep in the DNA of nerve ganglia, where it remains inactive for months or years. From time to time the virus reactivates, travels down the nerve, and starts an eruption. Common triggers include **stress**, dental procedures, infections, and trauma. Flare-ups usually become less severe over time.

Conventional medical treatment consists of antiviral drugs, such as Zovirax. Such medications can shorten the length and intensity of a herpes outbreak or, when taken consistently at lower dosages, reduce the frequency of flare-ups. In addition, they can reduce transmission of the disease.

Principal Proposed Natural Treatments

Several natural treatments have shown promise for treating herpes. Note, however, that while conventional treatments can reduce infectivity and thereby help prevent the spread of the disease, no natural treatment has been shown to do this. Keep in mind that common sense methods used to prevent herpes transmission are not entirely effective: many people are infectious even when they do not have obvious symptoms and use of a condom does not entirely prevent the spread of the virus. Therefore, if you are sexually active with a non-infected partner who wishes to remain that way, we strongly recommend that you use suppressive drug therapy.

Melissa officinalis (Lemon Balm)

More commonly known in the United States as lemon balm, *Melissa officinalis* is widely sold in Europe as a topical cream for the treatment of genital and oral herpes.

One double-blind, placebo-controlled study followed 66 people who were just starting to develop a cold sore (oral herpes). Treatment with melissa cream produced significant benefits on day 2, reducing intensity of discomfort, number of blisters, and the size of the lesion. (The researchers specifically looked at day 2 because, according to them, that is when symptoms are most pronounced.)

Another double-blind study followed 116 individuals with oral or genital herpes. Participants used either melissa cream or placebo cream for up to 10 days. The results showed that use of the herb resulted in a significantly better rate of recovery than those given placebo.

For more information, including dosage and safety issues, see the full **Melissa** article.

Aloe Vera

The succulent aloe plant is famous as a treatment for burns and minor wounds. However, while there is little evidence it is effective for those purposes, two studies suggest that aloe has potential value in the treatment of herpes infections.

A 2-week, double-blind, placebo-controlled trial enrolled 60 men with active genital herpes. Participants applied aloe cream (0.5% aloe) or placebo cream 3 times daily for 5 days. Use of aloe cream reduced the time necessary for lesions to heal and also increased the percentage of individuals who were fully healed by the end of 2 weeks.

A previous double-blind, placebo-controlled study by the same author enrolling 120 men with genital herpes found that aloe cream was more effective than pure aloe gel or placebo. The author theorized that the oily constituents in the cream improved aloe absorption.

For more information, including dosage and safety issues, see the full **Aloe** article.

L-Lysine

Another famous treatment for herpes involves the amino acid L-lysine. Taken regularly in sufficient doses, lysine supplements appear to reduce the number and intensity of herpes flare-ups. However, a study evaluating lysine taken only at the onset of a herpes attack found no benefit. (Consider using melissa for this latter purpose.)

One double-blind, placebo-controlled study followed 52 participants with a history of herpes flare-ups. While receiving 3 g of L-lysine every day for 6 months, the treatment group experienced an average of 2.4 fewer herpes flare-ups than the placebo group—a significant difference. The lysine group's flare-ups were also significantly less severe and healed faster.

Another double-blind, placebo-controlled crossover study on 41 subjects also found improvements in the frequency of attacks. Interestingly, this study found that 1,250 mg of lysine daily worked, but 624 mg did not.

Other studies, including one that followed 65 individuals, found no benefit, but they used lower dosages of lysine.

For more information, including dosage and safety issues, see the full **Lysine** article.

Zinc

Zinc lozenges or nasal sprays are thought to be effective for fighting the viruses that cause **colds**. A recent study suggests that topical zinc may be helpful for herpes infections of the mouth and face as well. In this trial, 46 individuals with cold sores were treated with a zinc oxide cream or placebo every 2 hours until cold sores resolved. The results showed that individuals using the cream experienced a reduction in severity of symptoms and a shorter time to full recovery.

Other Proposed Natural Treatments

Eleutherococcus, incorrectly called *Russian* or *Siberian ginseng*, has shown promise for the treatment of herpes. A 6-month, double-blind trial of 93 men and women with recurrent genital herpes infections found that treatment with eleutherococcus (2 g daily) reduced the frequency of infections by almost 50%.

A double-blind trial of 149 individuals with recurrent oral herpes compared the effectiveness of cream containing Zovirax against cream containing the herbs **sage** and rhubarb, and cream containing sage alone. The combination of sage and rhubarb proved to be equally effective to Zovirax cream; sage by itself was less effective, if at all.

One study suggests that topical treatment with a **vitamin C** solution may speed healing of oral herpes outbreaks. Oral vitamin C combined with bioflavonoids has also shown some promise for genital herpes.

The results of a small single-blind, controlled study suggests that the honeybee product **propolis** cream might cause attacks of genital herpes to heal faster.

Other herbs and supplements sometimes recommended for herpes infections, but that lack meaningful supporting evidence, include **adenosine monophosphate**, **astragalus**, **cat's claw**, **elderberry**, **kelp**, **sandalwood**, **tea tree oil**, and **witch hazel**.

A product containing vitamins and minerals as well as the herbs paprika, **rosemary**, **peppermint**, milfoil, **hawthorn**, and **pumpkin seed** has been used in Scandinavia for many years as a treatment for various mouth-related conditions. However, a double-blind study of 50 people with recurrent oral herpes failed to find 4 months' treatment with this product more effective than placebo.

Similarly, a 1-year, double-blind, placebo-controlled

study of 50 individuals with recurrent genital herpes failed to find the herb **echinacea** helpful for reducing the rate of flare-ups.

High Cholesterol

RELATED TERMS: *Hyperlipidemia*

PRINCIPAL PROPOSED NATURAL TREATMENTS: *Artichoke Leaf, Fiber, Soy, Stanols, Vitamin B₃ (Niacin)*

OTHER PROPOSED NATURAL TREATMENTS: *Achillea wilhelmsii, Alfalfa, Ashwagandha, Black Cohosh, Black Tea, Broccoli and Cabbage, Caigua, Calcium, Carob, Chitosan, Chromium, Cinnamon, Cordyceps, Creatine, Fenugreek, Flaxseed, Flaxseed Oil, Gamma Oryzanol, Garlic, Genistein, Green Tea, Guggul, He Shou Wu, L-Carnitine, Lecithin, Lifestyle Changes, Maitake, Mesoglycan, Multivitamin/Mineral Supplement, Pantethine, Policosanol, Probiotics, Red Yeast Rice, Spirulina, Tocotrienols*

One of the most significant discoveries in preventive medicine is that elevated levels of cholesterol in the blood accelerate **atherosclerosis**, a condition commonly known as *hardening of the arteries*. Along with **high blood pressure**, inactivity, **smoking**, and **diabetes**, high cholesterol has proven to be one of the most important promoters of **heart disease, strokes**, and **peripheral vascular disease** (blockage of circulation to the extremities, usually the legs).

Cholesterol does not directly clog arteries like grease clogs pipes. The current theory is that elevated levels of cholesterol irritate the walls of blood vessels and cause them to undergo harmful changes. Because most cholesterol is manufactured by the body itself, dietary sources of cholesterol (such as eggs) are not usually the most important problem. The relative proportion of unsaturated fats (from plants) and saturated fats (mainly from animal products) in the diet is more significant.

When the consequences of elevated cholesterol were first being researched, total cholesterol was the only measurement considered. Today, the overall *lipid profile* is taken into account. LDL ("bad") cholesterol, HDL ("good") cholesterol, and **triglycerides** are the most common other measurements related to cholesterol. Lipoprotein A and oxidized LDL cholesterol are drawing increasing attention as well.

This change in emphasis has thrown some long-standing recommendations into confusion. For example, reducing total fat intake generally decreases total cholesterol and on this basis medical authorities long ago adopted a policy of recommending low-fat diets. However, when you take into account other lipid measurements, it is now clear that reducing fat intake is not the clear blessing it first appeared to be. Cutting down on fat improves total and LDL cholesterol levels, but it worsens HDL and triglyceride levels; the net effect is unclear. At present, it is not clear what proportion and type of fat, carbohydrate, and protein form the ideal diet from a cholesterol perspective; there is no question, however, that losing weight is extremely important and if you are overweight and lose weight your cholesterol profile is very likely to improve.

Increasing exercise and losing weight may produce adequate improvements in the lipid profile. If such lifestyle changes are not effective, however, there are many highly effective drugs to choose from. Medications in the **statin family** are most effective and they have been shown to prevent heart attacks and reduce mortality. Other useful conventional options include Zetia (ezetimibe), **fibrate drugs**, and various forms of the vitamin niacin (discussed below).

Principal Proposed Natural Treatments

There are several herbs and supplements that appear to help lower cholesterol levels. For some (such as stanols/sterols, vitamin B₃, fiber, and soy), the evidence is sufficiently strong to have produced mainstream acceptance.

Note: If your primary problem is elevated triglycerides, see the **High Triglycerides** article.

Stanols/Sterols

Stanols are substances that occur naturally in various plants. Their cholesterol-lowering effects were first observed in animals in the 1950s. Since then, a substantial amount of research suggests that plant stanols (usually modified into stanol esters) can help to lower cholesterol in individuals with normal or mildly to moderately elevated cholesterol levels. Stanols are available in margarine spreads, salad dressings, and dietary supplement tablets. Related substances called *plant sterols* appear to have equivalent effects and in this article we will refer to sterols and stanols and their esters somewhat interchangeably.

Plant stanol esters reduce serum cholesterol levels by inhibiting cholesterol absorption. Because they are structurally similar to cholesterol, stanols (and sterols) can displace cholesterol from the "packages" that deliver cholesterol for absorption from the intestines to the bloodstream. The displaced cholesterol is not absorbed and is excreted from the body; the stanols themselves are ultimately not absorbed either.

Numerous double-blind, placebo-controlled studies, ranging in length from 30 days to 12 months, have found stanol esters and their chemical relatives effective for improving cholesterol levels. The combined results suggest that these substances can reduce total cholesterol and LDL ("bad") cholesterol by about 10 to 15%. Stanol esters did not have any significant effect on HDL ("good") cholesterol or triglycerides in most of these studies.

Individuals taking statin drugs may benefit from using stanols/sterols as well. According to one study, if you are on statins and start taking sterol ester margarine as well, your cholesterol will improve to the same extent as if you doubled the statin dose. Stanols or sterols also appear to enhance the effects of cholesterol-lowering diets.

In addition, three studies found stanols or sterols to be helpful for lowering cholesterol levels in people with type 2 (adult-onset) diabetes.

For more information, including dosage and safety issues, see the full **Stanols** article.

Niacin (Vitamin B$_3$)

The common vitamin niacin, also called *vitamin B$_3$*, is an accepted medical treatment for elevated cholesterol with solid science behind it. Several well-designed, double-blind, placebo-controlled studies have found that niacin reduced LDL cholesterol by approximately 10% and triglycerides by 25%, and raised HDL cholesterol by 20 to 30%. Niacin also lowers levels of lipoprotein A—another risk factor for atherosclerosis—by about 35%. Furthermore, long-term use of niacin has been shown to significantly reduce death rates from cardiovascular disease.

Niacin appears to be a safe and effective treatment for high cholesterol in people with diabetes as well, and (contrary to previous reports) does not seem to raise blood sugar levels. Unfortunately, niacin, if taken in sufficient quantities to lower cholesterol, can cause an annoying flushing reaction and occasionally liver inflammation. Close medical supervision is essential when using niacin to lower cholesterol.

Combining high-dose niacin with statin drugs (the most effective medications for high cholesterol) further improves lipid profile by raising HDL ("good") cholesterol. Unfortunately, there are real concerns that this combination therapy could cause a potentially fatal condition called *rhabdomyolysis*.

A growing body of evidence, however, suggests that the risk is relatively slight in individuals with healthy kidneys. Furthermore, even much lower doses of niacin than the usual dose given to improve cholesterol levels (100 mg versus 1,000 mg or more) may provide a similar benefit. At this dose, the risk of rhabdomyolysis should be decreased.

Nonetheless, it is not safe to try this combination except under close physician supervision. Rhabdomyolysis can be fatal.

For more information, including dosage and safety issues, see the full **Vitamin B$_3$** article.

Soluble Fiber

Water-soluble fiber supplements (such as **beta glucan** or psyllium) appear to lower cholesterol and the FDA has permitted products containing this form of fiber to carry a "heart-healthy" label. Many forms are available, ranging from oat bran to expensive fiber products sold through multilevel marketing firms. A good dose of oat bran is 5 to 10 g with each meal and at bedtime, and psyllium is taken at 10 g with each meal. However, eating a diet high in fresh fruits and vegetables and whole grains may be even better because of the many healthful nutrients such a diet contains.

Soy Protein

Soy protein appears to lower total cholesterol by about 9%, LDL ("bad") cholesterol by 13%, and triglycerides by 10%. The FDA has allowed foods containing soy protein to make the "heart-healthy" claim on the label. One study suggests that substituting as little as 20 g daily of soy protein for animal protein can significantly improve cholesterol levels.

Although it was once thought that isoflavones are the active ingredients in soy responsible for improving cholesterol profile, on balance evidence suggests otherwise.

For more information, including dosage and safety issues, see the full **Soy** article.

Artichoke Leaf

Although primarily used to stimulate gallbladder function, artichoke leaf may be helpful for high cholesterol as well.

In a double-blind, placebo-controlled study of 143 individuals with elevated cholesterol, artichoke leaf extract significantly improved cholesterol readings. Total cholesterol fell by 18.5% as compared to 8.6% in the placebo group; LDL cholesterol fell by 23% versus 6%; and the LDL to HDL ratio decreased by 20% versus 7%.

Artichoke leaf may work by interfering with cholesterol synthesis. A compound in artichoke called *luteolin* may play a role in reducing cholesterol.

For more information, including dosage and safety issues, see the full **Artichoke** article.

Other Proposed Natural Treatments

There are several other promising alternative treatments for high cholesterol. Approaches that specifically lower triglycerides (such as **fish oil**) are discussed in the High Triglycerides article.

According to numerous studies performed by a single research group, the substance policosanol can markedly improve cholesterol profile. However, these researchers own the patent on policosanol, which raises questions of conflict of interest. In 2006, the first reputable independent study of policosanol failed to find even minimal benefit; it is now unclear whether policosanol can be considered an evidence-based treatment. See the full **Policosanol** article for more information.

Red yeast rice is a traditional Chinese medicinal substance that is made by fermenting a type of yeast called *Monascus purpureus* over rice. It contains cholesterol-lowering chemicals in the **statin family**, including one identical to the drug lovastatin. Like statin drugs, red yeast rice appears to be effective for reducing cholesterol. Presumably it also presents the same safety risks as statins, compounded by the uncertainty regarding how *much* active drug any particular batch of red yeast rice contains. For more information, including complete dosage and safety issues, see the full **Red Yeast Rice** article.

In a 12-month study of 223 postmenopausal women, **calcium** supplements (calcium citrate at a dose of 1 g daily) significantly improved the ratio of HDL ("good") cholesterol to LDL ("bad") cholesterol. This appears to have been primarily due to a meaningful rise in HDL levels.

Krill are tiny shrimp-like crustaceans that flourish in the Antarctic Ocean and provide food for numerous aquatic animals. **Krill oil**, similar but not identical to fish oil, may improve cholesterol profile.

One double-blind study found evidence that **cinnamon**, taken at doses of 1 to 6 g daily, improved tryglycerides, LDL cholesterol, and total cholesterol, without worsening HDL cholesterol.

Inconsistent evidence hints that **flaxseeds** might reduce LDL cholesterol and, overall, slow down atherosclerosis. **Flaxseed oil** may be helpful as well, although evidence is again inconsistent. It may be the generic fiber and not the other specific ingredients in flaxseed that benefit cholesterol levels. Purified lignans (found in flaxseed) might *not* be helpful.

A growing body of evidence suggests that increased consumption of nuts, such as almonds, walnuts, pecans, and macadamia nuts, may improve lipid profile and reduce heart disease risk.

Some but not all studies suggest that "friendly" bacteria (**probiotics**) might be able to reduce cholesterol levels. So-called prebiotics, substances that enhance the growth of friendly bacteria, have shown inconsistent benefit in studies as well.

Both **black tea** and a special enriched **green tea** extract (high in theaflavin) have shown promise for lowering cholesterol. Green tea itself may not be helpful. A subsequent study found possible minimal enhancement in weight loss.

Other preliminary double-blind trials suggest potential benefit with the Iranian herb *Achillea wilhelmsii*, the Peruvian herb Caigua (*Cyclanterha pedata*), **carob fiber**, the Chinese caterpillar/fungus **cordyceps**, *Ipomoea batatas* (sweet potato), and a drink containing broccoli and cabbage.

Chitosan, a type of insoluble fiber derived from crustacean shells, has been proposed for reducing cholesterol levels, but current evidence suggests that if it does offer any benefits, they are minimal at best.

Weaker, and in some cases inconsistent, evidence

suggests potential benefit with berberine (found in **golden-seal**, **Oregon grape**, and **barberry**), grape polyphenols, **alfalfa**, **beta-hydroxy-beta-methylbutyrate (HMB)**, **conjugated linoleic acid (CLA)**, **L-carnitine**, **mesoglycan**, and **blue-green algae**.

Studies on whether the mineral **chromium** can improve cholesterol levels have returned mixed results. However, this mineral may offer benefit for people taking drugs in the **beta-blocker** family. These medications, used for high blood pressure and other conditions, sometimes reduce HDL cholesterol levels. Chromium supplements may offset this side effect.

One study provides preliminary evidence that the herb **black cohosh** may improve lipid profiles in post-menopausal women.

Rice bran oil, like other vegetable oils, appears to favorably change lipid profile as well as reduce heart disease risk in other ways. Weaker evidence suggests that **gamma oryzanol**, a substance found in rice bran oil, can also improve lipid profiles.

Substances related to vitamin E called *tocotrienols* are sometimes promoted as improving cholesterol levels, but the evidence regarding whether they really work remains inconsistent at best.

Other herbs and supplements sometimes recommended for high cholesterol include **ashwagandha**, **fenugreek**, **He shou wu**, and **maitake**, but there is as yet no real evidence that they work.

A number of studies published in the 1980s and 1990s reported that **garlic** preparations can lower cholesterol.

However, several more recent and generally better-designed studies have found that if any benefits exist, they are so small as to be of little help in real life.

Although **lecithin** is commonly believed to reduce cholesterol levels, evidence indicates that it does not work.

Similarly, **guggul**, the sticky gum resin from the mukul myrrh tree, has been widely marketed as a cholesterol-reducing herb. However, while preliminary studies found evidence of benefit, they all suffered from significant design flaws; a well-designed study did not find guggul effective.

Vitamin C, **cranberry**, and **elderberry** have failed to prove effective in studies thus far.

One study failed to find special fats called *medium-chain triacylglycerols* (MCTs) more effective for reducing cholesterol than ordinary unsaturated fats.

Unexpected results in a single trial hint that the sports supplement **pyruvate** might negate some of the beneficial effects of exercise on HDL levels.

Herbs and Supplements to Use Only with Caution

Various herbs and supplements may interact adversely with drugs used to treat high cholesterol. For more information on this potential risk, see the individual drug article in the Drug Interactions section of this book.

High Homocysteine

RELATED TERMS: *Hyperhomocysteinemia*

PRINCIPAL PROPOSED NATURAL TREATMENTS: *Folate, Vitamin B$_6$, Vitamin B$_{12}$*

OTHER PROPOSED NATURAL TREATMENTS: *Trimethylglycine (TMG), Phosphatidylcholine*

Beginning in the late 1990s, medical researchers began to suspect that high levels of homocysteine (a substance produced when the body breaks down the amino acid methionine) may accelerate **atherosclerosis**, the primary cause of **heart attacks**, **strokes**, and **intermittent claudication**. During a brief period, it was widely proclaimed that homocysteine was an even more important risk factor for heart disease than **cholesterol**.

However, it currently appears that reducing homocysteine provides minimal benefits, if any.

Most of the supporting evidence for a homocysteine–atherosclerosis connection comes from observational studies that found an association between high levels of homocysteine and increased atherosclerosis. Observational studies, however, do not show cause and effect. It is quite possible that unknown underlying factors increase homocysteine levels and also accelerate atherosclerosis, rather than that high homocysteine *causes* accelerated atherosclerosis. Only intervention trials (studies where people are actually given a treatment) can show whether a treatment is effective.

Several massive studies of this type were initiated in response to the observational data. The results of three such trials have now been reported, involving a total of more than 10,000 people. In these studies, high doses of supplementary vitamin B_6, vitamin B_{12}, and folate were used to lower homocysteine levels. *None* of these studies found significant benefit for preventing stroke, heart attack, or heart-related death.

A smaller study failed to find that these same homocysteine-lowering vitamins preserved mental function in people with loss of mental function caused by atherosclerosis in the brain. On one of the few positive notes, one substantial trial found that use of these homocysteine-lowering nutrients helped prevent restenosis (recurrent vessel clogging) after angioplasty.

Besides atherosclerosis, correlations have also been found between high homocysteine levels and numerous other diseases, including **Alzheimer's disease**, **osteoporosis**, **complications of pregnancy**, deep venous thrombosis, and pulmonary embolism. Again, however, most of the supporting evidence for a connection comes from observational studies and, therefore, does not prove that high homocysteine actually causes these illnesses.

One study found that in people who had already had a stroke and were partially paralyzed, supplementation with vitamin B_{12} and folate reduced the risk of falls leading to hip fractures. Participants were elderly Japanese with high levels of homocysteine and low levels of folate and B_{12}. It is not clear how the treatment produced this benefit: it might have reduced the tendency for recurrent strokes, strengthened bones, improved balance, or produced benefit by some other means.

People with **diabetes** or inflammatory bowel disease (**Crohn's disease** or **ulcerative colitis**) and those undergoing kidney dialysis may be at higher than normal risk for elevated homocysteine levels. A simple blood test can determine homocysteine levels. Both conventional and alternative practitioners use the natural substances described in the next section to treat elevated homocysteine.

Principal Proposed Natural Treatments

Three nutrients act together to help the body reduce homocysteine levels: vitamin B_6, vitamin B_{12}, and folate. Many Americans are at least marginally deficient in vitamin B_6. Vitamin B_{12} deficiency occurs primarily in seniors as well as people who take drugs that suppress stomach acid. Folate deficiency is thought to have become fairly uncommon in the U.S. due to the enrichment of grains that began in the late 1990s. However, it appears that the dose of folate required to achieve maximum homocysteine reduction was 800 mcg daily, higher than the usual nutritional recommendations.

Nonetheless, as noted above, studies utilizing high doses of these vitamins for lowering homocysteine and, therefore, preventing cardiovascular disease have generally failed to find benefit. For more information on these nutrients, including dosage and safety issues, see the full **Vitamin B_6**, **Vitamin B_{12}**, and **Folate** articles.

Other Proposed Natural Treatments

Some people develop extraordinarily high levels of homocysteine due to a genetic defect. The supplement **trimethylglycine** (TMG) is an FDA-approved treatment for this condition. TMG also seems to be effective for milder forms of high homocysteine. However, the nutrients mentioned in the previous section are less expensive and probably equally, if not more, effective at lowering homocysteine. Furthermore, TMG might raise cholesterol levels, thereby potentially undoing whatever benefit (if any) that might result from lowering homocysteine.

Phosphatidylcholine might also reduce homocysteine.

One study failed to find **soy isoflavones** helpful for reducing homocysteine levels.

High Triglycerides

RELATED TERMS: *Triglycerides, High; Hypertriglyceridemia*

PRINCIPAL PROPOSED NATURAL TREATMENTS: *Fish Oil, Niacin*

OTHER PROPOSED NATURAL TREATMENTS: Achillea wilhelmsii, *Chromium, Combined Vitamin C and Vitamin E, Creatine, Fenugreek, Flax Oil, Pantethine, Soy, Walnut Oil*

Triglycerides belong to a group of fat-related substances called *lipids.* An increase in levels of certain lipids—a condition called *hyperlipidemia*—contributes to heart disease.

To test for hyperlipidemia, physicians rely on blood tests called *lipid profiles* that measure triglycerides as well as two types of the lipid cholesterol: low-density lipoprotein (LDL) or "bad" cholesterol and high-density lipoprotein (HDL) or "good" cholesterol.

In many people with hyperlipidemia, elevation of LDL predominates. Drugs in the **statin family** work particularly well at treating this form of hyperlipidemia. (For information on natural treatments for this condition, see the **High Cholesterol** article.)

In some people with hyperlipidemia, however, high triglyceride levels are the primary problem. These people are just as much at risk for heart disease as people with elevated LDL cholesterol. Furthermore, if triglyceride levels get high enough, the pancreas may become inflamed, causing a dangerous condition called *pancreatitis.* Skin lesions called *xanthomas* may occur as well.

Common causes of elevated triglyceride levels include genetic predisposition, diabetes, excessive alcohol intake, and various medications (including **estrogen, tamoxifen, glucocorticoids, thiazide diuretics,** and some **beta-blockers**).

People with high triglycerides may not respond well to statin drugs. Instead, they may need to use high-dose **niacin** or drugs in the **fibrate family**. Exercise (with or without weight loss) also lowers triglycerides, sometimes dramatically. Diet is less effective and, in fact, a low-fat, high-carbohydrate diet may actually raise triglyceride levels.

Principal Proposed Natural Treatments

Fish oil has shown distinct promise for treating hypertriglyceridemia and a slightly modified form of fish oil (ethyl-omega-3 fatty acids) has been approved by the U.S. Food and Drug Administration (FDA) as a treatment for this condition. More than 2,000 people have participated in well-designed studies of fish oil for reducing triglyceride levels. Most studies ran from about 7 to 10 weeks.

Although not all studies have been positive, on balance it appears that fish oil supplements can reduce triglycerides by about 25 to 30%. However, the standard drug **gemfibrozil** appears to lower triglycerides to a greater extent than fish oil. **Note**: In some studies, use of fish oil has markedly raised LDL ("bad") cholesterol.

Fish oil has been studied for reducing triglyceride levels specifically in people with **diabetes** and it appears to do so safely and effectively. Furthermore, in people using statin drugs to control lipid levels, the addition of fish oil appears to improve results.

Fish oil is a source of omega-3 fatty acids, healthy fats that the body needs as much as it needs vitamins. The most important omega-3 fatty acids found in fish oil are named EPA (eicosapentaenoic acid) and DHA (docosahexaenoic acid). According to some, but not all, studies, EPA may have a greater triglyceride-lowering effect than DHA.

For more information, including dosage and safety issues, see the full **Fish Oil** article.

Other Proposed Natural Treatments

Numerous studies indicate that **soy** can reduce total and LDL cholesterol, especially when it replaces animal protein in the diet and on this basis it has been approved for a "heart healthy" label by the FDA. Soy also appears to modestly improve triglyceride levels.

The supplement **pantethine** is widely promoted as a natural treatment for hypertriglyceridemia. However, the evidence that it works rests on small studies with somewhat inconsistent results.

In people with type 2 diabetes, use of **chromium** may reduce triglyceride levels, according to some but not all preliminary trials.

However, chromium does not appear to be effective for reducing triglyceride levels in people *without* diabetes.

Other herbs and supplements that have shown promise for reducing triglyceride levels include **fenugreek**, **creatine**, and *Achillea wilhelmsii*.

The drug **tamoxifen** has a tendency to raise triglyceride levels. In an open study, simultaneous use of **vitamin C** (500 mg daily) and **vitamin E** (400 mg daily) counteracted this side effect.

The supplement **flax oil** contains omega-3 fatty acids similar but not identical to those found in fish oil. It has been proposed as an alternative to fish oil because it does not cause fishy burps. However, evidence suggests that flax oil is not as effective as fish oil for reducing triglycerides.

Walnut oil has shown some promise for reducing triglycerides.

Most natural treatments used to reduce cholesterol have the potential to reduce triglyceride levels as well. For more information on these many options, see the full **High Cholesterol** article.

HIV Support

RELATED TERMS: *Acquired Immunodeficiency Syndrome, AIDS, Human Immunodeficiency Virus*

PRINCIPAL PROPOSED NATURAL TREATMENTS: *None*

OTHER PROPOSED NATURAL TREATMENTS:

For Inhibiting Viral Replication: *Aloe, Astragalus, Bacailin, Boxwood Extract, Curcumin, Elderberry, Propolis, Reishi, Schisandra, Spirulina*

For Enhancing the Immune System: *Carnitine, Coenzyme Q_{10}, DHEA, Echinacea, Fish Oil, Ginseng, Licorice, Lipoic Acid, Maitake, Massage Therapy,* Momordica charantia, *N-Acetyl Cysteine, Omega-6 Fatty Acids, Proteolytic Enzymes, Trichosanthin, Whey Protein*

For Fighting Weight Loss: *Glutamine, Medium-chain Triglycerides (MCTs), Whey Protein*

For Treating Other Symptoms as well as Opportunistic Infections: *Bovine Colostrum, Chinese Herb Combinations, Cinnamon, DHEA, Tea Tree Oil*

For Treating Medication Side Effects: *Carnitine, CoenzymeQ$_{10}$, Glutamine, Vitamin B$_{12}$, Zinc*

For General Nutrition Support: *Beta-carotene, Iron, Multivitamins, Niacin, Selenium, Vitamin A, Vitamin B$_1$, Vitamin B$_2$, Vitamin B$_6$, Vitamin B$_{12}$, Vitamin C, Vitamin E, Zinc*

Natural Treatments to Avoid: *Garlic, St. John's Wort*

Note: *None of these treatments has been proven effective as yet for the uses cited above.*

Human immunodeficiency virus, or HIV, is the virus responsible for AIDS (acquired immunodeficiency syndrome). This virus progressively destroys or damages cells in the immune system, making its host vulnerable to certain cancers and infections. Opportunistic infections—caused by microorganisms that do not ordinarily cause illness in healthy people—can have serious or even fatal effects in people with AIDS.

Within a month or two of exposure, infection with HIV may cause short-term flu-like symptoms, followed by a symptom-free period lasting months to years during which the virus continues to multiply. After this stage, people with HIV may develop swollen lymph nodes, recurrent herpes sores, diarrhea, weight loss, and/or chronic yeast infections (oral or vaginal)—a state previously called *AIDS-related complex* or ARC. Children may experience delayed development or fail to thrive. The infection is called *AIDS* when the number of immune cells known as CD4+, or helper T-cells, drops below a certain level, or when opportunistic diseases such as *Pneumocystis carinii* pneumonia develop. Today, both ARC and AIDS are collectively called *symptomatic HIV infection*. This condition is increasingly rare in the developed world due to the success of pharmaceutical treatments and, for many people, HIV infection is a manageable, if challenging, chronic illness.

HIV is spread most commonly through unsafe sexual practices or by intravenous drug abuse. Mothers can infect their babies before or during birth, or later through breast-feeding.

The most effective treatment for HIV is called *HAART*, or *highly active antiretroviral therapy*. This approach generally involves the combined use of three or more drugs, taken from various families of antiretroviral drugs, including nonnucleoside reverse transcriptase inhibitors (NNRTIs), nucleoside reverse transcriptase inhibitors (NRTIs), fusion inhibitors, and protease inhibitors. Taken together, these medications can prevent the development of AIDS indefinitely. HAART, however, causes numerous side effects. Surveys have shown that people with HIV often take natural remedies in addition to conventional medications, in hopes of reducing side effects and enhancing efficacy. If you have HIV, it is particularly important to talk with your doctors about any natural substances you're taking and to be alert to possible interactions. Most importantly, people with HIV should not use St. John's wort or garlic, and even vitamin C may pose risks (see Natural Treatments to Avoid, below).

Proposed Natural Treatments for HIV

Among the many proposed natural treatments for HIV, none has more than preliminary supporting evidence.

Inhibiting Viral Replication

No natural remedies rival the effectiveness of antiretroviral drugs for inhibiting HIV replication in the body. However, preliminary research suggests that an extract of the leaves and stems of the boxwood shrub may have at least some efficacy. Many other herbs and supplements have been proposed as well, but there is little evidence as yet that they work.

➢ Boxwood

In a double-blind, placebo-controlled study of 145 people with HIV, French researchers studied the effects of two doses of a preparation made from the evergreen boxwood (*Buxus sempervirens*). The preparation was given in doses of 990 mg and 1,980 mg per day for periods ranging from 4 to 64 weeks.

When participants started the study, they had no symptoms of HIV and had never taken antiretroviral drugs. They were kept off anti-HIV drugs during the study (this was before the use of anti-HIV drugs became widespread). At the end, researchers found that among those taking the lower dose, fewer people developed AIDS, symptomatic HIV, or CD4+ counts below 200 compared with those taking the higher dose or placebo. Additionally, by the end of their treatment period, fewer people in the low-dose group had a large increase in the amount of HIV virus they carried compared to the other two groups.

The researchers had originally planned the study to continue for 18 months (78 weeks). However, as the study progressed, a review committee decided to halt the study early when the average participant had taken boxwood or placebo for only 37 weeks. The review committee felt it was unethical to continue to have some people take placebo, given the positive results among those taking the extract. Nonetheless, further research is necessary to confirm the effectiveness of boxwood extract for HIV, particularly in combination with proven antiviral drugs, which have now become the standard of care for HIV infection.

No severe side effects were reported in this study and the people taking boxwood had the same overall rate of side effects as those taking placebo.

However, there are some safety concerns with this herb. A substance called *cycloprotobuxine* is believed to be one of the active ingredients in boxwood. High doses of this substance can cause vomiting, diarrhea, muscular spasms, and paralysis. **Warning**: For this reason, the herb should only be taken under medical supervision! Safety in pregnant or nursing women, young children, or people with liver or kidney disease has not been established. In addition, touching fresh boxwood leaves can occasionally cause skin irritation.

Note: Only a special boxwood extract has been studied as a treatment for HIV infection. Do not try to use raw boxwood leaf, as it might not be safe.

➢ *Other Proposed Natural Treatments*

One of the constituents of the herb **aloe**, acemannan, has shown some promise in test tube and animal studies for stimulating immunity and inhibiting the growth of viruses, including the HIV. These findings have led to trials of acemannan (or whole aloe) for the treatment of HIV infection. However, a double-blind, placebo-controlled trial of acemannan failed to find any benefits for people with severe HIV infection. (Interestingly, there is some question whether the effects seen in these studies were actually due to acemannan itself or a contaminant called *aloeride*.)

Other substances that have been investigated for possible HIV suppression include **astragalus**, **bacailin** (Chinese skullcap), **curcumin**, **elderberry**, **propolis**, **schisandra**, **spirulina**, and **reishi**. However, as with aloe, the evidence that they work is primarily limited to test tube and animal studies; whether these results translate into real improvement among people with HIV has yet to be determined.

The herb St. John's wort contains a substance called *hypericin* which has been investigated for possible anti-HIV effects. However, contrary to popular belief, neither hypericin nor St. John's wort are at all useful for treating HIV. In addition, St. John's wort seriously impairs the activity of standard HIV medications and might lead to treatment failure. (See Natural Treatments to Avoid, below.)

Enhancing the Immune System

In test-tube studies, a number of substances have been found to improve measures of immunity in HIV infection, for example, by elevating CD4+ counts, changing the ratio between CD4+ cells and other immune cells, increasing amounts of other immune chemicals, or enhancing the body's ability to attack invading substances. However, there is relatively little information on whether they can actually help people with HIV infection.

➢ NAC

One of the natural substances most widely used by people with HIV in hopes of enhancing immune system function is the antioxidant **N-acetyl cysteine** (NAC), but evidence that it helps is somewhat conflicting.

NAC is a specially modified form of the dietary amino acid cysteine. NAC supplements help the body make the important antioxidant enzyme **glutathione**. Early human trials, including a double-blind study of 45 people, suggest that NAC may increase levels of CD4+ cells in healthy people and slow CD4+ cell decline in people with HIV. Another study of NAC combined with selenium had mixed results, affecting T-cell counts in some people but not others. However, preliminary results of yet another study found that NAC had no effect on CD4+ counts or the amount of HIV virus in the blood. **Whey protein** also contains cysteine and may increase glutathione levels, but there is no evidence as yet of any meaningful benefit.

➢ Other Proposed Natural Treatments

Other natural treatments that are sometimes recommended to boost immunity in HIV include **andrographis**, trichosanthin (compound *Q*), **lipoic acid**, **coenzyme Q$_{10}$**, **maitake**, a component of **licorice** known as *glycyrrhizin*, the herb *Momordica charantia* (also called *bitter melon*), **echinacea**, **ginseng**, **omega-6 fatty acids**, **carnitine**, **DHEA**, and **proteolytic enzymes**. However, there is no real evidence as yet that these treatments actually work. **Garlic** is sometimes recommended as well; however, for safety reasons it should be avoided in HIV infection. (See Natural Treatments to Avoid, below.)

Fish oil is also sometimes recommended for enhancing immunity in HIV infection. However, one 6-month, double-blind study found that a combination of the omega-3 fatty acids in fish oil plus the amino acid arginine was no more effective than placebo in improving immune function in people with HIV.

Study results are mixed on whether **massage therapy** can improve measures of immune function in people with HIV.

Treating Other Symptoms of HIV as Well as Opportunistic Infections

Besides the treatments mentioned earlier, a number of natural remedies have been proposed for symptoms of HIV or common opportunistic infections.

Bovine colostrum has been suggested as a treatment for the chronic diarrhea that commonly occurs in people with HIV or AIDS, but the evidence that it works is weak at best.

Tea tree oil and **cinnamon** have been suggested as treatments for thrush (oral candida infection).

Dehydroepiandrosterone (DHEA) is a hormone that seems to decrease in people with AIDS, possibly because of malnutrition and/or stress. One small double-blind trial suggests that DHEA (50 mg per day) may improve mood and fatigue scores in people with HIV; another small trial found inconclusive results. A more substantial (145-participant) double-blind study found that DHEA at a dose of 100 to 400 mg daily improved symptoms of dysthymia (minor **depression**) in people with HIV, without significant adverse effects.

Chinese herbal combinations have been investigated for the treatment of HIV, but the results have not been very promising. In a 12-week, double-blind, placebo-controlled trial, 30 HIV-infected adults with

CD4+ counts of 200 to 500 were given a Chinese herbal formula containing 31 herbs. The results hint that use of the herbal combination might have improved various symptoms compared to placebo, but none of the differences were statistically significant. Interestingly, people who believed they were taking the real treatment showed significant benefit regardless of whether they were in the placebo group or the real treatment group.

In another double-blind, placebo-controlled trial, 68 HIV-infected adults were given either placebo or a preparation of 35 Chinese herbs for a period of 6 months. The results indicate that use of Chinese herbs did not improve symptoms or objective measurements of HIV severity. In fact, people using the herbs reported *more* digestive problems than those given placebo.

Fighting Weight Loss

Undesired weight loss is a frequent symptom of HIV and AIDS. Sometimes weight loss is so extreme that the person seems to "waste away"—hence the name *AIDS wasting syndrome*, which is technically defined as the loss of more than 10% of body weight combined with either chronic diarrhea or weakness and fever. Many factors can contribute to this weight loss, including loss of appetite, nausea, malabsorption of nutrients, and mouth sores.

Supplemental MCTs and glutamine may be helpful for this symptom, although there is no definitive evidence as yet that they work.

➤ *MCTs*

Fat malabsorption is particularly common in HIV infection, and can lead to both diarrhea and weight loss. A particular type of fat known as *medium-chain triglycerides* (MCTs) is more easily absorbed than ordinary fats (long-chain triglycerides) and may help decrease diarrhea and wasting. Two small double-blind studies have found that MCTs are more easily absorbed than long-chain triglycerides in people with HIV or AIDS. However, there is no direct evidence as yet that MCTs actually help people gain weight.

In both of the studies described above, participants consumed nothing but a special nutritional formula containing MCTs. Taking MCTs in this way requires medical supervision to determine the dose.

People with HIV or diabetes should not use MCTs (or any other supplement) without a doctor's supervision. For more information, including dosage and safety issues, see the full **MCTs** article.

➤ *Glutamine*

Another promising treatment for wasting is the amino acid **glutamine**, a substance that plays a role in maintaining the health of the immune system, digestive tract, and muscle cells. Although research is still preliminary, one double-blind, placebo-controlled study found that a combination of glutamine and antioxidants (**vitamins C and E**, **beta-carotene**, **selenium**, and N-acetyl cysteine) led to significant weight gain in people with HIV who had lost weight.

Another small double-blind trial found that combination treatment with glutamine, **arginine**, and **beta-hydroxy beta-methylbutyrate** (HMB) could increase muscle mass and possibly improve immune status.

➤ *Other Natural Treatments*

Whey protein is sometimes recommended for weight gain in HIV, but evidence that it works is preliminary at best. One study found that while exercise improved weight gain, whey protein alone or in combination with exercise offered no benefit. Fish oil might be helpful for weight gain, however.

Treating Medication Side Effects

Several natural treatments have been proposed to treat side effects from various medications used in the treatment of HIV.

Reverse transcriptase inhibitors, such as lamivudine and zidovudine, may damage mitochondria, the energy-producing subunits of cells. The supplement CoQ_{10} has been tried for minimizing side effects attributed to mitochondrial damage. In one study, use of CoQ_{10} improved sense of well-being in asymptomatic people with HIV infection; however, it actually worsened pain symptoms in people with peripheral neuropathy.

Taking AZT can lead to **zinc** deficiency, which may interfere with immune function. One partially blinded study found that zinc supplements may benefit people on AZT. In the zinc-treated group, body weight increased or stabilized, CD4+ count rose, and participants had significantly fewer opportunistic infections.

Carnitine has also been proposed as a treatment for AZT side effects, based on very early evidence that it may keep AZT from damaging muscle cells.

Based on highly preliminary evidence, **vitamin B_{12}** has been suggested as a preventive for blood abnormalities caused by AZT.

In one well-designed double-blind study, use of the amino acid glutamine at a dose of 30 g daily significantly reduced the diarrhea caused by the protease inhibitor **nelfinavir**. Presumably, glutamine would be helpful for other protease inhibitors as well.

It has been suggested that the supplement NAC might help prevent side effects from the antibiotic trimethoprim-sulfamethoxazole (TMP-SMX). However, two controlled studies found that NAC did not significantly decrease adverse reactions to TMP-SMX. Note, however, that TMP-SMX is known to decrease **folate** levels in the body, and folate supplements might therefore be useful.

The herb **milk thistle** is sometimes recommended for preventing liver problems related to use of HIV medications. While there is no direct evidence that it is helpful for this purpose, there is fairly good evidence at least that use of milk thistle does not *adversely* affect blood levels of indinavir.

General Nutrition Support

People infected with HIV may be particularly vulnerable to malnutrition because of decreased appetite, poor absorption, or possibly increased requirements for specific nutrients. Studies have found deficiencies of **vitamins A, B_1, B_6, B_{12}, and E, beta-carotene, choline**, folate, selenium, and zinc to be common among people with HIV infection. Many deficiencies become more common as the disease worsens. This suggests, but does not prove, that taking supplements of these nutrients may be helpful.

Note: One study evaluated whether use of a **multivitamin** tablet might reduce infectivity of African women with HIV and unexpectedly found the opposite: multivitamin tablets increase the levels of HIV virus present in the genital area. The reason for this surprising finding is unknown. It is not clear whether the same response would occur among people living in developed countries who, presumably, have better underlying nutrition.

❧ *Vitamin A, Beta-carotene, and Mixed Carotenoids*

Vitamin A and beta-carotene are described together here because the body uses beta-carotene to produce vitamin A. Substances called *carotenoids* are closely related to vitamin A; this family includes **lutein** and **lycopene**.

Vitamin A deficiency may be linked to lower CD4+ counts as well as higher death rates among people in-

fected with HIV. A few preliminary studies have raised hopes that beta-carotene supplements might increase or preserve immune function or decrease symptoms among people with HIV. One small double-blind study suggested that taking beta-carotene might raise white blood cell count in people with HIV. However, two subsequent larger controlled trials found no significant differences between those taking beta-carotene or placebo in white blood cell count, CD4+ count, or other measures of immune function.

Two observational studies lasting 6 to 8 years suggest that higher intakes of vitamin A or beta-carotene may be helpful, but they also found that caution is in order with regard to dosage. This group of researchers generally linked higher intake of vitamin A or beta-carotene to lower risk of AIDS and lower death rates, with an important exception: people with the highest intake of either nutrient (more than 11,179 IU per day of beta-carotene, more than 20,268 IU per day of vitamin A) did worse than those who took somewhat less.

Note: Keep in mind also that excessive dosages of vitamin A can be toxic to the liver. Consult with your physician on the right dose for you. For other dosage and safety issues, see the full articles on **beta-carotene** and **vitamin A**.

Despite hopes that vitamin A given to pregnant, HIV-positive women might decrease the infection rate of their babies, two double-blind studies have found no significant differences between babies whose mothers took vitamin A and babies whose mothers took placebo. In any case, vitamin A is not considered safe in pregnancy; beta-carotene is preferred.

One double-blind study found statistically weak evidence that use of mixed carotenoids by AIDS patients might prolong life.

❧ *B Vitamins*

An observational study found that HIV-positive men with the highest intakes of vitamin B_1, B_2, B_6, and niacin had significantly longer survival rates, while a similar study found that those taking the most B_1 or niacin had a significantly lower rate of developing AIDS.

Vitamin B_{12} deficiencies in people infected with HIV have been linked to neurologic symptoms, including slower processing of information in studies of cognitive functioning; early research suggests that restoring B_{12} levels to normal may decrease these symptoms. B_{12}-deficiency has also been linked to lower CD4+ counts and more rapid development of AIDS.

Vitamin B_6–deficiency has been linked to impaired immune function in one study of people with HIV infection.

Note: Excessive intake of vitamin B_6 can cause neurologic problems. Consult with your physician on the right dose for you. For other dosage and safety issues, see the full **Vitamin B_6** article.

≽ Vitamins C and E

Massive doses of vitamin C have at times been popular among people with HIV based on highly preliminary evidence. An observational study linked high doses of vitamin C with slower progression to AIDS. High intake of vitamin E was also linked to decreased risk of progression to AIDS in a different observational study.

However, a double-blind study of 49 people with HIV who took combined vitamins C and E or placebo for 3 months did not show any significant effects on the amount of HIV virus detected or the number of opportunistic infections. It has been suggested that vitamin E may enhance the antiviral effects of AZT, but evidence for this is minimal.

≽ Choline

The substance choline has been newly added to the list of essential nutrients. Evidence suggests that people with HIV who are low in choline may experience more rapid disease progression.

≽ Iron

A study of 71 HIV-positive children noted a high rate of **iron** deficiency. One observational study of 296 men with HIV infection linked high intake of iron to a decreased risk of AIDS 6 years later.

Note: Do not take iron supplements unless you know that you are iron-deficient.

≽ Selenium

Selenium is required for a well-functioning immune system. Observational studies have linked higher levels of selenium in the blood with higher CD4+ counts and reduced risk of mortality from HIV disease. Selenium deficiency may also increase the infectiousness of women with HIV. In one double-blind, placebo-controlled study, use of selenium at a dose of 200 mcg decreased anxiety in patients undergoing HAART.

However, in a controlled study of 52 people with HIV, selenium did not improve the clinical conditions or raise CD4+ counts any more than no treatment. A study of selenium combined with NAC had mixed results, affecting T-cell counts in some people but not others.

Selenium has also been proposed as a preventive or treatment for cardiomyopathy, a disorder of the heart muscle that can affect people with AIDS, but evidence so far is weak.

≽ Zinc

Some but not all studies have found that HIV-positive people tend to be deficient in zinc, with levels dropping lower in more severe disease. But does this mean that taking zinc will help? The answer is not clear.

Higher zinc levels have been linked to better immune function and higher CD4+ cell counts, whereas zinc deficiency has been linked to increased risk of dying from HIV. One preliminary study among people taking AZT found that 30 days of zinc supplementation led to decreased rates of opportunistic infection over the following 2 years.

However, other research has linked higher zinc intake to more rapid development of AIDS. In another study of HIV-positive people, those with higher zinc intake or those taking zinc supplements in any dosage had a greater risk of death within the following 8 years.

≽ Multivitamins

Because so many nutrients are affected by HIV infection and treatments, multivitamin supplements are a logical choice.

Researchers interviewed 296 men with HIV but not AIDS about their diets and multivitamin use, then followed their progress for 6 years. Those who took a daily multivitamin had a significantly lower risk of developing AIDS during the study. In a similar study, HIV-positive men who took supplements of vitamin B_1, B_2, or B_6, at levels higher than the Recommended Dietary Allowance (RDA) early in the course of their disease had lower death rates 8 years later.

Natural Treatments to Avoid

People using HIV medications should not take **St. John's wort**. In a study of healthy volunteers, St. John's wort was found to decrease the blood concentration of indinavir, one of the most widely used **protease inhibitors**, by 49 to 99%. This could lead to treatment failure as well as the emergence of resistant strains of the HIV virus. St.

John's wort also appears to interact with non-nucleoside reverse transcriptase inhibitors (NNRTIs), such as nevirapine.

Garlic may also combine poorly with certain HIV medications. Two people with HIV experienced severe gastrointestinal toxicity from the protease inhibitor ritonavir after taking garlic supplements and another study found that garlic might interfere with the action of the protease inhibitor saquinavir, reducing blood levels of the medication.

One study found, rather surprisingly, that vitamin C at a dose of 1 g daily substantially reduced blood levels of indinavir.

Other possible harmful effects discussed elsewhere in this article include worsening of peripheral neuropathy symptoms by CoQ_{10} and increase of infectivity attributable to use of multivitamins. If you have HIV, talk with your doctor before using any herb or supplement, no matter how harmless it may seem. Given the large numbers of drugs, herbs, and supplements taken by many people with HIV, the possibility of interactions is high.

Hypertension

RELATED TERMS: *High Blood Pressure*

PRINCIPAL PROPOSED NATURAL TREATMENTS: *Biofeedback, Coenzyme Q_{10} (CoQ$_{10}$), Stevia*

OTHER PROPOSED NATURAL TREATMENTS: *Ayurvedic Herbal Combinations, Bacailin, Barberry, Calcium, Chocolate, Cordyceps, Fiber, Fish Oil, Garlic, Glucomannan, Grape Juice, Hibiscus,* Achillea wilhelmsii, *Maca, Magnesium, Melatonin, Olive Leaf, Milk Fermented by Probiotics, Potassium, Vitamin C*

HERBS AND SUPPLEMENTS TO USE ONLY WITH CAUTION: Citrus Aurantium, *Soy Isoflavones, Vitamin C Plus OPCs, Vitamin E*

Most people can't tell when their blood pressure is high, which is why hypertension is called the *silent killer*. In this case, what you don't know can hurt you. Elevated blood pressure can lead to a greatly increased risk of **heart attack**, **stroke**, and many other serious illnesses. Along with **high cholesterol** and **smoking**, hypertension is one of the most important causes of atherosclerosis. In turn, atherosclerosis causes heart attacks, strokes, and other diseases of impaired circulation.

The mechanism by which high blood pressure produces atherosclerosis is somewhat similar to what happens in a hose fitted with a high-pressure nozzle. All such nozzles come with a warning label that states, "Make sure to discharge pressure in hose after using." Unfortunately, many people frequently fail to pay attention to the warning and leave the hose puffed up with full pressure overnight. This rather common practice does not produce any immediate consequences. The hose doesn't develop leaks at the seams or burst outright on the first occasion you leave it untended. However, a garden hose that is frequently left under pressure will begin to age more rapidly than it would otherwise. Its lining will begin to crack, its flexibility will diminish, and within a season or two the hose will be sprouting leaks in all directions.

Similarly, when blood vessels are exposed to constantly high pressure, a similar process is set in motion. Blood pressures as elevated as 220/170 (systolic pressure/diastolic pressure), quite common during activities such as weight lifting, do no harm. Only when excessive pressure is sustained day and night do blood vessel linings begin to be injured and undergo those unhealthy changes known as *atherosclerosis*.

Thus, although it is important to lower blood pressure with all deliberate speed, only rarely does it need to be lowered instantly. In most situations, you have plenty of time to work on bringing down your blood pressure. However, that doesn't mean that you should ignore it.

Over time, high blood pressure can damage nearly every organ in the body.

The best way to determine your blood pressure is to take several readings at different times during the day and on different days of the week. Blood pressure readings will vary quite a bit from moment to moment; what matters most is the average blood pressure. Thus, if many low readings balance out a few high readings, the net result may be satisfactory. However, it is essential not to ignore a high value by saying, "I was just stressed then." Stress is part of life, and if it raises your blood pressure once, it will do so again. To come up with an accurate number, you must include every measurement in your calculations.

In most cases, the cause of hypertension is unknown. The kidneys play an important role in controlling blood pressure, and the level of squeezing tension in the blood vessels makes a large contribution as well.

Lifestyle changes can dramatically reduce blood pressure. Aerobic exercise is clearly helpful, and one study found that engaging in aerobic exercise 60 to 90 minutes weekly may be sufficient for producing maximum benefits. Another study found that taking four 10-minute "exercise snacks" of brisk walking per day significantly improves blood pressure. **Stopping smoking** and **losing weight** are also highly effective.

For many years doctors advised patients with hypertension to cut down on salt in the diet. Today, however, the value of this stressful dietary change has undergone significant questioning. Considering how rapidly our knowledge is evolving, we suggest consulting your physician to learn the latest recommendations.

If lifestyle changes fail to reduce blood pressure or if you can't make these alterations, many effective drugs are available. Sometimes you need to experiment with a few to find one that agrees with you.

Principal Proposed Natural Treatments

There are no herbs or supplements for hypertension with solid scientific support. The supplement CoenzymeQ$_{10}$ and extracts from the herb *Stevia rebaudiana* have shown some promise in preliminary trials. Fairly good evidence supports use of biofeedback, but the benefits seen are quite small.

CoenzymeQ$_{10}$

The supplement coenzyme Q$_{10}$ (CoQ$_{10}$) has shown promise as a treatment for high blood pressure, but the evidence that it works is not yet strong.

An 8-week, double-blind, placebo-controlled study of 59 men already taking medication for high blood pressure found that 120 mg daily of CoQ$_{10}$ reduced blood pressure by about 9% as compared to placebo.

In addition, a 12-week, double-blind, placebo-controlled study of 83 people with isolated systolic hypertension (a type of high blood pressure in which only the "top" number is high) found that use of CoQ$_{10}$ at a dose of 60 mg daily improved blood pressure measurements to a similar extent.

Also, in a 12-week, double-blind, placebo-controlled trial of 74 people with diabetes, use of CoQ$_{10}$ at a dose of 100 mg twice daily significantly reduced blood pressure as compared to placebo.

Antihypertensive effects were also seen in earlier smaller trials, but most of them were not double-blind, and therefore mean little.

For more information, including dosage and safety issues, see the full **CoQ$_{10}$** article.

Stevia

The herb stevia is best known as a sweetener. Its active ingredients are known as *steviosides*. In a 1-year, double-blind, placebo-controlled study of 106 people with moderate hypertension (approximately 165/103), steviosides at a dose of 250 mg 3 times daily reduced blood pressure by approximately 10%. Full benefits took months to develop. However, this study is notable for finding no benefits at all in the placebo group. This is unusual and tends to cast doubt on the results.

Benefits were also reported in a 2-year, double-blind, placebo-controlled study of 174 people with milder hypertension (average initial BP of approximately 150/95). This study used twice the dose of the previous study: 500 mg 3 times daily. A reduction in blood pressure of approximately 6 to 7% was seen in the treatment group as compared to the placebo group, beginning within 1 week and enduring throughout the entire 2 years. At the end of the study, 34% of those in the placebo group showed heart damage from high blood pressure (left ventricular hypertrophy), while only 11.5% of the stevioside group did, a difference that was statistically significant. No significant adverse effects were seen.

However, once again, no benefits at all were seen in the placebo group. This is a red flag for problems in study design. Both these studies were performed in China, a country that has a documented history of questionable medical study results.

For more information, including dosage and safety issues, see the full **Stevia** article.

Biofeedback

Biofeedback, a technique for gaining conscious control over involuntary bodily functions, has shown considerable promise for the treatment of mild hypertension. One review of the literature found 23 controlled trials on the subject of acceptable quality. Taken as a whole, these studies suggest that biofeedback can reduce blood pressure by approximately 5%, a modest but useful improvement.

For more information, see the **Biofeedback** article.

Other Proposed Natural Treatments

Numerous natural treatments have shown some promise for hypertension.

The Iranian herb *Achillea wilhelmsii* was tested in a double-blind trial of 60 men and women with mild hypertension. The results showed that treatment with an *A. wilhelmsii* extract significantly reduced blood pressure readings. In a double-blind study of 43 men and women with hypertension, use of a proprietary **Ayurvedic herbal combination** containing *Terminali arjuna* and about 40 other herbs proved approximately as effective for controlling blood pressure as the drug methyldopa.

Although the research record is mixed, it appears that **fish oil** may reduce blood pressure at least slightly. Fish oil contains two major active ingredients, DHA (docosahexaenoic acid) and EPA (eicosapentaenoic acid). Some evidence suggests that it is the DHA in fish oil, but not the EPA, that is responsible for this benefit.

Several studies have found that **glucomannan**, a dietary fiber derived from the tubers of *Amorphophallus konjac*, may improve high blood pressure. Other forms of fiber may be helpful as well.

Milk fermented by certain **probiotics** (friendly bacteria) may provide at least a small blood pressure–lowering effect.

People who are deficient in **calcium** may be at great risk of developing high blood pressure. Among people who already have hypertension, increased intake of calcium intake might slightly decrease blood pressure, according to some but not all studies.

Study results are mixed on whether **magnesium** or **potassium** supplements can improve blood pressure. At most, the benefit is quite small.

In a 30-day, double-blind, placebo-controlled study of 39 people taking medications for hypertension, treatment with 500 mg of **vitamin C** daily reduced blood pressure by about 10%. Smaller benefits were seen in studies of people with normal blood pressure or borderline hypertension. One double-blind study compared 500 mg, 1,000 mg, and 2,000 mg of vitamin C, and found an equivalent level of benefit in all three groups. (Because of the lack of a placebo group, this study cannot be used as proof of effectiveness, only as a demonstration of the equivalence of the doses.) However, other studies have failed to find evidence of benefit with vitamin C. This mixed evidence suggests, on balance, that if vitamin C does have any blood pressure–lowering effect, it is at most quite modest. Unexpectedly, one study found that a combination of vitamin C (500 mg daily) and grape seed **OPCs** (1,000 mg daily) slightly *increased* blood pressure. Whether this was a fluke of statistics or a real combined effect remains unclear.

Several flawed studies hint that the herb **garlic** may lower blood pressure slightly, perhaps by 5 to 10%.

One small study found possible benefit with sweetie fruit (a hybrid between grapefruit and pummelo), apparently due to its **citrus bioflavonoid** content. Tomato extract, rich in **lycopene**, has also shown promise.

Two small double-blind, placebo-controlled studies found evidence that **melatonin** taken at 2.5 to 3 mg before bedtime may slightly reduce nighttime blood pressure.

Other preliminary studies suggest possible benefit with **beta-hydroxy-beta-methylbutyrate** (HMB), **blue-green algae** products, **chitosan**, cocoa, concord grape juice, green coffee bean extract, various forms of the herb **hawthorn**, **hibiscus**, **kelp**, and **soy protein** (but see note about soy isoflavones below). However, for none of these is the supporting evidence reliable.

Getting adequate **vitamin D** may help prevent the development of hypertension.

The vitamin **folate** may help decrease blood pressure (as well as provide other heart healthy effects) in smokers.

The herbs **astragalus, bacailin, barberry,** *Coleus forskohlii,* **maitake, maca, olive leaf** and the supplements **beta-carotene, cordyceps, flaxseed oil,** and **taurine** are sometimes recommended for high blood pressure, but as yet there is no meaningful evidence that they work.

One study quoted as showing that a **Traditional Chinese herbal formula** can reduce blood pressure actually failed to find any effect on blood pressure.

Hatha yoga and **Tai Chi** have shown some potential benefit for high blood pressure.

Hyperthyroidism

In a 12-week study of 140 men and women with stage I hypertension, **chiropractic spinal manipulation** plus dietary change did not produce any greater benefit than dietary change alone.

Finally, because atherosclerosis is the main harm caused by hypertension, treatments discussed in the **Atherosclerosis** article should be considered as well.

Herbs and Supplements to Use Only with Caution

There is one highly credible case report of severe, dangerous hypertension caused by consumption of **soy isoflavones** during the course of a clinical trial on this supplement. This is most likely a rare, highly individual response, but if it could occur with one person, it could occur with another as well.

As noted above, in one study, a combination of vitamin C and grape seed OPCs mildly increased blood pressure. In another study, use of vitamin E raised blood pressure in people with type 2 diabetes.

The herb *citrus aurantium* (bitter orange) may increase blood pressure.

In addition, various herbs and supplements may interact adversely with drugs used to treat hypertension. For more information on this potential risk, see the individual drug article in the Drug Interactions section of this book.

Hyperthyroidism

RELATED TERMS: *Graves' Disease; Thyroid Hormone, Excess; Thyrotoxicosis*

PRINCIPAL PROPOSED NATURAL TREATMENTS: *None*

OTHER PROPOSED NATURAL TREATMENTS: *Bugleweed, L-Carnitine, Motherwort*

HERBS AND SUPPLEMENTS TO AVOID: *Ashwaghanda, Bladderwrack, Kelp*

Hyperthyroidism is a condition in which the thyroid gland releases excessive amounts of thyroid hormone. Symptoms include the following:

➤ **Weight loss**
➤ **Fatigue**
➤ **Fast heart rate**
➤ **Heart palpitations**
➤ **Intolerance to heat**
➤ **Insomnia**
➤ **Anxiety**
➤ **Frequent bowel movements**
➤ **Scant menstruation**
➤ **Bone thinning**
➤ **Hair loss**
➤ **Changes in the appearance of the eye (bulging or staring)**
➤ **Goiter (a visible enlargement of the neck caused by a swollen thyroid gland)**

The most common form of hyperthyroidism is Graves' disease. In this condition, the body manufactures antibodies that have the unintended effect of stimulating the thyroid gland. (In another condition, **Hashimoto's thyroiditis**, the body produces antibodies that decrease thyroid output.) In addition, benign tumors of the thyroid can secrete excessive thyroid hormone on their own (cancerous tumors seldom do). Viral infection of the thyroid (subacute thyroiditis) causes short-lived hyperthyroidism followed by a more prolonged period of **hypothyroidism**.

Medical treatment of hyperthyroidism is highly effective. In most cases of ongoing hyperthyroidism, radioactive iodine is used to destroy thyroid tissue. This approach is both safe and effective, because almost all the iodine in the body ends up in the thyroid and, therefore, the radioactive treatment does not damage any other tissues. Other approaches to hyperthyroidism include drugs to block the effects of high thyroid hormone or to slow thyroid hormone production, as well as, in relatively rare cases, surgery.

Proposed Natural Treatments

Physician supervision is necessary to determine why the thyroid is overactive in order to design a specific treatment plan. None of the treatments discussed in this section actually get to the root of the problem, nor have they been proven effective. Self-treatment of hyperthyroidism is not recommended.

Test tube and animal studies suggest that the herb **bugleweed** may reduce thyroid hormone by decreasing levels of TSH (the hormone that stimulates the thyroid gland) and by impairing thyroid hormone synthesis. In addition, bugleweed may block the action of thyroid-stimulating antibodies found in Graves' disease.

The supplement **L-carnitine** has shown promise for treating a special form of hyperthyroidism that may occur during the treatment of benign goiter. People with benign goiter often take thyroid hormone pills as treatment. Sometimes successful treatment of this condition requires taking slightly more thyroid hormone than the body needs, resulting in symptoms of mild hyperthyroidism. A double-blind, placebo-controlled trial found evidence that use of the supplement L-carnitine could alleviate many of these symptoms. This 6-month study evaluated the effects of L-carnitine in 50 women who were taking thyroid hormone for be-

nign goiter. The results showed that a dose of 2 g or 4 g of carnitine daily protected participants' bones and reduced other symptoms of hyperthyroidism. Carnitine is thought to affect thyroid hormone by blocking its action in cells.

For many people, the most problematic symptom of high thyroid is rapid or **irregular heartbeat**. In cases of temporary high thyroid levels (as in the viral infection form noted above) conventional treatment may involve simply protecting the heart. Germany's Commission E (the herbal regulating body in that country) has authorized use of the herb **motherwort** as part of an overall treatment plan for an overactive thyroid (hyperthyroidism). Motherwort is said to calm the heart; however, there is no meaningful evidence to indicate that it is effective for the heart-related symptoms of hyperthyroidism (or any other heart-related symptoms).

Herbs and Supplements to Avoid

According to one study in animals, the herb **ashwaghanda** may raise thyroid hormone levels. For this reason, it should not be used by people with hyperthyroidism.

Taking excessive **kelp**, **bladderwrack**, or other forms of seaweed can cause hyperthyroidism by overloading the body with iodine.

Hypothyroidism

RELATED TERMS: *Hashimoto's Thyroiditis; Thyroid Hormone, Low; Thyroiditis, Hashimoto's*

PRINCIPAL PROPOSED NATURAL TREATMENTS: *Armour Thyroid*

OTHER PROPOSED NATURAL TREATMENTS: *Bacopa monniera (Brahmi), Selenium, Traditional Chinese Herbal Medicine, Vitamin B$_3$, Zinc*

HERBS AND SUPPLEMENTS TO USE ONLY WITH CAUTION: *Bladderwrack, Genistein, Iodine, Iron, Isoflavones, Kelp, Soy*

In hypothyroidism, the thyroid gland fails to produce adequate levels of thyroid hormone. Symptoms include the following:

- Sluggishness
- Sensitivity to cold
- Weight gain
- Depression
- Dry skin
- Loss of hair
- Excessive menstruation
- Hoarseness
- Goiter (a visible enlargement of the neck caused by a swollen thyroid gland)

Hashimoto's thyroiditis is the most common natural cause of low thyroid hormone levels. In this autoimmune condition, the body develops antibodies that attack and gradually destroy the thyroid. A viral infection of the thyroid can also decrease thyroid hormone production, but the effect is generally mild and temporary. Finally, **iodine** deficiency can cause hypothyroidism, but this seldom occurs in the developed world where iodine is routinely added to salt.

Besides these natural causes, there is a still more common cause of hypothyroidism—medical treatment for *hyper*thyroidism (excessive production of thyroid hormone production). People with certain forms of hyperthyroidism receive treatment with radioactive iodine to inactivate the thyroid gland. This treatment causes hypothyroidism, which requires lifelong treatment with thyroid replacement therapy.

Until the 1990s, doctors commonly diagnosed hypothyroidism by conducting lab tests to measure thyroid hormone levels in the blood (the T_4 level). Unfortunately, normal thyroid levels vary widely between people, so this method couldn't always correctly identify the disease. A much better lab test, which became available in the 1990s, involves measurement of a hormone called *TSH, or thyroid stimulating hormone.*

TSH is released by the pituitary gland in order to control the thyroid gland. The pituitary gland constantly measures the level of thyroid hormone in the blood and adjusts TSH levels as necessary to get it right. When thyroid hormone levels are high, it turns TSH levels down. When thyroid hormone levels are too low, the pituitary raises TSH levels to stimulate the thyroid. If the thyroid gland does not respond by raising thyroid hormone levels, the pituitary turns up the TSH levels even higher. When TSH levels are higher than normal limits, this means that the thyroid gland is having trouble producing enough thyroid hormone for the body's needs: in other words, the person has entered a hypothyroid state or is about to enter such a state. This method of determining thyroid status has proved very reliable. In other words, the pituitary gland knows what it's talking about.

Medical treatment for low-thyroid conditions is safe and very effective. Treatment involves use of a hormone called *levothyroxine*, or T_4. The body actually uses two forms of thyroid, T_4 and T_3, but in most cases the body easily and automatically converts T_4 to T_3 in the right proportions. The dosage of drug is adjusted by monitoring TSH levels. When the pituitary gland is satisfied, the dose is most likely correct.

Other Proposed Treatments

So-called natural thyroid hormone is popular among people interested in alternative medicine. Sold by prescription only under the name Armour Thyroid®, this extract of pig thyroid contains both T_4 and T_3 (see previous section for description). There is no doubt that Armour Thyroid is as effective as standard synthetic thyroid hormone and it is a satisfactory choice for those who prefer to use natural treatments. However, there is no evidence that Armour Thyroid is any more effective than standard medications and there are some concerns that variations in stomach absorption may produce slightly erratic results. One double-blind study failed to find a combination of synthetic T_3 and T_4 more effective than synthetic T_4 as a treatment for hypothyroidism in regard to well-being, quality of life, or mental function. Another double-blind study also failed to find discernible improvements in mood, fatigue, well-being, or mental function; however, for reasons that are unclear, patients given T_3 plus T_4 were significantly more likely to prefer the new treatment to their previous care than those who were continued on T_4. Unless this was merely a statistical accident, people were apparently able to detect some subtle benefit with the combined treatment that they couldn't quite put their finger on.

Besides Armour Thyroid, there are no natural therapies with documented efficacy for the treatment of hypothyroidism. Treatments that sometimes recommended but lack any meaningful scientific support include **Bacopa monniera** (brahmi), **selenium**, **traditional Chinese herbal medicine**, **vitamin B$_3$**, and **zinc**.

Far too frequently, people with low thyroid levels consume seaweed or iodine supplements in hopes that they will help. However, while iodine deficiency does indeed cause low thyroid levels, taking iodine won't help at all if you're not deficient in it, and the vast majority of people living in the developed world have plenty of iodine. In fact, excessive iodine intake can occasionally cause hypothyroidism. This is a classic case of "more is not better." (For more information, see Herbs and Supplements to Use Only with Caution below.)

The Theory of Widespread Marginal Hypothyroidism

There is very little doubt that many cases of marginal hypothyroidism go unidentified and that occasional tests for thyroid adequacy should be part of routine medical care. However, some proponents of alternative medicine go further and suggest that undiagnosed hypothyroidism is a serious epidemic, causing a high percentage of all the illnesses afflicting modern man. (One of the most famous books on this theory is titled *Solved: The Riddle of Illness* by Stephen E. Langer, M.D., and James F. Scheer.) Supposedly, laboratory tests for thyroid hormone levels are not reliable and many people have marginally low thyroid levels despite normal lab readings.

These thyroid enthusiasts recommend that people use measurements of basal body temperature and not blood tests to determine whether thyroid levels are adequate. Basal body temperature is measured by placing a thermometer under the armpit before arising in the morning. According to proponents of the marginal hypothyroidism theory, a measurement of lower than about 97.5° Fahrenheit indicates a problem. People with basal body temperature readings below this level and symptoms consistent with hypothyroidism are advised to use Armour Thyroid (or various other animal-source thyroid gland supplements that can be obtained with a bit of work). The net result is supposed to be a great improvement in overall health and the resolution of many illnesses.

However, there are a number of problems with this theory. One is that the majority of women have basal body temperature readings below 97.5 in the period prior to ovulation, a fact used in the sympto-thermal method of natural family planning. Many healthy men have normal basal body temperatures below 97.5 as well. Since symptoms consistent with hypothyroidism (such as fatigue, depression, weight gain) occur in a great many people, this approach is guaranteed to recommend that enormous numbers of people take thyroid supplements.

Furthermore, the basal body temperature method was developed in the days before TSH levels could be measured. Back then, doctors could only measure T_4 levels and, as noted above, there is too great a variation in the normal level of T_4 for such tests to be reliable. However, now that the TSH test has become available, the situation has changed. TSH measurements indicate the body's own determination of its thyroid hormone level. It is difficult to justify ignoring the body's own opinion in favor of an arbitrary reading on a thermometer. Indeed, when people with normal TSH levels are given thyroid medication, the body responds by lowering its own production of thyroid hormone, essentially fighting this supposedly natural therapy.

Nonetheless, the enthusiasm for thyroid medication continues unabated, and some alternative medicine physicians continue to maintain that thyroid hormone supplementation is useful even in the presence of a normal TSH test. In 2001, a double-blind, placebo-controlled, crossover trial attempted to evaluate the validity of this theory. Researchers enrolled 22 people with symptoms consistent with hypothyroidism but normal TSH measurements, as well as 19 healthy people. About half of each group was given standard synthetic thyroid hormone (thyroxine 100 mcg—this is T_4 as described above) for 12 weeks and placebo for another 12 weeks; the other half received placebo for the first period and thyroid hormone for the second. Improvement was measured through questionnaires evaluating general health, emotional well-being, and mental function.

The results showed that participants with symptoms of low thyroid hormone improved significantly. However, those taking placebo improved just as much! In other words, thyroid hormone proved no more effective than placebo. (Interestingly, the healthy participants showed little response to either placebo or thyroid hormone.)

This study indicates that synthetic human thyroid hormone supplementation (T_4) is not helpful for people with normal TSH but symptoms that are reminiscent of low thyroid hormone. Unfortunately, it did not evaluate the effectiveness of the animal-source thyroid recommended by proponents of the hypothyroid theory and, therefore, does not entirely settle the controversy.

Herbs and Supplements to Use Only with Caution

As noted above, supplementation with iodine will not help the thyroid gland except in people who are iodine-deficient. In fact, in Japan, excessive use of seaweed (such as **kelp** or **bladderwrack**) is a fairly common cause of hypothyroidism.

For this reason, people with low thyroid hormone levels should not consume excessive amounts of these iodine-rich foods.

Soy and its **isoflavones** (such as **genistein**) appear to have numerous potential effects involving the thyroid gland. When given to people with impaired thyroid function, soy products have been observed to reduce absorption of thyroid medication. In addition, some evidence hints that soy isoflavones may directly inhibit the function of the thyroid gland, although this inhibition may only be significant in people who are deficient in iodine. However, to make matters more confusing, studies of healthy humans and animals given soy isoflavones or other soy products have generally found that soy either had no effect on thyroid hormone levels, or actually increased levels.

The bottom line: In view of soy's complex effects regarding the thyroid, people with impaired thyroid function should not take large amounts of soy products except under the supervision of a physician.

Iron supplements may also interfere with thyroid hormone absorption.

Immune Support

RELATED TERMS: *Immunity, Boosting; Infections, Frequent; Weak Immunity*

The body must contend with constant attacks by microscopic organisms. In order to defend against this onslaught, it deploys a wide range of defenses that together are called the *immune system*.

People with diseases that cause immune deficiency, such as **AIDS**, fall victim to infectious microorganisms that a healthy person could ward off easily. However, even healthy people get sick from time to time, victims of infections that manage to sneak by the defenses. And some apparently healthy people nonetheless get sick quite often.

If you fall into this latter category, you may wish to find treatments that can strengthen your immune system. Unfortunately, this is easier said than done. To explain why it is so difficult to improve resistance to illness, we need to delve a bit deeper into the nature of immunity.

The Immune System

The immune system consists primarily of various types of white blood cells and the chemicals that they manufacture (such as antibodies). In certain conditions, such as AIDS, many of these white blood cells are damaged or dead. In such cases, the term *immune deficiency* is clearly appropriate. The circumstance is analogous to an army that lacks, say, guns.

However, careful examination of most people who get frequent colds (or bladder infections or herpes attacks, for example) fails to turn up any visible deficits in the immune system. They have all the immune cells and antibodies they need in roughly the right amounts

and all the various parts appear to work just fine. So why do such people get sick so often? The short answer is: We don't know.

One can hypothesize that in some people the immune system fails to function properly for a relatively subtle, invisible reason, much as a well-equipped army might lose its fighting form due to apathy or disunity. However, keep in mind that even people who develop frequent colds manage to fight off thousands of other infections every day. (If they didn't, they would be dead.)

For this reason, an alternate hypothesis comes to mind: that over-susceptibility to a particular type of infection may be caused by something more specific than general immune weakness. As an example, chronically inflamed mucous membranes might lead to frequent colds, since an inflamed mucous membrane may be more porous to cold viruses. Similarly, a woman's bladder wall might allow particularly easy attachment of bacteria, leading to frequent bladder infections.

In reality, though, these are all speculations. We truly do not know why some people frequently develop minor infections. For this reason, it is very difficult to find a way to fix the problem.

Immunomodulation

Many natural products are said to boost general immunity. However, while we can scientifically study the effect of a single treatment on a single illness, at the present state of knowledge there is no way we can even *know* that a treatment strengthens the immune system in general.

Scientists can measure the effects of an herb on individual white blood cell types and note changes in activity, but they don't know how to interpret the results of those measurements as a whole. After all, the immune system is a *system*, and systems are notoriously complicated to analyze. Current knowledge does not allow us to predict the ultimate effect of fine changes in the parts.

To acknowledge this limitation, scientists tend to use the term *immunomodulatory* rather than *immune-stimulating* when they refer to a substance that causes measurable alterations in immune function. This terminology notes a change (modulation), but does not jump to conclusions regarding whether that change is good, bad, or indifferent.

Hundreds or thousands of herbs have immunomodulatory effects, so many that we will make no attempt to list them here. In many cases, these may represent nothing more than the body's reaction to the herb as a foreign presence—an immune reaction to the herb itself, in other words, with no special benefits. In some cases, observed immunomodulatory effects *could* indicate an alteration in immune function with potential benefits under certain conditions, but it is as yet impossible to know.

Theoretically, it is possible that some natural substance could boost all aspects of immunity. However, if it did, it would be a highly dangerous substance! The immune system is balanced on a knife edge. An immune system that is too relaxed fails to defend us from infections; an immune system that is too active attacks healthy tissues, causing autoimmune diseases. A universal immune booster might cause **lupus**, **Crohn's disease**, **asthma**, **Graves' disease**, **Hashimoto's thyroiditis**, **multiple sclerosis**, or **rheumatoid arthritis**, among other problems.

Rather than an immune booster, one might rather prefer a treatment that somehow fine-tunes the immune system. Does such a treatment exist? No one really knows, although claims abound.

Preventing or Treating Infectious Illnesses with Natural Medicine

Herbs and Supplements

There is no doubt that good general nutrition is necessary for strong immunity. However, excessive intake of some nutrients (**zinc**, for example) may weaken immunity. For information on which nutrients might be worth taking to improve your nutrition, see the article on **general nutritional support**. In that section, we also discuss some specific scientific evidence indicating that multivitamin/multimineral supplements may help certain people stay well.

A number of herbs and supplements have shown promise for preventing or treating certain specific infections. For more information, see the articles on **bladder infection**, **colds and flus**, **diarrhea**, **fungal infection**, **herpes infection**, **middle ear infection**, and **vaginal yeast infection**.

Immunizations are a widely used method for strengthening the immune response to specific illnesses, such as **influenza**. However, some people (especially seniors) may not respond adequately to immunizations. Certain natural products, such as **ginseng**, **vitamin E**, and **multivitamin/multimineral supplements** may enhance the response.

Echinacea is widely hyped as an immune strengthening herb, but current evidence suggests that regular use of echinacea does *not* help prevent colds or other infections. (Echinacea *does*, however, appear to be helpful for colds that have already begun.)

Lifestyle Issues

There is little doubt that if you live a healthy lifestyle with good nutrition and plenty of exercise, you'll approach more closely a state of optimum health. Keep in mind, however, that the key is moderation. Too much exercise (as in marathon running) can weaken the immune system, leading to infections. (If you wish to engage in heavy endurance exercise, **vitamin C**, **beta-sitosterol**, and **glutamine** have shown some promise for preventing the "post-marathon sniffle.")

Although it is commonly said that high levels of sugar intake weaken immunity, there is no meaningful evidence to support this view. Similarly, while severe **alcohol abuse** clearly damages immune function, there is no evidence that moderate alcohol consumption increases risk of infections.

Does getting cold cause colds? Possibly, but it hasn't been proven.

There is also no reliable evidence that reducing intake of dairy products will prevent respiratory infections.

Finally, contrary to popular belief, early antibiotic treatment of children with **ear infections** does not seem to damage the child's immunity and thereby cause a greater rate of ear infections.

Immune Support

Alternative Therapies

Various alternative therapies are said to be able to enhance overall health and thereby prevent illness in general. These include methods such as **acupuncture**, **Ayurveda**, **chiropractic spinal manipulation**, **naturopathy**, **Reiki**, **Tai Chi**, **Therapeutic Touch**, **traditional Chinese herbal medicine**, and **yoga**. However, there is as yet little to no meaningful scientific evidence to indicate that these methods have any specific positive effect on immunity.

Impotence

RELATED TERM: *Erectile Dysfunction*

PRINCIPAL PROPOSED NATURAL TREATMENTS: *Carnitine, L-Arginine, Ginseng*

OTHER PROPOSED NATURAL TREATMENTS: *Acupuncture, Ashwagandha,* Avena sativa, Butea superba, *Catuaba, Cordyceps, Damiana, Dehydroepiandrosterone (DHEA), Diindolylmethane (DIM),* Eleutherococcus, *Ginkgo, Horny Goat Weed* (Epimedium grandiflorum), *L-citrulline, Maca* (Lepidium meyenii), Macuna pruriens, *Melatonin, Molybdenum, Muira Puama (Potency Wood),* Polypodium vulgare, *Pygeum,* Rhodiola rosea, *Saw Palmetto, Schisandra, Suma, Traditional Chinese Herbal Medicine,* Tribulus terrestris, *Velvet Antler, Zinc*

HERBS AND SUPPLEMENTS TO USE ONLY WITH CAUTION: *Androstenedione, Licorice, Yohimbe, Soy or Soy Isoflavones*

Impotence, or erectile dysfunction, is the inability to achieve an erection. Impotence may occur for any of at least 15 possible causes, including diabetes, drug side effects, pituitary tumors, hardening of the arteries, hormonal imbalances, and psychological factors. A few of these conditions respond to specific treatment. For example, if a blood pressure drug is causing impotence, the best approach is to change drugs. If a pituitary tumor is secreting the hormone prolactin, treating that tumor may result in immediate improvement. However, in most cases, conventional treatment of impotence is nonspecific.

The drugs Viagra and Cialis have revolutionized treatment for erectile dysfunction. These medications work by increasing tissue sensitivity to the blood vessel–dilating substance nitric oxide (NO) in the penis. Older methods include mechanical devices that utilize a vacuum to produce an erection, drugs for self-injection, and implantation of penile prostheses.

Proposed Treatments for Impotence

Korean Red Ginseng

Two double-blind, placebo-controlled trials, involving a total of about 135 people, have found evidence that Korean red ginseng may improve erectile function.

In the better of the two trials, 45 participants received either placebo or Korean red ginseng at a dose of 900 mg 3 times daily for 8 weeks. After a 1-week period of no treatment, the two groups were switched. The results indicate that while using Korean red ginseng men experienced significantly better sexual function than while they were taking placebo.

For more information, including safety issues, see the full **Ginseng** article.

L-Arginine

The substance nitric oxide (NO) plays a role in the development of an erection. Drugs like Viagra increase the body's *sensitivity* to the natural rise in NO that occurs with sexual stimulation. A simpler approach might be to *raise* NO levels and one way to accomplish this involves use of the amino acid L-arginine. Oral arginine supplements may increase nitric oxide levels in the penis and elsewhere. Based on this, L-arginine has been advertised as "natural Viagra." However, there is as yet little evidence that it works. Drugs based on raising nitric oxide levels in the penis have not worked out for pharmaceutical developers; the body seems to simply adjust to the higher levels and maintain the same level of response.

The main support for the use of arginine in erectile dysfunction comes from a small double-blind trial in which 50 men with erectile dysfunction received either 5 g of L-arginine or placebo daily for 6 weeks. More men in the treated group experienced improvement in sexual performance than in the placebo group.

A double-blind crossover study of 32 men found no benefit with 1,500 mg of arginine given daily for 17 days; the much smaller dose and shorter course of treatment may explain the discrepancy between these two trials.

Arginine has also been evaluated in combination with the drug yohimbine (made from the herb **yohimbe**). A double-blind, placebo-controlled trial of 45 men found that one-time use of this combination therapy an hour or two prior to intercourse improved erectile function, especially in those with only moderate erectile dysfunction scores. Arginine and yohimbine were both taken at a dose of 6 g.

Note: Do not use the drug yohimbine (or the herb yohimbe) except under physician supervision, as it presents a number of safety risks.

For more information, including dosage and safety issues, see the full L-arginine article.

Carnitine

In a 6-month, double-blind trial of 120 men, average age 66, carnitine (propionyl-L-carnitine 2 g/day plus acetyl-L-carnitine 2 g/day) and testosterone (testosterone undecanoate 160 mg/day) were separately compared to placebo. The results indicated that both carnitine and testosterone improve erectile function; however, while testosterone significantly increased prostate volume, carnitine did not.

Another double-blind, placebo-controlled study found that propionyl-L-carnitine at 2 g/day enhanced the effectiveness of sildenafil (Viagra) in 40 men with diabetes who had previously failed to respond to sildenafil on at least eight occasions.

In another double-blind study, a combination of the propionyl and acetyl forms of carnitine enhanced the effectiveness of Viagra in men who suffered from erectile dysfunction caused by prostate surgery.

Carnitine has also shown promise for treating male infertility. For more information, including dosage and safety issues, see the full **Carnitine** article.

Other Treatments

A proprietary combination therapy containing arginine along with *Ginkgo biloba*, ginseng, and vitamins and minerals has shown some promise in an unpublished study.

In a 3-week, double-blind, placebo-controlled trial, 20 men with erectile dysfunction received either placebo or a special form of **magnet therapy** called *pulsed electromagnetic field therapy* (PEMF). PEMF was administered by means of a small box worn near the genital area and kept in place as continuously as possible over the study period; neither participants nor observers knew whether the device was actually activated or not. The results showed that use of PEMF significantly improved sexual function compared to placebo.

A double-blind, placebo-controlled study enrolled 40 men with difficulty achieving or maintaining an erection who also had low measured levels of **DHEA**. The results showed that DHEA at a dose of 50 mg daily improved sexual performance; however, the authors failed to provide a statistical analysis of the results, making the meaningfulness of this study impossible to determine.

Severe **zinc** deficiency is known to negatively affect sexual function. Since marginal zinc deficiency is relatively common, it is logical to suppose that supplementation with zinc may be helpful for some men. However, this hypothesis has only been studied in men receiving kidney dialysis. The results were promising.

The herb *Butea superba* has shown some promise for erectile dysfunction, according to a 3-month, randomized, double-blind study performed in Thailand.

One animal study suggests that **melatonin** might have some potential value in the treatment of impotence.

Oligomeric proanthocyanidin complexes (OPCs) have also shown some promise for erectile dysfunction, alone or in combination with arginine.

Based on exceedingly preliminary evidence, the herb **maca** (*Lepidium meyenii*) has been advertised as "herbal Viagra." In one study in rats, use of maca enhanced male sexual function. There is one published human trial as well. In this small, 12-week, double-blind, placebo-controlled study, use of maca at 1,500 mg or 3,000 mg increased male libido. While this was an interesting finding, the study did not report benefits in male sexual function—just in desire. Since loss of sexual function is a more common problem in men than loss of sexual desire, these results do not justify the herbal Viagra claim. Contrary to some reports, maca does not appear to affect testosterone levels.

Many other herbs are also reputed to improve sexual function in men, including **ashwagandha**, *Avena sativa* (oat straw), catuaba, **cordyceps**, **damiana**, **diindolyl-methane (DIM)**, *Eleutherococcus* (so-called Siberian ginseng), **L-citrulline**, *Macuna pruriens*, **molybdenum**, **muira puama** (potency wood), **pygeum**, *Polypodium vulgare*, **Rhodiola rosea**, **saw palmetto**, **schisandra**, **suma**, **traditional Chinese herbal medicine**, and *Tribulus terrestris*. However, there is as yet no real evidence that they offer any benefits.

Numerous case reports and uncontrolled studies had indicated that the herb *Ginkgo biloba* offers dramatic benefits for male (and female) sexual problems caused by antidepressants. However, as always, double-blind, placebo-controlled studies are necessary to truly establish efficacy. (For the reasons why, see **Why Does This Book Rely on Double-blind Studies?**.) When studies of this type were performed, it became clear that people had been misled about ginkgo's efficacy by the power of suggestion: ginkgo failed to improve sexual function to any greater extent than placebo.

In a small single-blind study, **acupuncture** proved superior to fake acupuncture for treatment of erectile dysfunction. However, because the treating practitioners administrating the control treatment were aware that they were providing sham acupuncture, it is quite likely that they unconsciously communicated lack of confidence as they provided it; this is an inherent limitation of single-blind studies.

Deer or antelope **velvet antler** is a popular treatment for sexual dysfunction. However, the one double-blind study performed on the subject failed to find benefit.

Herbs and Supplements to Use Only with Caution

The U.S. Food and Drug Administration (FDA) warned consumers not to purchase or consume several brands of dietary supplements after samples were found adulterated with the prescription drug tadalafil (Cialis), an analogue of sildenafil (Viagra). The products named in the warning are SIGRA, STAMINA Rx, STAMINA Rx for Women, Y-Y, Spontane ES, and Uroprin (all manufactured by NVE, Inc., and distributed by Hi-Tech). (See http://www.fda.gov/bbs/topics/ANSWERS/2003/ANS01235.html.)

The herb **yohimbe** is the source of the drug yohimbine, which has been shown to be modestly better than placebo for impotence. However, due to many drug interactions and other risks, we do not recommend using yohimbine except under the supervision of a physician. Because there is no agency regulating herbal product quality and labeling, the herb yohimbe presents even more risks, such as unpredictable yohimbine content.

Soy or soy **isoflavones**, as well as the herb **licorice**, may reduce testosterone levels in men. For this reason, men with impotence, **infertility**, or decreased libido may want to avoid these natural products.

One case report suggests that a product containing the herb *Epimedium grandiflorum* (horny goat weed) caused rapid heart rate and symptoms similar to mania.

The supplement **androstenedione**, often taken for male sexual dysfunction in the belief that it increases testosterone levels, actually appears to increase estrogen levels in men and might, therefore, increase problems with erectile function.

Inflammatory Bowel Disease

The term inflammatory bowel disease (IBD) refers to two disorders that involve inflammation of the intestines: **Crohn's disease** and **ulcerative colitis**. These are each discussed in their own articles.

Another condition called *irritable bowel syndrome* (IBS) is sometimes confused with IBD. However, IBS is a less serious illness that does not involve inflammation.

Insect Bites

Insect Bites

RELATED TERMS: *Insect Repellents*

PRINCIPAL PROPOSED NATURAL TREATMENTS: *None*

OTHER PROPOSED NATURAL TREATMENTS:

Insect Repellent (Topical): *Proprietary Product Containing Soybean Oil and Germanium Oil, Proprietary Bath Lotions, Essential Oils (Citronella Grass, Ocimum americanum, Citrus hystrix, Lemongrass, Turmeric, and Vanilla), Garlic*

Insect Repellent (Local): *Citronella Candles and Incense*

Insect Repellent (Oral): *Garlic*

Insect Bites (Treatment): *Topical Creams Containing Such Herbs as Aloe, Calendula, Chamomile, Goldenseal, Licorice, and Marshmallow*

PROBABLY NOT EFFECTIVE TREATMENTS: *Sonic Wrist Strap Repellents, Vitamin B$_1$*

Insects are the most successful group of creatures on earth, greatly outdoing mammals in number of species and sheer mass of life. Furthermore, despite great effort, human attempts to eliminate certain insects, such as mosquitoes, have utterly failed. In insects, it appears, humans have met their match.

When it comes to the more mundane level of avoiding insect bites, however, our species is doing a bit better. The chemical DEET (N,N-diethyl-3-methylbenzamide), found in almost all insect repellents, is highly successful especially against mosquitoes, flies, fleas, and ticks.

Contrary to popular belief, DEET appears to be a very safe substance when used in a normal fashion. After many decades of use by millions of people, use of DEET has been associated with only a small number of adverse reactions and those side effects that have been reported seem to represent unusual personal responses rather than toxicity in the ordinary sense.

Medical treatment for bites that have already occurred consists primarily of soothing topical treatments.

Proposed Natural Treatments

Due to fears about the safety of DEET (probably unfounded), many natural products have been marketed as safer substitutes. However, while some of these may be effective to a certain extent, none matches the power of the chemical.

One of the best of these appears to be a proprietary product containing soybean oil and geranium oil. In a small but well-designed study, this product, when applied to the skin, prevented insects from biting for an average of about 90 minutes. This benefit was equivalent to that of a low-strength DEET repellent (4.75%). However, researchers found that high-strength DEET repellents (24%) provided about 300 minutes of protection.

Proprietary bath lotions marketed to repel insects do not appear to provide more than a slight level of bite protection (unless DEET is added to them).

Various **essential oils**, applied topically, have also shown promise for preventing insect bites, but the supporting evidence remains preliminary. Some commonly used essential oils include the oil of **eucalyptus**, citronella grass (*Cymbopogon winterianus*), clove, hairy basil (*Ocimum americanum*), kaffir lime (*Citrus hystrix*), lemongrass, patchuli, pine, **turmeric**, and vanilla. Citronella candles and incense appear to reduce the number of bites by less than 50%.

The herb **garlic**, when taken by mouth, may act as a mild insect repellent. A 20-week, double-blind, placebo-controlled trial followed 80 Swedish soldiers and measured the number of tick bites received during the garlic and the placebo treatments. The results showed a modest but statistically significant reduction in tick bites when soldiers consumed 1,200 mg of garlic daily. However, another study failed to find one-time use of garlic helpful for repelling mosquitoes.

Wristbands impregnated with mosquito repellents do not appear to offer more than marginal efficacy. Sonic mosquito repellents do not appear to work at all. Oral **vitamin B$_1$** also appears to be completely ineffective.

For people who have already been bitten, topical creams containing such herbs as **aloe**, **calendula**, **chamomile**, **goldenseal**, **licorice**, and **marshmallow** are often recommended, but there is no evidence that they are effective.

Insomnia

RELATED TERMS: *Sleeplessness*

PRINCIPAL PROPOSED NATURAL TREATMENTS: *Melatonin, Valerian (Alone or Combined with Hops or Melissa)*

OTHER PROPOSED NATURAL TREATMENTS: *5-Hydroxytryptophan (5-HTP), Acupuncture or Acupressure, Ashwagandha, Astragalus, Biofeedback, Chamomile, He Shou Wu, Hops, Kava, Lady's Slipper Orchid, Magnesium, Passionflower, Relaxation Therapies, St. John's Wort, Skullcap*

According to recent reports, many people today have a serious problem getting a good night's sleep. Our lives are simply too busy for us to get the 8 hours we really need. To make matters worse, many of us suffer from insomnia. When we do get to bed, we may stay awake thinking for hours. Sleep itself may be restless instead of refreshing.

Most people who sleep substantially less than 8 hours a night experience a variety of unpleasant symptoms. The most common are headaches, mental confusion, irritability, malaise, immune deficiencies, depression, and fatigue. Complete sleep deprivation can lead to hallucinations and mental collapse.

The best way to improve sleep involves making lifestyle changes: eliminating caffeine and sugar from your diet, avoiding stimulating activities before bed, adopting a regular sleeping time, and gradually turning down the lights. More complex behavioral approaches to improving sleep habits can be adopted as well.

Many drugs can also help with sleep. Such medications as Sonata, Lunesta, Ambien, Restoril, Ativan, and Xanax are widely used for sleep problems. Of these, only Lunesta has been tested for long-term use. All of these medications are in essence tranquilizers and, therefore, have potential for dependence and abuse; the newer sleep-inducing drug Rozerem (ramelteon) acts like an enhanced version of the supplement melatonin (see below) and is not thought to have such potential.

Antidepressants can also be used to correct sleep problems. Low doses of certain antidepressants immediately bring on sleep because their side effects include drowsiness. However, this effect tends to wear off with repeated use. For chronic sleeping problems, full doses of antidepressants can sometimes be helpful. Antidepressants are believed to work by actually altering brain chemistry, which produces a beneficial effect on sleep. Trazadone and ami-

triptyline are two of the most commonly prescribed antidepressants when improved sleep is desired, but most other antidepressants can be helpful as well.

Principal Proposed Natural Treatments

Although the scientific evidence isn't yet definitive, the herb valerian and the hormone melatonin are widely accepted as treatments for certain forms of insomnia.

Valerian

Valerian has a long traditional use for insomnia and today it is an accepted over-the-counter treatment for insomnia in Germany, Belgium, France, Switzerland, and Italy. However, the evidence that it really works remains inconsistent and incomplete.

Valerian is most commonly recommended to be used as needed for occasional insomnia. However, the results of the largest and best designed study suggest that it may be more useful for long-term improvement of sleep. This 28-day, double-blind, placebo-controlled study followed 121 people with histories of significant sleep disturbance. This study looked at the effectiveness of 600 mg of an alcohol-based valerian extract taken 1 hour before bedtime.

Valerian didn't work right away. For the first couple of weeks, valerian and placebo were running neck and neck. However, by day 28 valerian had pulled far ahead. Effectiveness was rated as good or very good by participant evaluation in 66% of the valerian group and in 61% by doctor evaluation, whereas in the placebo group, only 29% were so rated by participants and doctors.

This study appears to provide good evidence that valerian is effective for insomnia. However, it has one confusing aspect: the 4-week delay before effects were seen. In another placebo-controlled study, valerian produced immediately noticeable effects on sleep and that is what most practitioners believe to be typical. Why valerian took so long to work in this one study has not been explained. Other studies, most of relatively low quality, found immediate benefits as well. And to make matters even more complex, three more recent studies of valerian failed to find any benefit at all, including one in which 135 people were given valerian and 135 given placebo. The explanation for these contradictions remains unclear.

Other studies have compared valerian (either alone or in combination with **hops** or **melissa**) against benzodiazepine drugs. Most of these studies found the herbal treatment approximately as effective as the drug, but due to the absence of a placebo group these results are less than fully reliable.

Mixed results like these suggest that valerian is at most modestly helpful for improving sleep. For more information, including dosage and safety issues, see the full **Valerian** article.

Melatonin

The body uses melatonin as part of its normal control of the sleep-wake cycle. The pineal gland makes serotonin and then turns it into melatonin when exposure to light decreases. Strong light (such as sunlight) slows melatonin production more than weak light does and a completely dark room increases the amount of melatonin made more than a partially darkened room does. Taking melatonin as a supplement seems to stimulate sleep when the natural cycle is disturbed. It may also have a direct sedative effect.

Although not all studies were positive, reasonably good evidence indicates that melatonin is helpful for insomnia related to **jet lag**, according to a major review published in 2001. One of the best supporting studies was a double-blind, placebo-controlled study that enrolled 320 travelers crossing 6 to 8 time zones. The participants were divided into four groups and given a daily dose of 5 mg of standard melatonin, 5 mg of slow-release melatonin, 0.5 mg of standard melatonin, or placebo. The group that received 5 mg of standard melatonin slept better, took less time to fall asleep, and felt more energetic and awake during the day than the other three groups.

Mixed results have been seen in studies involving the use of melatonin for ordinary insomnia, insomnia in swing-shift workers, and insomnia in elderly people.

A 4-week, double-blind trial evaluated the benefits of melatonin for children with difficulty falling asleep. A total of 40 children who had experienced this type of sleep problem for at least a year were given either placebo or melatonin at a dose of 5 mg. The results showed that use of melatonin significantly helped participants fall asleep more easily. Benefits were also seen in a similar study of 62 children with this condition. **Note:** The long-term safety of melatonin usage has not been established. Do not give your child melatonin except under physician supervision.

Many individuals stay up late on Friday and Saturday nights and then find it difficult to go to sleep at a reasonable hour on Sunday. A small double-blind, placebo-controlled study found evidence that use of melatonin 5.5 hours before the desired Sunday bedtime improved the ability of participants to fall asleep.

Benefits were seen in a small double-blind trial of patients in a pulmonary intensive care unit. It is famously difficult to sleep in an ICU, and the resulting sleep deprivation is not helpful for those recovering from disease or surgery. In this study of 8 hospitalized individuals, 3 mg of controlled-release melatonin significantly improved sleep quality and duration.

Blind people often have trouble sleeping on any particular schedule, because there are no light cues available to help them get tired at night. A small double-blind, placebo-controlled crossover trial found that the use of melatonin at a dose of 10 mg per day was able to synchronize participants' sleep schedules.

Some individuals find it impossible to fall asleep until early morning, a condition called *delayed sleep phase syndrome* (DSPS). Melatonin may be beneficial for this syndrome.

In addition, people trying to quit using sleeping pills in the benzodiazepine family may find melatonin helpful. A double-blind, placebo-controlled study of 34 individuals who regularly used such medications found that melatonin at a dose of 2 mg nightly (controlled-release formulation) could help them discontinue the use of the drugs.

Note: There can be risks in discontinuing benzodiazepine drugs. Consult your physician for advice.

For more information, including dosage and safety issues, see the full Melatonin article.

Other Proposed Natural Treatments

Acupressure or **acupuncture** may be helpful for insomnia, but the supporting evidence remains weak. A single-blind, placebo-controlled study involving 84 nursing home residents found that real acupressure was superior to sham acupressure for improving sleep quality. Treated participants fell asleep faster and slept more soundly.

Another single-blind, controlled study reported benefits with acupuncture, but failed to include a proper statistical analysis of the results. For this reason, no conclusions can be drawn from the report. In a third study, 98 people with severe kidney disease were divided into three groups: no extra treatment, 12 sessions of fake acupressure (not using actual acupuncture points), or 12 sessions of real acupressure. Participants receiving real acupressure experienced significantly improved sleep as compared to those receiving no extra treatment. However, fake acupressure was just as effective as real acupressure.

Numerous controlled studies have evaluated **relaxation therapies** for the treatment of insomnia. These studies are difficult to summarize because many involved therapy combined with other methods, such as **biofeedback**, sleep restriction, and paradoxical intent (trying not to sleep). The type of relaxation therapy used in the majority of these trials was progressive muscle relaxation (PMR). Overall, the evidence indicates that relaxation therapies may be somewhat helpful for insomnia, although not dramatically so. For example, in a controlled study of 70 people with insomnia, participants using progressive relaxation showed no meaningful improvement in the time taken to fall asleep or the duration of sleep, but they reported feeling more rested in the morning. In another study, 20 minutes of relaxation practice was required to increase sleeping time by 30 minutes.

One small double-blind study found a particular **Ayurvedic** herbal combination helpful for insomnia.

Herbs used for anxiety are commonly recommended for insomnia as well. As noted above, hops and lemon balm have been studied in combination with valerian. One double-blind study found that the antianxiety herb **kava** taken alone may aid sleep for people whose insomnia is associated with anxiety and tension. However, a fairly large study failed to find kava helpful for ordinary insomnia. (**Note**: There are serious concerns that kava may occasionally cause severe liver disorders.)

One tiny study hints that the fragrance of lavender **essential oil** might aid sleep.

Slight evidence hints that **magnesium** might be helpful for insomnia in seniors.

The herb **St. John's wort** and the supplement **5-HTP** have shown promise as treatments for **depression**. Because prescription antidepressants can aid sleep, these natural substances have been suggested for insomnia as well. However, there is no direct evidence that they are effective. A double-blind trial of 12 non-insomniacs found no sleep-promoting benefit with St. John's wort.

Other herbs reputed to offer both antianxiety and anti-insomnia benefits include **ashwagandha, astragalus, chamomile, He shou wu, lady's slipper, passionflower**, and **skullcap**. However, there is again no supporting evidence to indicate that any of these really work.

A number of supplements might offer benefits for improving mental function during periods of sleep deprivation. See the **Enhancing Memory and Mental Function** article for more information.

Intermittent Claudication

RELATED TERMS: *Peripheral Vascular Disease*
PRINCIPAL PROPOSED NATURAL TREATMENTS: *Arginine, Ginkgo, Inositol Hexaniacinate, L-Carnitine, Mesoglycan, Policosanol*
PROBABLY INEFFECTIVE TREATMENTS: *Beta-carotene, Vitamin E*

The arteries supplying the legs with blood may become seriously blocked in advanced stages of **atherosclerosis** (commonly, if somewhat incorrectly, known as *hardening of the arteries*). This can lead to severe, crampy pain when you walk more than a short distance because the muscles are starved for oxygen. This condition is called *intermittent claudication*. The intensity of intermittent claudication is often measured in the distance a person can walk without pain.

Conventional treatment for intermittent claudication consists of measures to combat atherosclerosis, the drug Trental (pentoxifylline), and other medications. In advanced cases, surgery to improve blood flow may be necessary.

Principal Proposed Natural Treatments

A number of natural treatments may be helpful for intermittent claudication, but it isn't clear whether it is safe to combine them with the medications that may be prescribed at the same time. Medical supervision is definitely necessary for this serious disease.

Ginkgo

According to eight double-blind, placebo-controlled trials, ginkgo can significantly increase pain-free walking distance, presumably by increasing circulation.

One study enrolled 111 patients and followed them for 24 weeks. Participants were measured for pain-free walking distance by walking up a 12% slope on a treadmill at two miles an hour. At the beginning of treatment, both the placebo and ginkgo (120 mg) groups were able to walk about 350 feet without pain.

At the end of the trial, although both groups had improved (the power of placebo is amazing!), the ginkgo group had improved significantly more, showing about a 40% increase in pain-free walking distance as compared to only a 20% improvement in the placebo group.

Similar improvements were also seen in a double-blind, placebo-controlled trial of 60 individuals who had achieved maximum benefit from physical therapy.

Taking a higher dose of ginkgo may provide enhanced benefits in intermittent claudication. A 24-week, double-blind, placebo-controlled study of 74 individuals found that ginkgo at a dose of 240 mg per day was more effective than 120 mg per day.

For more information, including dosage and safety issues, see the full **Ginkgo** article.

L-Carnitine

The vitamin-like substance L-carnitine also appears to be of some benefit in intermittent claudication. Although it does not increase blood flow, carnitine appears to increase walking distance by improving energy utilization in the muscles.

A 12-month, double-blind, placebo-controlled trial of 485 individuals with intermittent claudication evaluated the potential benefits of a special form of carnitine called *propionyl-L-carnitine*. Participants with relatively severe disease showed a 44% improvement in walking distance as compared to placebo. However, no improvement was seen in those with mild disease. Benefits were seen in most, but not all, other studies using L-carnitine or propionyl-L-carnitine.

For more information, including dosage and safety issues, see the full **Carnitine** article.

Inositol Hexaniacinate

The supplement inositol hexaniacinate, a special form of vitamin B_3, appears to be helpful for intermittent claudication. Double-blind studies involving a total of about 400 individuals have found that it can improve walking distance for people with intermittent claudication. For example, in one study, 100 individuals were given either placebo or 4 g of inositol hexaniacinate daily. Over a period of 3 months, participants improved significantly in the number of steps they could take on a special device before experiencing excessive pain.

For more information, including dosage and safety issues, see the full **Vitamin B_3** article.

Policosanol

A waxy substance extracted from sugarcane, policosanol is best known as a treatment for high cholesterol. However, it seems to be helpful for intermittent claudication as well, according to several studies performed by a single Cuban research group.

A 2-year, double-blind, placebo-controlled study of 56 individuals found that treatment with policosanol (10 mg twice daily) improved walking distance by more than 50% at 6 months, and the benefits increased over the course of the study.

Similar results were seen in a 6-month, double-blind, placebo-controlled study of 62 individuals.

In addition, a small double-blind trial found policosanol more effective than the drug lovastatin for treating intermittent claudication.

Policosanol's benefits in this condition are presumed due to its effects on platelet aggregation. It seems to prevent platelet aggregation to about the same extent as aspirin at 100 mg per day.

Some policosanol products on the market use beeswax as the source instead of sugarcane. However, there is some controversy over whether these products are actually effective. For more information, including dosage and safety issues, see the full **Policosanol** article.

Mesoglycan

Mesoglycan is a substance found in many tissues in the body, including the joints, intestines, and the lining of blood vessels. A 20-week, double-blind, placebo-controlled trial that enrolled 242 individuals evaluated the effects of mesoglycan in intermittent claudication. Significantly more participants in the mesoglycan group responded to treatment (defined as a greater than 50% improvement in walking distance) than in the placebo group. For more information, including dosage and safety issues, see the full **Mesoglycan** article.

Arginine

The supplement arginine may be able to improve walking distance for people with intermittent claudication. In a double-blind study of 41 individuals, 2 weeks of treatment with a high dose of arginine improved walking dis-

tance by 66%; no benefits were seen in the placebo group or a low-dose arginine group.

Good results were also seen in another study, although its convoluted design makes interpreting the results somewhat difficult.

For more information, including dosage and safety issues, see the full **Arginine** article.

Antioxidants

A double-blind, placebo-controlled trial of 1,484 individuals with intermittent claudication found no benefit from **vitamin E** (50 mg daily), **beta-carotene** (20 mg daily), or a combination of the two.

Herbs and Supplements to Use Only with Caution

Various herbs and supplements may interact adversely with drugs used to treat intermittent claudication. For more information on this potential risk, see the individual drug article in the Drug Interactions section of this book.

Interstitial Cystitis

PRINCIPAL PROPOSED NATURAL TREATMENTS: *None*

OTHER PROPOSED NATURAL TREATMENTS: *Arginine, Dietary Changes, Glycosaminoglycans, Quercetin, TENS*

Interstitial cystitis (IC) is a severe, chronic inflammation of the bladder that's both disruptive and painful. Many more women than men suffer from the condition—of the 700,000 people with IC, 90% are female.

The symptoms of IC are notoriously variable and can differ from one person to another or for one person from day to day. People with IC usually have an urgent and frequent need to urinate. They may experience recurring discomfort, tenderness, pressure, or intense pain in the bladder and surrounding pelvic area. This pain often intensifies as the bladder fills and may be exacerbated by sexual intercourse.

Certain foods may trigger symptoms; the most commonly mentioned include tomatoes, vinegar, spicy

foods, coffee, chocolate, alcohol, and fruits and vegetables particular to the individual.

IC is generally diagnosed after other conditions with similar symptoms, such as **bladder infection**, **herpes**, and **vaginal infection**, have been excluded.

The cause of IC is unknown. Although its symptoms resemble a bladder infection, IC does not appear to be caused by bacteria. One theory proposes that IC is caused by an infectious agent that simply hasn't been detected yet. A different theory holds that IC is an autoimmune reaction; still another, that it is related to allergies. Because it varies so much in symptoms and severity, IC may be not one disease but several.

A variety of treatments are often tried alone or in combination before one is found that works. Oral antihistamines, such as hydroxyzine (Atarax) and certirizine (Zyrtec), may provide relief and the drowsiness they produce often wears off over time. Other medications used for IC include pentosan polysulfate sodium (Elmiron), pyridium, and anti-inflammatory drugs.

Distending the bladder by filling it to capacity with water for 2 to 8 minutes is frequently useful, but although the beneficial effects may persist for months, symptoms usually return eventually. In some cases, medications such as dimethyl sulfoxide and heparin may be introduced into the bladder with a catheter; actual surgical alteration of the bladder is rarely used to treat IC.

Proposed Natural Treatments

There are no well-documented natural treatments for interstitial cystitis, but a few supplements have shown promise.

Quercetin

Quercetin is a bioflavonoid that may have anti-inflammatory properties. A small double-blind, placebo-controlled trial found that a supplement containing quercetin reduced symptoms of interstitial cystitis.

Arginine

The amino acid **arginine** helps the body make nitric oxide, a substance that relaxes smooth muscles like those found in the bladder. Based on this mechanism, arginine has been proposed as a treatment for IC.

A 3-month, double-blind trial of 53 individuals with interstitial cystitis found only weak indications that arginine might improve symptoms of interstitial cystitis.

Several participants dropped out of the study; when this was properly taken into account using a statistical method called *ITT analysis*, no benefit at all could be proven.

A very small double-blind study also failed to find arginine more effective than placebo.

Glycosaminoglycans

There is some evidence that in interstitial cystitis the surface layer of the bladder is deficient in protective natural substances called *glycosaminoglycans*. This in turn might allow the bladder to become inflamed; it might also initiate autoimmune reactions.

Based on these highly preliminary findings, using of supplemental glycosaminoglycans in the form of mesoglycan or **chondroitin sulfate** have been suggested for interstitial cystitis. However, there is no reliable evidence as yet that they really work.

TENS

Transcutaneous electrical stimulation, or TENS, is primarily used (with mixed results) in the treatment of muscular pain. It has also been tried in interstitial cystitis, but thus far the evidence that it works is highly preliminary.

Diet

Although there is no solid scientific evidence that dietary changes can relieve IC, many people find that certain foods increase their symptoms. The most frequently cited offenders are coffee, chocolate, ethanol, carbonated drinks, citrus fruits, and tomatoes. Based on these reports, it may be worthwhile to experiment with your diet.

Intestinal Gas

RELATED TERMS: *Flatulence; Bloating, Intestinal*

PRINCIPAL PROPOSED NATURAL TREATMENTS: *None*

OTHER PROPOSED NATURAL TREATMENTS: *Activated Charcoal, Artichoke Leaf, Beta-galactosidase, Boldo, Carminative Herbs (Such as Chamomile, Coriander, Caraway, Cumin, Dill, Fennel, Garlic, Ginger, Parsley, and Spearmint), Peppermint Oil, Probiotics, Turmeric, Yucca, Zinc*

The passing of intestinal gas is a normal process, but it can become unpleasant, uncomfortable, or embarrassing. Intestinal gas has two primary sources: bacteria in the intestines and air swallowed by mouth (aerophagia). Certain foods greatly increase the production of gas in the intestines by providing nutrients to gas-producing bacteria. Common gas-increasing foods include beans, beer, broccoli, cabbage, cauliflower, fructose, onions, prunes, red wine, and sorbitol. In general, high-fiber foods cause more gas than low-fiber ones and, for this reason, people who switch to a whole foods diet frequently experience more gas.

Certain medical conditions can also increase gas-related symptoms, including celiac sprue, colon cancer, **Crohn's disease**, fat malabsorption, irritable bowel syndrome, **lactose intolerance**, **pregnancy**, and **ulcerative colitis**. Finally, some people may experience significant gas discomfort without actually producing more gas than other people.

Treatment of excess gas begins with treating the underlying disease, if there is one. Beyond that, general steps include avoiding gas-producing foods and minimizing habits that cause aerophagia (such as gulping of beverages). Medications such as simethicone, metoclopramide, and antibiotics may also help, although the supporting evidence to indicate that they are effective remains incomplete.

Proposed Natural Treatments

There has been little meaningful scientific investigation of natural treatments to reduce gas in people who are otherwise healthy. However, some evidence supports the use of natural treatments for reducing gas production among those with irritable bowel syndrome (a cluster of nonspecific intestinal complaints) or dyspepsia (a cluster of nonspecific stomach-related complaints). It is likely, although not guaranteed, that the benefits seen in these studies would carry over to people without these conditions.

For example, a 4-week, double-blind, placebo-controlled study of 60 people with irritable bowel syndrome found that use of **probiotics** (friendly bacteria) reduced gas-related discomfort. Probiotics are presumed to work by replacing gas-producing bacteria with others that are less likely to create gas. **Note**: Initial use of probiotics reportedly can increase gas production for a short time.

Other treatments for irritable bowel syndrome, such as **peppermint oil** and **flaxseed**, may be helpful as well. For more information, see the full **Irritable Bowel Syndrome** article.

The herbs **turmeric**, **artichoke leaf**, and **boldo** have shown promise for reducing gas in people with dyspepsia. For more information, see the **Dyspepsia** article.

Beano, a product containing the enzyme alpha-galactosidase, is widely available for reducing gas caused by consuming beans. This enzyme breaks down some of the gas-producing carbohydrates in beans. However, a study designed to test this substance found only weak evidence of effectiveness.

Activated charcoal taken by mouth may reduce the amount of flatulence, although not all studies agree.

Certain herbs called *carminatives* are traditionally believed to aid the movement of gas. These include anise, **caraway**, cardamom, **chamomile**, coriander, cumin, dill, **fennel**, **garlic**, **ginger**, **parsley**, and spearmint.

In addition, numerous alternative therapies are said to help improve digestion and reduce gas, including **Chinese herbal medicine**, **intestinal cleansing**, and **food allergen identification and avoidance**. However, there is little supporting evidence for these approaches.

One study in dogs indicates that a combination of

charcoal, **yucca**, and **zinc** acetate significantly reduced the smell of intestinal gas, although not the amount that was released. Taken separately, charcoal was the most effective of these treatments. Garments containing activated charcoal have also shown promise for reducing the odor of flatulence.

Irritable Bowel Syndrome

RELATED TERMS: *Spastic Colon*

PRINCIPAL PROPOSED NATURAL TREATMENTS: *Flaxseed, Peppermint Oil, Probiotics, Traditional Chinese Herbal Medicine*

OTHER PROPOSED NATURAL TREATMENTS: *Acupuncture, Avoidance of Allergenic Foods,* Coleus forskohlii, *Digestive Enzymes (Including Bromelain and Other Proteolytic Enzymes), Fructo-oligosaccharides, Glutamine, Hypnotherapy, Melatonin, Slippery Elm*

The symptoms of irritable bowel syndrome (IBS) include one or more of the following: Alternating diarrhea and constipation, intestinal gas, bloating and cramping, abdominal pain, painful bowel movements, mucus discharge, and undigested food in the stool. Despite all these distressing symptoms, in IBS the intestines appear to be perfectly healthy when they are examined. Thus the condition belongs to a category of diseases that physicians call *functional*. This term means that while the function of the bowel seems to have gone awry, no injury or disturbance of its structure can be discovered.

The cause of IBS remains unknown. Medical treatment for IBS consists mainly of increased dietary fiber plus drugs that reduce bowel spasm. In addition, various forms of psychotherapy, including hypnosis, have been tried, with some success.

Principal Proposed Natural Treatments

Peppermint

Peppermint oil is widely used for IBS. While the research evidence is a bit inconsistent, 8 out of 12 placebo-controlled studies found peppermint oil more effective than placebo. However, most studies were small.

For more information, including dosage and safety issues, see the full **Peppermint** article.

Probiotics

Several double-blind trials indicate that various probiotics ("friendly" bacteria) may be helpful for IBS

For example, in a 4-week, double-blind, placebo-controlled trial of 60 individuals with IBS, probiotic treatment with *L. plantarum* reduced intestinal gas significantly. The benefits persisted for an additional year after treatment was stopped. A similar study of 40 people also found benefits with *L. plantarum*.

However, there have been negative results as well.

For more information, see the full **Probiotics** article.

Flaxseeds

In a double-blind study, 55 people with chronic constipation caused by IBS received either ground flaxseed or psyllium seed (a well-known treatment for constipation) daily for 3 months. Those taking flaxseed had significantly fewer problems with constipation, abdominal pain, and bloating than those taking psyllium. The flaxseed group had even further improvements in constipation and bloating while continuing their treatment in the 3 months after the double-blind study ended. The researcher concluded that flaxseed relieved constipation more effectively than psyllium.

For more information, see the **Flaxseed** article.

Chinese Herbal Medicine

Chinese herbal medicine is traditionally practiced in a highly individualized way, with herbal formulas tailored to the exact details of each person's case. In a double-blind, placebo-controlled trial, 116 people with IBS were randomly assigned to receive individualized Chinese herbal treatment, a "one-size-fits-all" Chinese herbal formulation, or placebo. Treatment consisted of 5 capsules 3 times daily, taken for 16 weeks. The results showed that both forms of active treatment were superior to placebo, significantly reducing IBS symptoms.

However, the individualized treatment was no more effective than the "generic" treatment.

For more information on this complex medical system, including important safety issues, see the **Traditional Chinese Herbal Medicine** article.

Other Proposed Natural Treatments

One study found evidence that pancreatic digestive enzymes (including **proteolytic enzymes** plus other enzymes called *lipases*) might be helpful for reducing the flare-up of IBS symptoms that may follow a fatty meal.

An herbal combination containing **candytuft**, **matricaria flower**, **peppermint leaves**, **caraway**, **licorice root**, and **lemon balm** has shown some promise for IBS.

One small double-blind placebo-controlled trial tested **melatonin** for people with IBS and sleep disturbances. Interestingly, though melatonin did not help the sleep disturbances, it did reduce abdominal pain. Benefits were also seen in another small study, again unrelated to improvements in sleep.

The herbs *Coleus forskohlii* and **slippery elm** as well as the supplement **glutamine** are also sometimes recommended for IBS, but there is no meaningful evidence as yet that they are helpful.

One double-blind study failed to find either the herb fumitory or an herbal relative of **turmeric** helpful for IBS.

The prebiotic supplement **fructo-oligosaccharides** has been advocated as a treatment for IBS. However, in a 12-week, double-blind, placebo-controlled study of 98 people, treatment at a dose of 20 g daily slightly worsened symptoms initially and then produced no effect. One study did find benefit with a combination prebiotic–probiotic formula.

Food allergies may play a role in IBS and diets based on identifying and eliminating allergenic foods might offer some benefit.

Hypnotherapy has shown some promise for IBS as well.

Acupuncture has been proposed as a treatment for IBS. However, study results have thus far failed to show it effective. For example, a 13-week study of 60 people with IBS found fake acupuncture just as beneficial as traditional acupuncture. Two other studies also failed to find benefit.

Jet Lag

PRINCIPAL PROPOSED NATURAL TREATMENTS: *Melatonin*

OTHER PROPOSED NATURAL TREATMENTS: *Nicotinamide Adenine Dinucleotide* (*NADH*)*, Tyrosine, Natural Treatments for Insomnia*

The body has an internal clock of sorts that follows the rhythms of night and day. Airplane travel confuses this clock, causing the phenomenon known as *jet lag*. If you've ever crossed several time zones, you've probably experienced jet lag to some degree. You may have felt exhausted in the morning and wide awake at night, and between those times experienced symptoms such as fatigue, loss of concentration, dizziness, lightheadedness, irritability, nausea, and headache.

Ordinarily, the body clock resets itself within a few days. It is possible to speed up this natural process by deliberately using stimuli to indicate to your body when you want it to wake up and when it should fall asleep. Common methods involve social activity and outdoor exercise during the daylight, combined with meal times appropriate to the new time zone. It is also generally considered important to stay awake upon arrival in the new time zone until night falls. Use of sleeping pills may be helpful at first, so you don't stay awake staring at the walls. In addition, some physicians are experimenting with wakefulness drugs used for narcolepsy, such as modafinil, to help travelers stay active and alert on arrival.

Principal Proposed Natural Treatments

Melatonin is a natural hormone that plays a role in the day–night cycle (the circadian rhythm). During daylight, the pineal gland in the brain produces an important neurotransmitter called *serotonin*. But at night, the pineal gland stops producing serotonin and instead makes melatonin. This melatonin release helps trigger sleep.

The amount of melatonin production varies according to the intensity of light to which you're exposed; for example, your body produces more melatonin in a completely dark room than in a dimly lit one.

This cyclic pattern of melatonin release helps set the body's biologic clock. Melatonin supplements taken by mouth can be used to *reset* this clock, an effect of potential benefit in jet lag.

According to a review published in 2001, reasonably good evidence indicates that melatonin is indeed effective for this purpose. One of the best supporting studies was a double-blind, placebo-controlled study that enrolled 320 travelers crossing six to eight time zones. The participants were divided into four groups and given a daily dose of 5 mg of standard melatonin, 5 mg of slow-release melatonin, 0.5 mg of standard melatonin, or placebo. The results of this large study were promising. The group that received 5 mg of standard melatonin slept better, took less time to fall asleep and felt more energetic and awake during the day than the other three groups.

For more information, including dosage and safety issues, see the full **Melatonin** article.

Other Proposed Natural Treatments

Nicotinamide adenine dinucleotide (NADH) is a chemical that the body manufactures on its own to serve a variety of biologic purposes. In a double-blind, placebo-controlled trial, 35 people taking an overnight flight across four time zones were given either 20 mg of NADH or placebo sublingually (under the tongue) on the morning of arrival. Participants were twice given tests of wakefulness and mental function: first at 90 minutes and then at 5 hours after landing. People given NADH scored significantly better on these tests than those given placebo.

Tyrosine is an amino acid found in meat proteins. A double-blind, placebo-controlled study that enrolled 20 U.S. Marines suggests that tyrosine supplements can improve alertness during periods of sleep deprivation. In this study, the participants were deprived of sleep for a night and then tested frequently for their alertness throughout the following day as they worked. Compared to placebo, 10 to 15 g of tyrosine given twice daily seemed to provide a "pick-up" for about 2 hours.

Similar benefits were seen with 2 g of tyrosine daily in a double-blind, placebo-controlled trial of 21 military cadets exposed to physical and psychological stress, including sleep deprivation. These findings suggest that tyrosine could be helpful for jet lag.

Besides these supplements, all the natural treatments used for insomnia may be helpful for getting a good night's sleep on the first night of travel. See the full **Insomnia** article for more information.

Kidney Stones

RELATED TERMS: *Calcium Oxalate Stones, Nephrolithiasis, Renal Calculi, Urinary Calculi, Urolithiasis*

PRINCIPAL PROPOSED NATURAL TREATMENTS: *Citrate*

OTHER PROPOSED NATURAL TREATMENTS: *Goldenrod (and Other Diuretic Herbs, such as Buchu, Cleavers, Dandelion, Juniper, Parsley, Horsetail, and Rosemary), Fish Oil, Gamma-linolenic Acid (GLA), Magnesium, Pumpkin Seeds, Rose Hips, Vitamin B$_6$*

HERBS AND SUPPLEMENTS TO USE ONLY WITH CAUTION: *Calcium, Grapefruit Juice, Vitamin C*

If you've ever passed a kidney stone, you do not want to repeat the experience! The sharp and irregular stones travel down the slender tube (ureter) leading from the kidney to the bladder, and from the bladder to the urethra, following the path by which urine exits the body. While tiny stones may pass unnoticed, a larger stone can induce some of the worst pain that humans experience.

Most kidney stones are composed of calcium and oxalic acid, substances present in the urine that can crystallize inside the kidneys. Although these chemicals occur in everyone's urine, our natural biochemistry is usually able to prevent them from crystallizing. However, sometimes these protective methods fail and a stone develops. This article focuses mainly on these *calcium oxalate stones*.

Less commonly, kidney stones may be made from calcium and phosphate, from another substance called *struvite* (usually the result of an infection) or, rarely, from uric acid or cystine.

It isn't known why some people develop kidney stones and others do not. However, once you've had a stone, you are fairly likely to develop another.

Low fluid intake greatly increases the risk of developing virtually all types of stones. For this reason, individuals at risk of developing stones are often advised to increase their fluid intake. However, while there is evidence that fluids in the form of coffee, tea, beer, and wine can decrease risk of kidney stone development, apple juice and grapefruit juice may have the opposite effect.

High intakes of sodium and protein (particularly animal protein) may also increase the risk of calcium oxalate stones, although some studies have found that protein has no such effect. Oxalate-rich foods, such as spinach and cocoa, may also increase the risk of developing calcium oxalate stones. Indirect evidence suggests that regular use of cranberry concentrate tablets might also increase risk of kidney stones. In addition, vitamin D affects calcium levels in the body, and prolonged use of extremely excessive doses of vitamin D has been known to cause kidney stones. Strangely, however, high-calcium foods don't seem to increase the risk of calcium oxalate stones (see Other Proposed Treatments for Kidney Stones below).

Conventional treatment for kidney stones varies depending on symptoms as well as the location and chemical composition of the stones. For those who pass a stone spontaneously, the main treatments are painkillers and fluids. The chemical composition of passed stones can be analyzed to determine their cause. Other stones may be detected earlier, when they are still in the kidney. Treatment depends on their location and symptoms. Those causing problems may be treated with *extracorporeal shock-wave lithotripsy*, a technique that can break up these stones from outside the body, allowing them to pass more easily. Occasionally, however, surgery may be necessary.

"Silent" stones, or those causing no symptoms, are often treated with preventive measures alone. These methods include increasing fluids, modifying the diet, and taking drugs or supplements to alter the chemistry of the urine.

Principal Proposed Natural Treatments

Citrate

Citrate, or citric acid, is an ordinary component of our diet, present in high amounts in citrus fruits. Citrate binds with calcium in the urine, thereby reducing the amount of calcium available to form calcium oxalate stones. It also prevents tiny calcium oxalate crystals from growing and massing together into larger stones. Finally, it makes the urine less acidic, which inhibits the development of both calcium oxalate and uric acid stones.

➢ *What Is the Scientific Evidence for Citrate?*

One form of citrate supplement, potassium citrate, was approved by the FDA in 1985 for the prevention of two kinds of kidney stones: calcium stones (including calcium oxalate stones) and uric acid stones.

In a 3-year, double-blind study of 57 people with a history of calcium stones and low urinary citrate levels, those given potassium citrate developed fewer kidney stones than they had previously. In comparison, the group given placebo had no change in their rate of stone formation.

Potassium-magnesium citrate was studied in a 3-year trial involving 64 participants with a history of calcium oxalate stones. During the study, new stones formed in only 12.9% of those taking the potassium-magnesium citrate supplement, compared to 63.6% of those taking placebo. Benefits have been seen in other small studies as well.

Citrate is available in the form of calcium citrate. Besides increasing citrate in the urine, this supplement has the advantage of being a readily absorbed form of calcium for those seeking to increase their calcium intake for other health reasons. However, calcium citrate has not yet been studied as a preventive for kidney stones.

Some physicians have proposed drinking citrus juices as a means of increasing urinary citrate levels. Like potassium citrate, orange juice decreases urinary acidity and raises urinary citrate, but it also raises urinary oxalate, which might tend to work against its beneficial effects. Lemon juice may be preferable, as it has almost five times the citrate of orange juice. A small study found that drinking 2 liters of lemonade daily doubled urinary citrate in people with decreased urinary citrate. Avoid regular consumption of grapefruit juice, though: in one large-scale study, women drinking 8 ounces of grapefruit juice daily increased their risk of stones by 44%.

It was first thought that citrate supplements were only helpful against kidney stones in individuals who didn't excrete the normal amount of citrate in their urine. However, some researchers now suggest that citrate treatment may also be useful for those at risk for stones whose citrate excretion is normal.

⇒ *Dosage*

The proper dosage of citrate depends on the chemical form and should be individualized under medical supervision.

⇒ *Safety Issues*

Potassium citrate can irritate the gastrointestinal tract, causing upset stomach or bloating in 9 to 17% of people. Potassium-magnesium citrate may potentially cause the same problem, although one study found it to be no more irritating than placebo.

Supplements containing potassium have the potential to raise blood levels of potassium too high, primarily in people with impaired kidneys or those taking a **potassium-sparing diuretic**, such as triamterene. Taking too much citrate can also result in overly alkaline blood, again particularly in people with kidney disease.

Citrate-induced reduction of urinary acidity can lead to decreased blood levels and effectiveness of numerous drugs, including **lithium**, **methotrexate**, **oral diabetes drugs**, **aspirin** and other salicylates, and **tetracycline antibiotics**. In addition, the urinary antiseptic methenamine is less effective in alkaline urine. Conversely, the blood levels of other drugs could increase, possibly increasing risk of toxicity. These drugs include stimulants, such as **ephedrine** and methamphetamine, as well as the drugs flecainide and mecamylamine.

Other Proposed Natural Treatments

Magnesium, in the form of magnesium oxide or magnesium hydroxide, may help to prevent calcium oxalate stone development. Magnesium inhibits the growth of these stones in the test tube and decreases stone formation in rats. However, human studies on magnesium have shown mixed results. In one 2-year open study, 56 participants taking magnesium hydroxide had fewer recurrences of kidney stones than 34 participants not given magnesium. In contrast, a double-blind (hence, far more

reliable) study with 124 participants found that magnesium hydroxide was essentially no more effective than placebo.

Two studies performed in Thailand hint that **pumpkin seeds** might help prevent kidney stones among children at high risk for developing them. However, this research only looked at chemical changes in the urine suggestive of a possible preventive effect, not actual reduction of stones. Furthermore, the design of the studies did not reach modern standards.

The herb **rose hips** might also improve the chemical composition of urine and thereby reduce kidney stone risk. However, rose hips are very high in **vitamin C**, and vitamin C itself has shown potential risks in people with a tendency toward stones (see Safety Issues below)

Vitamin B$_6$ might help prevent calcium oxalate stones in certain individuals. Deficiencies in this vitamin increase the amount of oxalate in the urine of animals and humans, and a small uncontrolled study found that supplementation decreased oxalate excretion in people with a history of stones. In addition, a 14-year observational study of more than 85,000 women with no history of kidney stones found that women with high intakes of B$_6$ developed fewer stones than those with the lowest intake. On the other hand, a large-scale observational study of more than 45,000 men found no link between B$_6$ and stones. Keep in mind that observational studies are notorious for producing misleading results. Only double-blind trials can actually provide evidence of benefit. (For information on why this is so, see **Why Does This Book Rely on Double-blind Studies?**.) Several supplements, including **fish oil**, **GLA**, **glycosaminoglycans** (GAGs), and **vitamin A**, are also sometimes recommended for kidney stones, but there is only extremely preliminary evidence that they are helpful.

A variety of herbs are often recommended for kidney stones, on the theory that they increase urine flow and this will help pass kidney stones. These include asparagus, birch leaf, bishop's weed fruit, **buchu**, **cleavers**, couch grass, **dandelion**, **goldenrod**, **juniper**, **rosemary**, **horsetail**, java, lovage, **parsley**, petasites, shiny restharrow, and **stinging nettle** herb and root combinations. However, there is no meaningful evidence that they are really effective.

One study claimed to find trigger point injection (a form of treatment somewhat related to **acupuncture**) helpful for reducing the pain of kidney stones, but because it lacked a placebo group the results mean very little.

Herbs and Supplements to Use Only with Caution

According to some, but not all research, use of **vitamin C** supplements can slightly raise levels of oxalate in the urine, which could in turn increase risk of kidney stones. However, large-scale observational studies have found that people who consume large amounts of vitamin C have no increased risk or even a decreased risk of kidney stone formation. Nonetheless, it seems that in certain people, high vitamin C intake can lead to a rapid increase in urinary oxalate, and in one case stones developed within a few days. **The bottom line**: People with a history of kidney stones should probably limit vitamin C supplements to about 100 mg daily.

Calcium supplements also present concerns, because they could conceivably increase formation of calcium oxalate or other calcium-based stones. Observational studies and other forms of preliminary evidence do suggest that use of calcium supplements may slightly increase kidney stone risk. Interestingly, though, increased intake of calcium from *food* does not seem to be associated with increased risk of kidney stones and could even help prevent them. Therefore, individuals with a history of kidney stones might be best advised to get their calcium from food rather than supplements. Alternatively, one study suggests that if calcium supplements are taken with food, no harm results. Furthermore, use of calcium as calcium citrate may present no increased risk, presumably because the citrate portion of the supplement has activity against kidney stones.

As noted above, regular consumption of grapefruit juice may significantly increase risk of stones.

Lactose Intolerance

PRINCIPAL PROPOSED NATURAL TREATMENTS: *Lactase*

OTHER PROPOSED NATURAL TREATMENTS: *Calcium, Probiotics*

Sugar comes in many forms. One type of sugar, lactose, occurs primarily in milk. Nature gives young children the ability to digest lactose, because they need to do so when they nurse. However, as people grow up, they often lose the lactose-digesting enzyme known as *lactase*. The result is a condition called *lactose intolerance*. Symptoms include intestinal cramps, gas, and diarrhea following consumption of lactose-containing foods.

Principal Proposed Natural Treatments

Lactose intolerance is most prevalent in people of Hispanic, African, Asian, Middle Eastern, or Native American descent, although Caucasians can develop it as well. Treatment consists primarily of avoiding foods containing lactose, such as milk and ice cream. Use of lactase supplements may help people who are lactose intolerant handle more lactose than otherwise. Also, special milk products are available from which the lactose has been removed (often through the use of lactase).

Other Proposed Natural Treatments

Aside from lactase, there are no effective natural treatments for lactose intolerance. Despite some positive anecdotes, scientific evidence suggests that use of **probiotics**, such as *Lactobacillus acidophilus*, will not improve symptoms. However, natural medicine does have one contribution to make to people who are lactose intolerant: reminding them to take calcium supplements. People who avoid lactose-containing foods often do not get enough calcium in their diets and may, therefore, be at increased risk of osteoporosis and other health problems. Calcium supplements should correct this problem. For detailed information on the proper dosages and types of calcium to use, see the full **Calcium** article.

Many people confuse milk allergy with lactose intolerance. The two conditions are not related. Milk allergy involves an allergic reaction to the protein component of milk, and lactase supplements will not help. For more information on natural approaches to food allergies, see the **Food Allergy** article.

Liver Cirrhosis

RELATED TERMS: *Alcoholic Liver Cirrhosis, Biliary Cirrhosis, Cirrhosis of the Liver*

PRINCIPAL PROPOSED NATURAL TREATMENTS: *Milk Thistle*

OTHER PROPOSED NATURAL TREATMENTS: *Antioxidants, Ayurvedic Herbal Combinations, BCAAs, Calcium and Vitamin D, OPCs, Phosphatidylcholine, SAMe, Taurine*

HERBS AND SUPPLEMENTS TO USE ONLY WITH CAUTION: *Barberry, Beta-carotene, Blue-green Algae, Borage, Chaparral, Coltsfoot, Comfrey, Germander, Germanium, Greater Celandine, Kava, Kombucha, Mistletoe, Pennyroyal, Pokeroot, Sassafras, Skullcap, Spirulina, Traditional Chinese Herbal Medicine, Vitamin A, Vitamin B$_3$, Vitamin K*

The liver is a marvelously sophisticated chemical laboratory, capable of carrying out thousands of chemical transformations on which the body depends. The liver produces important chemicals from scratch, modifies others to allow the body to use them better, and neutralizes an enormous range of toxins. Without a functioning liver, you can't live for very long.

Unfortunately, a number of influences can severely damage the liver. **Alcoholism** is the most common. Alcohol is a powerful liver toxin that harms the liver in three stages: alcoholic fatty liver, **alcoholic hepatitis**, and alcoholic cirrhosis. Although the first two stages of injury are usually reversible, alcoholic cirrhosis is not. Generally, more than 10 years of heavy alcohol abuse is required to cause liver cirrhosis. Other causes include **hepatitis C** infection, primary biliary cirrhosis, and **liver damage** caused by occupational chemicals and drugs.

A cirrhotic liver is firm and nodular to the touch, and in advanced cases is shrunken in size. These changes reflect severe damage to its structure. A high percentage of liver cells have died and fibrous scar-like tissue permeates the organ.

A cirrhotic liver cannot perform its chemical tasks, leading to wide-ranging impairment of bodily functions, such as the development of jaundice (yellowing of the skin due to unprocessed toxins), mental confusion, emaciation, and skin changes. In addition, the fibrous tissue impedes blood that is supposed to pass through the liver. This leads to abdominal swelling as fluid backs up (ascites) and to bleeding in the esophagus as veins expand to provide an alternative fluid path. Ultimately, coma develops, often triggered by internal bleeding or infection.

Treatments for liver cirrhosis begin with stopping the use of alcohol and all other liver-toxic substances. A number of treatments such as **potassium-sparing diuretics** can ameliorate symptoms to some extent, but they do not cure the disease.

The liver is too complex for a man-made machine to duplicate its functions, so there is no equivalent of kidney dialysis for liver cirrhosis. Only a liver transplant can help. Unfortunately, this is a very difficult operation, with a high failure rate. In addition, the supply of usable livers is inadequate to meet the need.

Note: Individuals with cirrhosis of the liver should not take any medications, herbs, or dietary supplements without first consulting a physician. The liver is in charge of processing many substances taken into the body and, when it is severely damaged, as in liver cirrhosis, ordinarily benign substances may become toxic.

Principal Proposed Natural Treatments

The herb milk thistle might offer various liver-protective benefits. In Europe, it is used to treat **viral hepatitis**, alcoholic fatty liver, alcoholic hepatitis, liver cirrhosis, and drug- or chemical-induced **liver toxicity**. An intravenous preparation made from milk thistle is used as an antidote for poisoning by the liver-toxic deathcap mushroom, *Amanita phalloides*. However, the supporting evidence for its use in any of these conditions remains far from definitive.

A double-blind, placebo-controlled study of 170 individuals with alcoholic or non-alcoholic cirrhosis found that, in the group treated with milk thistle, the 4-year survival rate was 58% as compared to only 38% in the placebo group. This difference was statistically significant.

A double-blind, placebo controlled trial that enrolled 172 individuals with cirrhosis for 4 years also found reductions in mortality, but they just missed the conventional cutoff for statistical significance. And a 2-year, double-blind, placebo-controlled study of 200 individuals with alcoholic cirrhosis found no reduction in mortality attributable to the use of milk thistle.

Other double-blind studies of cirrhotic individuals have found improvements in tests of liver function, although one did not.

For more information, including dosage and safety issues, see the full **Milk Thistle** article.

Other Proposed Natural Treatments

SAMe: May Improve Survival in Liver Cirrhosis

Individuals with liver cirrhosis have difficulty synthesizing the substance SAMe (S-adenosylmethionine) from the amino acid **methionine**. For this reason, supplemental SAMe (best known as a treatment for **depression** and **osteoarthritis**) has been tried as a treatment for cirrhosis. However, as yet the evidence that it works is not strong.

A 2-year, double-blind, placebo-controlled trial followed 117 people with alcoholic liver cirrhosis. Overall, those given SAMe didn't do significantly better than those given placebo. However, when the results were re-evaluated to eliminate individuals with severe liver cirrhosis, a significant reduction in mortality and liver transplantation was seen with SAMe.

SAMe has also shown a bit of promise for primary biliary cirrhosis, though evidence is not consistent.

For more information, including dosage and safety issues, see the full **SAMe** article.

Branched-chain Amino Acids: Might Be Helpful for Hepatic Encephalopathy

In advanced liver cirrhosis, individuals experience severe mental confusion and may slip into a coma. This condition is called *hepatic encephalopathy*. One of the primary causes of hepatic encephalopathy is excessive ammonia levels in the body.

There is some reason to believe that special amino acids called *branched-chain amino acids* (BCAAs) might be helpful for individuals with hepatic encephalopathy, based on how they are metabolized in the body. However, the evidence that BCAAs actually help is not yet conclusive. Furthermore, individuals with cirrhosis of the liver should not increase amino acid or protein intake except under physician supervision.

For more information, including dosage and safety issues, see the full **BCAAs** article.

Oligomeric Proanthocyanidins: Might Help Prevent Internal Bleeding

Individuals with cirrhosis are susceptible to internal bleeding. Highly preliminary evidence suggests that oligomeric proanthocyanidins (OPCs) might help prevent this problem.

OPCs are best documented as a treatment for **venous insufficiency** (closely related to **varicose veins**), where they are thought to work in part by stabilizing blood vessels. Individuals with cirrhosis have what amounts to internal varicose veins caused by the shunting of fluid around the damaged liver. For more information, including dosage and safety issues, see the full **OPCs** article.

Other Natural Treatments That Might Help

One small study suggests that the supplement **carnitine** might be helpful for people with hepatic encephalopathy.

The amino acid **taurine** might help reduce muscle cramps in individuals with cirrhosis. (However, see the warning in the BCAA section.)

One study suggests that protein from vegetable sources might be preferable to protein from animal sources for people with liver cirrhosis, presumably due to differences in amino acid content.

Preliminary evidence from animal studies suggest that the supplement **phosphatidylcholine** might help prevent alcoholic liver cirrhosis. The supplement **ornithine alpha-ketoglutarate** (OKG) has shown promise for treating hepatic encephalopathy, a life-threatening complication of cirrhosis.

Vitamin K has shown a bit of promise for helping prevent liver cancer in people with cirrhosis of the liver.

An **Ayurvedic herbal combination** has been studied for the treatment of cirrhosis, but current evidence supporting its use remains incomplete and contradictory.

Antioxidants have been proposed for the treatment of primary biliary cirrhosis, based on the theory that free radicals play a role in the disease process. However, despite apparent promise seen in open trials, a double-blind, placebo-controlled study of 61 subjects failed to find that combination of **vitamins A, C, and E, selenium, methionine,** and **CoenzymeQ$_{10}$** produced any benefit in terms of fatigue or other liver-related symptoms.

The bones of individuals with biliary cirrhosis often become thin. Taking **calcium** and **vitamin D** supplements might help. Antioxidants such as vitamin C, vitamin E, and **lipoic acid** have been tried for biliary cirrhosis, with promising results in very preliminary trials.

Herbs and Supplements to Use Only with Caution

Many natural products have the capacity to harm the liver. Furthermore, because of the generally inadequate regulation of dietary supplements that exists at the time of this writing, there are real risks that herbal products, at the least, may contain liver-toxic contaminants even if the actual herbs listed on the label are safe. For this reason, we recommend that people with liver disease do not use any medicinal herbs except under the supervision of a physician. Here, we list some specific information to aid in your decision-making process.

Vitamin A and **beta-carotene** supplements might cause alcoholic liver disease to develop more rapidly.

All forms of **vitamin B₃** may damage the liver when taken in high doses, including niacin, niacinamide (nicotinamide), and inositol hexaniacinate. (Nutritional supplementation at the standard daily requirement level should not cause a problem.)

A great many herbs and supplements have known or suspected liver-toxic properties, including but not limited to **barberry**, borage, chaparral, **coltsfoot**, **comfrey**, **germander**, germanium (a mineral), **greater celandine**, certain **green tea** extracts, **kava**, **kombucha**, **mistletoe**, **pennyroyal**, **pokeroot**, **sassafras**, and various herbs and minerals used in **traditional Chinese herbal medicine**. In addition, herbs that are not liver-toxic in themselves are sometimes adulterated with other herbs of similar appearance that are accidentally harvested in a misapprehension of their identity (for example, germander found in **skullcap** products). Furthermore, blue-green algae species such as **spirulina** may at times be contaminated with liver-toxic substances called *microcystins*, for which no highest safe level is known. Some articles claim that the herb **echinacea** is potentially liver-toxic, but this concern appears to have been based on a misunderstanding of its constituents. Echinacea contains substances in the pyrrolizidine alkaloid family. However, while many pyrrolizidine alkaloids are liver-toxic, those found in echinacea are not believed to have that property.

Whole **valerian** contains liver-toxic substances called *valepotriates*; however, valepotriates are thought to be absent from most commercial valerian products and case reports suggest that even very high doses of valerian do not harm the liver.

Liver Disease, General

RELATED TERMS: *Liver Support; Liver-toxic Herbs; Herbs, Liver-toxic; Gilbert's Syndrome; Cholestasis*

PRINCIPAL PROPOSED NATURAL TREATMENTS: *Milk Thistle, SAMe*

OTHER PROPOSED NATURAL TREATMENTS: *Andrographis, Artichoke Leaf, Beet Leaf, Betaine (Trimethylglycine, or TMG), Choline, Dandelion, Inositol, Lecithin, Licorice, Lipoic Acid, Liver Extracts, Noni, Phyllanthus, Picrorhiza kurroa, Schisandra, Taurine, Thymus Extract, Turmeric*

HERBS AND SUPPLEMENTS TO USE ONLY WITH CAUTION: *Beta-carotene, Blue-green Algae, Chaparral, Coltsfoot, Comfrey, Germander, Germanium, Green Tea Extracts, Greater Celandine, Kava, Kombucha, Mistletoe, Pennyroyal, Pokeroot, Sassafras, Skullcap, Spirulina, Traditional Chinese Herbal Medicine, Vitamin A, Vitamin B₃*

The liver is a marvelously sophisticated chemical laboratory, capable of carrying out thousands of chemical transformations on which the body depends. The liver produces important chemicals from scratch, modifies others to allow the body to use them better, and neutralizes an enormous range of toxins.

However, this last function of the liver, neutralizing toxins, is also the organ's Achilles' heel. The process of rendering toxins harmless to the body at large may bring harm to the liver itself.

Alcohol is the most common chemical responsible for toxic damage to the liver, causing fatty liver, **alcoholic hepatitis,** and, potentially, **cirrhosis of the liver.** Exposure to industrial chemicals may harm the liver. Many prescription medications may damage the liver as well, including cholesterol-lowering drugs in the **statin family** and high-dose **niacin** (also used to reduce cholesterol levels.) The over-the-counter drug **acetaminophen** (Tylenol) is highly toxic to the liver when taken to excess. Finally, numerous natural herbs and supplements contain chemicals that may cause or accelerate harm to the liver. (See Herbs and Supplements to Use Only with Caution below.)

Chemicals aren't the only source of harm to the liver. Viruses may infect it, causing **viral hepatitis**; hepatitis C, in particular, may become chronic and gradually destroy the liver. In addition, during **pregnancy,** the liver may become backed up with bile, a condition called *cholestasis of pregnancy.*

Conventional treatment of liver disease depends on the source of the problem. People who abuse alcohol will at the very least avoid further liver damage by stopping alcohol use, and, in cases short of liver cirrhosis, full liver recovery may be expected. When drugs are at fault, it may be possible to switch to a different drug.

Conventional treatment of liver injury caused by chronic viral hepatitis involves sophisticated immune-regulating therapies and has become fairly successful. In extreme cases of liver injury, a liver transplant may be necessary.

Principal Proposed Natural Treatments

Natural treatments for alcoholic hepatitis, cirrhosis, and viral hepatitis are each discussed in their own articles. In this article, we discuss natural treatments for other forms of liver disease. In addition, we address the herbs and supplements that may harm the liver and that, therefore, should not be take by people who already have liver disease.

Milk Thistle

The herb milk thistle has shown promise for a wide variety of liver conditions and, for this reason, it is often said to have general liver protective properties.

Some evidence suggests benefit for viral hepatitis (especially chronic hepatitis), cirrhosis of the liver, alcoholic hepatitis, and liver toxicity caused by industrial chemicals, mushroom poisons, and medications. However, as yet the evidence that milk thistle really works remains incomplete and contradictory.

For example, a double-blind, placebo-controlled study performed in 1981 followed 106 Finnish soldiers with alcoholic liver disease over a period of 4 weeks. The treated group showed a significant decrease in elevated liver enzymes and improvement in liver histology (appearance of cells under a microscope), as evaluated by biopsy in 29 subjects.

Two similar studies provided essentially equivalent results. However, a 3-month, randomized, double-blind study of 116 people showed little to no additional benefit, perhaps because most participants reduced their alcohol consumption and almost half stopped drinking entirely. Another study found no benefit in 72 patients followed for 15 months.

Study results similarly conflict on whether milk thistle is helpful in liver cirrhosis.

A double-blind, placebo-controlled study of 170 people with alcoholic or non-alcoholic cirrhosis found that in the group treated with milk thistle the 4-year survival rate was 58% as compared to only 38% in the placebo group. This difference was statistically significant.

A double-blind, placebo-controlled trial that enrolled 172 people with cirrhosis for 4 years also found reductions in mortality, but they just missed the conventional cutoff for statistical significance. Yet another study, a 2-year, double-blind, placebo-controlled trial of 200 people with alcoholic cirrhosis, found no reduction in mortality attributable to the use of milk thistle.

Other double-blind studies of people with cirrhosis have found improvements in tests of liver function, although one did not.

Milk thistle is also used in a vague condition known as *minor hepatic insufficiency,* or *sluggish liver.* This term is mostly used by European physicians and American naturopathic practitioners—conventional physicians in America don't recognize it. Symptoms are supposed to include aching under the ribs, fatigue, unhealthy skin appearance, general malaise, constipation, premenstrual syndrome, chemical sensitivities, and allergies.

For more information, including dosage and safety issues, see the full **Milk Thistle** article.

SAMe

The body manufactures S-adenosylmethionine (SAMe) for use in converting certain chemicals to other chemicals (specifically, through the processes of transmethylation and transsulfuration). Some evidence suggests that SAMe taken as an oral supplement may have value in the treatment of various liver diseases, including chronic viral hepatitis, liver cirrhosis, jaundice of pregnancy, and liver toxicity caused by drugs or chemicals.

Perhaps the best evidence regards cholestasis (backup of bile in the liver) caused by serious liver disease. In a 2-week, double-blind study of 220 people with cholestasis, use of SAMe (1,600 mg daily) significantly improved liver-related symptoms as compared to placebo. Most participants in this study had chronic viral hepatitis.

Another large study evaluated the potential benefits of SAMe for the treatment of people with alcoholic liver cirrhosis. This 2-year, double-blind, placebo-controlled study of 117 people failed to find SAMe helpful for the group as a whole. However, in a subgroup of people with less advanced disease, treatment with SAMe appeared to reduce the number of people who needed a liver transplant or who died.

Gilbert's syndrome is an unexplained but harmless condition in which levels of bilirubin rise in the body, causing an alarming yellowing of the skin (jaundice). Weak evidence hints that SAMe may help reduce bilirubin levels in this condition.

For more information, including dosage and safety issues, see the full **SAMe** article.

Other Proposed Natural Treatments

Very preliminary evidence suggests that the supplement **betaine** (trimethylglycine, or TMG—not to be confused with **betaine hydrochloride**) may be helpful for treating fatty liver caused by alcohol and other causes, and also for protecting the liver from toxins in general.

Despite early promise, the herb **phyllanthus** does not appear to be helpful for viral hepatitis.

Numerous other herbs and supplements have shown a bit of promise in test-tube studies for protecting the liver, including **andrographis, artichoke leaf,** beet leaf, **choline, dandelion, inositol, lecithin, licorice, lipoic acid,** liver extracts, *Picrorhiza kurroa,* **schisandra, taurine, thymus extract,** and **turmeric,** along with hundreds of others. However, it is a long way from test-tube studies to effects in people, and none of these treatments should be regarded as having proven or even probable liver-protective properties.

Herbs and Supplements to Use Only with Caution

Many natural products have the capacity to harm the liver. Furthermore, due to the generally inadequate regulation of dietary supplements that exists at the time of this writing, there are real risks that herbal products, at least, may contain liver-toxic contaminants even if the actual herbs listed on the label are safe. For this reason, we recommend that people with liver disease do not use any medicinal herbs except under the supervision of a physician. Here, we list some specific information to aid in your decision-making process.

High doses of the supplements **beta-carotene** and **vitamin A** are thought to accelerate the progression of alcoholic liver disease in people who abuse alcohol. (Nutritional supplementation at the standard daily requirement level should not cause a problem.)

All forms of **vitamin B$_3$,** including niacin, niacinamide (nicotinamide), and inositol hexaniacinate, may damage the liver when taken in high doses. (Again, nutritional supplementation at the standard daily requirement level should not cause a problem.)

A great many herbs and supplements have known or suspected liver-toxic properties, including but not limited to chaparral, **coltsfoot, corydalis, comfrey, germander,** germanium (a mineral), **greater celandine,** certain **green tea** extracts, **kava, kombucha, mistletoe, noni, pennyroyal, pokeroot, sassafras,** and various herbs and minerals used in **traditional Chinese herbal medicine.** In addition, herbs that are not toxic to the liver in themselves are sometimes adulterated with other herbs of similar appearance that are accidentally harvested in a misapprehension of their identity (for example, germander found in **skullcap** products). Furthermore, blue-green algae species such as **spirulina** may at times be contaminated with liver-toxic substances called *microcystins,* for which no highest safe level is known.

Some articles claim that the herb **echinacea** is potentially toxic to the liver, but this concern appears to have been based on a misunderstanding of its constituents. Echinacea contains substances in the pyrrolizidine alkaloid family. However, while many pyrrolizidine alkaloids are toxic to the liver, those found in echinacea are not believed to have that property.

Whole **valerian** contains liver-toxic substances called *valepotriates*; however, valepotriates are thought to be absent from most commercial valerian products and case reports suggest that even very high doses of valerian do not harm the liver.

Lupus

RELATED TERMS: *Systemic Lupus Erythematosus; SLE*

PRINCIPAL PROPOSED NATURAL TREATMENTS: *Dehydroepiandrosterone (DHEA)*

OTHER PROPOSED NATURAL TREATMENTS: *Beta-carotene, Cordyceps, Fish Oil, Flaxseed, Food Allergen Identification and Avoidance, Magnesium, Pantothenic Acid, Selenium, Vitamin B$_3$, Vitamin B$_{12}$, Vitamin E*

NATURAL PRODUCTS TO AVOID: *Alfalfa*

Systemic lupus erythematosus (also known as SLE, or just lupus) is an autoimmune disease that primarily affects women of childbearing age. Its cause is unknown, but is believed to involve both genetic inheritance and factors in the environment. Whatever the cause, people with SLE develop antibodies against substances in their own bodies, including their DNA. These antibodies cause widespread damage and are believed to be primarily responsible for the many symptoms of this disease.

SLE may begin with such symptoms as fatigue, weight loss, fever, malaise, and loss of appetite. Other common early symptoms include muscle pain, joint pain, and facial rash. As SLE progresses, symptoms may develop in virtually every part of the body. Kidney damage is one of the most devastating effects of SLE, but many other serious problems may develop as well, including seizures, mental impairment, anemia, and inflammation of the heart, blood vessels, eyes, and digestive tract.

Conventional treatment for SLE revolves around a variety of anti-inflammatory drugs. In mild cases, taking nonsteroidal anti-inflammatory drugs (NSAIDs) may help; more severe forms of SLE require long-term use of corticosteroid anti-inflammatory drugs, such as prednisone. The side effects of these medications can be quite serious themselves. So-called cytotoxic agents (azathioprine, cyclophosphamide, and chlorambucil) might also be helpful, but they have many side effects as well.

Close physician supervision is always required with lupus due to the risk of complications in so many organs.

Principal Proposed Natural Treatments

A meaningful body of evidence tells us that the hormone dehydroepiandrosterone (DHEA) may be helpful for the treatment of lupus, when used as a part of a comprehensive, physician-directed treatment approach.

DHEA is the most abundant steroid hormone found in the bloodstream. Your body uses DHEA as the starting material for making the sex hormones testosterone and estrogen. DHEA has been tried as a treatment for a variety of medical conditions, including **osteoporosis**, but it is showing its greatest promise in the treatment of SLE.

A 12-month, double-blind, placebo-controlled trial of 381 women with mild or moderate lupus evaluated the effects of DHEA at a dose of 200 mg daily. Although many participants in both groups improved (the power of placebo is often amazing), DHEA was more effective than placebo, reducing many symptoms of the disease.

Similarly, in a double-blind, placebo-controlled study of 120 women with SLE, use of DHEA at a dose of 200 mg daily significantly decreased symptoms and reduced the frequency of disease flare-ups.

A smaller study found equivocal evidence that a lower dose of DHEA (30 mg daily for women over 45, and 20 mg daily for women under 45) might also work.

Positive results were also seen in earlier, smaller studies.

For more information, including dosage and safety issues, see the full **DHEA** article.

Other Proposed Natural Treatments

Flaxseed contains lignans and alpha-linolenic acid, substances with a wide variety of effects in the body. In particular, flaxseed may antagonize the activity of a substance called *platelet-activating factor* (PAF) that plays a role in SLE kidney disease (lupus nephritis). Preliminary evidence suggests that flaxseed might help prevent or treat lupus nephritis.

Fish oil contains omega-3 fatty acids, which have some anti-inflammatory effects. Fish oil has been found useful in **rheumatoid arthritis**, a disease related to SLE. The results of two small double-blind studies suggest that fish oil might be useful for SLE as well. However, current evidence suggests that fish oil is *not* effective for lupus nephritis.

Other treatments sometimes recommended for SLE include **beta-carotene, cordyceps, magnesium, selenium, vitamin B$_3$, vitamin B$_{12}$, vitamin E, pantothenic acid**, and **food allergen identification and avoidance**. However, there is no meaningful evidence as yet that these treatments work for lupus.

One study failed to find **copper** supplements helpful for lupus symptoms.

Herbs and Supplements to Avoid

The herb **alfalfa** contains a substance called *L-canavanine*, which can worsen SLE or bring it out of remission. People with SLE should avoid alfalfa entirely.

Various herbs and supplements may interact adversely with drugs used to treat lupus. For more information on this potential risk, see the individual drug article in the Drug Interactions section of this book.

Macular Degeneration

RELATED TERMS: *Maculopathy*

PRINCIPAL PROPOSED NATURAL TREATMENTS: *Zinc with or without Antioxidants; Carotenoids (such as Lutein and Zeaxanthin)*

OTHER PROPOSED NATURAL TREATMENTS: *Bilberry, Ginkgo, Low Glycemic Index Diet, OPCs*

PROBABLY NOT EFFECTIVE TREATMENTS: *Vitamin E Alone*

The lens of the eye focuses an image of the world on a portion of the retina called the *macula*, the area of finest visual perception. Gradual deterioration of the macula is called *macular degeneration*. After cataracts, damage to the macula is the second most common cause of visual impairment in those over 65. **Smoking, high blood pressure**, and **atherosclerosis** are associated with progressive damage to the macula. Ultraviolet light may also play a role by creating harmful free radicals in the eye.

In the most common form of macular degeneration (dry macular degeneration), a substance known as *lipofuscin* accumulates in the lining of the retina. A much less common form of macular degeneration involves the abnormal growth of blood vessels (wet macular degeneration). This can be treated very successfully, if attended to soon enough, but may lead to irreversible blindness if left untreated. For this reason, medical consultation in all cases of macular degeneration (or any other type of vision loss) is essential.

Principal Proposed Natural Treatments

Note: The treatments described in this section are intended as supports to standard ophthalmalogical care, not as a substitute for it. All studies refer primarily to the more common type of macular degeneration: dry macular degeneration.

Zinc and Antioxidants

Growing evidence suggests that a mixture of zinc and antioxidants can prevent or slow the progression of early macular degeneration of the most common type.

A double-blind, placebo-controlled trial evaluated

the effects of zinc with or without antioxidants on macular degeneration in 3,640 individuals in the early stage of the disease. Participants were randomly assigned to receive one of the following treatments: antioxidants (**vitamin C** at 500 mg, **vitamin E** at 400 IU, and **beta-carotene** at 15 mg), zinc (80 mg) and **copper** (2 mg), **antioxidants** plus zinc, or placebo. The results indicate that zinc alone or, even better, zinc plus antioxidants, significantly slowed the progression of the disease.

Note: Zinc at doses of 80 mg and higher daily can be harmful. One of the problems is that high-dose zinc supplementation impairs copper absorption. That's why extra copper was provided in the study described above. However, there may be other risks as well. Physician supervision is advised. For other dosage and safety issues, see the full **Zinc** article.

Smaller studies of zinc for macular degeneration have found mixed results.

Note that it's not clear how much the antioxidants in the mixture contributed to the benefits. A 4-year, double-blind, placebo-controlled trial of 1,193 people with macular degeneration failed to find vitamin E alone helpful for preventing or treating macular degeneration.

Lutein and Other Carotenoids

Observational studies suggest that higher intake of dietary carotenoids is associated with a lower incidence of macular degeneration. Carotenoids are a group of substances that are found in many fruits and vegetables, especially yellow-orange and dark green ones. Beta-carotene is the most famous carotenoid. However, observational studies prove little about cause and effect. To determine whether carotenoids can actually prevent or treat macular degeneration, double-blind, placebo-controlled studies are necessary. (For information on why this is the case, see **Why Does This Book Rely on Double-blind Studies?**.) One such study failed to find any benefit with beta-carotene (taken along with vitamin E and vitamin C).

The less well-known carotenoids lutein and zeaxanthin have also been investigated for a possible role in preventing macular degeneration (as well as **cataracts**). These carotenoids, principally found in corn and dark green leafy vegetables, are found in high concentrations in the eye. It has been suggested that they may protect the macula from light-induced damage by dyeing it yellow, thereby acting as a kind of natural sunglasses. They also act in the usual antioxidant fashion by neutralizing free radicals. Hopes were somewhat dampened by one observational study that failed to find much association between the extent of macular degeneration and the intake of either lutein or zeathanthin. However, they rose again after the completion of a preliminary double-blind, placebo-controlled trial of lutein. This study enrolled 90 people with dry macular degeneration and followed them for 12 months. The participants received either lutein (10 mg), lutein plus antioxidants and a multivitamin/mineral supplement, or placebo. At the end of the study period, participants who had taken lutein alone or lutein plus the other nutrients showed improvements in vision, while no change in vision was seen in the placebo group.

While these are promising findings, further study is needed to establish the apparent benefit of lutein for macular degeneration. For more information, see the full **Lutein** article.

Other Proposed Natural Treatments

Like carotenoids, flavonoids are found in many plants and may offer a variety of beneficial effects. Weak but interesting evidence suggests that **bilberry** and **OPCs**, both rich in flavonoids, may prevent or treat macular degeneration.

The herb *Ginkgo biloba* also contains many flavonoids and is additionally thought to increase circulation. In a 6-month, double-blind, placebo-controlled study of 20 people with macular degeneration, use of ginkgo at a dose of 160 mg daily resulted in improved visual acuity. Furthermore, positive results were seen in a 24-week, double-blind study of 99 people with macular degeneration that compared ginkgo extract at a dose of 240 mg per day against ginkgo at a dose of 60 mg per day. Vision improved in both groups, but to a greater extent with the higher dose. This study would have been more meaningful if it had included a placebo group, but nonetheless, "dose-related" effects of this type hint that a treatment may really work.

Weak evidence hints that moderate wine consumption might help prevent macular degeneration. Similarly weak evidence suggests possible benefit with a **low glycemic index diet**.

One controlled study that unfortunately failed to use a placebo group appeared to find benefit with a combination of **acetyl-L-carnitine**, **fish oil**, and **CoenzymeQ_{10}**.

Male Infertility

RELATED TERMS: *Sperm Motility*

PRINCIPAL PROPOSED NATURAL TREATMENTS: *None*

OTHER PROPOSED NATURAL TREATMENTS: *Antioxidants, Carnitine, Coenzyme Q_{10} (CoQ_{10}), Lycopene, Maca* (Lepidium meyenii), *Panax ginseng, Selenium, Vitamin B_{12}, Vitamin C, Vitamin E, Zinc plus Folate*

HERBS AND SUPPLEMENTS TO USE ONLY WITH CAUTION: *Andrographis, Licorice, Melatonin, Stevia, Soy*

Male infertility, the inability of a man to produce a pregnancy in a woman, is often caused by measurable deficits in sperm function or sperm count. In about half of all cases, however, the source of the problem is never discovered.

The good news is that, without any treatment at all, about 25% of supposedly infertile men bring about a pregnancy within a year of the time they first visit a physician for treatment. In other words, infertility is often only low fertility in disguise.

Proposed Treatments for Male Infertility

Carnitine

Growing, if not entirely consistent, evidence suggests that various forms of the supplement **L-carnitine** may improve sperm function.

For example, in one double-blind study, 60 men with abnormal sperm function were given either carnitine (as L-carnitine 2 g/day and acetyl-L-carnitine 1 g/day) or placebo for 6 months. The results showed significant improvement in sperm function in the treated group as compared to the placebo group.

A similarly sized 6-month, double-blind, placebo-controlled study, this one involving men with low sperm counts, found benefits with carnitine (again as L carnitine 2 g/day and acetyl-L-carnitine at 1 g/day) taken alone or carnitine combined with the anti-inflammatory drug cinnoxicam.

In addition, a 2-month, double-blind, placebo-controlled, crossover study of 100 men with various forms of infertility found probable benefits with 2 g daily of L-carnitine.

Zinc Plus Folate

A 26-week, double-blind, placebo-controlled trial compared the effects of treatment with zinc (66 mg of zinc sulfate, supplying 15 mg of zinc), folate (5 mg), and zinc plus folate against placebo. A total of 108 fertile men and 103 men with impaired fertility ("subfertile men") participated in the study. The two supplements combined significantly improved the sperm count and the percentage of healthy sperm in the subfertile men; neither supplement alone produced this effect, and there was little effect of the combined therapy on fertile men.

Another study also found potential benefit with zinc plus folate.

For more information on dosage and safety issues, see the full articles on **folate** and **zinc**.

Vitamin B_{12}

Mild vitamin B_{12} deficiencies are relatively common in people over 60. Such deficiencies lead to reduced sperm counts and lowered sperm mobility. Thus vitamin B_{12} supplementation has been tried for improving fertility in men with abnormal sperm production.

In one double-blind study of 375 infertile men, supplementation with vitamin B_{12} produced no benefits on average in the group as a whole. However, in a particular subgroup of men with sufficiently low sperm count and sperm motility, B_{12} appeared to be helpful. Such "dredging" of the data is suspect from a scientific point of view, however, and this study cannot be taken as proof of effectiveness.

For more information, including dosage and safety issues, see the full **Vitamin B_{12}** article.

Antioxidants

Free radicals, dangerous chemicals found naturally in the body, may damage sperm. For this reason, a number of studies have evaluated the benefits of **antioxidants** for male infertility.

In a double-blind, placebo-controlled study of 110

men whose sperm showed subnormal activity, daily treatment with 100 IU of vitamin E resulted in improved sperm activity and increased rate of pregnancy in their partners. For more information, including dosage and safety issues, see the full **Vitamin E** article.

Preliminary studies suggest that vitamin C may improve sperm count and function. However, a recent double-blind study of 31 individuals that tested both vitamin C and vitamin E found no benefit. The dosages studied ranged from 200 to 1,000 mg daily. For more information, including dosage and safety issues, see the full **Vitamin C** article.

Other Herbs and Supplements

Highly preliminary evidence suggests improvements in sperm function or pregnancy rates with **Panax ginseng**, **lycopene**, **coenzyme Q_{10}**, and **selenium**.

A special extract of the algae *Haematococcus* (*Haematococcus* spp.) is said to stabilize the sperm cell membrane and one double-blind study reported on the manufacturer's website claims to have found benefits in terms of sperm quality and actually fertility.

The herb *Lepidium meyenii* (**maca**) is claimed to enhance fertility, but the supporting evidence is limited to animal studies and one tiny uncontrolled study in humans conducted by a single research group. Contrary to what is stated on numerous websites, maca does not appear to raise testosterone levels.

In a double-blind trial of 28 men with impaired sperm activity, use of docosahexaenoic acid (DHA), a component of **fish oil**, failed to improve sperm health.

Another double-blind study failed to find **L-arginine** effective for improving pregnancy rates.

One very small study failed to find **magnesium** helpful for infertility.

Many other substances have been suggested as treatments for poor sperm function and infertility, including the herbs **ashwagandha**, *Eleutherococcus*, **pygeum**, **saw palmetto**, and **suma**, as well as the supplements **SAMe** and **calcium**, but there is no meaningful supporting evidence for these treatments.

In addition, all of the treatments listed in the article on **impotence** have also been proposed as treatments for male infertility, though not necessarily with any supporting evidence.

Herbs and Supplements to Use Only with Caution

Soy or **soy isoflavones**, as well as the herb **licorice**, may reduce testosterone levels in men. For this reason, men with impotence, infertility, or decreased libido may want to avoid these natural products.

According to a preliminary double-blind study, the supplement **melatonin** affects testosterone and estrogen metabolism in men and, when taken at a dose of 3 mg daily for 6 months, may impair sperm function.

Preliminary evidence from animal studies hints that use of some forms of **peppermint** at high doses might impair fertility.

There is contradictory evidence from animal studies on whether the herb **andrographis** may impair fertility. The same is true of the herb **stevia**.

Menopausal Symptoms (Other Than Osteoporosis)

RELATED TERMS: *Hot Flashes/Flushes*

PRINCIPAL PROPOSED NATURAL TREATMENTS: *Black Cohosh, Isoflavones, Soy*

OTHER PROPOSED NATURAL TREATMENTS: *Acupuncture, Alfalfa, Chasteberry, DHEA, Dong Quai, Estriol, Evening Primrose Oil, Flaxseed, Gamma Oryzanol, Grass Pollen, Licorice, Progesterone Cream, Red Clover, St. John's Wort, Suma, Traditional Chinese Herbal Medicine, Vitamin C, Vitamin E*

The hormonal changes of menopause can produce a wide variety of symptoms, ranging from hot flashes and vaginal dryness to anxiety, depression, and insomnia. Many of these symptoms are undoubtedly caused by the natural decrease in estrogen production that occurs at menopause; however, the human body is so complex that other hormonal factors undoubtedly also play a role.

Menopause is not a disease. It is clearly a natural process, but one that many women prefer not to experience. No longer do women accept as merely part of life the decrease in libido, pain during intercourse, years of hot flashes, and other uncomfortable problems that may accompany menopause. This raises an important point: How close to nature do we want to live? One of the most valued ideals of alternative medicine is the desire to trust nature, but sometimes we may want to draw a line. For example, in a state of nature, infant and maternal mortality is high. This process of survival of the fittest helps humanity as a species to be stronger, but it is not something that a compassionate society can tolerate. Thus, no matter what our ideals, we frequently find ourselves tampering with nature. The treatment of menopause is simply one example among many.

Estrogen-replacement therapy can alleviate many of the problems associated with menopause. However, it creates counterbalancing risks. The most frightening issue is the increased risk of breast cancer that appears to be associated with replacement estrogen. In addition, estrogen therapy can cause blood clots in the legs and appears to raise the risk of heart disease rather than prevent it (as previously thought). The decision whether to use estrogen-replacement therapy for menopausal symptoms should involve a careful examination of the risks and benefits in consultation with a physician.

Principal Proposed Natural Treatments

Several natural treatments may reduce menopausal symptoms. However, we do not know for sure whether any of these reduce the risk of osteoporosis. See the full article on **osteoporosis** for more detailed information on natural ways to prevent bone loss.

Soy and Soy (or Other Source) Isoflavones

Both **soy** and **red clover** contain **phytoestrogens** (naturally occurring substances with estrogen-like actions) called *isoflavones*. It is thought that the isoflavones in these herbs may offer some benefits of estrogen with less risk. However, the current evidence base for this hypothesis is incomplete.

Improvements as compared to placebo have been seen regarding hot flashes as well as other symptoms such as vaginal dryness and mood have been seen in many studies of soy, mixed soy isoflavones, and the isoflavone **genistein** alone. However, about as many studies have failed to find significant benefit as compared to placebo with soy or concentrated isoflavones.

In addition, isoflavones from red clover have shown inconsistent results in studies, with the best and largest study finding no benefit.

What can one make of this mixed evidence? One problem here is that placebo treatment has a strong effect on menopausal symptoms. In such circumstances, statistical noise can easily drown out the real benefits of a treatment under study. Unlike estrogen, which has such a powerful effect on hot flashes and other menopausal symptoms that its benefits are almost always clear in studies, soy or concentrated isoflavones likely have a more modest effect, one that does not always show itself above the background noise of statistical variation. It has also been suggested that the placebo used in many of these studies, polyunsaturated fatty acids, may have efficacy of its own; this would tend to hide actual benefits.

Evidence regarding whether soy or soy isoflavones are helpful for osteoporosis remains conflicting. On balance, it is probably fair to summarize current evidence as indicating that isoflavones (either as soy, genistein, mixed isoflavones, or tofu extract) have a modestly beneficial effect on bone density.

Interestingly, one small but long-term study suggests that **progesterone cream** (another treatment proposed for use in preventing or treating osteoporosis) may *decrease* the bone-sparing effect of soy isoflavones.

For more information, including dosage and safety issues, see the full **Isoflavones** article.

Black Cohosh

The herb black cohosh is widely used for treatment of menopause, but the evidence that it works remains incomplete and inconsistent.

The best study was a 12-week, double-blind, placebo-controlled trial of 304 women with menopausal symptoms. This study appeared to find that black cohosh was more effective than placebo. The best evidence was for a reduction in hot flashes. However, the statistical procedures used in the study were unusual and open to question.

Previous smaller studies have found improvements not only in hot flashes but also in other symptoms of menopause. For example, in a double-blind, placebo-controlled study, 97 menopausal women received black cohosh, estrogen, or placebo for 3 months. The results indicated that the herb reduced overall menopausal symptoms (such as hot flashes) to the same extent as the drug. Microscopic analysis of cells showed that unlike estrogen, black cohosh did not affect the cells of the uterus. This is a positive result, as estrogen's effects on the uterus are potentially harmful. However, black cohosh did have an estrogen-like effect on the cells of the vagina. This also is a positive result, because it suggests that black cohosh might reduce vaginal thinning. Finally, the study found hints that black cohosh might help protect bone. However, a great many of the study participants dropped out, making the results less than reliable.

A study reported in 2006 found that black cohosh has weak estrogen-like effects on vaginal cells and possible positive effects on bone (specifically, stimulating new bone formation).

One interesting double-blind study evaluated a combination therapy containing black cohosh and **St. John's wort** in 301 women with general menopausal symptoms as well as depression. The results showed that use of the combination treatment was significantly more effective than placebo for both problems.

In contrast, there have been several studies that failed to find benefit. For example, in a 12-month, double-blind, placebo controlled study of 350 women, participants were given either black cohosh, a supplement containing 10 herbs, the multibotanical plus soy, standard hormone replacement therapy, or placebo. The results showed significant benefits as compared to placebo for hormone replacement therapy, but only slight, non-significant benefits with the other treatments. In addition, a double-blind study of 122 women failed to find statistically significant benefits with black cohosh as compared to placebo, as did a double-blind, placebo-controlled study of 124 women using a black cohosh/soy isoflavone combination. These negative outcomes were quite possibly due to the relatively small sizes of the black cohosh groups in these studies; in a condition such as menopausal symptoms, where the placebo effect is strong, and when the treatment is relatively weak, large numbers of participants are necessary to show benefit above and beyond the placebo effect.

Some interesting information has developed regarding *how* black cohosh might work. In the past, the herb was described as a phytoestrogen. However, subsequent evidence indicates that black cohosh is not a general phytoestrogen, but may act like estrogen in only a few parts of the body: the brain (reducing hot flashes), bone (potentially helping to prevent or treat osteoporosis), and possibly the vagina (alleviating dryness and thinning); it does not appear to act like estrogen in the breast or the uterus, which is good news, as estrogen is carcinogenic in those tissues. If this theory is true, black cohosh is a selective-estrogen receptor modifier (SERM) somewhat like the drug raloxifen (Evista). However, more evidence is needed to establish the facts of the matter.

For more information, including dosage and safety issues, see the full **Black Cohosh** article.

Other Proposed Natural Treatments

Grass pollen extracts have shown promise for treatment of benign prostate enlargement. Their benefits in that condition may result from a hormonal effect; on this basis grass pollens have been proposed for treatment of menopausal symptoms. One double-blind, placebo-controlled study followed 54 women with menopausal symptoms and found benefits with a supplement containing grass pollen extract.

For many years, the hormone progesterone (so-called natural progesterone, as distinguished from the synthetic progestins used instead of progesterone in birth control pills and hormone replacement therapy) was aggressively promoted by some alternative medicine practitioners as the true cure for osteoporosis. However, at that time there was no meaningful evidence that progesterone helps prevent osteoporosis—these claims were based largely on anecdotes, plausible reasoning, and "studies" that did not come close to modern scientific standards. When the subject was finally studied properly, the first results indicated that progesterone does not work for osteoporosis after all. However, it may work for other menopausal symptoms. A 1-year, double-blind, placebo-controlled study of 102 women found that cream containing 20 mg of the hormone progesterone (available over the counter) may be effective against hot flashes, though it did not appear to protect bone from breakdown. However another double-blind trial failed to find 32 mg daily effective for osteoporosis or any other menopause-related symptoms. See the **Progesterone** article for more information. The hormone **dehydroepi-androsterone** (DHEA) has been tested as a treatment for menopausal symptoms, with some promising results in a small, preliminary trial.

Evidence far too weak to be relied upon at all has been quoted in support of **gamma oryzanol**, **St. John's wort**, and **flaxseed** for menopausal symptoms. Other proposed treatments that lack meaningful supporting evidence include **vitamin C, bioflavonoids, licorice, suma**, and **chasteberry**.

Although **vitamin E** is often recommended for menopausal hot flashes, there is no real evidence that it is effective. One 9-week, double-blind, placebo-controlled trial evaluated vitamin E in more than 100 women with hot flashes associated with **breast cancer treatment**, but it found marginal benefits at best.

Two very small controlled studies provide weak evidence that **acupuncture** can improve menopausal symptoms.

Traditional Chinese herbal medicine has been proposed as a treatment for menopausal symptoms, but there is no meaningful evidence to indicate that it is effective. One study has been widely reported as proving the effectiveness of a particular Chinese herbal formula, but because it lacked a placebo group, it actually does not do so. Another study failed to find the Chinese herb *Pueraria lobata* helpful for menopausal symptoms.

Some evidence suggests that **evening primrose oil, dong quai**, and **ginseng** are not effective for menopausal symptoms.

The herb **alfalfa** contains strong phytoestrogens. This might make it helpful for menopause, but no studies have been reported.

One double-blind, placebo-controlled study failed to find **melatonin** more helpful than placebo for menopausal symptoms (actually, placebo did a little better than melatonin!). Another study failed to find that **ginkgo** improved mood, general energy level, or mental function in menopausal women.

Estriol: A Safer Form of Estrogen?

For over a decade, some alternative medicine practitioners have popularized the use of a special form of estrogen called *estriol*, claiming that, unlike standard estrogen, it doesn't increase the risk of cancer. However, this claim is unfounded.

There is no real doubt that estriol is effective. Controlled and double-blind trials have found oral or vaginal estriol effective for reducing hot flashes, night sweats, insomnia, vaginal dryness, recurrent **urinary tract infections**, and osteoporosis.

Estriol might cause less vaginal bleeding as a side effect than other forms of estrogen, but this has not been proven.

However, like other forms of estrogen, oral estriol stimulates the growth of uterine tissue. This leads to a risk of uterine cancer.

In a placebo-controlled study of 1,110 women, uterine tissue stimulation was seen among women given estriol orally (1 to 2 mg daily) as compared to those given placebo. Another large study found that oral estriol increased the risk of uterine cancer. In another study of 48 women given estriol 1 mg twice daily, uterine tissue stimulation was seen in the majority of cases.

In contrast, a 12-month, double-blind trial of oral estriol (2 mg daily) in 68 Japanese women found no effect on the uterus. It may be that the high levels of soy in the Japanese diet altered the results.

Additionally, test-tube studies suggest that estriol is just as likely to cause breast cancer as any other form of estrogen.

The bottom line: If you are considering using estriol, think of it as equivalent to any other form of estrogen.

Men's Health

Numerous conditions of particular relevance to men are discussed in the Collins Alternative Health Guide, including the following:

- Impotence (Erectile Dysfunction)
- Infertility
- Peyronie's Disease
- Preventing Heart Disease
- Prostate Enlargement
- Prostatitis
- Sports Supplements
- Stress

Menstrual Problems, General

A woman's menstrual cycle is controlled by a complex sequence of hormones. Various factors, not all of them understood, can lead to disturbances of menstruation. Relevant articles in the Collins Alternative Health Guide include the following:

> Amenorrhea (absence of menstrual periods)
> Cyclic mastitis (menstruation-related breast pain)

> Dysmenorrhea (menstrual pain)
> Premenstrual syndrome (PMS)

In addition, menstrual migraines (migraine headaches that occur in time with the menstrual cycle) are discussed in the **Migraine** article.

Migraine Headaches

PRINCIPAL PROPOSED NATURAL TREATMENTS: *5-Hydroxytryptophan (5-HTP), Butterbur, Feverfew, Magnesium*

OTHER PROPOSED NATURAL TREATMENTS: *Acupuncture, Biofeedback, Chiropractic, CoenzymeQ$_{10}$, Fish Oil, Food Allergen Avoidance, Magnet Therapy, Massage, Soy Isoflavones (Combined with Black Cohosh and Dong Quai), Vitamin B$_2$ (Riboflavin)*

The term *migraine* refers to a class of headaches sharing certain characteristic symptoms. Headache pain usually occurs in the forehead or temples, often on one side only and typically accompanied by nausea and a preference for a darkened room. Headache attacks last for several hours, up to a day, or more. They are usually separated by completely pain-free intervals. In some cases, headache pain is accompanied by a visual (or occasionally nonvisual) disturbance known as an *aura*. Migraines are classified as migraine with aura and migraine without aura.

Migraines can be set off by a variety of triggers, including fatigue, stress, hormonal changes, and foods, such as alcoholic beverages, chocolate, peanuts, and avocados. When people with migraine headaches first consult a physician, they are generally advised to identify such triggers and avoid them if possible. However, migraines quite frequently occur with no obvious avoidable triggering factor.

The underlying cause of migraine headaches has been a subject of continuing controversy for over a century. Opinion has swung back and forth between two primary beliefs: that migraines are related to epileptic seizures and originate in the nervous tissue of the brain, or that blood vessels in the skull cause headache pain when they dilate or contract (so-called vascular headaches). Most likely, several factors are involved and more than one stimulus can light the fuse that leads to a full-blown migraine attack.

Conventional treatment of acute migraines has lately been revolutionized by drugs in the triptan family. These medications can completely abort a migraine headache in many individuals. They work by imitating the action of serotonin on blood vessels, causing them to contract. However, while they are dramatically effective for the majority of people with migraines, a substantial minority do not respond, for reasons that are unclear.

People interested in prevention of migraines have a great variety of options, including ergot drugs, antidepressants, beta-blockers, calcium channel blockers, and antiseizure medications. Picking the best one is mostly a matter of trial and error. Most but not all people can find some medication that will work.

Principal Proposed Natural Treatments

Several herbs and supplements have shown considerable promise for helping to prevent migraines. Keep in mind that serious diseases may occasionally first present themselves as migraine-type headaches. If you suddenly start having migraines without a previous history, or if the pattern of your migraines changes significantly, it is essential to seek medical evaluation.

Butterbur

Two double-blind, placebo-controlled studies suggest that an extract of the herb butterbur may be helpful for preventing migraines.

Butterbur extract was tested as a migraine preventive in a double-blind, placebo-controlled study involving 60 men and women who experienced at least three migraines per month. After 4 weeks without any conventional medications, participants were randomly assigned to take either 50 mg of butterbur extract or placebo twice daily for 3 months. The results were positive: both the number of migraine attacks and the total number of days of migraine pain were significantly reduced in the treatment group as compared to the placebo group. Three out of four individuals taking butterbur reported improvement, as compared to only one out of four in the placebo group. No significant side effects were noted.

In another double-blind, placebo-controlled study performed by different researchers, 202 people with migraine headaches received either 50 mg twice daily of butterbur extract, 75 mg twice daily, or placebo. Over the 3 months of the study, the frequency of migraine attacks gradually decreased in all three groups. However, the group receiving the higher dose of butterbur extract showed significantly greater improvement than those in the placebo group. The lower dose of butterbur failed to prove significantly more effective than placebo.

Based on these two studies, it does appear that butterbur extract is helpful for preventing migraines and that 75 mg twice daily is more effective than 50 mg twice daily. However, further research is necessary to establish this with certainty.

For more information, including dosage and safety issues, see the full **Butterbur** article.

Feverfew

Five meaningful double-blind, placebo-controlled studies have been performed to evaluate feverfew's effectiveness as a preventive treatment for migraines, but the results have been inconsistent. The best of the positive trials used a feverfew extract made by extracting the herb with liquid carbon dioxide. Two other trials that used whole feverfew leaf also found it effective; however two studies that used feverfew extracts did not find benefit.

In a well-conducted 16-week, double-blind, placebo-controlled study of 170 people with migraines, use of a feverfew product made via liquid carbon-dioxide extraction resulted in a significant decrease in headache frequency as compared to the effect of the placebo treatment. In the treatment group, headache frequency decreased by 1.9 headaches per month, as compared to a reduction of 1.3 headaches per month in the placebo group. The average number of headaches per month prior to treatment was 4.76 headaches. A previous study using the same extract had failed to find benefit, but it primarily enrolled people who were less prone to migraines.

Two other studies used whole feverfew leaf and found benefit. The first followed 59 people for 8 months. For 4 months, half received a daily capsule of feverfew leaf and the other half received placebo. The groups were then switched and followed for an additional 4 months. Treatment with feverfew produced a 24% reduction in the number of migraines and a significant decrease in nausea and vomiting during the headaches. A subsequent double-blind study of 57 people with migraines found that use of feverfew leaf could decrease the severity of migraine headaches. Unfortunately, this trial did not report whether there was any change in the frequency of migraines.

One study using an alcohol extract failed to find benefit.

For more information, including dosage and safety issues, see the full **Feverfew** article.

Magnesium

Magnesium is another natural treatment that has shown promise for the prevention of migraine headaches. A 12-week, double-blind study followed 81 people with recurrent migraines. Half received 600 mg of magnesium daily (in the rather unusual form of trimagnesium dicitrate), and the other half received placebo. By the last 3 weeks of the study, the frequency of migraine attacks was reduced by 41.6% in the treated group, compared to 15.8% in the placebo group. The only side effects observed were diarrhea (18.6%) and digestive irritation (4.7%).

Similar results have been seen in other double-blind studies. There was one study that did not find a benefit, but it had many problems in its design.

Preliminary studies also suggest that magnesium may be helpful for migraines triggered by hormonal changes occurring with the menstrual cycle.

For more information, including dosage and safety issues, see the full **Magnesium** article.

5-HTP (5-Hydroxytryptophan)

The body manufactures 5-HTP on its way to making serotonin. When 5-HTP is taken as a supplement, the net result may be increased serotonin production. Since a number of drugs that affect serotonin are used to prevent migraine headaches, 5-HTP has been tried as well. Some evidence suggests that it may work when taken at a dosage of 400 to 600 mg daily. Lower doses may not be effective.

In a 6-month trial of 124 people, 5-HTP (600 mg daily) proved equally effective as the standard drug methysergide. The most dramatic benefits seen were a reduction in the intensity and duration of migraines. Since methysergide has been proven better than placebo for migraine headaches in earlier studies, the study results provide meaningful, although not airtight, evidence that 5-HTP is also effective.

Similarly good results were seen in another comparative study, using a different medication and 5-HTP (at a dose of 400 mg daily).

However, in one study, 5-HTP (up to 300 mg daily) was less effective than the drug propranolol. Also, in a study involving children, 5-HTP failed to demonstrate benefit. Other studies that are sometimes quoted as evidence that 5-HTP is effective for migraines actually enrolled adults or children with many different types of headaches (including migraines).

Putting all this evidence together, it appears possible that 5-HTP can help people with frequent migraine headaches if taken in sufficient doses, but further research needs to be done. In particular, we need a large double-blind study that compares 5-HTP against placebo over a period of several months.

For more information, including dosage and safety issues, see the full **5-HTP** article.

Other Proposed Natural Treatments

A 3-month, double-blind, placebo-controlled study of 55 people with migraines found that **vitamin B₂** at a daily dose of 400 mg significantly reduced the frequency and duration of migraine attacks. The majority of the participants experienced a greater than 50% decrease in the number of migraine attacks as well as the total days with headache pain. A subsequent study failed to find benefit with a combination of vitamin B₂, magnesium, and feverfew; however, it is possible that the 25 mg daily dose of vitamin B₂ used as the placebo confused the issue by providing some benefits on its own.

Another small double-blind, placebo-controlled trial hints that the supplement **coenzymeQ₁₀** (100 mg 3 times daily) may also help prevent migraines. In this study, about 50% of the people taking CoQ₁₀ had a significant decrease in migraine frequency, as compared to only 15% in the placebo group.

In a 24-week, double-blind study, 49 women with menstrual migraines received either placebo or **soy isoflavones** combined with **dong quai** and **black cohosh** extracts. Beginning at the twentieth week, use of the herbal supplement resulted in decreased severity and frequency of headaches as compared to placebo. It is not clear which of the ingredients in the combination was helpful; contrary to what is stated in this research report, the current consensus is that neither black cohosh nor dong quai are phytoestrogens, but they may have other effects.

Despite promising results in an earlier and widely publicized study, a much larger and longer study of **fish oil** for migraines failed to find benefit. In this 16-week, double-blind, placebo-controlled study of 167 individuals with recurrent migraines, use of fish oil did not significantly reduce headache frequency or severity. Another small double-blind, placebo-controlled study failed to find statistically significant evidence of benefit.

Calcium, chromium, folate, ginger, and **vitamin C** have also been reported to be helpful for migraines, but there is as yet no meaningful scientific evidence for any of these natural products.

Identifying and eliminating **allergenic foods** from your diet might be helpful for reducing the frequency of migraine attacks.

There is only incomplete, mixed evidence regarding the potential benefit of **chiropractic manipulation** or **acupuncture** for the treatment of or prevention of migraines.

Massage, biofeedback, and a form of **magnet therapy** called *PEMF* have also shown a bit of promise for migraines.

Herbs and Supplements to Use Only with Caution

Various herbs and supplements may interact adversely with drugs used to treat migraine headaches. For more information on this potential risk, see the individual drug article in the Drug Interactions section of this book.

Minor Burns

RELATED TERMS: *Superficial Burn, First-Degree Burn, Scald*

PRINCIPAL PROPOSED NATURAL TREATMENTS: *None*

OTHER PROPOSED NATURAL TREATMENTS: Aloe vera, *Arginine, Beta-carotene, Calendula, Chamomile, Comfrey, Copper, DHEA, Goldenseal, Gotu Kola, Honey, Ornithine Alpha-Ketoglutarate, Potato Peel, Selenium, Vitamin C, Vitamin E, Zinc*

Burns can be caused by heat, electricity, chemicals, and sun exposure. They vary in severity from causing minor pain to being life-threatening. First-degree burns are the mildest type, only damaging the top layer of skin. The skin gets red, painful, and tender. Though the skin may swell, no blisters form and the area turns white when touched.

Second-degree burns cause damage to deeper layers of the skin. The skin looks much like a first-degree burn except that blisters form at the surface. The blisters may be red or whitish and are filled with a clear fluid. Third-degree burns are the worst type of burn, extending through all layers of the skin and causing nerve damage. Because of this nerve damage, third-degree burns generally aren't painful and have no feeling when touched— an ominous sign. The skin may be white, blackened, or bright red. Blisters may also be present.

Only first-degree burns should be self-treated. More severe burns require a doctor's supervision to prevent infection and scarring. Third-degree burns and extensive second-degree burns can cause permanent injury or death.

The best treatment for minor burns is to cool the burn as quickly as possible by immersing the area in cold water. The burned area should be kept clean until it heals.

Proposed Natural Treatments

Although there are no well-established natural treatments for minor burns, several preliminary studies suggest a few options for reducing pain and speeding healing.

A series of studies done in India found that a combination of raw honey and gauze was significantly better than conventional types of bandages for superficial burns treated at a hospital. The burns covered with honey healed faster and with less frequent infection than the burns covered with other types of bandages. Other studies of varying quality have also found evidence of benefit.

Potato peel has also been used successfully in developing countries as a replacement for more expensive conventional bandages.

Highly preliminary studies suggest the herb *Gotu kola* may speed healing of burns and reduce scarring.

Aloe vera is often recommended as a treatment for minor burns; however, no evidence exists to support this claim and some studies have actually found it ineffective. Other popular topical burn treatments include **calendula**, **chamomile**, **goldenseal**, and **comfrey**.

Oral or topical **vitamin C**, **vitamin E**, and **beta-carotene**, alone or in combination, might be helpful for preventing sunburn. However, the evidence at this time is preliminary and contradictory.

Finally, there is some evidence that hospitalized individuals with severe burns may benefit from nutritional support with certain supplements, including **ornithine alpha-ketoglutarate (OKG)**, **arginine**, **zinc**, **copper**, **selenium**, and **dehydroepiandrosterone (DHEA)**.

Minor Injuries

RELATED TERMS: *Bruises, Contusions, Injuries, Joint Injuries, Ligament Injuries, Muscle Injuries, Sports Injuries, Sports and Fitness Support: Minor Sports Injuries, Sprains, Strains*

PRINCIPAL PROPOSED NATURAL TREATMENTS: *Proteolytic Enzymes*

OTHER PROPOSED NATURAL TREATMENTS: *Homeopathic Arnica, Bioflavonoids (Citrus Bioflavonoids and Oxerutins), Calcium and Vitamin D, Comfrey (Topical Only), Creatine, Horse Chestnut, OPCs, Vitamin C*

This article addresses injuries such as bruises, minor fractures, and sprains. Other forms of minor injury such as **minor burns**, **minor wounds**, **back pain**, and more chronic **soft tissue injuries** are discussed in their own articles.

Unless you never leave your couch, you are likely to injure yourself sometime. Although minor injuries such as bruises and sprains will heal without treatment, they can be quite unpleasant.

Conventional treatment for minor sprains and strains involves anti-inflammatory drugs, icing, and, in some cases, physical therapy. Bruises are sometimes treated with ultrasound, although there is no meaningful evidence that it really helps.

Principal Proposed Natural Treatments

Proteolytic enzymes help you digest the proteins in food. Your pancreas produces the proteolytic enzymes trypsin and chymotrypsin, and others, such as papain and bromelain, are found in foods. Proteolytic enzymes are primarily used as digestive aids for people who have trouble digesting proteins. When taken by mouth, proteolytic enzymes appear to be absorbed internally to a certain extent and might reduce inflammation and swelling. Several small studies have found proteolytic enzyme combinations helpful for the treatment of minor injuries. However, by far the best and largest trial failed to find benefit.

Most studies involved proteolytic enzymes combined with **citrus bioflavonoids**, also thought to decrease swelling.

A double-blind, placebo-controlled study of 44 individuals with sports-related ankle injuries found that treatment with a proteolytic enzyme and bioflavonoid combination resulted in faster healing and reduced the time away from training by about 50%. Based on these and other results, a very large (721-participant) double-blind, placebo-controlled trial of people with an ankle sprain was undertaken. It compared placebo against bromelain, trypsin, or **rutin** (a bioflavonoid), separately or in combination. None of the treatments alone or together proved more effective than placebo.

Three other small double-blind studies, involving a total of about 80 athletes, found that treatment with proteolytic enzymes significantly speeded healing of bruises and other mild athletic injuries as compared to placebo. In another double-blind trial, 100 people were given an injection of their own blood under the skin to simulate bruising following an injury. Researchers found that treatment with a proteolytic enzyme combination significantly speeded up recovery. However, most of these studies were performed decades ago and fall beneath modern standards in design and reporting.

For more information, including dosage and safety issues, see the full articles on **proteolytic enzymes** and **bromelain**.

Other Proposed Natural Treatments

Oligomeric proanthocyanidins (OPCs), substances found in grape seed and pine bark, have shown promise for the treatment of minor injuries. A 10-day, double-blind, placebo-controlled study enrolling 50 participants found that OPCs improved the rate at which edema disappeared following sports injuries. It is also relevant that a double-blind, placebo-controlled study of 63 women with breast cancer found that 600 mg of OPCs daily for 6 months reduced postoperative edema and pain. Similarly, in a double-blind, placebo-controlled study of 32 people who had cosmetic surgery on the face, swelling disappeared much faster in the treated group.

Preliminary evidence from a somewhat poorly reported double-blind trial of 40 college football players suggests that a combination of **vitamin C** and citrus bioflavonoids taken before practice can reduce the severity of athletic injuries.

Another small placebo-controlled study suggests that an oral combination product containing vitamin C, **calcium, potassium**, proteolytic enzymes, rutin, and OPCs can slightly accelerate healing of skin wounds.

A double-blind study of people recovering from minor injuries, including minor surgery, found that the bioflavonoid-like substances called *oxerutins* have similar effects.

The herb **horse chestnut** is thought to have properties similar to those of citrus bioflavonoids. The active ingredient in horse chestnut is a substance called *aescin*. One double-blind study of 70 people found that about 10 g of 2% aescin gel, applied externally to bruises in a single dose 5 minutes after the bruises were induced, reduced their tenderness.

The herb **comfrey** is unsafe for internal use due to the presence of liver-toxic pyrrolizidine alkaloids. However, topical use is believed to be safe. In a double-blind, placebo-controlled study of 142 people suffering from an ankle sprain, use of comfrey gel resulted in more rapid recovery than placebo gel, according to measurements of pain, swelling, and mobility.

The supplement **creatine** has shown some promise for preventing the muscle weakness that commonly occurs when a limb is immobilized following injury or surgery. However, one study failed to find creatine helpful for restoring strength following arthroscopic knee surgery.

The supplement **glucosamine** may be helpful for people who experience knee pain due to cartilage injury.

A small double-blind, placebo-controlled study suggests that use of calcium (1 g daily) plus **vitamin D** (800 IU daily) may speed bone healing after fracture in people with **osteoporosis**.

One study found that use of **relaxation therapies** to manage stress reduced the number of injury and illness days among competitive athletes.

One study failed to find that onion extract can help reduce scarring in the skin.

Homeopathic forms of the herb arnica are popular as a treatment for injuries as a treatment for injuries as well, but studies suggest that it is only a placebo.

Minor Wounds

RELATED TERMS: *Lacerations, Scrapes, Cuts*

PRINCIPAL PROPOSED NATURAL TREATMENTS: *Careful Wound Cleaning*

OTHER PROPOSED NATURAL TREATMENTS: **Aloe vera,** *Amino Acid Cream, Bee Propolis, Calendula, Cartilage, Essential Oils, Chamomile, Chitosan, Garlic, Goldenseal, Gotu Kola, Honey, Royal Jelly, St. John's Wort, Vitamin A, Vitamin C, Vitamin E, Zinc*

Minor cuts are an ordinary fact of life and nearly always heal on their own. There is no evidence that antibacterial gels and creams will help wounds heal faster or prevent infection. In fact, by keeping the air away from a wound, these treatments might actually interfere with healing.

The best approach to minor wounds is also the simplest and most natural: clean the wound well and keep it clean and exposed to the air. If signs of infection develop, such as redness, oozing, or swelling, a physician should be consulted.

Proposed Natural Treatments for Minor Wounds

Application of honey (or concentrated sugar preparations) to wounds appears to prevent infection and possibly speed healing. Contrary to what is stated in some alternative medicine sources, honey is thought to work primarily through its high sugar content, which directly kills microorganisms, rather than by means of trace substances contained in it.

Highly preliminary evidence suggests that the herb **gotu kola** might have general wound-healing properties, as well as help to prevent or treat **keloid scars** (a particular type of scar that is enlarged and bulging).

A small double-blind, placebo-controlled trial found that the amino acids cysteine, **glycine**, and threonine applied as a combination cream could help the healing of leg ulcers. A variety of nutrients, including **vitamins A, C, and E**, and **zinc**, taken both orally and topically, have also been tried as a treatment for minor wounds and creams containing A and E are common staples in the hospital. A number of topical herbs have been tried as well, including **calendula, cartilage, chamomile, chitosan, goldenseal**, royal jelly, and **St. John's wort**, but there is no real evidence as yet that any of these approaches provide any benefits.

Numerous herbs (and their **essential oils**) have antibacterial properties and, for this reason, might theoretically be helpful for preventing wound infection. However, this has not been proven. In addition, if a wound is serious enough that infection is a real risk, physician supervision is essential.

The gel of the *Aloe vera* plant has a long folk history in the treatment of skin conditions. There is some evidence from human and animal studies that aloe might be helpful for wound healing, but one study found that aloe gel actually slowed the healing of surgical wounds.

Animal studies suggest that the honeybee product **propolis** applied topically may be of benefit in healing wounds.

Mitral Valve Prolapse

RELATED TERMS: *Dysautonomia, Mitral Valve Prolapse Syndrome, MVP*

PRINCIPAL PROPOSED NATURAL TREATMENTS: *Magnesium*

OTHER PROPOSED NATURAL TREATMENTS: *5-Hydroxytryptophan (5-HTP), Acetyl-L-carnitine, Acupuncture, Arginine, CoenzymeQ$_{10}$, Creatine, Gamma-linolenic Acid, Hawthorn, Hops, Kava, L-carnitine, Lemon Balm, Lipoic Acid, Melatonin, Multivitamin/Multimineral Supplements, OPCs, Passionflower, Taurine, Valerian, Vitamin B$_1$, Vitamin E*

Mitral valve prolapse (MVP) affects about 2% of people in the United States. (Past estimates were higher due to errors in diagnosis.) As the name suggests, MVP involves prolapse of one of the valves of the heart, the mitral valve.

The mitral valve sits at the opening between the left atrium and left ventricle, and opens and closes so that blood flows only in one direction (atrium to ventricle). In MVP, the mitral valve fails to make a proper snug fit and instead billows (prolapses) back into the atrium, making a sound that can be heard through a stethoscope.

MVP is generally benign. Sometimes, however, the mitral valve fits so poorly that a large amount of blood leaks back from the ventricle to the atrium. This is called *mitral regurgitation* and it can be dangerous, eventually requiring surgery.

In the past, a set of symptoms called *dysautonomia* was thought to frequently occur in association with MVP. Dysautonomia involves malfunction of the autonomic nervous system (the part of the nervous system that is not under conscious control). MVP plus dysautonomia used to be called the *Mitral Valve Prolapse Syndrome*. Symptoms were said to include:

➤ **Chest pain with no apparent medical cause**
➤ **Panic attacks/anxiety**
➤ **Heart palpitations**
➤ **Sweating**
➤ **Dizziness**
➤ **Lightheadedness**
➤ **Weakness**
➤ **Balance problems**
➤ **Hypersensitive startle reflex**
➤ **Shortness of breath**
➤ **Numbness or tingling in the fingers or toes**
➤ **Hyperventilation**
➤ **Sensitivity to caffeine and other stimulants**

However, recent evidence indicates that symptoms of dysautonomia occur with no greater frequency in people with MVP than in people without MVP. In other words, there is probably no connection between the two conditions. People who were previously diagnosed with MVP Syndrome are now said to have two separate conditions: MVP plus symptoms of dysautonomia. The cause of these dysautonomic symptoms is not clear, but probably involves a response to stress.

Conventional treatment for MVP involves regular monitoring for mitral regurgitation, along with maintenance of normal weight and blood pressure to avoid excess strain on the valve. In addition, people with MVP are given antibiotics prior to surgical or dental procedures. Those procedures may release bacteria into the bloodstream and, in people with MVP, bacteria may stick to the valves and cause infection (a condition called *endocarditis*). Antibiotic treatment can prevent this.

People with MVP who also have symptoms of dysautonomia may be separately treated for those symptoms as well.

Principal Proposed Natural Treatments

Low levels of magnesium can cause some symptoms similar to dysautonomia. One study evaluated 141 people with MVP and dysautonomia and found that 60% of them had low levels of magnesium in the blood. This subgroup of people with low magnesium were then enrolled in a 10-week, double-blind, placebo-controlled crossover trial. (They received placebo or magnesium supplements for 5 weeks and then were "crossed over" to the other group.) People receiving magnesium experienced a significant reduction in dysautonomic symptoms, such as chest pain, palpitations, anxiety, and shortness of breath.

Note that it is unlikely that these people suffered from magnesium deficiency. Magnesium deficiency is thought to be a rare condition. More likely, low magnesium levels are a consequence of some other factor that also causes dysautonomia symptoms. Regardless, magnesium supplementation could help treat such symptoms. However, more studies are necessary to validate this promising possibility.

For more information, including dosage and safety issues, see the full **Magnesium** article.

Other Proposed Natural Treatments

Various herbs and supplements that are hypothesized to help the heart in miscellaneous ways (such as treating congestive heart failure or preventing coronary artery disease) are often recommended for MVP as well, on general principles. These include **arginine**, **coenzymeQ$_{10}$**, **creatine**, **hawthorn**, **L-carnitine**, **OPCs**, **taurine**, **vitamin B$_1$**, and **vitamin E**. However, there is no scientific reason to believe that any of these natural treatments would help MVP.

A variety of other natural treatments are used to treat anxiety-related dysautonomia symptoms. These include the following:

- **5-hydroxytryptophan (5-HTP)**
- **Acupuncture**
- **Hops**
- **Kava**
- **Lemon balm**
- **Melatonin**
- **Multivitamin/multimineral supplements**
- **Passionflower**
- **Valerian**

Natural treatments used for stress may be helpful as well.

A serious form of autonomic nervous system dysfunction can occur in people with diabetes. The supplements **lipoic acid**, **acetyl-L-carnitine**, and **gamma-linolenic acid** (GLA) have shown some promise for this condition and, for this reason, have been recommended for the treatment of the dysautonomic symptoms noted above.

Herbs and Supplements to Use Only with Caution

Numerous herbs and supplements may interact adversely with drugs used to treat mitral valve prolapse. For more information on this potential risk, see the individual drug article in the Drug Interactions section of this book.

Multiple Sclerosis

RELATED TERM: *MS*

PRINCIPAL PROPOSED NATURAL TREATMENTS: *None*

OTHER PROPOSED NATURAL TREATMENTS: *Bee Venom, Evening Primrose Oil, Fish Oil, Ginkgo, Linoleic Acid, Magnet Therapy, Neural Therapy, Phenylalanine, Reflexology, Threonine, Vitamin B$_{12}$, Vitamin D*

Multiple sclerosis (MS) is a disease affecting the fatty sheath that covers nerve fibers in the brain and spinal cord. This sheath, made of a substance called *myelin*, normally insulates the nerve fibers, allowing nerve impulses to move swiftly and efficiently between brain, spinal cord, and body. In MS, patchy areas of this insulating material are destroyed and replaced by scar tissue, which results in the slowing or blocking of nerve signals. People with MS may experience symptoms such as blurred vision, muscle weakness and spasticity, difficulty walking, poor coordination, bladder problems, numbness, and fatigue. In its most common form, the disease begins between the ages of 20 and 40 with an initial attack of symptoms followed by partial or complete remission. Further attacks usually follow and can eventually lead to progressive disability. Another form of the disease progresses more quickly.

Although the cause of MS isn't known for sure, scientists generally assume that MS is an autoimmune disease in which the immune system attacks the body's own myelin cells. Scientists theorize that something, perhaps a toxin or virus, triggers this autoimmune response in susceptible people. Not everyone appears to be equally susceptible. Gene studies suggest that genetics plays a role in who gets the disease, but other factors seem to be important as well. For example, MS tends to be more common the farther one goes from the equator. The disease is also more prevalent in societies with greater dietary intake of meat and animal fat, lower intake of unsaturated fats compared to saturated fats, and lower intake of fish. Not everyone agrees that all of these factors actually contribute to the disease. Some factors may simply be statistically associated with the actual cause.

There is no cure as yet for MS, but several new drugs—including two forms of the substance interferon (Avonex and Betaseron) and an unrelated drug, glatiramer acetate (Copaxone)—appear able to reduce the frequency of relapses in people with certain forms of MS and slow the rate of progression of the disease. Other medications reduce the severity of acute attacks or treat specific symptoms such as muscle spasticity.

Proposed Natural Treatments

While there are no well-documented natural treatments for multiple sclerosis, there are a few options that may provide some help.

There is some evidence that changing the type and amount of fat in the diet might alter the course of MS. Based on observations from population studies linking diets lower in fat or saturated fat to lower rates of MS, physician R.L. Swank developed a special low-fat diet for MS in which unsaturated fats replace most saturated fat. This approach, called the *Swank diet*, has been used by many people with MS. When he analyzed the long-term effects of the diet on his patients, Swank found that those adhering closely to the diet for 20 to 34 years developed significantly less disability than those who ate more saturated fat. Because these were not controlled trials, they do not actually prove that the Swank diet works. Nonetheless, the possible connection between MS and fatty acids continues to arouse interest and a variety of essential fatty acids have been proposed as possible treatments for MS (see below). Although a link between fat intake and MS is intriguing, research has not yet provided clear-cut evidence that any of these treatments help.

Linoleic Acid

One of the omega-6 essential fatty acids, linoleic acid, is found in high concentration in sunflower and safflower oil as well as in lower concentrations in most other vegetable oils. Several researchers have investigated whether linoleic acid in the form of sunflower seed oil can help MS, but the results of their research were equivocal.

Three groups of investigators performed double-blind studies, using olive oil as a placebo, to see if linoleic acid supplements could affect the symptoms or course of MS. Two of these studies (one involving 75 people, the other 116) found that those taking linoleic acid had shorter and less-severe attacks of MS compared to those taking placebo. However, in the 2 years of the trials, the frequency of attacks and overall levels of disability were not significantly affected. The third study of 76 people found that linoleic acid had no effects on either MS attacks or degrees of disability over 2 1/2 years, as compared to olive oil.

Another researcher suggests that these studies may have been too short—that it may take far longer than 2 years for linoleic acid to exert its effects on myelin. Olive oil also contains important fatty acids; others have wondered if the olive oil could have been an effective treatment on its own, thereby obscuring the benefits of linoleic acid. Finally, yet another researcher carefully examining the study reports found that linoleic acid might have been effective in those individuals with less severe MS symptoms.

Although interesting, this type of after-the-fact analysis must be interpreted with caution. More studies are needed to confirm whether linoleic acid, taken early in the course of MS or at other times, has the power to prevent, delay, or improve disability.

➤ Dosage

In the three double-blind studies described above, participants received 17 to 20 g of linoleic acid per day, the equivalent of 1 ounce of sunflower seed oil.

➤ Safety Issues

As a nutrient found in food, linoleic acid is considered to be safe. However, maximum safe dosages for young children, pregnant or nursing women, or people with severe liver or kidney disease have not been determined.

Other Essential Fatty Acids

There has been much excitement about other essential fatty acids as treatments for MS, including those found in fish oil (omega-3) and evening primrose oil (omega-6). However, current evidence does not yet support this concept.

Blood tests among people with MS have found lower levels of omega-3 fatty acids in their body fluids and tissues compared to those without MS. This hints, but does not prove, that taking extra omega-3 fatty acids might help. Only double-blind, placebo-controlled studies can show that treatments actually work. (For reasons why, see **Why Does This Book Rely on Double-blind Studies?**.) Unfortunately, the only meaningful double-

blind study of fish oil for MS failed to find evidence of benefit. In this 2-year study of 292 people with MS, comparing fish oil's omega-3 fatty acids with an olive oil placebo, there were no significant differences between the two groups. Another study did find possible benefit with fish oil as compared to olive oil in the relapsing-remitting form of MS. When used in combination with a low-fat diet, participants given fish oil showed benefits on some measures. However, the study was small, and the results far from definitive.

Similarly, while some researchers have suggested that gamma-linolenic acid (GLA) might be beneficial in MS, so far what little evidence there is remains more negative than positive.

For more information, including dosage and safety issues, see the **GLA** and **fish oil** articles.

Threonine

Early evidence suggests that threonine, a naturally occurring amino acid, might be able to decrease the muscle spasticity that often occurs with MS.

Two small double-blind studies found a modest but statistically significant improvement in muscle spasticity among people who took threonine compared to those who took a placebo. In one study of 26 people with MS, the improvement was so slight after 8 weeks of treatment that it was detectable by doctors but not by the participants themselves. In the other, both researchers and a few of the 33 participants noticed improvement after 2 weeks of treatment, with some individuals reporting fewer spasms and milder pain. Interestingly, this shorter trial that showed more improvement also used lower doses—6 g daily of L-threonine as opposed to 7.5 g daily of threonine. No significant side effects were noted in either study.

Vitamin B$_{12}$

Because several studies have found MS to be occasionally associated with vitamin B$_{12}$ deficiency and lack of B$_{12}$ can cause neurological problems on its own, some doctors recommend that people with MS be screened for this condition. One highly preliminary study suggested that massive doses of B$_{12}$ could improve certain test results ("evoked potentials"), but not disability, in people with chronic progressive MS. A double-blind study of 50 people with MS found that high doses of injected **hydroxocobalamin**, a form of B$_{12}$, did not affect the course of disease or number of relapses.

For more information, including dosage and safety issues, see the **Vitamin B$_{12}$** article.

Vitamin D

Our bodies normally obtain vitamin D in one of two ways: through our diet or through exposure of our skin to the sun. More than one group of researchers has noted that areas with less sunshine tend to have a higher incidence of MS, unless the residents eat more fish that is rich in vitamin D. This has led to a theory that vitamin D might confer some protection against MS. So far, no human studies have adequately tested this hypothesis, although one poorly designed study did investigate a combination of calcium, magnesium, and vitamin D given in the form of cod liver oil and found hints of benefit.

For more information, including dosage and safety issues, see the **Vitamin D** article.

Phenylalanine and TENS

Phenylalanine is an essential amino acid, meaning that we need it for life and our bodies can't manufacture it from other chemicals. We normally obtain all the phenylalanine we need for nutritional purposes from high-protein foods. Supplemental phenylalanine has been studied for MS only in combination with another treatment: transcutaneous electrical nerve stimulation (TENS), a portable electrical device used to decrease pain and muscle spasticity.

Two small double-blind trials compared phenylalanine to placebo among a total of 16 people with MS being treated with TENS. In both studies, those treated with phenylalanine and TENS experienced less muscle spasticity, fewer bladder symptoms, and less depression after 4 weeks of treatment than those treated with TENS and placebo. These findings are somewhat difficult to interpret, but tend to suggest that phenylalanine may be helpful in MS. For more information, including dosage and safety issues, see the full **Phenylalanine** article.

Other Proposed Natural Treatments

A special form of **magnet therapy** called *pulsed electromagnetic field therapy* (PEMF) has shown some promise for MS. In a 2-month, double-blind, placebo-controlled study, 30 people with multiple sclerosis applied a real or a fake PEMF device to one of three acupuncture points on the shoulder, back, or hip. The study found statistically significant improvements in the treatment group, most notably in bladder control, hand function, and muscle spasticity.

A small double-blind trial suggests that neural therapy, a treatment related to **acupuncture**, might be helpful for MS. In addition, weak evidence hints that **reflexology** might be helpful.

Use of bee stings or injected bee venom for MS has generated a great deal of interest over the years, despite a lack of reliable research supporting its use. The one meaningful study, reported in 2005, failed to find any benefit whatsoever.

Other treatments sometimes suggested for MS include **adenosine monophosphate** (AMP), **biotin**, **glycine**, **proteolytic enzymes**, **selenium**, **vitamin B$_1$**, **vitamin C**, and **vitamin E**, but little to no evidence supports these recommendations.

Although **ginkgo** is sometimes suggested as a treatment for MS, one double-blind study that examined ginkgolide B (a chemical in ginkgo) found no evidence of benefit. Another study failed to find **creatine** helpful.

Nausea

RELATED TERMS: *Car Sickness, Motion Sickness, Sea Sickness*

PRINCIPAL PROPOSED NATURAL TREATMENTS:

   Various Forms of Nausea: *Acupressure/Acupuncture, Ginger*

   Morning Sickness: *Vitamin B$_6$*

OTHER PROPOSED NATURAL TREATMENTS:

   Post-Surgical Nausea: *Peppermint*

   Morning Sickness: *Low-fat Diet, Vitamin C, Vitamin K*

Nausea can be caused by many factors, including stomach flu, viral infections of the inner ear (labyrinthitis), motion sickness, **pregnancy**, and **chemotherapy**. If you are continually nauseous, it can be more disabling than chronic pain. Successful treatment can make an enormous difference in your quality of life.

The sensation of nausea can originate in either the nervous system or the digestive tract itself. Most conventional treatments for nausea, such as Dramamine and Compazine, act on the nervous system, but products like Pepto-Bismol soothe the digestive tract directly.

Principal Proposed Natural Treatments

The herb ginger has become a widely accepted treatment for nausea of various types. Vitamin B_6 may be helpful for the nausea of pregnancy.

Ginger

Limited scientific evidence suggests that the herb ginger can be helpful for various forms of nausea.

≫ Nausea and Vomiting of Pregnancy

Four double-blind, placebo-controlled studies enrolling a total of 246 women found ginger more effective than placebo for treatment of morning sickness.

For example, a double-blind, placebo-controlled trial of 70 pregnant women evaluated the effectiveness of ginger for morning sickness. Participants received either placebo or 250 mg of powdered ginger 3 times daily for a period of 4 days. The results showed that ginger significantly reduced nausea and vomiting. No significant side effects occurred.

Benefits were also seen in a double-blind, placebo-controlled trial of 27 women and in a poorly designed double-blind, placebo-controlled trial of 26 women.

One study of 138 women and another of 291 women found ginger as effective for morning sickness as vitamin B_6. Unfortunately, neither of these studies used a placebo group. Since there is only one study indicating that vitamin B_6 is effective (see below), it isn't quite ready to be used as a "gold standard" treatment. Comparing one unproven treatment to another without using a placebo group leaves much to be desired.

Note: Ginger has not been proven safe for pregnant women.

≫ Motion Sickness

A double-blind, placebo-controlled study of 79 Swedish naval cadets found that 1 g of ginger could decrease vomiting and cold sweating without significantly decreasing nausea and vertigo. Benefits were also seen in a double-blind study of 36 individuals given ginger, dimenhydrinate, or placebo.

In addition, a double-blind comparative study that followed 1,489 individuals aboard a ship found ginger to be equally effective as various medications (cinnarizine, cinnarizine with domperidone, cyclizine, dimehydrinate with caffeine, meclizine with caffeine, and scopolamine). Another double-blind study found equivalent benefit of ginger at a dose of 500 mg every 4 hours and dimenhydrinate (100 mg every 4 hours) in a group of 60 passengers aboard a ship. Similar results were also seen in a small double-blind study involving children.

However, a 1984 study funded by NASA found that ginger was not any more effective than placebo at reducing the symptoms of nausea caused by a vigorous nausea-provoking method. Negative results were also seen in another study that used a strong nausea stimulus.

Put all together, these studies paint a picture of a treatment that is somewhat effective for motion sickness but cannot overcome severe nausea.

≫ Post-surgical Nausea

A British double-blind study compared the effects of ginger, placebo, and the drug metoclopramide in the treatment of nausea following gynecological surgery. The results in 60 women showed that both treatments produced similar benefits compared to placebo.

A similar British study followed 120 women receiving gynecological surgery. Whereas nausea and vomiting developed in 41% of participants given placebo, in the groups treated with ginger or metoclopramide (Reglan), these symptoms developed in only 21% and 27%, respectively. Benefits were also seen in a double-blind study of 80 people.

However, three other studies enrolling a total of about 400 people failed to find ginger more effective than placebo.

A 2004 article that reviewed all this evidence concluded that, on balance, evidence suggests that ginger is *not* effective for post-surgical nausea.

Warning: Do not use ginger either before or immediately after surgery or labor and delivery without a physician's approval. Not only is it important to have an empty stomach before undergoing anesthesia, there are theoretical concerns that ginger may affect bleeding.

For more information, including additional dosage and safety issues, see the full **Ginger** article.

≫ Other Forms of Nausea

One study failed to find ginger helpful for reducing nausea caused by the cancer chemotherapy drug **cisplatin**.

Acupressure/Acupuncture

A single acupuncture point—P6—has traditionally been thought to be helpful for relief of various forms of nausea and vomiting. This point is located on the inside of the forearm, about 2 inches above the wrist crease. Most studies have investigated the effects of pressure on this point (acupressure) rather than needling. The most common methods involve a wristband with a pearl-sized bead in it situated over P6. The band exerts pressure on the bead while it is worn, and the user can press on the bead for extra stimulation.

Although the research record is mixed, on balance it appears that P6 stimulation offers benefits for various types of nausea. This approach has been studied in anesthesia-induced nausea, the nausea and vomiting of pregnancy, and other forms of nausea.

≫ Anesthesia-induced Nausea

General anesthetics and other medications used for **surgery** frequently cause nausea.

At least eight controlled studies enrolling a total of more than 750 women undergoing gynecologic surgery found that P6 stimulation reduced post-surgical nausea as compared to placebo.

On the negative side, a double-blind, placebo-controlled study of 410 women undergoing gynecological surgery failed to find P6 acupressure more effective than fake acupuncture. (Both were more effective than no treatment). A small trial of acupuncture in gynecological surgery also failed to find benefit, as did three studies of acupressure for women undergoing C-section.

Studies of acupuncture or acupressure in other forms of surgery have produced about as many negative results as positive ones.

≫ Nausea and Vomiting of Pregnancy

Several controlled studies have evaluated the benefits of acupressure or acupuncture for morning sickness. The results for acupressure have generally been more positive than for acupuncture.

For example, a double-blind, placebo-controlled study of 97 women found evidence that wristband acupressure may work. Participants wore either a real wristband or a phony one that appeared identical. Both real and fake acupressure caused noticeable improvement in more than half of the participants. However, women using the real wristband showed better results in terms of the duration of nausea. Intensity of the nausea symptoms was not significantly different between groups.

These results are consistent with previous studies of acupressure for morning sickness. However, two studies failed to find benefit for severe morning sickness.

However, one large trial of *acupuncture* instead of acupressure failed to find benefit. This single-blind, placebo-controlled study of 593 pregnant women with morning sickness compared the effects of traditional acupuncture, acupuncture at P6 only, acupuncture at "wrong" points (sham acupuncture), and no treatment. Women in all three treatment groups (including the fake acupuncture group) showed significant improvements in nausea and dry retching compared to the no-treatment group. However, neither form of real acupuncture proved markedly more effective than fake acupuncture.

≫ Other Forms of Nausea

Studies are conflicting on whether acupressure is helpful for motion sickness.

A single-blind, placebo-controlled trial of 104 people undergoing high-dose **chemotherapy** for breast cancer found that electrical stimulation on P6 significantly reduced episodes of vomiting. Similar improvements were found in a pilot study. In a small sham-controlled study, acupressure wristbands showed promise, although the benefit seen just missed the conventional cutoff for statistical significance. Another study failed to find benefit.

For more information, including safety issues, see the full **Acupuncture** article.

Vitamin B$_6$

A large double-blind study (with almost 350 people) suggests that 30 mg daily of vitamin B$_6$ can reduce the sensation of nausea in morning sickness. For more information, including dosage and safety issues, see the full **Vitamin B$_6$** article.

Other Proposed Natural Treatments

Preliminary studies suggest **peppermint** oil may be able to reduce post-operative nausea. **Multivitamin/mineral tablets** have also shown promise, possibly due to their vitamin B$_6$ content.

On the basis of studies conducted in the 1950s, a combination of **vitamin K** (at the enormous dose, for vitamin K, of 5 mg daily) and **vitamin C** (25 mg daily) is sometimes recommended for morning sickness.

Nausea of Pregnancy

RELATED TERMS: *Hyperemesis Gravidarum, Morning Sickness*
PRINCIPAL PROPOSED NATURAL TREATMENTS: *Acupressure/Acupuncture, Ginger, Vitamin B$_6$*
OTHER PROPOSED NATURAL TREATMENTS: *Red Raspberry, Vitamin C, Vitamin K*

Nausea afflicts the majority of women during the first trimester of pregnancy. However, this is also the precise period in which drug therapy is most worrisome due to the extreme vulnerability of the fetus at that time. For this reason, conventional medicine has to some extent welcomed alternative medicine's quest for safe, natural treatment options.

Principal Proposed Natural Treatments

Two natural therapies, vitamin B$_6$ and ginger, have some evidence supporting their use in the treatment of nausea in pregnancy. In addition, acupuncture/acupressure may be helpful.

For natural treatments relevant to other aspects of pregnancy, see the articles on **Pregnancy and Support**, **Breastfeeding Support**, **Preeclampsia**, and **Herbs and Supplements to Avoid in Pregnancy and Breastfeeding**.

Vitamin B$_6$

For many years, conventional practitioners have recommended vitamin B$_6$ supplements to treat morning sickness. In 1995, a large double-blind, placebo-controlled study validated this use. In this trial, a total of 342 pregnant women were given placebo or 30 mg of vitamin B$_6$ daily. Participants then graded their symptoms by noting the severity of their nausea and recording the number of vomiting episodes. The women in the B$_6$ group experienced significantly less nausea than the placebo group, suggesting that regular use of B$_6$ can be helpful for morning sickness. However, despite the benefits for nausea, vomiting episodes were not significantly reduced.

At this dose (30 mg daily), vitamin B$_6$ is believed to be entirely safe. For more information, including dosage and safety issues, see the full **Vitamin B$_6$** article.

Ginger

Ginger is a nausea remedy recommended by many physicians as well as by traditional healers from a number of countries. In 2001, a relatively well-designed double-blind, placebo-controlled trial of 70 pregnant women evaluated the effectiveness of ginger for morning sickness. Participants received either placebo or 250 mg of powdered ginger 3 times daily for a period of 4 days. The results showed that ginger significantly reduced nausea and vomiting. No significant side effects occurred.

Benefits were also seen in an earlier double-blind, placebo-controlled trial of 27 women, and in a poorly designed double-blind, placebo-controlled trial of 26 women.

One study of 138 women and another of 291 women found ginger equally effective for morning sickness as vitamin B$_6$. Neither of these studies used a placebo group.

For more information, including dosage and safety issues, see the full article on **Ginger**.

Acupressure/Acupuncture

Several studies have evaluated treatment on a single acupuncture point—P6—traditionally thought to be effective for relief of nausea and vomiting. This point is located on the inside of the forearm, about 2 inches above the wrist crease. Most trials have investigated the effects of pressure on this point (acupressure), rather than needling. The most common means used involve a wristband with a pearl-sized bead in it, situated over P6. It exerts pressure by itself while it is worn, and the user can also press on it for extra stimulation.

A double-blind, placebo-controlled study of 97 women that was reported in 2001 found evidence that wristband acupressure may help relieve symptoms of morning sickness. Participants wore either a real wristband or a phony one that appeared identical. Both real and fake acupressure caused noticeable improvement in more than half of the participants. However, women using the real wristband showed significantly greater improvement. Benefits were also reported the same year in a double-blind, placebo-controlled study of 60 women.

These results are consistent with previous studies that also found benefit. Furthermore, a double-blind, placebo-controlled study of 60 pregnant women found that 10 minutes of self-applied manual acupressure on either P6 or a sham point 4 times daily improved symptoms. However, two studies failed to find benefit for severe morning sickness.

For more information, including safety issues, see the full **Acupuncture** article.

Other Proposed Natural Treatments

Multivitamin/mineral tablets have shown promise for morning sickness, possibly due to their vitamin B_6 content.

A combination of **vitamin K** (at a dose of 5 mg—enormously higher than nutritional needs) and **vitamin C** (25 mg) is sometimes recommended for morning sickness, based on an uncontrolled study conducted in the 1950s. **Red raspberry** is also frequently recommended, but there is no evidence that it works.

Neck Pain

RELATED TERMS: *Cervicalgia, Cervical Pain*

PRINCIPAL PROPOSED NATURAL TREATMENTS: *None*

OTHER PROPOSED NATURAL TREATMENTS: *Acupuncture, Biofeedback, Boswellia, Butterbur, Chiropractic, Chondroitin, Ginger, Glucosamine, Hypnosis, Massage, Osteopathic Manipulation, Prolotherapy, Proteolytic Enzymes, Relaxation Therapies, Turmeric, White Willow*

Neck pain is a common condition, affecting millions of Americans. In many cases, x-rays do not show anything visibly wrong with the neck, suggesting that the problem is a relatively subtle one involving soft tissues. (Conversely, x-rays of people without neck pain often show arthritis; this suggests that even when positive x-ray results are found in people with neck pain, they may be unrelated.) Subtle or not in origin, the discomfort of neck pain can be severe and lead to real disability.

The cause of soft-tissue neck pain is not known. Symptoms may follow a whiplash injury, or simply arise, apparently, from bad posture or chronic tension.

Note: It is unclear that *any* conventional medicine intervention for neck pain or whiplash speeds recovery or produces any other long-term benefit.

Proposed Natural Treatments

Although several alternative treatments for neck pain have shown promise, none possess meaningful scientific substantiation.

Acupuncture

A 1999 review of the literature found one double-blind and eight single-blind, placebo-controlled trials of **acupuncture** for various forms of neck pain, enrolling a total of more than 250 participants. The results of these small trials are almost equally balanced: about as many found acupuncture superior to placebo as found it no better than placebo.

A subsequent study of 177 people with chronic neck pain compared acupuncture to placebo acupuncture as well as massage. The results after five sessions showed no significant difference between real and fake acupuncture. Three smaller studies published after 1999 also failed to find any meaningful superiority of real acupuncture over fake acupuncture. In addition, one study failed to find laser acupuncture any more effective than fake laser acupuncture for treatment of whiplash.

Chiropractic

Millions of Americans report that **chiropractic spinal manipulation** has relieved their neck pain, but there is as yet little scientific evidence supporting the use of spinal manipulation for this purpose. Most studies have found manipulation (with or without related therapies such as mobilization or massage) to be no more effective than placebo or no treatment. One large study (almost 200 participants) found that a special exercise program called *MedX* was more effective than chiropractic spinal manipulation.

Other Treatments

Osteopathic manipulation, a form of treatment often compared to chiropractic, is widely believed to help neck pain, but there is as yet no meaningful scientific evidence to support its use for this condition. Many people with neck pain use **massage therapy** for relief, but, again, scientific support is lacking, and one study found fake laser acupuncture more effective than massage for neck pain.

A treatment called **prolotherapy**, as well as the herb **white willow**, have shown promise for **back pain** and might be useful for neck pain as well.

In one study, an ambitious holistic treatment regimen for neck pain (including **craniosacral osteopathy** along with Rosen Bodywork and Gestalt Psychotherapy) failed to prove more effective than no treatment.

Other herbs and supplements sometimes recommended for neck pain, either on the basis of their use for related conditions, or because of their known medical properties, include **boswellia**, **butterbur**, **chondroitin**, **ginger**, **glucosamine**, **proteolytic enzymes**, and **turmeric**.

Biofeedback, **hypnosis**, and **relaxation therapies** may offer help for pain in general.

Night Vision (Impaired)

PRINCIPAL PROPOSED NATURAL TREATMENTS: *Bilberry*

OTHER PROPOSED NATURAL TREATMENTS: *Black Currant, Oligomeric Proanthocyanidins (OPCs),*
Vitamin A, Zinc

The ability to see in poor light depends on the presence of a substance in the eye called *rhodopsin*, or *visual purple*. It is destroyed by bright light but rapidly regenerates in the dark. However, for some people, the adaptation to darkness or the recovery from glare takes an unusually long time. There is no medical treatment for this condition.

Principal Proposed Natural Treatments

The herb bilberry, a close relative of the American blueberry, is the most commonly mentioned natural treatment for impaired night vision. This use dates back to World War II, when pilots in Britain's Royal Air Force reported that a good dose of bilberry jam just before a mission improved their night vision, often dramatically. After the war, medical researchers investigated the constituents of bilberry and found a group of active chemicals called *anthocyanosides*. These naturally occurring antioxidants appear to have numerous potentially important actions within the eye.

However, neither anecdote nor basic scientific evidence of this type can prove a treatment effective. Only double-blind, placebo-controlled studies can do that. (To learn why this is so, see **Why Does This Book Rely on Double-blind Studies?**.) The current evidence from studies of this type is more negative than positive, with all of the most recent studies finding no benefit.

For example, a double-blind crossover trial of 15 individuals found no short- or long-term improvements in night vision attributable to bilberry. Similarly negative results were seen in a double-blind, placebo-controlled crossover trial of 18 subjects and another of 16 subjects. Earlier studies had reported some benefit, but they were less rigorous in design.

Thus, at present, bilberry cannot be recommended as a treatment for improving night vision. For more information, including dosage and safety issues, see the full **Bilberry** article.

Other Proposed Natural Treatments

Evidence from a small double-blind, placebo-controlled study suggests that anthocyanosides from black currant might have some benefit for night vision.

Oligomeric proanthocyanidins (OPCs) have also been recommended for improving night vision, although the evidence that they help is far too weak to rely upon at all.

There is no question that deficiencies of **vitamin A** and **zinc** can also negatively affect night vision. However, there is no reason to believe that taking *extra* amounts of these nutrients will enhance vision.

Nosebleeds

RELATED TERMS: *Epistaxis*

PRINCIPAL PROPOSED NATURAL TREATMENTS: *Citrus Bioflavonoids*

OTHER PROPOSED NATURAL TREATMENTS: *Bilberry, Bromelain, Oligomeric Proanthocyanidins (OPCs), Proteolytic Enzymes, Shepherd's Purse, Vitamin C*

Who among us has never had a nosebleed? Whether a dab of blood on a tissue or a terrifying flood, a nosebleed can arise from many causes: dry winter air, colds, injuries, or the common if unsavory habit of picking one's nose. In many cases, no cause can be identified with certainty.

Sometimes nosebleeds arise more frequently because of faulty or weak *collagen*, a strengthening protein present in blood vessel walls and the surrounding connective tissue. Collagen problems may lead to nosebleeds in people who take corticosteroids and those with a condition called *fragile capillaries*. Corticosteroids, including nasal steroids used for allergies, can thin the collagen in the mucous membranes lining the nose. In fragile capillaries, weak or defective collagen in blood vessel walls may contribute to bleeding. People with such collagen problems may have problems with bleeding gums, heavy menstrual periods, and bruising in addition to nosebleeds.

Rarely, the cause of nosebleeds and other bleeding lies in the blood itself. Anything that reduces blood clotting may lead to nosebleeds. Drugs such as warfarin (Coumadin) or heparin, or regular use of aspirin, decrease the blood's tendency to clot. **Caution**: If you are taking such medications and begin to experience nosebleeds, talk to your doctor. Even natural substances such as ginkgo, policosanol, high-dose vitamin E, and garlic may increase the tendency to bleed.

Conventional treatments for nosebleeds include various maneuvers for stopping acute bleeding, followed by the diagnosis and treatment of any underlying problems. Sometimes a physician can prevent future nosebleeds by cauterizing the blood vessel responsible.

Principal Proposed Natural Treatments

One supplement that may help prevent nosebleeds is citrus bioflavonoids. Bioflavonoids (or flavonoids) are plant substances that bring color to many fruits and vegetables. Citrus fruits are a rich source of bioflavonoids, including diosmin, hesperidin, rutin, and naringen.

A double-blind, placebo-controlled study of 96 people with fragile capillaries found that a combination of the bioflavonoids diosmin and hesperidin decreased symptoms of capillary fragility, such as nosebleeds and bruising. In this 6-week trial, participants—41% of whom had problems with nosebleeds—took 2 tablets daily of the bioflavonoid combination or placebo. Those who received bioflavonoids had significantly greater improvements in both their symptoms and their capillary strength compared to those taking placebo. Unfortunately, the researchers didn't state how much the nosebleeds improved.

For more information, including dosage and safety issues, see the full **Citrus Bioflavonoids** article.

Other Proposed Natural Treatments

Oligomeric proanthocyanidins (OPCs) are bioflavonoid-like compounds found in large amounts in grape seed and grape extract products. Test-tube studies have found that OPCs protect collagen, partly by inhibiting an enzyme that breaks it down. One rather poorly designed double-blind study of 37 people—most of whom had fragile capillaries—found that OPCs were more effective than placebo in decreasing capillary fragility; however, the study authors left many questions unanswered in their report, making it hard to determine how seriously to take their results, and they did not address nosebleeds specifically.

Related chemicals called *anthocyanosides* are present in high concentrations in the herb **bilberry**. Like OPCs, anthocyanosides may strengthen capillaries through their effects on collagen. **Proteolytic enzymes** (such as **bromelain**) are also thought to possibly help stabilize capillaries. However, no studies have directly addressed the potential value of either of these treatments for nosebleeds.

Vitamin C is vital for the development of normal collagen. People with scurvy (severe vitamin C deficiency) may bleed easily from the nose, as well as developing spontaneous bruises and other bleeding symptoms. However, there is no evidence as yet that vitamin C supplementation helps to decrease nosebleeds in the absence of true scurvy, a condition that is rare today.

The herb shepherd's purse (*Capsella bursae pastoris*) has been traditionally used as a topical application to control nosebleeds, although scientific evidence of its effectiveness is lacking. The herb should not be used during pregnancy because it is thought to stimulate uterine contractions.

Nutrition for Cigarette Smokers

PRINCIPAL PROPOSED NATURAL TREATMENTS: *Quitting Smoking*

OTHER PROPOSED NATURAL TREATMENTS: *Folate, Multivitamin and Mineral Supplements, Vitamin C, Vitamin E*

HERBS AND SUPPLEMENTS TO AVOID: *High-dose Beta-carotene*

Cigarette smoking is one of the biggest risk factors for cancer and heart disease. The more cigarettes a person smokes and the longer it's kept up, the greater the risk of dying from cancer, heart attack, or stroke. Probably less well known is that smokers are also much more likely to catch colds and other infections.

Of course, the best remedy for these risks and problems is quitting smoking, but that's not easy for many people. Because cigarette smoking poses such a public health risk, many studies have attempted to discern whether vitamin supplementation among smokers might help avert cancer and heart disease. However, the results have not been particularly promising and one supplement, beta-carotene, may actually be dangerous for smokers.

Proposed Natural Treatments

People who smoke often have deficiencies in numerous nutrients, including **zinc**, **calcium**, **folate**, **vitamins C** and **E**, **beta-carotene**, lycopene, and essential fatty acids in the omega-3 and omega-6 families. There are many possible causes for this depletion, including free radicals in cigarette smoke that destroy natural antioxidants; however, for some nutrients the most important single cause might be poor diet rather than smoking itself (smokers have, on average, a less well-balanced diet than non-smokers).

In addition, some evidence suggests that folate or vitamin C supplements may improve arterial function in smokers, thereby potentially helping to prevent heart disease.

High doses of vitamin E have not proven helpful for preventing heart disease or lung cancer in smokers. However, vitamin E consumption has shown some promise for reducing risk of prostate cancer in smokers.

For all these reasons, many smokers undoubtedly benefit from general nutritional support in the form of a multivitamin/mineral tablet. However, high doses of the antioxidant vitamin beta-carotene may not be helpful for smokers and could even cause harm (see next section).

Beta-Carotene: A Supplement to Avoid

Although nutritional doses of the antioxidant nutrient beta-carotene help to supply needed vitamin A, there is evidence that smokers should avoid high doses of beta-carotene.

An enormous double-blind, placebo-controlled study called the Alpha-Tocopherol, Beta-Carotene Cancer Prevention (ATBC) enrolled 29,133 Finnish male smokers and examined the effects of vitamin E and beta-carotene supplements on lung cancer rates among them. The results showed that 20 mg of beta-carotene daily for 5 to 8 years *increased* the risk of lung cancer by 18%.

In addition, a statistical analysis of the ATBC study, including 1,862 smokers with heart problems, found that individuals taking either beta-carotene or a beta-carotene/vitamin E combination had significantly increased risk of fatal heart attack compared to those taking placebo. Another statistical review of the study analyzed the effects of beta-carotene on individuals with angina pectoris, one of the first symptoms of heart disease. Results indicated that beta-carotene was associated with a slight increase in angina.

Another large double-blind, placebo-controlled trial enrolling 18,314 smokers, former smokers, and workers exposed to asbestos studied the effects of a different combination, beta-carotene and vitamin A, on lung cancer and cardiovascular disease. Evidence from the trial suggests that 30 mg of beta-carotene and 25,000 IU of vitamin A taken together daily have no beneficial effects and may be harmful. Individuals taking the supplements had a 28% higher incidence of lung cancer than the placebo group; a 17% higher death rate from lung cancer; and a 26% higher death rate from cardiovascular disease. The trial was stopped 21 months early based on these findings.

The bottom line on beta-carotene: Although nutritional dosages of beta-carotene (in the neighborhood of 3 mg daily for adults) are probably healthful, smokers should avoid doses of beta-carotene greater than in the range of 20 to 30 mg daily.

Obsessive-Compulsive Disorder

RELATED TERM: *OCD*

PRINCIPAL PROPOSED NATURAL TREATMENTS: *None*

OTHER PROPOSED NATURAL TREATMENTS: *Inositol, St. John's Wort, 5-HTP, Magnet Therapy*

Obsessive-compulsive disorder (OCD) is a psychological condition that involves recurrent and persistent thoughts or images (obsessions) that are experienced as intrusive and cause distress. These obsessions are not simply excessive worries about real-life problems, but take on an unrealistic quality. In order to combat their obsessions, people with OCD engage in repetitive behaviors (compulsions), often following rigid self-imposed rules.

The cause of OCD is not known. Antidepressant drugs that affect serotonin levels, such as selective serotonin reuptake inhibitors (SSRIs), often relieve symptoms significantly, but the reasons for this are not clear. Psychotherapeutic and behavioral methods may also help.

Proposed Natural Treatments

The supplement **inositol** is thought to increase the body's sensitivity to serotonin and on that basis it has been studied for use in a number of psychological conditions, including OCD.

In a small double-blind trial, use of inositol at a dose of 18 g daily for 6 weeks significantly improved symptoms of OCD as compared to placebo. However, some evidence suggests that inositol does not increase the effectiveness of standard drugs for OCD.

One study found that people with OCD have lower than normal levels of **vitamin B_{12}**. This suggests, but absolutely does not prove, that vitamin B_{12} supplements might be helpful for the condition.

The herb **St. John's wort** has antidepressant properties and is thought to affect serotonin levels. On this basis, it has been tried for OCD, but as yet there is no reliable evidence that it is effective. On a similar basis, the supplement **5-HTP** has been suggested as a treatment for OCD, but again there is no meaningful evidence to turn to.

A form of **magnet therapy** called *r*TMS has shown

promise for the treatment of depression. However, a double-blind, placebo-controlled study of 18 people with OCD found no evidence of benefit through the use of rTMS.

Herbs and Supplements to Use Only with Caution

Various herbs and supplements may interact with drugs used to treat OCD. For more information on these potential risks see the individual drug article in the Drug Interactions section of this book.

Osteoarthritis

PRINCIPAL PROPOSED NATURAL TREATMENTS:

Reducing Symptoms and Slowing the Progression of the Disease: Chondroitin Sulfate, Glucosamine

Reducing Symptoms Only: S-Adenosylmethionine (SAMe), Avocado/Soybean Unsaponifiables, Cetylated Fatty Acids, Acupuncture

OTHER PRSOPOSED NATURAL TREATMENTS:

Herbs and Supplements: Ayurveda, Boswellia, Cat's Claw, Chinese Herbal Medicine, Devil's Claw, Ginger, Green-lipped Mussel, Methyl Sulfonyl Methane (MSM), Multimineral Supplement, Niacinamide, Proteolytic Enzymes, Rose Hips, Velvet Antler, White Willow, Zinc

Therapies: Bee Venom, Magnet Therapy, Prolotherapy, Yoga

PROBABLY INEFFECTIVE TREATMENTS: *Mesoglycan, Vitamin E*

In osteoarthritis, the cartilage in joints has become damaged, disrupting the smooth gliding motion of the joint surfaces. The result is pain, swelling, and deformity.

The pain of osteoarthritis typically increases with joint use and improves at rest. For reasons that aren't clear, although x-rays can find evidence of arthritis, the level of pain and stiffness experienced by people does not match the extent of injury noticed on x-rays.

Many theories exist about the causes of osteoarthritis, but we don't really know what causes the disease. Osteoarthritis is often described as "wear and tear" arthritis. However, evidence suggests that this simple explanation is not correct. For example, osteoarthritis frequently develops in many joints at the same time, often symmetrically on both sides of the body, even when there is no reason to believe that equal amounts of wear and tear are present. Another intriguing finding is that osteoarthritis of the knee is commonly (and mysteriously) associated with osteoarthritis of the hand. These factors, as well as others, have led to the suggestion that osteoarthritis may actually be a body-wide disease of the cartilage.

During one's lifetime, cartilage is constantly being turned over by a balance of forces that both break down and rebuild it. One prevailing theory suggests that osteoarthritis may represent a situation in which the degrading forces get out of hand. Some of the proposed natural treatments for osteoarthritis described later may inhibit enzymes that damage cartilage.

When the cartilage damage in osteoarthritis begins, the body responds by building new cartilage. For several years, this compensating effort can keep the joint functioning well. Some of the natural treatments described below appear to work by assisting the body in repairing cartilage. Eventually, however, building forces cannot keep up with destructive ones and what is called *end-stage osteoarthritis* develops. This is the familiar picture of pain and impaired joint function.

The conventional medical treatment for osteoarthritis consists mainly of anti-inflammatory drugs, such as naproxen and Celebrex. The main problem with anti-inflammatory drugs is that they can cause ulcers. Another possible problem is that they may actually speed the progression of osteoarthritis by interfering with cartilage repair and promoting cartilage destruction. In contrast, two of the treatments described below might actually slow the course of the disease, although this has not been proven.

Principal Proposed Natural Treatments

Several natural treatments for osteoarthritis have a meaningful though not definitive body of supporting evidence indicating that they can reduce pain and improve function. In addition, there is some evidence that glucosamine and chondroitin might offer the additional benefit of helping to prevent progressive joint damage.

Glucosamine

Inconsistent evidence hints that glucosamine can reduce symptoms of mild to moderate arthritis; a small amount of evidence indicates that regular use can slow down the gradual worsening of arthritis that normally occurs with time.

➤ Symptom Relief

Glucosamine is widely accepted as a treatment for osteoarthritis. However, the supporting evidence that it works is somewhat inconsistent, with several of the most recent studies failing to find benefit. Two types of studies have been performed: those that compared glucosamine against placebo and those that compared it against standard medications.

In the placebo-controlled category, one of the best trials was a 3-year, double-blind study of 212 people with osteoarthritis of the knee. Participants receiving glucosamine showed reduced symptoms as compared to those receiving placebo.

Benefits were also seen in other double-blind, placebo-controlled studies, enrolling a total of more than 800 people and ranging in length from 4 weeks to 3 years.

Other double-blind studies enrolling a total of more than 400 people compared glucosamine against ibuprofen and found glucosamine equally effective as the drug.

However, more recent studies have not been so promising. In four studies involving a total of almost 500 people, use of glucosamine failed to improve symptoms to any greater extent than placebo. A fifth study evaluated the effects of *stopping* glucosamine after taking it for 6 months. In this double-blind study of 137 people with osteoarthritis of the knee, participants who stopped using glucosamine (and, unbeknownst to them, took placebo instead) did no worse than people who stayed on glucosamine. In addition, a very large (1,583-participant) study failed to find either glucosamine (as glucosamine hydrochloride) or glucosamine plus chondroitin more effective than placebo. It appears that most of the positive studies were funded by manufacturers of glucosamine products and most of the studies performed by neutral researchers failed to find benefit.

The supplement **methyl sulfonyl methane** (MSM) has been widely included along with glucosamine in natural arthritis products since at least 2001, but the first meaningful supporting evidence that it might actually have any effect did not emerge until 2004. In a double-blind, placebo-controlled study, 118 people with mild-to-moderate osteoarthritis of the knee were given either glucosamine (500 mg 3 times daily), MSM (500 mg 3 times daily), a combination of glucosamine and MSM, or placebo. The study ran for 12 weeks. The results showed that both MSM and glucosamine improved arthritis symptoms as compared to placebo and that the combination of MSM and glucosamine was even more effective than either supplement separately.

➤ Slowing the Disease

A 3-year, double-blind, placebo-controlled study of 212 individuals found indications that glucosamine may protect joints from further damage. Over the course of the study, individuals given glucosamine showed some actual improvement in pain and mobility, while those given placebo worsened steadily. Furthermore, x-rays showed that glucosamine treatment prevented progressive damage to the knee joint.

A separate 3-year study enrolling 202 people confirmed these results.

➤ How Does Glucosamine Work?

Glucosamine appears to stimulate cartilage cells in the joints to make proteoglycans and collagen, two proteins essential for the proper function of joints. Glucosamine may also help prevent collagen from breaking down.

For more information, including dosage and safety issues, see the full **Glucosamine** article.

Chondroitin Sulfate

As described in the previous section, the supplement chondroitin is often combined with glucosamine. Several studies have evaluated chondroitin used alone, as well, with generally positive results, both for improving symptoms and slowing the progression of the disease.

➤ Symptom Relief

According to some but not all double-blind, placebo-controlled studies chondroitin may relieve symptoms of osteoarthritis.

One study enrolled 85 people with osteoarthritis of the knee and followed them for 6 months. Participants received either 400 mg of chondroitin sulfate twice daily or placebo. At the end of the trial, doctors rated the improvement as good or very good in 69% of those taking chondroitin sulfate but in only 32% of those taking placebo.

Another way of comparing the results is to look at maximum walking speed among participants. Whereas individuals in the chondroitin group were able to improve their walking speed gradually over the course of the trial, walking speed did not improve at all in the placebo group. Additionally, there were improvements in other measures of osteoarthritis, such as pain level, with benefits seen as early as 1 month. This suggests that chondroitin was able to stop the arthritis from gradually getting worse.

Good results were seen in a 12-month, double-blind trial that compared chondroitin against placebo in 104 individuals with arthritis of the knee, as well as in a 12-month trial of 42 participants.

Another interesting study evaluated intermittent or "on and off" use of chondroitin. In this study, 120 people received either placebo or 800 mg of chondroitin sulfate daily for two separate 3-month periods over a year. The results showed that even when taken this way, used of chondroitin improved symptoms.

Benefits were also seen in two short-term trials involving a total of about 240 individuals.

Generally positive results were also seen in other studies, including one that found chondroitin about as effective as the anti-inflammatory drug diclofenac.

However, a very large (1,583-participant) and well-designed study failed to find either chondroitin or glucosamine plus chondroitin more effective than placebo. It has been suggested that chondroitin, like glucosamine, may primarily show benefit in studies funded by manufacturers of chondroitin products.

➤ Slowing the Disease

Growing evidence tells us that, like glucosamine, chondroitin slows the progression of arthritis.

An important feature of the study of 42 individuals mentioned previously was that the individuals taking a placebo showed progressive joint damage over the year, but among those taking chondroitin sulfate no worsening of the joints was seen. In other words, chondroitin sulfate seemed to protect the joints of osteoarthritis sufferers from further damage.

A longer and larger double-blind, placebo-controlled trial also found evidence that chondroitin sulfate can slow the progression of osteoarthritis. One hundred and nineteen people were enrolled in this study, which lasted a full 3 years. Thirty-four of the participants received 1,200 mg of chondroitin sulfate per day; the rest received placebo. Over the course of the study researchers took x-rays to determine how many joints had progressed to a severe stage.

During the 3 years of the study only 8.8% of those who took chondroitin sulfate developed severely damaged joints, whereas almost 30% of those who took placebo progressed to this extent.

Similar long-term benefits were seen in two other studies, enrolling a total of more than 200 people.

Additional evidence comes from animal studies. Researchers measured the effects of chondroitin sulfate (administered both orally and via injection directly into the muscle) in rabbits, in which cartilage damage had been induced in one knee by the injection of an enzyme. After 84 days of treatment, the damaged knees in the animals that had been given chondroitin sulfate had significantly more cartilage left than the knees of the untreated animals. Taking chondroitin sulfate by mouth was as effective as taking it through an injection.

Looking at the sum of the evidence, it does appear that chondroitin sulfate may actually protect joints from damage in osteoarthritis.

For more information, including dosage and safety issues, see the full **Chondroitin** article.

SAMe

A substantial body of scientific evidence indicates that S-adenosylmethionine (SAMe) can relieve symptoms of arthritis. Numerous double-blind studies involving more than a thousand participants in total suggest that it is approximately as effective for this purpose as standard anti-inflammatory drugs. However, there is no meaningful evidence that SAMe slows the progression of the disease.

One of the best double-blind studies enrolled 732 patients and followed them for 4 weeks. Over this period, 235 of the participants received 1,200 mg of SAMe per day, while a similar number took either placebo or 750 mg daily of the standard drug naproxen. The majority of these patients had experienced moderate symptoms of osteoarthritis of either the knee or of the hip for an average of 6 years.

The results indicate that SAMe provided as much pain-relieving effect as naproxen and that both treatments were significantly better than placebo. However, differences did exist between the two treatments. Naproxen worked more quickly, producing readily apparent benefits at the 2-week follow-up, whereas the full effect of SAMe was not apparent until 4 weeks. By the end of the study, both treatments were producing the same level of benefit.

In a double-blind study that compared SAMe against the new anti-inflammatory drug Celebrex (celecoxib), once more the drug worked faster than the supplement, but in time both were providing equal benefits.

Evidence regarding slowing the progression of arthritis is at present limited to studies involving animals rather than people.

For more information, including dosage and safety issues, see the full **SAMe** article.

Avocado/Soybean Unsaponifiables

Special extracts of avocado and soybeans called *avocado/soybean unsaponifiables* (ASUs) have been investigated as a treatment for osteoarthritis, with very promising results in studies enrolling a total of several hundred people.

For example, in a double-blind trial, 260 individuals with arthritis of the knee were given either placebo or ASU at 300 or 600 mg daily. The results over 3 months showed that use of ASU significantly improved arthritis symptoms as compared to placebo. There was no significant difference seen between the two doses tested.

Thus far, however, it does not appear that ASU can slow the progression of osteoarthritis.

For more information, including dosage and safety issues, see the full **ASUs** article.

Cetylated Fatty Acids

A type of naturally occurring fatty acid called *cetylated fatty acids* have shown growing promise for osteoarthritis. It is used both as a topical cream and as an oral supplement.

Three double-blind placebo-controlled studies have found cetylated fatty acids helpful for osteoarthritis. Two involved a topical product and one used an oral formulation.

In one the studies using the cream, 40 people with osteoarthritis of the knee applied either cetylated fatty acid or placebo to the affected joint. The results over 30 days showed greater improvements in range of motion and functional ability among people using the real cream than those using the placebo cream. In another 30-day study, also enrolling 40 people with knee arthritis, use of cetylated fatty acid cream improved postural stability, presumably due to decreased pain levels. In addition, a 68-day, double-blind, placebo-controlled study of 64 people with knee arthritis tested an oral cetylated fatty acid supplement (the supplement also contained lesser amounts of **lecithin** and **fish oil**). Participants in the treatment group experienced improvements in swelling, mobility, and pain level as compared to those in the placebo group. Inexplicably, the study report does not discuss whether or not side effects occurred. While this is a promising body of research, it is far from definitive. Current advertising claims for cetylated fatty acids go far beyond the existing evidence. For example, a number of websites claim that cetylated fatty acids are more effective than glucosamine or chondroitin. However, no comparison studies have been performed upon which such a claim could be rationally based.

For more information, including dosage and safety issues, see the full **Cetylated Fatty Acid** article.

Acupuncture

A review published in 2001 evaluated the results of studies of **acupuncture** for osteoarthritis of the knee. The reviewers found seven studies they rated as meaningful, involving a total of 393 participants. Although not all studies were positive, overall the reviewers concluded that "strong evidence" indicates that acupuncture is more effective for knee arthritis than sham acupuncture. Benefits were seen in two other studies published subsequent to this review.

Acupuncture has also been studied for the treatment of arthritis in the hip. A single-blind, controlled trial of 67 people with osteoarthritis of the hip found that acupuncture significantly improved symptoms, with relief lasting for months after the end of treatment. One small study found acupuncture more effective than advice and exercises for hip pain. However, yet another study

Osteoarthritis

found that insertion of needles at random spots in the general vicinity of the hip was just as effective as traditional acupuncture. Larger trials will be necessary to fully sort out acupuncture's effectiveness for hip pain.

Acupuncture for osteoarthritis in various joints as also been compared to anti-inflammatory drugs, steroid injections, and diazepam (Valium) with mixed results.

Other Proposed Natural Treatments

Other Treatments

A 6-week, double-blind, placebo-controlled study of 247 individuals with osteoarthritis of the knee evaluated a combination herbal product containing **ginger** and the Asian spice galanga (*Alpinia galanga*). The results showed that participants in the ginger/galanga group improved to a significantly greater extent than those receiving placebo. However, despite news reports claiming that this study proves ginger effective for osteoarthritis, it only provides information on the effectiveness of the herbal combination. The two double-blind studies performed on ginger alone were small, and produced contradictory results.

The herb **white willow** contains the aspirin-like substance salicin. A 2-week, double-blind, placebo-controlled trial of 78 individuals with arthritis found evidence that willow extracts can relieve osteoarthritis pain. However, another double-blind study enrolling 127 people with osteoarthritis found white willow less effective than a standard anti-inflammatory drug and no more effective than placebo. Again, the likely explanation for these contradictory results is that white willow at usual doses provides relatively modest benefits.

As noted above, the supplement methyl sulfonyl methane (MSM) has shown promise for osteoarthritis when taken along with glucosamine. Besides that study, benefits were also seen in a 12-week double-blind placebo-controlled trial of 50 people with osteoarthritis, utilizing MSM at a dose of 3 g twice daily.

Other treatments with incomplete supporting evidence from double-blind trials include **Ayurvedic herbal combination therapy, boswellia, cat's claw**, a proprietary complex of minerals with or without cat's claw, **devil's claw, proteolytic enzymes, rose hips, soy** protein, and **vitamin B₃**.

Traditional Chinese herbal medicine has also shown some promise for osteoarthritis. However, one study that compared a commonly used Chinese herbal product (Duhuo Jisheng Wan) to the drug diclofenac found that the herb worked more slowly than the drug, yet produced about an equal rate of side effects.

Growing but not yet definitive evidence suggests that the natural substance hyaluronic acid may help reduce osteoarthritis symptoms when it is injected directly into an affected joint. However, there is no reason to believe that *oral* hyaluronic acid should help.

Incomplete and inconsistent evidence from human and animal studies only weakly suggests that **green-lipped mussel** might alleviate osteoarthritis symptoms.

One double blind study involving dogs found some evidence of benefit with elk **velvet antler**.

Numerous other herbs and supplements sometimes recommended for osteoarthritis include **beta-carotene, boron, cartilage, chamomile, copper, dandelion, D-phenylalanine, feverfew, molybdenum, selenium, turmeric**, and **yucca**. However, there is little to no evidence as yet that these treatments are effective.

Other studies provide evidence that certain supplements proposed for osteoarthritis do *not* work. For example, a 2-year, double-blind study of 136 people with knee arthritis found **vitamin E** ineffective for either reducing symptoms or slowing the progression of the disease. In addition, a 6-month, double-blind, placebo-controlled trial of 77 people with osteoarthritis failed to find any symptomatic benefit with vitamin E. Similarly, in a large (almost 400-participant) 5-year, double-blind, placebo-controlled study, use of injected **mesoglycan** failed to slow the progression of osteoarthritis.

Prolotherapy is a special form of injection therapy that is popular among some alternative practitioners. A double-blind, placebo-controlled study evaluated the effects of 3 prolotherapy injections (using a 10% dextrose solution) at 2-month intervals in 68 people with osteoarthritis of the knee. At 6-month follow-up, participants who had received prolotherapy showed significant improvements in pain at rest and while walking, reduction in swelling, episodes of "buckling," and range of flexion, as compared to those who had received placebo treatment. The same research group performed a similar double-blind trial of 27 individuals with osteoarthritis in the hands. The results at 6-month follow-up showed that range of motion and pain with movement improved significantly in the treated group as compared to the placebo group.

Several double-blind, placebo-controlled studies suggest that pulsed electromagnetic field therapy, a special form of **magnet therapy**, can improve symptoms of osteoarthritis. One small study provides extremely weak supporting evidence for the more ordinary form of magnet therapy: static magnets. A subsequent much larger study of static magnets failed to find real magnets more effective than placebo magnets, but a manufacturing error may have obscured genuine benefits (some people in the placebo group were accidentally given active magnets).

Limited evidence supports the use of bee venom injections for osteoarthritis. **Hatha yoga** has also shown some promise.

Herbs and Supplements to Use Only with Caution

Various herbs and supplements may interact adversely with drugs used to treat osteoarthritis. For more information on this potential risk, see the individual drug article in the Drug Interactions section of this book.

Osteoporosis

PRINCIPAL PROPOSED NATURAL TREATMENTS: *Calcium and Vitamin D, Genistein and Other Isoflavones, Strontium, Vitamin K, Ipriflavone*

OTHER PROPOSED NATURAL TREATMENTS: *Black Cohosh, Black Tea, Boron, Dehydroepiandrosterone (DHEA), Estriol, Fish Oil, Gamma-linolenic Acid (GLA), Reducing High Homocysteine with Folate and Vitamin B_{12}, Magnesium, Manganese, Progesterone, Silicon, Trace Minerals*

HERBS AND SUPPLEMENTS TO USE ONLY WITH CAUTION: *Vitamin A*

Many factors are now known or suspected to accelerate the rate of bone loss. These include smoking, alcohol, low calcium intake, excessive phosphorus intake (such as found in soft drinks), lack of exercise, various medications, and several medical illnesses. Excessive consumption of vitamin A may also increase risk of osteoporosis and rapid weight loss may increase the risk in postmenopausal women. Raw food vegetarians are also likely to have significant bone thinning.

In general, women are far more prone to osteoporosis than men and, for this reason, the following discussion focuses almost entirely on them.

Hormone replacement therapy prevents or reverses osteoporosis in women. However, now that long-term use of hormone replacement therapy has been found to be unsafe, conventional medical treatment for osteoporosis in women centers mainly on drugs in the bisphosphonate family, such as Fosamax (taken along with calcium and vitamin D—see below).

Weight-bearing exercise, such as walking, is also strongly recommended.

Principal Proposed Natural Treatments

There is good evidence that people with osteoporosis or who are at risk for it should take calcium and vitamin D supplements regardless of what other treatments they may be using.

Substances called *isoflavones* found in soy and other plants may be helpful for osteoporosis (as well as general **menopausal symptoms**). Vitamin K and a new supplement called *strontium ranelate* have also shown promise. A semisynthetic isoflavone called *ipriflavone* has shown considerable promise for osteoporosis, but safety concerns have decreased its popularity.

Calcium and Vitamin D

Calcium is necessary to build and maintain bone. You need vitamin D, too, as the body cannot absorb calcium without it. Many people do not get enough calcium in their daily diet and, although your body can manufacture vitamin D when exposed to the sun, supplemental vitamin D may be necessary in this age of sunblock.

According to most but not all studies, calcium supplements (especially as calcium citrate, and taken with vitamin D) are slightly helpful for in preventing and slowing down bone loss in post-menopausal women. However, the effect is relatively minor and may not be strong enough to reduce the rate of osteoporotic fractures.

One study found benefits for male seniors using a calcium- and vitamin D–fortified milk product. However, there are some concerns that excessive calcium intake could raise risk of prostate cancer in men. See the **Calcium** article for more information.

Any improvements in bone rapidly disappear once the supplements are stopped. People who religiously continue calcium use may do better than those who forget from time to time.

Vitamin D alone may offer some mild bone-protective benefits as well.

Use of calcium supplements early in life might put calcium "in the bank" and prevent problems later, especially when children also engage in physical exercise; however, study results are somewhat contradictory.

Vitamin D and calcium taken together may also have a modestly protective effect against the severe bone loss caused by **corticosteroid** drugs, such as prednisone.

Certain other supplements may enhance the effects of calcium and vitamin D. One study found that adding various trace minerals (**zinc** at 15 mg, **copper** at 2.5 mg, and **manganese** at 5 mg) produced further improvement. However, copper by itself may not be helpful.

There is some evidence that essential fatty acids may also enhance the effectiveness of calcium. In one study, 65 postmenopausal women were given calcium along with either placebo or a combination of omega-6 fatty acids (from **evening primrose oil**) and omega-3 fatty acids (from **fish oil**) for a period of 18 months. At the end of the study period, the group receiving essential fatty acids had higher bone density and fewer fractures than the placebo group. In contrast to this, however, a similar 12-month, double-blind trial of 42 postmenopausal women found no benefit from essential fatty acids. The explanation for the discrepancy may lie in the differences between the women studied. The first study involved women living in nursing homes, while the second studied healthier women living on their own. The second group of women may have been better nourished and already receiving sufficient essential fatty acids in their diet.

Finally, vitamin K may also enhance the effect of calcium (see below).

Interestingly, vitamin D may offer another benefit for osteoporosis in seniors: most though not all studies have found that vitamin D supplementation improves balance in seniors (especially female seniors) and reduces risk of falling. Since the most common adverse consequence of osteoporosis is a fracture due to a fall, this could offer a meaningful benefit.

For more information, including dosage and safety issues, see the full articles on **calcium** and **vitamin D**.

Genistein and other Isoflavones

Soy contains substances called *isoflavones* that produce effects in the body somewhat similar to the effects of estrogen. Although study results are not entirely consistent, growing evidence suggests that **genistein** and other isoflavones can (like estrogen) help prevent bone loss.

For example, in a 1-year, double-blind, placebo-controlled study, 90 women aged 47 to 57 were given genistein at a dose of 54 mg/day, standard hormone replacement therapy (HRT), or placebo. The results showed that genistein prevented bone loss in the back and hip to approximately the same extent as HRT. No adverse effects on the uterus or breast were seen.

In a 1-year, double-blind, placebo-controlled study of 203 postmenopausal Chinese women, use of soy isoflavones at a dose of 80 mg daily had mildly positive protective effects on bone mass in the hip. This supplement contained 46.4% daidzein, 38.8% glycetein, and 14.7% genistein.

Another study evaluated an isoflavone supplement made from **red clover** (containing 6 mg biochanin A, 16 mg formononetin, 1 mg genistein, and 0.5 mg daidzein daily). In this 1-year, double-blind, placebo-controlled study of 205 people, use of red clover isoflavones significantly reduced loss of bone in the lumbar spine.

Benefits were also seen in a 1-year, double-blind, placebo-controlled study using an extract made from the soy product tofu.

Interestingly, unlike estrogen, which primarily helps prevent the destruction of bone, some evidence suggests that isoflavones may also assist in creating new bone.

In about one out of three people, intestinal bacteria convert some soy isoflavones into a substance called *equol*. Isoflavones may have a greater bone-protecting effect in such equol producers.

For more information, including dosage and safety issues, see the full **Soy** article.

Strontium

The mineral strontium (as strontium ranelate) is showing increasing promise as an aid in the treatment of osteoporosis.

The best and largest study on strontium was a double-blind, placebo-controlled study of 1,649 postmenopausal women with osteoporosis. In this 3-year study, a dose of strontium ranelate at 2 g daily significantly increased bone density in the spine and hip and significantly decreased the rate of vertebral fractures.

While some treatments for osteoporosis act to increase bone formation and others decrease bone breakdown, some evidence suggests that strontium ranelate has a dual effect, providing both these benefits at once.

There is one major caveat, however: at present all major controlled clinical trials of strontium ranelate have involved some of the same researchers. Entirely independent confirmation is needed. It is not clear to what extent the "ranelate portion" of strontium ranelate is necessary for this benefit, or whether other strontium salts would work as well.

Note: The strontium used in these studies is not the same as the radioactive strontium that was such a concern during the decades of above-ground atomic testing.

For more information, including dosage and safety issues, see the full **Strontium** article.

Vitamin K

Increasing evidence indicates that vitamin K may help prevent osteoporosis. It may work by reducing bone breakdown, rather than by enhancing bone formation.

The best evidence for a beneficial effect comes from a 3-year, double-blind, placebo-controlled trial of 181 women. Participants, postmenopausal women between the ages of 50 and 60, were divided into three groups: placebo, calcium plus vitamin D plus magnesium, or calcium plus vitamin D plus magnesium plus vitamin K (at a dose of 1 g daily). Researchers monitored bone loss by using a standard DEXA bone density scan. The results showed that the study participants using vitamin K along with the other nutrients lost less bone than those in the other two groups.

In another study, 66 Indonesian women with osteoporosis were treated with either calcium plus vitamin K or calcium plus placebo. The trial lasted 48 weeks. At the end, the results showed that calcium plus vitamin K was more effective in improving bone density in the lumbar spine than calcium plus placebo.

While these two studies don't provide definitive proof, they do strongly suggest that women at risk for osteoporosis should consider taking vitamin K along with other nutrients.

For more information, see the full **Vitamin K** article.

Ipriflavone

Ipriflavone is a semisynthetic variation of soy isoflavones. Ipriflavone appears to help prevent osteoporosis by interfering with bone breakdown. Estrogen works in much the same way, but ipriflavone does not appear to produce estrogenic effects anywhere else in the body other than in

bone. For this reason, it probably doesn't increase the risk of breast or uterine cancer. However, it also doesn't reduce the hot flashes, night sweats, mood changes, or vaginal dryness of menopause. In addition, it may cause health risks of its own.

Numerous double-blind, placebo-controlled studies involving a total of more than 1,700 participants have examined the effects of ipriflavone on various forms of osteoporosis. Overall, it appears that ipriflavone can stop the progression of osteoporosis and perhaps reverse it to some extent.

For example, a 2-year, double-blind study followed 198 postmenopausal women who had evidence of bone loss. At the end of the study, there was a gain in bone density of 1% in the ipriflavone group compared to a loss of 0.7% in the placebo group.

Conversely, the largest and longest study of ipriflavone found no benefit. In this 3-year trial of 474 postmenopausal women, no differences in extent of osteoporosis were seen between ipriflavone and placebo groups. However, for reasons that aren't clear, the researchers in this study gave women only 500 mg of calcium daily. All other major studies of ipriflavone gave participants 1,000 mg of calcium daily. It's possible that ipriflavone requires the higher dose of calcium to work properly.

Ipriflavone may also be helpful for preventing osteoporosis in women who are taking Lupron or corticosteroids, medications that accelerate bone loss. (However, the combined use of ipriflavone and drugs that suppress the immune system, such as corticosteroids, presents risks.)

There is some evidence that combining ipriflavone with estrogen may improve anti-osteoporosis benefits. However, we do not know whether such combinations increase or decrease the other benefits and adverse effects of estrogen-replacement therapy.

Finally, for reasons that are not at all clear, ipriflavone appears to be able to reduce pain in osteoporosis-related fractures that have already occurred.

For more information, including dosage and safety issues, see the full **Ipriflavone** article.

Other Proposed Natural Treatments

Observational studies hint that **high homocysteine** might increase risk of osteoporosis. One double-blind study found evidence that supplemental **folate** and **vitamin B$_{12}$** (known to reduce homocysteine) might reduce risk of osteoporotic fractures.

Some evidence suggests that the hormone **DHEA**

may be helpful for preventing or treating osteoporosis, especially in postmenopausal women over 70. One study found weak evidence that DHEA might be helpful for preventing the osteoporosis that sometimes develops in women with **anorexia nervosa**.

Very preliminary evidence suggests that **black tea**, which is quite similar but not identical to **green tea**, may help protect against osteoporosis.

Similarly weak evidence hints that the herb **black cohosh** might help prevent osteoporosis.

According to one very preliminary study but not another, **boron** may be helpful for preventing osteoporosis. However, there are some concerns that boron supplements may raise levels of the body's own estrogen, especially in women on estrogen-replacement therapy and, therefore, might present an increased risk of cancer. If you want to increase your boron intake, the best way might be to eat more fruits and vegetables.

One study widely advertised as showing that **silicon** is helpful for osteoporosis actually failed to show much of anything.

Although it has long been believed that consuming too much protein (especially animal-based protein) increases the risk of osteoporosis, the balance of available evidence suggests the reverse: if anything, high intake of protein appears to help strengthen bone. One study found that calcium supplements may do a better job of strengthening bones in people with relatively high protein intake than those with lower intake.

One study failed to find **arginine** supplements helpful for enhancing bone density.

The Progesterone Story

Many books promote the idea that natural **progesterone** prevents or even reduces osteoporosis. In this case, the term *natural* indicates that we are using the same progesterone found in the body. It is still made synthetically, but it is called *natural progesterone* to distinguish it from its chemical cousins known as *progestins*. Generally, prescription "progesterone" is actually a progestin.

The progesterone/osteoporosis story began with test tube and other preliminary studies suggesting that progesterone or progestins can stimulate the activity of cells that build bone. Subsequently, a poorly designed and uncontrolled study (really a series of case histories from one physician's practice) purportedly demonstrated that progesterone cream can slow or even reverse osteoporosis.

However, a 1-year, double-blind trial of 102 women given either progesterone cream (providing 20 mg progesterone daily) or placebo cream, along with calcium and multivitamins, found no evidence of any improvements in bone density attributable to progesterone.

Furthermore, in a 3-year study of 875 women, combination treatment with estrogen and oral progesterone was no more effective for osteoporosis than estrogen alone.

The Estriol Story

For over a decade, some alternative medicine practitioners have popularized the use of a special form of estrogen called *estriol*, claiming that, unlike standard estrogen, it doesn't increase the risk of cancer. However, this claim is unfounded.

Controlled trials performed in Japan have found that estriol helps prevent bone loss in menopausal women, although one small study found no benefit.

However, like other forms of estrogen, oral estriol stimulates the growth of uterine tissue. This leads to a risk of uterine cancer.

In a placebo-controlled study of 1,110 women, uterine tissue stimulation was seen among women given estriol orally (1 to 2 mg daily) as compared to those given placebo. Another large study found that oral estriol increased the risk of uterine cancer. In another study of 48 women given estriol at a dose of 1 mg twice daily, uterine tissue stimulation was seen in the majority of cases.

In contrast, a 12-month, double-blind trial of oral estriol (2 mg daily) in 68 Japanese women found no effect on the uterus. It may be that the high levels of soy in the Japanese diet altered the results. Additionally, test-tube studies suggest that estriol is just as likely to cause breast cancer as any other form of estrogen.

The bottom line: If you use estriol, you should consider it like any other form of estrogen.

Herbs and Supplements to Use Only with Caution

While the evidence is not yet strong, some research suggests that excessive intake of **vitamin A** may increase the risk of osteoporosis.

Various herbs and supplements may interact adversely with drugs used to treat osteoporosis. For more information on this potential risk, see the individual drug article in the Drug Interactions section of this book.

Pancreatitis

Pancreatitis

RELATED TERMS: *Acute Pancreatitis, Chronic Pancreatitis*

PRINCIPAL PROPOSED NATURAL TREATMENTS: *Digestive Enzymes*

OTHER PROPOSED NATURAL TREATMENTS: *Multivitamin/Multimineral Supplements*

Antioxidants: *Beta-carotene, Grapeseed Extract (a Source of OPCs), Lipoic Acid, Methionine, Milk Thistle, Selenium, Vitamin C, Vitamin E*

The pancreas is an organ that creates enzymes necessary to properly digest starch, protein, and fat. In addition, cells responsible for creating insulin are also found in the pancreas. Pancreatitis is a condition in which the pancreas is inflamed. When pancreatitis is prolonged, pancreatic function declines, leading to malabsorption of nutrients and, possibly, mild diabetes.

Pancreatitis occurs in three forms: acute (short-term) pancreatitis, recurrent acute pancreatitis, and chronic pancreatitis.

Acute pancreatitis is a painful condition, but with treatment it ordinarily resolves in 3 to 7 days. Causes include alcohol abuse, gallstones, extremely high blood levels of triglycerides, direct trauma to the pancreas, abdominal surgery and procedures, kidney failure, infection, and certain medications.

The treatment of acute pancreatitis consists primarily of resting the pancreas by discontinuing all eating and drinking. Intravenous fluids are used to maintain fluid balance.

Recurrent acute pancreatitis involves multiple bouts of acute pancreatitis, sometimes in the context of a more mild, chronic condition. Each bout is treated as described above.

Chronic pancreatitis is a more gradual process that leads to partial or complete pancreatic failure. Its most common cause is alcohol abuse, although the condition may also occur for other reasons or for no known reason at all. Chronic pancreatitis causes many symptoms, including most prominently abdominal pain, weight loss, diarrhea because of undigested fat, and mild diabetes. Treatment primarily involves use of digestive enzymes and, if necessary, insulin, as well as dietary changes and pain medication. If alcohol abuse contributed to chronic pancreatitis, it's important to stop drinking.

Principal Proposed Natural Treatments

Digestive enzymes are the mainstay of treatment for chronic pancreatitis and all of these can be considered natural products. The digestive enzymes prescribed by physicians for pancreatitis are not necessarily more powerful than their dietary supplement equivalent and some experimentation with different products might lead to the best results. Excessive consumption of digestive enzymes can cause harm, however, and for this reason doctor's supervision is strongly recommended.

Other Proposed Natural Treatments

Chronic pancreatitis leads to malabsorption of fat, which can in turn lead to deficiencies of fat-soluble vitamins, such as **vitamin A** and **vitamin E**. In addition, chronic pancreatitis might impair absorption of vitamin B_{12} and possibly other nutrients as well. While it is not clear that these deficiencies are severe enough to cause harm, it makes sense for people with pancreatitis to consider taking a multivitamin/mineral supplement as nutritional insurance.

Antioxidants are substances that help the body neutralize free radicals. Free radicals are dangerous, naturally occurring substances that are thought to play a role in pancreatitis, as well as many other conditions. A small double-blind, placebo-controlled trial of people with pancreatitis (chronic as well as recurring acute), examined the effectiveness of an antioxidant supplement providing 9,000 IU beta-carotene, 540 mg vitamin C, 270 IU vitamin E, 600 mcg selenium, and 2,000 mg methionine daily. The results showed improvement both in symptoms and laboratory signs of disease severity.

Other natural supplements with antioxidant properties sometimes recommended for chronic pancreatitis include grapeseed extract (a source of **OPCs**), **lipoic acid**, and **milk thistle**.

Parasites, Intestinal

RELATED TERMS: *Giardia, Intestinal Parasites, Pinworms, Worms*

PRINCIPAL PROPOSED NATURAL TREATMENTS: *None*

OTHER PROPOSED NATURAL TREATMENTS: *Anise, Berberine (Found in Barberry, Goldenseal, Goldenthread, and Oregon Grape), Black Walnut Fruit, Cloves, Curled Mint, Essential Oils, Garlic, Gentian, Grapefruit Seed Extract, Lapacho, Neem, Olive Leaf, Oregano, Propolis, Pumpkin Seed, Sweet Annie, Tansy,* Terminalia arjuna, *Thyme, Wormseed, Wormwood*

The human intestines play host to an enormous variety of bacteria and fungi. Most of these are harmless or even helpful. However, other microscopic organisms can also take up residence in the intestines. Such organisms are called *intestinal parasites.*

Common parasites include amoebas (especially *Entamoeba histolytica*), cryptosporidium, giardia (*Giardia lamblia*), hookworm (*Ancylostoma duodenale* and *Necator americanus*), pinworm (*Enterobius vermicularis*), roundworm (*Ascaris lumbricoides*), and tapeworm (*Taenia species*).

Intestinal parasites can cause a wide variety of symptoms, including gas, bloating, diarrhea, abdominal cramping, bloody stools, itching in the anus, weight loss, and many others. Some parasites are no more than a nuisance, while others can cause serious disease and even death.

Conventional treatment for parasites begins with careful identification of the particular parasite involved, followed by the use of medications capable of destroying the infestation. Careful attention to hygiene while camping or traveling in developing countries can help prevent future infections with parasites.

Proposed Natural Treatments

Intestinal parasites are hardy organisms not easily killed. Traditional remedies used for parasites are generally fairly toxic. Until recently, conventional treatments for parasites were also quite toxic. However, now that safe drugs have been developed, it can be said as a general rule that conventional therapies for parasites are less toxic and almost certainly more effective than natural remedies.

Despite this, many natural products are marketed for the treatment of parasites. The profusion of such offerings is due primarily to a particular current of thought among some alternative practitioners that states that parasites are the underlying cause of many illnesses. Most such natural products are made of herbs that kill parasites in the test tube. However, it is a long way from a test tube study to meaningful effects in humans and there is no reliable meaningful evidence that any of these natural therapies are useful in a practical sense. Some herbs commonly mentioned for the treatment of parasitic infections include anise, black walnut fruit, cloves, curled mint, **essential oils**, **garlic**, **gentian**, grapefruit seed extract, **lapacho**, **neem**, **olive leaf**, **oregano**, **propolis**, **pumpkin seed**, sweet Annie, tansy, *Terminalia arjuna*, thyme, wormseed, and **wormwood**.

The substance berberine has shown some promise for the treatment of parasites and it was, for a time, evaluated as a potential new anti-parasitic drug. Berberine is found in **barberry**, **goldenseal**, goldenthread, **Oregon grape**, and other herbs, and for this reason these herbs are commonly mentioned as useful for the treatment of parasitic infections. However, the only studies relevant to these herbs used purified chemical berberine; to obtain the same amount of berberine in the form of an herb, you would have to consume massive (and possibly toxic) quantities.

Parkinson's Disease

RELATED TERMS: *Paralysis Agitans*

PRINCIPAL PROPOSED NATURAL TREATMENTS: *CDP-Choline (Also Called Citicholine), Coenzyme Q_{10}*

OTHER PROPOSED NATURAL TREATMENTS: *5-Hydroxytryptophan (5-HTP), Alexander Technique, D-Phenylalanine, Glutathione, L-Methionine, Magnet Therapy, NADH, Phosphatidylserine, Policosanol, SAMe, Vitamin C, Vitamin E*

HERBS AND SUPPLEMENTS TO USE ONLY WITH CAUTION: *5-Hydroxytryptophan (5-HTP), Amino Acids (Such as BCAAs, Methionine, and Phenylalanine), Iron, Kava, SAMe, Vitamin B_6*

Parkinson's disease is a chronic disorder typically affecting people over age 55. The condition is caused by the death of nerve cells in certain parts of the brain, leading to characteristic problems with movement. These include a "pill rolling" tremor in the hands (so called because it appears that the individual is rolling a small object between thumb and forefinger), difficulty initiating walking, a shuffling gait, decreased facial expressiveness, and trouble talking. Thinking ability may become impaired in later stages of the disease and depression is common.

Although the underlying cause of Parkinson's disease is unknown, many researchers believe that free radicals may play a role in destroying at least some of the nerve cells.

The nerve cells that are affected in Parkinson's disease work by supplying the neurotransmitter dopamine to another part of the brain. Most treatments for Parkinson's disease work by artificially increasing the brain's dopamine levels. Simply taking dopamine pills won't work, however, because the substance cannot travel from the bloodstream into the brain. Instead, most people with Parkinson's disease take **levodopa** (L-dopa), which can pass into the brain and be converted there into dopamine. Many people take levodopa with carbidopa, a drug that increases the amount of levodopa available to make dopamine.

At first, levodopa produces dramatic improvement in symptoms; however, over time, levodopa becomes less effective and more likely to produce side effects. Other drugs may be useful as well, including bromocriptine, trihexyphenidyl, entacapone, tolcapone, selegiline, and pergolide. There are also surgical treatments that can decrease symptoms, such as pallidotomy and deep brain stimulation.

Principal Proposed Natural Treatments

CDP-Choline

Short for cytidinediphosphocholine, CDP-choline (sometimes called *citicholine*) is a substance that occurs naturally in the human body. It is closely related to **choline**, a nutrient commonly put in the B vitamin family. For reasons that are not completely clear, CDP-choline seems to increase the amount of dopamine in the brain. On this basis, it has been tried for Parkinson's disease.

In a 4-week, single-blind study of 74 people with Parkinson's disease, researchers tested whether oral CDP-choline might help levodopa be more effective. Researchers divided participants into two groups: one group received their usual levodopa dose, the other received half their usual dose without knowing which dosage they were getting. All the participants took 400 mg of oral CDP-choline 3 times daily.

Even though 50% of the participants were taking only half their usual dose of levodopa, both groups scored equally well on standardized tests designed to evaluate the severity of Parkinson's disease symptoms.

Support for the use of CDP-choline also comes from studies in which the supplement was administered by injection.

In general, CDP-choline appears to be safe. The study of oral CDP-choline for Parkinson's disease reported only a few brief, nonspecific side effects such as nausea, dizziness, and fatigue. In a study of 2,817 elderly people who took oral CDP-choline for up to 60 days for problems other than Parkinson's disease, side effects were few and mild and reported in only about 5% of participants. Two-thirds of these side effects were gastrointestinal (nausea, stomach pain, and diarrhea) and none required stopping CDP-choline. The dose in this study was 550 to 650 mg per day, about half the dose used for Parkinson's disease.

Coenzyme Q$_{10}$

The supplement coenzyme Q$_{10}$ (CoQ$_{10}$) has shown promise in the treatment of Parkinson's disease.

In a double-blind trial, 28 people with Parkinson's disease were given either placebo or 360 mg of CoQ$_{10}$ daily, along with conventional care. The results indicated that use of the supplement produced a mild improvement in symptoms.

A previous study found suggestions that CoQ$_{10}$ may help slow the progression of Parkinson's disease. In this 16-month, double-blind, placebo-controlled trial, 80 people with Parkinson's disease were given either CoQ$_{10}$ (at a dose of 300, 600, or 1,200 mg daily) or placebo. Participants in this trial had early stages of the disease and did not yet need medication. The results suggested that CoQ$_{10}$, especially at the highest dose, might have slowed disease progression. However, various statistical technicalities made the results inconclusive.

For more information, including dosage and safety issues, see the full **CoQ$_{10}$** article.

Other Proposed Natural Treatments

Several other natural products have been studied for preventing or treating Parkinson's disease, with mixed results.

SAMe

Whether a symptom of the disease or a response to disability, depression affects many people with Parkinson's disease and long-term use of levodopa may contribute to this problem. Research suggests that levodopa can deplete the brain of a substance called *S-adenosylme-thionine* (SAMe for short). As SAMe has been found in a number of small studies to have antidepressant effects, it is possible that depleting it might trigger depression.

Researchers conducted a trial to determine if taking SAMe supplements could decrease depression in 21 individuals with Parkinson's disease who were taking levodopa. In this double-blind study, each participant received either a combination of oral and injected SAMe or placebo daily for 30 days, followed by the alternate treatment for another 30 days. Although other symp-

toms of Parkinson's didn't change, 72% of people taking SAMe felt that their depression was improved after 2 weeks, while only 30% noted improvement with placebo. It is not yet known if oral SAMe alone would have similar effects.

Although SAMe might appear to be an excellent accompaniment to levodopa, there is another side to the issue. During treatment with levodopa, SAMe participates in breaking it down and gets used up in the process. It is possible that taking extra SAMe could lead to decreased effectiveness of levodopa. In the short-term study described above, SAMe did not interfere with levodopa's effects, but longer-term use might do so.

The bottom line: If you have Parkinson's disease, it's safest to use SAMe—if at all—only under the supervision of a physician.

For more information, including dosage and safety issues, see the full **SAMe** article.

Phosphatidylserine

Phosphatidylserine (PS for short) is a major component of cell membranes. Several studies have found PS supplementation effective for improving mental function in individuals with **Alzheimer's disease**. One trial examined its use in 62 people, all of whom had both Parkinson's disease and Alzheimer's-type dementia. The results appeared to indicate some benefit, but due to the incompleteness of the report on this trial, it is difficult to draw conclusions.

For more information, including dosage and safety issues, see the full **Phosphatidylserine** article.

Vitamin E

Because of indications that free radicals play a role in causing Parkinson's disease, treatment with high doses of vitamin E has been tried to see if it can slow down the progression of Parkinson's disease. However, a large study yielded disappointing results. In this trial, 800 individuals newly diagnosed with Parkinson's disease took 2,000 IU of tocopherol (synthetic vitamin E) or placebo daily for an average of 14 months. Vitamin E had no effects in delaying symptoms of the disease—nor did it reduce side effects of levodopa.

For more information, including dosage and safety issues, see the full **Vitamin E** article.

Vitamin C

One problem with levodopa treatment for Parkinson's disease is the so-called on-off effect, in which a person taking levodopa will move more freely for some hours, followed by sudden "freezing up." Vitamin C has been tried as a remedy for "on-off effects" in a small double-blind study, but the results were so minimal that the researchers didn't feel justified in recommending it.

For more information, including dosage and safety issues, see the full **Vitamin C** article.

Other Treatments

The herb *Mucuna pruriens* contains L-dopa. One very small study reportedly found evidence that use of the herb as an L-dopa source offers advantages over purified L-dopa given as a medication itself.

Other proposed natural treatments for Parkinson's disease have minimal or conflicting evidence supporting them, including **NADH**, **glutathione**, **policosanol**, and the amino acids **D-phenylalanine** and **L-methionine**. Caution is advised with the latter three, as they might affect the function of levodopa. (See Herbs and Supplements to Use Only with Caution, below.)

Weak evidence hints that the supplement **5-HTP** might be helpful for depression in people with Parkinson's disease. However, 5-HTP should not be combined with the drug carbidopa. (See Herbs and Supplements to Use Only with Caution below.)

A 2-month, double-blind, placebo-controlled trial of 18 people found that rTMS (a special form of **magnet therapy**) improved Parkinson's symptoms. Benefits were seen in another small controlled study as well.

A postural training method called *Alexander technique* has shown some promise.

In two studies, **acupuncture** failed to provide much benefit for Parkinson's disease.

Herbs and Supplements to Use Only with Caution

If you have Parkinson's disease, it is best to avoid taking the herb **kava**. Preliminary reports suggest that kava may counter the effects of dopamine and possibly reduce the effectiveness of medications for Parkinson's.

Other substances may also interact with Parkinson's drugs. **Iron** supplements can interfere with absorption of levodopa and carbidopa, and should not be taken within 2 hours of either medication. Amino acid supplements, such as **branched-chain amino acids** (BCAAs), can temporarily decrease levodopa's effectiveness, as may methionine and phenylalanine, two amino acids studied for treatment of Parkinson's disease.

Vitamin B$_6$ in doses higher than 5 mg per day might also impair the effectiveness of levodopa and should be avoided. However, if you take levodopa–carbidopa combinations, this restriction may not necessarily apply. Talk with your physician about an appropriate dose of vitamin B$_6$.

The supplement 5-HTP has a potentially dangerous interaction with carbidopa. Using the two substances together may increase your chance of developing symptoms resembling those of the disease **scleroderma**.

As noted above, SAMe could conceivably impair the effectiveness of levodopa.

One report suggests that by amplifying the action of levodopa, policosanol might increase side effects called *dyskinesias*.

Very weak evidence hints that prolonged (many years) intake of high levels of iron and **manganese** might increase risk of developing Parkinson's disease.

Periodontal Disease

RELATED TERM: *Gum Disease*

PRINCIPAL PROPOSED NATURAL TREATMENTS: *None*

OTHER PROPOSED NATURAL TREATMENTS: *Bloodroot; Calcium; Caraway; Coenzyme Q_{10} (CoQ_{10}); Cranberry Juice; Folate Mouthwash; GLA; Green Tea Chew Candy; Herbal Mouthwash Containing Chamomile, Echinacea, Myrrh, Mint, Sage, and Ratania; Magnesium; Oligomeric Proanthocyanidins (OPCs); Macleya cordata (Plume Poppy) and Prunella vulgaris; Propolis; Sea Cucumber; Tea Tree Oil; Vitamin B_{12}; Vitamin C; Witch Hazel; Xylitol; Zinc*

Periodontal disease begins with gum inflammation and progresses to pockets of infection, bone loss, and loosening of the teeth. It is present in 90% of individuals over the age of 65.

Conventional prevention and treatment include regular flossing, using mouthwash that contains extracts of the herb thyme (such as thymol, found in Listerine), and using special tooth-brushing appliances. If the condition becomes advanced, special deep-cleaning techniques and even surgery may be necessary.

Proposed Natural Treatments for Periodontal Disease

One double-blind study of 89 people tested a European herbal mouthwash (used with a special gum irrigator) containing **chamomile, echinacea,** myrrh, **mint, sage,** and ratania. The herbal preparation proved more effective than a conventional mouthwash.

Oligomeric proanthocyanidins (OPCs) have antioxidant and anti-inflammatory properties. A 14-day, double-blind, placebo-controlled trial of 40 people evaluated the potential benefits of a chewing gum product containing 5 mg of OPCs from pine bark. Use of the OPC gum resulted in significant improvements in gum health and reductions in plaque formation; no similar benefits were seen in the placebo group.

A double-blind study of 30 people found weak evidence that use of borage oil (a source of **GLA**) at a dose of 3,000 mg daily may reduce gingival inflammation. The study also examined **fish oil** at a dose of 3,000 mg daily, or combined fish oil and borage oil at the dose of 1,500 mg each, but failed to find significant benefits with these treatments as compared to placebo.

Other natural dental products that have shown promise in small double-blind studies include a toothpaste containing *Macleya cordata* (plume poppy) and *Prunella vulgaris* (also known as heal-all or self-heal), a chew candy containing **green tea,** an irrigation fluid containing **propolis** extract, a toothpaste containing sea cucumber, and a gel containing **tea tree oil**.

Preliminary studies suggest that **folate** mouthwash may help in periodontal disease. Oral folate supplementation does not appear to be especially effective. However, one small double-blind study found potential benefit with a mixed B-complex supplement (containing 50 mg of each of **thiamin, riboflavin, niacinamide, pantothenate,** and **pyridoxine;** 50 mcg each of **biotin** and **vitamin B_{12};** and 400 mcg of folate).

One test tube study suggests that **cranberry** juice might be useful for treating or preventing gum disease. However, there is one kink to work out before cranberry could be practical for this purpose: the sweeteners added to cranberry juice aren't good for your teeth, but without them cranberry juice is very bitter.

The supplement **coenzymeQ_{10}** is sometimes claimed to be an effective treatment for periodontal disease. However, the studies on which this idea is based are too flawed to be taken as meaningful.

Xylitol is a naturally occurring sugar that appears to help suppress the development of **cavities** when it is used in gum, candy, or toothpaste. Highly preliminary evidence suggests that it may help prevent gum disease, as well.

Other treatments sometimes proposed for periodontal disease, but that lack meaningful scientific support, include **bioflavonoids, bloodroot, calcium, caraway, magnesium, vitamin C, witch hazel,** and **zinc**.

Peyronie's Disease

PRINCIPAL PROPOSED NATURAL TREATMENTS: *Acetyl-L-Carnitine, Para-Aminobenzoic Acid (PABA)*

OTHER PROPOSED NATURAL TREATMENTS: *Gotu Kola, Vitamin E*

Peyronie's disease is a condition in which a plaque (a thickened, hardened piece of tissue) forms on one side of the penis. If the plaque becomes large enough, it reduces flexibility of the penis. During erection, the less-flexible part of the penis expands to a lesser extent, causing the penis to bend. Pain may occur as well. Severe curvature of the penis can make intercourse difficult or even impossible.

The cause of Peyronie's disease is unknown, but it may involve injury to the penis that causes local bleeding, which in turn leads to the formation of fibrous tissue. However, the majority of cases occur without any obvious preceding injury.

People with Peyronie's disease may have a generalized tendency to form fibrous tissue, as shown by a higher-than-average incidence of **Dupuytren's contracture** (a condition in which fibrous tissue develops in the hands among men with Peyronie's). The condition also appears to be partially heritable.

Treatment of Peyronie's disease consists first and foremost of watchful waiting. In many cases, the disease never becomes severe enough to cause serious difficulty. Pain on erection generally decreases with time and in some cases the extent of curvature also decreases.

When the condition is too severe to ignore, there are a variety of methods that may be tried, including injection of various drugs into the fibrous plaque, use of radiation therapy, and surgery. Of all these, only surgery is widely accepted as effective. However, because it can cause complications such as shortening of the penis, it is usually reserved for serious cases.

Principal Proposed Natural Treatments

Acetyl-L-Carnitine

L-carnitine is an amino acid the body uses to turn fat into energy. It is not usually considered a nutrient because the body can manufacture all it needs. Two forms of L-carnitine—acetyl-L-carnitine and propionyl-L-carnitine—have been tried as treatments for Peyronie's disease.

A 3-month, double-blind study compared the effectiveness of acetyl-L-carnitine to the drug tamoxifen in 48 men with Peyronie's disease. Acetyl-L-carnitine (at a dose of 1 g daily) reduced penile curvature while tamoxifen did not; in addition, the supplement reduced pain and slowed disease progression to a greater extent than tamoxifen.

Another study evaluated the potential benefits of combination therapy with propionyl-L-carnitine and an injected medication (verapamil). In this trial, 60 people with severe Peyronie's disease were given verapamil injections plus 3 months of treatment with either propionyl-L-carnitine (2 g per day) or tamoxifen. Use of propionyl-L-carnitine plus verapamil significantly reduced penile curvature, plaque size, and the need for surgery, while tamoxifen plus verapamil had little effect.

These studies remain preliminary, but their results are definitely encouraging. For more information, see the full **L-carnitine** article.

Paraminobenzoic Acid

Para-aminobenzoic acid (PABA) has been suggested for a variety of diseases in which abnormal fibrous tissue is involved, including Peyronie's disease. However, there has only been one reported double-blind study. (For more information on why such studies are essential, see **Why Does This Book Rely on Double-blind Studies?**) This trial enrolled 103 men with Peyronie's disease and followed them for 1 year. The results showed that use of PABA at a dose of 3 g 4 times daily significantly slowed the progression of Peyronie's disease; it did not, however, reduce pre-existing plaque.

For more information, including dosage and safety issues, see the full **PABA** article.

Other Proposed Natural Treatments

Vitamin E has also been advocated for the treatment of Peyronie's disease, as well as for the related condition Dupuytren's contracture, but there is as yet no meaningful evidence that it is effective.

The herb **gotu kola** is used to treat various conditions in which fibrous scar tissue causes problems and for that reason it has been advocated for Peyronie's disease. However, again there is no meaningful evidence that it is effective.

Herbs and Supplements to Use Only with Caution

Various herbs and supplements may interact adversely with drugs used to treat Peyronie's disease. For more information on this potential risk, see the individual drug articles in the Drug Interactions section of this book.

Phlebitis

RELATED TERMS: *Deep Vein Thrombosis, Saphenous Thrombophlebitis, Superficial Phlebitis, Thrombophlebitis*
PRINCIPAL PROPOSED NATURAL TREATMENTS: *None*
OTHER PROPOSED NATURAL TREATMENTS: *Bromelain, Horse Chestnut, Mesoglycan*

The term *phlebitis* refers to an inflammation of a vein, usually in the leg, frequently accompanied by blood clots that adhere to the wall of the vein. When the affected vein is close to the surface, the condition is called *superficial phlebitis*. This condition usually resolves on its own without further complications. However, when phlebitis occurs in a deep vein, a condition called *deep vein thrombosis* (DVT), a clot could dislodge from the vein and lodge in the lungs. This is a life-threatening condition.

Symptoms of superficial phlebitis include pain, swelling, redness, and warmth around the affected vein. The vein feels hard to the touch because of the clotted blood.

Deep vein thrombosis is harder to diagnose. It can occur without any symptoms until the clot reaches the lungs. However, in about half of the cases, there are warning symptoms including swelling, pain, and warmth in the entire calf, ankle, foot, or thigh (depending on where the involved vein is located). Although these symptoms can also be caused by more benign conditions, deep vein thrombosis is such a life-threatening disorder that physician consultation is necessary.

Risk factors for any type of phlebitis include recent surgery or childbirth, varicose veins, inactivity, or sitting for long periods (such as on a long airplane ride). Prolonged placement of intravenous catheters can also cause phlebitis, possibly requiring antibiotic treatment.

Conventional treatments for superficial phlebitis include analgesics for pain, warm compresses, and compression bandages or stockings to increase blood flow. In more severe cases, anticoagulants or minor surgery may be required.

Deep vein thrombosis requires more aggressive treatment, including hospitalization, strong anticoagulants, and a variety of possible surgical procedures.

Proposed Natural Treatments for Phlebitis

There are no well-established natural treatments for phlebitis at this time.

Note: Because phlebitis is a potentially life-threatening disorder, you should seek a doctor's advice before attempting any natural treatments.

Bromelain

Bromelain is an enzyme found in the stems of pineapple. Because it has anti-inflammatory properties and may be able to prevent blood platelet aggregation, it has been suggested as a treatment for phlebitis. However, there is no good evidence as yet supporting this use.

Mesoglycan

Mesoglycan is a type of substance found in the tissues of the body, including blood vessels. It is closely related to the anticoagulant drug heparin. Preliminary evidence suggests that mesoglycan might be helpful in treating phlebitis, although not all studies agree.

Other Natural Treatments

Horse chestnut is often used for chronic venous insufficiency and varicose veins, conditions related to phlebitis. For this reason, horse chestnut is sometimes recommended for phlebitis as well, but there is as yet no real evidence that it works.

Photosensitivity

Photosensitivity

RELATED TERMS: *Erythropoietic Protoporphyria, Photoallergy, Photodermatitis, Phototoxicity, Polymorphous Light Eruptions, Porphyria Cutanea Tarda*

PRINCIPAL PROPOSED NATURAL TREATMENTS: *Beta-carotene*

OTHER PROPOSED NATURAL TREATMENTS: *AMP, EGCG (from Green Tea), Nicotinamide, Vitamin B_6, Vitamin C, Vitamin E*

HERBS AND SUPPLEMENTS TO USE ONLY WITH CAUTION: *Artichoke, Celery, Chrysanthemum, Dandelion, Dill, Endive, Essential Oils, Fennel, Fig, Lettuce, Lime, Marigold, Parsley, Parsnip, St. John's Wort, Sunflower*

Everyone will burn if exposed to enough ultraviolet radiation from the sun or other sources. However, some people burn particularly easily or develop exaggerated skin reactions to sunlight. Doctors call this condition photosensitivity. For some people, consuming certain medications or plant products—or rubbing them on their skin—can cause photosensitivity. Similar reactions are seen in diseases such as some forms of porphyria (a group of usually hereditary metabolic disorders) or **lupus**. In another condition, called *polymorphous light eruptions* (PLEs), dramatic rashes can develop after fairly limited sun exposure.

The most important step toward treating photosensitivity is to identify whether an external substance is causing the reaction and then eliminate it if possible. Antibiotics are among the most common photosensitizing drugs. Many other natural substances can also cause this reaction. Another commonsense step is to use sunscreen and wear protective clothing or simply to stay out of the sun.

Some types of photosensitivity may respond to specific treatments such as oral beta-carotene, steroids, or other medications.

Principal Proposed Natural Treatments

Beta-carotene, a plant pigment giving color to carrots and yams, may be beneficial for at least two kinds of photosensitivity: polymorphous light eruptions and photosensitivity caused by certain types of porphyria. It is the best-studied supplement for photosensitivity, although only four studies on it have been placebo-controlled and these had conflicting results. According to one theory, beta-carotene prevents skin damage by

neutralizing free radicals, harmful chemicals created in the skin by the action of radiation.

One characteristic of beta-carotene is that it gives a deep yellow color to human skin when taken in high doses for several months. Since supplementation must go on for a while to see results, this side effect makes it difficult to conduct a truly double-blind study in which neither researchers nor the participants know who is taking the active compound and who is taking placebo. (For reasons why double-blinding is so important, see **Why Does This Book Rely on Double-blind Studies?**.) Once people begin to turn yellow, they are likely to figure out what they're taking, possibly affecting the study outcome. Therefore, even the results of placebo-controlled studies of beta-carotene are open to question.

That said, three controlled trials of beta-carotene for polymorphous light eruptions found mixed results. A 10-week study in 50 people with PLE given beta-carotene plus canthaxanthin (another carotene) or placebo found evidence of significant benefit. However, in two other controlled trials of beta-carotene alone, lasting 12 to 15 weeks (the number of participants was not reported), modest benefits were seen in one study and no benefits at all in the other.

Many uncontrolled studies have reported that beta-carotene extends the time that people with erythropoietic protoporphyria (EPP) can safely spend in the sun. However, studies that lack a control group, as these did, are notorious for producing over-optimistic results, and an 11-month controlled trial found no benefit. A few case reports suggest beta-carotene may also be helpful in another kind of porphyria called *porphyria cutanea tarda*.

For more information, including dosage and safety issues, see the full **Beta-carotene** article.

Other Proposed Natural Treatments

Many, though not all, studies suggest that various antioxidants, including **vitamin C, lycopene**, mixed **carotenoids, green tea**, and **vitamin E** (taken orally or used topically) may help prevent **sunburn** in people without photosensitivity.

On this basis, a variety of antioxidants have been tried for photosensitivity as well. In a double-blind, placebo-controlled trial of 12 people with EPP, 1 g of vitamin C taken orally daily appeared to help reduce symptoms. However, the study was too small for the results to be statistically significant.

A small double-blind, placebo-controlled trial of individuals with PLE found no benefit with combined vitamin C (3 g per day) and vitamin E (1,500 IU per day).

In an uncontrolled study of AMP in 21 people with porphyria cutanea tarda, many showed decreased photosensitivity, much to the surprise of the investigator.

Two cases of EPP were also reportedly improved by **vitamin B₆**. In addition, **nicotinamide**—another B vitamin—was found to help prevent PLEs in an uncontrolled (and, therefore, highly unreliable) study of 42 people.

Herbs and Supplements to Use Only with Caution

A number of common herbs and plant products are known to provoke extreme reactions to sunlight in some individuals. One of the more well-known culprits is **St. John's wort**, which has caused fatal photosensitivity reactions in cattle that grazed on it. In one study of highly sun-sensitive people, double doses of the herb produced mild increases in reaction to ultraviolet radiation. There is also one report of a severe skin reaction in an individual who used St. John's wort and then received ultraviolet therapy for psoriasis. In addition, topical St. John's wort apparently caused severe sunburn in one individual. For this reason, photosensitive people should probably avoid St. John's wort.

Photosensitivity can also result from touching or eating other plants, including celery, dill, **fennel**, fig, lime, **parsley**, and parsnip, as well as arnica, **artichoke**, chrysanthemum, **dandelion**, lettuce, endive, marigold, and sunflower. Lest you swear off gardening or salads altogether, be aware that most people do not react to these plants. **Essential oils** of plants may be more problematic than the whole plant itself.

Preeclampsia and Pregnancy-Induced Hypertension

RELATED TERMS: *Eclampsia, Gestational Hypertension, Hypertension of Pregnancy, PIH, Toxemia (Pregnancy)*

PRINCIPAL PROPOSED NATURAL TREATMENTS: *Calcium*

OTHER PROPOSED NATURAL TREATMENTS: *Arginine, Evening Primrose Oil, Folate, Lycopene, Magnesium, N-acetylcysteine, Omega-3 Fatty Acids, Vitamin C and Vitamin E in Combination, Zinc*

Pregnant women occasionally experience an increase in blood pressure known as *gestational hypertension* or *pregnancy-induced hypertension* (PIH). In a more severe condition called *preeclampsia*, a rise in blood pressure is accompanied by protein in the urine and sometimes by sudden weight gain, swelling in the face or hands, and other symptoms. When left untreated, preeclampsia can lead to seizures (called *eclampsia*) or liver, kidney, or bleeding problems in the mother and distress or growth retardation in the fetus. Unless preeclampsia is mild, doctors usually seek to deliver the baby early.

Principal Proposed Natural Treatments

Although there are no fully established natural treatments for the prevention of preeclampsia or PIH, calcium has shown significant promise.

A meta-analysis (statistical review) of 11 studies of calcium supplementation in pregnancy, involving a total of more than 6,000 women, found that calcium slightly reduced the risk of preeclampsia and hypertension, particularly in two groups of women: those at high risk for hypertension and/or those with low calcium intakes.

However, by far the largest single study in the meta-analysis found no benefits. In this double-blind study, researchers gave either 2 g of calcium or placebo daily to 4,589 women from weeks 13 to 21 of their pregnancy onward. In the end, researchers found no significant decreases in rates of hypertension or preeclampsia—not even when they looked specifically at women whose daily calcium consumption mirrored that of women in developing countries.

The meta-analysis included this negative study in its calculations, but still found that calcium seemed to be helpful.

In a subsequent double-blind, placebo-controlled study published in 2006 and conducted by the World Health Organization, calcium supplements (1.5 g per day) were tried in 8,325 pregnant women whose calcium intake was inadequate. Calcium failed to reduce the incidence of preeclampsia. However, it did appear to reduce the severity of preeclampsia episodes that did develop.

The bottom line: Calcium might be of some benefit for those pregnant women who are at high risk for hypertension or deficient in calcium. However, for well-nourished, low-risk women, effects are likely to be minimal or nil.

All of the above refers to preventing preeclampsia. One double-blind, placebo-controlled study suggests that calcium supplements are *not* effective for treating preeclampsia that has already developed.

Note: Calcium appears to offer the additional benefit of reducing blood levels of lead during pregnancy.

For more information, including dosage and safety issues, see the full **Calcium** article.

Other Proposed Natural Treatments

Antioxidants are substances that fight free radicals, dangerous naturally occurring molecules that may play a role in preeclampsia. For various theoretical reasons, it has been proposed that use of antioxidants by pregnant women may help stop preeclampsia from developing. One double-blind, placebo-controlled study found evidence that a combination of the antioxidant **vitamin E** (400 IU daily) and **vitamin C** (1,000 mg daily) reduced incidence of preeclampsia. Benefits were seen in another study of this combination as well. Additionally, a double-blind trial found potential preventive effects with the antioxidant substance **lycopene** (taken at 2 mg twice daily). However, researchers caution that further study is necessary: many other treatments have shown initial promise for preventing preeclampsia, but lost luster when subsequent studies were performed. The most prominent of these once-promising substances include **folate**, **magnesium**, **omega-3 fatty acids** (fish oil), and **zinc**. Furthermore, a large follow-up studies of vitamin E and vitamin C failed to find any benefit.

Other studies have looked at possible treatments preeclampsia once it has already occurred. Results are somewhat positive, though mixed on the potential benefits of **arginine** for this purpose. **Evening primrose oil** has failed to prove helpful as has a combination of vitamin C, vitamin E, and the drug allopurinol. However, magnesium, taken by injection but not orally, appears to provide meaningful benefits.

One study failed to find n-acetylcysteine helpful for severe preeclampsia.

Pregnancy Support

SEE ALSO: *Breast-feeding Support*

HERBS AND SUPPLEMENTS TO AVOID DURING PREGNANCY AND BREAST-FEEDING:

NAUSEA AND VOMITING OF PREGNANCY PREECLAMPSIA

PRINCIPAL PROPOSED NATURAL TREATMENTS:

Anemia: *Iron (If Deficient)*

Hemorrhoids: *Citrus Bioflavonoids, Oxerutins*

Prevention of Neural Tube Defects: *Folate*

Varicose Veins: *Citrus Bioflavonoids, Gotu Kola, Horse Chestnut, Oxerutins*

OTHER PROPOSED NATURAL TREATMENTS:

Assisting or Initiating Childbirth: *Acupuncture, Aromatherapy, Castor Oil, Hypnotherapy, Massage, Proteolytic Enzymes, Red Raspberry*

Constipation: *Dandelion, Fiber Supplements, Flaxseed, Glucomannan, Lactulose*

Diabetes in Pregnancy: *Chromium, Vitamin B_6*

Gingivitis: *Folate*

Jaundice of Pregnancy: *S-Adenosylmethionine (SAMe)*

Leg Cramps: *Calcium, Magnesium, Vitamin B_1 Plus Vitamin B_6*

Prevention of Low Birth Weight: *B Vitamins, Calcium, Fish Oil, Folate, Iron, Magnesium, Vitamin D, Zinc*

Prevention of Miscarriage: *Vitamin B_{12}*

Prevention of Prematurity: *Calcium, Fish Oil, Iron, Magnesium, Zinc*

Support of Healthy Mental Function in Infant: *Fish Oil*

Pregnancy is a time of dramatic transitions. Body systems that once sustained a single human now support two. Organs, blood vessels, body chemistry, and even the solid supporting structures of a woman's body all go through changes; in the meantime, the fetus's body grows from a tiny bundle of cells to a full-sized baby.

It's no wonder that women feel the desire for remedies to help with these transitions. Since ancient times, women have tried herbs and other natural treatments to ease discomfort or assist with pregnancy, childbirth, and breast-feeding. However, pregnancy is also a circumstance when the potential risk of any treatment rises dramatically. Seemingly benign medications—even natural ones—have been found to cause birth defects or increase the risk of complications. Some traditional remedies, such as blue cohosh for labor stimulation, must be discarded for safety reasons.

Thorough study is needed before any treatment can be considered absolutely safe in pregnancy—and in many cases, this research has not yet been completed. It's important to talk with your doctor before deciding to use any treatment, whether it is natural or conventional.

Principal Proposed Natural Treatments

Many natural treatments have shown promise for conditions related to pregnancy. In this section, we discuss those with the most scientific support. However, treatments for **nausea and vomiting of pregnancy** and **preeclampsia** are not discussed here; instead, they are addressed in separate articles. **Breast-feeding support** also has an article of its own.

Note: The safety of the following treatments has not been confirmed, except for nutrients such as vitamins and minerals, for which appropriate dosages for pregnancy have been established. For more information on potentially harmful natural treatments, see **Herbs and Supplements to Avoid during Pregnancy and Breast-feeding**.

Varicose Veins

Increased pressure from the expanding abdomen and other factors can lead to pooling of fluid in the legs, a condition called *venous insufficiency* (closely related to varicose veins).

Venous insufficiency/varicose veins occur outside pregnancy as well and a wide variety of natural treatments have shown promise in their treatment, including buckwheat, **butcher's broom**, **citrus bioflavonoids**, **gotu kola**, **horse chestnut**, **OPCs**, and red vine leaf. These are discussed in the **Venous Insufficiency** article.

Only one natural treatment, oxerutins, has been studied in a double-blind trial enrolling *pregnant* women with venous insufficiency. In this study of 69 women, researchers found oxerutins more effective than placebo.

For more information, see the full **Oxerutin** article.

Hemorrhoids

Hemorrhoids are actually varicose veins in or around the anus. Oxerutins and citrus bioflavonoids have been studied for hemorrhoids during pregnancy.

A double-blind study enrolling 97 pregnant women found oxerutins (1,000 mg daily) significantly better than placebo at reducing the pain, bleeding, and inflammation of hemorrhoids. Evidence for citrus bioflavonoids is limited to one open trial. Other natural treatments for varicose veins are often recommended for hemorrhoids as well, although research on their use for this condition in pregnancy is lacking.

For more information, see the article on **hemorrhoids**.

Anemia

Iron supplements can be key in treating anemia in pregnancy, but may not be good for you or your baby if you are not anemic. If you are not anemic, talk to your doctor before taking iron supplements.

Interestingly, one study suggests that **iron** plus **folate** is more effective for the treatment of iron-deficiency anemia in pregnancy than iron alone, even in women who do not appear to be folate-deficient.

Prevention of Neural Tube Defects

Folate supplements can help prevent a serious and common type of birth defect known as *neural tube defects* (NTDs).

One preliminary study of 859 babies suggests that zinc may help prevent NTDs as well, but evidence so far is weak.

Other Proposed Natural Treatments

Other natural remedies have been recommended for treating discomforts and complications of pregnancy or decreasing risks to the baby.

Assisting Childbirth
⇒ *Castor Oil*

Castor bean oil was noted by the ancient Egyptians to stimulate labor, and it is still used by some conventional physicians and midwives to induce contractions—for example, if labor does not occur spontaneously after the waters have broken. A recent controlled trial in 100 pregnant women compared oral castor oil to no treatment and found that 57.7% of those given castor oil began labor within 24 hours, compared to only 4.2% of those without treatment. Other preliminary studies also suggest that castor oil may help. Unfortunately, castor oil is a strong laxative, and diarrhea is a nearly universal effect—not a particularly pleasant experience during childbirth.

In addition, considering how common this treatment is, research on its safety and effectiveness is surprisingly scant. One case of a potentially fatal complication linked to use of castor oil has been reported, though some have questioned whether the castor oil was responsible. In addition, an observational study of South African women found that those self-treating with castor oil and/or other traditional herbs had a higher incidence of meconium (fetal feces) in the amniotic fluid, a sign of fetal distress.

⇒ *Acupuncture*

Acupuncture has shown some promise for reducing pain in labor, but the quality of most of the supporting evidence is relatively poor.

A study of 45 pregnant women found that women who received acupuncture on the mathematically calculated birth "due date" gave birth sooner than those who did not.

⇒ *Other Natural Treatments*

One double-blind, placebo-controlled trial evaluated the effects of **red raspberry** in 192 pregnant women. Treatment (placebo or 2.4 g of raspberry leaf daily) began at 32 weeks of pregnancy and was continued until the onset of labor. The results failed to show any statistically meaningful differences between the groups. Red raspberry did not significantly shorten labor, reduce pain, or prevent complications.

Blue cohosh is a toxic herb and should not be used. One published case report documents profound heart failure in a baby born to a mother who used blue cohosh to induce labor. Severe medical consequences were also seen in a child whose mother took both black and blue cohosh.

Proteolytic enzymes may reduce inflammation and discomfort following episiotomy.

Hypnotherapy and **massage therapy** have shown some promise for assisting labor. In a large controlled trial (more than 600 participants), lavender oil **aromatherapy** failed to improve pain after childbirth.

Constipation

Constipation frequently occurs during pregnancy, for reasons that are not entirely clear.

Fiber supplements, such as psyllium seed, are commonly recommended for the treatment of constipation in pregnancy because of their apparent safety. **Flaxseed** is another high-fiber seed and alternative practitioners often recommend it. However, flaxseed contains estrogen-like substances that might pose hazards to the fetus; one study found an effect on reproductive organs and function in baby rats whose mothers ate large amounts of flaxseed during pregnancy.

Other natural remedies for constipation during pregnancy include **dandelion root** and a combination of **glucomannan** and lactulose. However, there is no meaningful evidence to indicate that they are effective.

Note: Avoid use of powerful laxatives, including natural remedies such as buckthorn, cascara, rhubarb, castor bean oil, and **senna**, as these can induce uterine contractions. (See the Assisting Childbirth section above.) The traditional remedy **yellow dock**, though milder, might warrant similar caution.

Leg Cramps

Pregnant women sometimes experience painful leg cramps. A double-blind study of 73 women with this symptom found that **magnesium** was significantly more effective than placebo in decreasing their distress.

Calcium has also been studied for this problem, but research so far gives little indication that it helps. A combination of **vitamins B_1** and **B_6** has also been sug-

gested for leg cramps, but evidence that it helps remains minimal.

Prevention of Prematurity

Interesting though not entirely consistent evidence suggests that use of **fish oil** or its constituents by pregnant women might help prevent premature births. Double-blind studies have evaluated the minerals calcium, zinc, and magnesium for this purpose as well, but the results have been mixed. A number of trials suggest that anemia is linked to prematurity; however, evidence as to whether iron supplements can help remains inconclusive. Several studies have evaluated folate but did not find it effective for preventing premature birth.

One study failed to find **vitamin C** helpful for preventing premature birth. However, another study found that vitamin C (100 mg/day after 20 weeks of pregnancy) helped prevent early rupture of the chorioamniotic membrane ("the water breaking"). Another study found that use of vitamin E (400 IU/day) and vitamin C (500 mg/day) after premature water breaking helped hold off delivery by several days.

Prevention of Low Birth Weight

Babies born below a specific weight (5-1/2 pounds)—called *low birth weight*—are at greater risk for complications.

A recent meta-analysis of 7 controlled studies looked at the effects of calcium supplementation on birth weight. These studies predominantly focused on preventing hypertension and/or preeclampsia in the mother, both of which can result in low-birth-weight babies. Overall, calcium appeared to decrease the percentage of babies weighing less than 5 pounds 8 ounces. However, other analysts looking at a somewhat different group of studies came to the opposite conclusion.

Quite a few double-blind studies have examined zinc as well as magnesium for preventing low birth weight, with mixed results. Results have been similarly mixed in other controlled trials of folate and fish oil or one of its fatty acids. **Vitamin D** and **B vitamins** have also been proposed, but so far evidence of their usefulness is weak.

Several decades ago, iron was believed to be helpful in preventing low birth weight. However, a recent large-scale unblinded study of well-nourished women found that routine iron supplements in pregnancy had no effect on birth weight. In addition, as previously noted, iron supplementation in pregnant women who are not anemic may not be good for either mother or baby.

In a double-blind, placebo-controlled study of 1,877 women, use of combined **vitamin E** and vitamin C failed to prove helpful.

Other Uses of Natural Treatments

A lesser-known problem in pregnancy is an increased tendency toward swollen or bleeding gums—a condition known as *gingivitis*. Two small double-blind studies suggest that folate mouthwash may help. However, folate supplements do not appear to be especially effective against gingivitis.

A condition called *intrahepatic cholestasis* may occur during pregnancy, causing jaundice and other complications. Preliminary evidence suggests that the supplement **SAMe** might be helpful.

One placebo-controlled study of 30 women suggests that the mineral **chromium** may be useful for *gestational diabetes*, the term for **diabetes** that occurs during

pregnancy. Vitamin B_6 has also been proposed for this condition, but evidence in support of its effectiveness is minimal.

Use of fish oil or its constituents DHA and EPA by pregnant women might help support healthy cognitive and visual function in their children.

Low levels of **vitamin B_{12}** may increase risk of miscarriage and B_{12} supplements may help.

Two studies suggest that acupuncture and associated therapies can help "turn" a breech presentation.

One study failed to find docosahexaenoic acid (DHA, from fish oil) helpful for preventing postpartum depression.

Herbs and Supplements to Avoid During Pregnancy

For information on this important topic, see **Herbs and Supplements to Avoid during Pregnancy and Breast-feeding**.

Premenstrual Syndrome

RELATED TERMS: PMS

PRINCIPAL PROPOSED NATURAL TREATMENTS: *Calcium, Chasteberry*

OTHER PROPOSED NATURAL TREATMENTS: *Chiropractic, Ginkgo, Gamma-linolenic Acid (GLA), Grass Pollen (Plus Grass Pistils and Royal Jelly), Inositol, Krill Oil, Magnesium, Massage, Multivitamin and Mineral Supplement, Oligomeric Proanthocyanidins (OPCs), Progesterone Cream, Soy Isoflavones (Plus Dong Quai and Black Cohosh), Vitamin E*

PROBABLY INEFFECTIVE TREATMENTS: *Vitamin B_6*

Many women experience a variety of unpleasant symptoms in the week or two before menstruating. These include irritability, anger, headaches, anxiety, depression, fatigue, fluid retention, and breast tenderness. When emotional symptoms related to depression predominate in PMS, the condition is sometimes called *premenstrual dysphoric disorder* (PMDD). These symptoms undoubtedly result from hormonal changes of the menstrual cycle, but apart from that general statement, medical researchers do not know the cause of PMS or how to treat it.

Conventional treatments for PMS and PMDD include antidepressants, beta-blockers, diuretics, oral contraceptives, and other hormonally active formulations. Of all these, antidepressants in the SSRI family (such as Prozac) are perhaps the most effective.

Principal Proposed Natural Treatments

There is fairly good evidence that calcium supplements can significantly reduce all the major symptoms of PMS. There is also some evidence for the herbs chasteberry and ginkgo. Vitamin B_6 is widely recommended as well, but its scientific record is mixed at best.

Calcium

A large double-blind, placebo-controlled study found positive results using calcium for the treatment of PMS symptoms. Participants took 300 mg of calcium (as calcium carbonate) 4 times daily. Compared to placebo, calcium significantly reduced mood swings, pain, bloating, depression, back pain, and food cravings.

Similar findings were also seen in earlier preliminary studies of calcium for PMS.

For more information, including dosage and safety issues, see the full **Calcium** article.

Chasteberry

The herb chasteberry is widely used in Europe as a treatment for PMS symptoms. More than most herbs, chasteberry is frequently called by its Latin names: *Vitex* or *Vitexagnus-castus.*

A double-blind, placebo-controlled study of 178 women found that treatment with chasteberry over three menstrual cycles significantly reduced PMS symptoms. The dose used was one tablet 3 times daily of a chasteberry dry extract. Women in the treatment group experienced significant improvements in symptoms, including irritability, depression, headache, and breast tenderness.

Unfortunately, there is little corroborating evidence as yet for this one well-designed study. A previous double-blind trial compared chasteberry to vitamin B_6 (pyridoxine) instead of placebo. The two treatments proved equally effective. However, because vitamin B_6 itself has not been shown effective for PMS (see below), these results mean little.

Even better evidence indicates that chasteberry can help the **cyclic breast tenderness** often, but not necessarily, connected with PMS.

For more information, including dosage and safety issues, see the full **Chasteberry** article.

Vitamin B_6

Vitamin B_6 has been used for PMS for many decades by both European and U.S. physicians. However, the results of scientific studies are mixed at best. The most recent and best-designed double-blind study, enrolling 120 women, found no benefit. In this trial, three prescription drugs were compared against vitamin B_6 (pyridoxine, at 300 mg daily) and placebo. All study participants received 3 months of treatment and 3 months of placebo. Vitamin B_6 proved to be no better than placebo.

Approximately a dozen other double-blind studies have investigated the effectiveness of vitamin B_6 for PMS, but none were well designed and the results were mixed. Some books on natural medicine report that the negative results in some of these studies were due to insufficient B_6 dosage, but in reality there was no clear link between dosage and effectiveness.

It has been suggested that the combination of B_6 and magnesium might be more effective than either treatment alone, but this remains to be proven (see below).

For more information, including dosage and safety issues, see the full **Vitamin B_6** article.

Other Proposed Treatments for PMS

Ginkgo

One double-blind, placebo-controlled study evaluated the benefits of *Ginkgo biloba* extract for women with PMS symptoms. This trial enrolled 143 women, 18 to 45 years of age, and followed them for two menstrual cycles. Each woman received either the ginkgo extract (80 mg twice daily) or placebo on day 16 of the first cycle. Treatment was continued until day 5 of the next cycle and resumed again on day 16 of that cycle. As compared to placebo, ginkgo significantly relieved major symptoms of PMS, especially breast pain and emotional disturbance.

For more information, including dosage and safety issues, see the full **Ginkgo** article.

Magnesium

Preliminary studies suggest that magnesium may also be helpful in PMS. A double-blind, placebo-controlled study of 32 women found that magnesium taken from day 15 of the menstrual cycle to the onset of menstrual flow could significantly improve premenstrual mood changes.

Another small double-blind preliminary study found that regular use of magnesium could reduce symptoms of PMS-related fluid retention. In this study, 38 women were given magnesium or placebo for 2 months. The results showed no effect after one cycle, but by the end of two cycles, magnesium significantly reduced weight gain, swelling of extremities, breast tenderness, and abdominal bloating.

In addition, one small double-blind study (20 participants) found that magnesium supplementation might help prevent menstrual **migraines**.

For more information, including dosage and safety issues, see the full **Magnesium** article.

As mentioned earlier, preliminary evidence suggests that combining vitamin B$_6$ with magnesium might improve the results.

Additional Treatments

Several double-blind, placebo-controlled studies, enrolling a total of about 400 women, found evidence that **multivitamin and mineral supplements** may be helpful for PMS. It is not clear which ingredients in these supplements played a role.

Preliminary double-blind trials also suggest that **vitamin E** may be helpful for PMS.

A product containing **grass pollen**, royal jelly (a product made by bees), and the pistils (seed-bearing parts) of grass has been proposed for use in PMS. In a double-blind, placebo-controlled crossover trial of 32 women, use of the product for two menstrual cycles appeared to significantly improve PMS symptoms as compared to use of placebo.

A double-blind, placebo-controlled study of 30 women with complaints of premenstrual fluid retention found that use of oligomeric proanthocyanidins (OPCs) at a dose of 320 mg daily significantly reduced the *sensation* of fluid retention in the leg; however, actual leg swelling as measured was not significantly improved.

One poorly designed human trial hints that **krill oil** may be helpful for some PMS symptoms.

In a 24-week, double-blind study, 49 women with menstrual migraines received either placebo or a combination supplement containing **soy isoflavones**, **dong quai**, and **black cohosh** extracts. The treatment proved at least somewhat more effective than placebo. Soy isoflavones alone have also shown some potential benefit.

Evening primrose oil, a source of the omega-6 fatty acids, was once thought to be helpful for cyclic breast pain. However, it probably does not work for this purpose. It has also been proposed as a treatment for general PMS symptoms, but there is only minimal supporting evidence.

Highly preliminary evidence suggests that **St. John's wort** might be helpful for mood changes in PMS.

One study often cited as evidence that **massage therapy** is helpful for PMS was fatally flawed by the absence of a control group. However, a better-designed trial compared reflexology (a special form of massage involving primarily the foot) against fake reflexology in 38 women with PMS symptoms and found evidence that real reflexology was more effective.

A small crossover trial of **chiropractic manipulation** for PMS symptoms found equivocal results at best.

Progesterone cream is sometimes recommended for PMS, but there is no meaningful evidence that it is effective.

One study failed to find the supplement **inositol** helpful for PMS.

Prostatitis

RELATED TERMS: *Acute Bacterial Prostatitis, Chronic Prostatitis, Prostatodynia, Prostatalgia, Chronic Pelvic Pain Syndrome (In Men)*

PRINCIPAL PROPOSED NATURAL TREATMENTS: *None*

OTHER PROPOSED NATURAL TREATMENTS: *Acupuncture, Biofeedback, Bromelain, Buchu, Couch Grass, Cranberry, Echinacea, Eleutherococcus, Garlic, Goldenseal, Grass Pollen Extract, Lapacho, Marshmallow, Multivitamin/Mineral Supplements, Pipsissewa, Proteolytic Enzymes, Pygeum, Quercetin, Saw Palmetto, Vitamin C, Watermelon Seed, Zinc*

Prostatitis is inflammation of the prostate. The prostate is a walnut-sized gland in men that surrounds the urethra. It produces a fluid that is part of semen.

There are three main types of prostatitis: acute bacterial, chronic bacterial, and chronic non-bacterial.

Acute bacterial prostatitis is the easiest form to treat,

but it is also the least common. Symptoms include chills, fever, pain in the lower back and genital area, urinary frequency and urgency (often at night), burning or painful urination, and body aches. Examination of the urine shows white blood cells. Antibiotic treatment is highly successful for this form of prostatitis.

Chronic bacterial prostatitis resembles acute prostatitis, but it is milder and may go on for a long time (months or years). It is believed that chronic bacterial prostatitis is caused by a problem in the prostate that makes the gland a focus for infection. Antibiotic treatment usually relieves symptoms, but they often come back after treatment is stopped.

Chronic non-bacterial prostatitis, also known as *chronic pelvic pain syndrome* or *prostatodynia*, is the most common form of prostatitis. Unfortunately, it is also the least understood and the hardest to treat. Symptoms include urinary urgency, urinary frequency (especially at night), pain or burning while urinating, difficulty urinating, lower abdominal pain or pressure, rectal or perineal discomfort, lower back pain, painful ejaculation, and impotence. These symptoms may wax and wane for no obvious reason. Conventional medicine lacks a specific treatment for chronic non-bacterial prostatitis. Supportive treatments may be used, including stool softeners, pain medications, and warm sitz baths.

Proposed Natural Treatments for Prostatitis

Quercetin belongs to a class of water-soluble plant coloring agents called *bioflavonoids*, which have anti-inflammatory and antioxidant properties. Bioflavonoids have been investigated for a wide variety of medical uses. A study published in 1999 suggests that quercetin may be helpful for chronic non-bacterial prostatitis. In this double-blind trial, 30 men with fairly severe chronic non-bacterial prostatitis were given either quercetin (500 mg twice daily) or placebo for a month. The results showed that participants given quercetin improved to a significantly greater extent than those in the placebo group. The greatest gains were seen in reduction of pain.

A special **grass pollen** extract has also shown promise. In a 6-month, double-blind study of 60 men with non-bacterial prostatitis, use of the grass pollen extract was more effective than placebo.

Grass pollen is better known as a treatment for **benign prostatic hypertrophy** (BPH). All the other commonly used natural treatments for this condition have also been suggested for prostatitis. However, while there is reasonably good supporting evidence that some of these help BPH, the evidence regarding their use in prostatitis remains weak. For example, uncontrolled trials and other highly preliminary forms of evidence hint that the herb **pygeum** might be helpful for prostatitis. Also, an open-controlled trial (using a no-treatment group) found indications that **saw palmetto** might be helpful for prostatitis; however, an open comparative study found the drug finasteride more effective than the herb for this purpose.

Other herbs and supplements sometimes recommended for prostatitis, but that lack almost any supporting evidence, include **bromelain**, **buchu**, couch grass, **cranberry**, **echinacea**, **eleutherococcus**, **garlic**, **goldenseal**, **lapacho**, **marshmallow**, **multivitamin/mineral supplements**, pipsissewa, **proteolytic enzymes**, **vitamin C**, watermelon seed, and **zinc**. **Acupuncture** and **biofeedback** have been tried as well.

Herbs and Supplements to Use Only with Caution

Various herbs and supplements may interact adversely with drugs used to treat prostatitis. For more information on this potential risk, see the individual drug articles in the Drug Interactions section of this book.

Psoriasis

PRINCIPAL PROPOSED NATURAL TREATMENTS: *Oregon Grape*

OTHER PROPOSED NATURAL TREATMENTS: *Acupuncture, Aloe Vera Cream, Capsaicin Cream, Cetylated Fatty Acids, Fish Oil, Folate (to Reduce Side Effects of Methotrexate), Fumaric Acid, Hypnotherapy, Seal Oil, Vitamin A, Vitamin D*

Up to 2% of Americans suffer from psoriasis, a skin condition that leads to an intensely itchy rash with clearly defined borders and scales that resemble silvery mica. The fingernails are also frequently involved, showing pitting or thickening.

Medical treatment for psoriasis includes applications of topical steroids and peeling agents that expose the underlying skin for the steroid to contact. Ultraviolet light can also be used, sometimes combined with coal tar applications or medications called *psoralens*. Synthetic relatives of vitamin A and vitamin D are also used.

Principal Proposed Natural Treatments

Evidence from two double-blind, placebo-controlled trials and one comparative trial suggest that cream made from the herb Oregon grape (*Mahonia*) may help reduce symptoms of psoriasis, although it does not seem to be as effective as standard medications.

In a double-blind study published in 2006, 200 people were given either a cream containing 10% Oregon grape extract or placebo twice a day for 3 months. The results indicate that the people using Oregon grape experienced greater benefits than those in the placebo group and the difference was statistically significant. The treatment was well tolerated, although in a few people it caused rash or burning sensation.

Benefits were also seen in a double-blind, placebo-controlled study of 82 people with psoriasis. However, the study design had a significant flaw: the treatment salve was darker in color than the placebo, possibly allowing participants to guess which was which.

Another study found that dithranol, a conventional drug used to treat psoriasis symptoms, was more effective than Oregon grape. Regrettably, the authors fail to state whether this study was double-blind. Forty-nine participants applied one treatment to their left side and the other to their right for 4 weeks. Skin biopsies were then analyzed and compared with samples taken at the beginning of the study. The physicians evaluating changes in skin tissue were unaware which treatments had been used on the samples. Greater improvements were seen in the dithranol group.

A large open study in which 443 participants with psoriasis used Oregon grape topically for 12 weeks found the herb to be helpful for 73.7% of the group. Without a placebo group, it's not possible to know whether Oregon grape was truly responsible for the improvement seen, but the trial does help to establish the herb's safety and tolerability.

Laboratory research suggests Oregon grape has some effects at the cellular level that might be helpful in psoriasis, such as slowing the rate of abnormal cell growth and reducing inflammation.

For more information, including dosage and safety issues, see the full **Oregon grape** article.

Other Proposed Natural Treatments for Psoriasis

Aloe

Aloe vera cream may be helpful for psoriasis, according to a double-blind study performed in Pakistan that enrolled 60 men and women with mild to moderate symptoms of psoriasis. Participants were treated with either topical *Aloe vera* extract (0.5%) or a placebo cream, applied 3 times daily for 4 weeks. Aloe treatment produced significantly better results than placebo, and these results were said to endure for almost a year after treatment was stopped. The study authors also reported a high level of complete "cure," but what exactly they meant by this was not reported clearly.

However, a follow-up study of 40 people that attempted to replicate these results failed to find aloe more effective than placebo. For more information, including dosage and safety issues, see the full **Aloe** article.

Cayenne

Capsaicin is the "hot" in cayenne pepper. Creams made from capsaicin are used to treat a number of pain-related conditions. Some evidence indicates that capsaicin cream may be helpful for psoriasis as well. A double-blind, placebo-controlled trial of almost 200 people found that use of topical capsaicin can improve itching as well as overall severity of psoriasis. Benefits were also seen in a smaller double-blind trial.

For more information on capsaicin cream, see the **Cayenne** article.

Fish Oil

The evidence regarding fish oil's effectiveness for psoriasis remains incomplete and contradictory.

An 8-week, double-blind study followed 28 people with chronic psoriasis. Half received 10 capsules of fish oil daily, and the other half received a placebo. By the end of the study, researchers saw significant improvement in itching, redness, and scaling, but not in the size of the psoriasis patches. However, another double-blind study followed 145 people with moderate to severe psoriasis for 4 months and found no benefit as compared to placebo.

For more information, including dosage and safety issues, see the full **Fish Oil** article.

Other Natural Treatments

Based on very preliminary evidence, **shark cartilage** and **cetylated fatty acids** have also been proposed for treatment of psoriasis.

Beta-carotene, barberry, burdock, chromium, cleav- ers, *Coleus forskohlii*, **goldenseal**, topical **licorice** cream, **milk thistle, red clover, selenium, taurine, vitamin E, yellow dock**, and **zinc** are also sometimes mentioned as possible treatments for psoriasis. However, as yet there is no meaningful evidence that they work.

A somewhat toxic natural substance called *fumaric acid* is sometimes recommended for psoriasis as well. **Vitamin A** or special forms of **vitamin D** taken at high levels may improve symptoms, but these are dangerous treatments that should be used only under the supervision of a physician.

People using the drug **methotrexate** for psoriasis frequently develop nausea, mouth sores, and other side effects. Evidence indicates that taking **folate** supplements may help.

Seal oil has shown a hint of promise for treatment of psoriatic arthritis (a type of joint pain and inflammation that can occur in association with psoriasis).

Although case reports suggest that **acupuncture** might be useful for psoriasis, a controlled trial failed to find acupuncture more effective than fake acupuncture.

One study found that **hypnosis** may improve psoriasis symptoms.

Herbs and Supplements to Use Only with Caution

Various herbs and supplements may interact adversely with drugs used to treat psoriasis. For more information on this potential risk, see the individual drug article in the Drug Interactions section of this book.

Raynaud's Phenomenon

PRINCIPAL PROPOSED NATURAL TREATMENTS: *None*

OTHER PROPOSED NATURAL TREATMENTS: *Acupuncture, Arginine, Biofeedback, Fish Oil, Ginkgo, Gamma-Linolenic Acid (GLA), Inositol Hexaniacinate, Vitamin C*

Raynaud's phenomenon is a little understood condition in which the fingers and toes show an exaggerated sensitivity to cold. Classic cases show a characteristic white, blue, and red color sequence as the digits lose blood supply and then rewarm. Some people develop only one or two of these signs.

The cause of Raynaud's phenomenon is unknown. It can occur by itself as primary Raynaud's (also called

Raynaud's disease) or as a consequence of other illnesses, such as **scleroderma**. In the latter case, it is called *secondary Raynaud's*.

Conventional treatment consists mainly of reassurance and the recommendation to avoid exposure to cold and the use of tobacco (which can worsen Raynaud's). In severe cases, a variety of drugs can be tried.

Proposed Natural Treatments

Preliminary evidence supports the use of several natural supplements in the treatment of Raynaud's phenomenon. Most of the positive evidence regards primary Raynaud's.

In a 17-week, double-blind, placebo-controlled trial of 35 people with Raynaud's, **fish oil** (taken at a dose that provided a total of 3.96 g of EPA and 2.64 g of DHA daily) reduced reaction to cold among those with primary Raynaud's disease, but did not seem to help those with Raynaud's caused by other illnesses.

In an 84-day, double-blind, placebo-controlled study of 23 people with primary Raynaud's, use of **inositol**

hexaniacinate significantly reduced the frequency of attacks.

The herb **Ginkgo biloba** has been found to increase circulation in the fingertips and thus has been proposed as a treatment for Raynaud's. A 10-week, double-blind, placebo-controlled trial of 22 people with primary Raynaud's found that use of ginkgo at the very high dose of 120 mg 3 times daily reduced the number of Raynaud's attacks.

One very small double-blind study found suggestions that **evening primrose oil** might help primary or secondary Raynaud's.

A double-blind, placebo-controlled crossover trial of 10 individuals failed to find **arginine** at 8 g daily helpful for primary Raynaud's.

A small double-blind trial tested the effects of a single dose of 2 g vitamin C on Raynaud's caused by scleroderma and found no benefit.

Current evidence suggests that **biofeedback** is at most no more than marginally effective for Raynaud's. The same is true of **acupuncture**.

Restless Legs Syndrome

PRINCIPAL PROPOSED NATURAL TREATMENTS: *None*

OTHER PROPOSED NATURAL TREATMENTS: *Folate, Iron, Magnesium, Vitamin B$_{12}$, Vitamin C, Vitamin E*

People with restless legs syndrome (RLS) often feel an intense urge to move their legs, particularly when sitting still or trying to fall asleep. Unlike those with nighttime leg cramps—a different condition—people with RLS don't experience pain. Instead, they may describe an uncomfortable "creepy-crawly sensation" inside their legs. Walking relieves the symptoms, but as soon as people settle down again, the urge to move recurs. The feeling is sometimes described as "wanting to ride a bicycle under the covers."

RLS tends to run in families, often emerging or worsening with age. People with RLS frequently have another condition as well, called *periodic leg movements in sleep* (PLMS). People with PLMS kick their legs frequently during the night, disrupting their own sleep and that of their bed partner.

Since RLS is occasionally linked to other serious diseases, it's advisable to see a doctor if you have its symptoms.

Conventional medical treatment for RLS usually involves taking a levodopa–carbidopa combination, better known as a treatment for Parkinson's disease. The drug quinine has been used in the past, but one double-blind study found no benefit.

Because of this and a risk of dangerous side effects, quinine is no longer used for this purpose.

Proposed Natural Treatments

Preliminary evidence suggests that symptoms of RLS may be relieved by supplementation with one of several minerals or vitamins, including magnesium, folate, iron, and vitamin E. However, as yet there are no double-blind studies to support these treatments and, therefore, their use remains speculative.

Magnesium

Preliminary studies suggest that supplemental **magnesium** may be helpful for RLS, even when magnesium levels are normal. An open study of 10 people with insomnia related to RLS or periodic leg movements in sleep found that their sleep improved significantly when they took magnesium nightly for 4 to 6 weeks. However, open studies are extremely unreliable, because they do not factor out the placebo effect and no double-blind studies on magnesium for RLS have been reported.

Folate

Based on numerous case reports of improvement, **folate** is also sometimes recommended for RLS. Symptoms decreased in one study of 45 patients given 5 to 30 mg of folate daily. However, again this was not a double-blind experiment and therefore the meaningfulness of the results are questionable. Keep in mind that such high doses of folate should be administered only under medical supervision.

Folate taken in nutritional doses may be of benefit to pregnant women with RLS who are deficient in this vitamin.

Iron

A number of studies have linked RLS to low levels of **iron** in the blood. In one analysis of the medical records of 27 people with RLS, those with the most severe symptoms had lower-than-average levels of serum ferritin, one measure of iron deficiency. In another study in which 18 elderly people with RLS were compared with 18 elderly people without the condition, those with RLS also had reduced levels of serum ferritin. When 15 of these people were given iron, all but one experienced a reduction in symptoms. Those with the lowest initial ferritin levels improved the most. However, once more, these were not double-blind studies and, therefore, their results cannot be trusted.

In contrast to these results, a double-blind study of 28 people found that iron didn't relieve RLS any better than placebo. However, in this particular study, participants had normal levels of iron on average. The study didn't effectively measure whether iron might help RLS among people with iron deficiency.

One theory holds that mild iron deficiency may cause RLS by decreasing the amount of a neurotransmitter called *dopamine*. This theory is supported by findings that conventional drugs which increase dopamine activity (such as the Parkinson's disease medication mentioned above) can also alleviate RLS.

The bottom line: Iron supplements might be useful for people with RLS who are also deficient in iron, but this has not been proven. Still, if you're deficient in iron, that's a situation worth correcting. Note that tests for anemia won't necessarily pick up the low-grade iron deficiency that is linked to RLS. For that purpose, you'll need tests that specifically evaluate iron levels, such as ferritin, serum iron, and total iron-binding capacity.

Vitamin E

Vitamin E has also been proposed for this condition. In one report, seven out of nine people with RLS given 400 to 800 IU daily of vitamin E experienced virtually complete control of symptoms, while the other two had partial relief. Other anecdotal reports suggest that vitamin C may be useful, and that **vitamin B$_{12}$** may benefit people with RLS who are deficient in this nutrient. However, while these reports may sound good, again they mean next to nothing because they were not double-blind studies.

Rheumatoid Arthritis

PRINCIPAL PROPOSED NATURAL TREATMENTS: *Fish Oil*

OTHER PROPOSED NATURAL TREATMENTS: *Boswellia, Bromelain, Cat's Claw, Curcumin (Turmeric), Devil's Claw, Folate, Food Allergen Avoidance, Gamma-Linolenic Acid (GLA), Magnet Therapy, Olive Oil, Tripterygium wilfordii, Vegetarian Diet, Vitamin B$_6$, Vitamin E, Zinc*

Rheumatoid arthritis (RA) is an autoimmune disease in the general family of **lupus**. For reasons that are not understood, in rheumatoid arthritis the immune system goes awry and begins attacking innocent tissues, especially cartilage in the joints. Various joints become red, hot, and swollen under the onslaught. The pattern of inflammation is usually symmetrical, occurring on both sides of the body. Other symptoms include inflammation of the eyes, nodules or lumps under the skin, and a general feeling of malaise.

Rheumatoid arthritis is more common in women than in men and typically begins between the ages of 35 and 60. The diagnosis is made by matching the pattern of symptoms with certain characteristic laboratory results.

Medical treatment consists mainly of two categories of drugs: anti-inflammatory drugs in the ibuprofen family (nonsteroidal anti-inflammatory drugs, or NSAIDs) and drugs that may be able to put rheumatoid arthritis into full or partial remission, the so-called disease-modifying antirheumatic drugs (DMARDs).

Anti-inflammatory drugs relieve symptoms of rheumatoid arthritis but do not change the overall progression of the disease, whereas the DMARDs seem to affect the disease itself. A good analogy might be the various options available to "treat" a house "suffering" from a severe termite infestation. You could remove heavy furniture, tiptoe about instead of holding public dances, and put large beams under the joists. However, none of these methods would do anything to stop the gradual destruction of your house. These methods are like NSAIDs and other supportive techniques in that they treat only the symptoms.

A more definitive approach would be to hire an exterminator and kill the termites. In medical terms, this would be described as a disease-modifying treatment. Because medical treatments for chronic diseases are seldom as completely effective as this example, a closer analogy might be spraying a chemical that slows the spread of termites but does not stop them.

In rheumatoid arthritis, the drugs believed to alter the course of the disease (to slow it down or stop it) include antimalarials (hydroxychloroquine and chloroquine), sulfasalazine, TNF inhibitors (etanercept, infliximab, and adalimumab), interleukin-1 receptor antagonists, leflunomide methotrexate, gold compounds, D-penicillamine and cytotoxic agents (azathioprine, cyclophosphamide, and cyclosporine). They are unrelated to one another but work somewhat similarly in practice.

Unfortunately, most of the drugs in this category can cause severe side effects. Because of this toxicity, for years a so-called pyramid approach was taken with people with rheumatoid arthritis. Physicians started with NSAIDs to help with the pain and inflammation and progressed to successively stronger and more toxic medications only when the basic treatments failed. Natural treatments such as those described here might also be useful in early stages.

However, over the last few years, research has found that severe joint damage occurs very early in rheumatoid arthritis. This evidence has caused many authorities to suggest early, aggressive treatment with disease-modifying drugs to prevent joint damage. Nonetheless, this approach has not been universally adopted, and some physicians still prescribe NSAIDs for early stages of rheumatoid arthritis. The treatments described here may be reasonable alternative options.

Principal Proposed Natural Treatments

Rheumatoid arthritis is a difficult disease and no alternative approach solves it easily. Even if you choose to use alternative methods, you should maintain regular visits to a rheumatologist to watch for serious complications. Finally, keep in mind that medical treatment may be able to slow the progression of rheumatoid arthritis. It is not likely that any of the alternative options have the same power.

Fish oil is the only natural treatment for rheumatoid arthritis with significant documentation. According to the results of at least 13 double-blind, placebo-controlled studies involving a total of more than 500 participants, supplementation with omega-3 fatty acids can significantly reduce the symptoms of rheumatoid arthritis. However, unlike some of the standard treatments, fish oil has not been shown to slow the progression of rheumatoid arthritis. It has been suggested that omega-3 supplementation is more effective when omega-6 intake (particularly arachidonic acid) is kept low, as occurs with a vegetarian diet. The benefits of fish oil may also be enhanced by simultaneous use of olive oil.

For more information, including dosage and safety issues, see the full **Fish Oil** article.

Flaxseed oil has been offered as a more palatable substitute for fish oil, but it doesn't seem to work.

Other Proposed Natural Treatments

Boswellia

Boswellia serrata is a shrub-like tree that grows in the dry hills of the Indian subcontinent. It is the source of a resin called *salai guggal*, which has been used for thousands of years in Ayurvedic medicine, the traditional medicine of the region. It is very similar to a resin from a related tree, *Boswellia carteri*, which is also known as *frankincense*. Both substances have been used historically for arthritis.

Recent research has identified boswellic acids as the likely active ingredients in boswellia. In animal studies, boswellic acids have shown anti-inflammatory effects, but their mechanism of action seems to be quite different from that of standard anti-inflammatory medications.

An issue of *Phytomedicine* that was devoted to boswellia briefly reviewed previously unpublished studies on the herb. A pair of placebo-controlled trials involving a total of 81 people with rheumatoid arthritis found significant reductions in swelling and pain over the course of 3 months. Furthermore, a comparative study of 60 participants over 6 months found the boswellia extract relieved symptoms about as well as oral gold therapy. However, keep in mind that while gold shots can induce remission in rheumatoid arthritis, we have no evidence that boswellia can do the same.

Another double-blind study found no difference between boswellia and placebo. The bottom line is that we need more research to know for sure whether boswellia is an effective treatment for rheumatoid arthritis.

For more information, including dosage and safety issues, see the full **Boswellia** article.

Devil's Claw

The herb devil's claw may be beneficial in rheumatoid arthritis. One double-blind study followed 89 people with rheumatoid arthritis for 2 months. The group given devil's claw showed a significant decrease in pain intensity and an improvement in mobility.

Another double-blind study of 50 people with various types of arthritis showed that 10 days of treatment with devil's claw provided significant pain relief.

For more information, including dosage and safety issues, see the full **Devil's Claw** article.

Other Herbs and Supplements

Preliminary evidence, including small double-blind trials, support the use of the following herbs and supplements for the treatment of rheumatoid arthritis: **gamma-linolenic acid** (GLA, found in evening primrose oil and borage oil), **cat's claw** (*Uncaria tomentosa*), and the **Chinese herb** *Tripterygium wilfordii* (either applied topically or taken orally).

Note: *Tripterygium wilfordii* is believed to be unsafe for pregnant or nursing women, and may present risks in other groups as well.

Highly preliminary evidence suggests potential benefits with the following herbs and supplements: **methyl sulfonyl methane** (MSM), **yucca**, and a mixture of poplar, ash, and **goldenrod**.

Vitamin E may reduce pain in rheumatoid arthritis, but it does not seem to reduce inflammation. Some evidence suggests that adding vitamin E, or vitamin E plus other antioxidants, to standard rheumatoid arthritis therapy might improve results.

Individuals taking the drug **methotrexate** for treatment of rheumatoid arthritis may benefit by taking **folate** supplements. Folate appears to reduce methotrexate side effects, including mouth sores, nausea, and liver inflammation. In addition, folate supplements may help reverse a more subtle methotrexate side-effect: a rise in blood levels of **homocysteine**. Elevated levels of homocysteine are thought to increase risk of heart-disease.

The following treatments are also sometimes proposed as effective for rheumatoid arthritis, but there is as yet little to no scientific evidence for or against their use: **adrenal extract**, **beta-carotene**, **betaine hydrochloride**, **boron**, **burdock**, **cayenne**, **chamomile**, **copper**, **feverfew**, **folate**, **ginger**, **L-histidine**, **horsetail**, **magnesium**, **manganese**, **molybdenum**, **pantothenic acid**, **D-phenylalanine**, *Perilla frutescens*, **pregnenolone**, **proteolytic enzymes**, sea cucumber, and **vitamin C**.

Current evidence regarding **green-lipped mussel** for rheumatoid arthritis is more negative than positive.

One study failed to find **vitamin B$_6$** at a dose of 50 mg daily helpful for rheumatoid arthritis, despite a general B$_6$ deficiency seen in people with this condition. **Zinc** supplements have been evaluated as a treatment for rheumatoid arthritis, but overall the study results have not been encouraging. Other treatments that have as yet generally failed to prove effective in small double-blind trials include **selenium**, collagen, **probiotics**, **white willow**, and an **Ayurvedic herbal mixture** containing extracts of **ashwagandha**, boswellia, **ginger**, and **turmeric**. Two studies commonly cited as evidence that turmeric alone is useful for rheumatoid arthritis actually fail to provide any meaningful supporting evidence.

Other Alternative Therapies

Adopting a vegetarian diet may help mild rheumatoid arthritis. Identifying and avoiding **food allergens** has also been tried, but one controlled trial found no clear evidence of benefit with a low saturated fat, hypoallergenic diet.

Magnet therapy has shown some promise for rheumatoid arthritis.

A double-blind, placebo-controlled study tested the effect of treatment on a single **acupuncture** point in 56 people with rheumatoid arthritis, but failed to find benefit. However, using a single acupuncture point to treat a complex disease such as rheumatoid arthritis must be regarded as highly questionable; normal acupuncture treatment would involve many points.

Herbs and Supplements to Use Only with Caution

Various herbs and supplements may interact adversely with drugs used to treat rheumatoid arthritis. For more information on this potential risk, see the individual drug article in the Drug Interactions section of this book.

Rosacea

RELATED TERMS: *Acne Rosacea*

PRINCIPAL PROPOSED NATURAL TREATMENTS: *Chrysanthemum Indicum (Topical)*

OTHER PROPOSED NATURAL TREATMENTS: *Aloe, Apple Cider Vinegar, Aromatherapy, Betaine Hydrochloride, Burdock, Chamomile, Chinese Herbal Medicine, Digestive Enzymes, Food Allergen Avoidance, Green Tea (Topical), Niacinamide (Topical), Red Clover, Rose Hips, Selenium, Vitamin B–Complex, Vitamin C, Vitamin D, Vitamin E, Yellow Dock, Zinc*

Rosacea is a chronic skin condition that affects the skin of the face (generally, to the greatest extent near the center), the eyelids, and, sometimes, the neck, and upper back and chest. Symptoms mostly occur in sun-exposed areas, and consist of redness, acne-like pustules and papules (but not comedones, or blackheads), visible blood vessels (telangiectasias), and swelling of the skin. Dramatic facial flushing may occur after consuming alcohol, hot drinks, or spicy foods, or after exposure to excessive sunlight or extremes of hot or cold. In the eye, acne rosacea produces symptoms known as blepharitis. Over time, rosacea may cause the nose to become enlarged.

Treatment of rosacea involves avoiding stimuli that worsen the disease, as well as using medications similar to those used for acne. Laser treatment can remove unsightly blood vessels and reduce flushing.

Proposed Natural Treatments for Rosacea

A substantial (246-participant) 12-week, double-blind study found that a cream containing 1% *Chrysanthellum indicum* significantly improved rosacea symptoms as compared to placebo.

Weaker evidence hints that cream containing **niacinamide** might be helpful.

One preliminary study, available as yet only in abstract form, found some evidence that a cream made from **green tea** may provide benefits as well.

Some alternative practitioners believe that rosacea is

caused by poor digestion and recommend use of **betaine hydrochloride** or apple cider vinegar to increase stomach acid. In addition, they may recommend **digestive enzymes**. However, there is no meaningful scientific evidence to indicate that use of these treatments will reduce symptoms of rosacea.

Other natural treatments sometimes recommended for rosacea, but that also lack scientific support, include **aloe, aromatherapy, burdock, chamomile, Chinese herbal medicine, food allergen avoidance, red clover, rose hips, selenium, vitamin B–complex, vitamins C, D,** and **E, yellow dock,** and **zinc.**

For rosacea symptoms that affect the eye, see the article on **Blepharitis.**

Herbs and Supplements to Use Only with Caution

Various herbs and supplements might interact adversely with drugs used to treat rosacea. For more information, see the individual drug article in the Drug Interactions section of this book.

Scar Tissue

RELATED TERMS: *Keloid Scars*

PRINCIPAL PROPOSED NATURAL TREATMENTS: *None*

OTHER PROPOSED NATURAL TREATMENTS: *Acupuncture, Allantoin, Aloe Vera, Coconut Oil, Collagen, Elastin, Gotu Kola, Jojoba Oil, Lavender Oil, Magnet Therapy, Massage, Selenium, Snail Extract, Tamanu Oil, Vitamin A, Vitamin C, Vitamin E, Zinc*

When the body repairs a wound, it often does so by creating fibrous scar tissue. Internal scars, such as may develop following surgery, can cause significant pain. Surface scars are generally painless, but they may be cosmetically unpleasant. In some cases, scars on the skin can develop into a special form of oversized scar called a *keloid.* Keloids are generally red or pink and often form a ridge several millimeters above the skin. These scars occur when the body continues to fill the scar with collagen after it has healed. Darker-skinned people are more likely to develop keloids than those with lighter skin.

Conventional treatment of any type of scar is less than entirely satisfactory. Keloids and other scars on the skin may be reduced in size by freezing (cryotherapy), steroid injections, radiation therapy, or surgical removal. However, a new, even more visible scar may develop in the place of the one that was removed. Similarly, removal of painful internal scars may lead to the new formation of painful scar tissue.

Proposed Natural Treatments

The herb **gotu kola** is said to help remove keloid scars. When used for this purpose, it is taken orally, applied to the skin, or injected into the scar. However, there is no reliable evidence that it is effective.

According to some schools of **acupuncture**, surface scars impede the flow of "energy" and thereby cause various illnesses. Acupuncture treatment of both surface and internal scars is said either to shrink them or, at least, to reduce their effects. However, there is no meaningful scientific evidence to indicate that acupuncture offers any benefits for scars.

Other natural treatments proposed for scars, but again without reliable supporting evidence, include: *Aloe vera,* allantoin, coconut oil, collagen, elastin, jojoba oil, lavender oil, **massage, magnet therapy, selenium,** snail extract, tamanu oil, **vitamin A, vitamin C, vitamin E,** and **zinc.**

Schizophrenia

PRINCIPAL PROPOSED NATURAL TREATMENTS: *Glycine*

OTHER PROPOSED NATURAL TREATMENTS: *Coenzyme Q_{10} (CoQ_{10}), D-Serine, Eicosapentaenoic Acid (EPA), Folate, Gingko, Melatonin, Milk Thistle, rTMS, Vitamin B_3 (Niacin), Vitamin B_6, Vitamin C, Several Natural Treatments for Tardive Dyskinesia*

HERBS AND SUPPLEMENTS TO AVOID: *Chromium Picolinate, Dong Quai, Kava, Phenylalanine, St. John's Wort, Yohimbe*

Schizophrenia is a chronic, severe, disabling brain disease. People with schizophrenia often suffer terrifying symptoms such as hearing internal voices not heard by others or believing that other people are reading their minds, controlling their thoughts, or plotting to harm them. These symptoms may leave them fearful and withdrawn. Their speech and behavior can be so disorganized that they may be incomprehensible or frightening to others. Schizophrenia increases a person's risk of suicide, self-mutilation, substance abuse, and other social problems such as unemployment, homelessness, and incarceration.

Schizophrenia is found all over the world. The severity of the symptoms and the long-lasting, chronic pattern of schizophrenia often cause a high degree of disability. Approximately 1% of the population develops schizophrenia during their lifetime; more than 2 million Americans suffer from the illness in a given year. Although schizophrenia affects men and women with equal frequency, the disorder often appears earlier in men. Men are usually affected in their late teens or early twenties, while women are generally affected in their twenties to early thirties.

Researchers aren't sure what causes schizophrenia. Problems with brain structure and chemistry are thought to play a role. There appears to be a strong genetic component to schizophrenia, but some researchers believe that environmental factors may contribute. They theorize that a viral infection in infancy and/or extreme stress may trigger schizophrenia in people who are predisposed to it.

Conventional drug treatment for schizophrenia is moderately effective. While it seldom produces a true cure, it can enable a person with schizophrenia to function in society.

Principal Proposed Natural Treatments

Untreated schizophrenia is a very dangerous disease for which there is effective treatment and, for this reason, it is not ethical to perform studies that compare a hypothetical new treatment against placebo. Therefore, studies of natural treatments for schizophrenia have looked at their potential benefit for enhancing the effects of standard treatment (or minimizing its side effects). No natural treatments have been studied as sole therapy for schizophrenia.

Up until recently, all common medications used for schizophrenia fell into a class called **phenothiazines.** These drugs are most effective for the *positive* symptoms of schizophrenia, such as hallucinations and delusions. (Such symptoms are called *positive* because they indicate the *presence* of abnormal mental functions, rather than the *absence* of normal mental functions.) In general, however, these medications are less helpful for the *negative* symptoms of schizophrenia, such as apathy, depression, and social withdrawal.

The supplement glycine might be of benefit here. A clinical trial enrolled 22 participants who continued to experience negative symptoms of schizophrenia despite standard therapy. In this double-blind, placebo-controlled, crossover study, volunteers were randomly assigned to receive either 0.8 g of glycine per kg of body weight (about 60 g per day) or placebo for 6 weeks, along with their regular medications. The groups were then switched after a 2-week "wash-out" period during which they all received placebo.

Significant improvements (about 30%) in symptoms such as depression and apathy were seen with glycine when compared to placebo. As a bonus, glycine also reduced some of the side effects caused by the prescription drugs. Furthermore, the benefits appeared to continue for another 8 weeks after the glycine was discontinued.

No changes were seen in positive symptoms (for instance, hallucinations), but it isn't possible to tell whether that is because these symptoms were already being controlled by prescription medications or whether glycine simply has no effect on that aspect of schizophrenia.

Four other small double-blind, placebo-controlled clinical trials of glycine together with standard drugs for schizophrenia (including the newer drugs olanzapine and risperidone) also found it to be helpful for negative symptoms.

However, one small double-blind, placebo-controlled trial (19 participants) suggests that adding glycine to the drug clozapine may not be a good idea. In this study, glycine was found to reduce the benefits of clozapine without helping to relieve the participants' negative symptoms. Lack of benefit, although no actual harm, was seen in two other double-blind, placebo-controlled trials of glycine and clozapine.

Curiously, a natural substance (sarcosine) that *blocks* the action of glycine has also shown promise for schizophrenia.

For more information, including dosage and safety issues, see the full **Glycine** article.

Other Proposed Natural Treatments

Numerous other natural therapies have shown promise for aiding various aspects of treatment for schizophrenia, but in most cases the current supporting evidence is weak at best.

Enhancing Drug Action

Four out of five published double-blind, placebo-controlled studies indicate that EPA (eicosapentaenoic acid, a major constituent of **fish oil**) may enhance the effectiveness of drug treatment for schizophrenia. However, all of these studies were quite small.

A small 6-week, double-blind, placebo-controlled study evaluated the potential effectiveness of the supplement **DHEA** taken at a dose of 100 mg daily for enhancing the effectiveness of drug treatment for schizophrenia. The results indicated that use of DHEA led to improvement in various symptoms, especially negative symptoms (see discussion of glycine, above, for definition).

Preliminary evidence suggests that **ginkgo** and the amino acid D-serine may also enhance the effectiveness of various anti-psychotic drugs.

Tardive Dyskinesia

Tardive dyskinesia (TD) is a potentially permanent side effect of drugs used to control schizophrenia and other psychoses. This late-developing (tardy, or tardive) complication consists of annoying, mostly uncontrollable movements (dyskinesias). Typical symptoms include repetitive sucking or blinking, slow twisting of the hands, or other movements of the face and limbs. TD can cause tremendous social embarrassment to particularly vulnerable people.

Several natural treatments have shown promise for preventing or treating TD. For more information, see the **Tardive Dyskinesia** article.

Other Drug Side Effects

Vitamin B_6 might also reduce symptoms of akathesia, a type of restlessness associated with phenothiazine antipsychotics.

One small double-blind study found that use of DHEA reduced the Parkinson-like movement disorders that may occur in people taking phenothiazine drugs.

According to studies performed in China, the herb ginkgo may reduce various side effects caused by drugs used to treat schizophrenia.

Preliminary studies suggest that phenothiazine drugs might deplete the body of **coenzyme Q_{10}** (CoQ_{10}). While there is as yet no evidence that taking CoQ_{10} supplements provides any specific benefit for people using phenothiazines, supplementing with CoQ_{10} might be a good idea on general principles.

The herb **milk thistle** might protect against the liver toxicity sometimes caused by phenothiazine drugs.

Other Options

Preliminary evidence suggests that a special form of **magnet therapy** called *repetitive transcranial magnetic stimulation* (rTMS) may be useful for schizophrenia. However, not all studies have found benefits above the placebo effect, and in any case rTMS is not yet available outside a research setting.

A study of 19 people with schizophrenia who had disturbed sleep patterns found that 2 mg of controlled-release **melatonin** improved sleep.

High doses of various vitamins, including **vitamin A, vitamin B_1, vitamin B_3** (niacin), **vitamin B_6, vitamin B_{12}, vitamin E, folate**, and **vitamin C**, have all been suggested for the treatment of schizophrenia, but the evidence that they offer any real benefit remains incomplete and contradictory at best.

Sciatica

Herbs and Supplements to Avoid

There are some indications that using the supplement **phenylalanine** while taking antipsychotic drugs might increase the risk of developing tardive dyskinesia.

Antipsychotic drugs can cause dystonic reactions—sudden intense movements and prolonged muscle contraction of the neck and eyes. There is some evidence that the herb **kava** can increase the risk or severity of this side effect.

Phenothiazine drugs can cause increased sensitivity to the sun. Various herbs, including **St. John's wort** and **dong quai**, can also cause this problem. Combined treatment with herb and drug might increase the risk further.

St. John's wort might also interact adversely with the newer antipsychotic drugs in the clozapine family. If you take one of these drugs and then start taking St. John's wort, your blood levels of the drug may fall. However, if you are already taking both the herb and the drug, and then you stop St. John's wort, the level of drug in your body could reach the toxic point.

The supplement **chromium** is often sold in the form chromium picolinate. Because picolinate can alter levels of various neurotransmitters (substances that the brain uses to function), there are theoretical concerns that it could cause problems for people with schizophrenia.

The herb **yohimbe** is relatively toxic and can cause problems if used incorrectly. Phenothiazine medications may increase the risk of this toxicity.

Sciatica

RELATED TERMS: *Sciatic Pain*

PRINCIPAL PROPOSED NATURAL TREATMENTS: *None*

OTHER PROPOSED NATURAL TREATMENTS: *Acupuncture, Alexander Technique, Biofeedback, Chiropractic, Feldenkrais, Massage, Pilates, Prolotherapy, Tai Chi, Yoga*

Sciatica is irritation of the sciatic nerve, a major nerve that passes down the back of each thigh. The sciatic nerve originates in the lower spine and travels deep in the pelvis to the lower buttocks. From there it passes along the back of each upper leg and divides at the knee into branches that go to the feet. Sciatica typically causes pain that shoots down the back of one thigh or buttock.

Anything that causes irritation or puts pressure on the sciatic nerve can cause sciatica. The most common cause is probably a sprain or strain of muscles or ligaments in the area and, for this reason, sciatica is often associated with low back pain. The cushions between the bones of the spine—the disks—can also cause sciatica when they bulge out of place or degenerate. Other causes of sciatica include spinal stenosis (narrowing of the spinal canal in the lumbar area), spondylolisthesis (slippage of a bone in the low back), and, very rarely, benign or malignant tumors.

Diagnosis of sciatica is made by symptoms, neurologic evaluation, and tests, such as nerve conduction study, x-ray, and MRI scan. Common symptoms include the following:

➤ **Burning, tingling, or a shooting pain down the back of one leg**
➤ **Pain in one leg or buttock that is worse with sitting, standing up, coughing, sneezing, or straining**
➤ **Weakness or numbness in one leg or foot**

More serious symptoms that sometimes occur in sciatica include difficulty walking, standing, or moving; increasing weakness or numbness in the leg or foot; and loss of bowel or bladder control.

In most cases, sciatic pain resolves on its own without specific treatment. Bed rest, although still sometimes recommended, is probably not helpful. However, physical therapy techniques and steroid injections have shown promise. If permanent nerve damage is threatened, surgery may be necessary.

Attacks of sciatica tend to recur. Certain common

sense steps that may help prevent recurrences include the following:

➤ When lifting, hold the object close to your chest, maintain a straight back, and use your leg muscles to slowly rise.

➤ Practice good posture to reduce pressure on your spine.

➤ If possible, avoid sitting or standing in one position for prolonged periods.

➤ Use a low back support during prolonged sitting. Rest one foot on a low stool if standing for long periods.

➤ Sleep on a firm mattress.

➤ Exercise regularly, at least 30 minutes most days of the week. Good choices include walking, swimming, or exercises recommended by your doctor or physical therapist.

➤ Consider job retraining if your work requires a lot of heavy lifting or sitting.

Proposed Natural Treatments

Acupuncture has shown promise for sciatica, but the research evidence supporting its use remains highly preliminary. Similarly, **biofeedback**, **chiropractic**, **massage**, and **prolotherapy**, while sometimes advocated for sciatic pain, have not been proven effective.

Alexander Technique, Feldenkrais, Pilates, **Tai Chi**, and **yoga** are thought to improve posture and movement habits. On this basis, these methods are advocated for preventing or treating sciatica, but again, proof of effectiveness is lacking.

For other approaches that might be useful for sciatica, see the articles on **low back pain** and **soft tissue pain**.

Scleroderma

RELATED TERMS: *Systemic Sclerosis, SSc*

PRINCIPAL PROPOSED NATURAL TREATMENTS: *None*

OTHER PROPOSED NATURAL TREATMENTS: *Acupuncture; Beta-carotene; Boswellia; Danshen Root; Gotu Kola; Methyl Sulfonyl Methane (MSM); Para-aminobenzoic Acid (PABA); Selenium; Thymus Extract; Vitamin C; Vitamin E; Treatments for Raynaud's Phenomenon, Rheumatoid Arthritis, and Esophageal Reflux*

HERBS AND SUPPLEMENTS TO AVOID: *L-tryptophan, Combination Therapy with 5-HTP and the Drug Carbidopa*

S cleroderma, technically called *systemic sclerosis* or *SSc*, is a disease of unknown cause that affects the connective tissues of the skin and various organs. Common symptoms include thickening and tightening of the skin (beginning with the extremities), Raynaud's phenomenon (a condition characterized by an exaggerated reaction in the fingertips to cold exposure), joint pain (especially in the fingers and knees), esophageal reflux (heartburn), calcium deposits under the skin, and telangiectasias (mats of enlarged small blood vessels). Scleroderma can lead to serious complications, such as fibrosis of the lungs, heart, and kidneys; for this reason, medical supervision is essential. There is no cure as yet for scleroderma, although

drugs may be used to alleviate the various individual symptoms of the disease.

Proposed Natural Treatments

The supplement **PABA** has been suggested as a treatment for scleroderma. A 4-month, double-blind study of 146 people with longstanding, stable scleroderma failed to find any evidence of benefit. However, half of the participants in this trial dropped out before the end, making the results unreliable.

The herb **gotu kola** has a long history of use for various skin conditions; for this reason, it has been tried as a treatment for scleroderma. However, as yet there is no meaningful evidence that it is effective. Other herbs and supplements proposed for treatment of scleroderma (but that do not have any significant supporting evidence) include **boswellia, thymus extract, MSM,** antioxidants (such as the antioxidant vitamins **vitamin C, vitamin E,** and **beta-carotene,** and the mineral **selenium,** which supports the body's own antioxidant defense system), and danshen root. (One study failed to find vitamin C helpful for the treatment of Raynaud's phenomenon associated with scleroderma.)

One highly preliminary study suggests that **acupuncture** might have value for this condition.

Finally, several herbs and supplements have shown promise for treating the individual symptoms of scleroderma. For more information, see the articles on **Raynaud's phenomenon, rheumatoid arthritis,** and **esophageal reflux.**

Herbs and Supplements to Avoid

Combination therapy with the supplement **5-HTP** and the drug **carbidopa** has reportedly caused skin changes similar to those that occur in scleroderma. Furthermore, **L-tryptophan,** a supplement closely related to 5-HTP, has been taken off the market because it caused numerous cases of eosinophilia-myalgia syndrome, which is sometimes regarded as a close relative of scleroderma. It is thought that this outbreak was due to a contaminant in a certain batch of the supplement, but some controversy about this explanation remains.

Finally, various herbs and supplements may interact adversely with drugs used to prevent or treat scleroderma. For more information on this potential risk, see the appropriate individual drug articles in the Drug Interactions section of this book.

Seasonal Affective Disorder

RELATED TERMS: *SAD, Seasonal Depression, Winter Depression*
PRINCIPAL PROPOSED NATURAL TREATMENTS: *None*
OTHER PROPOSED NATURAL TREATMENTS: *Melatonin, Negative Ions, St. John's Wort, Vitamin B₁₂, Vitamin D*

In late fall, when the days get shorter, some people develop a special form of depression called *seasonal affective disorder,* or SAD. This condition should not be confused with mild winter blues. It is a real illness, as severely debilitating as any other form of clinical **depression.**

Symptoms are generally worst in January and February, and begin to disappear as the days lengthen in the spring. SAD occurs most often in adolescents and women, but it is not limited to those groups. Up to 25% of the population may suffer from a mild version of SAD and perhaps 5% experience the full disorder.

The cause of SAD is not known, but is believed to relate to the daily biological clock and the way it responds to sunlight. The hormones melatonin and serotonin are thought to be involved, although exactly in what manner remains unclear.

Conventional treatment for SAD focuses on increasing exposure to light. Making sure to get outside during the brightest part of the day may help significantly.

Bright artificial light sources (phototherapy) are also helpful. Antidepressant drugs may be used if these treatments prove ineffective.

Proposed Natural Treatments

Vitamin D

The body creates **vitamin D** when it is exposed to the sun and during the winter vitamin D levels drop. For this reason, it seems logical that vitamin D supplements might help people with SAD. One double-blind, placebo-controlled trial conducted during winter on 44 people without seasonal affective disorder found that vitamin D supplements produced improvements in various measures of mood. However, a double-blind, placebo-controlled study of 2,217 women over 70 failed to find benefit. It has been suggested that phototherapy for SAD works by raising vitamin D levels, but current evidence indicates that this hypothesis is incorrect.

Melatonin

The hormone **melatonin** plays a major role in the daily biological clock. Our bodies are designed to manufacture melatonin at night and stop making it when the sun comes out. One study found that people with SAD had higher levels of melatonin than those without the condition. On this basis, it would seem that supplemental melatonin should worsen SAD symptoms. However, the evidence for such an effect is inconsistent. Some researchers have proposed that interaction between SAD and melatonin might be more complex than merely high or low levels and that, when taken at certain times of day, melatonin might help the condition. A very small study found that when melatonin was given in the afternoon, it produced some benefit for people with SAD. However, a study of melatonin used in the early morning or the late evening failed to find any benefit.

Vitamin B$_{12}$

A small study failed to find **vitamin B$_{12}$** helpful for SAD.

St. John's Wort

The herb St. John's wort has shown considerable promise for treating depression in general. However, the evidence that the herb is helpful for SAD consists only of studies too preliminary to prove much.

Note: Combining St. John's wort with bright light therapy might not be safe. A substance called *hypericin*, found in most St. John's wort products, may cause the body to become hypersensitive to light, increasing risk of damage to the skin and eyes. See the full article on **St. John's wort** for more information.

Negative Ions

For reasons that are not at all clear, use of a device that produces negative ions may help SAD symptoms, according to two preliminary controlled studies.

Seborrheic Dermatitis

RELATED TERMS: *Dandruff, Seborrhea*

PRINCIPAL PROPOSED NATURAL TREATMENTS: *Aloe*

OTHER PROPOSED NATURAL TREATMENTS: *Folate, Tea Tree Oil, Vitamin B$_6$*

Seborrheic dermatitis is an inflammation of the upper layers of the skin that causes scales on the scalp, face, and other parts of the body. When it affects newborns, it's called *cradle cap.*

Seborrheic dermatitis starts gradually. In adults, it often first appears as a condition similar to dandruff, but involving more inflammation of the scalp; itching, burning, or hair loss may occur. Seborrhea may also affect the skin behind the ears, on the eyebrows, on the bridge of the nose, around the nose, or on the trunk.

Besides inflammation of the scalp, newborns with cradle cap might get red bumps on their faces, scaling behind the ears, or a persistent diaper rash. Older children with seborrheic dermatitis may develop a thick, flaky rash.

Seborrhea tends to run in families and often worsens during cold weather. Researchers don't know what causes it and they haven't found a cure, but there are ways to control the condition. Special shampoos containing selenium sulfide, pyrithione zinc, salicylic acid, sulfur, or tar may be helpful for adult dandruff associated with seborrhea.

Corticosteroids may be used for intensely inflammatory lesions; but milder treatments, such as salicylic acid in mineral oil or medicated baby shampoo, are used to treat young children and infants who have scalp rashes.

Principal Proposed Natural Treatments

There is some evidence that the herb aloe might offer some relief to people with seborrheic dermatitis.

The gel inside the cactus-like leaves of the aloe plant (*Aloe vera*) has traditionally been used to treat burns and cuts. While it may not be effective for this purpose, a recent study indicates that aloe may help relieve the symptoms of seborrheic dermatitis.

In this double-blind, placebo-controlled study, 44 adults with seborrheic dermatitis applied either an aloe ointment or a placebo cream to affected areas 2 times daily for 4 to 6 weeks. Compared to the placebo group, those who used aloe reported that their symptoms improved significantly (62% versus 25%). Doctors who examined the participants also concluded that those using aloe had a significant decrease in scaliness, itching, and number of affected areas.

For more information, including dosage and safety issues, see the full **Aloe** article.

Other Proposed Natural Treatments

In a 4-week, placebo-controlled study of 126 people with mild to moderate dandruff, use of 5% **tea tree oil** shampoo significantly reduced dandruff symptoms. Unfortunately, this study was not double-blind: the researchers knew which participants were receiving tea tree oil and which were receiving placebo. For this reason, its results can't be taken as completely reliable. (For more information on why double-blinding matters, see **Why Does This Book Rely on Double-blind Studies?**.)

One small double-blind study found benefit for dandruff with an extract made from the traditional Mexican herb *Solanum chrysotrichum*.

Highly preliminary studies in the 1950s and '60s suggest that **folate** taken orally, or **vitamin B_6** applied topically, may relieve some symptoms.

Essential fatty acids, **zinc**, **iron**, and **vitamins A, E, D, B_1, B_2**, and **C** have also been suggested as treatments for seborrheic dermatitis but there is no real evidence as yet that they work.

Seniors' Health

RELATED TERMS: *Aging, Life Extension*

Many seniors today are interested in natural medicine options. In this article, we discuss the issues of particular importance to this age group.

Natural Treatments Advocated for Seniors in General

Marginal nutritional deficiencies occur more often in older people than in most other age groups. For this reason, many seniors could benefit from enhancing nutrition. For information on this topic, see the **General Nutritional Support** article.

Some proponents of alternative medicine advocate products and treatments for the purpose of life extension. However, despite some promising results in test tube and other preliminary studies, there is no meaningful evidence that any alternative treatment can prolong life.

Numerous natural supplements have been promoted as fountains-of-youth for seniors, said to enhance life in multiple ways, including restoring youthful levels of energy, well-being, and mental function. However, there is again no evidence to indicate that any of these are effective. One such hormone, the widely hyped DHEA, has actually been fairly convincingly shown ineffective for this purpose.

A study published in 1990 created hopes that the human growth hormone (somatotropin or HGH) could increase strength and reverse many symptoms of aging in men. However, subsequent evidence suggests that HGH is not useful for this purpose. In any case, despite widespread marketing, HGH cannot be successfully used as an oral supplement because it is destroyed by stomach acid. (In the positive trial just described, it was administered intravenously.) Various amino acids and other supplements are marketed as HGH-releasers on the premise that they cause the body to increase HGH production. However, there is no reliable evidence that they actually do so to any meaningful extent; in any case, since HGH itself is no fountain-of-youth, this potential effect is of little significance.

Anabolic hormones have also failed to prove useful for enhancing strength in older people. The supplements creatine and HMB (hydroxymethyl butyrate) have shown a bit of promise for this purpose, but the evidence for benefit remains weak.

Note that there is one natural approach guaranteed to enhance strength in seniors: exercise. There is little doubt that increasing exercise is one of the most health-positive steps available for people of any age.

Finally, some evidence suggests that **vitamin D** supplements may improve balance (technically, reduce body sway) in frail seniors and thereby help prevent falls. However, not all studies have found benefits.

Natural Treatments for Specific Conditions of Relevance to Seniors

Even though natural treatments have not been shown helpful for fighting the effects of aging in general, they have shown considerable promise for treating specific health conditions of relevance to older individuals. For information, see the following articles:

For Men
- Aging Skin
- Alzheimer's Disease and Related Conditions
- Back Pain
- Cancer Prevention
- Cancer Treatment
- Cataracts
- Diverticular Disease
- Enhancing Memory and Mental Function
- Fatigue
- General Well-being
- Heart Attack
- Heart Disease Prevention
- Immune Support
- Insomnia
- Macular Degeneration
- Osteoarthritis
- Prostate Cancer
- Prostate Enlargement (BPH)
- Sciatica
- Sexual Dysfunction

For Women
- Aging Skin
- Alzheimer's Disease and Related Conditions
- Back Pain
- Cancer Prevention
- Cancer Treatment
- Cataracts
- Diverticular Disease
- Enhancing Memory and Mental Function
- Fatigue
- General Wellbeing
- Heart Attack
- Heart Disease Prevention
- Immune Support
- Insomnia
- Macular Degeneration
- Menopausal Symptoms
- Osteoarthritis
- Osteoporosis
- Sciatica
- Sexual Dysfunction
- Varicose Veins

Safety Concerns

Many people implicitly believe that "natural" means "safe." However, there is no scientific reason to believe that this should be the case. Many of today's drugs are highly safe, while some herbs and supplements present real safety risks. For information on any issues relevant to any particular substance, see its entry in the Collins Alternative Health Guide, Herbs & Supplements.

Perhaps the biggest issue of concern is interactions between natural supplements and medications. For more information on possible interactions with medications you are taking, see the Drug Interactions section of the Collins Alternative Health Guide.

Sexual Dysfunction in Women

RELATED TERMS: *Antidepressant-induced Sexual Dysfunction, Female Sexual Arousal Disorder, Hypoactive Sexual Desire Disorder, Low Libido in Women*

PRINCIPAL PROPOSED NATURAL TREATMENTS: *None*

OTHER PROPOSED NATURAL TREATMENTS: *Combination Herb/Supplement Therapies, Dehydroepiandrosterone (DHEA), Diindolylmethane (DIM), Horny Goat Weed, Maca, Molybdenum, Rhodiola rosea, Topical Treatment Containing GLA, Vitamin C*

PROBABLY NOT EFFECTIVE TREATMENTS: Ginkgo biloba *for Antidepressant-induced Sexual Dysfunction*

Although male sexual problems have long been the subject of intensive medical research, the equivalent problems in women have received relatively little attention until recently. The tremendous commercial success of the drug Viagra has lately prompted pharmaceutical companies to focus attention on finding a comparable treatment for women.

Loss of libido, painful intercourse, and difficulty achieving orgasm trouble many women. In most cases, the cause is unknown. Possible identifiable causes include side effects from drugs such as antidepressants or sedatives, hormonal insufficiency, or adrenal insufficiency.

Current conventional treatments for sexual dysfunction in women are limited, except when a simple fixable cause is present (such as use of an antidepressant in the SSRI category).

Proposed Natural Treatments

Although there is no good evidence for natural treatments for sexual dysfunction, several substances have shown promising results in preliminary trials. These include DHEA, yohimbine, and arginine.

DHEA

Some evidence suggests that the hormone dehydroepiandrosterone (DHEA) may be helpful for improving sexual function in older women, but not in younger women.

DHEA is produced by the adrenal glands. Levels of DHEA decline naturally with age and fall precipitately in cases of adrenal failure. Because both elderly people and those with adrenal insufficiency report a drop in libido, several studies have examined whether supplemental DHEA can increase libido in these groups.

A 12-month, double-blind, placebo-controlled trial evaluated the effects of DHEA (50 mg daily) in 280 individuals between the ages of 60 and 79. The results showed that women over age 70 experienced an improvement in libido and sexual satisfaction. No benefits were seen in younger women. Two other trials did not find benefit, but they enrolled many fewer people and ran for a shorter period of time.

In addition, two small double-blind, placebo-controlled studies tested whether a one-time dose of DHEA at 300 mg could increase ease of sexual arousal in pre- or postmenopausal women respectively. The results again indicate that DHEA is effective for older women but not for younger women.

One 4-month, double-blind, placebo-controlled study of 24 women with adrenal failure found that 50 mg per day of DHEA (along with standard treatment for adrenal failure) improved libido and sexual satisfaction. DHEA is not usually prescribed to individuals with adrenal failure, but this study suggests that it should be.

For more information, including dosage and safety issues, see the full **DHEA** article.

Combination Products

A double-blind, placebo-controlled trial evaluated a combination therapy containing the amino acid **arginine**; the herbs **ginseng**, **ginkgo**, and **damiana**; and multivitamins and minerals. Researchers enrolled a total of 77 women between the ages of 22 and 71 years and followed them for 4 weeks. All participants complained of poor sexual function.

The results showed superior sexual satisfaction scores in the treatment group compared to the placebo group. Some of the specific benefits seen included enhanced libido, increased frequency of intercourse and orgasm, greater vaginal lubrication, and augmented clitoral sensation.

Yohimbine is a drug derived from the bark of the **yohimbe** tree. Studies have only used the standardized drug, not the actual herb. One small double-blind, crossover study of yohimbine combined with arginine found an increase in measured physical arousal among 23 women with female sexual arousal disorder as compared to placebo. However, the women themselves did not report any noticeable effects. Only the combination of yohimbine and arginine produced results; neither substance was effective when taken on its own.

An open trial of yohimbine alone to treat sexual dysfunction induced by the antidepressant fluoxetine (Prozac) found improvement in 8 out of 9 people, 2 of whom were women. However, in the absence of a placebo group, these results can't be taken as reliable; in addition, there are concerns about the safety of combining yohimbe with antidepressants.

Note: Yohimbine and the herb yohimbe are relatively dangerous substances in general. They should only be used under physician supervision.

The other constituents used in these combination therapies may also present some risks (see the full articles for safety issues).

Other Treatments

One double-blind, placebo-controlled study found evidence that use of **vitamin C** led to an increase in intercourse frequency in healthy women, presumably because it increased libido.

A very small double-blind trial reported that a proprietary topical treatment containing **GLA** and a variety of additional supplements and herbs improved sexual function in woman with female sexual arousal disorder.

A highly preliminary study has been used to claim that the herb ephedra is helpful for women with sexual dysfunction. However, this trial was very small, enrolled women without sexual problems, and only examined sexual responsiveness to visual stimuli. In another study, ephedrine improved female sexual dysfunction caused by SSRI antidepressants, but so did placebo and there was no significant difference between the benefits seen with the two treatments. **Note:** There are serious health risks associated with ephedra. For this reason, we do not recommend that women with sexual dysfunction use ephedra. For more information on the health risks of this herb, see the full **Ephedra** article.

Numerous case reports and uncontrolled studies raised hopes that the herb *Ginkgo biloba* might be an effective treatment for antidepressant-induced sexual dysfunction. However, as always, double-blind, placebo-controlled studies are necessary to truly establish efficacy (see **Why Does This Book Rely on Double-blind Studies?**). When double-blind studies were finally performed, the results indicated that ginkgo is no more effective than placebo.

Other treatments often proposed for treating female sexual dysfunction, but that lack any meaningful supporting evidence, include **horny goat weed**, **maca**, **molybdenum**, **diindolylmethane** (DIM), and *Rhodiola rosea*.

Shingles

RELATED TERMS: Herpes zoster, *Post-herpetic Neuralgia*

PRINCIPAL PROPOSED NATURAL TREATMENTS: *Capsaicin, Proteolytic Enzymes*

OTHER PROPOSED NATURAL TREATMENTS: *Acupuncture, Adenosine Monophosphate (AMP), Vitamin B$_{12}$, Vitamin E*

*H*erpes zoster (shingles) is an acute, painful infection caused by the varicella-zoster virus, the organism that causes chicken pox. It develops many years after the original chicken pox infection, typically in the elderly or those with compromised immune systems. The first sign may be a tingling feeling, itchiness, or shooting pain on an area of skin. A rash may then appear, with raised dots or blisters forming. When the rash is at its peak, rash symptoms can range from mild itching to extreme pain. People with shingles on the upper half of the face should seek medical attention, as the virus may cause damage to the eyes.

Shingles usually resolves without complications within 3 to 5 weeks. However, in some people, especially seniors, the pain may persist for months or years. This condition is known as *post-herpetic neuralgia* (PHN). It is thought to be caused by a continuing irritation of the nerves after the infection is over.

Conventional medical treatment for shingles includes antiviral drugs (acyclovir, famicyclovir, valacyclovir). When used properly, these lead to faster resolution of symptoms, including lesions and acute neuralgia, and may reduce the incidence and severity of PHN. **Steroids** (prednisone) and **tricyclic antidepressants** (amitriptyline) are also prescribed to lessen shingles symptoms and the former might help prevent PHN.

Individuals who do develop PHN may be treated with steroids, antidepressants, and topical creams (see capsaicin, below). In severe cases, nerve blocks might be used.

Principal Proposed Natural Treatments

For the initial attack of shingles, proteolytic enzymes may be helpful. Capsaicin cream is an FDA-approved treatment for PHN.

Proteolytic Enzymes

There is some evidence that proteolytic enzymes may be helpful for the initial attack of shingles.

Proteolytic enzymes are produced by the pancreas to aid in digestion of protein and certain foods also contain these enzymes. Besides their use in digestion, these enzymes may have some effects in the body as a whole when taken orally. The most-studied proteolytic enzymes include papain (from papaya), **bromelain** (from pineapple), and **trypsin** and **chymotrypsin** (extracted from the pancreas of various animals).

A double-blind study of 190 people with shingles compared proteolytic enzymes to the standard antiviral drug acyclovir. Participants were treated for 14 days and their pain was assessed at intervals. Although both groups had similar pain relief, the enzyme-treated group experienced fewer side effects.

Similar results were seen in another double-blind study in which 90 people were given either an injection of acyclovir or enzymes, followed by a course of oral medication for 7 days.

Proteolytic enzymes are thought to benefit cases of shingles by decreasing the body's inflammatory response and regulating immune response to the virus.

For more information, including dosage and safety issues, see the full **Proteolytic Enzymes** article.

Capsaicin: Useful for Post-herpetic Neuralgia

Capsaicin, the "hot" in hot peppers, has been found effective for treating the pain related to PHN and has been approved by the FDA for that purpose. Capsaicin is thought to work by inhibiting chemicals in nerve cells that transmit pain (for further detail on how this works, see the **Cayenne** article).

Topical capsaicin cream is available in two strengths: 0.025 and 0.075%. Both preparations are indicated for use in neuralgia. The cream should be applied sparingly to the affected area 3 to 4 times daily. Treatment should continue for several weeks as the benefit may take a while to develop. Capsaicin creams are approved over-the-counter drugs and should be used as directed.

Over-the-counter creams containing concentrated capsaicin are recognized as safe, but caution should be used near the eyes and mucous membranes. Mild to moderate burning may occur at first, but it decreases over time.

Other Proposed Natural Treatments

Adenosine monophosphate (AMP), a natural by-product of cell metabolism, has been studied as a possible treatment for initial shingles symptoms as well as PHN prevention.

In a double-blind, placebo-controlled study of 32 people with shingles, AMP was injected 3 times a week for 4 weeks. At the end of the 4-week treatment period, 88% of those treated with AMP were pain-free versus only 43% in the placebo group; all participants still in pain were then given AMP and no recurrence of pain was reported in 3 to 18 months of follow-up. However, this was a highly preliminary study and more evidence is needed before AMP can be considered a proven treatment for shingles.

Oral AMP has not been tried for this condition. **Note**: Do not self-inject AMP products meant for oral consumption.

Vitamins E and **B$_{12}$** have also been suggested as possible treatments for PHN, but the evidence that they work is extremely weak.

A single-blind, placebo-controlled study of 62 people with post-herpetic neuralgia failed to find any benefit with **acupuncture** treatment.

Sickle Cell Disease

PRINCIPAL PROPOSED NATURAL TREATMENTS: *Zinc*

OTHER PROPOSED NATURAL TREATMENTS: *Alpha-Linolenic Acid, Beta-carotene, Coenzyme Q_{10}, Fish Oil, Folate, Garlic, Green Tea, Lipoic Acid, Magnesium, Oligomeric Proanthocyanidins (OPCs), Suma, Vitamin B_2, Vitamin B_6, Vitamin B_{12}, Vitamin C, Vitamin E*

Sickle cell disease is an inherited blood disorder. Normally, red blood cells are disc-shaped and flexible. In sickle cell disease, however, hemoglobin (the chemical within red blood cells that carries oxygen around the body) is abnormal. This defect causes red blood cells to collapse into a crescent, or sickle, shape.

These abnormal blood cells are destroyed at an unusually high rate, causing a shortage of red blood cells (anemia). In addition, they can suddenly clump together and clog up small blood vessels throughout the body. This clumping causes what is called a *sickle cell crisis*.

When blood vessels are blocked by sickle-shaped red blood cells, parts of the body are deprived of oxygen. This can cause severe pain and damage to the organs and tissues that are deprived.

Common triggers of sickle cell crisis include smoking, exercise, exposure to high altitudes, fever, infection, dehydration, and the drop in oxygen or changes in air pressure that can occur during airplane travel.

Diagnosis of sickle cell disease and sickle cell trait (a condition in which a person has one of the two genes necessary to develop sickle cell disease) can be done through blood testing, using a technique called *hemoglobin electrophoresis*. Treatment involves managing the anemia, chronic pain, and organ damage caused by sickle cell disease. In addition, the drug hydroxyurea can reduce occurrences of sickle cell crisis. Of course, it is also important to minimize exposure to conditions or situations that can trigger sickle cell crisis.

Principal Proposed Natural Treatments

Children with sickle cell disease often do not grow normally. Zinc deficiency can also cause growth retardation and there is some evidence that people with sickle cell disease are more likely than others to be deficient in the mineral zinc. For this reason, zinc supplementation at nutritional doses has been suggested for children with sickle cell disease.

In a placebo-controlled study, 42 children (ages 4 to 10) with sickle cell disease were given either zinc supplements (10 mg of zinc daily) or placebo for a period of 1 year. Results showed that by the end of the study, the participants given zinc showed enhanced growth compared to those given placebo. Curiously, researchers did not find any solid connection between the severity of zinc deficiency and the extent of response to treatment.

Zinc is thought to have a stabilizing effect on the cell membrane of red blood cells in people with sickle cell disease. For this reason, it has been tried as an aid for preventing sickle cell crisis. In a double-blind, placebo-controlled study of 145 people with sickle cell disease conducted in India, participants received either placebo or about 50 mg of zinc 3 times daily. During 18 months of treatment, the zinc-treated subjects had an average of 2.5 crises, compared to 5.3 for the placebo group. However, zinc didn't seem to reduce the severity of a crisis, as measured by the number of days spent in the hospital for each crisis.

Sickle cell disease can also cause skin ulcers (nonhealing sores). In a 12-week, placebo-controlled trial, use of zinc at 88 mg 3 times per day for 12 weeks enhanced the rate of ulcer healing.

Warning: The high dosages of zinc used in the last two studies can cause dangerous toxicity and should be taken—if at all—only under the supervision of a doctor. The nutritional dose described in the first study, however, is safe.

For more information, including detailed dosage and safety issues, see the full **Zinc** article.

Other Proposed Natural Treatments

A 1-year-long, double-blind, placebo-controlled crossover study of 82 people with sickle cell disease tested a combination herbal treatment made from plants indigenous to Nigeria. The results indicate that use of the herbal mixture reduced the incidence of sickle cell crisis.

A very small double-blind, placebo-controlled trial

found intriguing evidence that **fish oil** may reduce the frequency of painful sickle cell episodes, possibly by reducing the tendency of the blood to clot.

Numerous other herbs and supplements have been suggested for people with sickle cell disease, including alpha-linolenic acid, **beta-carotene**, **coenzyme Q₁₀**,

folate, **garlic**, **green tea**, **lipoic acid**, **magnesium**, **oligomeric proanthocyanidins (OPCs)**, **suma**, vitamin B$_2$, vitamin B$_6$, vitamin B$_{12}$, vitamin C, and vitamin E, but as yet the supporting evidence for these treatments remains far too preliminary to be relied upon at all.

Sjogren's Syndrome

RELATED TERMS: *Sicca, Xerostomia*

PRINCIPAL PROPOSED NATURAL TREATMENTS: *Herb–Vitamin–Mineral Combination, N-Acetyl Cysteine*

OTHER PROPOSED NATURAL TREATMENTS: Aloe vera, *Bovine Colostrum, Citrus Bioflavonoids, Dandelion, Dehydroepiandrosterone (DHEA), Echinacea, Fish Oil, Gamma-linolenic Acid, Garlic, Inositol, Magnesium, Methionine, Olive Leaf Extract, Red Clover, Vitamin A, Vitamin C, Vitamin E, Zinc*

Sjogren's syndrome is an autoimmune condition in which the immune system destroys moisture-producing glands, such as tear glands and salivary glands. When Sjogren's syndrome occurs by itself, it is called *primary Sjogren's syndrome*. When it occurs in the context of other autoimmune conditions, such as **rheumatoid arthritis** or **systemic lupus erythematosus** (lupus), it is called *secondary Sjogren's syndrome*.

Sjogren's is most common in women aged 40 to 60. Symptoms include dry eyes (sicca), dry mouth (xerostomia), difficulty swallowing, loss of taste and smell, swollen salivary glands, severe dental cavities caused by dry mouth, oral yeast infections (thrush), and vaginal dryness. Fatigue and joint pain may occur as well, ranging in intensity from mild to disabling. Sjogren's can also affect the kidneys, digestive tract, lungs, liver, pancreas, or other internal organs.

As with other autoimmune diseases, symptoms of Sjogren's tend to wax and wane. The disease is diagnosed by blood tests as well as examination of the eyes and mouth. Treatment primarily involves use of artificial tears, artificial saliva, and vaginal lubricants to relieve dryness. In some cases, anti-inflammatory or immune-suppressant drugs may be used.

Principal Proposed Natural Treatments

N-acetyl Cysteine

N-acetyl cysteine (NAC) is a specially modified form of the dietary amino acid cysteine. When taken orally,

NAC helps the body make the important antioxidant enzyme **glutathione**. It is also thought to help loosen secretions and, for this reason, it has been tried as a treatment for Sjogren's syndrome.

In a double-blind, placebo-controlled crossover trial of 26 people with Sjogren's syndrome, use of NAC at a dose of 200 mg 3 times per day improved eye-related symptoms. The supplement also showed some promise for mouth-related symptoms, but the effects were less clear-cut. While these are promising results, a much larger trial would be necessary to fully document the potential benefits of this treatment approach.

For more information, see the full **NAC** article.

Herb–Vitamin–Mineral Combination

A product containing vitamins and minerals as well as the herbs paprika, **rosemary**, **peppermint**, milfoil, **hawthorn**, and **pumpkin seed** has been used in Scandinavia for many years as a treatment for various mouth-related conditions. A double-blind, placebo-controlled study of 44 people found that 4 months' treatment with this combination improved some signs and symptoms of Sjogren's syndrome, including rate of salivary flow. A larger study is needed to fully explore the potential benefits of this treatment.

Other Proposed Natural Treatments

Colostrum is the fluid that a woman's breasts produce during the first day or two after she has given birth. Very preliminary evidence suggests that oral hygiene products containing **bovine colostrum** (colostrum from cows) may provide beneficial effects for the mouth symptoms of Sjogren's syndrome.

One small study found preliminary evidence that toothpaste containing **betaine** may be helpful for dry mouth symptoms of Sjogren's syndrome.

Gamma-linolenic acid (GLA), an essential fatty acid in the omega-6 family, has been tried as a treatment for the fatigue often associated with Sjogren's. However, in a 6-month, double-blind, placebo-controlled trial of 90 people, use of GLA failed to prove more effective than placebo. One small double-blind study, however, found that a combination of GLA and the omega-6 fatty acid linoleic acid (found in many vegetable oils) may improve eye symptoms in Sjogren's.

A 6-month study failed to find benefits with **DHEA** at a dose of 200 mg daily.

Numerous other natural products are widely recommended for Sjogren's syndrome, but they lack supporting scientific evidence. These include *Aloe vera*, **citrus bioflavonoids**, **dandelion**, **echinacea**, **fish oil**, **garlic**, **inositol**, **magnesium**, **methionine**, **olive leaf extract**, **red clover**, **vitamin A**, **vitamin C**, **vitamin E**, and **zinc**.

Herbs and Supplements to Use Only with Caution

One case report weakly hints that the herb echinacea might potentially trigger dangerous symptoms (specifically, critical hypokalemic renal tubular acidosis) in people with Sjogren's.

Numerous herbs and supplements may interact adversely with drugs used to treat Sjogren's syndrome. For more information, see the individual drug articles in the Drug Interactions section of this book.

Soft Tissue Pain

RELATED TERMS: *Musculoskeletal Pain; Pain, Muscle; Pain, Soft Tissue*

PROPOSED NATURAL TREATMENTS: *Acupuncture, Biofeedback, Boswellia, Butterbur, Chiropractic, Devil's Claw, Hypnosis, Magnet Therapy, Massage, D-phenylalanine, Prolotherapy, Proteolytic Enzymes, Relaxation Therapy, White Willow*

When specific causes of symptoms aren't known, doctors sometimes refer to conditions simply by naming the symptoms. Such is the case for so-called soft tissue pain. The term *soft tissue pain* simply refers to discomfort somewhere in the interconnected system of muscles, tendons, and ligaments, as opposed to the bones, and says nothing about the particular cause.

The most commonly used conventional treatments for soft tissue pain consist primarily of drugs that relieve pain and/or inflammation in general, such as ibuprofen and acetaminophen, as well as muscle relaxants. Physical therapy methods are commonly recommended for selected forms of soft tissue pain, but there is little to no reliable scientific evidence that they help. Other methods, such as therapeutic exercises, may help, but most reported studies are significantly flawed by the lack of a credible placebo treatment. (For why

this is important, see **Why Does This Book Rely on Double-blind Studies?**.)

A similar lack of reliable evidence exists regarding other non-surgical, non-drug methods used to control soft tissue pain, such as injection therapy, radiofrequency denervation, and transcutaneous electrical nerve stimulation (TENS).

Surgery may be useful for certain selected forms of soft tissue pain, although again the supporting research evidence is generally very incomplete.

Proposed Natural Treatments

Natural treatments for the following forms of soft tissue pain are discussed in their own articles:

➢ **Back Pain**
➢ **Bursitis**

➤Fibromyalgia
➤Neck Pain
➤Rotator Cuff Injury
➤Sciatic Pain
➤Sports Injuries
➤Sprains
➤Tendonitis
➤Tension Headache
➤TMJ

Alternative therapies that may be useful for soft tissue pain in general include **acupuncture**, **biofeedback**, **chiropractic**, **hypnosis**, **magnet therapy**, **massage**, **prolotherapy**, and **relaxation therapy**.

Herbs and supplements that may have a general pain-relieving effect include **boswellia**, **butterbur**, **devil's claw**, **D-phenylalanine**, **proteolytic enzymes**, and **white willow**.

Sports and Fitness Support: Enhancing Performance

RELATED TERM: *Ergogenic Aids*

PRINCIPAL PROPOSED NATURAL TREATMENTS: *Creatine, HMB*

OTHER PROPOSED NATURAL TREATMENTS: *Acupuncture, Arginine, Branched-Chain Amino Acids (BCAAs), Caffeine, Carnitine, Chromium, Citrulline, Ciwujia, Coenzyme Q_{10}, Cordyceps, Deer Antler, Dehydroepiandrosterone (DHEA), Dihydroxyacetone Pyruvate (DHAP), Gamma Oryzanol, Ginseng, Glutamine, Guarana, Human Growth Hormone Enhancers, Inosine, Ipriflavone, Iron, Lipoic Acid, Magnesium, Ma Huang (Ephedra), Medium-Chain Triglycerides (MCTs), Multivitamin, NADH, Policosanol, Ornithine Alpha-Ketoglutarate (OKG), Panax notoginseng, Pantothenic Acid/Pantethine, Phosphate, Phosphatidylserine, Rhodiola rosea, Ribose, Schisandra, Suma, Tribulus terrestris, TMG, Whey Protein*

HERBS AND SUPPLEMENTS TO USE ONLY WITH CAUTION: *Androstenedione, Boron, Vanadium*

In the competitive world of sports, the smallest advantage can make an enormous difference in the outcome of a contest. A substance that improves an athlete's strength, speed, or endurance is called an *ergogenic aid*.

The most effective ergogenic aids are both dangerous and illegal: stimulants, anabolic steroids, and human growth hormone. Numerous natural options are marketed as alternatives. In this article, we explore the many supplements used in the hopes of improving sports performance.

For additional sports-related articles, see **Sports and Fitness Support: Enhancing Recovery**.

Principal Proposed Natural Treatments

Two natural supplements have shown meaningful promise as ergogenic aids: creatine and HMB.

Creatine

Creatine, one of the best-selling and best-documented supplements for enhancing athletic performance, is a naturally occurring substance that plays an important role in the production of energy in the body. The body converts creatine to phosphocreatine, a form of stored energy used by muscles. In theory, taking supplemental creatine will build up a reserve of phosphocreatine in the muscles to help them perform on demand. Supplemental creatine may also help the body make new phosphocreatine faster when it has been used up by intense activity.

However, the balance of current evidence suggests that that if creatine supplements have any benefit for sports performance, it is slight, and limited to highly specific forms of exercise.

Several small double-blind studies have found that

creatine can improve performance in exercises that involve repeated short bursts of high-intensity activity with intervening rest periods of adequate length.

For example, a double-blind, placebo-controlled study investigated creatine and swimming performance in 18 men and 14 women. Men taking the supplement had significant increases in speed when doing six bouts of 50-meter swims started at 3-minute intervals, compared to men taking placebo. However, their speed did not improve when swimming 10 sets of 25-yard lengths started at 1-minute intervals. Researchers theorize that the shorter rest time between laps was not enough for the swimmers' bodies to resynthesize phosphocreatine.

Interestingly, none of the women enrolled in the study showed any improvement with the creatine supplement. The authors of this study noted that women normally have more creatine in their muscle tissue than men do, so perhaps creatine supplementation (at least at this level) is not of benefit to women, as it appears to be for men. Further research is needed to fully understand the difference between the genders in response to creatine.

In an earlier double-blind study, 16 physical education students carried out ten 6-second bursts of extremely intense exercise on a stationary bicycle, separated by 30 seconds of rest. The results showed that the students who took 20 g of creatine for 6 days were better able to maintain cycle speed throughout the repetitions. Many other studies showed similar improvements in performance capacity involving repeated bursts of action. However, there have been negative results as well; in general, minimal to no benefits have been seen in studies involving athletes engaged in normal sports rather than contrived laboratory tests.

In contrast, studies of endurance or non-repetitive aerobic burst exercise generally have not shown benefits from creatine supplementation. Therefore, creatine probably won't help you with marathon running or single sprints.

Besides repetitive burst exercise, creatine has also shown promise for increasing isometric exercise capacity (pushing against a fixed resistance), in some, but not all studies. In addition, two double-blind, placebo-controlled studies, each lasting 28 days, provide some evidence that creatine as well as creatine plus HMB (see below) can increase lean muscle and bone mass. However, one double-blind trial failed to find creatine helpful for enhancing general fitness, including resistance exercise performance, in male seniors.

The contradictory results seen in these small trials suggest that creatine offers at most a very modest sports performance benefit. For more information, including dosage and safety issues, see the full **Creatine** article.

Hydroxymethyl Butyrate

Technically beta-hydroxy beta-methylbutyric acid, HMB is a chemical that occurs naturally in the body when the amino acid leucine breaks down. Leucine is found in particularly high concentrations in muscles. During athletic training, damage to the muscles leads to the breakdown of leucine as well as increased HMB levels. Some evidence suggests that taking HMB supplements might signal the body to slow down the destruction of muscle tissue. On this basis, HMB has been studied as a sports performance supplement for enhancing strength and muscle mass.

According to many (but not all) of the small double-blind trials that have been reported, HMB appears to improve muscle-growth response to weight training.

For example, in a controlled study, 41 male volunteers aged 19 to 29 were given either 0, 1.5, or 3 g of HMB daily for 3 weeks. The participants also lifted weights 3 days a week according to a defined (rather severe) schedule. The results suggested that HMB can enhance strength and muscle mass in direct proportion to intake.

In another controlled study reported in the same article, 32 male volunteers took either 3 g of HMB or placebo daily, and then lifted weights for 2 or 3 hours daily, 6 days a week for 7 weeks. The HMB group saw a significantly greater increase in bench-press strength than the placebo group. However, there was no significant difference in body weight or fat mass by the end of the study.

Similarly, a double-blind, placebo-controlled trial of 39 men and 36 women found that over 4 weeks, HMB supplementation improved response to weight training.

Two placebo-controlled studies of women found that 3 g of HMB had no effect on lean body mass and strength in sedentary women, but it did provide an additional benefit when combined with weight training. In addition, a double-blind study of 31 men and women, all 70 years old, undergoing resistance training found significant improvements in fat-free mass attributable to the use of HMB (3 g daily).

However, there have been negative studies as well.

All of these studies were small and therefore, their results are ultimately not terribly reliable. Larger studies will be necessary to truly establish whether HMB is helpful for power athletes working to enhance strength and muscle mass.

For more information, including dosage and safety issues, see the full **HMB** article.

Other Proposed Natural Treatments

Numerous other supplements are marketed as ergogenic aids, said to improve speed, strength, or endurance. Unfortunately, the evidence that they work is marginal at best, and in many cases the best available evidence indicates that these substances are *not* effective.

Ginseng

There are three different herbs commonly called *ginseng*: Asian or Korean ginseng (*Panax ginseng*), American ginseng (*Panax quinquefolius*), and Siberian "ginseng" (*Eleutherococcus senticosus*). The latter is actually not ginseng at all, but the Russian scientists responsible for promoting it believe that it functions identically. According to some experts, a fourth herb, ciwujia, is actually *Eleutherococcus*, while others claim it is a related but different species.

Panax ginseng has shown some promise as a mild ergogenic aid, but published evidence remains at best incomplete and contradictory. Other forms of ginseng generally lack any meaningful supporting evidence.

For example, an 8-week, double-blind, placebo-controlled trial evaluated the effects of *Panax ginseng* with and without exercise in 41 people. The participants were given either ginseng or placebo, and then underwent exercise training or remained untrained throughout the study. The results showed that ginseng improved aerobic capacity in people who did not exercise, but offered no benefit in those who did exercise.

In a 9-week, double-blind, placebo-controlled trial of 30 highly trained athletes, treatment with *Panax ginseng* or *Panax ginseng* plus **vitamin E** produced significant improvements in aerobic capacity. Another double-blind, placebo-controlled trial of 37 participants also found some benefit. Also, a double-blind, placebo-controlled study of 120 people found that ginseng gradually improved reaction time and lung function over a 12-week treatment period among participants from 40 to 60 years old. (No benefits were seen in younger people.)

On the other hand, in an 8-week, double-blind trial that followed 31 healthy men in their twenties, no benefit with *Panax ginseng* could be demonstrated. Many other small trials of *Panax ginseng* have failed to find evidence of benefit.

These mixed outcomes suggest that *Panax ginseng* is only slightly effective at best.

A double-blind study of 20 endurance athletes over an 8-week period failed to find evidence of benefit with a standard eleutherococcus formulation. Lack of benefit was also seen in another small double-blind, crossover trial. Furthermore, in a small double-blind, placebo-controlled trial of endurance athletes, use of eleutherococcus actually increased physiologic signs of stress during intensive training. Ciwujia has not yet been studied in meaningful double-blind trials.

For more information, including dosage and safety issues, see the full **Ginseng** and **Eleutherococcus** articles.

Medium-chain Triglycerides

Medium-chain triglycerides (MCTs) are fats with an unusual chemical structure that allows the body to digest them easily. Most fats are broken down in the intestine and reassembled into a special form that can be transported in the blood. But MCTs are absorbed intact and taken to the liver, where they are used directly for energy. In this sense, they are processed very similarly to carbohydrates. For that reason, MCTs have been proposed as an alternative to "carbo-loading" (consumption of a large quantity of carbohydrates prior to intense physical exercise) for providing a concentrated source of easily utilized energy.

A number of double-blind studies have evaluated MCTs' effects on high-intensity or endurance exercise performance, but the results have been thoroughly inconsistent. This is not surprising because all of the studies were too small to properly eliminate the effects of chance.

For more information, including dosage and safety issues, see the full **MCTs** article.

Iron

The majority of athletes are probably not iron-deficient and you shouldn't take iron supplements if you already have enough iron in your body. However, if you are deficient in this essential mineral, iron supplements may enhance athletic training.

A double-blind, placebo-controlled trial of 42 non-anemic women with evidence of slightly low iron reserves found that iron supplements significantly increased the benefits gained from exercise. Participants were put on a daily aerobic training program for the latter 4 weeks of this 6-week trial. At the end of the trial, those receiving iron showed significantly greater gains in speed and endurance than those given placebo.

In addition, a double-blind, placebo-controlled study of 40 non-anemic elite athletes with mildly low iron stores found that 12 weeks of iron supplementation enhanced aerobic performance.

Benefits with iron supplementation for marginally iron-depleted athletes were observed in other double-blind trials as well. However, several other studies failed to find significant improvements. These contradictory results suggest that the benefits of iron supplements for non-anemic, iron-deficient athletes is small at most.

For more information, including dosage and safety issues, see the full **Iron** article.

Colostrum

Colostrum is the fluid that new mothers' breasts produce during the first day or two after birth. Colostrum contains growth factors, such as IGF-1, that could enhance muscle development and, on this basis, it has been tried as a sports supplement.

An 8-week, double-blind study found that use of colostrum enhanced sprinting performance. Other double-blind studies found improvements in rowing performance and vertical jump, respectively.

In addition, a small double-blind study found that colostrum, as compared to **whey protein**, increased lean mass in healthy men and women undergoing aerobic and resistance training. However, no improvements in performance were seen in this trial.

Finally, in a double-blind, placebo-controlled study, use of colostrum over an 8-week training period did not improve performance on an exercise-to-exhaustion test; however, it did improve performance on a repeat bout 20 minutes later.

Interestingly, research suggests that the growth factor IGF-1 in colostrum is not directly absorbed into the body, yet consumption of colostrum nonetheless increases IGF-1 levels in the blood, perhaps by stimulating its natural release.

For more information, including dosage and safety issues, see the full **Colostrum** article.

Pyruvate (Dihydroxyacetone Pyruvate, DHAP)

Pyruvate supplies the body with pyruvic acid, a natural compound that plays important roles in the manufacture and use of energy. Pyruvate supplements have become popular with bodybuilders and other athletes based on slim evidence that pyruvate can improve body composition. However, at the present time, the evidence regarding pyruvate as an ergogenic aid is weak and contradictory at best. One study failed to find that pyruvate supplements improved body composition or exercise performance; furthermore, pyruvate appeared to negate the beneficial effect of exercise on **cholesterol profile**.

For more information, including dosage and safety issues, see the full **Pyruvate** article.

Policosanol

Policosanol is a mixture of waxy substances manufactured from sugarcane. It contains octacosanol, which is also made from wheat germ oil. Both are marketed as performance-enhancing dietary supplements said to increase muscle strength and endurance and improve reaction time and stamina. However, the only evidence for policosanol as a performance enhancer comes from one small double-blind trial with marginal results.

Phosphatidylserine

Phosphatidylserine (PS) is a phospholipid and a major component of cell membranes. Good evidence suggests that PS can improve mental function, especially in the elderly. However, PS has also been marketed as a sports supplement, said to help bodybuilders and power athletes develop larger and stronger muscles.

This claim is based on modest evidence indicating that PS slows the release of cortisol following heavy exercise. Cortisol is a hormone that causes muscle tissue to break down. For reasons that are unclear, the body produces increased levels of cortisol after heavy exercise. Strength athletes who believe natural cortisol release works against their efforts to rapidly build muscle mass hope that PS will help them advance more quickly. However, only two double-blind, placebo-controlled studies of PS as a sports supplement have been reported and neither one found effects on cortisol levels. Of these small trials, one found a possible ergogenic benefit and the other did not.

For more information, including dosage and safety issues, see the full **Phosphatidylserine** article.

Branched-chain Amino Acids: Leucine, Isoleucine, and Valine

Amino acids are molecules that form proteins when joined together. Three of them—leucine, isoleucine, and valine—are called *branched-chain amino acids* (BCAAs), describing the shape of the molecules. Muscles have a particularly high BCAA content.

Both strength training and endurance exercise use greater amounts of BCAAs than normal daily activities, perhaps increasing an athlete's need for dietary intake of these amino acids. Sports such as mountaineering and skiing may cause even greater depletion of BCAAs because of metabolic changes that occur at higher altitudes. Athletes have tried BCAA supplements to build muscle, improve performance, postpone fatigue, and cure over-training syndrome (prolonged fatigue and other symptoms caused by excessive exercise). However, most of the evidence suggests that BCAAs are not helpful for these purposes.

Whey protein is rich in BCAAs and, on this basis, it has also been proposed as a bodybuilding aid. However, there is no evidence that whey protein is more effective for this purpose than any other protein. One small double-blind study found evidence that both casein and whey protein were more effective than placebo at promoting muscle growth after exercise, but whey was no more effective than the far less expensive casein.

For more information, including dosage and safety issues, see the full **Branched-chain Amino Acids** article.

Other Amino Acids

Besides BCAAs, athletes use a number of other amino acids, sometimes individually and sometimes in combination. Amino acids believed by some to have ergogenic effects include **arginine**, **glutamine**, and ornithine (ornithine and glutamine combined form **ornithine alpha-ketoglutarate**, or OKG), as well as the branched-chain amino acids leucine, isoleucine, and valine, discussed above.

However, evidence supporting the use of amino acids as ergogenic aids is sparse to nonexistent. The few clinical trials performed generally don't show positive results.

Chromium

The mineral **chromium** has been sold as a "fat burner" and is also said to help build muscle tissue. However, studies evaluating its benefits as a performance enhancer or an aid to bodybuilding have yielded almost entirely negative results.

Coenzyme Q$_{10}$

Coenzyme Q$_{10}$ (CoQ$_{10}$, ubiquinone) is a natural substance that plays a fundamental role in the mitochondria, the parts of the cell that produce energy from food. On this basis, CoQ$_{10}$ has been proposed as a performance enhancer for athletes. However, most clinical trials have found no significant improvement with CoQ$_{10}$.

For more information, including dosage and safety issues, see the full **Coenzyme Q$_{10}$** article.

Inosine

Inosine is an important chemical found throughout the body. It plays many roles, one of which is helping to make ATP, the body's main form of usable energy. Based primarily on this fact, inosine supplements have been proposed as an energy booster for athletes. However, most of the available evidence suggests that it doesn't work.

For more information, including dosage and safety issues, see the full **Inosine** article.

Ribose

Ribose is a carbohydrate that is also vital for the manufacture of ATP. Ribose has shown some promise for improving exercise capacity in people with certain enzyme deficiencies and other rare conditions that cause muscle pain during exertion. On this basis, it has been touted as an athletic performance enhancer; however, five small double-blind, placebo-controlled trials in humans failed to find any benefit. In one of these studies, dextrose (a form of ordinary sugar), proved effective while ribose did not.

For more information, including dosage and safety issues, see the full **Ribose** article.

Gamma Oryzanol

Very preliminary evidence suggests that gamma oryzanol, a substance derived from rice bran oil, may increase endorphin release and aid muscle development. These findings have created interest in using gamma oryzanol as a sports supplement. However, a 9-week, double-blind, placebo-controlled trial of 22 weight-trained males found no difference between placebo or 500 mg daily of gamma oryzanol in terms of performance, body composition, or hormone levels.

For more information, including dosage and safety issues, see the full **Gamma Oryzanol** article.

Trimethylglycine

Trimethylglycine (TMG) is a naturally occurring compound that may help to prevent **atherosclerosis** and is therefore sometimes taken as a supplement. In the course of its metabolism in the body, TMG is turned into another substance, dimethylglycine (DMG).

In Russia, DMG is used extensively as an athletic performance enhancer and it has recently become popular among American athletes. TMG is cheaper and it may have the same effects as DMG as it changes into DMG in the body. However, there is no evidence that DMG is effective, and some evidence that it is not.

For more information, including dosage and safety issues, see the full **Trimethylglycine** article.

DHEA

Athletes have used DHEA on the belief that (like phosphatidylserine) it might limit the body's response to cortisol and thereby cause an increase in muscle tissue growth. However, study results have conflicted on whether or not DHEA really interferes with cortisol. Furthermore, studies of DHEA as an aid to increasing muscle mass or enhancing sports performance have produced mixed results at best.

For more information, including dosage and safety issues, see the full **DHEA** article.

Tribulus Terrestris

Tribulus terrestris is a tropical plant with a long history of medicinal use. It has been tried for low libido in both men and women and for impotence and female infertility.

One theory regarding how *T. terrestris* might help with sexual problems is that a component from the plant called *protodioscine* is converted to the hormone DHEA in our bodies. DHEA is used by the body as a building block for both testosterone and estrogen (as well as other hormones). This finding has led bodybuilders and strength athletes to try *T. terrestris* for increasing muscular development. So far, however, the scientific evidence seems to be against it. This is not surprising because DHEA itself has not been found effective as a sports supplement.

One study involving 15 men compared the effects of *T. terrestris* (3.21 mg per kilogram of body weight—for example, 292 mg daily for a 200-pound man) against placebo on body composition and endurance among men engaged in resistance training. At the end of the 8-week study, the only significant difference between the treatment and placebo groups was that the placebo group showed greater gains in endurance.

For more information, including dosage and safety issues, see the full *Tribulus terrestris* article.

Phosphate

Phosphate has been studied as an ergogenic aid to improve aerobic capacity and endurance with greatly mixed results. One unanswered question is whether the findings in some studies resulted from the ingestion of phosphate or from the other compounds the phosphate was mixed with, such as sodium or calcium. Because the trials performed so far have used inconsistent methods and measurements, it isn't possible to know yet whether or not phosphate has any potential benefit as a sports supplement.

Commercial Preparations

A small double-blind study of a mixture of various herbs and supplements marketed as SPORT found no evidence that it can improve sports performance in trained athletes.

Stimulants: Ma Huang and Caffeine

A number of plant-derived stimulants are used by some athletes to improve their performance, including ephedrine from the Chinese herb ma huang (also called *ephedra*) and caffeine from coffee, tea, **maté**, cola, or **guarana** (a plant native to South America). Both ephedrine and caffeine are central nervous system stimulants. Caffeine also appears to change the way your body burns calories, possibly allowing it to burn fats first and preserve muscle glycogen for later in the competition—sort of like "saving the best for last."

Caffeine does appear to improve performance during endurance-type exercises.

Note: The International Olympic Committee has set a tolerance limit for caffeine in the urine at 12 mcg/ml. If you're competing in a sport that follows similar regulations, you may want to have a cup of coffee or tea, but don't drink the whole pot.

Ephedrine's value in enhancing sports performance has not been established; at the same time, there are serious safety issues associated with its use (see the Safety Issues section in the full article on **ephedra**). Some sports federations have determined that specific amounts of ephedrine in an athlete's system are grounds for disqualification.

Other

One small double-blind trial found that use of the herb *Rhodiola rosea* improved endurance exercise performance. However, another study failed to find benefit with a combination of **cordyceps** and rhodiola.

One small study found endurance exercise benefits with *Panax notoginseng*.

One small trial suggests that **acupuncture** may enhance peak performance capacity.

A small double-blind study failed to find any performance or training-enhancing benefits with a newly marketed silicate product. **N-acetylcysteine** (NAC), **fish oil**, **soy isoflavones**, astaxanthin, and **tyrosine** have also failed to show benefit in preliminary trials.

Numerous other natural substances have been marketed as ergogenic aids, despite an almost complete lack of evidence that they help, including **carnitine**, cordyceps, **deer antler**, **ipriflavone**, **lipoic acid**, **NADH**, and **suma**. One study found that **L-citrulline**, another purported ergogenic aid, actually *decreases* exercise capacity.

Many websites advertise products that they claim act like human growth hormone, often called *HGH enhancers*. However, these products are entirely speculative because there are no natural treatments proven to raise human growth hormone levels.

Similarly, there are no herbs or supplements known to act as "natural anabolic steroids." (See also the discussion of androstenedione in the Not Recommended Treatments section below.)

One small study failed to find benefit with a liquid **multivitamin/mineral supplement**.

Not Recommended Treatments

Three commonly recommended supplements fall in the "not recommended for athletes" category: vanadium, boron, and androstenedione.

The mineral vanadium has been suggested for use by bodybuilders based on its effects on insulin, but there is no evidence that it helps. A double-blind, placebo-controlled study involving 31 weight-trained athletes found no benefit of supplementation at more than 1,000 times the nutritional dose. Furthermore, there are serious safety concerns about taking vanadium at such high doses. See the full article on **vanadium** for more information.

The mineral boron has been proposed as a sports supplement because it is thought to increase testosterone levels. However, studies performed thus far have failed to provide meaningful evidence that it helps increase muscle mass or enhances performance. Furthermore, clinical studies suggest that boron supplementation is more likely to increase estrogen than testosterone. Increased estrogen is not likely to have a sports performance benefit in men, while in women it might increase risk of breast cancer. Therefore, we don't recommend taking supplemental boron as a sports supplement. See the full article on **boron** for more information.

The hormone androstenedione is said to enhance athletic performance and strength by increasing testosterone production, thereby building muscle. However, in double-blind studies, when androstenedione was given to men, it neither altered total testosterone levels, nor improved sports performance, strength, or lean body mass. It did, however, increase estrogen levels, an effect that would not be considered favorable. Interestingly, androstenedione does appear to raise testosterone levels in women, but it is not clear whether this would produce favorable results. For more information, see the full **androstenedione** article.

Sports and Fitness Support: Enhancing Recovery

PRINCIPAL PROPOSED NATURAL TREATMENTS: *Vitamin C*

OTHER PROPOSED NATURAL TREATMENTS: *Beta-carotene, Beta-sitosterol, Bromelain, Glucosamine, Glutamine, Horse Chestnut, Oligomeric Proanthocyanidins (OPCs), Selenium, Thymus Extract, Vitamin E*

In the competitive world of sports, the smallest advantage can make an enormous difference in the outcome of a contest. A supplement that could improve an athlete's strength, speed, or endurance could make the difference between tenth place and first place in a race. Supplements advocated for these purposes are discussed in the article **Sports and Fitness Support: Enhancing Performance**.

Supplements could conceivably play another helpful role for athletes: aiding recovery from the "side effects" of intense exercise. While exercise of moderate intensity is almost undoubtedly a purely positive activity, high-intensity endurance exercise, such as running marathons, can cause respiratory infections. In addition, all forms of exercise, when carried to the extremes common among serious athletes and bodybuilders, can cause severe muscle soreness, which may in turn get in the way of training. Herbs and supplements advocated for these problems are the subject of this article.

For information on natural treatments intended to aid recovery from *injuries* caused by sports.

Principal Proposed Natural Treatments

Extremely intense exercise, such as training for and running in a marathon, is known to lower immunity and endurance athletes frequently get sick after maximal exertion. Vitamin C might help prevent this, although not all studies agree.

According to a double-blind, placebo-controlled study involving 92 runners, taking 600 mg of vitamin C for 21 days prior to a race made a significant difference in the incidence of sickness afterwards. Within 2 weeks after the race, 68% of the runners taking placebo developed symptoms of a **common cold**, versus only 33% of those taking the vitamin C supplement. As part of the same study, non-runners of similar age and gender to those running were also given vitamin C or placebo. Interestingly, for this group, the supplement had no apparent effect on the incidence of upper respiratory infections. Vitamin C seemed to be specifically effective in this capacity for those who exercised intensively.

Two other studies found that vitamin C could reduce the number of colds experienced by groups of people involved in rigorous exercise in extremely cold environments. One study involved 139 children attending a skiing camp in the Swiss Alps, while the other enrolled 56 military men engaged in a training exercise in Northern Canada during the winter months. In both cases, the participants took either 1 g of vitamin C or placebo daily at the time their training program began. Cold symptoms were monitored for 1 to 2 weeks following training and significant differences in favor of vitamin C were found.

However, one very large study of 674 U.S. Marine recruits in basic training found no such benefit. The results showed no difference in the number of colds between the treatment and placebo groups.

What's the explanation for this discrepancy? There are many possibilities. Perhaps basic training in the Marines is significantly different from the other forms of exercise studied. Another point to consider is that the Marines didn't start taking vitamin C right at the beginning of training, but waited 3 weeks. The study also lasted a bit longer than the positive studies mentioned

above—it continued for 2 months. Maybe vitamin C is more effective at preventing colds in the short term. Of course, another possibility is that it doesn't really work. More research is needed to know for sure.

For more information, including dosage and safety issues, see the full **Vitamin C** article.

Other Proposed Natural Treatments

Like vitamin C, the amino acid **glutamine** may be helpful for preventing the infections that occur after severe exercise.

Glutamine is an important fuel source for some of our immune system cells. Some evidence suggests that athletes who have trained very hard have lower-than-normal levels of glutamine in their blood. One double-blind clinical trial involving 151 athletes found that supplementation with 5 g of glutamine immediately after heavy exercise, followed by another 5 g 2 hours later, reduced the incidence of infections quite significantly. Only 19% of those taking glutamine reported infections, while 51% of the placebo group succumbed to illness.

Weaker evidence suggests that **beta-sitosterol** might also offer some promise for this purpose.

However, **thymus extract**, another proposed immune booster for athletes, does not seem to work, according to a double-blind, placebo-controlled trial of 60 athletes.

Exercising increases the presence of free radicals, naturally occurring substances that can damage tissue. Some researchers have theorized that such damage may in part cause the muscle soreness, and perhaps muscle deterioration, that can accompany a strenuous workout. Based on this theory, but little direct evidence, various **antioxidants** have been proposed to help prevent athletic muscle soreness or muscle damage including the following:

- **Astaxanthin**
- **Beta-carotene**
- **Coenzyme Q_{10}**
- **Oligomeric proanthocyanidins (OPCs)**
- **Selenium**
- **Vitamin C**
- **Vitamin E**

One double-blind trial compared vitamin C, vitamin E, and placebo for muscle soreness in 24 male volunteers. Vitamin C was found to relieve muscle soreness, while vitamin E did not. Two other studies failed to find vitamin C combined with vitamin E effective. Another study failed to find benefit with the algae-derived **carotenoid astaxanthin**.

The supplement **bromelain**, used for sports injuries, has also been proposed for reducing muscle soreness after exercise. A double-blind, placebo-controlled trial compared bromelain against ibuprofen, but found no benefit with either.

The supplement **phosphatidylserine** has also failed to prove effective for reducing muscle soreness after exercise, as has **chondroitin** and **magnet therapy**.

Athletes who train excessively may experience a condition called *overtraining syndrome*. Symptoms include depression, fatigue, reduced performance, and physiologic signs of stress. Numerous supplements have been suggested as treatments for this condition, most prominently antioxidants, **branched-chain amino acids** (BCAAs), and glutamine, but none have yet been proven effective.

Strep Throat

RELATED TERMS: *Streptococcal Pharyngitis, Rheumatic Fever, Streptococcal Pharyngitis*

PRINCIPAL PROPOSED NATURAL TREATMENTS: *None*

OTHER PROPOSED NATURAL TREATMENTS: *Throat Coat Tea (Symptoms Only)*, Pelargonium sidoides *(For Non-dangerous Forms of Sore Throat Only)*

Most cases of sore throat are caused by viruses, generally the same viruses that cause colds. One familiar type of sore throat, however, is caused by bacteria in the streptococcus family: streptococcal pharyngitis, commonly known as strep throat. It is relatively common in children.

Symptoms of strep throat include intense throat pain (generally developing suddenly), difficulty swallowing, and fever ranging from 101° to 104° degrees Fahrenheit. In children, headache, abdominal pain, nausea, and vomiting may also occur. The back of the throat generally (but not always) becomes beefy red in color, possibly with white or red dots. However, none of these signs or symptoms is absolutely characteristic of strep throat and, in some cases, none of these symptoms is present. Ultimately, diagnosis of strep throat must be made through a laboratory examination of material swabbed from the back of the throat.

The primary significance of strep throat is not the throat infection itself, but rather a delayed complication called *rheumatic fever*. Strep throat itself will disappear in 3 to 5 days even without treatment. However, when a certain group of streptococcal bacteria are involved, called *Group A beta-hemolytic streptococci*, there is risk of a severe, dangerous complication developing about 1 to 5 weeks later, when all seems to be well. This is the feared sequellae of strep throat known as rheumatic fever.

The initial attack of rheumatic fever involves five major signs and symptoms:

> **Carditis: inflammation of the heart, often causing a heart murmur**
> **Chorea: rapid, purposeless, nonrepetitive movements that are not under conscious control**
> **Migratory polyarthritis: severe joint pain, redness, and swelling that moves from joint to joint**
> **Subcutaneous nodules: nodules under the skin**
> **Erythema marginatum: a serpentine, flat rash**

These symptoms will eventually subside. However, when they are gone, the valves of the heart may be permanently damaged, necessitating open heart surgery.

About 3% of untreated Group A beta-hemolytic strep throat cases lead to rheumatic fever. Children ages 4 to 15 are most at risk. Adults with strep throat may develop rheumatic fever, but the chance is extremely low. Rheumatic fever is rare in the U.S. because of prompt treatment of strep throat, but it is not rare in developing countries, where it is one of the leading causes of heart disease.

The cause of rheumatic fever is interesting. It is thought that certain strains of strep bacteria contain glycoproteins that, from the perspective of the immune system, resemble glycoproteins found in the heart, joints, and/or nerve tissue. When the body makes antibodies to attack the strep bacteria, those antibodies also damage the body.

The only known way to prevent rheumatic fever in people with strep throat involves using antibiotics at relatively high doses and for a prolonged period of time. The goal is to entirely eradicate the invading bacteria, so that the body does not feel a need to make antibodies against it.

Proposed Natural Treatments

The unique relationship of rheumatic fever and strep throat is confusing and may lead you to use alternative treatments for it in a way that is not helpful.

Here's how the misconception usually goes: For most diseases, when symptoms abate, the risk is over. Based on this natural understanding of illness, many people use herbs or other natural treatments for strep throat, then feel safe when throat pain and fever disappear.

However, for strep throat, the situation is different. As discussed above, symptoms of strep throat disappear on their own, without treatment, in 3 to 5 days. The big risk comes 1 to 5 weeks later, when rheumatic fever may strike. Antibiotic treatment for strep throat is not primarily intended to treat the strep throat itself (although it does that), but rather to prevent rheumatic fever. There are no herbs or supplements known to prevent rheumatic fever.

Some people try to treat strep throat with herbs believed to stimulate the immune system, such as echina-cea. However, this approach has a serious problem: if echinacea did manage to increase the immune system's activity, the result would be to increase the intensity of rheumatic fever, not decrease it! Remember that rheumatic fever is caused, in a sense, by an overactive immune system, not an underactive one.

The bottom line: Strep throat caused by Group A beta-hemolytic streptococcus cannot be treated with alternative medicine. Conventional diagnosis and treatment is necessary to ensure safety.

However, if tests are done and a case of strep throat does not appear to be caused by Group A beta-hemolytic strep, other forms of treatment may be appropriate.

The herb *Pelargonium sidoides* might actually shorten the duration of non–Group A strep infection, according to a double-blind, placebo-controlled study of 143 children. Whether it is helpful as supplementary treatment to antibiotics for children undergoing treatment for Group A strep remains unknown.

The popular herb tea Throat Coat might help sooth sore throat discomfort. Throat Coat contains herbs traditionally thought to soothe inflamed mucous membranes. One small double-blind study did indeed find that Throat Coat was superior to a placebo for this purpose. It seems reasonable to use Throat Coat along with conventional treatment even for Group A strep infections. However, this tea contains licorice, which can be toxic if taken to excess.

See also all treatments discussed under **Colds and Flus**.

Stress

PRINCIPAL PROPOSED NATURAL TREATMENTS: *Ginseng (Panax Species)*

OTHER PROPOSED NATURAL TREATMENTS: *Adrenal Extract, Alternative Therapies (such as Biofeedback, Guided Imagery, Hypnotherapy, Massage, Relaxation Therapy, Tai Chi, and Yoga), Ashwagandha, Astragalus,* Eleutherococcus senticosus, *Kava, Maitake, Multivitamin/Mineral Supplements, Phosphatidylserine, Reishi, Rhodiola, Schisandra, Shiitake, Suma, Theanine from Black Tea, Tyrosine, Valerian*

The effects of stress on your health can be far-reaching. Some of the conditions often associated with stress include **insomnia**, **high blood pressure**, **tension headaches**, **anxiety**, **depression**, **decreased mental function**, and drug or **alcohol abuse**. Stress is known to cause changes in the body's chemistry, altering the balance of hormones in our systems in ways that can lower our resistance to disease. As a result, we can

Stress

become more susceptible to **colds and flus** and other types of illness. Too much stress sometimes brings on outbreaks of **cold sores** or genital **herpes** for people who carry these viruses in their systems. Other chronic diseases such as **irritable bowel syndrome**, **asthma**, **inflammatory bowel disease**, and **rheumatoid arthritis** may also flare up during times of stress.

If it's possible to avoid situations that cause you to feel tense, unhappy, or worn down, that's obviously to your benefit. However, it isn't always possible to live a stress-free existence. Work deadlines, family demands, relationship problems, traffic jams, missed appointments, forgotten birthdays, personality conflicts, college exams—all of these things, and many more, can be sources of stress. Furthermore, though most of us associate stress with unpleasant events, even wonderful events in our lives, like weddings, vacations, and holidays, can be genuinely stressful.

Not everyone responds to these situations by getting "stressed out." There are those apparently unflappable folks whose pulse rate wouldn't even go up during an earthquake and then there are those for whom being five minutes late constitutes reason for a state of total panic. How you manage the stress in your life can determine the impact it will have on you.

There are many different methods of dealing with stress. The basics for good health that we all know (but often forget) help in coping with stress: eating a balanced diet and getting adequate rest help your body adapt and respond to the events in your life. Ironically, stress can interfere with your ability to take care of yourself in this way. When you're worrying so much you can't sleep, getting adequate rest becomes impossible. Stress can affect your eating habits too. So what else can you do? Exercise, meditation, and biofeedback are all widely accepted stress management tools that might help you break out of a stress-induced downward spiral.

For some people, stressful circumstances can trigger symptoms severe enough to warrant seeking medical attention. Conditions associated with stress, such as insomnia, anxiety, depression, and **panic attacks**, may become severe enough to require medications.

Principal Proposed Natural Treatments

One proposed natural approach to treating the physical consequences stress involves the use of so-called *adaptogens*. The term *adaptogen* refers to a hypothetical treatment described as follows: An adaptogen helps the body adapt to stresses of various kinds, whether

heat, cold, exertion, trauma, sleep deprivation, toxic exposure, radiation, infection, or psychological stress. Furthermore, an adaptogen should cause no side effects, be effective in treating a wide variety of illnesses, and help return an organism toward balance no matter what may have gone wrong.

However, physical exercise is the only indubitable example of an adaptogen. There is no solid evidence that any substance functions in this way. However there is a bit of suggestive evidence for the herb *Panax ginseng* and it is discussed in this section.

Panax Ginseng

Most of the evidence cited to indicate that *Panax ginseng* has adaptogenic effects comes from animal studies involving ginseng extracts injected into the abdomen. Such studies are of questionable relevance to the oral use of ginseng by people; furthermore, the majority of these studies were performed in the former Soviet Union and failed to reach acceptable scientific standards. However, a few potentially meaningful studies in humans have found effects that are at least consistent with the possibility of benefits in stressful situations.

➤ *Animal Studies*

According to a number of animal studies, most of which were poorly designed and reported, *Panax ginseng* injections into the blood stream or abdomen can increase stamina, improve mental function, protect against radiation, infections, toxins, exhaustion, and stress, and activate white blood cells. However, when ginseng is injected into the abdomen or bloodstream, it enters the body directly without going through the digestive tract. This mode of administration is strikingly different from taking ginseng by mouth.

A smaller number of animal studies (again, most of them poorly designed) have looked at the potential benefits of ginseng administered orally and often reported benefit. In addition, studies in mice found that consuming ginseng before exposure to a virus significantly increased the survival rate and number of antibodies produced.

➤ *Human Studies*

Human studies of *Panax ginseng* have only indirectly examined its potential benefits as an adaptogen. For example, a double-blind, placebo-controlled study found evidence that *Panax ginseng* may improve immune system response. This trial enrolled 227 participants at three medical offices in Milan, Italy. Half were given ginseng at a dosage of 100 mg daily and the other half received placebo. Four weeks into the study, all participants received influenza vaccine.

The results showed a significant decline in the frequency of colds and flus in the treated group compared to the placebo group (15 versus 42 cases). Also, antibody levels in response to the vaccination rose higher in the treated group than in the placebo group.

These findings have been taken by some researchers to support their belief that ginseng has an adaptogenic effect. However, the study might instead simply indicate a general form of **immune support** unrelated to stress.

Other studies have looked at *Panax ginseng's* effects on overall mental function, **general wellbeing**, and **sports performance**. While it is true that positive results in such studies might tend to hint at an adaptogenic effect, the results were in general too mixed to provide conclusive evidence for benefit.

The bottom line: It is not clear that *Panax ginseng* offers general benefits for stress.

For more information, including dosage and safety issues, see the full **Ginseng** article.

Other Proposed Natural Treatments

Multivitamins Plus Minerals

Surprisingly, a treatment as simple as **multivitamin-mineral tablets** may be helpful for stress.

In a double-blind, placebo-controlled study, 300 men and women were given either a multivitamin-mineral tablet or placebo for 30 days. The results showed that people taking the nutritional supplement experienced less anxiety overall and an enhanced ability to cope with stressful circumstances. The supplement used in this study supplied the following nutrients and dosages: **vitamin B_1**, 10 mg; **vitamin B_2**, 15 mg; **vitamin B_6**, 10 mg; **vitamin B_{12}**, 10 mcg; **vitamin C**, 1,000 mg; **calcium**, 100 mg; and **magnesium**, 100 mg.

Benefits were seen in another double-blind, placebo-controlled trial that enrolled 80 healthy male volunteers. The supplement used in this trial was similar but not identical.

It's not clear how these nutrients help stress, but considering that many of us would benefit from general nutritional supplementation in any case, it might be worth trying.

Eleutherococcus senticosus

In the 1940s, Dr. Brekhman, the same scientist who first dubbed *Panax ginseng* an adaptogen, decided that a much less expensive herb, *Eleutherococcus senticosus*, is also an adaptogen. A thorny bush that grows much more rapidly than true ginseng, this plant later received the misleading name of "Siberian" or "Russian ginseng." Its chemical makeup, however, is completely unrelated to that of *Panax ginseng*.

As with *Panax ginseng*, many animal studies finding adaptogenic benefits with eleutherococcus have been reported, but most were relatively poorly designed and used injections rather than oral administration of the herb, making the results not particularly relevant to the normal human usage of the herb.

Numerous human trials of eleutherococcus have been reported as well, some involving enormous numbers of participants. However, most of these were not double-blind and many were not even controlled, making the results nearly meaningless. (For information on why double-blind, placebo-controlled studies are essential to establish the effectiveness of a treatment, see **Why Does This Book Rely on Double-blind Studies?**.)

Again, as with *Panax ginseng*, a few reasonably well-designed studies in humans have been reported that may have indirect bearing on the herb's potential adaptogenic properties. For example, in one double-blind trial, participants took either 10 ml of extract of eleutherococcus or placebo 3 times daily for a 4-week period. Blood samples were analyzed to determine changes in immune cells. A statistically significant increase in numbers of cells important to immune functions was observed in the treatment group as compared to the placebo group.

This study has been widely advertised as proving the eleutherococcus strengthens immunity. However, mere changes in immune cell profile do not at all automatically translate into enhanced immunity. (See the **Immune Support** article for more information on why this is so.) More meaningful data was obtained in a double-blind, placebo-controlled study involving 93 people who experience recurrent flare-ups of herpes. Use of eleutherococcus significantly reduced the severity, frequency, and duration of herpes outbreaks relative to placebo during the 6-month trial. This study does suggest a possible immune strengthening effect.

Like *Panax ginseng*, eleutherococcus has also been studied for potential sports performance enhancement benefits, but published studies have not been encouraging. One small double-blind, placebo-controlled trial of endurance athletes actually found that use of eleutherococcus may increase physiologic signs of stress during intensive training.

For more information, including dosage and safety issues, see the full **Eleutherococcus** article.

Other Possible Adaptogens

Three small double-blind trials suggest that the herb **rhodiola** (*Rhodiola rosea*) may improve mental alertness in people undergoing sleep deprivation or other stressful circumstances.

Numerous other herbs are said to be adaptogens as well. These include **ashwagandha, astragalus, maitake, reishi,** shiitake, **suma,** and **schisandra.** However, there is little to no real evidence as yet that they have adaptogenic effects.

One study failed to find greater adaptogenic effects with fish oil as compared to placebo.

Other Options

Preliminary double blind trials suggest that the amino acid **tyrosine** may improve memory and mental function under conditions of sleep deprivation or other forms of stress.

One double-blind study found that use of vitamin C at doses of 3,000 mg daily (slow release) reduced both physical and emotional responses to stress.

In a small double-blind study, theanine, a constituent of **black tea,** reduced the body's reaction to acute physical stress.

According to another small double-blind trial, a mixture of **soy phosphatidylserine** and **lecithin** may decrease the physiological response to mental stress.

A proprietary **Ayurvedic** herbal formula containing *Bacopa monniera* and almost 30 other ingredients has shown some promise for treating symptoms of stress. In a 3-month, double-blind, placebo-controlled trial of 42 people in high-stress jobs who complained of fatigue, participants using the herbal formula reported fewer stress-related problems. Also, in a 3-month, double-blind, placebo-controlled study of 50 adult students, this formula appeared to improve memory and attention and reduce other signs of stress.

In naturopathic medicine, **adrenal extract** is often recommended for treatment of stress, but there is no evidence that it is effective.

Many people report that they experience stress relief through the use of alternative therapies such as **biofeedback, guided imagery, hypnotherapy, massage, relaxation therapy, Tai chi,** and **yoga.** One study failed to find regular massage more effective for controlling stress than use of a relaxation tape.

For other natural treatments relevant to stress, see the discussion in the articles on **insomnia** and **anxiety.**

Strokes

RELATED TERMS: *Cerebral Vascular Accident, CVA, Transient Ischemic Attack, TIA*

PRINCIPAL PROPOSED NATURAL TREATMENTS:

   Prevention: *Policosanol; All Herbs and Supplements Used for High Cholesterol, High Blood Pressure, or Atherosclerosis*

   Treatment: *Glycine, Vinpocetine*

OTHER PROPOSED NATURAL TREATMENTS: *Acupuncture, Bilberry, Beta-carotene, Feverfew, Fish Oil, Garlic, Ginger, Ginkgo, Quercetin, Vitamin E, White Willow*

HERBS AND SUPPLEMENTS TO USE ONLY WITH CAUTION: *Ephedra, Iron*

OTHER NATURAL TREATMENTS TO AVOID: *Chelation Therapy*

Strokes occur when part of the brain suddenly loses its blood supply and dies. The underlying cause is generally atherosclerosis, a condition in which the walls of blood vessels become thickened and irregular. As atherosclerosis progresses, blood flow through important arteries becomes restricted to a much smaller passage than nature designed. This narrow passage can then suddenly become blocked, often by a blood clot. When this happens, brain cells downstream of the blockage are suddenly deprived of oxygen (cerebral ischemia).

Brain cells require a constant supply of oxygen to survive. Within seconds, they begin to malfunction, and within minutes they die.

In so-called transient ischemic attacks (TIAs), the blockage to blood flow is temporary and symptoms rapidly disappear. However, in a true stroke, officially called a *cerebral vascular accident* (CVA), the blockage lasts long enough to cause cell death in a significant section of the brain. Less commonly, strokes are caused by bleeding into the brain, known as a *hemorrhagic stroke*.

The symptoms of a stroke depend on the area of the brain affected. Paralysis of one limb or one side of the face is common. Loss of speech or sensation may also occur.

Much of the loss that occurs in a stroke is permanent, but some recovery usually does occur in time. There are two main causes of this recovery. The first involves the body's ability to grow new blood vessels. Nerve cells on the margins of the dead area may cling to survival, functioning imperfectly on whatever oxygen drifts over to them. Eventually, new blood vessel growth enables the nerve cells to recover perfectly.

The second cause of recovery involves the brain's remarkable ability to adapt to difficult circumstances: to a lesser or greater extent, surviving parts of the brain can take over tasks once performed by brain cells that have died.

Conventional treatment for a stroke has several phases, but the most important is prevention. Stopping smoking, losing weight, reducing cholesterol levels, and controlling blood pressure fight atherosclerosis and thereby reduce the risk of stroke. Also, physicians may recommend use of blood-thinning drugs such as aspirin to prevent the blood clots that so frequently are the final step to a stroke. Furthermore, if there is evidence that the main blood vessels leading to the brain are seriously narrowed, surgery or angioplasty may be considered to widen those vessels.

Treatment of a stroke that has just occurred involves maintaining life during the immediate recovery period and limiting the spread of brain damage (if possible). Finally, physical and occupational therapists help the stroke survivor to adapt.

Principal Proposed Natural Treatments

There are a number of alternative options that may be useful for preventing or even possibly treating strokes. The best documented are those that fight atherosclerosis.

Stroke Prevention

Meaningful evidence tells us that numerous herbs and supplements are helpful for improving the **cholesterol profile**, which in turn should decrease **atherosclerosis** and help prevent strokes. Weaker evidence supports the use of other herbs and supplements for lowering **blood pressure** or for treating atherosclerosis in general. For detailed information, see the full articles on those topics.

See also the article on **chelation therapy** for reasons to avoid this controversial alternative treatment.

⮞ *Policosanol*

Various herbs and supplements with blood-thinning properties have been suggested to be used instead of or along with aspirin as a means of preventing blood clots. The best evidence regards the supplement policosanol and, for that reason, it is discussed here. Additional options with less supporting evidence are outlined on the Other Proposed Natural Treatments section below.

Several double-blind, placebo-controlled trials indicate policosanol significantly reduces the blood's tendency to clot. In one double-blind, placebo-controlled study of 43 participants, use of policosanol at 20 mg per day proved approximately as effective as 100 mg of aspirin; in addition, when the two treatments were taken in combination, the effect was greater than with either treatment alone. Furthermore, as described in the article on policosanol, this supplement appears to reduce cholesterol levels, making it potentially an all-around stroke-preventing treatment. However, while long-term use of aspirin has been shown to reduce stroke risk, there have not been any equivalent studies of policosanol. In addition, combined treatment with policosanol and aspirin (or related drugs) could conceivably thin the blood *too* much, resulting in dangerous bleeding events.

For more information, including dosage and safety issues, see the full **Policosanol** article.

Stroke Treatment

As we described above, cells at the margin of a stroke may cling to life until new blood vessels form to supply them with full circulation. Certain herbs and supplements might facilitate this by increasing blood flow or alternatively by reducing brain-cell oxygen requirements.

Although the evidence remains preliminary, two supplements have shown some promise for this purpose: vinpocetine and glycine.

≫ *Vinpocetine*

In a single-blind, placebo-controlled trial, 30 participants who had just experienced a stroke received either placebo or vinpocetine along with conventional treatment for 30 days. Three months later, evaluation showed that participants in the vinpocetine group were significantly less disabled.

A few other studies, some of poor design, also provide suggestive evidence that vinpocetine may be helpful for strokes. However, at present this body of evidence remains far from conclusive.

Note: There are concerns that vinpocetine could interact harmfully with standard drugs used to thin the blood. For more information, including dosage and safety issues, see the full **Vinpocetine** article.

≫ *Glycine*

The supplement glycine has also been proposed as a treatment for limiting permanent stroke damage. However, at present the supporting evidence is largely limited to one moderate-sized Russian trial. In this double-blind, placebo-controlled study, 200 participants received glycine within 6 hours of an acute stroke. The results indicate that use of glycine at 1 g daily for 5 days led to less long-term disability than placebo treatment.

However, paradoxically, there are potential concerns that high-dose glycine could actually *increase* harm caused by strokes and drugs that block glycine have been investigated as treatments to limit stroke damage. The authors of the Russian study on strokes described above make an argument that the overall effect of supplemental glycine is protective; nonetheless, until this controversy is settled, prudence suggests that you should not take glycine following a stroke except on physician advice.

For more information, including additional dosage and safety issues, see the full **Glycine** article.

Other Proposed Natural Treatments

Evidence suggests that high consumption of fish or **fish oil** reduces stroke incidence. This is believed to occur as a result of a number of effects, including impairment of blood clots, improvement of cholesterol profile, and other unidentified means.

Many other herbs and supplements may also reduce the blood's tendency to clot and thereby help prevent strokes, including **bilberry**, **feverfew**, **garlic**, **ginger**, **ginkgo**, **quercetin**, **vitamin E**, and **white willow**. How-

ever, the supporting evidence for these supplements remains weak at best, and the mere fact that they thin the blood does not prove that they will reduce stroke risk. For example, while vitamin E is known to reduce blood clotting and is also a strong antioxidant, several large studies have failed to find vitamin E helpful for stroke prevention.

Similarly, the herb white willow has been advocated as a substitute for aspirin because it contains salicin, a substance very much like aspirin. However, willow in usual doses doesn't appear to impair blood coagulation to the same extent as aspirin and, for that reason, it is probably not equally effective.

Besides vitamin E, other antioxidants such as **beta-carotene** have been proposed for stroke prevention, but there is no evidence that they are effective.

Acupuncture is widely used in China for enhancing recovery from strokes. However, while some studies have suggested benefits, the best-designed and largest studies have not been promising. For example, in a single-blind, placebo-controlled trial of 104 people who had just experienced strokes, 10 weeks of twice-weekly acupuncture did not prove more effective than fake acupuncture. Similarly negative results were seen in a single-blind, controlled study of 150 people recovering from stroke, which compared acupuncture (including electro-acupuncture), high-intensity muscle stimulation, and sham treatment. All participants received 20 treatments over a 10-week period. Neither acupuncture nor muscle stimulation produced any benefits. In addition, a 10-week study of 106 people, which provided a total of 35 traditional acupuncture sessions to each participant, also failed to find benefit. The few studies that did report improvements due to acupuncture were very small and some did not use a placebo group.

The semisynthetic substance citicholine (closely related to the nutrient **choline**) has shown some promise for aiding recovery from strokes.

Herbs and Supplements to Use Only with Caution

If you are at risk for a stroke, it might be advisable to avoid excessive intake of **iron**. Some evidence suggests that high iron levels may increase stroke risk and worsen strokes that do occur.

In addition, people susceptible to stroke should exercise great caution regarding the herb **ephedra**. Ephedra contains ephedrine, a drug that raises blood pressure and stimulates the heart and has caused heart attacks and strokes. Certain preparations of ephedra may present an additional risk beyond ephedrine's effects on the circulatory system: direct toxicity to nerves.

Finally, numerous herbs and supplements may interact adversely with drugs used to prevent or treat strokes. For more information on this potential risk, see the individual drug articles in the Drug Interactions section of this book.

Sunburn

PRINCIPAL PROPOSED NATURAL TREATMENTS: *EGCG, Vitamin C, Vitamin E*

OTHER PROPOSED NATURAL TREATMENTS: Aloe vera, *Beta-carotene and Other Carotenoids, OPCs, Jojoba, Poplar Bud*

We're all familiar with sunburn—the short-term skin inflammation caused by overexposure to the sun. Besides the familiar redness, pain, blistering, and flaking, overexposure to sunlight can lead to long-term skin damage, including premature aging and an increased risk of skin cancer.

The chief culprit in sunburn is not the sun's heat but its ultraviolet radiation, which occurs in the forms UVA and UVB. This radiation acts on substances in our skin to form chemicals called *free radicals*. These free radicals appear to be partly responsible for the short-term damage of sunburn and perhaps for long-term damage from the sun as well.

Conventional approaches to sunburn focus on prevention: staying out of the sun (especially when the sun is strongest), wearing protective clothing, and using sunscreen. Sunscreen blocks much of the radiation from our skin and helps prevent inflammation. A recent study of 1,383 Australians suggests that regular sunscreen use may also diminish the number of tumors caused by one form of skin cancer, squamous cell carcinoma.

Many drugs and herbs may increase your sensitivity to the sun. Some of the drugs that increase sun sensitivity are sulfa drugs, tetracycline, phenothiazines, and piroxicam. Herbs which might increase sensitivity to the sun include **St. John's wort** and **dong quai**. Particular care should be taken when combining any of these substances, as they could amplify each other's effects.

Principal Proposed Natural Treatments

Several studies have found that vitamins C, vitamin E, and EGCG (a bioflavonoid present in green tea) may help to prevent sunburn when used either topically or orally. Many manufacturers already add vitamin E to sunscreens.

Vitamins C and E

Antioxidants such as vitamins C and E neutralize free radicals in the blood and in other parts of our bodies. Test tube and animal studies suggest that they perform the same job in the skin. Levels of these antioxidants in skin cells decrease after exposure to ultraviolet radiation, suggesting they may be temporarily depleted.

In several animal studies, vitamins C and E applied topically to the skin helped to protect against ultraviolet damage. One study found that topical vitamin E seemed to work best against UVB, topical vitamin C protected more against UVA, and the two vitamins together worked better than either one by itself. Vitamin E was effective even when applied to mouse skin 8 hours after ultraviolet exposure had occurred. Combining the vitamins with sunscreen yielded the best result, adding to the UV-protection offered by sunscreen alone.

In addition, preliminary evidence from a small double-blind, placebo-controlled trial suggests that a face cream containing vitamin C could improve the appearance of sun-damaged skin.

Oral use of combined vitamins C and E may offer very modest benefit as well. One double-blind study of 10 people found that 2 g of vitamin C and 1,000 IU of vitamin E taken for 8 days resulted in a modest decrease in skin reddening induced by ultraviolet light. A 50-day placebo-controlled study of 40 people found that high doses of these vitamins in combination provided a

Sunburn

minimal but statistically significant sun-protection factor of about 2. (Compare this to the sun protection factor of 15 to 45 in many sunscreens.) One study found benefits with a combination of vitamins E and C, selenium, OPCs, and carotenoids. However, so far research hasn't found that vitamin E and C, taken separately, are any more helpful than placebo.

For more information, including dosage and safety issues, see the full articles on **vitamin C** and **vitamin E**.

EGCG

Green tea contains a potent antioxidant known as *epigallocatechin gallate*, or **EGCG**. According to several studies, mice given green tea to drink or receiving topical applications of green tea were protected against skin inflammation and carcinogenesis caused by exposure to UVB. Benefits were also seen in two preliminary human trials.

The typical proposed dose of EGCG is 3 mg per square inch of skin.

Other Proposed Natural Treatments

Beta-carotene and Mixed Carotenoids

Beta-carotene belongs to a large family of natural chemicals known as *carotenoids*. Other members of this family include lutein, lycopene, and zeaxanthin. Widely found in plants, carotenoids are a major source of the red, orange, and yellow hues seen in many fruits and vegetables. Beta-carotene is important nutritionally because the body uses it to produce vitamin A.

Beta-carotene, alone or in combination with lutein and other carotenoids, may be able to reduce the effects of sunburn, but study results are mixed.

In a double-blind study, 20 young women took 30 mg daily of beta-carotene or placebo for 10 weeks before a 13-day stretch of controlled sun exposure at a sea-level vacation spot. Those who'd taken the beta-carotene before and during the sun exposure experienced less skin redness than those taking placebo, even when both groups used sunscreen.

A 12-week, double-blind, placebo-controlled study found beta-carotene (at 24 mg daily) and a mixture of beta-carotene, lutein, and lycopene (at 8 mg each daily) equally protective against sun-induced skin redness.

Two open studies of mixed carotenoids found similar results. These trials, one of 20 and one of 22 people, found that after taking mixed carotenoids for 12 to 24 weeks, participants could tolerate more ultraviolet radiation before developing skin redness. Vitamin E (500 IU per day) taken along with beta-carotene in one of the studies didn't significantly affect the results. Another study found benefits with tomato paste (rich in lycopene). However, since these studies weren't double-blind, the results are not very reliable.

Not every study has found beta-carotene or mixed carotenoids to be helpful. In a double-blind trial of 16 older women, high doses of beta-carotene taken for 23 days didn't provide any more protection than placebo against simulated sun exposure. Another 10-week study found that high doses of beta-carotene provided greater protection against natural sunshine than placebo, but the benefits, though statistically significant, were too minor to matter. Completely negative results were seen in a 4-week uncontrolled study of high doses of mixed carotenoids.

Other Natural Treatments

The substances collectively called **OPCs**, found in pine bark and grape seed, have shown some promise for sunburn protection.

Although research information is lacking, topical jojoba, poplar bud (*Populi gemma*), and **Aloe vera** are sometimes recommended for soothing sunburn pain and itch. However, one small study found that applying aloe vera gel after UVB exposure had no effect on skin redness.

Surgery Support

RELATED TERMS: *Anesthesia, Lymphedema, Operations, Postoperative Recovery*

PRINCIPAL PROPOSED NATURAL TREATMENTS: *Acupuncture/Acupressure, Bioflavonoids, Oxerutins and other OPCs, Proteolytic Enzymes*

OTHER PROPOSED NATURAL TREATMENTS: *Arnica, Bee Propolis, Ginger, Horse Chestnut, Hypnotherapy, Magnet Therapy, Multivitamin and Mineral Supplements, Peppermint, Relaxation and Guided Imagery*

HERBS AND SUPPLEMENTS TO USE ONLY WITH CAUTION: *Garlic, Ginkgo, St. John's Wort, Vitamin E*

Surgery, even relatively minor surgery, is a significant trauma to the body. The surgical incision itself can cause swelling (edema), pain, and bruising; anesthesia frequently causes nausea and bloating. Certain surgeries that damage the body's lymphatic system, such as radical mastectomy, can cause a specific form of long-lasting swelling called *lymphedema*.

Modern surgery involves numerous sophisticated nondrug techniques to help wounds heal rapidly and completely. Various medications can be used to help offset the side effects of anesthesia.

Principal Proposed Natural Treatments

A variety of herbs, supplements, and other alternative therapies have shown promise for problems encountered following surgery. However, keep in mind that many such substances have shown the potential to increase risk of bleeding during or after surgery. (See Herbs and Supplements to Use Only with Caution below.) Furthermore, it is not at present possible to determine all the potential interactions between herbs and drugs used for anesthesia. For this reason, herbs and supplements should only be used for surgical support under the supervision of a physician.

Proteolytic Enzymes

According to most but not all studies, proteolytic enzymes may help reduce pain, bruising, and swelling after surgery.

A double-blind, placebo-controlled trial of 80 people undergoing knee surgery found that treatment with mixed proteolytic enzymes after surgery significantly improved rate of recovery, as measured by mobility and swelling.

Another double-blind, placebo-controlled trial eval-

uated the effects of a similar mixed proteolytic enzyme product in 80 individuals undergoing oral surgery. The results showed reduced pain, inflammation, and swelling in the treated group as compared to the placebo group. Benefits were also seen in another trial of mixed proteolytic enzymes for dental surgery, as well as in one study involving only bromelain.

Other double-blind, placebo-controlled studies have found bromelain helpful in nasal surgery, cataract removal, and foot surgery. However, a study of 154 individuals undergoing facial plastic surgery found no benefit.

Note: Bromelain thins the blood and could increase risk of bleeding during or after surgery. For this reason, physician supervision is essential.

For more information, including dosage and safety issues, see the full articles on **bromelain** and **proteolytic enzymes**.

Oxerutins and Other Bioflavonoids

Oxerutins have been widely used in Europe since the mid-1960s, primarily as a treatment for **varicose veins**. Derived from a naturally occurring bioflavonoid called *rutin*, oxerutins were specifically developed to treat varicose veins and related venous problems. However, they may also be helpful for treating swelling following surgery. Closely related bioflavonoids from citrus fruit may be helpful as well.

Women who have undergone surgery for breast cancer may experience a lasting and troublesome side effect: swelling in the arm caused by damage to the lymph system. Along with the veins, the lymphatic system is responsible for returning fluid to the heart. When this system is damaged by breast cancer surgery, fluid accumulates in the arm. Three small double-blind, placebo-controlled studies enrolling a total of more than 100 people have examined the effectiveness of oxerutins in lymphedema following breast cancer surgery, with generally good results.

For example, in a small 6-month, double-blind study, oxerutins reduced swelling and improved comfort and mobility as compared to placebo. Another study found benefit with a combination formula containing oxerutins, **ginkgo**, and the drug heptaminol.

The citrus bioflavonoids diosmin and hesperidin have also shown promise for lymphedema following breast cancer surgery, as has a product containing hesperidin plus a bioflavonoid-rich extract of the herb **butcher's broom**. **Note**: Do not use bioflavonoid combinations containing tangeretin if you are taking tamoxifen for breast cancer.

Oxerutins might also be helpful for the ordinary swelling that occurs after any type of surgery. In one double-blind trial, researchers gave oxerutins or placebo for 5 days to 40 people recovering from minor surgery or other minor injuries and found oxerutins significantly helpful in reducing swelling and discomfort.

For more information, including dosage and safety issues, see the full articles on **oxerutins** and **citrus bioflavonoids**.

OPCs

OPCs (oligomeric proanthocyanidins), substances found in grape seed and pine bark, may be helpful for recovery from surgery as well. Like oxerutins, to which they are chemically related, OPCs are thought to work by reducing leakage from capillaries.

A double-blind, placebo-controlled study of 63 women with breast cancer found that 600 mg of OPCs daily for 6 months reduced postoperative symptoms of lymphedema. Additionally, in a double-blind, placebo-controlled study of 32 people who were followed for 10 days after a face-lift, swelling disappeared much faster in the treated group.

For more information, including dosage and safety issues, see the full **OPCs** article.

Acupuncture/Acupressure

Acupuncture and acupressure are two related forms of treatment that involve stimulating certain locations on the body, known as *acupuncture points*. Numerous studies have evaluated treatment on a single acupuncture point—P6—for the relief of nausea following anesthesia. This point is located on the inside of the forearm, about 2 inches above the wrist crease.

Many controlled studies involving more than 2,000 people have tested the potential benefits of stimulation at P6 in people undergoing surgery. In most of these trials, treatment was carried out through the surgery itself, as well as afterwards. The results of these many trials, involving various types of surgery and diverse forms of acupuncture/acupressure, thoroughly contradict one another. On balance, however, it appears that acupuncture/acupressure may reduce post-surgical nausea to at least some extent beyond that of the placebo effect.

Acupuncture has also been explored as a means of reducing pain after surgery, but there have been more negative than positive results.

Contrary to popular belief, acupuncture does *not* appear to be helpful for providing or enhancing anesthesia itself.

For more information, see the full **Acupuncture** article.

Other Proposed Natural Treatments

The herb **ginger** is thought to have anti-nausea effects and in studies has been given to people prior to surgery in order to prevent the nausea that many people experience when they awaken from anesthesia. However, despite some early positive results, the preponderance of evidence indicates that ginger is not helpful for this purpose.

Warning: Do not use ginger either before or immediately after surgery, or labor and delivery, without a physician's approval. Not only is it important to have an empty stomach before undergoing anesthesia, there are theoretical concerns that ginger may affect bleeding.

Preliminary evidence suggests that peppermint oil may be helpful for post-operative flatulence and nausea.

A preliminary controlled study found that the honeybee product **propolis** mouthwash following oral surgery significantly speeded healing time as compared to placebo.

One small double-blind, placebo-controlled study found that **magnet therapy** patches of the "unipolar" variety reduced pain and swelling after suction lipectomy.

In a double-blind, placebo-controlled study of 37 people undergoing surgery for **carpal tunnel syndrome**, an ointment made from the herb arnica (combined with **homeopathic** arnica tablets) appeared to slightly reduce post-surgical pain.

Horse chestnut has effects similar to OPCs (discussed above) and has also shown promise for reducing postoperative swelling.

In two studies, the sports supplement **creatine** has been tried as an aid to strengthen recovery after knee surgery but no benefits were seen.

Good nutrition is essential to recovery from any physical trauma. For this reason, use of a **multivitamin and mineral supplement** in the weeks leading up to surgery, and for some time afterwards, might be advisable.

A placebo-controlled study failed to find that onion extract can help reduce skin scarring following surgery.

One study found that **massage therapy** reduced post-operative pain.

At least 20 controlled studies, enrolling a total of more than 1,500 people, have evaluated the potential benefit of **hypnosis** for people undergoing surgery. Their combined results suggest that hypnosis may provide benefits both during and after surgery, including: reducing anxiety, pain, and nausea, normalizing blood pressure and heart rate, minimizing blood loss, and speeding recovery and shortening hospitalization. Unfortunately, many of these studies were of very poor quality.

Relaxation therapy techniques, such as meditation and guided imagery, have also shown promise for relieving some of the discomforts of surgery.

Herbs and Supplements to Use Only with Caution

Numerous herbs and supplements have the potential to cause problems during or after surgery, including some of those discussed in this article. For this reason, we strongly suggest that you do not use any herb or supplement in the week leading up to surgery, except under physician's supervision.

For example, the herb **garlic** significantly thins the blood and case reports suggest that garlic can increase bleeding during or after surgery. For this reason, it is probably advisable to avoid garlic supplements prior to surgery and not to restart it after surgery until all risk of bleeding is past.

Use of the herb ginkgo has also been associated with serious bleeding complications related to surgery.

Many other herbs and supplements have also shown potential for increasing risk of bleeding. Most prominent among these are high-dose **vitamin E** and **policosanol**. Others include bromelain, **chamomile, devil's claw, dong quai, feverfew, fish oil**, ginger, horse chestnut, **ipriflavone, mesoglycan**, papaya, **PC-SPES, phosphatidylserine, red clover, reishi, vitamin A**, and **white willow**.

In addition, one report suggests that use of **St. John's wort** may interact with anesthetic drugs.

Tardive Dyskinesia

RELATED TERMS: *Tardive Dyskinesis*

PRINCIPAL PROPOSED NATURAL TREATMENTS: *Vitamin E*

OTHER PROPOSED NATURAL TREATMENTS: *BCAAs, Choline, DMAE, GLA, Lecithin, Manganese, Melatonin, Niacin, Vitamin B$_6$, Vitamin C*

HERBS AND SUPPLEMENTS TO USE ONLY WITH CAUTION: *Phenylalanine*

Tardive dyskinesia (TD) is a potentially permanent side effect of drugs used to control schizophrenia and other psychoses. This late-developing (tardy, or tardive) complication consists of annoying, mostly uncontrollable movements (dyskinesias). Typical symptoms include repetitive sucking or blinking, slow twisting of the hands, or other movements of the face and limbs. TD can cause tremendous social embarrassment to particularly vulnerable individuals.

Several different theories have been proposed for the development of TD. According to one, long-term treatment with antipsychotic drugs causes the brain to become overly sensitive to the neurotransmitter dopamine, resulting in abnormal movements. According to another, imbalances among different neurotransmitters can cause or aggravate symptoms. In a third theory, TD may arise in part from damage to the brain caused by free radicals generated by schizophrenia treatments. All of these theories may contain some truth.

Unfortunately, discontinuing medication that caused TD usually doesn't help and may even worsen the dyskinesia as well as the underlying schizophrenia. Drugs such as L-dopa and oxypertine may improve TD but present their own significant risk of side effects. Fortunately, newer medications for schizophrenia that are less likely to cause TD have been developed in recent years.

Principal Proposed Natural Treatments

Vitamin E is an antioxidant, a substance that works to neutralize free radicals in the body. As noted above, it has been suggested that free-radicals may play a role in TD. If this is true, it makes sense that vitamin E might help prevent or treat the condition.

Between 1987 and 1998, at least five double-blind studies were published which indicated that vitamin E was beneficial in treating TD. Although most of these studies were small and lasted only 4 to 12 weeks, one 36-week study enrolled 40 people. Three small double-blind studies reported that vitamin E was not helpful. Nonetheless, a statistical analysis of the double-blind studies done before 1999 found good evidence that vitamin E was more effective than placebo. Most studies found that vitamin E worked best for TD of more recent onset.

However, in 1999, the picture on vitamin E changed with the publication of one more study—the largest and longest to date. This double-blind study included 107 participants from nine different research sites who took 1,600 IU of vitamin E or placebo daily for at least 1 year. In contrast to most of the previous studies, this trial failed to find vitamin E effective for decreasing TD symptoms.

Why the discrepancy between this study and the earlier ones? The researchers, some of whom had worked on the earlier, positive studies of vitamin E, were at pains to develop an answer. They proposed a number of possible explanations. One was that the earlier studies were too small or too short to be accurate and that vitamin E really didn't help at all. Another was the most complicated: that vitamin E might help only a subgroup of people who had TD—those with milder TD symptoms of more recent onset—and that fewer of these people had participated in the latest study. They also pointed to changes in schizophrenia treatment since the last study was done, including the growing use of antipsychotic medications that do not cause TD.

The bottom line: The effectiveness of vitamin E for a given person is simply not known. Given the lack of other good treatments for TD, and the general safety of the vitamin, it may be worth discussing with your physician.

For more information, including dosage and safety issues, see the full **Vitamin E** article.

Other Proposed Natural Treatments for Tardive Dyskinesia

Choline and Related Substances

According to one theory, TD symptoms may be caused or aggravated by an imbalance between two neurotransmitters, dopamine and acetylcholine. The nutrient **choline** and several related substances—**lecithin**, CDP-choline, and **DMAE**—have been suggested as possible treatments, with the goal of increasing the amount of acetylcholine the body produces. Lecithin and CDP-choline are broken down by the body to produce choline, and choline provides one of the building blocks for acetylcholine. DMAE (2-dimethylaminoethanol, sometimes called *deanol*) may also increase production of acetylcholine, although this has been questioned.

Although a variety of small studies have been conducted on these substances, evidence for their effectiveness is mixed at best. Three small double-blind studies of lecithin had conflicting results: one found lecithin more helpful than placebo, one found it to be barely superior, and one found it no better than placebo. In two small double-blind trials of choline itself, some people experienced decreased TD symptoms on choline compared to placebo but other people did not, and several people grew worse.

CDP-choline, a natural substance closely related to choline, has also been the subject of a couple of small studies with mixed results. An open study of 10 people found it helpful for TD, but a tiny double-blind study did not find any evidence of benefit.

The substance DMAE is better studied than these other cholinergic treatments for TD—but the preponderance of evidence suggests it is not effective. Of 12 double-blind studies reviewed, only one found DMAE to be significantly effective when compared with placebo. A meta-analysis of proposed treatments for TD found DMAE to be no more effective than placebo.

Other Natural Treatments

A 6-week, double-blind, placebo-controlled study of 22 individuals with schizophrenia and TD found that **melatonin** at a dose of 10 mg/day significantly improved TD symptoms.

One small pilot study suggests that **vitamin B₆** may be helpful for the treatment of TD. In this 4-week, double-blind, crossover trial of 15 people, treatment with vitamin B₆ significantly improved TD symptoms as compared to placebo. Benefits were seen after 1 week of treatment.

Preliminary evidence suggests that **branched-chain amino acids** (BCAAs) might decrease TD symptoms. Other proposed treatments include **niacin** and **manganese**, but so far evidence for their effectiveness is weak at best. Two double-blind trials of evening primrose oil, which contains large amounts of the essential fatty acid **gamma-linolenic acid** (GLA), found that it was not significantly more effective than placebo at reducing TD.

Prevention: High-dose Vitamins?

An informal 20-year study of more than 60,000 people treated with antipsychotic drugs plus high doses of vitamins found that only 34 of them (0.5%) developed TD. This is far fewer than might be expected: the estimated rate of TD among people treated with traditional antipsychotic medications is 20 to 25%. These results were based on reports from 80 psychiatrists who routinely used high-dose vitamins along with drugs to treat people with schizophrenia. Vitamins typically included **vitamin C**, niacin, vitamin B₆, and vitamin E in varying dosages. However, because the study design was very informal, it is not possible to draw firm conclusions from its results.

Herbs and Supplements to Use Only with Caution

There is some concern that the amino acid **phenylalanine**, present in many protein-rich foods, may worsen TD. In a double-blind study of 18 people with schizophrenia, those who took phenylalanine supplements had more TD symptoms than those who took placebo.

Other herbs and supplements may interact adversely with drugs used to treat schizophrenia. For more information, see the individual drug article in the Drug Interactions section of this book.

Temporomandibular Joint Syndrome

RELATED TERMS: *TMJ Syndrome*

PRINCIPAL PROPOSED NATURAL TREATMENTS: *None*

OTHER PROPOSED NATURAL TREATMENTS: *Acupuncture, Capsaicin Cream, Chiropractic, Chondroitin, EMG Biofeedback, Glucosamine, Massage, Prolotherapy*

Temporomandibular joint (TMJ) syndrome is a disorder involving the two joints (one on each side) that attach the lower jaw to the skull. These two joints open and close the mouth and are located directly in front of each of the ears. In TMJ syndrome, the area around the temporomandibular joints becomes chronically tender and inflamed. Symptoms include the following:

> Pain in the temporomandibular joint
> Popping, clicking, or grating in the temporomandibular joint while eating and/or drinking
> A sensation of the jaw "catching" or "locking" briefly, while attempting to open or close the mouth, or while chewing
> Difficulty opening the mouth completely
> Pain in the jaw

> Facial pain
> Muscle pain and/or spasm in the area of the temporomandibular joint
> Headache
> Ear pain
> Neck and/or shoulder pain

TMJ syndrome often occurs in people who have had accidents or injuries involving their jaw, but many others have had no such incident. It is believed that grinding the teeth or clenching the jaw in response to stress may trigger the condition in many cases. Other possible causes include arthritis of the temporomandibular joint, facial bone defects, and misalignments of the jaw or of the bite.

The underlying cause of TMJ syndrome is not known. In most cases, the joint appears to be healthy, suggesting that it is the soft tissue around the joint rather than the joint itself that has the problem. However, some cases of TMJ syndrome may be caused by TMJ arthritis, TMJ dislocation, or other forms of true joint injury.

Treatment of TMJ includes stress management, avoidance of certain foods that trigger discomfort (such as gum or beef jerky), and anti-inflammatory medications. The older antidepressant drug amitriptyline, taken in low doses, as well as the muscle relaxant cyclobenzaprine may help as well.

According to a few controlled trials, some people with more severe forms of TMJ may benefit from the use of a dental appliance. Finally, on rare occasions, surgery may be necessary.

Proposed Natural Treatments

The supplement **glucosamine**, taken alone or in combination with **chondroitin**, has shown considerable promise for the treatment of osteoarthritis. Because osteoarthritis of the temporomandibular joint can play a role in some cases of TMJ syndrome, researchers have begun to investigate the potential role of these supplements in treating the condition. Promising results were seen in a double-blind study that compared glucosamine to ibuprofen in the treatment of 45 people with TMJ arthritis. Over the 3-month study period, the supplement proved equal in effectiveness to the drug. However, because this study lacked a placebo group, it cannot be taken as fully reliable. Another double-blind study, this one involving glucosamine without chondroitin, did have a placebo group, but too many participants dropped out to allow meaningful conclusions to be drawn.

EMG biofeedback is a form of **biofeedback therapy** that involves teaching a person to gain conscious control of muscle tension. A meta-analysis (formal statistical review) of published studies suggests that EMG biofeedback might be helpful for TMJ pain. However, the reviewers noted that the evidence is as yet incomplete, and more (and better quality) research is needed.

Similarly, while preliminary controlled trials suggest that **acupuncture** may be helpful for TMJ syndrome, more research is needed.

A cream made from **cayenne** and other hot peppers (capsaicin cream) has shown promise for a variety of painful conditions. However, one study failed to find capsaicin cream more effective than placebo cream for TMJ syndrome.

Other treatments sometimes recommended for TMJ, but that lack reliable scientific support, include **chiropractic**, **massage**, and **prolotherapy**.

Tendonitis

RELATED TERMS: *Achilles' Tendonitis, Golfer's Elbow, Iliotibial Band Tendonitis, Lateral Epicondylitis, Medial Epicondylitis, Peripatellar Tendonitis, Rotator Cuff Tendonitis, Tendinitis, Tennis Elbow*

PRINCIPAL PROPOSED NATURAL TREATMENTS: *Acupuncture*

OTHER PROPOSED NATURAL TREATMENTS: *Arnica, Boswellia, Bromelain, Chondroitin, Citrus Bioflavonoids, Creatine, Devil's Claw, Glucosamine, Horse Chestnut, Manganese, Massage, Oligomeric Proanthocyanidin Complexes (OPCs), Oxerutins, Prolotherapy, Proteolytic Enzymes, Vitamin C, White Willow*

The tendons are one of the body's weakest links. While muscle and bone heal well after injury, the fibrous tissue that connects muscle to bone has a relatively poor blood supply and, for that reason, it recovers only slowly.

Inflammation in the tendon or its sheath is called *tendonitis*. Symptoms include tenderness, redness, swelling, and pain on exertion. These symptoms may last for months or years. Tendonitis occurs most commonly in the following areas: elbow (lateral epicondylitis or medial epicondylitis, also known as *tennis elbow* and *golfer's elbow*), knee (*peripatellar tendonitis*), hip (*iliotibial band tendonitis*), shoulder (*rotator cuff tendonitis*), lower calf (*Achilles' tendonitis*), forearm, and thumb.

Overuse of a tendon (repetitive strain injury) is the most common cause of tendonitis. This form of injury frequently occurs in computer keyboard users, people who perform manual labor, and athletes (such as tennis elbow and golfer's elbow). Acute injury to a tendon, such as an excessive stretch, can also cause tendonitis.

Conventional treatment consists primarily of avoiding the movement that caused the injury and allowing the body to heal on its own. Non-steroidal anti-inflammatory drugs (such as ibuprofen) may help reduce pain, but have not been shown to speed recovery. Steroid injection into the affected tendon is thought to help in certain cases, but the scientific basis for this commonly used method remains weak at best. The role of physical therapy in recovery from tendonitis also has not been well evaluated from a scientific perspective. A technique called *extracorporeal shockwave therapy* does not appear to work.

Principal Proposed Natural Treatments

Although the evidence remains incomplete and somewhat inconsistent, **acupuncture** treatment has shown considerable promise for the treatment of tendonitis. Most studies have evaluated the effect of acupuncture on tennis elbow (lateral epicondylitis).

For example, a placebo-controlled, single-blind trial of 45 people with tennis elbow compared the effectiveness of real and sham acupuncture given twice weekly for 10 weeks. The results showed significant improvement in pain intensity and ability to use the elbow among those who received real acupuncture. Good results were also seen in a placebo-controlled study of 48 people with tennis elbow.

Another study compared superficial insertion of acupuncture needles (sham treatment insertion) with normal deep insertion in 82 people with tennis elbow. The results showed greater improvement among the participants treated with deep acupuncture, at least in the short term. However, the difference was only temporary; by the 3-month follow-up, both groups were hurting to the same extent.

Benefits have also been seen in studies of people with tendonitis in the shoulder. For example, a trial of 52 people with rotator cuff (shoulder) tendonitis found acupuncture more effective than sham acupuncture. Another study compared superficial to deep-insertion acupuncture in 44 participants with shoulder pain and also found relative benefits. In this trial, the results of deep acupuncture endured for at least 3 months.

Laser acupuncture is a widely used substitute for needle acupuncture, but it may not be effective. A double-blind study of 49 people with tennis elbow failed to find 10 treatments with laser acupuncture more effective than the same number of treatments using fake laser acupuncture.

Other Proposed Natural Treatments

A form of **massage** called *deep transverse friction massage* has shown some promise for tendonitis, but as yet the research record is too weak to draw conclusions.

The supplements **glucosamine** and **chondroitin** are widely used for the treatment of **osteoarthritis**. Evidence suggests that they may work by enhancing the production of substances that keep cartilage healthy and flexible. On this basis, they have also been recommended for treating or preventing tendonitis. However, there is as yet no direct evidence that they work.

The herb **white willow** contains a substance called *salicin*, which is quite similar to aspirin. It seems likely that appropriate doses of the herb might offer some symptomatic relief for tendonitis.

Other natural treatments sometimes recommended for tendonitis, but which lack scientific substantiation for that purpose, include **prolotherapy** and the following herbs and supplements

- **Arnica**
- **Boswellia**
- **Bromelain**
- **Citrus bioflavonoids**
- **Creatine**
- **Devil's claw**
- **Horse chestnut**
- **Manganese**
- **Oligomeric proanthocyanidin complexes (OPCs)**
- **Oxerutins**
- **Proteolytic enzymes**
- **Vitamin C**

Tension Headache

RELATED TERM: *Headache, Tension*

PRINCIPAL PROPOSED NATURAL TREATMENTS: *Acupuncture, Chiropractic*

OTHER PROPOSED NATURAL TREATMENTS:

Body-Mind Therapies: *Biofeedback, Hypnosis, Relaxation Therapies, 5-HTP, Aromatherapy, Butterbur, Massage, Osteopathic Manipulation, Prolotherapy, Therapeutic Touch*

HERBS AND SUPPLEMENTS TO AVOID: *Kava*

Modern life is stressful, and tension headaches are one result of that stress. People with such headaches often describe a sensation like a tight band around the head; this band may in fact exist as a contracted muscle. Other characteristics of tension headache include aching, dull, or throbbing pain, usually concentrated in the forehead, temples, or base of the skull. Symptoms may overlap those of **migraine**, **cluster**, or sinus headaches, and medical advice may be necessary to distinguish among them.

Medical treatment for tension headaches generally involves the use of **nonsteroidal anti-inflammatory drugs** and possibly muscle relaxants. Physicians may also recommend physical therapy techniques in hopes of addressing the causes of tension headaches, such as muscle tension in the neck or jaw.

Principal Proposed Natural Treatments

Both acupuncture and chiropractic have undergone significant evaluation as treatments for tension headaches.

Acupuncture

Placebo-controlled studies of acupuncture for tension headaches have yielded mixed results. One study compared six sessions of traditional acupuncture against sham acupuncture in 18 people with chronic tension headache. The real treatment caused a 31% reduction in pain and was found to be significantly more effective than placebo.

In addition, a study of 29 students suffering from various types of headaches found that a single acupuncture treatment decreased the number of days during which headaches occurred, as well as total use of medications. A statistically insignificant reduction in the number of days of attacks was seen in the placebo group.

However, a study of 39 participants with tension headache found no convincing evidence that acupuncture was helpful. In addition, a single-blind study of 50 participants with tension headache found that a special brief style of acupuncture treatment given once a week for 6 weeks did not reduce headache frequency. Several other trials also failed to find evidence of benefit with various forms of acupuncture.

For more information on this method, see the full **Acupuncture** article.

Chiropractic Spinal Manipulation

Neck tension can cause tension and pain in the head. Such *cervicogenic headaches* overlap closely with tension headaches. Chiropractic spinal manipulation has shown some promise for these conditions, but the evidence is incomplete and somewhat contradictory.

In a controlled trial of 150 participants, investigators compared spinal manipulation to the drug amitriptyline for the treatment of chronic tension–type headaches. By the end of the 6-week treatment period, participants in both groups had improved similarly. However, 4 weeks after treatment was stopped, people who had received spinal manipulation showed statistically significantly better reduction in headache intensity and frequency and used fewer over-the-counter medications than those who had used the amitriptyline.

In another positive trial, 53 participants with cervicogenic headaches received chiropractic spinal manipulation or laser acupuncture plus massage. Chiropractic manipulation was more effective.

However, a similar study of 75 participants with recurrent tension headaches found no difference between the two groups. Other, smaller studies of spinal manipulation have been reported as well, with mixed results.

In a more recent controlled trial, 200 people with cervicogenic headaches were randomly assigned to receive one of four therapies: manipulation, a special exercise technique, exercise plus manipulation, or no therapy. Each participant received at least eight to 12 treatments over a period of 6 weeks. All three treatment approaches produced better results than no treatment, and approximately the same effect as each other. While these results may sound promising, in fact they prove nothing at all, since any treatment whatsoever will generally produce better results than no treatment due to the power of suggestion. Ordinarily, researchers get around this problem by using double-blind, placebo-controlled trials. (For more information on this important subject, see **Why Does This Book Rely on Double-blind Studies?**) While it isn't possible to do a truly double-blind trial of chiropractic, the better trials noted previously used a form of placebo treatment, making them more reliable than this one.

For more information on this method, see the full **Chiropractic** article.

Other Proposed Natural Treatments

A number of other alternative treatments have undergone some evaluation for their usefulness in the treatment of tension headaches.

Several techniques in the category of body-mind medicine have shown promise for the treatment of tension headaches. These include **hypnosis**, **biofeedback**, and **relaxation techniques**, often used in combination with each other.

A topical ointment known as Tiger Balm is a popular remedy for headaches, muscle pain, and other conditions. Tiger Balm contains the aromatic substances camphor, menthol, cajaput, and clove oil, making it a form of **aromatherapy**. A double-blind study enrolling 57 people with acute tension headache compared Tiger Balm (applied to the forehead) against placebo ointment, as well as against the drug **acetaminophen** (Tylenol). The placebo ointment contained mint essence to make it smell similarly to Tiger Balm. Real Tiger Balm proved more effective than placebo. In addition, it was just as effective as acetaminophen and more rapid acting.

Another form of aromatherapy, **peppermint oil** applied to the forehead, has also shown promise, but current studies remain highly preliminary.

Therapeutic touch (TT) is a form of "energy healing" popular in the American nursing community. In a blinded study, 60 participants with tension headaches were randomly assigned to receive either therapeutic touch or a placebo form of the therapy. The true therapy proved to be more effective than placebo.

A study of 28 people with tension headaches compared one session of **osteopathic manipulation** to two forms of sham treatment and found evidence that real treatment provided a greater improvement in headache pain.

Prolotherapy, **massage**, and reflexology (a special form of massage) have all been recommended for the treatment of tension headaches, but there is little evidence to support their use.

The herb **butterbur** is thought to have antispasmodic and anti-inflammatory properties, making it potentially useful for tension headaches.

The supplement **5-HTP** has shown some promise for migraine headaches. However, an 8-week, double-blind, placebo-controlled trial of 65 people with tension headaches found that 5-HTP did not significantly reduce the number of headaches experienced. It did, however, reduce participants' need to use other pain-relieving medications.

Herbs and Supplements to Avoid

The herb **kava** is sometimes suggested as a muscle relaxant and stress reducer. However, there is no meaningful evidence that kava is effective for tension headaches (or any form of muscle tension), and it has been taken off the market in many countries for safety reasons: its use has been linked with severe liver damage.

Finally, numerous herbs and supplements may interact adversely with prescription drugs used to treat tension headaches. For more information on this potential risk, see the individual drug articles in the Drug Interactions section of this book.

Tinnitus

RELATED TERM: *Ears (Ringing)*

PRINCIPAL PROPOSED NATURAL TREATMENTS: *None*

OTHER PROPOSED NATURAL TREATMENTS: *Acupuncture, Biofeedback, Glutamic Acid, Hypnosis, Ipriflavone, Massage, Melatonin, Oxerutins, Periwinkle, Vitamin A Combined with Vitamin E, Vitamin B$_{12}$, Zinc*

PROBABLY NOT EFFECTIVE TREATMENTS: Ginkgo biloba

Tinnitus is the technical term for ringing in the ear, although it may actually involve sounds better described as buzzing, roaring, or hissing. The noise can be intermittent or continuous and can vary in pitch and loudness. Most people have experienced tinnitus occasionally for a minute or two. However, some people have tinnitus continuously, over long periods of time. It can range from a minor annoyance to a serious and nearly intolerable condition.

Exposure to loud noise can lead to tinnitus, as can ear obstructions, ear infections, otosclerosis (abnormal bone growth in the ear), head injuries, or heart and blood vessel disorders. In some cases, treating the underlying disorder will relieve the tinnitus; however, in many cases the cause either can't be found or can't be treated.

One approach involves covering up the noise to make it more tolerable; this includes hearing aids, tinnitus maskers (devices worn in the ear that emit pleasant sounds), or simply playing music to cover the noise. Avoiding loud noises, nicotine, aspirin, caffeine, and alcohol may help, since these often aggravate tinnitus.

Drugs such as carbamazepine, benzodiazepines, and tricyclic antidepressants may be tried, although none of these have been proven effective for tinnitus.

Proposed Natural Treatments

There are no well-documented natural treatments for tinnitus.

Several studies have evaluated *Ginkgo biloba* extract for treating tinnitus, but the results have been conflicting. While some small studies found benefit, by far the largest and best-designed of these trials found no benefit. In this double-blind, placebo-controlled trial, 1,121 individuals with tinnitus were given 12 weeks of treatment with standardized ginkgo at a dose of 50 mg 3 times daily. The results showed no difference between the treated and the placebo group.

A separate set of researchers performed an additional study on ginkgo for tinnitus, and then additionally conducted a meta-analysis (statistically rigorous review) of the published data. Their conclusion: The evidence is strong enough to state that ginkgo does *not* benefit tinnitus.

One double-blind, placebo-controlled study found that **zinc** deficiency was common in people with tinnitus. Zinc supplements appeared to help, but the study was too small to provide statistically meaningful results. In contrast, another small double-blind, placebo-controlled study of people with tinnitus did not discover frequent zinc deficiency and failed to find any benefit with zinc supplements.

Vitamins A and **E** in combination, **vitamin B$_{12}$**, glutamic acid, **ipriflavone**, **oxerutins**, and periwinkle have also been suggested for the treatment of tinnitus, but as yet the supporting evidence for their use remains far too weak to rely upon.

Melatonin may improve sleep in people with tinnitus; however, it doesn't appear to have any effect on the tinnitus itself.

Several studies of **acupuncture** for tinnitus failed to find benefit. **Biofeedback**, **massage therapy**, and **hypnosis** have also been tried, but the results have been mixed at best.

Tooth Decay Prevention

RELATED TERMS: *Cavities, Prevention; Dental Caries; Caries, Prevention*

PRINCIPAL PROPOSED NATURAL TREATMENTS: *Xylitol*

OTHER PROPOSED NATURAL TREATMENTS: *Black Tea, Cranberry, Myrrh, Probiotics, Propolis, Sanguinaria, Sorbitol*

Cavities, technically called *dental caries*, are caused by a bacteria called *Streptococcus mutans*. This bacteria lives in the mouth and thrives on sugar and other carbohydrates. In the presence of carbohydrates, *S. mutans* produces acids that dissolve the enamel of teeth, causing cavities.

Strong evidence indicates that fluoride toothpastes help prevent cavities. Fluoride rinses may help as well. The benefits of water fluoridation are less clear. There is little scientific support for the use of professionally applied fluoride varnishes.

Principal Proposed Natural Treatments

Double-blind studies enrolling almost 4,000 people, mostly children, have found that the natural sugar xylitol can prevent cavities. These trials used xylitol-sweetened gum, candies, or toothpaste. The best evidence regards xylitol gum.

In one of the largest of these trials, researchers tested gum sweetened with various concentrations of xylitol and/or sorbitol against gum sweetened with sucrose and a control group receiving no gum. This 40-month trial was completed by 861 children. Gum containing 100% xylitol reduced the incidence of cavities the most. However, all of the xylitol and sorbitol gum groups showed significant reductions in cavities as compared to the control group. In contrast, the children receiving sucrose-sweetened gum had a slight increase in cavities compared to the control group.

A double-blind, placebo-controlled study of 1,677 children compared a standard fluoride toothpaste with a similar toothpaste that also contained 10% xylitol. Over the 3-year study period, children given the xylitol-enriched toothpaste developed significantly fewer cavities than those in the fluoride-only group. Studies in

adults and children have shown similar results for xylitol gum and candy.

Another series of studies suggests that children acquire cavity-causing bacteria from their mothers and that regular use of xylitol by a mother of a newborn child may provide long lasting protection to the child as well.

Xylitol is thought to prevent cavities by inhibiting the growth of the *Streptococcus mutans* bacteria.

For more information, including dosage and safety issues, see the full **Xylitol** article.

Other Proposed Natural Treatments

Another sugar substitute called *sorbitol* may work as well as xylitol for the prevention of cavities in children. However, xylitol appears to work better than sorbitol for preventing cavities in adults.

Friendly bacteria (**probiotics**) have been proposed for the prevention of cavities, on the ground that they can fight harmful cavity-causing bacteria. The best evidence regards a probiotic product called *Lactobacillus* GG (LGG). In a double-blind, placebo controlled trial, 594 children aged 1 to 6 years old were given either normal milk or milk to which LGG had been added, for a period of 7 months. The results showed significantly fewer cavities in the children receiving LGG.

One very preliminary study found suggestive evidence that use of a toothpaste containing the herb **sanguinaria** (bloodroot) plus fluoride is more effective for cavity prevention than fluoride alone.

Very weak evidence hints that **cranberry** juice might help prevent cavities.

Other natural treatments advocated for preventing cavities, but that lack reliable scientific support, include **black tea**, myrrh, and **propolis**.

Ulcerative Colitis

RELATED TERMS: *Inflammatory Bowel Disease (Ulcerative Colitis, Crohn's Disease)*

PRINCIPAL PROPOSED NATURAL TREATMENTS: *Nutritional Support, Aloe, Fish Oil, Probiotics*

OTHER PROPOSED NATURAL TREATMENTS: *Blue-green Algae, Boswellia, Bromelain, Evening Primrose Oil, Food Allergen Avoidance, Glutamine, Mesoglycans, Wheat Grass Juice*

Ulcerative colitis is a disease of the colon that is closely related to **Crohn's disease**. The two are grouped in a category called *inflammatory bowel disease* (IBD) because they both involve inflammation of the digestive tract.

The major symptoms of ulcerative colitis include abdominal pain and bloody diarrhea. When the disease becomes severe, fever, weight loss, dehydration, and anemia may develop. Sometimes, constipation develops instead of diarrhea. Arthritis, skin sores, and liver inflammation may occur as well.

One of the most feared consequences of ulcerative colitis is dramatic dilation of the colon, which can lead to fatal perforation of the colon. Ulcerative colitis also leads to a greatly increased risk of colon cancer.

Ulcerative colitis tends to wax and wane, with periods of remission punctuated by severe flare-ups. Medical treatment aims at reducing symptoms and inducing and maintaining remission.

Sulfasalazine is one of the most common medications for ulcerative colitis. Given either orally or as an enema, it can both decrease symptoms and prevent recurrences. **Corticosteroids**, such as prednisone, are used similarly in more severe cases, sometimes combined with other immunosuppressive drugs, such as azathioprine and **cyclosporine**. Partial removal of the colon may be necessary in severe cases.

Principal Proposed Natural Treatments

People with ulcerative colitis can easily develop deficiencies in numerous nutrients. Chronic bleeding leads to iron deficiency. Malabsorption, decreased appetite, drug side effects, and increased nutrient loss through the stool may lead to mild or profound deficiencies of protein, **vitamins A, B$_{12}$, C, D, E, and K, folate, calcium, copper, magnesium, selenium, and zinc**. If you have ulcerative colitis, supplementation to restore adequate body stores of these nutrients is highly advisable and may improve specific symptoms as well as overall health. We recommend working closely with your physician to identify any nutrient deficiencies and evaluate the success of supplementation in correcting them.

Essential Fatty Acids

Fish oil and evening primrose oil contain healthy fats called *essential fatty acids*. According to some, though not all, of the small, double-blind, placebo-controlled trials reported, fish oil might be helpful for reducing *symptoms* of active ulcerative colitis. Evening primrose oil has also shown promise. However, larger studies will be necessary to discover for certain whether fish oil or evening primrose oil really help.

Regular use of fish oil alone, or in combination with gamma-linolenic acid (found in evening primrose oil), has not been found effective for *preventing* disease flare-ups in people whose ulcerative colitis has gone into remission.

For more information, including dosage and safety issues, see the **Fish Oil** and **Evening Primrose Oil** articles.

Probiotics

Friendly bacteria, or probiotics, might be helpful in ulcerative colitis.

A double-blind trial of 116 people with ulcerative colitis compared probiotic treatment against a relatively low dose of the standard drug mesalazine. The results suggest that probiotic treatment might be equally effective as low-dose mesalazine for controlling symptoms and maintaining remission. Evidence of benefit was seen in other trials as well.

Probiotics might be useful for people with ulcerative colitis who have had part or all of the colon removed. Such individuals frequently develop a complication called *pouchitis*, inflammation of part of the remaining intestine. Two double-blind, placebo-controlled studies found that probiotics can help prevent pouchitis and also reduce relapses in people who already have it. The probiotic mixture used in these trials contained four strains of *Lactobacillus*, three strains of *Bifidobacterium*, and one strain of *Streptococcus salivarius*.

In addition, some evidence hints that probiotics might reduce the joint pain that commonly occurs in people with inflammatory bowel disease.

For more information, including dosage and safety issues, see the **Probiotics** article.

Aloe

In a double-blind, placebo-controlled trial, 44 people hospitalized with severe active ulcerative colitis were given oral aloe gel or placebo twice daily for 4 weeks. The results showed that aloe was more effective than placebo in inducing full or partial remission of symptoms.

For more information, including dosage and safety issues, see the full **Aloe** article.

Other Proposed Natural Treatments

A double-blind, placebo-controlled study of 24 people with ulcerative colitis examined the effects of wheat grass juice taken at a dose of 100 cc daily for one month.

According to various measures of disease severity, participants given wheat grass juice improved to a greater extent than those given placebo. However, wheat grass juice is rather bitter and it seems unlikely that the study could truly be blind, meaning that participants and doctors didn't know who was getting the wheat grass juice and who was getting the placebo. Indeed, when researchers polled the participants, a majority of those given wheat grass juice correctly identified it. For this reason, as well as its small size, the results of the study are not convincing.

Glutamine, **boswellia**, **bromelain**, **blue-green algae**, **colostrum**, and **mesoglycan** (glycosaminoglycans) have been suggested for the treatment of ulcerative colitis, but the evidence that they work remains highly preliminary at best.

There are also weak indications that **allergies** to foods such as milk may play a role in ulcerative colitis.

Herbs and Supplements to Use Only with Caution

Various herbs and supplements may interact adversely with drugs used to treat ulcerative colitis. For more information on this potential risk, see the individual drug article in the Drug Interactions section of this book.

Ulcers

PRINCIPAL PROPOSED NATURAL TREATMENTS: *Probiotics (As an Adjunct to Standard Therapy)*

OTHER PROPOSED NATURAL TREATMENTS: *Aloe, Beeswax Extract (Related to Policosanol)*, Bacopa monniera, *Butterbur, Cayenne, Colostrum, Cranberry, Deglycyrrhizinated Licorice (DGL), Fish Oil, Garlic, Rhubarb, Turmeric, Vitamin B$_{12}$*

The highly concentrated acid produced by the stomach is quite capable of burning a hole through the tissue of the stomach and duodenum (part of the small intestine). That it usually does not do so is a tribute to the effectiveness of the methods that the body uses to protect itself. However, sometimes these protective mechanisms fail and the ever-present acid begins to produce an ulcer.

Ulcer pain is caused by stomach acid coming into contact with unprotected tissue. Eating generally decreases ulcer pain temporarily because food neutralizes the acid. As soon as the food begins to be digested, the pain returns.

Conventional medical treatment for ulcers has gone through a slow revolution. A few decades ago, the prescribed response to ulcers was a bland diet—one low in spices and high in dairy products, which were believed to coat the stomach. However, eventually it was discovered that spicy foods are innocent and that milk itself is somewhat ulcer forming! The only other option at that time was surgery.

Next came **antacids** containing magnesium and aluminum (such as Maalox). However, these were seldom strong enough to allow the ulcer to heal fully. Ulcer treatment took a big step forward with the development of Tagamet (cimetidine), followed by Zantac (ranitidine), Pepcid (famotidine), and others. These **H_2-blocking drugs** dramatically lower the stomach's production of acid. Later, a new class of even more potent acid suppressors appeared, the **proton-pump inhibitors**, led by Prilosec (omeprazole).

When stomach acid is suppressed, ulcer pain rapidly diminishes and the ulcer heals. For a time, these drugs were regarded as the definitive answer to ulcers. This early enthusiasm began to fade when it became clear that ulcers frequently returned after the drugs were stopped. In the late 1980s, a new explanation for this problem began to surface. First regarded as a wacky theory, it has now become the accepted explanation.

We now believe that ulcers are caused by the bacteria *Helicobacter pylori*. Apparently, this previously ignored organism has the capacity to infect the stomach and, by so doing, weaken the stomach lining. Only when antibiotics to kill *H. pylori* are combined with stomach acid suppressants do ulcers go away and stay away. However, it isn't easy to kill *H. pylori*; antibiotic treatment is not always successful and it has side effects. Friendly bacteria (probiotics) may help this treatment work better.

Principal Proposed Natural Treatments

Probiotics are bacteria that are healthy for you. The most famous probiotic is *Lactobacillus acidophilus*, found in yogurt. There are many other probiotics as well. Evidence suggests that various probiotics in the *Lactobacillus* family can inhibit the growth of *H. pylori*. While this effect does not appear to be strong enough for probiotic treatment to eradicate *H. pylori* on its own, preliminary studies (one of which was double-blind) suggest that probiotics may help standard antibiotic therapy work better, improving the rate of eradication and reducing side effects.

For more information, including dosage and safety issues, see the full **Probiotics** article.

Other Proposed Natural Treatments

Individuals who take H_2 blockers or proton pump inhibitors for ulcers may not be able to properly absorb **vitamin B_{12}** and might therefore benefit from B_{12} supplements.

The most famous supplement used for ulcer disease is a special form of licorice known as **deglycyr-rhizinated licorice** (DGL). However, the studies that supposedly showed it effective were not double-blind and they involved a combination product that also contained antacids. Very preliminary evidence does suggest that DGL might help protect the stomach from damage caused by **non-steroidal anti-inflammatory drugs**.

A collection of substances extracted from beeswax has been studied as a treatment for preventing and treating ulcers, with promising results. Known as *D-002*, this product is chemically related to **policosanol**.

Fish oil in combination with antibiotic therapy has been tried as a treatment for eradicating *H. pylori*, but it did not prove particularly effective.

Highly preliminary studies suggest that various bioflavonoids including **citrus bioflavonoids** can inhibit the growth of *H. pylori*. All fruits and vegetables provide bioflavonoids, but these substances can also be taken as supplements.

The herb **cranberry** is thought to help prevent **bladder infections** by preventing adhesion of bacteria to the bladder. Preliminary evidence suggests that it might also help prevent the adhesion of *H. pylori* to the stomach wall. Theoretically, this could reduce the risk of ulcers, but as yet the only direct evidence regarding this potential benefit comes from a study that was somewhat poorly designed and reported.

Neither **garlic** nor **cayenne** appear to be helpful against *H. pylori*. However, some evidence suggests that cayenne can protect the stomach against damage caused by anti-inflammatory drugs.

Colostrum and **butterbur** might also help protect the stomach lining.

Bacopa monniera, **betaine hydrochloride, cat's claw, glutamine, marshmallow, MSM, reishi, selenium, suma, vitamin A, vitamin C**, and **zinc** have also been suggested as aids to ulcer healing, but there is as yet no meaningful scientific evidence that they are effective.

Contrary to some reports, the herb **turmeric** does

not appear to be effective for treating ulcers and it might increase the risk of developing ulcers if taken at excessive doses.

Rhubarb and **aloe** have been suggested as treatments for bleeding ulcers. However, this condition is sufficiently dangerous that conventional medical treatment is far more appropriate.

Herbs and Supplements to Use Only with Caution

Various herbs and supplements may interact adversely with drugs used to treat ulcers. For more information on this potential risk, see the individual drug article in the Drug Interactions section of this book.

Urticaria

RELATED TERMS: *Angioedema, Dermographism, Hives, Prickly Heat*

PRINCIPAL PROPOSED NATURAL TREATMENTS: *None*

OTHER PROPOSED NATURAL TREATMENTS: *Acupuncture, Food Allergen Elimination Diet, Quercetin, Vitamin B_{12}, Vitamin C*

Urticaria, commonly called *hives*, is an inflammation of the surface layers of the skin and is characterized by small, itchy red or white welts (called *wheals*). Urticaria is usually caused by an allergic reaction; however, the allergenic trigger is often unknown. When a cause can be identified, it is frequently something taken by mouth, such as shellfish or other fish, dairy products, peanuts or other legumes, chocolate, fresh fruit, or medications. Sometimes other allergens, such as pollens, molds, or animal dander, can produce hives. Hives can also be caused by heat (cholinergic urticaria or "prickly heat"), cold (cold urticaria), pressure (dermographism and pressure urticaria), light (solar urticaria), exercise, and certain infections such as hepatitis B.

In most acute cases, urticaria disappears within hours or days without any treatment. Sometimes, however, it may continue for a prolonged period or recur frequently. Such chronic cases are often very difficult to treat.

Urticaria is closely related to another condition called *angioedema*, which involves swelling in the deeper layers of the skin. When swelling occurs in the throat or tongue, angioedema can be life-threatening.

Urticaria and angioedema are also closely related to anaphylaxis, an extremely dangerous condition that can lead to death within minutes or hours. Anaphylaxis is an overwhelming allergic reaction that may lead to swelling of internal organs, collapse of blood circulation, shock, or suffocation. It may be caused by all the same factors that trigger hives; one of the most well-known causes is bee sting allergy.

Conventional treatments for urticaria and angioedema include avoidance of triggering factors and use of antihistamines and, occasionally, corticosteroids. When breathing is threatened, epinephrine shots and possibly hospitalization may be needed.

Proposed Treatments for Urticaria

Food Allergen Elimination Diet

Because urticaria may be caused by food allergies, food allergen elimination diets have been tried as a treatment for chronic symptoms.

There are many forms of the elimination diet. One of the most common involves starting with a highly restricted diet consisting only of foods that are seldom allergenic, such as rice, yams, and turkey. Other proponents of the elimination diet allow a greater range of foods at the outset. If dietary restriction leads to resolution or improvement of symptoms, foods are then reintroduced one by one to see which, if any, will trigger urticaria. (For more information see the article on **food allergies**.)

The results of preliminary studies suggest that the elimination diet can be effective in some cases of chronic or recurrent urticaria. However, this is an arduous approach that is not for the faint of heart. Various forms of allergy testing have been advocated to make matters easier; the idea is to identify specific offending foods only, rather than eliminating practically everything. Unfortunately, food allergy testing appears to be somewhat unreliable when it comes to identifying foods that cause urticaria.

Acupuncture

In China, urticaria is often treated with **acupuncture**; however, the evidence that acupuncture works for this condition is far too weak to rely upon at all.

Other Natural Treatments

Vitamins C and B$_{12}$ and the flavonoid **quercetin** have also been suggested, but there is no evidence as yet that they really work for treating urticaria.

Uveitis

RELATED TERMS: *Acute Anterior Uveitis, Anterior Uveitis, Irido-cyclitis, Iritis*

PRINCIPAL PROPOSED NATURAL TREATMENTS: *None*

OTHER PROPOSED NATURAL TREATMENTS: *Turmeric, Vitamin E Combined with Vitamin C*

The term *uveitis* means "inflammation of the uvea." The uvea is the middle layer of the tissues surrounding the eyeball, stretching from the iris at the front of the eye all the way back to a lining beneath the retina at the back of the eye. The three main types of uveitis are named based on where inflammation occurs:

➤ *Iritis* (or *anterior uveitis*) for inflammation toward the front of the eye
➤ *Cyclitis* (or *intermediate uveitis*) for inflammation along the body of the eye
➤ *Choroiditis* (or *posterior uveitis*) for inflammation in the rear of the eye

Uveitis can also be called *acute* or *chronic*, depending on whether it is short or long in duration.

Uveitis usually occurs in only one eye. In the most common forms of uveitis, the eye is reddened and the redness reaches into the area just next to the iris. The affected pupil may be smaller than the other and its shape may be irregular. Vision is often blurred or misty and blinking will not clear it. Deep, aching pain generally accompanies uveitis.

Uveitis can begin after injury to the eye or eye surgery, but it can also start with no obvious trigger. While the underlying cause of uveitis is unknown, autoimmune processes are thought to play a role.

If left untreated, uveitis can cause permanent damage to vision, including blindness. For this reason, medical examination and treatment is mandatory. The diagnosis of uveitis is made by means of a special medical tool called a *slit lamp*. Treatment involves medications to reduce inflammation and control pressure in the eye.

Other Proposed Natural Treatments

No natural treatment can *substitute* for standard medical care for uveitis. However, two natural substances taken together, **vitamin C** and **vitamin E**, have shown promise when used in *addition* to standard treatment.

In a double-blind trial of 145 people undergoing treatment for acute anterior uveitis, participants were additionally given either placebo or combined treatment with vitamin C (500 mg twice daily) and vitamin E (100 mg twice daily). People receiving the real treatment had better visual acuity at the end of the 8-week study period. Researchers hypothesized that free radicals (a class of dangerous, naturally occurring chemicals) play a role in the eye injury caused by uveitis. Vitamin C and vitamin E are antioxidants and tend to neutralize free radicals. While further study is necessary to corroborate these results, it appears plausible at least that use of these antioxidants may help keep the eye healthy while it recovers from the condition.

Other antioxidants besides vitamins E and C have also been recommended for acute uveitis, but there is as yet no real evidence that they are helpful. These include **beta-carotene, bilberry, citrus bioflavonoids, lipoic acid, lutein, OPCs, selenium,** and **vitamin A.**

Antioxidants are also often recommended for chronic uveitis (again, alongside conventional care). One study examined the potential benefits of an anti-oxidant extract made from the herb turmeric, and appeared to find benefit. However, this study lacked a placebo group and therefore cannot be taken as reliable.

Finally, websites discussing natural treatments for uveitis make numerous other recommendations, based on pure speculation. The list includes the following:

- Fish oil
- Flax oil
- Manganese
- Vitamin B complex (a mixture of vitamins B_1, B_2, B_3, B_6, and B_{12}, pantothenic acid, biotin, and folate, possibly along with inositol and choline)
- Olive leaf extract
- Red clover
- Zinc

Vaginal Infection

RELATED TERMS: *Bacterial Vaginosis; Candida; Candidal Yeast Infection;* Gardnerella; Trichomonas; *Vaginal Yeast Infection; Vaginitis; Yeast Infection, Vaginal*

PRINCIPAL PROPOSED NATURAL TREATMENTS: *None*

OTHER PROPOSED NATURAL TREATMENTS: *Boric Acid, Essential Oils, Garlic, Goldenseal, Probiotics,* Solanum nigrescens, Tabeuia avellanedae, *Tea Tree Oil, Vitamin C*

There are three main causes of vaginal infections: the fungus (yeast) *Candida albicans,* the parasite *Trichomonas vaginalis,* and the bacterial organism *Gardnerella vaginalis.*

Factors that can contribute to vaginal infections include antibiotics (which kill friendly bacteria, allowing yeast to grow); corticosteroids and HIV (which suppress the immune system); oral contraceptives and pregnancy (which alter the vaginal environment by changing hormone levels); and diabetes (increased sugar levels provide a friendly environment for yeast).

Conventional medical treatment for vaginal infections caused by candida include vaginal suppositories containing antifungal medications or, in some cases, oral antifungal medications. Women with diabetes often find that yeast infections are less common when their blood sugar levels are well controlled.

Trichomonas infections are treated with oral metronidazole and *Gardnerella* infections with oral or vaginal metronidazole or vaginal clindamycin. So-called non-specific vaginitis is usually caused by *Garnerella,* but there are other causes.

Proposed Natural Treatments

There are some promising natural treatments for vaginal infections caused by candida and other organisms, but the scientific evidence for them is not yet strong.

Probiotics (friendly bacteria), such as acidophilus, are normally found in the vagina. When colonies of these organisms are present, it is difficult for unfriendly organisms such as candida to become established. Probiotic supplements can help restore a normal balance of vaginal organisms, which could, in theory, reduce the chance of developing a vaginal infection. For this reason, women have been advised to use yogurt or other products containing acidophilus, both orally and in vaginal suppositories, to prevent or treat yeast infections. However, evidence that probiotics really help remains incomplete and inconsistent. A fairly large study (278 participants) failed to find *Lactobacillus* helpful for preventing yeast infections caused by antibiotics.

Tea tree oil, an essential oil from the plant *Melaleuca alternifolia,* possesses antibacterial and antifungal properties and appears to spare friendly bacteria in the *Lactobacillus* family. Tea tree oil has been tried for various forms of vaginal infection, but again there is little scientific evidence as yet that it works. In an open trial, 96 women with trichomonal vaginitis were treated with tampons saturated in tea tree oil and left in the vagina for 24 hours, followed by daily vaginal douches with a tea tree oil solution. The researcher reported good results with this regimen in 3 to 4 weeks. However, because this was not a double-blind trial, its results mean little.

A double-blind study of 100 women found **vitamin C** vaginal tablets (250 mg) at most marginally helpful for non-specific vaginitis.

Boric acid is a chemical substance with antiseptic properties. A double-blind comparison study of 108 women with yeast infections found that 92% of those who used boric acid suppositories nightly for 2 weeks experienced full recovery, as compared to 64% of those given suppositories of the somewhat outdated antifungal drug nystatin. However, there are safety concerns with boric acid. If taken internally, it is quite toxic. For this reason, it should not be applied to open wounds. In addition, it should not be used by pregnant women, nor be applied to the skin of infants.

A single-blind trail of 100 women with candida vaginitis compared nystatin suppositories against suppositories made from the plant *Solanum nigrescens* and found equivalent benefits. However, this plant can be toxic and should not be used except under physician supervision.

Test-tube studies have found antifungal properties in numerous herbs, including the tropical tree *Tabeuia avellanedae*, **garlic** extracts, the plant alkaloid berberine sulfate (found in **goldenseal**), and **essential oils** of various plants, including cinnamon, eucalyptus, lemongrass, **oregano**, palmarosa, and peppermint. However, it is a long way from test-tube studies to proof of safety and effectiveness in people.

Varicose Veins

PRINCIPAL PROPOSED NATURAL TREATMENTS: *Butcher's Broom, Gotu Kola, Horse Chestnut, Oligomeric Proanthocyanidins (OPCs), Oxerutins and Other Bioflavonoids, Red Vine Leaf (Grape Leaf)*

OTHER PROPOSED NATURAL TREATMENTS: *Bromelain, Calendula, Collinsonia, Comfrey, Mesoglycan, Witch Hazel*

Walking upright has given our leg veins a difficult task. Although they lack the strong muscular lining of arteries, they must constantly return a large volume of blood to the heart. The movements of the legs act as a pump to push the blood upward while flimsy valves stop gravity from pulling it back down.

However, over time these valves often begin to fail. The blood then begins to pool in the deep veins of the leg, stretching the vein wall and injuring its lining. This situation is called *venous insufficiency*. Typically, the legs begin to feel heavy, swollen, achy, and tired. *Varicose veins*, a condition closely related to venous insufficiency, occur when veins near the surface of the skin are damaged. They visibly dilate and become distorted, resulting in a cosmetically unpleasant appearance.

Varicose veins affect women about two to three times as often as men. Occupations involving prolonged standing also increase the incidence of venous insufficiency.

Pregnancy and **obesity** do so as well because the increase of pressure in the abdomen makes it more difficult for the blood to flow upward.

Conventional medical treatment of venous insufficiency consists mainly of reducing weight, elevating the legs, and wearing elastic support hose. Unsightly damaged veins can be destroyed by injection therapy or be surgically removed.

Principal Proposed Natural Treatments

When it comes to natural products, some illnesses are far more responsive than others. While there are no well documented natural therapies for **asthma** (as an example), more than half a dozen natural therapies have meaningful supporting evidence as treatments for venous insufficiency/varicose veins.

These treatments have much in common. All of

them appear to work by strengthening the walls of veins and other vessels, with the net effect of reducing fluid leakage. Studies indicate that use of such products reduces leg swelling and pain. However, there is no meaningful evidence that any natural product can cure unsightly varicose veins that already exist, or prevent new ones from developing.

Warning: Symptoms similar to those caused by varicose veins can actually be due to more dangerous conditions such as **phlebitis** or thrombosis. Medical evaluation is necessary prior to self-treating with the natural supplements described here.

Horse Chestnut

The most popular herbal treatment for venous insufficiency is horse chestnut.

More than 800 people have been involved in double-blind, placebo-controlled studies of horse chestnut for treating venous insufficiency. One of the largest of these trials followed 212 people over a period of 40 days using a crossover design. Participants initially received either horse chestnut or placebo and then were crossed over to the other treatment (without their knowledge) after 20 days. Horse chestnut treatment significantly reduced leg edema, pain, and the sensation of heaviness when compared to placebo.

However, the design of this study was not quite up to modern standards. A better-designed double-blind study of 74 people also found benefit.

Good results were also seen in a partially double-blinded, placebo-controlled study that compared the effectiveness of horse chestnut versus compression stockings in 240 people over a course of 12 weeks (horse chestnut and placebo were blinded, but not the compression stockings). Compression stockings worked faster to lessen swelling, but by 12 weeks the results were equivalent between the two treatments and both were better than placebo.

Unlike many herbs, the active ingredients in horse chestnut have been identified to a reasonable degree of certainty. They appear to be a complex of related chemicals known collectively as *aescin*. Aescin reduces the rate of fluid leakage from stressed and irritated vessel walls. We don't really know how it does this, but the most prominent theory proposes that aescin plugs leaking capillaries, prevents the release of enzymes that break down collagen and open holes in capillary walls, and forestalls other forms of vein damage.

For more information, including dosage and safety issues, see the full **Horse Chestnut** article.

Oxerutins and Other Bioflavonoids

Oxerutins have been widely used in Europe since the mid-1960s but this supplement remains hard to find in North America. Derived from a naturally occurring bioflavonoid called *rutin*, oxerutins were specifically developed to treat varicose veins and related venous problems. It is not clear whether this particular derivative of rutin is more effective than other bioflavonoids used for these conditions, but oxerutins are by far the best studied.

About 20 double-blind, placebo-controlled studies, enrolling a total of more than 2,000 participants, have examined oxerutins' effectiveness for treating varicose veins and venous insufficiency. Virtually all have found oxerutins significantly more effective than placebo, giving substantial relief from swelling, aching, leg pains, and other uncomfortable symptoms, while causing no significant side effects. Together, these studies make a strong case for the use of oxerutins in these conditions.

For example, a 12-week, double-blind, placebo-controlled study enrolled 133 women with moderate, chronic venous insufficiency. Half received 1,000 mg oxerutins daily and the rest took placebo. All participants were also fitted with standard compression stockings and wore them for the duration of the trial. The researchers measured subjective symptoms, such as aches and pains, as well as objective measures of edema in the leg.

Those who took oxerutins experienced significantly less lower-leg edema than the placebo group. Furthermore, these better results lasted through a 6-week follow-up period, even though participants were no longer taking oxerutins. The stockings, on the other hand, produced no lasting benefit after participants stopped wearing them. They gave symptomatic relief while they were worn, but they didn't improve capillary circulation in a lasting way, as oxerutins apparently did.

Several other double-blind, placebo-controlled studies have also found benefits with oxerutins. Additionally, there is some evidence that troxerutin—one of the compounds in the standardized mixture sold as oxerutins—may be effective when taken alone, though perhaps not as effective as the standard mixture of oxerutins.

Oxerutins are closely related to the natural flavonoid rutin, which is found primarily in citrus fruits and buckwheat. Two double-blind, placebo-controlled studies suggest that buckwheat tea might also be effective against varicose veins, presumably because of its rutin content. Other citrus-derived bioflavonoids, such as diosmin, hesperidin, and hidrosmin, may also be effective. (See also

Varicose Veins

discussion of a combination treatment containing hesperidin methyl chalcone, below.)

For more information, including dosage and safety issues, see the full articles on **citrus bioflavonoids** and **oxerutins**.

OPCs

Grape seed and pine bark contain high levels of special bioflavonoids called *oligomeric proanthocyanidin complexes* (OPCs). Similar substances are found in cranberry, bilberry, blueberry, hawthorn, and other plants.

OPCs are interesting antioxidant chemicals that appear to have the ability to improve collagen (a type of strengthening tissue found in many parts of the body), reduce capillary leakage, and control inflammation.

Placebo-controlled studies (most of them double-blind) involving a total of about 400 participants suggest that OPCs provide significant benefit for varicose veins. For example, a double-blind study comparing grape seed OPCs against placebo in 71 individuals showed improvement in 75% of the treated group, as compared to 41% in the control group. Similarly, a 2-month, double-blind, placebo-controlled trial of 40 individuals with chronic venous insufficiency found that 100 mg 3 times daily of OPCs from pine bark significantly reduced edema, pain, and the sensation of leg heaviness. Another double-blind, placebo-controlled study of 20 individuals also found OPCs from pine bark effective.

In addition, evidence from small double-blind trials suggest OPCs might be more effective for venous insufficiency than either diosmin or horse chestnut.

For more information, including dosage and safety issues, see the full **OPCs** article.

Gotu Kola

There is significant scientific evidence for the effectiveness of the herb gotu kola in varicose veins/venous insufficiency.

A vacuum suction chamber has been used in some gotu kola studies to evaluate the rate of fluid leakage in venous insufficiency. It produces swelling when applied to the skin of the ankle. When leg veins are leaking a lot of fluid, this swelling takes longer to disappear.

In one study of people with venous insufficiency, 2 weeks of treatment with gotu kola extracts was shown to reduce the time necessary for the swelling to disappear.

A placebo-controlled study (whether it was double-blind was not stated) of 52 patients with venous insuf-ficiency compared the effects of gotu kola extract at 180 mg daily and 90 mg daily against placebo. After 4 weeks of treatment, researchers observed improvement in various measurements of vein function in all treated patients, but not in the placebo group. They also found that the higher dose was more effective than the lower dose. This kind of dose responsiveness is generally taken as good evidence that a treatment is actually effective.

Another study of double-blind design followed 87 people with varicose veins and compared the benefits of gotu kola at 60 mg and 30 mg daily against placebo. Again, the results showed improvements in both treated groups, but greater improvement at the higher dose.

A double-blind study of 94 people with venous insufficiency of the lower limb compared the benefits of gotu kola extract at 120 mg daily and 60 mg daily against placebo. The results also showed a significant dose-related improvement in the treated groups in symptoms such as subjective heaviness, discomfort, and edema.

A 1992 review of all the gotu kola studies available concluded that gotu kola extract provides a dose-related improvement in venous insufficiency symptoms, reducing foot swelling, ankle edema, and fluid leakage from the veins.

For more information, including dosage and safety issues, see the full **Gotu Kola** article.

Red Vine Leaf

Extracts of red vine leaf (*Folia vitis viniferae*, or grape leaf) have also been tried as a treatment for chronic venous insufficiency. One 12-week, double-blind, placebo-controlled study followed 219 individuals with chronic venous insufficiency. In this study, daily doses of 360 mg and 720 mg red vine leaf extract both proved significantly more effective than placebo in reducing edema as well as improving pain and other symptoms. The researchers concluded that the higher dosage resulted in a slightly greater, more sustained improvement. Benefits were also seen in a much smaller study.

The usual dose of red vine leaf is 360 mg or 720 mg taken once daily.

In the double-blind study just described, side effects were largely limited to mild gastrointestinal distress and occasional reports of headaches. Blood tests and physical examination did not reveal any harmful effects. However, comprehensive safety studies have not yet been performed and red vine leaf is not at present recommended for pregnant or nursing women, or individuals with severe liver or kidney disease.

Butcher's Broom

Butcher's broom (*Ruscus aculeatus*) is so named because its branches were a traditional source of broom straw used by butchers. This Mediterranean evergreen bush has a long history of traditional use in the treatment of urinary conditions. More recent European interest has focused on the possible value of butcher's broom in the treatment of hemorrhoids and varicose veins.

A well-designed and reported double-blind trial evaluated the effectiveness of a standardized butcher's broom extract in 166 women with chronic venous insufficiency. For a period of 12 weeks, participants received either placebo or butcher's broom (one tablet twice daily containing 36.0 to 37.5 mg of a methanol dry extract concentrated at 15–20:1). The results showed that leg swelling (the primary measurement used) decreased significantly in the butcher's broom group as compared to the placebo group.

Similar results were seen in a 12-week, double-blind, placebo-controlled trial with 148 participants. Studies of a combination treatment containing butcher's broom are mentioned below.

For more information, including dosage and safety issues, see the full **Butcher's Broom** article.

Other Proposed Natural Treatments

At least 20 double-blind, placebo-controlled studies have evaluated the efficacy of a popular European treatment containing butcher's broom extract combined with the bioflavonoid hesperidin methyl chalcone as well as **vitamin C**. Although not all studies were positive and many suffered from design flaws, in general it appears that this combination treatment is more effective than placebo.

A substance extracted from pig intestines known as **mesoglycan** has been investigated in Italy as a remedy for varicose veins and related conditions. In the best of the reported trials, 183 individuals with leg ulcers due to poor vein function were treated with either placebo or mesoglycan (first by injection and then orally) for 24 weeks. The results of this double-blind study suggest that mesoglycan significantly improved the rate at which the leg ulcers healed.

Bromelain is not actually a single substance, but rather a collection of protein-digesting enzymes found in pineapple juice and in the stems of pineapple plants. Although there is no direct evidence on its use for varicose veins, bromelain has anti-edema effects similar to treatments used for varicose veins, suggesting that it might be helpful.

The herb collinsonia, or stone root, has a long traditional history of use as an oral treatment for varicose veins and hemorrhoids, but it has not been scientifically evaluated to any meaningful extent. The same is true for topical **witch hazel**, **comfrey**, and **calendula**.

Vertigo

RELATED TERMS: *Dizziness, Benign Positional Vertigo, Meniere's Disease, Benign Paroxysmal Positional Vertigo, Vertiginous Syndrome*

PRINCIPAL PROPOSED NATURAL TREATMENTS: *None*

OTHER PROPOSED NATURAL TREATMENTS: *Ginkgo, Ginger, Hypnosis, Oxerutins, Vitamin B$_6$*

Vertigo is closely related to dizziness, but involves the perception of actually seeing the room spin about you, similar to what happens when you spin around rapidly and then stop. Often, vertigo is accompanied by nausea and a loss of balance. Vertigo may pass quickly or it may last for hours or even days.

There are many possible causes of vertigo, including motion sickness, infection in the inner ear, vision problems, head injury, insufficient blood supply to the brain, and brain tumors. A condition called *benign paroxysmal positional vertigo* leads to attacks of vertigo triggered by certain head positions; its cause is believed to be deposits of calcium in the inner ear. Another condition, *Meniere's disease*, is characterized by sudden, intense attacks of vertigo often accompanied by nausea and vomiting, along with ringing in the ears and progressive deafness. Its cause is unknown.

Conventional treatments for vertigo depend upon the cause and severity of the condition. Drugs for motion sickness and mild vertigo of any cause include meclizine, dimenhydrinate, and perphenazine. Scopolamine is prescribed for severe motion sickness. Benign paroxysmal positional vertigo is often treated through a series of exercises which help to alleviate symptoms. For Meniere's disease, changes in diet are often recommended (including limiting sodium, sugar, and alcohol intake), sometimes in combination with diuretic drugs.

Proposed Natural Treatments

Several natural treatments have been tried for vertigo; however, the scientific evidence for these treatments is very preliminary at this time. **Note**: Treatments (such as **ginger**) used specifically for motion sickness are discussed in the **Motion Sickness** article.

A double-blind, placebo-controlled study of 67 people with vertigo found that 160 mg of *Ginkgo biloba* extract per day significantly reduced symptoms compared to placebo. At the end of the 3-month study, 47% of the ginkgo group had completely recovered, as compared to only 18% of the placebo group. For more information, including dosage and safety issues, see the full **Ginkgo** article.

The supplements **oxerutins** and **vitamin B$_6$** are sometimes recommended for vertigo; however, the evidence supporting these treatments is extremely preliminary.

Hypnosis has been tried for vertigo resulting from head trauma, with some apparent success.

Viral Hepatitis

PRINCIPAL PROPOSED NATURAL TREATMENTS: *Milk Thistle, Traditional Chinese Herbal Medicine*

OTHER PROPOSED NATURAL TREATMENTS: *Astragalus, Ayurvedic Herbs, Cordyceps, Lecithin, Licorice, Liver Extracts, Phosphatidylcholine,* Phyllanthus amarus, *Reishi, SAMe, Schisandra, Taurine, Thymus Extract, Vitamin C, Whey Protein*

HERBS AND SUPPLEMENTS TO USE ONLY WITH CAUTION: *Barberry, Beta-carotene, Blue-green Algae, Borage, Chaparral, Coltsfoot, Comfrey, Germander, Germanium, Greater Celandine, Kava, Kombucha, Mistletoe, Pennyroyal, Pokeroot, Sassafras, Skullcap, Spirulina, Traditional Chinese Herbal Medicine, Vitamin A, Vitamin B$_3$*

Hepatitis is an infection of the liver caused by one of several viruses, the most common of which are named *hepatitis* A, B, and C. Hepatitis A is spread mainly through contaminated food and water, whereas hepatitis B is tra　　itted by sexual contact and use of contaminated nec　　s. The route of transmission of hepatitis C is not completely clear but is believed to be similar to that of hepatitis B.

When you first develop hepatitis, it is called *acute hepatitis*. Hepatitis can also become a long-term disease known as *chronic hepatitis*. All forms of hepatitis cause jaundice, liver tenderness, and severe fatigue. Hepatitis A is the mildest form and seldom causes symptoms continuing longer than a couple of months. Hepatitis B and C

produce more severe symptoms, which last two or three times longer and can go on to become chronic.

Chronic hepatitis consists of persistent liver infection and inflammation that lingers long after the primary symptoms of the disease have disappeared. It can produce subtle symptoms of liver tenderness and continued fatigue and over time can gradually destroy the liver. Chronic hepatitis also appears to increase the risk of liver cancer.

The best treatment for hepatitis is prevention. You can avoid hepatitis A by practicing good hygiene and using the conventional preventive treatment, known as immune globulins, while traveling in areas where the disease is common. Hepatitis B can be prevented by immunization and the same precautions taken against **HIV** infection. HIV precautions almost certainly decrease the transmission of hepatitis C as well.

Conventional medicine has little in the way of treatment for the initial hepatitis infection once it has started. Treatment for chronic hepatitis is developing but is still quite imperfect. The most effective methods involve varieties of interferon.

Principal Proposed Natural Treatments

Traditional Chinese Herbal Medicine

Viral hepatitis has long been a serious problem in China and other parts of Asia and, for this reason, many herbal formulas to treat it have been devised. The traditional Chinese herbal combination *Shosaiko-to* (Minor Bupleurum) has been approved as a treatment for chronic hepatitis by the Japanese Health Ministry. However, a search of the literature uncovered only one large-scale, double-blind, placebo-controlled study supporting its effectiveness. In this 24-week trial, the efficacy of Shosaiko-to was tested in 222 people with chronic active hepatitis using a double-blind, placebo-controlled crossover design. Results showed that use of Shosaiko-to significantly improved liver function measurements compared to placebo. Although these results are promising, an absence of long-term evaluation limits their meaningfulness. (Researchers only followed participants for 3 months.) Other Chinese herbal remedies have been tested as adjuncts to conventional interferon treatment with some promising results. However, published trials are of generally poor quality.

Other combination Chinese herbal therapies have also shown a bit of promise for the treatment of chronic hepatitis, including those named *Bing Gan Tang, Yi Zhu decoction, Fuzheng Jiedu Tang,* and *Jianpi Wenshen recipe.* However, the quality of most of these studies was again quite poor. **Note**: There are many incidents in which use of Chinese herbs appears to have *caused* liver injury. For this reason, we do not recommend using Chinese herbs for hepatitis, except under the supervision of a physician.

A well-designed, double-blind, placebo-controlled study evaluated a mixture of traditional Chinese herbs for people with hepatitis C and symptoms of fatigue. The tested mixture contained: Radix astragali (6%), Radix acanthopanax (8%), Radix bupleuir (8%), Radix et tuber curcumae (10%), Rhizoma polygonum (10%), Radix glycyrrhiza (4%), Radix isatis (14%), Radix paeoniae rubra (14%), Radix salviae (14%), and Herba taraxaci

(12%). However, it failed to prove more effective than placebo regarding symptoms or objective signs.

One Chinese herb widely advocated for chronic hepatitis B, *Sophorae flavescentis,* has not yet been shown effective, according to a comprehensive review of studies.

For more information, see the article on **traditional Chinese herbal medicine**.

Milk Thistle

The herb milk thistle may be useful as a supportive treatment for viral hepatitis, both chronic and acute. However, study results remain mixed.

A few preliminary double-blind, placebo-controlled studies of people with chronic hepatitis have found indication that use of milk thistle can bring about significant improvement in symptoms such as fatigue, reduced appetite, and abdominal discomfort. However, the most recent and best-designed study failed to find any benefit in chronic hepatitis C.

Other studies have evaluated milk thistle for the treatment of acute hepatitis, again with mixed results.

For more information, including dosage and safety issues, see the full **Milk Thistle** article.

Other Proposed Natural Treatments

Ayurvedic Medicine

Ayurvedic medicine, the ancient medical system of India, has many traditional treatments for hepatitis. Some of these have undergone scientific evaluation. One such is a combination treatment called *Kamalahar,* which contains *Tecoma undulata,* **Phyllanthus urinaria**, *Embelia ribes,* **Taraxacum officinale**, *Nyctanthes arbortistis,* and **Terminalia arjuna**. In a double-blind, placebo-controlled study, 52 people with acute hepatitis were randomly assigned to receive placebo or this combination herbal therapy at a dose of 500 mg 3 times daily for 15 days. The results indicate that the herbal combination improved liver function to a significantly greater extent than placebo.

Another combination therapy contains *Capparis spinosa, Cichorium intybus, Solanum nigrum, Terminalia arjuna, Cassia occidentalis,* **Achillea millefolium**, and *Tamarix gallica.* In a poorly reported, 5-week, double-blind, placebo-controlled study of 30 children with hepatitis A, use of this combination formula apparently improved the rate of recovery as compared to placebo. Benefits were also seen in a 6-week study of 34 people with acute hepatitis. A third double-blind, placebo-controlled study evaluated the effectiveness of this combination in the treatment of a variety of liver conditions, including chronic and acute hepatitis, and found some evidence of benefit.

Single herbs have been tried as well. In a double-blind trial of 33 people with acute viral hepatitis, use of the herb *Picrorhiza kurroa* at a dose of 375 mg 3 times daily significantly speeded recovery time as compared to placebo.

The herb *Phyllanthus amarus* has also been extensively studied as a treatment for chronic viral hepatitis, but it does not appear to be effective. Its close relative *Phyllanthus urinaris* has also failed to prove effective.

Note that at the present, the quality of the reported studies remains poor, and Ayurvedic herbs cannot be regarded as a proven treatment for viral hepatitis. For more information, see the **Ayurveda** article.

Other Herbs and Supplements

Chronic hepatitis can cause cholestasis (backup of bile in the liver). In a 2-week, double-blind study of 220 individuals with cholestasis, use of the supplement **SAMe** at a dose of 1,600 mg daily significantly improved liver-related symptoms as compared to placebo. Most participants in this study had chronic viral hepatitis.

The supplement **phosphatidylcholine** has shown some promise for hepatitis. In one double-blind study, it enhanced the effect of interferon in people with chronic hepatitis C, but not in those with chronic hepatitis B. However, in an open study phosphatidylcholine failed to produce improvements in individuals with acute hepatitis.

One study failed to find **N-acetylcysteine** at a dose of 600 mg daily helpful for acute viral hepatitis.

In Japan, an injectible combination of **licorice** (the herb, not the candy) and certain amino acids is used for chronic hepatitis. However, it is not clear whether oral licorice has a similar effect; furthermore, the high dosages used for treatment of chronic hepatitis may cause an elevation of blood pressure and other serious medical problems. **Warning**: Do not inject preparations of licorice designed for oral use.

Thymus extract has been tried as a treatment for hepatitis B and C. However, the results of small double-blind trials have not been positive.

Other common natural medicine recommendations for hepatitis include **astragalus, cordyceps, reishi, schisandra, taurine, vitamin C,** and **whey protein**. However, there is as yet no meaningful scientific evidence that these approaches really work.

Herbs and Supplements to Use Only with Caution

Many natural products have the capacity to harm the liver. Furthermore, due to the generally inadequate regulation of dietary supplements that exists at the time of this writing, there are real risks that herbal products, at least, may contain liver-toxic contaminants even if the actual herbs listed on the label are safe. For this reason, we recommend that people with liver disease do not use any medicinal herbs except under the supervision of a physician. Here, we list some specific information to aid in your decision-making process.

All forms of **vitamin B₃** may damage the liver when taken in high doses, including niacin, niacinamide (nicotinamide), and inositol hexaniacinate. (Nutritional supplementation at the standard daily requirement level should not cause a problem.) A great many herbs and supplements have known or suspected liver-toxic properties, including but not limited to: **barberry,** borage, chaparral, **coltsfoot, comfrey, germander,** germanium (a mineral), **greater celandine, kava, kombucha, mistletoe, pennyroyal, pokeroot, sassafras,** and various herbs and minerals used in traditional Chinese herbal medicine. In addition, herbs that are not liver-toxic in themselves are sometimes adulterated with other herbs of similar appearance that are accidentally harvested in a misapprehension of their identity (for example, germander found in **skullcap** products). Furthermore, blue-green algae species such as **spirulina** may at times be contaminated with liver-toxic substances called *microcystins*, for which no highest safe level is known.

Some articles claim that the herb **echinacea** is potentially liver-toxic, but this concern appears to have been based on a misunderstanding of its constituents. Echinacea contains substances in the pyrrolizidine alkaloid family. However, while many pyrrolizidine alkaloids are liver-toxic, those found in echinacea are not believed to have that property.

Whole **valerian** contains liver-toxic substances called *valepotriates*; however, valepotriates are thought to be absent from most commercial valerian products and case reports suggest that even very high doses of valerian do not harm the liver.

Vitiligo

RELATED TERM: *Depigmentation*

PRINCIPAL PROPOSED NATURAL TREATMENTS: *Khellin, L-Phenylalanine*

OTHER PROPOSED NATURAL TREATMENTS: *Folate, Ginkgo, PABA,* Picrorhiza kurroa, *Vitamin B$_{12}$*

Vitiligo is a skin disease in which pigment-making cells, called *melanocytes*, are destroyed, leaving white irregular patches of skin where pigment used to be. The patches usually appear on the hands, feet, arms, face, and lips, but can also occur on the skin around the mouth, nose, eyes, and genitals. Hair growing from areas affected by vitiligo may also turn white. Although vitiligo in itself isn't painful, it can cause emotional distress.

Science hasn't identified the cause of vitiligo, but some researchers theorize that an autoimmune process plays a role. In an autoimmune disease, the body's immune system starts attacking innocent tissues. In vitiligo, antibodies may develop against melanocytes, ultimately destroying some of them. Vitiligo seems to be more common in people who have other autoimmune diseases; however, most people with vitiligo have no other autoimmune disease.

Most conventional vitiligo treatments combine ultraviolet light (UVA) exposure with oral or topical drugs that selectively sensitize the skin to UVA—such drugs are called *psoralens* because they are most commonly used to treat psoriasis. The results of this treatment are generally reasonably good. Another option is topical corticosteroids, which may be best for localized vitiligo. In severe cases, surgical procedures including skin grafting and melanocyte transplantation may be considered, although these approaches are still experimental.

Principal Proposed Natural Treatments

Most natural therapies for vitiligo also employ exposure to UVA or natural sunlight in conjunction with an oral or topical treatment.

Khellin

Khellin, an extract of the fruit of the Mediterranean plant khella (*Ammi visnaga*), is closely related to the standard psoralen drug methoxsalen. Both are used in conjunction with UVA to repigment vitiligo patches.

A double-blind, placebo-controlled study of 60 people indicated that the combination of oral khellin and natural sun exposure caused repigmentation in 76.6% of the treatment group; in comparison, no improvement was seen in the control group receiving sunlight plus placebo. A subsequent placebo-controlled study of 36 people found that a topical khellin gel plus UVA caused repigmentation in 86.1% of the treated cases, as opposed to 66.6% in the placebo group.

A typical oral dosage of khellin is 100 mg daily.

Khellin has no reported side effects when used topically. Oral doses, however, have caused various side effects ranging from nausea and vomiting to liver inflammation.

L-Phenylalanine

A handful of preliminary studies suggest that oral L-phenylalanine, a natural amino acid, might also be helpful for vitiligo. It too is combined with either sunlight or controlled ultraviolet light.

Of four studies on the subject, only one was double-blind. It found positive results; however, because only 24 people were enrolled, further research will be necessary to confirm its conclusions. The other studies were open, uncontrolled trials, and as such prove little.

For more information, including dosage and safety issues, see the full **Phenylalanine** article.

Other Proposed Natural Treatments for Vitiligo

A double-blind study of 52 people found that use of *Ginkgo biloba* extract (40 mg 3 times daily) helped slow the spread of vitiligo in people with limited, slowly spreading symptoms.

There is some evidence that people with vitiligo have lower than average levels of both **vitamin B$_{12}$** and **folate**. In addition, there is a particularly high incidence of vitiligo among individuals with pernicious anemia, a condition in which vitamin B$_{12}$ is poorly absorbed. However, this information does not prove that taking extra vitamin B_{12} and folate will help. Furthermore, a much larger study of 100 people found no significant association between vitiligo and low levels of either vitamin. One uncontrolled study does suggest that vitamin B_{12} and folate supplements might improve pigmentation in vitiligo, but because of its poor design the results prove little.

The herb *Picrorhiza kurroa* is used by Ayurvedic physicians to treat fever, dyspepsia, asthma, bronchitis, and liver disease. One poorly designed single-blind study suggests the herb might increase effectiveness of the standard drug methoxsalen.

Para-aminobenzoic acid (PABA) is best known as an active ingredient in sunblock. Based on a 1942 study,

oral PABA has been suggested as a vitiligo treatment. The study, however, lacked a control group, so the results aren't meaningful. Ironically, another study suggests that high oral doses of PABA can actually cause vitiligo.

As noted above, vitiligo is sometimes associated with pernicious anemia. Pernicious anemia in turn is often linked to low levels of stomach gastric acid, a condition called *achlorhydria*. For this reason, some physicians specializing in natural medicine recommend supplemental hydrochloric acid (HCl, often in the form of **betaine hydrochloride**) to augment low gastric acid, but there is no evidence as yet that it helps.

Warts

RELATED TERMS: *Common Warts, Condyloma Acuminata, Flat Warts, Plantar Warts, Verruca Vulgaris*

PRINCIPAL PROPOSED NATURAL TREATMENTS: *Hypnosis*

OTHER PROPOSED NATURAL TREATMENTS: *Aloe, Bloodroot, Colloidal Silver, Echinacea, Essential Oils, Greater Celandine, Neem, Tea Tree Oil, Zinc*

A wart is a non-cancerous skin growth that occurs when a virus called *human papillomavirus* (HPV) infects the surface layer of the skin. In most cases, warts have a roughened surface and a clearly defined boundary. They most commonly occur on the fingers, hands, and arms, but can occur almost anywhere. Warts on the bottom of the feet are called *plantar warts*, and those that occur in the genital area are called *genital warts*.

Warts are usually painless. However, when they occur in an area that causes them to be subjected to pressure or rubbing, such as the bottom of the foot (plantar warts), they can become extremely tender. Genital warts that occur on the cervix are associated with a significantly increased risk of **cervical dysplasia**.

Conventional treatment for warts primarily involves a variety of methods to directly remove them. Over-the-counter topical treatments containing salicylic acid gradually dissolve the wart, but may take many weeks to work. (**Note**: Do not use this method on genital warts.) Podophyllin, trichloroacetic acid (TCA), and cantharidin are other substances that may be applied

to a wart to remove it and which may be more effective, but they are generally only applied by a physician in an office setting. Other methods of wart-removal include freezing the wart with liquid nitrogen (cryotherapy), burning the wart, removing it with a laser, or cutting it out.

A completely different approach involves stimulating the immune system to destroy the wart. The drug Aldara (imiquimod) is the most common approach of this type, although injections of the immune-stimulating substance interferon are sometimes tried as well.

Principal Proposed Natural Treatments

Warts often disappear on their own, as if the body has gotten "fed up" and decided to mount an immune response to remove them. Some evidence indicates that the body can be encouraged to do so through the use of the power of suggestion.

Hypnotherapy may be regarded as the deliberate use of the power of suggestion for therapeutic benefit. In three controlled studies enrolling a total of 180 people with warts, use of hypnosis caused warts to regress to a significantly greater extent than no treatment, placebo treatment, or (in one of the studies) salicylic acid treatment. Another study found that fake treatment with an x-ray machine can cause children's warts to disappear. For more information, see the full **Hypnosis** article.

Other Proposed Natural Treatments

Numerous herbs and supplements are marketed as part of topical products said to help remove warts. However, there is no meaningful scientific evidence to indicate that any of them are effective.

One somewhat poorly conducted double-blind study hints that high (and potentially toxic) doses of the mineral **zinc**, taken orally, may be helpful for warts.

The herb **bloodroot** (*Sanguinaria canadensis*) is traditionally made into a paste and applied directly to the surface of a wart to dissolve it, in the manner of the topical treatments described above.

Other proposed topical treatments include **aloe, colloidal silver, greater celandine, neem, tea tree oil**, and other **essential oils**. These herbs are said to kill viruses. The herb **echinacea** is also sometimes recommended because it is thought to have immune-stimulating effects. However, there is no meaningful evidence that any of these approaches have any greater wart-removal powers than placebo therapy.

Weight Loss, Undesired

RELATED TERMS: *Appetite, Enhancing; Cachexia; Excessive Weight Loss; Weight Loss Caused by Illness*

PRINCIPAL PROPOSED NATURAL TREATMENTS: *Fish Oil*

OTHER PROPOSED NATURAL TREATMENTS: *Arginine, Beta-hydroxy-beta-methylbutyrate (HMB), Branched-chain Amino Acids (BCAAs), Creatine, Conjugated Linoleic Acid (CLA), Glutamine, Lipoic Acid, Medium-chain Triglycerides (MCTs), Melatonin, N-acetyl Cysteine (NAC), Ornithine Alpha-Ketoglutarate (OKG)*

While many more people suffer from excess appetite and would rather decrease it so they can **lose weight**, some people find that they have insufficient desire to eat food and thereby lose weight even though they don't want to. Mild weight loss can occur in relatively healthy people with stomach problems, such as **dyspepsia** or gastric atonia (sluggish action of the stomach). More severe loss of weight can occur among people who are receiving cancer chemotherapy or have serious diseases, such as **HIV, emphysema (COPD), Crohn's disease**, or **congestive heart failure**. In extreme cases, inadequate caloric and fat intake leads to a form of starvation (cachexia) that can hamper recovery and increase the risk of death.

Conventional treatment of undesired weight loss primarily involves concentrated protein–calorie supplements, often taken in liquid form. However, among people who have cancer, simply increasing nutritional intake may not help. Cancer can cause a condition called *tumor-induced weight loss* (TIWL), in which symptoms of starvation occur despite apparently adequate nutrition. The cause is thought to be a particular form of inflammation caused by the cancer. For this reason, nonsteroidal anti-inflammatory drugs have been tried for the treatment of TIWL, with some positive results. Progesterone-related drugs may be helpful for TIWL as well, for reasons that are not clear.

Note: This article does not cover psychological eating disorders, such as **bulimia** or **anorexia**.

Principal Proposed Natural Treatments

Fish oil contains omega-3 fatty acids, "good fats" that have many potential health-promoting properties. As noted above, cancer-induced weight loss involves inflammation and responds to treatment with anti-inflammatory drugs. Fish oil also has anti-inflammatory effects. According to some, though not all, studies, fish oil supplements can help people with cancer gain weight.

A typical dosage of fish oil used for cancer-induced weight loss is about 12 g daily. For more information, see the full **Fish Oil** article.

Other Proposed Natural Treatments

Fats are a concentrated form of energy and, for that reason, people with undesired weight loss are often encouraged to increase fat intake. People with cancer have an additional reason to consume more fat: cancer interferes with the normal process of fat storage, making it less efficient. Certain special fats may be particularly helpful for correcting this "fat deficiency," including **conjugated linoleic acid** (CLA) and **medium-chain triglycerides** (MCTs), along with fish oil as discussed above.

People with HIV/AIDS may have trouble *absorbing* fats. Two small double-blind studies have found that MCTs are more easily absorbed than ordinary fats in people with this condition.

However, there is no direct evidence as yet that MCTs actually help people with HIV infection gain weight. **Note**: In both of the studies noted here, participants consumed *nothing but* a special nutritional formula containing MCTs. Taking MCTs in this way requires medical supervision to determine the dose.

People with excessive weight loss due to serious illness may also need extra protein. Amino acids are the basic building blocks of proteins and may be easier to digest than whole proteins. Certain amino acid supplements have shown particular usefulness in treating cancer cachexia. One such is **branched chain amino acids** (BCAAs), a collection of the amino acids leucine, isoleucine, and valine. A double-blind study tested BCAAs on 28 people with cancer who had lost their appetites because of either the disease itself or its treatment. Appetite improved in 55% of those taking BCAAs (4.8 g daily) compared to only 16% of those who took placebo.

Promising results for both cancer-induced and HIV-induced weight loss have also been seen with the amino acids **arginine**, **glutamine**, and **ornithine alpha-ketoglutarate** (OKG).

Other treatments found useful for cancer- or HIV-induced weight loss include the antioxidants **lipoic acid** and **N-acetyl cysteine** (NAC), a cocktail containing the sports supplement **beta-hydroxy-beta-methylbutyrate** (HMB) combined with the amino acids arginine and glutamine, and the hormone **melatonin**.

Traditional remedies for mild, occasional loss of appetite involve the use of bitter-tasting herbs, such as gentian (sold as "bitters" in liquor stores), **devil's claw**, **goldenseal**, **hops**, and **horehound**.

In one study, use of the supplement **creatine** failed to help maintain muscle mass in people undergoing chemotherapy for colon cancer.

Herbs and Supplements to Use Only with Caution

Various herbs and supplements may interact adversely with drugs used to treat the underlying condition causing weight loss. For more information on this potential risk, see the individual drug article in the Drug Interactions section of this book.

Weight Loss Aids

RELATED TERMS: *Obesity, Overweight, Weight Control*

PRINCIPAL PROPOSED NATURAL TREATMENTS: *Chromium, Fiber, Pyruvate*

OTHER PROPOSED NATURAL TREATMENTS: *5-Hydroxytryptophan (5-HTP), Acupuncture, Ayurveda, Calcium, CLA, Coleus forskohlii, Combination Herb/Supplement Therapies, DHEA, Diacylglycerol, Ephedrine (Alone or with Caffeine), Evening Primrose Oil, Green Tea, Hydroxycitric Acid (HCA) (Garcinia cambogia), Hypnotherapy, L-Carnitine, Low-carb Diet, Low–glycemic Index Diet, MCTs, Spirulina, Vitamin C, Vitamin D*

Losing weight can be a lifelong challenge. Researchers who study obesity consider it a chronic health condition that must be managed much like high blood pressure or high cholesterol. That means there's no easy cure.

Losing just 5 to 10% of your total weight can lower **blood pressure**, improve **cholesterol profile**, prevent **diabetes**, improve blood sugar control if you already have diabetes, and reduce the risk of developing **osteoarthritis** of the knee.

A combination of improved diet and regular exercise might be the best way to lose weight and keep it off.

Although prior weight-loss drugs, such as amphetamines and fen-phen, have had a patchy safety record, sibutramine (Meridia) appears to be safe and modestly effective for weight loss. New drugs currently in development will likely offer greater benefits.

Principal Proposed Natural Treatments

Chromium

Chromium is a mineral the body needs in only small amounts, but it's important to human nutrition.

Although it has principally been studied for improving blood sugar control in people with diabetes, chromium has also been tried for reducing total weight and body fat percentage, with some success. Both of these potential benefits involve chromium's effects on insulin. Before we can explain how chromium may help, we need to provide some background information on how the body controls its blood sugar levels.

The body needs a constant level of glucose (sugar) in the blood. When you digest a carbohydrate meal, glucose levels rise. Protein meals have the same effect, although to a lesser extent. Your body responds by secreting insulin. Insulin causes the cells of your body to absorb glucose out of the blood, thereby reducing circulating blood sugar.

Once cells have taken in glucose, they can burn it for energy or convert it to a storage form. Liver and muscle cells can store a limited amount of glucose as glycogen. Fat cells can convert unlimited amounts of glucose into energy stored as fat.

The process also goes the opposite way. When your body has used up the food from its last meal, blood glucose levels drop. Just as the body doesn't like it when glucose levels are too high, low glucose levels also cause problems. So your body applies its control mechanisms to raise blood sugar levels. It does so by reducing its output of insulin and also by raising levels of another hormone called *glucagon*. The net effect is that energy storage depots are mobilized. Glycogen is converted back into glucose. In addition, fat cells release their contents into the bloodstream to supply an alternate energy source.

In summary, high insulin levels build fat, while low insulin levels break down fat.

Based on this push-pull effect, if you want to lose weight you'd probably rather keep your insulin levels low.

Dieting is the most obvious method of reducing insulin. When you don't take in enough calories to supply your body's daily needs, insulin levels fall and your body breaks down fat cells. Exercising is another method; by increasing your body's energy requirements, exercise causes insulin levels to fall and fat cells to break down.

But it's difficult to consistently use more energy than you take in. Hunger takes over and you start wanting to eat. If there were some way to trigger fat breakdown without going hungry, it would make weight loss much easier.

There's another important connection between insulin and weight to consider. Individuals who weigh too much often develop *insulin resistance*. In this condition, certain cells of the body become less sensitive to insulin. The body senses this, and increases insulin production until it overcomes the resistance. It is possible that fat cells respond to these increased levels of insulin by storing even more fat.

Chromium is thought to improve the body's responsiveness to insulin. Combining this fact with the insulin–weight connections just described, some researchers have proposed that chromium may assist in decreasing weight or improving body composition (the ratio of fatty tissue to lean tissue).

Their main argument goes like this: chromium increases insulin sensitivity. This causes levels of insulin to fall. With reduced amounts of insulin in the blood, fat cells are less inclined to store fat and weight loss may become easier.

In addition, there is some evidence that chromium partially blocks insulin's effects on fat cells, interfering with its fat-building effect. This could also promote weight loss.

However, there are several flaws in these arguments. For example, even very small amounts of insulin in the blood effectively suppress fat breakdown. Another problem is that during insulin resistance, fat cells also appear to become resistant to insulin. Insulin resistance, in other words, might be a natural method of keeping the lid on weight gain. Chromium supplements might have the undesired effect of increasing the ability of fat cells to respond to insulin, helping them store fat better!

However, theory only takes one so far. It is more important to review the results of studies in which people were given chromium supplements to reduce their weight.

➢ What Is the Scientific Evidence That Chromium Aids Weight Loss?

About 10 reasonably well-designed, double-blind, placebo-controlled trials have evaluated chromium's potential benefit for weight loss.

In the largest study, 219 people were given either placebo or 200 or 400 mcg of chromium picolinate daily. Participants were not advised to follow any particular diet. Over a period of 72 days, individuals taking chromium experienced significantly greater weight loss than those not taking chromium, more than 2-1/2 pounds versus about 1/4 pound. Interestingly, individuals taking chromium actually gained lean body mass, so the difference in loss of fatty tissue was greater: more than 4 pounds versus less than 1/2 pound. How-

ever, a very high dropout rate makes the results of this study somewhat unreliable.

In a smaller double-blind study by the same researcher, 130 moderately overweight individuals attempting to lose weight were given either placebo or 400 mcg of chromium daily. Although hints of benefit were seen, they were too slight to be statistically significant.

Several other small double-blind, placebo-controlled studies also failed to find evidence of benefit with chromium picolinate.

When larger studies find positive results and smaller studies do not, it often indicates that the treatment under study is only weakly effective. This may be the case with chromium as a weight-loss treatment.

For more information, including dosage and safety issues, see the full **Chromium** article.

Pyruvate

Pyruvate supplies the body with pyruvic acid, a natural compound that plays important roles in the manufacture and use of energy. Theoretically, taking pyruvate might increase the body's metabolism, particularly of fat.

Several small studies enrolling a total of about 150 people have found evidence that pyruvate or DHAP (a combination of pyruvate and the related substance dihydroxyacetone) can aid weight loss and/or improve body composition.

For example, in a 6-week, double-blind, placebo-controlled trial, 51 people were given either pyruvate (6 g daily), placebo, or no treatment. All participated in an exercise program. In the treated group, significant decreases in fat mass (2.1 kg) and percentage body fat (2.6%) were seen, along with a significant increase in muscle mass (1.5 kg). No significant changes were seen in the placebo or nontreatment groups.

Another placebo-controlled study (blinding not stated) used a much higher dose of pyruvate, 22 to 44 g daily depending on total calorie intake. In this trial, 34 slightly overweight people were put on a mildly weight-reducing diet for 4 weeks. Subsequently, half were given a liquid dietary supplement containing pyruvate. Over the course of 6 weeks, people in the pyruvate group lost a small amount of weight (about 1-1/2 pounds) while those in the placebo group did not lose weight. Most of the weight loss came from fat.

Another interesting placebo-controlled study evaluated the effects of DHAP when people who had previously lost weight increased their calorie intake. Seventeen severely overweight women were put on a restricted diet as inpatients for 3 weeks, during which time they lost approximately 17 pounds. They were then given a high-calorie diet. Approximately half of the women also received 15 g of pyruvate and 75 g of dihydroxyacetone daily. The results found that after 3 weeks of this weight-gaining diet, individuals receiving the supplements gained only about 4 pounds, as compared to about 6 pounds in the placebo group. Close evaluation showed that pyruvate specifically blocked regain of fat weight.

While all these studies are intriguing, we really need large studies (100 participants or more) to establish the benefits of pyruvate for weight loss.

For more information, including dosage and safety issues, see the full **Pyruvate** article.

Fiber

Dietary fiber is important to many intestinal tract functions, including digestion and waste excretion. It also appears to have a mild cholesterol-lowering effect and might help reduce the risk of some kinds of cancer (although the current evidence is a bit contradictory).

Fiber might also be useful for losing weight. It's thought to work in a simple way by filling the stomach and causing a feeling of fullness, while providing little to no calories. Fiber might also interfere with absorption of fat.

There are two kinds of fiber: soluble fiber, which swells up and holds water, and insoluble fiber, which does not. Soluble fiber is found in psyllium seed (sold as a laxative), apples, and oat bran. Most other plant-based foods contain insoluble fiber.

Fiber supplements may contain a variety of soluble or insoluble fibers from grain, citrus, vegetable, and even shellfish sources.

Several double-blind, placebo-controlled studies have evaluated fiber supplements as a weight-loss aid. The results have been somewhat inconsistent, but in general it appears that some forms of fiber may slightly enhance weight loss.

In one of the largest studies, 97 mildly overweight women on a strict low-calorie diet were given either placebo or an insoluble fiber (type not stated) 3 times daily for 11 weeks. Women given fiber lost almost 11 pounds compared to about 7 pounds in the placebo group. Participants using the fiber reported less hunger.

Researchers weren't finished with their subjects! For an additional 16 weeks, their diet was changed to one that supplied more calories. As expected, participants regained some weight during this period. Nonetheless, by the end of the 16 weeks, individuals taking fiber were still 8 pounds lighter than at the beginning of the study, while those taking placebo were only 6 pounds lighter.

Another study evaluated whether the benefits of dietary fiber endure over 6 months of dieting. This double-blind trial of 52 overweight individuals found that use of an insoluble, dietary fiber product (made from beet, barley, and citrus) almost doubled the degree of weight loss as compared to placebo. Once more, participants using the fiber supplement reported less hunger.

Two other double-blind, placebo-controlled studies evaluated a similar insoluble fiber product. The first enrolled 60 moderately overweight women and put them on a 1,400-calorie diet along with placebo or fiber for a period of 2 months. The other study was similar, but enrolled only 45 women and followed them for 3 months. The results of both studies again showed improved weight loss and reduced feelings of hunger in the treated groups. However, a 24-week study of 53 moderately overweight individuals found no difference in effect between placebo and 4 g of insoluble fiber daily. Another study failed to find benefit with either of two soluble fiber supplements (methylcellulose or pectin plus beta glucan) in terms of weight, hunger, or satiety.

Glucomannan, a source of soluble dietary fiber from the tubers of *Amorphophallus konjac*, has also been tried for weight loss, with positive results in adults. In a double-blind, placebo-controlled trial of 20 overweight individuals, researchers found that use of glucomannan significantly improved weight loss over an 8-week period. Benefits were also seen in a double-blind, placebo-controlled trial of 28 overweight individuals who had just experienced a heart attack. However, another trial studied the effectiveness of glucomannan as a weight-loss agent in 60 overweight children and found no benefit.

An 8-week, double-blind, placebo-controlled trial of 59 overweight people evaluated the effects of chitosan, a mostly insoluble fiber from crustaceans, taken at a dose of 1.5 g prior to each of the two biggest meals of the day. No special diets were assigned. The results showed that, on average, participants in the placebo group gained more than 3 pounds over the course of the study, while those taking chitosan lost more than 2 pounds. However, a subsequent 24-week, double-blind, placebo-controlled study of 250 people using the same dosage of chitosan failed to find benefit. Negative results were also seen in an 8-week, double-blind, placebo-controlled trial of 51 women given 1,200 mg twice daily and in a 28-day, double-blind trial of 30 overweight people using 1 g twice daily. The balance of these and other studies indicate that chitosan probably does not work. Further argument against the use of chitosan comes from the fact that chitosan supplements may at times contain toxic levels of arsenic.

A few trials have only evaluated effects on hunger and satiety rather than weight loss. One study found that the soluble fiber pectin (from apples) reduces hunger sensations. Another found that the soluble fiber guar gum slows stomach emptying and increases the sensation of fullness. However, a more recent study evaluated the effects of guar gum in 25 women undergoing a weight-loss program and found no influence on hunger.

⇒ Dosage
The optimum dose of fiber and the proper time to take it have not been determined.

In the first three studies described previously, insoluble fiber supplements were given 20 to 30 minutes prior to each meal at a dose of about 2.3 g, along with a large glass of water.

⇒ Safety Issues
Fiber supplements must be taken with water; otherwise they may block the digestive tract. Even when used properly, mild gastrointestinal side effects such as gas and bloating may occur.

As a kind of positive side effect, fiber supplements may reduce cholesterol and blood pressure levels.

For additional dosage information and other important safety issues, see the full articles on **chitosan** and **glucomannan**.

Other Proposed Treatments for Weight Loss

5-HTP (5-hydroxytryptophan)
The supplement **5-HTP** is thought to affect serotonin levels. Because serotonin is thought to play a role in weight regulation, 5-HTP has been investigated as a possible weight-loss aid. A total of four small, double-blind, placebo-controlled clinical trials have been reported.

The first of these, a double-blind, crossover study, found that use of 5-HTP (at a daily dose of 8 mg per kilogram body weight) reduced caloric intake despite the fact that the 19 participants made no conscious effort to eat less. Participants given placebo consumed about 2,300 calories per day, while those taking 5-HTP ate

only 1,800 calories daily. Use of 5-HTP appeared to lead to a significantly enhanced sense of satiety after eating. Over the course of 5 weeks, women taking 5-HTP effortlessly lost more than 3 pounds.

A follow-up study by the same research group enrolled 20 overweight women who were trying to lose weight. Participants received either 5-HTP (900 mg per day) or placebo for two consecutive 6-week periods. During the first period, there was no dietary restriction, while during the second participants were encouraged to follow a defined diet expected to lead to weight loss.

Participants receiving placebo did not lose weight during either period. However, those receiving 5-HTP lost about 2% of their initial body weight during the no-diet period and an additional 3% while on the diet. Thus, a woman with an initial weight of 170 pounds lost about 3-1/2 pounds after 6 weeks of using 5-HTP without dieting and another 5 pounds while dieting. Once again, participants taking 5-HTP experienced quicker satiety.

Similar benefits were seen in a double-blind study of 14 overweight women given 900 mg of 5-HTP daily.

Finally, a double-blind, placebo-controlled study of 20 overweight individuals with adult-onset diabetes found that use of 5-HTP (750 mg per day) without intentional dieting resulted in about a 4-1/2 pound weight loss over a 2-week period. Use of 5-HTP reduced carbohydrate intake by 75% and fat intake to a lesser extent.

Unfortunately, all these studies were performed by a single research group. In science, results aren't considered valid until they are independently replicated by different researchers. In addition, all these studies were small in size. For these reasons, further research is necessary before we can consider 5-HTP a proven weight-loss agent.

Garcinia cambogia
Hydroxycitric acid (HCA), a derivative of citric acid, is found primarily in a small, sweet, purple fruit called *Garcinia cambogia*, the Malabar tamarind. Although animal and test-tube studies as well as one human trial suggest that HCA might encourage weight loss, other studies have found no benefit. In an 8-week, double-blind, placebo-controlled trial of 60 overweight individuals, use of HCA at a dose of 440 mg 3 times daily produced significant weight loss as compared to placebo.

In contrast, a 12-week, double-blind, placebo-controlled trial of 135 overweight individuals, who were given either placebo or 500 mg of HCA 3 times daily, found no effect on body weight or fat mass. However, this study has been criticized for using a high-fiber diet, which is thought to impair HCA absorption.

Other small placebo-controlled studies found HCA had no effect on metabolism, appetite, or weight.

The bottom line: It is not yet clear whether *Garcinia cambogia* is an effective treatment for weight loss.

Caffeine and Ephedrine

Caffeine and ephedrine (found in ephedra, an herb also known as *ma huang*) are central nervous system stimulants. Considerable evidence suggests ephedrine/caffeine combinations can modestly assist in weight loss.

For example, in a double-blind, placebo-controlled trial, 180 overweight people were placed on a weight-loss diet and given either ephedrine–caffeine (20 mg/ 200 mg), ephedrine alone (20 mg), caffeine alone (200 mg), or placebo, 3 times daily for 24 weeks. The results showed that the ephedrine/caffeine treatment significantly enhanced weight loss, resulting in a loss of more than 36 pounds as compared to only 29 pounds in the placebo group. Neither ephedrine nor caffeine alone produced any benefit. Contrary to some reports, participants did not develop tolerance to the treatment. For the whole 6 months of the trial, the treatment group maintained the same relative weight loss advantage over the placebo group.

While this study only found benefit with caffeine–ephedrine and not with ephedrine alone, other studies have found that ephedrine alone also offers some weight loss benefits.

We don't know exactly how ephedrine–caffeine works. However, caffeine has actions that cause fat breakdown and enhance metabolism. Ephedrine suppresses appetite and increases energy expenditure. The combination appears to produce synergistic effects, with appetite suppression probably the most important overall factor.

Note: Ephedrine presents serious medical risks, and should only be used under physician supervision. See the full **Ephedra** article for more information.

Medium-chain Triglycerides

Some evidence suggests that **medium-chain triglyceride** (MCT) consumption might enhance the body's tendency to burn fat. This has led to investigations of MCTs as a weight-loss aid. However, the results of clinical trials thus far have been fairly unimpressive.

In a 4-week, double-blind, placebo-controlled trial, 66 women were put on a very low-carbohydrate diet to induce a state called *ketosis*. Half of the women received a liquid supplement containing ordinary fats; the other half received a similar supplement in which the ordinary fats were replaced by MCTs.

The results indicated that the MCT supplement significantly increased the rate of "fat burning" during the first 2 weeks of the trial and also reduced the loss of muscle mass. However, these benefits declined during the last 2 weeks of the trial, which suggests that the effects of MCTs are temporary.

In studies that involved substituting MCTs for ordinary fats in a low calorie diet have shown minimal relative benefits at best.

A related supplement called *structured medium- and long-chain triacylglycerols* (SMLCT) has been created to provide the same potential benefits as MCTs, but in a form that can be used as cooking oil. In a preliminary double-blind trial, SMLCT showed some promise as a "fat-burner."

Other Approaches to Weight Loss

A special type of fat known as *diacylglycerol* has shown promise as a weight loss aid. For example, in a 24-week, double-blind, placebo-controlled study, 131 overweight men and women were placed on a weight loss diet including, in part, supplementary foods containing either diacylglycerols or ordinary fats. The results showed that participants using diacylglycerols lost more weight. Benefits were seen in a smaller double-blind trial as well. Diacylglycerols appear to be safe.

Some evidence suggests that the supplements **creatine** and **colostrum** may each slightly improve body composition (fat to muscle ratio) as compared to placebo among individuals undergoing an exercise program.

It has been suggested that **calcium** supplements, or high-calcium diets, may slightly enhance weight loss, but current evidence is inconsistent and overall more negative than positive. It does appear to be the case that calcium absorption is impaired during weight loss, which suggests that one should take calcium supplements while intentionally losing weight.

A 6-month, double-blind study found that the supplement **DHEA** at a dose of 50 mg daily may help decrease abdominal fat and improve insulin sensitivity (thereby potentially helping to prevent diabetes) in seniors. However, another study failed to find DHEA at 40 mg twice daily helpful for weight loss in severely overweight adolescents

A supplement related to DHEA, 3-acetyl-7-oxo-dehydroepiandrosterone (also called *7-oxy* or *7-keto-*

DHEA), has shown a bit of promise for enhancing weight loss.

Results of two small, double-blind, placebo-controlled studies suggest that **vitamin C** supplements might aid in weight loss.

One small double-blind study indicates that a concentrated extract of the herb *Coleus forskohlii* might increase the rate of fat burning.

A double-blind, placebo-controlled trial that enrolled 158 moderately overweight volunteers tested a mixture of chromium, **cayenne**, inulin (a nondigestible carbohydrate), and **phenylalanine** (an amino acid), as well as other herbs and nutrients. All participants lost weight over the 4-week trial. Those using the supplement lost a bit more weight, but the difference was not mathematically significant. However, a bit of positive news came from close examination of results. Among those taking the supplement, a significantly higher percentage of the weight loss came from fat instead of muscle.

One study found benefit with a combination treatment containing niacin-bound chromium, *Gymnema sylvestre*, and HCA.

Weight-loss benefits were seen in a double-blind trial of 150 overweight people given either placebo or one of two doses of a combination therapy containing chitosan, chromium, and HCA. Benefits were also seen in a 45-day double-blind, placebo-controlled trial of 44 overweight people that tested a combination product containing **yerbe mate**, **guarana**, and **damiana**.

A double-blind, placebo-controlled study evaluated the effects of a mixture containing *Citrus aurantium* (bitter orange), caffeine, and **St. John's wort**. *Citrus aurantium* contains various stimulant chemicals related to nasal spray decongestants. The results suggest that this combination might assist weight loss, but the study was so small (23 participants divided into three groups) that the results mean little.

Ayurvedic herbs have shown some promise for weight loss. In a 3-month, double-blind, placebo-controlled study, 70 overweight individuals were divided into four groups: placebo, triphala guggul (a mixture of five Ayurvedic ingredients) plus Gokshuradi guggul (a mixture of eight Ayurvedic ingredients), triphala guggul plus Sinhanad guggul (a mixture of six Ayurvedic herbs), or triphala guggul plus Chandraprabha vati (a mixture of 36 Ayurvedic ingredients). Reportedly, all three Ayurvedic ingredients produced significant weight loss and improvements in cholesterol compared to placebo; furthermore, the improvements produced by each of the treatments were close to identical.

Studies attempting to determine whether **evening primrose oil** can aid in weight loss have yielded mixed results.

One study failed to find useful results with a combination of rhubarb, **ginger**, **astragulus**, red sage, and **turmeric**.

Beans partially interfere with the body's ability to digest carbohydrates, which is why they cause flatulence. Based on this, products containing the French white bean *Phaseolus vulgaris* have been widely marketed as weight loss aids. However, published studies have generally failed to find these "carbohydrate blockers" effective for this purpose. According to the manufacturer of a current product, more concentrated extracts of *Phaseolus vulgaris*, taken in higher doses, actually can work. Unfortunately, the evidence for this claim rests entirely on unpublished studies that we are unable to verify. Until these studies are published in a journal and subject to proper review, it will be difficult to know how reliable they may be.

Conjugated linoleic acid (CLA) is a mixture of different isomers, or chemical forms, of linoleic acid. CLA has been proposed as a fat-burning substance, but the evidence suggests that if it produces any benefit at all, the effect is minimal. **Note**: There are concerns that use of CLA by overweight people could raise insulin resistance and therefore increase risk of diabetes. In addition, use of CLA might impair endothelial function, and thereby increase cardiovascular risk.

One interesting study found that topical application of glycyrrhetinic acid, a constituent of **licorice**, can reduce fat thickness in the thigh.

A mixture of the herbs of *Magnolia officinalis* and *Phellodendron amurense* is said to help reduce stress-induced overeating, but the only supporting evidence for this claim is a study too small to provide meaningful results.

Hypnosis is popular as an aid to weight loss. However, a careful analysis of published studies suggests that the benefits are slight at best.

Although **acupuncture** is widely used for weight loss, as yet the evidence from published studies is incomplete and inconsistent.

One double-blind study failed to find capsaicin (the "hot" in **cayenne pepper**) helpful for preventing weight regain after weight loss, but it did seem to cause some increase in fat metabolism.

A rather theoretical study found that two ingredients in **green tea** may interact to increase metabolism and, on this basis, green tea became a popular weight control supplement. However, other evidence indicates that if green tea increases metabolism at all, the effect is extremely small. One double-blind study that evaluated the potential benefits of green tea for preventing weight regain after weight loss failed to find greater benefits with green tea than with placebo. In another study, use of green tea failed to produce significant weight loss in overweight women with polycystic ovary syndrome. However, a study using oolong tea enriched with green tea catechins found some apparent weight loss benefit.

Other supplements that have been studied but not found effective include spirulina, **L-carnitine**, and **oligomeric proanthocyanidin complexes** (OPCs) from grape seed.

An enormous number of other supplements are marketed for weight loss, but without meaningful supporting evidence.

For example, certain supplements are said to be lipotropic, meaning that they help your body metabolize fat or slow down the rate at which it's stored. **Vitamins B₅** and **B₆**, **biotin**, **choline**, **inositol**, **lecithin**, and **lipoic acid** are often placed in this category. However, there is no real evidence that they'll help you lose weight.

A number of amino acids are said to reduce hunger, including **phenylalanine**, **tyrosine**, **methionine**, and **glutamine**. Because the herb **kava** appears to be helpful for anxiety, it has been proposed as a treatment for mood-related overeating. The antidepressant herb St. John's wort has been recommended with much the same reasoning.

Seaweeds, such as **kelp**, **bladderwrack**, and sargassi, are often added to diet formulas, under the assumption that they will affect the thyroid gland through their **iodine** content. (An underactive thyroid can cause weight gain.) However, the effect of iodine on thyroid function depends on whether you are iodine-deficient. Excess iodine can actually suppress the action of the thyroid. The herb **guggul** (*Commiphora mukul*) is often claimed to enhance thyroid function and, for this reason, it is often sold as a weight-loss agent. However there is little evidence that it actually affects the thyroid, and a small double-blind trial found it no more effective than placebo for weight loss.

Numerous herbs and supplements with potential or known effects on insulin are widely added to weight-loss formulas, again, without any evidence that they are effective. These include **alfalfa**, *Anemarrhena asphodeloides*, **arginine**, *Azadirachta indica* (**neem**), **bilberry leaf**, **bitter melon** (*Momordica charantia*), *Catharanthus roseus*, *Coccinia indica*, *Cucumis sativus*, *Cucurbita ficifolia*, *Cuminum cyminum* (cumin), *Euphorbia prostrata*, **garlic**, **glucomannan**, *Guaiacum coulteri*, *Guazuma ulmifolia*, guggul, holy basil (*Ocimum sanctum*), *Lepechinia caulescens*, *Musa sapientum* L. (banana), nopal cactus (*Opuntia streptacantha*), onion, *Psacalium peltatum*, pterocarpus, *Rhizophora mangle*, **salt bush**, *Spinacea oleracea*, *Tournefortia hirsutissima*, *Turnera diffusa*, and **vanadium**.

Herbs with laxative or diuretic properties or reputations are also popular in weight-loss formulas, although they are unlikely to produce anything beyond a slight temporary effect. These include **barberry**, **buchu**, cascara sagrada bark, cassia powder, **cleavers**, corn silk, couchgrass, **dandelion root**, fig, **goldenrod**, hydrangea root, **juniper berry**, **peppermint**, prune, **senna leaf**, tamarind, turkey rhubarb root, and **uva ursi**.

Herbs supposed to "strengthen" the body in general are found in many diet formulas, including **ashwagandha**, **cordyceps**, *Eleutherococcus*, **fo-ti**, **ginseng**, **maitake**, **reishi**, **schisandra**, and **suma**.

Other herbs and supplements sometimes recommended for weight loss for reasons that are unclear include buckthorn, cayenne, chickweed, **coenzyme Q₁₀**, **cranberry**, **fennel**, **flaxseed**, **ginger**, **ginkgo**, **gotu kola**, **grape seed extract**, **hawthorn**, licorice, **milk thistle**, **parsley**, **passionflower**, **plantain**, **white willow**, **yellow dock**, **yucca**, and **zinc**.

Numerous dietary methods have been proposed for aiding weight loss. For information on two of the most popular "alternative" diets for weight loss, see the articles on **low-carbohydrate diets** and **low–glycemic index diets**. In general, it appears that all weight loss approaches are about equally helpful (provided that you stick to the rules!). One study found that reducing consumption of high sugar beverages appears to have a minor effect, if any.

Women's Health

Numerous conditions of relevance to women are discussed in the Collins Alternative Health Guide. Below, we list those that conventionally fall in the area of Women's Health.

Reproductive-age Women

According to a recent review, reasonably good evidence suggests that natural treatments can address three conditions of concern to reproductive-age women:

- *Dysmenorrhea*
- *Nausea of Pregnancy*
- *PMS*

In addition, natural medicine has shown considerable promise for the following:

- **Breast-feeding Support**
- **Chronic Venous Insufficiency (a condition related to varicose veins)**
- **Cyclic Breast Pain**
- **Pregnancy, Support**

Natural therapies have also been advocated for the following conditions:

- **Acne**
- **Amenorrhea**
- **Bladder Infections**

- **Breast Enhancement**
- **Brittle Nails**
- **Cervical Dysplasia**
- **Eating Disorders**
- **Infertility**
- **Rosacea**
- **Sexual Dysfunction**
- **Vaginal Infections**

See also **general nutritional support** for information on nutrients that may be helpful for overall health.

Menopausal Women

Natural medicine has shown promise for several conditions of particular relevance to menopausal women, including:

- **Aging Skin**
- **Bladder Infections**
- **Brittle Nails**
- **Chronic Venous Insufficiency (a condition related to varicose veins)**
- **Menopausal Symptoms**
- **Osteoporosis**
- **Sexual Dysfunction**
- **Vaginal Infections**

See also **general nutritional support** for information on nutrients that may be helpful for overall health.

HERBS AND SUPPLEMENTS

5-Hydroxytryptophan

SUPPLEMENT FORMS/ALTERNATE NAMES: *5-HTP*
PRINCIPAL PROPOSED USES: *Depression, Migraine Headaches, Other Types of Headaches*
OTHER PROPOSED USES: *Obesity (Weight Loss), Fibromyalgia, Anxiety, Insomnia*

Many antidepressant drugs work, at least in part, by raising serotonin levels. The supplement 5-hydroxytryptophan (5-HTP) has been tried in cases of depression for a similar reason: the body uses 5-HTP to make serotonin, so providing the body with 5-HTP might therefore raise serotonin levels.

As a supplement, 5-HTP has also been proposed for all the same uses as other antidepressants, including aiding weight loss, preventing migraine headaches, decreasing the discomfort of fibromyalgia, improving sleep quality, and reducing anxiety.

Sources

5-HTP is not found in foods to any appreciable extent. For use as a supplement, it is manufactured from the seeds of an African plant (*Griffonia simplicifolia*).

Therapeutic Dosages

A typical dosage of 5-HTP is 100 to 300 mg 3 times daily. Once 5-HTP starts to work, it may be possible to reduce the dosage significantly and still maintain good results.

Therapeutic Uses

The primary use of 5-HTP is for **depression**. Several small short-term studies have found that it may be as effective as standard antidepressant drugs. Since standard antidepressants are also used for **insomnia** and **anxiety**, 5-HTP has also been suggested as a treatment for those conditions, but there is only very preliminary evidence as yet that it works.

Similarly, antidepressant drugs are often used for **migraine headaches**. Some, but not all, studies suggest that regular use of 5-HTP may help reduce the frequency and severity of migraines, as well as help other types of headaches. Additionally, preliminary evidence suggests that 5-HTP can reduce symptoms of **fibromyalgia** and perhaps act as a **weight loss aid**.

What Is the Scientific Evidence for 5-Hydroxytryptophan?

Depression

Several small studies have compared 5-HTP to standard antidepressants. The best one was a 6-week study of 63 people given either 5-HTP (100 mg 3 times daily) or an antidepressant in the Prozac family (fluvoxamine, 50 mg 3 times daily). Researchers found equal benefit between the supplement and the drug. However, 5-HTP caused fewer and less severe side effects.

Migraine and Other Headaches

There is some evidence that 5-HTP may help prevent migraines when taken at a dosage of 400 to 600 mg daily. Lower doses may not be effective.

In a 6-month trial of 124 people, 5-HTP (600 mg daily) proved equally effective as the standard drug methysergide. The most dramatic benefits observed were reductions in the intensity and duration of migraines. Since methysergide has been proven better than placebo for migraine headaches in earlier studies, the study results provide meaningful, although not airtight, evidence that 5-HTP is also effective.

Similarly good results were seen in another comparative study, using a different medication and 5-HTP (at a dose of 400 mg daily).

However, in one study, 5-HTP (up to 300 mg daily) was less effective than the drug propranolol. Also, in a study involving children, 5-HTP failed to demonstrate benefit. Other studies that are sometimes quoted as evidence that 5-HTP is effective for migraines actually enrolled adults or children with many different types of headaches (including migraines).

Putting all this evidence together, it appears likely that 5-HTP can help people with frequent migraine headaches if taken in sufficient doses, but further research needs to be done. In particular, we need a large double-blind study that compares 5-HTP against placebo over a period of several months.

Finally, an 8-week, double-blind, placebo-controlled trial of 65 individuals (mostly women) with tension headaches found that 5-HTP at a dose of 100 mg 3 times daily did not significantly reduce the number of headaches experienced; however, it did reduce participants' need to use other pain-relieving medications.

Obesity (Weight Loss)

The drug fenfluramine was one member of the now infamous phen-fen treatment for weight loss. Although very successful, fenfluramine was later associated with damage to the valves of the heart and was removed from the market. Because fenfluramine raises serotonin levels, it seems reasonable to believe that other substances that affect serotonin might also be useful for weight reduction.

Four small double-blind, placebo-controlled clinical trials examined whether 5-HTP can aid weight loss. The first, a double-blind crossover study, found that use of 5-HTP (at a daily dose of 8 mg per kilogram body weight) reduced caloric intake despite the fact that the 19 participants made no conscious effort to eat less. Participants given placebo consumed about 2,300 calories per day, while those taking 5-HTP ate only 1,800 calories daily. Use of 5-HTP appeared to lead to a significantly enhanced sense of satiety after eating. Over the course of 5 weeks, women taking 5-HTP effortlessly lost more than 3 pounds.

A follow-up study by the same research group enrolled 20 overweight women who were trying to lose weight. Participants received either 5-HTP (900 mg per day) or placebo for two consecutive 6-week periods. During the first period, there was no dietary restriction, while during the second period participants were encouraged to follow a defined diet expected to lead to weight loss.

Participants receiving placebo did not lose weight during either period. However, those receiving 5-HTP lost about 2% of their initial body weight during the no-diet period and an additional 3% while on the diet. Thus, a woman with an initial weight of 170 pounds lost about 3-1/2 pounds after 6 weeks of using 5-HTP without dieting and another 5 pounds while dieting. Once again, participants taking 5-HTP experienced quicker satiety.

Similar benefits were seen in a double-blind study of 14 overweight women given 900 mg of 5-HTP daily.

Finally, a double-blind, placebo-controlled study of 20 overweight individuals with adult-onset diabetes found that use of 5-HTP (750 mg per day) without intentional dieting resulted in about a 4-1/2 pound weight loss over a 2-week period. Use of 5-HTP reduced carbohydrate intake by 75% and fat intake to a lesser extent.

Fibromyalgia

Antidepressants are the primary conventional treatment for fibromyalgia, a little-understood disease characterized by aching, tender muscles, fatigue, and disturbed sleep. One study suggests that 5-HTP may be helpful as well. In this double-blind trial, 50 subjects with fibromyalgia were given either 100 mg of 5-HTP or placebo 3 times daily for a month. Those receiving 5-HTP experienced significant improvements in all symptom categories, including pain, stiffness, sleep patterns, anxiety, and fatigue.

Anxiety

An 8-week, double-blind, placebo-controlled study compared 5-HTP and the drug clomipramine in 45 individuals suffering from anxiety disorders. The results showed that 5-HTP was effective, but clomipramine was more effective.

Safety Issues

No significant adverse effects have been reported in clinical trials of 5-HTP. Side effects appear to be generally limited to short-term, mild digestive distress and possible allergic reactions.

One potential safety issue with 5-HTP involves an interaction with a medication used for Parkinson's disease: carbidopa. Several reports suggest that the combination can create skin changes similar to those that occur in the disease scleroderma.

According to several reports, when dogs have consumed excessive amounts of 5-HTP, they developed signs of excess serotonin. In humans, this so-called serotonin syndrome includes such symptoms as confusion, agitation, rapid heart rate, high blood pressure, muscle jerks, loss of coordination, sweating, shivering, fever, and rapid breathing; coma and death are possible. Serotonin syndrome might also occur if 5-HTP is combined with drugs that raise serotonin levels, such as SSRIs (such as, Prozac), other antidepressants, or the pain medication tramadol.

There are some reasons for concern that 5-HTP could increase the risk of "infantile spasms" (technically, massive myoclonic seizure disorder) in developmentally disabled children.

Although safety in children has not been proven,

children have been given 5-HTP in studies without any apparent harmful effects. Safety in pregnant or nursing women and those with liver or kidney disease has not been established.

Peak X

One report in 1998 raised a potential safety concern with 5-HTP. Researchers discovered evidence of an unidentified substance called *peak* X in a limited number of 5-HTP products.

Peak X has a frightening history involving a supplement related to 5-HTP: tryptophan. The body turns tryptophan into 5-HTP and the two supplements have similar effects in the body. Until the late 1980s, tryptophan was widely used as a sleep aid. However, it was taken off the market when thousands of people using tryptophan developed a disabling and sometimes fatal blood disorder called *eosinophilia myalgia*. Peak X, introduced through a manufacturer's mistake, is thought to have been the cause, although not all experts agree.

Despite this one report, it seems unlikely that 5-HTP could present the same risk as tryptophan. It is manufactured completely differently; peak X has not been seen again in 5-HTP samples and no epidemic of eosinophilia myalgia has occurred with 5-HTP use.

Interactions You Should Know About

If you are taking:

➤ prescription antidepressants (including SSRIs, MAO inhibitors, or tricyclics), the pain drug tramadolor, or migraine drugs in the triptan family (such as sumatriptan): Do not take 5-HTP in addition except on a physician's advice.
➤ the Parkinson's disease medication carbidopa: Taking 5-HTP at the same time might cause skin changes similar to those that develop in the disease scleroderma.

Acerola

Malpighia glabra

PRINCIPAL PROPOSED USES: *Source of Vitamin C*
OTHER PROPOSED USES: *Antioxidant*

Acerola is a small tree that grows in dry areas of the Caribbean and Central and South America. Traditionally, its fruit has been used to treat diarrhea, arthritis, fevers, and kidney, heart, and liver problems. Acerola contains 10 to 50 times more vitamin C by weight than oranges. Other important substances found in acerola include **bioflavonoids**, **magnesium**, **pantothenic acid**, and **vitamin A**.

What Is Acerola Used for Today?

Acerola is primarily marketed as a source of vitamin C and bioflavonoids. Because of these constituents, it has substantial **antioxidant** properties. One study found that acerola significantly increased the antioxidant ac-

tivity of **soy** and **alfalfa**. It is not clear, however, that this rather theoretical finding indicates anything of significance to human health. Other powerful antioxidants such as **vitamin E** and **beta-carotene** have proved disappointing when they were subjected to studies that could discern whether their actions as antioxidants translated into actual health benefits.

Like many plants, acerola has antibacterial and antifungal properties, at least in the test tube. However, no studies in humans have been reported.

Dosage

A typical supplemental dosage of acerola is 40 to 100 mg daily.

Safety Issues

As a widely used food, acerola is believed to have a relatively high safety factor. However, it has been discovered that people who are allergic to latex may be allergic to acerola as well.

Maximum safe doses in young children, pregnant or nursing women, and people with severe liver or kidney disease have not been established.

Acidophilus and Other Probiotics

SUPPLEMENT FORMS/ALTERNATE NAMES: S. thermophilus, B. bifidus, L. reuteri, L. acidophilus,
L. bulgaricus, L. plantarum, *Probiotics*, Lactobacillus, Bifidobacterium, L. casei, Saccharomyces boulardii, S. salivarius, L. gasseri, Lactobacillus GG, Lactobacillus *LB*

PRINCIPAL PROPOSED USES: *Various Forms of Diarrhea, Including "Traveler' Diarrhea," Diarrhea Caused by Antibiotics, and Viral Diarrhea (in Children); Gastrointestinal Side Effects of Cancer Therapy; Irritable Bowel Syndrome*

OTHER PROPOSED USES: *Allergic Rhinitis, Canker Sores, Colds (Prevention), Colon Cancer (Prevention), Constipation (Chronic), Diverticular Disease, Eczema, High Cholesterol, Immune Support, Inflammatory Bowel Disease (Ulcerative Colitis and Crohn's Disease), Milk Allergies, Rheumatoid Arthritis, Ulcers, Vaginal Infection, Yeast Hypersensitivity Syndrome*

*L*actobacillus acidophilus is a "friendly" strain of bacteria used to make yogurt and cheese. Although we are born without it, acidophilus soon establishes itself in our intestines and helps prevent intestinal infections. Acidophilus also flourishes in the vagina, where it protects women against yeast infections.

Acidophilus is one of several microbes known collectively as *probiotics* (literally, "pro life," indicating that they are bacteria and yeasts that help rather than harm). Others include the bacteria *L. bulgaricus, L. reuteri, L. plantarum, L. casei, B. bifidus, S. salivarius,* and *S. thermophilus* and the yeast *Saccharomyces boulardii*. Your digestive tract is like a rain forest ecosystem with billions of bacteria and yeasts rather than trees, frogs, and leopards. Some of these internal inhabitants are more helpful to your body than others. Acidophilus and related probiotics not only help the digestive tract function, they also reduce the presence of less healthful organisms by competing with them for the limited space available. For this reason, use of probiotics can help prevent infectious diarrhea.

Antibiotics can disturb the balance of your "inner rain forest" by killing friendly bacteria. When this happens, harmful bacteria and yeasts can move in and flourish. This can lead to vaginal yeast infections. Conversely, it appears that the regular use of probiotics can help prevent vaginal infections and generally improve the health of the gastrointestinal system. Whenever you take antibiotics, you should probably take probiotics as well and continue them for some time after you are done with the course of treatment.

Sources

Although we believe that they are helpful and perhaps even necessary for human health, we don't have a daily requirement for probiotic bacteria. They are living creatures, not chemicals, so they can sustain themselves in your body unless something comes along to damage them, such as antibiotics.

Cultured dairy products such as yogurt and kefir are good sources of acidophilus and other probiotic bacteria.

Supplements are widely available in powder, liquid, capsule, or tablet form. Grocery stores and natural food stores both carry milk that contains live acidophilus.

Therapeutic Dosages

Dosages of acidophilus are expressed not in grams or milligrams, but in billions of organisms. A typical daily dose should supply about 3 to 5 billion live organisms. Other probiotic bacteria are used similarly. The typical dose of *S. boulardii* yeast is 500 mg twice daily (standardized to provide 3×10^{10} colony-forming units per gram), to be taken while traveling, or at the start of using antibiotics and continuing for a few days after antibiotics are stopped.

Because probiotics are not drugs, but rather living organisms that you are trying to transplant to your digestive tract, it is necessary to take the treatment regularly. Each time you do, you reinforce the beneficial bacterial colonies in your body, which may gradually push out harmful bacteria and yeasts growing there.

The downside of using a living organism is that probiotics may die on the shelf. In fact, a study reported in 1990 found that most acidophilus capsules on the market contained no living acidophilus. The situation has improved in subsequent evaluations, but still some products are substandard. The container label should guarantee living organisms at the time of purchase, not just at the time of manufacture. Another approach is to eat acidophilus-rich foods such as yogurt, in which the bacteria are most likely still alive.

To treat or prevent vaginal infections, mix 2 tablespoons of yogurt or the contents of a couple of capsules of acidophilus with warm water and use as a douche.

Finally, in addition to increasing your intake of probiotics, you can take fructo-oligosaccharides, supplements that can promote thriving colonies of helpful bacteria in the digestive tract. (Fructo-oligosaccharides are carbohydrates found in fruit. *Fructo* means "fruit" and an *oligosaccharide* is a type of carbohydrate.) Taking this supplement is like putting manure in a garden; it is thought to foster a healthy environment for the bacteria you want to have inside you. The typical daily dose of fructo-oligosaccharides is between 2 and 8 g.

Therapeutic Uses

Evidence from many but not all double-blind, placebo-controlled trials suggests that probiotics may be helpful for many types of **diarrhea** as well as **irritable bowel syndrome**.

Additionally, probiotics have shown significant, if not entirely consistent, promise for preventing or treating **eczema**, treating **ulcerative colitis**, and helping to prevent **colds**, possibly by **improving immunity**.

Although probiotics are widely used to prevent or treat **vaginal yeast infections**, evidence regarding potential benefit remains incomplete and inconsistent. One large, well-designed trial failed to find a *Lactobacillus* preparation helpful for preventing yeast infections caused by antibiotics.

The bacteria *Helicobacter pylori* is the main cause of **ulcers** in the stomach and duodenum. Antibiotics can kill *H. pylori*, but more than one must be used at the same time and, even then, the bacteria is not necessarily eradicated. Probiotics may be helpful. Evidence suggests that various probiotics can inhibit the growth of *H. pylori*. While this effect does not appear to be strong enough for probiotic treatment to eradicate *H. pylori* on its own, preliminary trials as well as two small double-blind trials suggest that various probiotics may help standard antibiotic therapy work better, reducing side effects and possibly increasing rate of eradication.

Some but not all preliminary double-blind trials suggest that probiotics might help prevent heart disease by reducing **cholesterol** levels.

Probiotics might be helpful for **allergic rhinitis** (hay fever).

There is some evidence that probiotics can help reduce symptoms of milk allergies when added to milk. In addition, milk fermented by probiotics may slightly improve blood pressure levels.

One double-blind, placebo-controlled study of 70 people with **chronic constipation** found some evidence of benefit with *Lactobacillus casei Shirota*.

Probiotic treatment has also been proposed as a treatment for **canker sores** and as a preventative measure against colon **cancer**, but there is no solid evidence that it is effective.

Probiotics have shown some promise for helping to prevent **cavities** by antagonizing cavity-causing bacteria.

Probiotics are often proposed for the treatment of a controversial condition known as *yeast hypersensitivity syndrome* (also known as chronic candidiasis, chronic candida, systemic candidiasis, or just **candida**). As described by some alternative medicine practitioners, yeast hypersensitivity syndrome is a common problem that consists of a population explosion of the normally benign *Candida* yeast that live in the vagina and elsewhere in the body, coupled with a type of allergic sensitivity to it. Probiotic supplements are widely recommended for this proposed condition because they establish large, healthy populations of friendly bacteria that compete with the *Candida* that is trying to take up residence. However, there is no evidence that yeast hypersensitivity is a common problem and virtually none that it exists at all.

In one small, 12-week study, *Lactobacillus* GG failed to prove more effective than placebo for the treatment of **rheumatoid arthritis**.

A year-long open trial of 150 women failed to find *Lactobacillus* probiotics effective for preventing **urinary tract infections** as compared to **cranberry** juice or no treatment. However, a large (453-participant), 3-month, double-blind, placebo-controlled study of a special healthy *E. coli* probiotic did find benefits.

What Is the Scientific Evidence for Acidophilus and Other Probiotics?

Traveler's Diarrhea

According to several studies, it appears that regular use of acidophilus and other probiotics can help prevent "traveler's diarrhea" (an illness caused by eating contaminated food, usually in developing countries). One double-blind, placebo-controlled study followed 820 people traveling to southern Turkey and found that use of *Lactobacillus* GG significantly protected against intestinal infection.

Other studies using *S. boulardii* have found similar benefits, including a double-blind, placebo-controlled trial enrolling 3,000 Austrian travelers. The greatest benefits were seen in travelers who visited North Africa and Turkey. The researchers noted that the benefit depended on consistent use of the product and that a dosage of 1,000 mg daily was more effective than 250 mg daily.

Infectious Diarrhea

Probiotics may also help prevent or treat acute infectious diarrhea in children and adults.

A review of the literature published in 2001 found 13 double-blind, placebo-controlled trials on the use of probiotics for acute infectious diarrhea in infants and children; 10 of these trials involved treatment and 3 involved prevention. Overall, the evidence suggests that probiotics can significantly reduce the duration of diarrhea and perhaps help prevent it. The evidence is strongest for the probiotic *Lactobacillus* GG and for infection with a particular virus called *rotavirus*.

For example, one double-blind, placebo-controlled trial of 269 children (ages 1 month to 3 years) with acute diarrhea found that those treated with *Lactobacillus* GG recovered more quickly than those given placebo. The best results were seen among children with rotavirus infection (rotavirus is a virus that can cause severe diarrhea in children). Similar results with *Lactobacillus* GG were seen in a double-blind study of 71 children.

In addition, a double-blind study evaluated the possible benefits of the probiotic *L. reuteri* in 66 children with rotavirus diarrhea. The study found that treatment shortened the duration of symptoms and, the higher the dose, the better the effect.

A double-blind, placebo-controlled study of 81 hospitalized children found that treatment with *Lactobacillus* GG reduced the risk of developing diarrhea, particularly rotavirus infection. A double-blind, placebo-controlled study found that *Lactobacillus* GG helped prevent diarrhea in 204 undernourished children.

Other studies, though not entirely consistent, generally indicate that the probiotics *B. bifidum*, *Streptococcus thermophilus*, *L. casei*, *Lactobacillus* LB, and *S. boulardii*—both individually and combined with *L. reuteri* and *L. chamnosus*—may also help prevent or treat diarrhea in infants and children. One study found that bacteria in the *B. bifidum* family can kill numerous bacteria that cause diarrhea.

Keep in mind that diarrhea in young children can be serious. If it persists for more than a day, you should consult a physician.

A large (211-participant) double-blind, placebo-controlled study found that adults with diarrhea can benefit from probiotic treatment as well. Another study found that regular use of probiotics could help prevent gastrointestinal infections in adults.

Antibiotic-Related Diarrhea

The results of many but not all double-blind and open trials suggest that probiotics, especially *S. boulardii* and *Lactobacillus* GG, may help prevent or treat antibiotic-related diarrhea (including the most severe form, *Clostridium difficle* disease).

For example, one study evaluated 180 people, who received either placebo or 1,000 mg of saccharomyces daily along with their antibiotic treatment and found that the treated group developed diarrhea significantly less often. A similar study of 193 people also found benefit. However, a study of 302 people found no benefit with *Lactobacillus* GG.

However, use of probiotics has not thus far shown any ability to help prevent the development of resistant bacterial strains that may arise during antibiotic treatment.

Note: Diarrhea that occurs in the context of antibiotics may be dangerous; for this reason, physician consultation is essential.

Other Forms of Diarrhea

Preliminary evidence suggests that probiotics may be helpful for reducing diarrheas and other gastrointestinal side effects caused by cancer treatment (radiation or chemotherapy).

Small double-blind studies suggest S. *boulardii* might be helpful for treating chronic diarrhea in people with HIV, hospitalized patients being tube-fed, and people with Crohn's disease.

Inflammatory Bowel Disease (Ulcerative Colitis and Crohn's Disease)

The conditions Crohn's disease and ulcerative colitis fall into the family of conditions known as inflammatory bowel disease. Chronic diarrhea is a common feature of these conditions.

A double-blind trial of 116 people with ulcerative colitis compared probiotic treatment against a relatively low dose of the standard drug mesalazine. The results suggest that probiotic treatment might be equally effective as low-dose mesalazine for controlling symptoms and maintaining remission. Evidence of benefit was seen in other trials as well.

One preliminary study found S. *boulardii* helpful for mild diarrhea in stable Crohn's disease. However, two studies failed to find benefit with *Lactobacillus* probiotics.

Probiotics might be useful for people with ulcerative colitis who have had part or all of the colon removed. Such people frequently develop a complication called *pouchitis*, inflammation of part of the remaining intestine. A 9-month, double-blind trial of 40 people found that a combination of three probiotic bacteria could significantly reduce the risk of a pouchitis flare-up in people with chronic pouchitis. Participants were given either placebo or a mixture of various probiotics, including four strains of *Lactobacilli*, three strains of *Bifidobacteria*, and one strain of *Streptococcus salivarius*. The results showed that treated people were far less likely to have relapses of pouchitis. Another study found that probiotics used right after surgery can help prevent pouchitis from developing at all.

Finally, some evidence hints that probiotics might reduce the joint pain that commonly occurs in people with either kind of inflammatory bowel disease.

Irritable Bowel Syndrome

People with irritable bowel syndrome (IBS) experience crampy digestive pain as well as alternating diarrhea and constipation and other symptoms. Although the cause of irritable bowel syndrome is not known, one possibility is a disturbance in healthy intestinal bacteria. Based on this theory, probiotics have been tried as a treatment for IBS.

In a 4-week, double-blind, placebo-controlled trial of 60 people with IBS, treatment with L. *plantarum* reduced intestinal gas significantly. The benefits persisted for an additional year after treatment was stopped.

In another 4-week, double-blind trial, 40 people with IBS again received either L. *plantarum* or placebo. The results showed improved overall symptoms in the treated group as compared to the placebo group.

Benefits were seen in four other small double-blind trials as well, using L. *plantarum*, L. *acidophilus*, L. *salivarus*, and *Bifidobacterium*, or proprietary probiotic combinations including various strains. Benefits have also been seen with a combination prebiotic/probiotic formula. However, some studies have failed to find probiotics more effective than placebo.

Eczema

Use of probiotics during pregnancy and after childbirth may reduce risk of childhood eczema. In a double-blind, placebo-controlled trial that enrolled 159 women, participants received either placebo or *Lactobacillus* GG capsules beginning 2 to 4 weeks before expected delivery. After delivery, breast-feeding mothers continued to take placebo or the probiotic for 6 months; formula-fed infants were given placebo or probiotic directly for the same period of time. The results showed that use of *Lactobacillus* GG reduced children's risk of developing eczema by approximately 50%.

Infants who already have eczema may benefit as well, according to six small double-blind trials.

Immunity

A number of studies suggest that various probiotics can enhance immune function. One 12-week, double-blind, placebo-controlled trial evaluated 25 healthy elderly people, half of whom were given milk containing a particular strain of *Bifidobacterium lactis*, the others milk alone. The results showed various changes in immune parameters which the researchers took as possibly indicating improved immune function. Another double-blind, placebo-controlled study of 50 people using *B. lactis* had similar results.

A 7-month, double-blind, placebo-controlled study of 571 children in daycare centers in Finland found that use of milk fortified with *Lactobacillus* GG reduced the number and severity of respiratory infections. Benefits were seen in three other large studies, in which probiotics combined with multivitamins and minerals helped prevent colds (or reduce their duration and severity) in adults. However, a smaller and shorter study failed to find any effect on respiratory infections.

One study found that *Lactobacillus* GG or *L. acidophilus* may improve the immune response to vaccinations.

Cholesterol

An 8-week, double-blind, placebo-controlled trial of 70 overweight people found that a probiotic treatment containing *S. thermophilus* and *Enterococcus faecium* could reduce LDL ("bad") cholesterol by about 8%. Similarly positive results were seen in other short-term trials of various probiotics. However, a 6-month, double-blind, placebo-controlled trial found no long-term benefit. Researchers speculate that participants stopped using the product regularly toward the later parts of the study.

Safety Issues

Probiotics may occasionally cause a temporary increase in digestive gas, but beyond that they do not present any known risks for most people. However, individuals who are immunosuppressed could conceivably be at risk for developing a dangerous infection with the probiotic organism itself; at least one person taking immunosuppressive medications has died in this manner.

Interactions You Should Know About

If you are taking **antibiotics**, it may be beneficial to take probiotic supplements at the same time and to continue them for a couple of weeks after you have finished the course of drug treatment. This will help restore the balance of natural bacteria in your digestive tract.

Adenosine Monophosphate

ALTERNATE NAMES/RELATED TERMS: *AMP*

PRINCIPAL PROPOSED USES: *None*

OTHER PROPOSED USES: *Cold Sores, Photosensitivity, Shingles and Post-herpetic Neuralgia*

Adenosine monophosphate (AMP) is a substance the body creates on the way to making adenosine triphosphate (ATP), a source of energy used throughout the body. ATP is so ubiquitous in the body it is sometimes called the body's "energy currency."

Based on highly preliminary evidence, AMP has been recommended as a treatment for **shingles** and **photosensitivity**.

Requirements/Sources

There is no nutritional requirement for AMP because the body manufactures it from scratch.

Therapeutic Dosages

A typical recommended dose of AMP is 100 to 200 mg daily. However, it is not clear that AMP can be absorbed orally and most studies have involved an injected form of the substance.

Therapeutic Uses

In adults, infection by the virus *Herpes zoster* can cause a condition known as *shingles*. The initial shingles attack generally abates in a couple of weeks, but symptoms can go on to become chronic. This condition is called *post-herpetic neuralgia* (PHN). Some evidence hints that people with *Herpes zoster* infection may have lower than normal levels of AMP. On this slim basis, AMP has been studied as a possible treatment for initial shingles symptoms as well as for preventing PHN.

In a double-blind, placebo-controlled study of 32 people with shingles, AMP was injected 3 times per week for 4 weeks. At the end of the 4-week treatment period, 88% of those treated with AMP were pain-free versus only 43% in the placebo group; all participants still in pain were then given AMP and no recurrence of pain was reported in 3 to 18 months of follow-up.

However, this was a preliminary study, and more evidence is needed before AMP can be considered a proven treatment for shingles or PHN. Furthermore, oral AMP has not been tried for this condition. It is questionable whether AMP taken orally actually makes it intact into the body.

Another study found weak evidence that injected AMP might be helpful for **cold sores**. However, this study was not a double-blind trial; it was an open study, in which the placebo effect and other confounding factors could have played a major role. For that reason, its results cannot be relied upon at all. (For information on why double-blind studies are essential to prove a treatment effective, see **Why Does This Book Rely on Double-blind Studies?**.)

Another open study hints that AMP, this time in an oral form, might be helpful for people with excessive sensitivity to the sun (photosensitivity) associated with a condition called *porphyria cutanea tarda*.

Safety Issues

In the human studies performed, use of oral AMP has not been associated with any side effects. However, it has been suggested that use of supplemental AMP could potentially decrease immunity.

Safety in young children, pregnant or nursing women, or people with severe liver or kidney disease has not been established.

Adrenal Extract

ALTERNATE NAMES/RELATED TERMS: *Glandular Extract, Adrenal*

PRINCIPAL PROPOSED USES: *Stress, "Adrenal Exhaustion"*

OTHER PROPOSED USES: *Allergies, Asthma, Fatigue, Rheumatoid Arthritis*

The adrenal gland, an endocrine gland situated near the kidneys, is divided into two parts. The inner portion (medulla) of the adrenal gland secretes epinephrine (adrenaline) and norepinephrine (noradrenaline). The outer portion (the cortex) manufactures the hormones cortisone and aldosterone. All these hormones are necessary for life.

Adrenal extracts are made from the adrenal glands of cows, pigs, or other animals. According to a theory prevalent in alternative medicine, the consumption of adrenal extracts can strengthen the function of an underperforming or exhausted adrenal gland. However, there is no scientific evidence to support this belief and no rational justification to indicate that it might be true.

Early in the twentieth century, physicians used glandular extracts as an actual source of hormones. For example, extracts of ovaries were used to supply female hormones such as progesterone. Similarly, animal adrenal glands may contain significant levels of adrenal hormones. This is the basis for some of the recommended uses of adrenal extracts, such as **allergies**, **asthma**, and **rheumatoid arthritis** (conditions that respond to cortisone). However, modern adrenal extracts are manufactured in such a way that they do not contain significant levels of adrenal hormones. Therefore, it is difficult to find any justification for their use along these lines.

Some manufacturers of glandular products claim that the animal version of an organ provides nutrients that support the corresponding organ in humans. However, there is no evidence that the human adrenal gland requires any nutrients that are uniquely available in animal adrenals.

It has been suggested by one manufacturer of glandular products that consuming extracts of an organ might offer benefit in an immune-related manner. According to this theory, some people may possess antibodies to certain of their own glands and the consumption of an animal version of the gland will divert these antibodies from their target. However, this explanation does not make a great deal of sense. Antibodies are primarily produced against proteins and, even if cow adrenal glands had the same proteins as human adrenal glands, which is unlikely, proteins are not absorbed whole into the bloodstream.

It may be that, on an unconscious level, those who recommend glandular extracts are being influenced by the ancient notion of *sympathetic magic*, the idea that eating a lion's heart, for example, will create courage. However, this is a pre-scientific form of thinking that is difficult to take seriously in the modern era.

Not only is the proposed action of adrenal glandular extracts questionable, their primary proposed purpose for use is questionable as well. Adrenal glandular extracts are most often recommended for treatment of a purported condition called *adrenal exhaustion*. In adrenal exhaustion, the adrenal glands are supposedly weakened by the chronic stresses of modern life and incapable of performing at full capacity. However, there is no believable scientific basis for believing this to be true. The notion of adrenal exhaustion developed as a result of studies done in the mid-twentieth century that involved extreme, life-threatening stress; the studies do not support the existence of a milder, common "adrenal fatigue." (And even if it did exist, there is no reason to think that adrenal extracts would help.)

Finally, there are no meaningful scientific studies that have found benefit with adrenal gland extracts in their modern, non-hormonal form. Only double-blind, placebo-controlled studies can show a treatment effective and, at present, none have been reported for adrenal extracts. (For information on why this type of study is essential, see **Why Does This Book Rely on Double-blind Studies?**)

Alfalfa

Medicago sativa

PRINCIPAL PROPOSED USES: *Nutritional Support*

OTHER PROPOSED USES: *Allergies, Diabetes, Lowering Cholesterol, Menopausal Symptoms*

Alfalfa is one of the earliest cultivated plants, used for centuries for feeding livestock. This probably is true in part because it is easy to grow, thrives in many varied climates throughout the world, and provides an excellent protein-rich food source for cattle, horses, sheep, and other animals. The name alfalfa comes from the Arabian *al-fac-facah*, for "father of all foods." Its high protein content and abundant stores of vitamins make it a good nutritional source for humans, too. Historic (but undocumented) medicinal uses of alfalfa include treatment of stomach upset, arthritis, bladder and kidney problems, boils, and irregular menstruation.

Requirements/Sources

Alfalfa sprouts appear on many salad bars and in the grocery's produce section. Bulk powdered herb or capsules and tablets containing alfalfa leaves or seeds are available in pharmacies and health food stores.

Therapeutic Dosages

A typical dose of alfalfa for tea is 1 to 2 teaspoons per cup, steeped in boiling water for 10 to 20 minutes. Tablets and capsules of whole alfalfa or alfalfa extracts should be taken according to the manufacturer's recommendations. Certain products are said to be free of canavanine (see Safety Issues) and other potentially harmful constituents, and may be preferable.

Therapeutic Uses

Alfalfa is high in vitamin content, providing beta-carotene, various B-vitamins, and vitamins C, E, and K,

Alfalfa

and can be used as a nutritional supplement. However, keep in mind that high doses of alfalfa may present some health risks (see Safety Issues below).

Numerous animal studies and preliminary human trials indicate that extracts from alfalfa seeds, leaves, and roots might be helpful for lowering **cholesterol** levels. However, there have not been any well-designed, double-blind, placebo-controlled trials demonstrating alfalfa useful for this (or any other) purpose.

Studies using mice to investigate alfalfa's traditional use for **diabetes** found that it improved some symptoms.

Alfalfa has also been investigated in the laboratory (but not yet evaluated in people) as a source of plant estrogens, which might make it helpful for **menopause**. Alfalfa may also have some use in fighting fungi. Rats fed a disease-causing fungus were able to eliminate more of the fungus from their systems when fed a diet high in alfalfa. It has been suggested that one of the saponins from alfalfa causes damage to the cell membranes of fungi.

Finally, alfalfa has been proposed as a treatment for hay fever, but there is no scientific evidence that it is helpful for this purpose.

Safety Issues

Alfalfa in its various forms may present some health risks. Powdered alfalfa herb, alfalfa sprouts, and alfalfa seeds all contain L-cavanine, a substance that may cause abnormal blood cell counts, spleen enlargement, or recurrence of lupus in patients with controlled disease. However, heating alfalfa may correct this problem.

Researchers investigating alfalfa seeds' ability to lower cholesterol levels discovered that it had another effect on the lab animals used for testing. In some of the monkeys, it caused a disease very similar to lupus. Further research on this effect revealed that monkeys that had abnormal blood cell counts when eating either alfalfa seeds or sprouts and then recovered when alfalfa was no longer part of their diet, developed the symptoms again when given an isolated component of alfalfa called *L-canavanine*. Alfalfa seeds and sprouts have a higher concentration of L-canavanine than the leaves or roots.

In a clinical trial of alfalfa seeds for lowering cholesterol involving only three human volunteers, one man who participated developed pancytopenia (an abnormally low number of all of the various types of blood cells) and enlargement of the spleen. Additionally, there are two published case reports of patients who had lupus which was controlled with drug therapy, suffering relapses after consuming alfalfa tablets. Again, L-canavanine is thought to be responsible for these effects.

When alfalfa seeds were autoclaved (heated to extremely high temperatures) and fed to monkeys for a year, no ill effects were seen and the monkeys' cholesterol levels decreased. It may be that the L-canavanine can be destroyed by extreme heat, while the saponins that seem to be responsible for the beneficial effects of alfalfa remain intact. If so, a heat-treated product might prove safe; however, much research remains to be done before we can know this for certain.

At present, it seems prudent that people who have been diagnosed with lupus, or those who suspect a predisposition to it based on family history, should probably avoid alfalfa. This includes the tablets used for supplements and the sprouts on the salad bar (go for the lettuce or the spinach instead).

Because of the estrogenic effects of some of alfalfa's components, alfalfa is not recommended for pregnant or nursing women or young children. In addition, the high vitamin K content in alfalfa could, in theory, make the drug warfarin (Coumadin) less effective.

Finally, a number of cases of food poisoning have been documented from fresh sprouts infected with bacteria that was present on the seeds prior to germination. Unfortunately, sprouts can appear fresh and yet host enough bacteria to cause illness in people who eat them. Some health care workers recommend that those at higher risk for such infections—young children, those with chronic diseases, and the elderly—avoid eating sprouts altogether.

Interactions You Should Know About

If you are taking **warfarin (Coumadin)**, the high vitamin K content of alfalfa might make it less effective.

Aloe

Aloe vera

PRINCIPAL PROPOSED USES:

Topical Aloe: *Burn Healing, Genital Herpes, Psoriasis, Seborrhea*

Oral Aloe: *Diabetes*

OTHER PROPOSED USES

Topical Aloe: *Cancer Treatment Support (preventing side effects of radiation therapy), Wound Healing*

Oral Aloe: *Asthma, HIV, Immune Support, Ulcers*

The succulent aloe plant has been valued since prehistoric times for the treatment of burns, wound infections, and other skin problems. Medicinal aloe is pictured in an ancient cave painting in South Africa and Alexander the Great is said to have captured an island off Somalia for the sole purpose of possessing the luxurious crop of aloe found there.

Most uses of aloe refer to the gel inside its cactus-like leaves. However, the skin of the leaves themselves can be condensed to form a sticky substance known as drug aloe or aloes. It is a powerful laxative, but it is seldom used because its effects are unpleasant. The uses described below are intended to refer only to aloe gel, not to drug aloe. However, to make matters trickier, some aloe gel products contain small amounts of drug aloe and it is possible that this contaminant is the actual source of benefits seen in some studies.

What Is Aloe Used for Today?

We suspect millions of people would swear by their own experience that applying aloe to the skin can drastically reduce the time it takes for **burns** (including **sunburn**) to heal. However, scientific evidence fails to support this belief. Studies suggest that aloe is not effective for treating sunburn and may actually impair the healing of second-degree burns.

Aloe also appears to be ineffective for treating the burn-like skin damage caused by **radiation therapy for cancer**. In a double-blind, placebo-controlled study of 194 women undergoing radiation therapy for breast cancer, use of aloe gel failed to protect the skin from radiation-induced damage. Lack of benefit was also seen

in an open trial of 225 women. One study evaluated aloe soap in 73 men and women undergoing radiation therapy for various forms of cancer and, overall, failed to find benefit except possibly at the highest doses. Another study failed to find aloe gel helpful for mouth inflammation caused by **radiation therapy** for head and neck cancer.

Besides its use for burns, aloe has been widely recommended for aiding **wound healing**. However, while the results of test tube and animal studies of aloe for wounds have been positive, one clinical report in people suggests that aloe can actually impair the healing of severe wounds.

Does topical aloe provide any benefit at all? There is some evidence (although quite incomplete) that it might help **genital herpes**, **psoriasis**, and **seborrhea**. See below for more information.

Aloe gel has also been tried as an oral treatment. Two studies suggest that that aloe gel taken orally might be helpful for **type 2 diabetes**. One study found possible benefits for **ulcerative colitis**.

Oral aloe is also sometimes recommended as an aid in the treatment of **asthma**, **stomach ulcers**, and **general immune support**, but there is no meaningful evidence that it is effective for any of these purposes.

One of the constituents of aloe gel, acemannan, has shown some promise in test tube and animal studies for stimulating immunity and inhibiting the growth of viruses. These finding have led to the suggestion that acemannan can help **HIV infection**. However, the one reported double-blind, placebo-controlled trial failed to show benefits.

What Is the Scientific Evidence for Aloe?

Genital Herpes

A 2-week, double-blind, placebo-controlled trial enrolled 60 men with active genital herpes. Participants applied aloe cream (0.5% aloe) or placebo cream 3 times daily for 5 days. Use of aloe cream reduced the time necessary for lesions to heal (4.9 days versus 12 days) and also increased the percentage of individuals who were fully healed by the end of 2 weeks (66.7% versus 6.7%).

A previous double-blind, placebo-controlled study by the same author enrolling 120 men with genital herpes found that cream made from aloe was more effective than pure aloe gel or placebo.

Seborrhea

Seborrhea is a fairly common skin condition, leading to oily, red, and scaly eruptions in such areas as the eyebrows, eyelids, nose, ear, upper lip, chest, groin, and chin. A double-blind, placebo-controlled study of 44 individuals found that 4 to 6 weeks of treatment with aloe ointment could significantly reduce symptoms of seborrhea.

Psoriasis

According to a double-blind study that enrolled 60 men and women with mild to moderate symptoms of psoriasis, aloe cream may be helpful for this chronic skin condition. Participants were treated with either topical aloe extract (0.5%) or a placebo cream, applied 3 times daily for 4 weeks. Aloe treatment produced significantly better results than placebo and these results were said to endure for almost a year after treatment was stopped. The study authors also reported a high level of complete "cure," but what exactly they meant by this was not reported clearly.

However, another study failed to replicate these results. Over four weeks of treatment, marked improvement was seen in 72.5% of skin patches treated with aloe, but 82% of those treated with placebo. This was a statistically significant difference *in favor* of placebo.

Further studies will be needed to sort out these contradictory results.

Diabetes

Evidence from two human trials suggests that aloe gel can improve blood sugar control in individuals with type 2 diabetes.

A single-blind, placebo-controlled trial evaluated the potential benefits of aloe in either 72 or 40 individuals with diabetes (the study report appears to contradict itself). The results showed significantly greater improvements in blood sugar levels among those given aloe over the 2-week treatment period.

Another single-blind, placebo-controlled trial evaluated the benefits of aloe in individuals who had failed to respond to the oral diabetes drug glibenclamide. Of the 36 individuals who completed the study, those taking glibenclamide and aloe showed definite improvements in blood sugar levels over 42 days as compared to those taking glibenclamide and placebo.

Although these are promising results, large studies that are double- rather than single-blind will be needed to establish aloe as an effective treatment for hypoglycemia.

Ulcerative Colitis

In a double-blind, placebo-controlled study of 44 people with active ulcerative colitis, use of oral aloe gel at a dose of 100 ml twice daily for 4 weeks appeared to improve both subjective symptoms and objective measurements of disease severity. About half of the people given aloe showed response to treatment; about 30% experienced full remission. Benefits occurred only rarely in the placebo group. However, this was a small study, and its results can't be taken as conclusive.

Dosage

Topical aloe vera cream typically contains 0.5% aloe and is applied three times daily.

For the treatment of diabetes, a dosage of 1 tablespoon of aloe juice twice daily has been used in studies.

Safety Issues

Other than occasional allergic reactions, no serious problems have been reported with aloe gel, whether used internally or externally. However, comprehensive safety studies are lacking. Safety in young children, pregnant or nursing women, or those with severe liver or kidney disease has not been established.

There is one report of an herb-drug interaction between aloe and the anesthesia drug sevoflurane, in which it appeared that aloe may have increased sevoflurane's "blood thinning" effect.

In addition, keep in mind that if aloe is used as a treatment for diabetes, and it works, blood sugar levels could fall too low, necessitating a reduction in medication dosage. Close monitoring of blood sugar levels is therefore advised.

Interactions You Should Know About

If you are using:

> Hydrocortisone cream: Aloe gel might help it work better.

> Medications for diabetes: Oral use of aloe vera might cause your blood sugar levels to fall too low.

Andrographis
Andrographis paniculata

PRINCIPAL PROPOSED NATURAL USES: *Colds (both Treatment and Prevention)*

OTHER PROPOSED NATURAL USES: *Heart Disease Prevention, Familial Mediterranean Fever, Immune Support, Liver Protection, Stimulating Gallbladder Contraction*

Andrographis is a shrub found throughout India and other Asian countries that is sometimes called *Indian echinacea*. It has been used historically in epidemics, including the Indian flu epidemic in 1919 during which andrographis was credited with stopping the spread of the disease.

What Is Andrographis Used for Today?

Over the last decade, andrographis (often combined with eleutherococcus) has become popular in Scandinavia as a treatment for **colds**. It is beginning to become available in the United States as well. Reasonably good evidence tells us that it can reduce the severity of cold symptoms. It may also help prevent colds.

Although we don't know how andrographis might work for colds, preliminary evidence suggests that it might stimulate immunity, potentially making it useful for **general immune support**.

Andrographis combined with **eleutherococcus, licorice**, and schisandra has shown promise for a genetic disease called *familial Mediterranean fever*.

Preliminary studies in animals weakly suggest that andrographis may offer benefits for preventing **heart disease**. In addition, highly preliminary studies suggest that andrographis may help protect the liver from toxic injury, perhaps more successfully than the more famous liver-protective herb **milk thistle**. It also appears to stimulate gallbladder contraction. Andrographis does not appear to have any antibacterial effects.

What Is the Scientific Evidence for Andrographis?

Reducing Cold Symptoms

A meta-analysis (statistically rigorous review of studies) published in 2004 found seven reasonable quality double-blind, controlled trials, enrolling a total of 896 participants, evaluating the use of andrographis for the treatment of acute respiratory infections. The combined results indicate that andrographis is more effective than placebo for reducing symptoms.

For example, a 4-day, double-blind, placebo-controlled study of 158 adults with colds found that treatment with andrographis significantly reduced cold symptoms. Participants were given either placebo or 1,200 mg daily of an andrographis extract standardized to contain 5% andrographolide. The results showed that by day 2 of treatment, and even more by day 4, individuals who were given the actual treatment experienced significant improvements in symptoms compared to participants in the placebo group. The greatest response was seen in earache, sleeplessness, nasal drainage, and sore throat, but other cold symptoms improved as well.

Three other double-blind, placebo-controlled studies, enrolling a total of about 400 people, evaluated an herbal combination treatment containing both andrographis and *Eleutherococcus senticosus*. Another study found this combination more effective than **echinacea** for colds in children.

Andrographis has also been compared to acetaminophen (Tylenol). In a double-blind study of 152 adults with sore throat and fever, participants received andrographis (in doses of 3 g per day or 6 g per day, for 7 days) or acetaminophen. The higher dose of andrographis (6 g) decreased symptoms of fever and throat pain to about the same extent as acetaminophen, but the lower dose of andrographis (3 g) was not as effective. There were no significant side effects in either group.

A Russian study of questionable quality apparently found andrographis approximately as effective as the drug amanditine for influenza infections.

Preventing Colds

According to one double-blind, placebo-controlled study, andrographis may increase resistance to colds. A total of 107 students, all 18 years old, participated in this 3-month-long trial that used a dried extract of andrographis. Fifty-four of the participants took two 100-mg tablets standardized to 5.6% andrographolide daily—considerably less than the 1,200 to 6,000 mg per day that has been used in studies on treatment of colds. The other 53 students were given placebo tablets with a coating identical to the treatment. Then, once a week throughout the study, a clinician evaluated all the participants for cold symptoms.

By the end of the trial, only 16 people in the group using andrographis had experienced colds, compared to 33 of the placebo-group participants. This difference was statistically significant, indicating that andrographis reduces the risk of catching a cold by a factor of two as compared to placebo.

Dosage

A typical dosage of andrographis is 400 mg 3 times a day. Doses as high as 1,000 to 2,000 mg 3 times daily have been used in some studies. Andrographis is usually standardized to its content of andrographolide, typically 4 to 6%.

Safety Issues

Andrographis has not been associated with any side effects in human studies. In one study, participants were monitored for changes in liver function, blood counts, kidney function, and other laboratory measures of toxicity. No problems were found.

However, some animal studies have raised concerns that andrographis may impair fertility. One study found that male rats became infertile when fed 20 mg of andrographis powder daily. In this case, the rats stopped producing sperm and showed physical changes in some of the testicular cells involved in sperm production. Researchers also detected evidence of degeneration of other anatomical structures in the testicles. However, another study showed no evidence of testicular toxicity in male rats that were given up to 1 g per kilogram body weight daily for 60 days, so this issue remains unclear; furthermore, a human trial using the widely tested andrographis-eleutherococcus combination found no adverse effect on male fertility measurements such as sperm quality and number.

One group of female mice also did not fare well on high dosages of andrographis. When fed 2 g per kilogram body weight daily for 6 weeks (thousands of times higher than the usual human dose), all female mice failed to get pregnant when mated with males of proven fertility. Meanwhile, of the control females, 95.2% got pregnant when mated with a similar group of male mice. Another study found a potential explanation for this in evidence that androphraphis relaxes the uterus. While andrographis is probably not a useful form of birth control, these results are worrisome regarding the use of androphraphis by pregnant women.

Finally, if androphraphis does indeed stimulate the immune system (a big "if"), this would lead to a whole host of potential risks. The immune system is balanced on a knife edge. An immune system that is too relaxed fails to defend us from infections, but an immune system that is too active attacks healthy tissues, causing autoimmune diseases. A universal immune booster might cause or exacerbate **lupus**, **Crohn's disease**, **asthma**, Graves' disease, **Hashimoto's thyroiditis**, **multiple sclerosis**, and **rheumatoid arthritis**, among other illnesses.

Safety in young children, nursing women, or those with severe liver or kidney disease has also not been established.

Also, because andrographis may stimulate gallbladder contraction, it should not be used by individuals with gallbladder disease except under physician supervision.

Androstenedione

PRINCIPAL PROPOSED USES: *Sports Performance Enhancement*

Androstenedione is a hormone produced naturally in the body by the adrenal glands, the ovaries (in women), and the testicles (in men). The body first manufactures **DHEA**, then turns DHEA into androstenedione, and finally transforms androstenedione into testosterone, the principal male sex hormone. Androstenedione is also transformed into estrogen.

Androstenedione is widely used by athletes who believe that it can build muscle and increase strength. However, there is no evidence that it works. Furthermore, androstenedione supplements may cause positive urine tests for illegal steroid use, due to the common presence of a contaminant (19-norandrostenedione).

Sources

Androstenedione is not an essential nutrient—your body manufactures it from scratch. It is found in meat and in some plants, but to get a therapeutic dosage, you will need to take supplements.

Therapeutic Dosages

The typical recommended dose of androstenedione is 100 mg 2 times daily with food.

Therapeutic Uses

Androstenedione is said to enhance **athletic performance** and strength by increasing testosterone production, thereby building muscle. However, in double-blind studies, when androstenedione was given to men, it did not alter total testosterone levels, nor improve sports performance, strength, or lean body mass. It did, however, increase estrogen levels, an effect that would not be considered favorable. Curiously, some evidence suggests that androstenedione does raise testosterone levels in women; again, this is not likely to produce favorable results and it could cause harm (see Safety Issues). The most consistent effect of androstenedione is to increase estrogen levels.

Safety Issues

There are concerns that androstenedione, like related hormones, might increase the risk of liver cancer and heart disease. In support of this last consideration, there is some evidence that androstenedione can adversely affect cholesterol levels. In addition, because androstenedione may raise testosterone levels in women, it could cause women to develop facial hair and other male-pattern appearance changes.

According to one case report, use of androstenedione was associated with loss of libido and decreased sperm count in a 29-year-old bodybuilder. While a single case report does not prove cause-and-effect, androstenedione's apparent ability to raise estrogen levels in men would be consistent with these symptoms.

Another case report suggests an additional potential complication with the use of androstenedione. A man who was using androstenedione to improve his physique experienced priapism (painful continuous erection) for more than 30 hours, requiring a visit to the emergency room. Previously, also while using androstenedione, he had experienced an episode lasting 2 to 3 hours that spontaneously resolved itself. It isn't certain that androstenedione was the cause, but this appears to be the most likely possibility.

Arginine

Arginine

SUPPLEMENT FORMS/ALTERNATE NAMES: *Arginine Hydrochloride, L-Arginine*

PRINCIPAL PROPOSED USES: *Angina, Congestive Heart Failure, Sexual Dysfunction in Men (Impotence), Intermittent Claudication, Sexual Dysfunction in Women*

OTHER PROPOSED USES: *Colds (Prevention), Cystic Fibrosis, Diabetes, Female Infertility, Heart Attack (aiding recovery), Interstitial Cystitis, Maintaining Effectiveness of Nitrate Drugs, Male Infertility, Osteoporosis, Preeclampsia, Raynaud's Phenomenon, Sickle Cell Disease, Surgery Support*

PROBABLY NOT EFFECTIVE USES: *Altitude Sickness*

Arginine is an amino acid found in many foods, including dairy products, meat, poultry, and fish. It plays a role in several important mechanisms in the body, including cell division, wound healing, removal of ammonia from the body, immunity to illness, and the secretion of important hormones.

The body also uses arginine to make nitric oxide (NO), a substance that relaxes blood vessels and also exerts numerous other effects in the body. Based on this, arginine has been proposed as a treatment for various cardiovascular diseases, including congestive heart failure and intermittent claudication, as well as impotence, female sexual dysfunction, interstitial cystitis and many other conditions. Arginine's potential effects on immunity have also created an interest in using it as part of an "immune cocktail" given to severely ill hospitalized patients and also for preventing colds.

Requirements/Sources

Normally, the body either gets enough arginine from food or manufactures all it needs from other widely available nutrients. Certain stresses, such as severe burns, infections, and injuries, can deplete your body's supply of arginine. For this reason, arginine (combined with other nutrients) is used in a hospital setting to help enhance recovery from severe injury or illness.

Arginine is found in dairy products, meat, poultry, fish, nuts, and chocolate.

Therapeutic Dosages

A typical supplemental dosage of arginine is 2 to 8 g per day. For congestive heart failure, higher dosages up to 15 g have been used in trials.

Warning: Do not try to self-treat congestive heart failure. If you have this condition, be sure to consult your physician before taking any supplements.

Therapeutic Uses

Small double-blind, placebo-controlled studies suggest that arginine might be helpful for the treatment of several seemingly unrelated conditions that are, in fact, all linked by arginine's effects on nitric oxide: **congestive heart failure**, **intermittent claudication**, **angina**, **impotence**, and **sexual dysfunction in women**.

Note: The first three conditions in this list are life-threatening. If you have angina, congestive heart failure, or intermittent claudication, do not attempt to treat yourself with arginine except under physician's supervision.

Arginine has been proposed for use after a **heart attack**, to aid recovery. In one study, arginine did not cause harm, and showed potential modest benefit. However, in another study, arginine failed to prove helpful for treatment of people who had just suffered a heart attack, and possibly increased post–heart-attack death rate.

One preliminary, double-blind study suggests that arginine supplementation might help prevent **colds**.

A small, double-blind, placebo-controlled study suggests that use of arginine (700 mg 4 times daily) may support transdermal **nitroglycerin** therapy for angina. Ordinarily, the drug nitroglycerin becomes less effective over time as the body develops a tolerance to it. However, arginine supplements appear to help prevent the development of tolerance.

The results of one controlled (but not blinded) study in women suggest that arginine might help standard **fertility therapy for women** (specifically, in vitro fertilization) work better. However, studies have not found any benefit in **male infertility**.

Weak evidence suggests that arginine might improve insulin action in people with type 2 (adult-onset) **diabetes**. Nutritional mixtures containing arginine have shown promise for enhancing recovery from **major surgery**, injury, or illness, perhaps by enhancing immunity. Highly preliminary evidence suggests that arginine might be worth investigating as a treatment for pulmonary hypertension in people with **sickle cell disease**.

Conflicting results have been seen in preliminary double-blind studies of arginine for **preeclampsia**. Preliminary double-blind studies have failed to find arginine helpful for **asthma**, cystic fibrosis, **interstitial cystitis**, kidney failure, **osteoporosis**, or **Raynaud's phenomenon**. One study found that an arginine-rich food bar did not help relax arteries or thin the blood in people with **high cholesterol**.

Arginine has been proposed for preventing **altitude sickness**, but the one reported study found harmful effects (increase in headache) rather than beneficial ones.

What Is the Scientific Evidence for Arginine?

Note: The first three conditions in this section are life-threatening. If you have angina, congestive heart failure, or intermittent claudication, do not attempt to treat yourself with arginine except under physician's supervision.

Congestive Heart Failure

Three small, double-blind, placebo-controlled studies enrolling a total of about 70 individuals with congestive heart failure found that oral arginine at a dose of 5 to 15 g daily could significantly improve symptoms as well as objective measurements of heart function.

Intermittent Claudication

People with advanced hardening of the arteries, or atherosclerosis, often have difficulty walking because of lack of blood flow to the legs, a condition known as intermittent claudication. Pain may develop after walking less than half a block.

In a double-blind study of 41 individuals, 2 weeks of treatment with a high dose of arginine improved walking distance by 66%; no benefits were seen in the placebo group or a low-dose arginine group.

Good results were also seen in another study, although its convoluted design makes interpreting the results somewhat difficult.

Angina

A double-blind study of 25 individuals with angina pectoris found that treatment with arginine at a dose of 6 g per day improved exercise tolerance, but not objective measurements of heart function.

A double-blind, placebo-controlled crossover trial of 36 individuals with heart disease found that use of arginine (along with antioxidant vitamins and minerals) at a daily dose of 6.6 g reduced symptoms of angina.

Impotence

The substance nitric oxide (NO) plays a role in the development of an erection. Drugs like Viagra increase the body's *sensitivity* to the natural rise in NO that occurs with sexual stimulation. A simpler approach might be to *raise* NO levels and one way to accomplish this involves use of the amino acid L-arginine. Oral arginine supplements may increase NO levels in the penis and elsewhere. Based on this, L-arginine has been advertised as "natural Viagra." However, there is as yet little evidence that it works. Drugs based on raising NO levels in the penis have not worked out for pharmaceutical developers; the body seems simply to adjust to the higher levels and maintain the same level of response.

Nonetheless, some small studies have found possible evidence of benefit.

In a double-blind trial, 50 men with erectile dysfunction received either 5 g of arginine per day or placebo for 6 weeks. More men in the treated group experienced improvement in sexual performance than in the placebo group.

A double-blind crossover study of 32 men found no benefit with 1,500 mg of arginine daily for 17 days. However, the lower dose of arginine as well as the shorter course of treatment may explain the discrepancy between these two studies.

Arginine has also been evaluated in combination with the drug yohimbine (as opposed to the herb **yohimbe**). A double-blind, placebo-controlled trial of 45 men found that one-time use of this combination therapy an hour or two prior to intercourse improved erectile function, especially in those with only moderate erectile dysfunction scores. Arginine and yohimbine were both taken at a dose of 6 g. **Note:** Do not use the drug yohimbine (or the herb yohimbe) except under physician supervision, as it presents a number of safety risks.

One study supposedly found that arginine plus **OPCs** can improve male sexual function, but because the study lacked a placebo group it did not, in fact, find anything at all. (For more information on why placebos are necessary, see **Why Does This Book Depend on Double-blind Studies?**.)

A small unpublished double-blind study listed on the manufacturer's website reported benefits with a proprietary combination of arginine and the herbs **ginseng**, **ginkgo**, and **damiana**, and **vitamins and minerals**.

Sexual Dysfunction in Women

Some postmenopausal women have difficulty experiencing sexual arousal. One small double-blind study of yohimbine combined with arginine found an increase in measured physical arousal among 23 women with this condition. However, the women themselves did not report any noticeable subjective effects, suggesting that the effect was slight. In addition, only the combination of yohimbine and arginine produced results; neither substance was effective when taken on its own. Slight benefits were also seen in a double-blind, placebo-controlled trial that evaluated a combination therapy containing arginine, along with the herbs **ginseng**, **ginkgo**, and **damiana**, and **vitamins and minerals**.

Interstitial Cystitis

Interstitial cystitis is a condition in which an individual feels like he or she has symptoms of a bladder infection, but no infection is present. Medical treatment for this condition is less than satisfactory.

A 3-month, double-blind trial of 53 individuals with interstitial cystitis found only weak indications that arginine might improve symptoms of interstitial cystitis. Several participants dropped out of the study; when this was properly taken into account using a statistical method called *ITT analysis*, no benefit at all could be proven.

A very small double-blind trial also failed to find evidence of benefit.

Colds

A 2-month, double-blind study involving 40 children with a history of frequent colds concluded that arginine seemed to provide some protection against respiratory infections. Of the children who were given arginine, 15 stayed well during the 60 days of the study. By contrast, only 5 of the children who took placebo stayed well, a significant difference.

Nutritional Support in Hospitalized Patients

Several nutritional products that contain arginine as well as other substances have been tried in hospital settings to enhance recovery following major surgery, ill-ness, or injury. These mixtures are delivered *enterally*, which means through a tube into the stomach. A review of 15 studies, about half of them double-blind and involving a total of 1,557 individuals, found that such products can reduce episodes of infection, time on ventilator machines, and length of stay in the hospital.

However, because of the many nutrients contained in these so-called *immunonutrient mixtures*, it is not clear whether arginine deserves the credit.

Safety Issues

At moderate doses (2 to 3 g per day), oral arginine appears to be safe and essentially free of side-effects, although minor gastrointestinal upset can occur. However, there are some potential safety issues regarding high-dose arginine. These cautions are based on findings from animal studies and hospital experiences of intravenous administration.

For example, arginine may stimulate the body's production of gastrin, a hormone that increases stomach acid. For this reason, there are concerns that arginine could be harmful for people with **ulcers** or who take drugs that are hard on the stomach. In addition, a double-blind trial found that arginine (30 g/day) may increase the risk of **esophageal reflux** (heartburn) by relaxing the sphincter at the bottom of the esophagus.

Arginine might also alter potassium levels in the body, especially in people with severe liver disease. This is a potential concern for individuals who take drugs that also alter potassium balance (such as **potassium-sparing diuretics** and **ACE inhibitors**), as well as those with severe kidney disease. If you fall into any of these categories, do not use high-dose arginine except under physician supervision.

Evidence that arginine can improve insulin sensitivity raises theoretical concerns that, if you have **diabetes** and take arginine, your blood sugar could fall too low. However, one study suggests that arginine is safe for use by people with stable type 2 (adult-onset) diabetes.

The amino acid **lysine** has been advocated for use in **oral or genital herpes**. According to the theory behind this recommendation, it is important to simultaneously restrict arginine intake. If true, this would tend to suggest that arginine supplements would be harmful for people with a tendency to develop herpes. However, there is no meaningful evidence to support this hypothesis.

Maximum safe doses in pregnant or nursing women, young children, and those with severe liver or kidney disease have not been established.

Interactions You Should Know About

If you are taking:

➤ Lysine to treat herpes: Arginine might counteract the potential benefit.
➤ Drugs that are hard on the stomach (such as nonsteroidal anti-inflammatory medications): Taking high doses of arginine might stress your stomach additionally.

➤ Medications that can alter the balance of potassium in your body (such as potassium-sparing diuretics [or ACE inhibitors]): High doses of arginine should be used only under physician supervision.
➤ Transdermal nitroglycerin: Arginine may help prevent the development of tolerance. (Note: Your doctor's supervision is essential.)

Arjun
Terminalia arjuna

PRINCIPALPROPOSED USES: *Angina*

OTHER PROPOSED USES: *High Cholesterol, Intestinal Parasites*

Arjun is a tree common in Central and South India. Its bark has a long history of use in **Ayurvedic medicine** (the traditional medicine of India) for the treatment of heart problems. Other uses of various parts of the Arjun tree include hemorrhage, diarrhea, irregular menstruation, skin ulcers, acne, wounds, and fractures.

What Is *Terminalia arjuna* Used for Today?

Evidence suggests that *Terminalia arjuna* may have blood vessel–relaxing properties. The herb has shown promise in the treatment of **angina**, a condition in which blood vessels in the heart cannot carry adequate oxygen to the heart muscle.

In addition, exceedingly weak evidence suggests that terminalia may have antimicrobial effects, providing benefits against amoebas and other microorganisms.

One study has been used to indicate that terminalia can **improve cholesterol levels**, but in fact it proves little because the study was not double-blind.

What Is the Scientific Evidence for *Terminalia arjuna*?

A 1-week, double-blind, placebo-controlled, crossover trial of 58 individuals evaluated the effectivness of terminalia for angina by comparing it against placebo and also against the standard drug isosorbide mononitrate.

The results indicated that the herb reduced anginal episodes and increased exercise capacity. It was more effective than placebo and approximately as effective as the medication.

A subsequent 3-month study compared the effectiveness of *Terminalia arjuna* against placebo in 40 people with a recent **heart attack**. All participants in this study suffered from a particular complication of a heart attack called *ischaemic mitral regurgitation*. The results showed that use of the herb improved heart function and reduced angina symptoms.

A combination Ayurvedic therapy containing terminalia and approximately 40 other herbs has also shown some promise for angina.

Dosage

A typical dosage of *Terminalia arjuna* is 500 mg 2 or 3 times daily.

Safety Issues

Use of terminalia has not been associated with any severe adverse effects. However, comprehensive safety studies have not been performed. Safety in young children, pregnant or nursing women, or people with severe liver or kidney disease has not been established.

Artichoke

Cynara scolymus

PRINCIPAL PROPOSED USES: *High Cholesterol, Dyspepsia (Indigestion)*

OTHER PROPOSED USES: *Liver Protection*

The artichoke is one of the oldest cultivated plants. It was first grown in Ethiopia and then made its way to southern Europe via Egypt. Its image is found on ancient Egyptian tablets and sacrificial altars. The ancient Greeks and Romans considered it a valuable digestive aid and reserved what was then a rare plant for consumption in elite circles. In sixteenth-century Europe, the artichoke was also considered a "noble" vegetable meant for consumption by the royal and the rich.

In traditional European medicine, the leaves of the artichoke (not the flower buds, which are the parts commonly cooked and eaten as a vegetable) were used as a diuretic to stimulate the kidneys and as a *choleretic* to stimulate the flow of bile from the liver and gallbladder. (Bile is a yellowish-brown fluid manufactured in the liver and stored in the gallbladder; it consists of numerous substances, including several that play a significant role in digestion.)

In the first half of the twentieth century, French scientists began modern research into these traditional medicinal uses of the artichoke plant. Their work suggested that the plant does indeed stimulate the kidney and gallbladder. Mid-century, Italian scientists isolated a compound from artichoke leaf called *cynarin*, which appeared to duplicate many of the effects of whole artichoke. Synthetic cynarin preparations were used as a drug to stimulate the liver and gallbladder and to treat elevated cholesterol from the 1950s to the 1980s; competition from newer pharmaceuticals has since eclipsed the use of cynarin.

What Is Artichoke Used for Today?

Artichoke leaf (as opposed to cynarin) continues to be used in many countries.

Germany's Commission E has authorized its use for "dyspeptic problems." *Dyspepsia* is a rather vague term that corresponds to the common word "indigestion," indicating a variety of digestive problems, including discomfort in the stomach, bloating, lack of appetite, nausea, and mild diarrhea or constipation. At least one substantial double-blind study indicates that artichoke leaf is indeed helpful for this condition.

Another fairly substantial study indicates that artichoke leaf may help lower **cholesterol**.

Based on a general notion that artichoke leaf is good for the liver, it has become a popular treatment for alcohol-induced hangovers. However, a small double-blind, placebo-controlled study failed to find it more effective than placebo.

A number of animal studies suggest that artichoke protects the **liver** from damage by chemical toxins. Artichoke's liver-protective effects, however, have never been proven in controlled clinical trials.

What Is the Scientific Evidence for Artichoke?

High Cholesterol

In a double-blind, placebo-controlled study of 143 people with high cholesterol, artichoke leaf extract significantly improved cholesterol readings. Total cholesterol fell by 18.5% as compared to 8.6% in the placebo group; LDL cholesterol by 23% versus 6%; and LDL-to-HDL ratios by 20% versus 7%.

An earlier double-blind, placebo-controlled study of 44 healthy people failed to find any improvement in cholesterol levels attributable to artichoke leaf. The researchers note, however, that study participants, on average, started the trial with lower than normal cholesterol levels (due to a statistical accident); improvement, therefore, couldn't be expected!

Artichoke leaf may work by interfering with cholesterol synthesis. Besides cynarin, a compound in artichoke called *luteolin* may play a role in reducing cholesterol.

Dyspepsia

In Europe, vague digestive symptoms are commonly attributed to inadequate flow of bile from the gallbladder. Evidence tells us that artichoke leaf does indeed stimulate the gallbladder, This by itself, however, does not prove artichoke helpful for dyspepsia. In 2003, however, a large (247-participant) double-blind study evaluated artichoke leaf as a treatment for dyspepsia. In this carefully conducted study, artichoke leaf extract proved significantly more effective than placebo for alleviating digestive symptoms.

A previous study of an herbal combination containing artichoke leaf also found benefits.

Dosage

Germany's Commission E recommends 6 g of the dried herb or its equivalent per day, usually divided into 3 doses. Artichoke leaf extracts should be taken according to label instructions.

Warning: People with gall bladder disease should use artichoke only under medical supervision (see Safety Issues below).

Safety Issues

Artichoke leaf has not been associated with significant side effects in studies so far, but full safety testing has not been completed. For this reason, it should not be used by pregnant or nursing women. Safety in young children or in people with severe liver or kidney disease has also not been established.

In addition, because artichoke leaf is believed to stimulate gallbladder contraction, individuals with gallstones or other forms of gallbladder disease could be put at risk by using this herb. Such individuals should use artichoke leaf only under the supervision of a physician. It is possible that increased gallbladder contraction could lead to obstruction of ducts or even rupture of the gallbladder.

Finally, individuals with known allergies to artichokes or related plants in the *Asteraceae* family, such as arnica or chrysanthemums, should avoid using artichoke or cynarin preparations.

Ashwagandha

Withania somniferum

PRINCIPAL PROPOSED USES: *Adaptogen (Improve Ability to Withstand Stress)*

OTHER PROPOSED USES: *Anxiety, Depression, Enhancing Mental Function, Immune Support, Infertility in Men or Women, Insomnia, Male Sexual Dysfunction, Reducing Cancer Risk, Sports Performance Enhancement*

Ashwagandha is sometimes called *Indian ginseng*, not because it's related botanically (it's closer to potatoes and tomatoes), but because its traditional uses were similar. Like ginseng, ashwagandha was thought to be a "tonic herb" capable of generally strengthening the body. On this basis it has been used in hopes of prolonging life, improving overall health, enhancing mental function, increasing fertility and libido, augmenting physical energy, and preventing infections.

In addition, as its species name *somniferum* suggests, ashwagandha been used traditionally for inducing sleep.

What Is Ashwagandha Used for Today?

Modern herbalists classify ashwagandha as an adaptogen, a substance said to increase the body's ability to withstand **stress** of all types. (See the article on **ginseng** for more information on adaptogens.) However, the evidence for an adaptogenic effect is limited to test tube and animal studies.

Other proposed uses of ashwagandha are based on even weaker evidence, including: preventing cancer, improving immunity, **enhancing mental function**, and combating **anxiety** and **depression**.

Some traditional uses of ashwagandha are also invoked today, such as **enhancing sexual function in men**, **increasing fertility in men or women**, **aiding sleep**, and **enhancing sports performance**; however, there is no supporting scientific evidence for these uses.

Dosage

A typical traditional dosage of ashwagandha is 1 to 2 g of the root (boiled in milk or water for 15 to 20 minutes) taken 3 times daily.

Safety Issues

Ashwagandha is believed to be safe; however, formal safety studies have not been reported. Therefore, it should not be used by pregnant or nursing women, young children, or those with severe kidney or liver disease.

According to one study in animals, ashwaghanda may raise thyroid hormone levels. For this reason, it should not be used by people with hyperthyroidism. In addition, based on traditional beliefs that ashwagandha has sedative effects, interactions with sedative drugs are a potential concern.

Interactions You Should Know About

If you are taking sedative drugs, you should not take ashwagandha at the same time except under your doctor's supervision.

Astragalus
Astragalus membranaceus

PRINCIPAL PROPOSED USES: *Strengthen Immunity (Against Colds, Flus, and Other Illnesses)*
OTHER PROPOSED USES: *AIDS, Atherosclerosis, Chemotherapy Side Effects, Chronic Active Hepatitis, Diabetes, Genital Herpes, Hypertension (High Blood Pressure), Hyperthyroidism, Insomnia*

Dried and sliced thin, the root of the astragalus plant is a common component of Chinese herbal formulas. According to tradition, astragalus "strengthens the spleen, blood and Qi, raises the yang Qi of the spleen and stomach, and stabilizes the exterior." Don't worry if you didn't understand what you just read, because without many months of training in **traditional Chinese herbal medicine**, there's no way you could have. Suffice it to say that the traditional understanding of the way astragalus works is different from the way it tends to be presented today.

What Is Astragalus Used for Today?

In the United States, astragalus has been presented as an **immune stimulant** useful for treating **colds and flus**. Many people have come to believe that they should take astragalus, like **echinacea**, at the first sign of a cold.

The belief that astragalus can strengthen immunity has a partial basis in traditional Chinese medicine. The expression noted above, "stabilize the exterior," means helping to create a "defensive shield" against infection. However, according to tradition, astragalus formulas should not be taken during the early stage of infections. To do so is said to resemble "locking the chicken-coop with the fox inside," causing the infection to be "driven deeper." Rather, astragalus is supposedly appropriate only for use while you're healthy, for the purpose of preventing future illnesses.

What Is the Scientific Evidence for Astragalus?

Although Chinese herbal tradition suggests that astragalus should generally be used in combination with other herbs, modern Chinese investigators have found various intriguing effects when astragalus is taken by itself. Extracts of astragalus have been found to stimulate parts of the **immune system** in mice and humans and to increase the survival time of mice infected with various diseases. Other highly preliminary research suggests that astragalus might be useful in treating **atherosclerosis**, **hyperthyroidism**, **hypertension**, **insomnia**, **diabetes**, chronic active **hepatitis**, genital **herpes**, **AIDS**, and increase the efficacy and/or reduce the side effects of

cancer chemotherapy. However, none of these possibilities can be regarded as proven.

Dosage

A typical daily dosage of astragalus involves boiling 9 to 30 g of dried root to make tea. Newer products use an alcohol-and-water extraction method to produce an extract standardized to astragaloside content, although there is no consensus on the proper percentage.

Safety Issues

Astragalus appears to be relatively nontoxic. High one-time doses, as well as long-term administration, have not caused significant harmful effects. Side effects are rare and generally limited to the usual mild gastrointestinal distress or allergic reactions. However, some Chinese herb manuals suggest that astragalus at 15 g or lower per day can raise blood pressure, while doses above 30 g may lower blood pressure.

As mentioned above, traditional Chinese medicine warns against using astragalus in cases of acute infections. Other traditional contraindications include "deficient yin patterns with heat signs" and "exterior excess heat patterns." Because understanding what these mean would require an extensive education in traditional Chinese herbal medicine, we recommend using astragalus only under the supervision of a qualified Chinese herbalist.

Safety in young children, pregnant or nursing women, or those with severe liver or kidney disease has not been established.

Barberry
Berberis vulgaris

PRINCIPAL PROPOSED USES: *None*

OTHER PROPOSED USES:

Oral: *Allergies, Constipation, Diarrhea, Dyspepsia, Heartburn, High Blood Pressure, High Cholesterol*

Topical: *Eczema, Psoriasis, Minor Wounds*

Barberry is a bush that grows wild in Europe and North America. It is closely related to **Oregon grape** (*Berberis aquifolium*). The root, stem, bark, and fruit of barberry are all used medicinally. Barberry was traditionally used as a treatment for digestive problems, including constipation, diarrhea, dyspepsia (stomach upset), heartburn, and loss of appetite. It was said to work by increasing the flow of bile, and on this basis it has also been used for liver and gallbladder problems. Topical preparations of barberry have been recommended for the treatment of eczema, psoriasis, and minor wounds.

What Is Barberry Used for Today?

There are no medically established uses of barberry. Only double-blind, placebo-controlled studies can establish a treatment effective and none have been performed on barberry. (For information on why this type of study is essential, see **Why Does This Book Rely on Double-blind Studies?**.)

Very weak evidence (too weak to be relied upon at all) hints that barberry root extracts may have anti-inflammatory, fever-reducing, and analgesic (pain-reducing) effects.

Similarly weak evidence hints that barberry fruit may have antihypertensive and **antihistaminic** effects.

Barberry, like **goldenseal** and Oregon grape, contains the chemical berberine. There has been some studies of purified berberine that might apply to barberry as well. Berberine inhibits the growth of many microorganisms, including fungi, protozoa, and bacteria.

On this basis, berberine has been proposed as a topical antiseptic for use in **minor wounds** and **vaginal infections**. Berberine has also shown potential as a treatment for various heart-related conditions, including reducing **high cholesterol** and **high blood pressure** and preventing **heart arrythmias**. However, it is not clear that barberry provides enough berberine to produce any of these potential benefits.

Topical formulations of the related plant Oregon grape have shown some promise for **psoriasis**, and barberry has been marketed for this condition as well. However, there is no direct evidence that it works.

Dosage

Barberry is traditionally used at a dose of 2 g 3 times daily or an equivalent amount in extract form. For treatment of psoriasis and other skin conditions, barberry is used in the form of a 10% cream, applied to the skin 3 times daily.

Safety Issues

One study suggests that topical use of berberine could cause **photosensitivity** (an increased tendency to react to sun exposure). Berberine-containing herbs should not be used by pregnant women because berberine may increase levels of bilirubin, potentially damaging the fetus, and might also cause genetic damage. Individuals who already have elevated levels of bilirubin (jaundice), or any other form of liver disease, should also avoid berberine-containing herbs.

Safety in young children and nursing women has not been established.

One study hints that berberine may decrease the efficacy of the drug tetracycline.

Interactions You Should Know About

If you are taking antibiotics in the **tetracycline** family, barberry might decrease their effectiveness.

Beano

ALTERNATE NAMES/RELATED TERMS: Alpha-galactosidase
PRINCIPAL PROPOSED USES: *Intestinal Gas*

Many foods can cause gassiness, including beans (legumes), broccoli, cabbage, onions, and whole grains. This occurs because these foods contain complex carbohydrates that are not entirely broken down in the digestive tract and instead serve as food for intestinal bacteria. These bacteria produce hydrogen and carbon dioxide gas as they digest the carbohydrates. While everyone develops intestinal gas to some extent, certain people have an intolerance of complex carbohydrates and develop relatively more severe symptoms. Use of alpha-galactosidase has been advocated as a treatment for both complex carbohydrate intolerance and ordinary gassiness. This enzyme helps break down complex carbohydrates. When taken as a supplement, it may enhance the digestive process and thereby deprive gas-producing bacteria of fuel to work on.

Requirements/Sources

Alpha-galactosidase is ordinarily manufactured by the body and is not a nutrient. It is found in particularly high quantities in the yeast *Aspergillus niger*, the source of commercial products.

Therapeutic Dosages

A typical supplemental dosage of alpha-galactosidase provides 450 GalU (galactosidase units) per meal.

Therapeutic Uses

Although alpha-galactosidase is widely marketed as an over-the-counter treatment to prevent **intestinal gas**, there is only limited evidence that it really works. In two preliminary double-blind, controlled trials enrolling a total of 39 people, use of alpha-galactosidase along with a meal of beans significantly reduced symptoms of excess gas. Two other relevant trials were also small and suffered from significant design flaws. Larger and more strictly designed studies will be necessary to determine whether alpha-galactosidase is truly an effective treatment for reducing intestinal gas.

Safety Issues

Although alpha-glucosidase appears to be safe for people in normal health, there are potential concerns involving people with **diabetes** as well as those with a rare condition named *galactosemia*.

Alpha-glucosidase breaks down complex carbohydrates into easily absorbed sugars. This may raise blood sugar levels in people with diabetes. Drugs that block alpha-glucosidase (alpha-glucosidase inhibitors) have proven benefit for people with diabetes. One study found that use of alpha-glucosidase supplements reduced the effectiveness of the diabetes drug acarbose, an alpha-glucosidase inhibitor drug. For this reason, people with diabetes who are using alpha-glucosidase inhibitors should avoid alpha-glucosidase supplements. In addition, it is theoretically possible that alpha-glucosidase might increase blood sugar levels in people with diabetes who are not taking alpha-glucosidase inhibitors, but this has not been thoroughly evaluated.

People with the genetic condition galactosemia should also avoid alpha-galactosidase as it could, in theory, worsen symptoms of the disease.

Safety in young children, pregnant or nursing women, or people with severe liver or kidney disease has not been established.

Interactions You Should Know About

If you are taking the drugs acarbose (Precose) or miglitol (Glyset) for treatment of diabetes, use of alpha-galactosidase may decrease their effectiveness.

Bee Pollen

PRINCIPAL PROPOSED USES: *None*

OTHER PROPOSED USES: *Allergies, Enhancing Memory, Enhancing Sports Performance, Respiratory Infections*

Bee pollen is the pollen collected by bees as they gather nectar from flowers for making honey. Like honey, bee pollen is used as a food by the hive. The pollen granules are stored in pollen sacs on the bees' hind legs. Beekeepers who wish to collect bee pollen place a screen over the hive with openings just large enough for the bees to pass through. As the bees enter the hive, the screen compresses their pollen sacs, squeezing the pollen from them. The beekeepers can then collect the pollen from the screen.

Although it has been recommended for a variety of uses, particularly for improving sports performance and relieving allergies, little to no scientific evidence backs up any of the claims about the therapeutic value of bee pollen.

Requirements/Sources

Bee pollen is not the sort of thing you will find in your everyday diet, unless you regularly eat the snack bars that include it. Tablets and some snack products containing bee pollen are available in pharmacies and health food stores.

Therapeutic Dosages

Athletes using bee pollen report consuming 5 to 10 tablets per day. Tablets can contain variable amounts of bee pollen, usually from 200 to 500 mg. The manufacturer's recommendations may provide more guidance.

Therapeutic Uses

Bee pollen has been touted as an energy enhancer and is sometimes used by athletes in the belief that it will **enhance performance** during competitions. However, there is no real evidence that bee pollen is effective and some evidence that it is not.

Bee pollen is also commonly taken to try to prevent **hay fever** on the theory that eating pollens will help you build up resistance to them. When used for this purpose, locally grown bee pollen is usually recommended;

however, be aware that it is possible to have a severe allergic reaction to the bee pollen itself. Other proposed uses of bee pollen include combating **age-related memory loss** and other effects of aging, and treating respiratory infections, endocrine disorders, and colitis. No scientific evidence supports any of these uses (see Safety Issues).

What Is the Scientific Evidence for Bee Pollen?

A few clinical trials have tested bee pollen's ability to increase energy or improve memory.

Sports Performance

According to a 1977 article in the *New York Times*, two studies on the use of bee pollen to improve sports performance found it to be of no significant benefit. Unfortunately, it has not been possible to obtain copies of the actual studies on which this article was based.

Both trials were said to be double-blind and placebo-controlled. The first, performed in 1975, involved 30 members of a university swim team. Participants were divided into 3 groups and given a daily dose of either 10 tablets of bee pollen, 10 placebo tablets, or 5 bee pollen and 5 placebo tablets. In 1976, the same experimental protocol was used, but this time with 60 participants: 30 swimmers, and 30 long-distance runners. Bee pollen did not significantly improve performance in either trial. A third study on bee pollen's effects on sports performance,

also difficult to obtain, reportedly found that breathing, heart rate, and perspiration returned to normal levels more quickly in track team members taking pollen than in those taking a placebo. However, reviewers criticized the methods used in this study. The runners may have known who was taking placebo and who was taking pollen, and this could have influenced the results.

Memory

The effects of pure bee pollen on memory have not been investigated, but clinical trials of a **Chinese herbal medicine** containing bee pollen have been conducted in China and Denmark. The improvements in memory seen in the Chinese study were not significant and in the more recent double-blind, placebo-controlled crossover study in Denmark, no improvements were found at all. The formula tested was only 14% bee pollen, so the results may not tell us very much about bee pollen's effectiveness.

Safety Issues

Several cases of serious allergic reactions to bee pollen have been reported in the medical literature, including anaphylaxis, an acute allergic response which can be life threatening. The anaphylactic reactions occurred within 20 to 30 minutes of ingesting fairly small amounts of bee pollen—in one case less than a teaspoon.

The majority of these case reports involved people with known allergies to pollen.

Bee Propolis

ALTERNATE NAMES/RELATED TERMS: *Bee Glue, Bee Putty, Propolis*

PRINCIPAL PROPOSED USES: *None*

OTHER PROPOSED USES:

   Topical Uses: *Genital Herpes, Skin Wounds, Oral Surgery, Tooth Decay, Vaginal Infections*

   Oral Uses: *Cancer Prevention, Giardiasis*

Although honey is perhaps the most famous bee product of interest to human beings, bees also make propolis, another substance that humans have used for thousands of years. Bees coat the hive with propolis in much the same way we use paint and caulking on our homes. People began using propolis more than 2,300 years ago for many purposes, the foremost

of which was applying it to wounds to fight infection. It is a resinous compound made primarily from tree sap and contains biologically active compounds called *flavonoids*, which come from its plant source. Propolis does indeed have antiseptic properties; the flavonoids in propolis may be responsible for its antimicrobial effects as well as other alleged health benefits.

Requirements/Sources

Propolis is available in a wide assortment of products found in pharmacies and health food stores, including tablets, capsules, powders, extracts, ointments, creams, lotions, and other cosmetics.

Therapeutic Dosages

Topical propolis ointments, creams, lotions, balms, and extracts are usually applied directly to the area being treated. However, we do not recommend applying bee propolis directly to the eyes (see Safety Issues).

Propolis intended for oral use comes in a wide variety of forms, including tablets, capsules, and extracts. Products vary so much that your best bet is to follow the directions on the label.

Therapeutic Uses

Test-tube studies have found propolis to be active against a variety of microorganisms, including bacteria, viruses, and protozoans. These findings have been the basis for most propolis research in humans and animals.

The results of a small controlled study suggests that propolis cream might cause attacks of **genital herpes** to heal faster.

A preliminary controlled study found that propolis mouthwash following oral **surgery** significantly speeded healing time as compared to placebo. Propolis extracts may also have value in treatment of severe periodontal disease, according to a study that evaluated the use of propolis extracts as part of an irrigation procedure performed twice weekly by dentists.

In one study, rats given propolis in their drinking water developed fewer cavities than rats given regular water. However, no human studies have been performed to see if we would also benefit.

Animal studies also suggest that topical propolis may be of benefit in **healing wounds**.

One group of researchers compared a propolis extract against the standard antiprotozoal drug tinidazole in 138 people infected with the parasite **giardiasis**. The extract appeared to work about as well as the drug therapy.

A number of clinical trials have tested the use of propolis for eye infections and vaginal infections. However, these were poorly designed; better trials are necessary before we can say for sure that propolis is an effective treatment for any of these conditions.

One isolated study, published only in abstract form, tested bee propolis in women with mild endometriosis and **infertility**. Reportedly, researchers found that use of bee propolis at a dose of 500 mg twice daily resulted in a pregnancy rate of 60%, as compared to 20% in the placebo group, a difference that was statistically significant. It is not clear why propolis should have this effect.

Finally, test-tube studies suggest that propolis has antioxidant, anti-inflammatory, and **cancer-preventing** properties. Again, without actual human studies, these results suggest the need for future research but do not prove propolis effective for any particular condition.

Safety Issues

Propolis is an ingredient commonly consumed in small quantities in honey. Safety studies have found it to be essentially nontoxic when taken orally; propolis also appears to be nonirritating when applied to the skin. However, allergic reactions to propolis are relatively common; it is a known "sensitizing agent," meaning it tends to induce allergies to itself when it is taken for an extended time.

Beta-Carotene

PRINCIPAL PROPOSED USES: *Providing the Nutritional Vitamin A Requirement*

OTHER PROPOSED USES: *Alcoholism, Cataract Prevention, Depression, Epilepsy, Exercise-Induced Asthma, Female Infertility, Headaches, Heartburn, HIV Support, Macular Degeneration Prevention, Male Infertility, Osteoarthritis, Parkinson's Disease, Photosensitivity, Psoriasis, Rheumatoid Arthritis, Schizophrenia, Sunburn Prevention*

PROBABLY INEFFECTIVE USES: *Cancer Prevention, Heart Disease Prevention*

Note: All the significant positive evidence for beta-carotene applies to food sources, not supplements.

Beta-carotene belongs to a family of natural chemicals known as **carotenoids**. Widely found in plants, carotenoids along with another group of chemicals, the bioflavonoids, give color to fruits, vegetables, and other plants.

Beta-carotene is a particularly important carotenoid from a nutritional standpoint, because the body easily transforms it to **vitamin A**. While vitamin A supplements themselves can be toxic when taken to excess, it is believed (although not proven) that the body will make only as much vitamin A out of beta-carotene as it needs. Assuming this is true, this built-in safety feature makes beta-carotene the best way to get your vitamin A.

Beta-carotene is also often recommended for another reason: it is an antioxidant, like **vitamin E** and **vitamin C**. In observational studies, high intake of carotenoids from food has been associated with reduced risk of various illnesses (including heart disease and cancer). However, observational studies are inherently unreliable, as described below. In intervention trials, beta-carotene supplements have not been found to offer any benefits; in fact, when taken in high doses for a long period of time, beta-carotene supplements might slightly increase the risk of heart disease and some forms of cancer.

Requirements/Sources

Although beta-carotene is not a required nutrient, vitamin A is essential for health and beta-carotene is converted into vitamin A in the body. The exact conversion factor varies with the circumstances; in general, 2 mcg of beta-carotene in supplement form is thought to be equivalent to 1 mcg of vitamin A. See the article on **vitamin A** for requirements based on age and sex.

Dark green and orange-yellow vegetables are good sources of beta-carotene. These include carrots, sweet potatoes, squash, spinach, romaine lettuce, broccoli, apricots, and green peppers.

Note: Plant **sterols**, used to treat **high cholesterol**, may impair absorption of beta-carotene.

Therapeutic Dosages

We are not sure at the present time whether it is advisable to take dosages of beta-carotene supplements much higher than the recommended allowance for nutritional purposes, which is about 1.5 to 1.8 mg daily in adults. Rather than taking doses higher than this, it is probably more advisable to increase your intake of fresh fruits and vegetables.

Therapeutic Uses

There are no well-documented therapeutic uses of beta-carotene, beyond supplying nutritional doses of vitamin A.

Numerous observational studies have found that a high intake of foods rich in carotenoids is associated with a lower incidence of lung cancer, other forms of **cancer** and **heart disease**. However, beta-carotene supplements have not been found to be helpful for preventing these conditions.

Similar evidence links high dietary intake of carotenoids to a lower incidence and/or slowed progression of **cataracts**, **macular degeneration**, and **osteoarthritis**, but again there is no reliable evidence that beta-carotene supplements are helpful for these conditions (except possibly for preventing cataracts in smokers).

Preliminary evidence raised hopes that beta-carotene supplements might increase or preserve immune function or decrease symptoms among people with **HIV**.

However, other studies found no benefit, and some evidence hints that too much beta-carotene might actually be harmful.

Beta-carotene supplements may be helpful for protecting the skin from **sunburn**, particularly in people with extreme **sensitivity to the sun**, but the evidence regarding this potential use is somewhat contradictory. One double-blind trial found that faithful daily use of sunscreen was more effective at preventing sun damage to the skin than oral beta-carotene plus sunscreen used as needed.

One preliminary study found evidence that beta-carotene might be helpful for cystic fibrosis, by helping prevent lung infections.

Another preliminary study suggests that beta-carotene might help prevent exercise-induced asthma.

Beta-carotene has been proposed as a treatment for **alcoholism, asthma, depression, epilepsy, headaches, heartburn, male infertility, female infertility, Parkinson's disease, psoriasis, rheumatoid arthritis**, and **schizophrenia**, but there is little to no evidence that it works.

There is some evidence that beta-carotene is not effective for **cervical dysplasia** or **intermittent claudication**.

What Is the Scientific Evidence for Beta-Carotene?

Cancer Prevention

The story of beta-carotene and cancer prevention is full of apparent contradictions. It starts in the early 1980s, when the cumulative results of many studies suggested that people who eat a lot of fruits and vegetables are significantly less likely to get cancer. A close look at the data pointed to carotenoids as the active ingredients in fruits and vegetables. It appeared that a high intake of dietary carotene might significantly reduce the risk of lung cancer, bladder cancer, breast cancer, esophageal cancer, and stomach cancer.

However, observational studies cannot prove cause and effect. It is always possible that individuals who consume a great deal of carotenoids in the diet are different in other ways; for example, they might exercise more or have healthier lifestyles in other regards.

This is not a purely theoretical issue. For example, based primarily on observational studies, hormone replacement therapy was promoted as a heart-protective treatment for postmenopausal women. However, when placebo-controlled studies were performed, hormone replacement therapy was shown to slightly increase the risk of heart disease. One possible explanation for this discrepancy is that the apparent benefits of hormone replacement therapy were due to the fact that women who used it tended to belong to a higher socioeconomic class than those who did not. (For a variety of reasons, some of which are not known, higher income is associated with improved health.)

Something similar appears to be the case with beta-carotene. Although individuals who consume foods high in beta-carotene appear to obtain some protection from heart disease and cancer, when researchers gave beta-carotene supplements to study participants, there was no protective effect.

Most studies enrolled people in high-risk groups, such as smokers, because it is easier to see results when you look at people who are more likely to develop cancer to begin with.

The anti-cancer bubble burst for beta-carotene in 1994 when the results of the Alpha-Tocopherol, Beta-Carotene (ATBC) study became available. These results showed that beta-carotene supplements did not prevent lung cancer, but actually increased the risk of getting it by 18%. This trial had followed 29,133 male smokers in Finland who took supplements of about 50 IU of vitamin E (alpha-tocopherol), 20 mg of beta-carotene (more than 10 times the amount necessary to provide the daily requirement of vitamin A), both, or placebo daily for 5 to 8 years. (In contrast to the results for beta-carotene, vitamin E was found to reduce the risk of cancer, especially prostate cancer.)

In January 1996, researchers monitoring the Beta-Carotene and Retinol Efficacy Trial (CARET) confirmed the prior bad news with more of their own: the beta-carotene group had 46% more cases of lung cancer deaths. This study involved smokers, former smokers, and workers exposed to asbestos. Alarmed, the National Cancer Institute ended the $42 million CARET trial 21 months before it was planned to end.

At about the same time, the 12-year Physicians' Health Study of 22,000 male physicians was finding that 50 mg of beta-carotene (about 25 times the amount necessary to provide the daily requirement of vitamin A) taken every other day had no effect—good or bad—on the risk of cancer or heart disease. In this study, 11% of the participants were smokers and 39% were ex-smokers.

Similarly, another study of beta-carotene supplements failed to find any effect on the risk of cancer in women.

Beta-Carotene

There are several possible explanations for these apparently contradictory findings. As noted above, it is possible that intake of carotenoids as such is unrelated to cancer and that some unrelated factor common to individuals with a high carotene diet is the cause of the benefits seen in observational trials.

Another possibility is that beta-carotene alone is not effective and the other carotenoids found in fruits and vegetables may be more important for preventing cancer than beta-carotene. One researcher has suggested that taking beta-carotene supplements depletes the body of these other beneficial carotenoids and thereby causes a harmful effect. In support of this theory, a large study found that consumption of fruits and vegetables is generally associated with lower lung cancer risk, but when beta-carotene is taken, this preventive effect disappears.

Heart Disease Prevention

The situation with beta-carotene and heart disease is rather similar to that of beta-carotene and cancer. Numerous studies suggest that carotenoids as a whole can help prevent heart disease. However, isolated beta-carotene may not help prevent heart disease and could actually increase your risk.

The same double-blind intervention trial involving 29,133 Finnish male smokers (mentioned under the discussion of cancer and beta-carotene) found 11% *more* deaths from heart disease and 15 to 20% *more* strokes in those participants taking beta-carotene supplements.

Similar poor results with beta-carotene were seen in another large, double-blind study of smokers. Beta-carotene supplementation was also found to increase the incidence of **angina** in smokers.

Osteoarthritis

A high dietary intake of beta-carotene is associated with a significantly slower progression of osteoarthritis, according to a study in which researchers followed 640 individuals over a period of 8 to 10 years. However, as with heart disease and cancer, we don't know whether beta-carotene is responsible for this effect.

HIV Support

One small, double-blind study suggested that beta-carotene supplements might raise white blood cell count in people with HIV. However, two subsequent larger controlled trials found no significant differences between those taking beta-carotene or placebo in white blood cell count, CD4+ count, or other measures of immune function.

Evidence from observational studies suggests that higher intakes of vitamin A or beta-carotene may be helpful; however, caution is in order regarding dosage. Researchers generally linked higher intake of vitamin A or beta-carotene to lower risk of AIDS and lower death rates, with an important exception: people with the highest intake of either nutrient (more than 11,179 IU per day of beta-carotene or more than 20,268 IU per day of vitamin A) did worse than those who took somewhat less.

Macular Degeneration and Cataracts

Despite promising results from observational studies, intervention trials of beta-carotene for these eye conditions have generally not shown benefit. Beta-carotene proved ineffective for preventing cataracts in one large study and, in another large study, beta-carotene supplements combined with vitamin E and C failed to prevent either macular degeneration or cataracts. On a more positive note, one large study found that beta-carotene supplements helped prevent cataracts in study participants who smoked; nonetheless, no benefit was seen in the group as a whole.

Cervical Dysplasia

According to a 2-year, double-blind, placebo-controlled study of 141 women with mild cervical dysplasia (a precancerous condition of the cervix), beta-carotene, taken at a dosage of 30 mg daily along with 500 mg of vitamin C, does not help to reverse the dysplasia. Negative results were seen in other trials of beta-carotene as well.

Intermittent Claudication

A double-blind, placebo-controlled trial of 1,484 individuals with intermittent claudication found no benefit from beta-carotene (20 mg daily), vitamin E (50 mg daily), or a combination of the two.

Safety Issues

At recommended dosages, beta-carotene is believed to be very safe. The only side effects reported from beta-carotene overdose are diarrhea and a yellowish tinge to the hands and feet. These symptoms disappear once you stop taking beta-carotene or reduce your dose.

However, long-term use of beta-carotene supplements, especially at doses considerably above the amount necessary to supply adequate vitamin A, might slightly increase the risk of heart disease and certain forms of cancer. The solution: eat plenty of fresh fruits and vegetables, and get your beta-carotene that way.

In addition, some evidence suggests that beta-carotene supplements might cause **alcoholic liver disease** to develop more rapidly in individuals who abuse alcohol.

Beta-Glucan

ALTERNATE NAMES/RELATED TERMS: *Oat bran*
PRINCIPAL PROPOSED USES: *High Cholesterol*
OTHER PROPOSED USES: *Immune Support*

The term *beta-glucan* refers to a class of soluble fibers found in many plant sources. The best-documented use of beta-glucan involves improving heart health; the evidence for benefit is strong enough that the FDA has allowed a "heart healthy" label claim for food products containing substantial amounts of beta-glucan. Much weaker evidence supports the potential use of certain beta-glucan products for modifying the activity of the immune system.

Requirements/Sources

Beta-glucan is not an essential nutrient. It is found in whole grains (especially oats, wheat, and barley) and fungi such as baker's yeast, *Coriolus versicolor,* and the medicinal mushrooms **maitake** and **reishi.**

Different food sources contain differing amounts of the various chemical constituents collectively called *beta-glucan.* Grains primarily contain beta-1,3-glucan and beta-1,4-glucan. Fungal sources contain a mixture of beta-1,3-glucan and beta-1,6-glucan. Purified products containing only the 1,3 form are also available.

Therapeutic Uses

A substantial, if not entirely consistent, body of evidence indicates that beta-glucan, or foods containing it (such as oats), can modestly improve **cholesterol profile.** The most consistent benefits have been seen regarding levels of total cholesterol and LDL ("bad") cholesterol. Modest improvements of up to 10% have been seen in studies. Possible improvements in HDL ("good") cholesterol have only been seen inconsistently. It is thought that beta-glucan reduces cholesterol levels by increasing excretion of cholesterol from the digestive

tract. This affects two forms of cholesterol: cholesterol from food and, more importantly, cholesterol from the blood "recycled" by the liver through the intestines.

Beta-glucan may also modestly improve **blood pressure levels,** though not all studies agree.

In addition, beta-glucan may help limit the rise in blood sugar that occurs after a meal; this could in theory, offer heart-healthy benefits, especially in people with **diabetes.**

The other primary proposed use of beta-glucan products involves effects on the immune system. Test-tube, animal, and a few controlled studies in humans suggest that beta-glucans can alter various measurements of immune function. In the alternative medicine literature, these effects are commonly summarized as indicating that beta-glucan is an "immune stimulant." This description, however, is an oversimplification. The immune system is extraordinarily complicated and as yet incompletely understood. At the current level of scientific understanding it is not possible to characterize the effects of beta-glucan more specifically than to say that it has *immunomodulatory* actions or that it is a *biological response modifier.* These intentionally unsensational terms indicate that we merely know beta-glucan affects (modulates) immune function, not that it improves immune function.

Some of the immune-related effects seen in studies include alterations in the activity of certain white blood cells and changes in the levels or actions of substances called *cytokines* that modulate immune function.

Based on these largely theoretical findings, as well a small number of very preliminary human trials, various beta-glucan products have been advocated for the treatment of conditions as diverse as **allergic rhinitis, cancer,** infections, and sepsis (overwhelming infection following major trauma, illness, or surgery). However, the evidence for actual clinical benefit remains highly preliminary.

One study failed to find that beta-1,3-glucan (in topical gel form) helpful for treatment of actinic keratosis, a form of sun-induced precancerous changes seen in **aging skin**.

Therapeutic Dosages

For improving total and LDL cholesterol, studies have found benefit with beta-glucan at doses ranging from 3 to 15 g daily. However, benefits have been seen more consistently at the higher end of this range and one carefully designed study found no benefit at 3 g daily.

Beta-glucan products can contain molecules of various average lengths (molecular weight). Some manufacturers claim superior benefits with either high or low molecular weight versions. However, one study failed to find any difference between high molecular weight and low molecular weight beta-glucan for normalizing cholesterol and blood sugar levels.

Safety Issues

Beta-glucan, as a substance widely present in foods, is thought to have a high margin of safety. However, if it really does activate the immune system, harmful effects are at least theoretically possible in people with conditions where the immune system is overactive. These include **multiple sclerosis, lupus, rheumatoid arthritis, asthma, inflammatory bowel disease**, and hundreds of others conditions. In addition, people taking immunosuppressant drugs following organ transplantation surgery could, in theory, increase their risk of organ rejection. However, there are no reports as yet to indicate that any of these hypothetical problems have actually occurred. Maximum safe doses in young children, pregnant or nursing women, or people with severe liver or kidney disease have not been established.

Betaine Hydrochloride

PRINCIPAL PROPOSED USES: *None*

OTHER PROPOSED USES: *Asthma, Digestive Problems, Excess Candida, Food Allergies, Hay Fever, Heartburn, Rheumatoid Arthritis, Ulcers, and many others*

When taken as a supplement, betaine hydrochloride provides extra hydrochloric acid in the stomach. A major branch of alternative medicine known as **naturopathy** has long held that low stomach acid is a widespread problem that interferes with digestion and the absorption of nutrients. Betaine hydrochloride is one of the most common recommendations for this proposed condition, along with the more folksy choice of apple cider vinegar.

Betaine without the hydrochloride molecule attached is also sold as a supplement. In this chemically very different form, it is called *trimethylglycine* (TMG). TMG is not acidic, and it has completely different properties.

Sources

Betaine hydrochloride is not an essential nutrient and no food sources exist.

Therapeutic Dosages

Betaine hydrochloride is typically taken in pill form at dosages ranging from 325 to 650 mg with each meal.

Therapeutic Uses

Based on theories about the importance of stomach acid to overall health, betaine hydrochloride has been recommended for a wide variety of problems, including **asthma, digestive problems**, excess **candida, food allergies, hay fever, lupus, rheumatoid arthritis**, and many other conditions. When one sees such broadly encompassing uses, it is not surprising to find that there is as yet no real scientific research on its effectiveness for any of these conditions.

Many naturopathic physicians also believe that betaine hydrochloride can heal **ulcers** and **esophageal reflux (heartburn)**. This sounds paradoxical, since conventional treatment for those conditions involves reducing stomach acid, while betaine hydrochloride increases it. However, according to one theory, lack of stomach acid leads to incomplete digestion of proteins and these proteins cause allergic reactions and other responses that lead to digestive problems, which in turn cause ulcers and heartburn. Again, scientific evidence is lacking.

Safety Issues

Betaine hydrochloride should not be used by those with ulcers or esophageal reflux (heartburn) except on the advice of a physician. This supplement seldom causes any obvious side effects, but it has not been put through rigorous safety studies. In particular, safety for young children, pregnant or nursing women, or those with severe liver or kidney disease has not been established.

Beta-Sitosterol

PRINCIPAL PROPOSED USES: *Benign Prostatic Hyperplasia (Prostate Enlargement)*
OTHER PROPOSED USES: *Immune Support, Sports and Fitness Support: Enhancing Recovery*

Numerous plants contain cholesterol-like compounds called sitosterols and their close relatives sitosterolins. A special mixture of these called **beta-sitosterol** is used for the treatment of **benign prostatic hyperplasia (BPH)**.

What Is Beta-Sitosterol Used for Today?

Some conditions are luckier than others. For some mysterious reason, there seem to be more useful herbal treatments for BPH than almost any other disease. Beta-sitosterol joins saw palmetto, pygeum, nettle, and grass pollen as a moderately well-documented treatment for BPH.

Based on highly preliminary evidence, it has been suggested that sitosterols may also help strengthen the immune system. In particular, one study suggests that beta-sitosterol can help prevent the temporary immune weakness that typically occurs during recovery from endurance exercise and can lead to a post-race infection.

What Is the Scientific Evidence for Beta-Sitosterol?

A review of the literature, published in 1999, found a total of four double-blind, placebo-controlled studies on beta-sitosterol for BPH, enrolling a total of 519 men. All but one of these studies found significant benefits in both perceived symptoms and objective measurements, such as urine flow rate.

The largest study followed 200 men with BPH for a period of 6 months. After the trial was completed, many of the participants were followed for an additional year, during which the benefits continued. Similar results were seen in a 6-month, double-blind trial of 177 individuals.

Beta-sitosterol binds to prostate tissue and affects the metabolism of prostaglandins, substances found in the body that affect pain and inflammation. However, it is not clear whether this is the correct explanation for how beta-sitosterol might help in BPH.

Dosage

The daily dosage of beta-sitosterol is 60 to 135 mg. Effects usually take 4 weeks to develop.

Safety Issues

Although detailed safety studies have not been performed, beta-sitosterol is believed to be safe. No significant side effects or drug interactions have been reported.

Bilberry

Vaccinium myrtillus

PRINCIPAL PROPOSED USES: *None*

OTHER PROPOSED USES: *Diabetes (Leaf Rather Than Fruit), Diabetic Retinopathy, Easy Bruising, Hemorrhoids, Minor Injuries, Surgery Support, Varicose Veins*

PROBABLY NOT EFFECTIVE USES: *Poor Night Vision*

Often called *European blueberry*, bilberry is closely related to American blueberry, cranberry, and huckleberry. Its meat is creamy white instead of purple, but it is traditionally used, like blueberries, in the preparation of jams, pies, cobblers, and cakes.

Bilberry fruit also has a long medicinal history. In the twelfth century, Abbess Hildegard of Bingen wrote of bilberry's usefulness for inducing menstruation. Over subsequent centuries, the list of uses for bilberry grew to include a bewildering variety of possibilities, from bladder stones to typhoid fever.

What Is Bilberry Used for Today?

The modern use of bilberry dates back to World War II, when British Royal Air Force pilots reported that a good dose of bilberry jam just prior to a mission improved their night vision, often dramatically. Subsequent investigation showed that bilberry contains biologically active substances known as anthocyanosides. Some evidence suggests that anthocyanosides may benefit the retina, as well as strengthen the walls of blood vessels, reduce inflammation, and stabilize tissues containing collagen (such as tendons, ligaments, and cartilage).

However, neither anecdote nor basic scientific evidence of this type can prove a treatment effective. Only double-blind, placebo-controlled studies can do that. Regarding night vision, the balance of the evidence suggests that bilberry is *not* helpful. Slight evidence hints that bilberry might be helpful for **diabetic retinopathy**. One double-blind study suggests that bilberry might be helpful for **hemorrhoids**.

Finally, because the anthocyanosides in bilberry resemble the oligomeric proanthocyanidin complexes (OPCs) found in grape seed and pine bark, bilberry has been recommended for all the same uses as those substances, including **easy bruising**, **varicose veins**, **minor injuries**, and **surgery support**.

Animal studies also suggest that bilberry leaves (rather than the fruit) may be helpful for improving blood sugar control in **diabetes** and for lowering blood triglycerides.

What Is the Scientific Evidence for Bilberry?

Night Vision

A double-blind crossover trial of 15 individuals found no short- or long-term improvements in night vision attributable to bilberry. Similarly negative results were seen in a double-blind, placebo-controlled crossover trial of 18 subjects and another of 16 subjects.

In contrast, two much earlier controlled, but not double-blind, studies of bilberry found that the herb temporarily improved night vision. However, the effect was not found to persist with continued use. A later double-blind, placebo-controlled study on 40 healthy subjects found that a single dose of bilberry extract improved visual response for 2 hours.

Visual benefits have also been reported in other small trials, but these studies did not use a placebo control group and are therefore not valid as evidence.

Hemorrhoids

In a 4-week, double-blind, placebo-controlled study of 40 people with hemorrhoids, oral use of bilberry extract significantly reduced hemorrhoid symptoms as compared to placebo.

Diabetic Retinopathy

A double-blind, placebo-controlled trial of bilberry extract in 14 people with diabetic retinopathy or hypertensive retinopathy (damage to the retina caused by diabetes or hypertension, respectively) found significant improvements in the treated group. However, the small size of this study makes the results less than fully reliable. Other studies are also cited as indicating benefits, but they were not double-blind and therefore mean little.

Dosage

The standard dosage of bilberry is 120 to 240 mg twice daily of an extract standardized to contain 25% anthocyanosides.

Safety Issues

Bilberry fruit is a food and, as such, is quite safe. Enormous quantities have been administered to rats without toxic effects. One study of 2,295 people given bilberry extract found a 4% incidence of side effects such as mild digestive distress, skin rashes, and drowsiness. Although safety in pregnancy has not been proven, clinical trials have enrolled pregnant women. Safety in young children, nursing women, or those with severe liver or kidney disease is not known. There are no known drug interactions. Bilberry does not appear to interfere with blood clotting.

Little is known about the safety of bilberry leaf. Based on animal evidence that it can reduce blood sugar levels in people with diabetes, it is possible that use of bilberry leaf by people with diabetes could require a reduction in drug dosage.

Interactions You Should Know About

If you are taking:

> medications to reduce blood sugar, bilberry leaf (not fruit) might amplify the effect, and you may need to reduce your dose of medication.

Biotin

SUPPLEMENT FORMS/RELATED TERMS: *Biocytin (Brewer's Yeast Biotin Complex)*
PRINCIPAL PROPOSED USES: *Supplementation During Pregnancy*
OTHER PROPOSED USES: *Brittle Nails, "Cradle Cap" in Children, Diabetic Neuropathy, Improving Blood Sugar Control in Diabetes, Support for Individuals on Anticonvulsants*

Biotin is a water-soluble B vitamin that plays an important role in metabolizing the energy we get from food. Biotin assists four essential enzymes that break down fats, carbohydrates, and proteins.

Biotin deficiency is rare, except, possibly, among pregnant women. All proposed therapeutic uses of biotin supplements are highly speculative.

Requirements/Sources

Although biotin is a necessary nutrient, we usually get enough from bacteria living in the digestive tract. Severe biotin deficiency has been seen in people who frequently eat large quantities of raw egg white. Raw egg white contains a protein that blocks the absorption of biotin. Fortunately, cooked egg white does not present this problem.

The official U.S. and Canadian recommendations for daily intake of biotin are as follows:

> Infants 0–5 months, 5 mcg
> 6–11 months, 6 mcg
> Children 1–3 years, 8 mcg
> 4–8 years, 12 mcg
> 9–13 years, 20 mcg
> Males and females 14–18 years, 25 mcg
> 19 years and older, 30 mcg
> Pregnant women, 30 mcg
> Nursing women, 35 mcg

Good dietary sources of biotin include brewer's yeast, nutritional (torula) yeast, whole grains, nuts, egg yolks, sardines, legumes, liver, cauliflower, bananas, and mushrooms.

There is some evidence that slight biotin deficiency may tend to occur during normal pregnancy. For this reason, pregnant women are advised to take a prenatal vitamin that contains the recommended amount of biotin.

Therapeutic Dosages

For people with diabetes, the usual recommended dosage of biotin is 7,000 to 15,000 mcg daily.

For treating "cradle cap" (a scaly head rash often found in infants), the usual dosage of biotin is 6,000 mcg daily, *given to the nursing mother* (not the child). A lower dosage of 3,000 mcg daily is used to treat brittle fingernails and toenails.

Therapeutic Uses

All the proposed uses of biotin discussed here are speculative, based on highly incomplete evidence.

Preliminary research suggests that supplemental biotin might help reduce blood sugar levels in people with either type 1 (childhood onset) or type 2 (adult onset) diabetes, and possibly reduce the symptoms of **diabetic neuropathy**. However, no double-blind, placebo-controlled studies have been reported on these potential uses of biotin. (For why double-blind trials are so important, see **Why Does This Book Rely on Double-blind Studies?**)

Even weaker evidence suggests that biotin supplements may be helpful for **brittle nails**. On the basis of virtually no evidence at all, biotin is also sometimes proposed for treating cradle cap in infants.

There are indirect indications that individuals taking antiseizure medications might benefit from biotin supplementation at nutritional doses. However, it has been suggested that biotin should be taken at least 2 hours before or after the medication dose, to avoid potential interference with its absorption. In addition, excessive biotin supplementation (above nutritional needs) should be avoided, because it might possibly interfere with seizure control. **Note**: All these proposed interactions are quite speculative and, even if they do exist, may not be important enough to make a difference in real life.

Safety Issues

Biotin appears to be quite safe. However, maximum safe dosages for young children, pregnant or nursing women, or those with severe liver or kidney disease have not been established.

Interactions You Should Know About

If you are taking **anticonvulsant medications**: You may need extra biotin, but do not take more than the dosage recommendations listed in the Requirements/Sources section. In addition, take it 2 to 3 hours apart from the medication.

Bitter Melon
Momordica charantia

PRINCIPAL PROPOSED USES: *Diabetes*

Widely sold in Asian groceries as food, bitter melon is also a folk remedy for diabetes, cancer, and various infections.

What Is Bitter Melon Used for Today?

Preliminary studies hint that bitter melon may improve blood sugar control in people with adult-onset (type 2) **diabetes**. However, because these studies were not double-blind, their results are not reliable.

In test-tube studies, a protein in bitter melon called *MAP-30* kills viruses and slows the growth of some cancer cells. However, it is a long way from the test tube to real people and there have not as yet been any human trials of bitter melon or its constituents for the treatment of cancer or viral diseases.

Dosage

The typical dosage of bitter melon is one small, unripe, raw melon or about 50 to 100 ml of fresh juice, divided into 2 or 3 doses over the course of the day. The only problem is that bitter melon tastes *extremely* bitter. Noted naturopath Michael Murray suggests that you should "simply plug your nose and take a 2-ounce shot."

Safety Issues

As a widely eaten food in Asia, bitter melon is often regarded as safe. However, it does appear to present some health risks. The most significant of these comes from the fact that it may work! Combining bitter melon with standard drugs may reduce blood sugar too well, possibly leading to dangerously low blood sugar levels. In fact, there are case reports of two children with diabetes who went into hypoglycemic coma after taking bitter melon. For this reason, if you already take drugs for diabetes, you should add bitter melon to your diet only with a physician's supervision. (And definitely don't stop your medication and substitute bitter melon instead. It is not as powerful as insulin or other conventional treatments.)

Other possible risks include impaired fertility, liver inflammation, and spontaneous abortion.

Safety in young children, nursing women, or those with severe kidney disease has not been established.

Interactions You Should Know About

If you are taking **medications to reduce blood sugar,** bitter melon might amplify the effect, and you may need to reduce your dose of medication.

Black Cohosh

Cimicifuga racemosa

PRINCIPAL PROPOSED USES: *Menopausal Symptoms*

OTHER PROPOSED USES: *Dysmenorrhea (Painful Menstruation), Osteoporosis, Premenstrual Syndrome (PMS)*

Black cohosh is a tall perennial herb originally found in the northeastern United States. Native Americans used it primarily for women's health problems, but also as a treatment for arthritis, fatigue, and snakebite. European colonists rapidly adopted the herb for similar uses. In the late nineteenth century, black cohosh was the principal ingredient in the wildly popular Lydia E. Pinkham's Vegetable Compound for menstrual cramps.

What Is Black Cohosh Used for Today?

Black cohosh's main use today is for the treatment of **menopausal symptoms.** Meaningful but far from definitive evidence indicates that black cohosh extract might reduce hot flashes as well as other symptoms of menopause.

In the past, black cohosh was believed to be a phytoestrogen, a plant-based substance that has actions similar to estrogen. However, as we describe below, growing evidence indicates that black cohosh does not have general estrogen-like actions. Rather, it may act like estrogen only in certain places: the brain (reducing hot flashes), bone (potentially fighting osteoporosis), and vagina (reducing vaginal dryness).

Black cohosh has also been tried for reducing hot flashes in women who have undergone surgery for **breast cancer,** but it does not appear to be effective for this purpose.

Finally, black cohosh is sometimes recommended as a kind of general women's herb, said to be effective for a variety of menstrual issues, such as **dysmenorrhea,** PMS, and irregular menstruation. However, there is as yet no meaningful evidence at all that it is effective for these conditions.

What Is the Scientific Evidence for Black Cohosh?

Menopausal Symptoms

The body of evidence regarding black cohosh for menopausal symptoms remains incomplete and inconsistent, though promising.

The best study was a 12-week, double-blind, placebo-controlled trial of 304 women with menopausal symptoms. This study appeared to find that black cohosh was more effective than placebo. The best evidence was for a reduction in hot flashes. However, the statistical procedures used in the study were unusual and open to question.

Previous smaller studies have found improvements not only in hot flashes but also in other symptoms of menopause. For example, in a double-blind, placebo-controlled study, 97 menopausal women received black cohosh, estrogen, or placebo for 3 months. The results indicated that the herb reduced overall menopausal symptoms (such as hot flashes) to the same extent as the drug. Microscopic analysis of cells showed that unlike estrogen, black cohosh did not affect the cells of the uterus. This is a positive result, as estrogen's effects on the uterus are potentially harmful. However, black cohosh did have an estrogen-like effect on the cells of the vagina. This is also a positive result, because it suggests that black cohosh might reduce vaginal thinning. Finally, the study found hints that black cohosh might help protect bone. However, a great many of the study participants dropped out, making the results less than reliable.

A study reported in 2006 found that black cohosh has weak estrogen-like effects on vaginal cells and possible positive effects on bone (specifically, stimulating new bone formation).

An earlier study also found multiple benefits with black cohosh, but its results are difficult to trust. This trial followed 80 women for 12 weeks and compared the effects of black cohosh, estrogen, and placebo. Again, black cohosh improved menopausal symptoms and vaginal cell health. However, in this study estrogen proved less effective than placebo. This result is so difficult to believe that it casts serious doubt on the meaningfulness of the results.

Several other studies are also often cited as evidence that black cohosh is useful for various symptoms of menopause, but in reality they prove nothing at all. These trials lacked a placebo group. Although women reported improvements in symptoms, there is no way to know whether black cohosh was responsible. Women given placebo reliably report improvements in menopausal symptoms too; a 50% reduction in hot flashes is fairly typical. Thus, it is possible that the benefits seen in these studies had nothing to do with black cohosh.

One interesting double-blind study evaluated a combination therapy containing black cohosh and **St. John's wort** in 301 women with general menopausal symptoms as well as depression. The results showed that use of the combination treatment was significantly more effective than placebo for both problems.

In contrast, several other studies failed to find benefit. For example, in a 12-month, double-blind, placebo controlled study of 350 women, participants were given either black cohosh, a multibotanical containing 10 herbs, the multibotanical plus soy, standard hormone replacement therapy, or placebo. The results showed significant benefits as compared to placebo for hormone replacement therapy, but only slight, non-significant benefits with the other treatments. In addition, a double-blind study of 122 women failed to find statistically significant benefits with black cohosh as compared to placebo, as did a double-blind, placebo-controlled study of 124 women using a black cohosh/soy isoflavone combination. These negative outcomes were possibly due to the relatively small sizes of the black cohosh groups; in a condition such as menopausal symptoms, where the placebo effect is strong, and when the treatment is relatively weak, large numbers of participants are necessary to show benefit above and beyond the placebo effect.

Putting all this information together, it is fair to say that black cohosh may be effective for reducing hot flashes; whether it is helpful for any other aspects of menopause remains unknown.

Some interesting information has developed regarding how black cohosh may work. In the past, the herb was described as a phytoestrogen, a plant-based chemical with estrogen-like effects. However, subsequent evidence indicates that black cohosh is not a general phytoestrogen, but may act like estrogen in only a few parts of the body: the brain (reducing hot flashes) and bone (potentially helping to prevent or treat osteoporosis), and, to some extent, in the vagina. It does not appear to act like estrogen in the breast or the uterus. If this theory is true, black cohosh is a selective-estrogen receptor modifier (SERM) somewhat like the drug raloxifen (Evista). However, more evidence is needed to establish the facts of the matter.

Breast Cancer Survivors

Women who have had treatment for breast cancer frequently experience hot flashes, often but not always due to the use of the estrogen-antagonist medications like **tamoxifen**. Estrogen treatment is not an option for this problem, as it might increase risk of cancer recurrence. Because black cohosh does not seem to have estrogen-like actions in the breast, researchers felt safe to try it in 85 women who had undergone treatment for breast cancer.

Unfortunately, the results were not encouraging: in this 2-month, double-blind, placebo-controlled trial, black cohosh did not reduce hot-flash symptoms.

Dosage

The most commonly used dosage of black cohosh is 1 or 2 20-mg tablets twice daily of a standardized extract, manufactured to contain 1 mg of 27-deoxyacteine per tablet.

Note: An analysis of 11 available black cohosh products found that 3 of them contained an Asian herb related to black cohosh rather than the proper herb.

Make sure not to confuse black cohosh with the toxic herb **blue cohosh** (*Caulophyllum thalictroides*).

Safety Issues

Black cohosh seldom produces any side effects other than occasional mild gastrointestinal distress. Studies in rats have found no significant toxicity when black cohosh was given at 90 times the therapeutic dosage for a period of 6 months. Since 6 months in a rat corresponds to decades in a human, this study appears to make a strong statement about the long-term safety of black cohosh.

Unlike estrogen, black cohosh does not stimulate breast-cancer cells growing in a test tube. However, black cohosh has not yet been subjected to large-scale studies similar to those conducted for estrogen. For this reason, safety for those with previous breast cancer is not known. Also, because of potential hormonal activity, black cohosh is not recommended for adolescents or pregnant or nursing women.

Black cohosh has been found to slightly lower blood pressure and blood sugar in certain animals. For this reason, it's possible that the herb could interact with drugs for high blood pressure or diabetes, but there are no reports of any such problems.

There are a few reports of a black cohosh product causing severe liver injury. However, it is not clear whether the cause was black cohosh itself, or a contaminant present in the product.

One highly preliminary study found that black cohosh might reduce the effectiveness of the chemotherapy drug **cisplatin**.

Safety in young children or those with severe liver or kidney disease is not known.

Interactions You Should Know About

If you are taking **cisplatin**, black cohosh might reduce its effectiveness.

Black Tea

Camellia sinensis

ALTERNATE NAMES/RELATED TERMS: *Theanine*
PRINCIPAL PROPOSED USES: *Heart Disease Prevention*
OTHER PROPOSED USES: *Cancer Prevention; Osteoporosis Prevention*

Black and green tea are made from the same plant, but black tea has been allowed to oxidize, altering its constituents. While green tea is high in catechins (especially epigallocatechin gallate, or EGCG), black tea contains relatively high levels of theaflavins, theanine, and thearubigens. Although **green tea** is more commonly presented as a healthful beverage, traditional black tea too might have health-promoting properties. However, there is no reliable evidence as yet for any of its proposed health benefits.

What Is Black Tea Used for Today?

According to some but not all observational studies, high consumption of black tea is associated with reduced risk of heart disease and heart disease death.

Unfortunately, observational studies are notoriously unreliable for proving the efficacy of a treatment. Some additional support comes from animal studies that hint black tea may help prevent **atherosclerosis**, the primary cause of heart disease. However, only double-blind, placebo-controlled studies can actually prove a treatment effective, and very few have been conducted on black tea. (For information about why such studies are essential, see **Why Does This Book Rely on Double-blind Studies?**.) One double-blind, placebo-controlled study found that black tea modestly improves cholesterol profile, but it enrolled too few participants (a total of 15) to provide trustworthy results.

A much larger study (more than 200 participants) evaluated a form of green tea enriched with black tea theaflavin. In this substantial 3-month study, use of the tea product resulted in significant reductions in LDL ("bad") cholesterol as compared to placebo. However, these results might not apply to black tea itself.

Theanine, a component of black tea, has been advocated as a **sports supplement**. Physical activity causes elevation of the stress hormone cortisol, which could, in theory, interfere with the benefits of exercise by slowing muscle growth. One study widely reported by tea advocates tested a mixture of theanine and several other herbs and supplements (*Magnolia officinalis, Epimedium koreanum*, **beta-sitosterol**, and **phosphatidylserine**).

The results appeared to indicate that use of this combination could decrease the cortisol response to exercise and, on this basis, theanine and the combination supplement are widely marketed as an aid to body building. However, this study suffers from a number of limitations. Perhaps the most important of these limitations is that presumably the body releases cortisol during exercise for a reason and preventing this response may not, in fact, produce health benefits. In addition, the study was not designed to look for particular benefits, such as improved muscle development.

Black tea might also help **prevent cancer**, though evidence from observational studies is thoroughly inconsistent. Weak observational study evidence additionally hints at benefits for **osteoporosis**.

Dosage

Optimal doses of black tea or its constituents are not known.

Safety Issues

As an extraordinarily widely consumed beverage, black tea is presumed to have a high safety factor. Its side effects would be expected to be similar to those of coffee—heartburn, gastritis, insomnia, anxiety, and heart arrhythmias (benign palpitations or more serious disturbances of heart rhythm). All drug interactions that can occur with caffeine would be expected to occur with black tea.

Interactions You Should Know About

If you are taking:

➤ **MAO inhibitors**: The caffeine in black tea could cause dangerous drug interactions.
➤ **Stimulant drugs such as Ritalin**: The stimulant effects of black tea might be amplified.
➤ **Drugs to prevent heart arrhythmias or to treat insomnia, heartburn, ulcers, or anxiety**: Black tea might interfere with their action.

Bladderwrack

Fucus vesiculosis

ALTERNATE NAMES/RELATED TERMS: *Black Tang, Cut Weed, Rockweed, Rockwrack, Seawrack*

PRINCIPAL PROPOSED USES: *None*

OTHER PROPOSED USES: *Atherosclerosis, Constipation, Heartburn, Hypothyroidism Caused by Iodine Deficiency, Immune Support*

Bladderwrack is a type of seaweed found on the coasts of the North Sea, the western Baltic Sea, and the Atlantic and Pacific Oceans. A common food in Japan, it is used as an additive and flavoring in various food products in Europe. Bladderwrack is commonly found as a component of kelp tablets or powders used as nutritional supplements. It is sometimes loosely called *kelp*, but that term technically refers to a different seaweed.

What Is Bladderwrack Used for Today?

Bladderwrack contains high concentrations of **iodine** and, for this reason, it has been recommended as a treatment for **hypothyroidism** (underactive thyroid gland). However, iodine will only help for the type of hypothyroidism caused by iodine deficiency, which is a relatively rare condition in the developed world. If your iodine levels are not low, taking extra amounts of iodine can cause your thyroid gland to become either over- or underactive, *causing* hypothyroidism or **hyperthyroidism**, respectively. Furthermore, the amount of iodine supplied by bladderwrack is unpredictable (see Safety Issues below).

A component of bladderwrack called *alginic acid* swells upon contact with water; when taken orally, it forms a type of seal at the top of the stomach and, for this reason, is used in over-the-counter preparations for heartburn. The same constituent gives bladderwrack laxative properties as well.

Other proposed uses of bladderwrack include treating **atherosclerosis** and **strengthening immunity**, but there is no meaningful evidence at present that it works for these purposes.

Dosage

It is important not to take bladderwrack in dosages providing more than the recommended daily intake of iodine. For more information on the appropriate intake for various groups of people, see the **Iodine** article. Products that provide bladderwrack should state the amount of iodine they provide; if they do not do so, they should not be used.

Safety Issues

Studies have found that levels of iodine vary widely among bladderwrack products. Because of this, if you use bladderwrack as a regular supplement, there is a real risk you may receive an overdose of iodine and develop hyperthyroidism or hypothyroidism.

Bladderwrack and other seaweed preparations can also worsen **acne** and decrease **iron** absorption.

Finally, bladderwrack, like other sea plants, can concentrate toxic heavy metals, such as arsenic, from the surrounding sea water. One report suggests that use of a bladderwrack product with a high heavy metal content is responsible for a case of kidney failure. Heavy metals present particular risks for pregnant or nursing women, children, individuals with kidney disease, or anyone using bladderwrack in high doses or over a long period of time.

Blessed Thistle

Cnicus benedictus

PRINCIPAL PROPOSED USES: *Dyspepsia, Poor Appetite*

Blessed thistle has a long history of use in European herbal medicine. All parts of the above-ground plant are used medicinally. The herb was used primarily for digestive problems, including heartburn, gastritis, burping, constipation, and flatulence. Blessed thistle was also used for liver and gallbladder diseases. Blessed thistle is also a component of the famous herbal combination therapy Essiac, widely used (though without scientific support) as a treatment for **cancer**.

What Is Blessed Thistle Used for Today?

Blessed thistle has been approved by Germany's Commission E as a treatment for loss of appetite and nonspecific indigestion (**dyspepsia**).

Blessed thistle contains the bitter constituent cnicin. Bitter substances are widely believed to promote appetite, though this has not been proven.

Cnicin does appear to have antimicrobial properties, killing bacteria and fungi in the test tube. These findings do not, however, indicate that blessed thistle can be used as an oral antibiotic. Antibiotics are substances that can be taken into the body at high enough doses to kill microbes throughout the system. In contrast, blessed thistle extracts, like those of many plants, appear to have antiseptic properties, meaning that they kill microbes on direct contact.

Dosage

A typical dose of blessed thistle is 2 g 2 or 3 times daily.

Safety Issues

Although comprehensive safety studies have not been performed, blessed thistle is believed to be safe. However, cross-reactions are possible among people allergic to plants in the daisy family.

Safety in young children, pregnant or nursing women, or people with severe liver or kidney disease has not been established.

Bloodroot

Sanguinaria canadensis

PRINCIPAL PROPOSED USES:

Topical Uses: *Periodontal Disease Prevention, Cavity Prevention, Warts*
Internal Uses: *Respiratory Illnesses*

Bloodroot is a perennial flowering herb that was widely used by Native Americans both as a reddish-orange dye and as a medicine. Some tribes drank bloodroot tea as a treatment for sore throats, fevers, and joint pain, while others applied the somewhat caustic sap to skin cancers.

European herbalists used bloodroot to treat respiratory infections, asthma, joint pain, warts, ringworm, and nasal polyps.

In the mid 1800s, a Dr. Fells of Middlesex Hospital in London developed a treatment consisting of a paste of bloodroot, flour, water, and zinc chloride applied directly to breast tumors and other cancers. Similar formulations were used in various locales up through the turn of the century. Today, bloodroot is still a common constituent of folk medicine "drawing salves" said to pull tumors out of the body.

What Is Bloodroot Used for Today?

Herbalists frequently recommend bloodroot pastes and salves for the treatment of **warts**. Bloodroot is an *escharotic*, that is to say a scab-producing substance, and it functions much like commercial wart plasters containing salicylic acid. Although there has not been any real scientific study of the use of bloodroot for warts, based on its escharotic effects, it could be helpful.

One constituent of bloodroot, sanguinarine, appears to possess topical antibiotic properties. On this basis, the FDA has approved the use of bloodroot in commercially available toothpastes and oral rinses to inhibit the development of dental plaque and **periodontal disease** (gingivitis). However, the evidence that it really helps remains incomplete and inconsistent. On a similar note, one very preliminary study found suggestive evidence that use of a toothpaste containing sanguinaria plus fluoride is more effective for **cavity prevention** than fluoride alone.

Bloodroot is also often combined with other herbs in cough syrups. Some herbalists recommend drinking bloodroot tea for respiratory ailments, but others consider the herb to be too unpredictable in its side effects.

Dosage

For the treatment of warts, bloodroot can be made into a paste and applied directly to the involved area. However, it's important to start slowly to see how sensitive you are. Excessive application can lead to severe burns. Once you've discovered your tolerance, you can apply the herb for a day or so, then remove it and wait for the scab to develop and then drop off. This process is repeated until the wart is gone.

Bloodroot tea for internal use is made by boiling 1 teaspoon of powdered root in a cup of water and taken 2 or 3 times daily.

Safety Issues

Oral bloodroot appears to be relatively safe and nontoxic. However, in large doses, it causes nausea and vomiting and even at lower dosages it has been reported to cause peculiar side effects in some people, such as tunnel vision and pain in the feet. For this reason, many herbalists recommend that it be used only under the supervision of a qualified practitioner.

Topical applications of bloodroot can cause severe burns if used too vigorously and for too long a time. Despite some reassuring evidence from animal studies, there are still theoretical concerns that bloodroot could be harmful during pregnancy. Safety in young children, nursing women, or those with severe liver or kidney disease has also not been established.

Blue Cohosh

Caulophyllum thalictroides

PRINCIPAL PROPOSED USES: *None*

OTHER PROPOSED USES: *Inducing Labor (not recommended), Regulating Menstrual Cycle (not recommended)*

Warning: *Blue cohosh is a toxic herb and the Collins Alternative Health Guide strongly recommends against using it.*

Blue cohosh is a flowering herb native to North America, growing in forested areas from the southeastern United States to Canada. Sometimes known as squaw root or papoose root, the herb may have been used medicinally by native Americans, although this belief is controversial. Other common names for the herb include yellow ginseng and blue ginseng. Blue cohosh should not be confused with the similarly named (but unrelated and much safer) black cohosh. Blue cohosh was used in the 1800s by European settlers and African Americans, primarily for gynecologic conditions. Blue cohosh also has a reputation as an herb that can induce abortions, although concerns regarding its efficacy and safety make this use extremely ill-advised. In addition, it has been used for the treatment of arthritis, cramps, epilepsy, inflammation of the uterus, hiccups, colic, and sore throat.

What Is Blue Cohosh Used for Today?

Blue cohosh is widely prescribed by herbalists and midwives today. A 1999 survey published in the *Journal of Nurse-Midwifery* found that 64% of certified nurse-midwives who prescribe herbal medicines use blue cohosh to induce labor. It has also been used for a wide variety of menstrual problems, including several for which it would not be logical to believe that the same treatment could help. For example, blue cohosh has been used to start menstrual periods that were late in coming and yet also to stop excessive or ongoing menstrual flow.

There is no credible evidence that blue cohosh is effective for any of the conditions for which it has been used. Furthermore, several published reports cite cases of serious side effects to infants apparently caused by blue cohosh (see Safety Issues below).

Dosage

Blue cohosh is usually used as a tincture. Common dosages range from 5 to 10 drops taken every 2 to 4 hours.

Safety Issues

There are many serious safety concerns with blue cohosh.

Some of the compounds found in blue cohosh, such as caulophyllosaponin, methylcytisin, and caulosaponin, appear to constrict coronary vessels, limiting blood flow to the heart and reducing its ability to pump. One published case report documents profound heart failure in a child born to a mother who used blue cohosh to induce labor. Severe medical consequences were seen in another child as well. Other blue cohosh constituents are known to interfere with the ability of a newly fertilized ovum to implant in the uterus, damage the uterus and thyroid, and cause severe birth defects in cattle and laboratory rats.

Given these reports, the availability of safe alternatives for stimulating labor, and the lack of studies to document the herb's efficacy and safety, the Collins Alternative Health Guide strongly advises against using blue cohosh.

Blue Flag

Iris versicolor or *Iris caroliniana Watson*

PRINCIPAL PROPOSED USES: *None*

OTHER PROPOSED USES: *Eczema, Menstrual Problems*

Grown throughout North America, the underground stem, or rhizome, of the eye-catching blue flag plant in the iris family was traditionally thought to have medicinal properties.

Historically, the plant has been used to treat constipation, dermatitis, and skin disease. Late nineteenth-century medical literature also referenced the plant as an emmenagogue, a type of herb believed helpful for inducing labor or treating menstrual problems of various types.

Blue flag contains furfural, a known mucous membrane irritant. It also contains isophthalic acid, iridin, beta-sitosterol, irigenin, irilone-4'-glucoside, and irisolone-4'-bioside. Iridin reportedly can be poisonous to humans and animals; however, there is some uncertainty as to whether the chemical of that name cited as toxic is identical to the substance found in blue flag.

What Is Blue Flag Used for Today?

Blue flag has no established medical uses and is not widely used today. However, some herbalists still recommend it for **menstrual problems**, as well as for various skin diseases such as **eczema**.

Dosage

Typical doses of blue flag are 0.6 to 2 g of the dried rhizome, or 1 to 2 ml of the liquid extract, 3 times daily.

Safety Issues

Safety studies of blue flag have not been performed and related species have been found toxic. It is also said to cause nausea and vomiting when taken at higher doses. For all these reasons, we recommend avoiding blue flag.

Boldo

Peumus boldus

PRINCIPAL PROPOSED USES: *None*

OTHER PROPOSED USES: *Constipation, Dyspepsia, Liver Protection*

Boldo (*Peumus boldus*) is an evergreen shrub native to South America. It grows about 6 to 20 feet high and has thick waxy leaves. Although boldo has a long history of use as a culinary spice and medicinal herb, and is still one of the most common medicinal plants used in Chile, it has only recently become the subject of scientific research.

The leaves of the boldo plant have traditionally been used as a treatment for liver and bladder disorders, as well as rheumatism. They have also been used for a wide variety of other ailments, including headache, earache, congestion, menstrual pain, and syphilis. Recent research suggests boldo may protect the liver from toxins, stimulate the gallbladder, and reduce inflammation.

What Is Boldo Used for Today?

Germany's Commission E has approved boldo for "spastic gastrointestinal complaints and dyspepsia." **Dyspepsia** is a rather vague term that corresponds to the common word "indigestion," indicating a wide variety of digestive problems, including stomach discomfort, lack of appetite, and nausea.

In Europe, dyspepsia is commonly attributed to inadequate flow of bile from the gallbladder. Although this connection has not been proven, boldo has been used as a treatment for dyspepsia based on how it affects the gallbladder. Boldo does not seem to increase bile production, but it may cause gallbladder contraction.

Boldo taken alone has not been well evaluated as a treatment for dyspepsia; however, a combination herbal treatment containing boldo (along with other herbs thought to stimulate the gallbladder) has been studied. In a double-blind, placebo-controlled trial, 60 people given either an artichoke leaf–boldo–celandine combination or placebo found improvements in symptoms of indigestion after 14 days of treatment. How this combination might be effective for treating dyspepsia is unclear.

Note: Celandine may present significant risk of liver toxicity.

Studies on animals have found that boldo may have some ability to **protect the liver** from toxins, perhaps due to the antioxidant effects of a boldo constituent called *boldine.*

Boldo also has anti-inflammatory properties, and, in addition, may act as a laxative. Finally the essential oils found in boldo have antimicrobial properties; this is true of many essential oils, however, and does not indicate that boldo can act as an antibiotic.

Dosage

Germany's Commission E recommends 3 g of the dried leaf or its equivalent per day for digestive complaints.

Safety Issues

Although comprehensive safety studies have not been completed, boldo leaf appears to be safe at normal doses. No side effects were reported in any of the animal studies. However, the plant's essential oils are very toxic and can cause kidney damage if taken in purified form or if very large amounts of the leaf are ingested. The safety of long-term use is also questionable.

Individuals with gallstones should only take boldo under a physician's supervision due to the risk of gallstones being expelled and becoming lodged in a bile duct or the intestines. Those with obstruction of the bile ducts should not use boldo at all, due to the risk of rupture.

Warning: Animal studies suggest that boldo can cause birth defects and spontaneous abortion. For this reason, pregnant women should not use boldo. Safety in nursing women, young children, and individuals with severe liver or kidney disease has not been established.

Boron

SUPPLEMENT FORMS/ALTERNATE NAMES: *Boron Chelate, Sodium Borate*

PRINCIPAL PROPOSED USES: *None*

OTHER PROPOSED USES: *Osteoarthritis, Osteoporosis, Prostate Cancer Prevention, Rheumatoid Arthritis, Sports Supplement*

Plants need boron for proper health, but it's not known whether humans do. However, boron does seem to assist in the proper absorption of calcium, magnesium, and phosphorus from foods and to slow the loss of these minerals through urination. Very preliminary evidence suggests that boron supplements may be helpful for osteoarthritis and osteoporosis.

Sources

No dietary or nutritional requirement for boron has been established and boron deficiency is not known to cause any disease. Good sources include leafy vegetables, raisins, prunes, nuts, non-citrus fruits, and grains.

A typical American daily diet provides 1.5 to 3 mg of boron.

Therapeutic Dosages

When used as a treatment for osteoarthritis or osteoporosis, boron is often recommended at a dosage of 3 mg per day, an amount similar to the average daily intake from food. However, food sources may be safer (see Safety Issues below).

Therapeutic Uses

Boron aids in the proper metabolism of vitamins and minerals involved with bone development, such as calcium, copper, magnesium, and vitamin D. In addition, boron appears to affect estrogen and possibly testosterone as well, hormones that affect bone health. On this basis, boron has been suggested for preventing or treating **osteoporosis**. However, there have been no clinical studies to evaluate the potential benefits of boron supplements for any bone-related conditions.

On the basis of similarly weak evidence, boron is often added to supplements intended for the treatment of **osteoarthritis**.

Boron has also been proposed as a **sports supplement**, based on its effects on hormones. However, studies have, as yet, failed to find evidence that it helps increase muscle mass or enhances performance.

One large observational study suggests that higher intake of boron may reduce risk of prostate **cancer**.

Finally, boron is sometimes recommended as a treatment for **rheumatoid arthritis**, but there is no evidence to support this use.

What Is the Scientific Evidence for Boron?

Osteoarthritis

In areas of the world where people eat relatively high amounts of boron—between 3 and 10 mg per day—the incidence of osteoarthritis is below 10%. However, in regions where there is less boron in the diet—1 mg or less per day—the incidence of arthritis is much higher. In addition, the joints of people with osteoarthritis have been found to contain less boron than people without the condition. These observations have given rise to the hypothesis that boron supplements might be helpful for people who already have arthritis symptoms.

However, the only direct evidence that it works comes from one highly preliminary study reported in 1990.

Osteoporosis

In one small study, 13 postmenopausal women were first fed a diet that provided 0.25 mg of boron for 119 days; then they were fed the same diet with a boron supplement of 3 mg daily for 48 days. The results revealed that boron supplementation reduced the amount of calcium lost in the urine. This suggests (but certainly doesn't prove) that boron can help prevent osteoporosis.

However, in a similar study, boron administration did not affect urine calcium loss. Another study found that boron fails to affect calcium loss among people who receive enough magnesium.

Safety Issues

Since the therapeutic dosage of boron is about the same as the amount you can get from food, it is probably fairly safe. Unpleasant side effects, including nausea and vomiting, are only reported at about 50 times the highest recommended dose.

One potential concern with boron regards its effect on hormones. In at least two small studies, boron was found to increase the body's own estrogen levels, especially in women on estrogen-replacement therapy. Because elevated estrogen increases the risk of breast and uterine cancer in women past menopause, this may be a matter of concern for those who wish to take supplemental boron. Further research is necessary to discover whether boron's apparent effect on estrogen is a real problem or not. At the present time, we would recommend getting your boron from fruits and vegetables: a large study found that high intake of boron from these sources did not affect breast cancer rates.

Interactions You Should Know About

If you are receiving **hormone-replacement therapy**, use of boron may not be advisable due to the risk of elevating estrogen levels excessively.

Boswellia

Boswellia serrata

ALTERNATE NAMES/RELATED TERMS: *Frankincense*

PRINCIPAL PROPOSED USES: *Asthma, Osteoarthritis, Rheumatoid Arthritis*

OTHER PROPOSED USES: *Bursitis, Crohn's Disease, Tendonitis, Ulcerative Colitis*

The gummy resin of the boswellia tree has a long history of use in Indian herbal medicine as a treatment for arthritis, bursitis, respiratory diseases, and diarrhea.

What Is Boswellia Used for Today?

Growing evidence suggests that boswellia has anti-inflammatory effects. On this basis, the herb has been tried for a number of conditions in which inflammation is involved, including painful conditions such as bursitis, **osteoarthritis**, **rheumatoid arthritis**, and **tendonitis**. For the same reason, it has also been tried for **asthma** and inflammatory bowel disease (**ulcerative colitis** or **Crohn's Disease**).

In addition, extracts of boswellia have been studied as an aid to standard care for malignant glioma (a type of incurable brain tumor). Use of boswellia appears to decrease symptoms, probably by decreasing inflammation in the brain (as well as through other mechanisms). However, this has not been proven and individuals with cancer should not use boswellia (or any other herb or supplement) except on physician's advice.

What Is the Scientific Evidence for Boswellia?

Rheumatoid Arthritis

According to a review of unpublished studies, preliminary double-blind trials have found boswellia effective in relieving the symptoms of rheumatoid arthritis. Two placebo-controlled studies, involving a total of 81 people with rheumatoid arthritis, reportedly found significant reductions in swelling and pain over the course of 3 months. In addition, a comparative study of 60 people over 6 months found that boswellia extract produced symptomatic benefits comparable to oral gold therapy. However, this review was rather sketchy on details.

A more recent double-blind, placebo-controlled study that enrolled 78 people with rheumatoid arthritis found no benefit. However, about half of the patients dropped out, which seriously diminishes the significance of the results.

Asthma

A 6-week, double-blind, placebo-controlled study of 80 people with relatively mild asthma found that treatment with boswellia at a dose of 300 mg 3 times daily reduced the frequency of asthma attacks and improved objective measurements of breathing capacity.

Osteoarthritis

In a double-blind study of 30 people with osteoarthritis of the knee, researchers compared boswellia against placebo. Participants received either boswellia or placebo for 8 weeks and were then switched over to the opposite treatment for an additional 8 weeks. The results showed significantly greater improvement in knee pain, knee mobility, and walking distance with boswellia compared to placebo.

Inflammatory Bowel Disease

An 8-week, double-blind, placebo-controlled trial of 102 people with Crohn's disease compared a standardized boswellia extract against the drug mesalazine. Participants taking boswellia fared at least as well as those taking mesalazine, according to a standard score of Crohn's disease severity. A small, poorly designed trial found some indications that boswellia might also offer benefit in ulcerative colitis.

Dosage

A typical dose of boswellia is 300 to 400 mg 3 times a day of an extract standardized to contain 37.5% boswellic acids. Some studies have used dosages as high as 1,200 mg 3 times daily.

Safety Issues

In clinical trials of pharmaceutical grade standardized boswellia extract, no serious side effects have been reported. Crude herb preparations, however, may not be as safe as the specially manufactured extract. Safety in young children, pregnant or nursing women, or individu-als with severe liver or kidney disease has not been estab-lished.

Brahmi

Bacopa monnieri

PRINCIPAL PROPOSED USES: *Enhancing Memory and Mental Function*
OTHER PROPOSED USES: *Allergies, Asthma, Depression, Hypothyroidism, Narcotic Addiction, Ulcers*

Bacopa monnieri is a creeping perennial with white or blue flowers that grows throughout much of Southern Asia. It has been used traditionally to treat **epilepsy, depression, insomnia,** and **schizophrenia.** In the traditional medicine of India, **Ayurveda,** *B. monnieri* is considered to fall in the *brahmi* category of herbs, a group of substances said to assist the mind and enhance awareness. From this comes *B. monnieri's* common name of brahmi, despite the fact that many other herbs fall into the brahmi category as well.

What Is *B. monnieri* Used for Today?

B. monnieri is widely marketed today as a "brain tonic" for enhancing memory and mental function. However, as discussed in the next section, the evidence that it works remains weak at best.

Even weaker evidence, far too preliminary to rely upon at all, hints that *B. monnieri* might have potential value for **allergies, asthma, narcotic addiction, hypothyroidism,** depression, and **ulcers.** However, far more research is necessary before anyone could responsibly promote *B. monnieri* for these conditions.

What Is the Scientific Evidence for *B. monnieri?*

Although several double-blind, placebo-controlled studies have evaluated the potential value of *B. monnieri* for enhancing mental function, the results are far from conclusive.

B. monnieri appears to have **antioxidant** properties in the brain, which could potentially lead to positive effects on mental function. However, a 12-week, double-blind, placebo-controlled trial of 76 individu-als that tested the potential memory-enhancing bene-fits of *B. monnieri* generally failed to find much evidence of benefit. The only significant improvement seen among all the many measures used was in one that evaluated retention of new information. While this may sound at least somewhat promising, in fact it means almost nothing. Here's why: When a study uses many different techniques to assess improvement, mere chance ensures that at least one of them will come up with results. Properly designed studies should focus on one test of benefit alone (the *primary outcome measure*) that is selected prior to running the trial. "Fishing" for results among multiple tests is a highly suspect method.

Nonetheless, if several independent studies use mul-tiple tests of improvement and the pattern of response is reliably maintained, then the results begin to appear more significant. Unfortunately, this does not seem to be the case with *B. monnieri.* In a previous double-blind, placebo-controlled study enrolling 46 individuals, use of *B. monnieri* over a 2-week period again produced bene-fits, but in an entirely different pattern. In yet another double-blind, placebo-controlled study, this one involv-ing 38 people, short-term use of *B. monnieri* failed to produce any measurable improvements in memory. In addition, use of combined *Ginkgo biloba* (120 mg) and *B. monnieri* (300 mg) has also failed to improve mental function. This type of inconsistency suggests that the limited benefits seen in some studies were due to chance.

Slightly more promising results have been seen in studies of a proprietary Ayurvedic mixture containing *B. monnieri* and about 30 other ingredients. However, these studies are generally not up to modern scientific stan-dards.

Dosage

The proposed active ingredients in *B. monnieri* are substances called bacosides. A typical dose of *B. monnieri* used in the studies described above was 300 to 450 mg daily of a concentrated alcohol extract standardized to bacoside content, equivalent to about 6 to 9 g of whole dried herb.

Safety Issues

There are no well known significant side effects associated with the use of *B. monnieri*. However, comprehensive safety studies have not been reported. Safety in young children, pregnant or nursing women, or people with severe liver or kidney disease has not been established.

Branched-Chain Amino Acids

SUPPLEMENT FORMS/ALTERNATE NAMES: *BCAAs (Combined) or Leucine, Isoleucine, and Valine (Separately)*

PRINCIPAL PROPOSED USES: *Amyotrophic Lateral Sclerosis (ALS, Lou Gehrig's Disease), Loss of Appetite (in people with Cancer)*

OTHER PROPOSED USES: *Severe Liver Disease, such as Cirrhosis; Muscular Dystrophy; Recovery From Surgery; Recovery from Traumatic Brain Injury; Tardive Dyskinesia; Sports Performance Enhancement*

Branched-chain amino acids (BCAAs) are naturally occurring molecules (leucine, isoleucine, and valine) that the body uses to build proteins. The term "branched chain" refers to the molecular structure of these particular amino acids. Muscles have a particularly high content of BCAAs.

For reasons that are not entirely clear, BCAA supplements may improve appetite in cancer patients and slow the progression of amyotrophic lateral sclerosis (ALS, or Lou Gehrig's disease, a terrible condition that leads to degeneration of nerves, atrophy of the muscles, and eventual death).

BCAAs have also been proposed as a supplement to boost athletic performance.

Requirements/Sources

Dietary protein usually provides all the BCAAs you need. However, physical stress and injury can increase your need for BCAAs to repair damage, so supplementation may be helpful.

BCAAs are present in all protein-containing foods, but the best sources are red meat and dairy products. Chicken, fish, and eggs are excellent sources as well. Whey protein and egg protein supplements are another way to ensure you're getting enough BCAAs. Supplements may contain all three BCAAs together or simply individual BCAAs.

Therapeutic Dosages

The typical dosage of BCAAs is 1 to 5 g daily.

Therapeutic Uses

Preliminary evidence suggests that BCAAs may improve appetite in people undergoing treatment for **cancer**. There is also some evidence that BCAA supplements may reduce symptoms of **amyotrophic lateral sclerosis** (ALS, or Lou Gehrig's disease); however, not all studies have had positive results.

Preliminary evidence from a series of small studies suggests that BCAAs might decrease symptoms of **tardive dyskinesia**, a movement disorder caused by long-term usage of antipsychotic drugs. BCAAs have also shown a bit of promise for enhancing recovery from traumatic brain injury.

Because of how they are metabolized in the body, BCAAs might be helpful for individuals with severe liver disease (such as **cirrhosis**).

BCAAs have also been tried for aiding muscle recovery after bed rest (such as may follow **surgery**).

Although there is a little supportive evidence, on balance, current research does not indicate that BCAAs are effective as a **sports supplement**.

BCAAs have also as yet failed to prove effective for muscular dystrophy.

What Is the Scientific Evidence for Branched-Chain Amino Acids?

Appetite in Cancer Patients

A double-blind study tested BCAAs on 28 people with cancer who had lost their appetites due to either the disease itself or its treatment. Appetite improved in 55% of those taking BCAAs (4.8 g daily) compared to only 16% of those who took placebo.

Amyotrophic Lateral Sclerosis (Lou Gehrig's Disease)

A small, double-blind study found evidence that BCAAs might help protect muscle strength in people with Lou Gehrig's disease. Eighteen individuals were given either BCAAs (taken 4 times daily between meals) or placebo and followed for 1 year. The results showed that people taking BCAAs declined much more slowly than those receiving placebo. In the placebo group, 5 of 9 participants lost their ability to walk, 2 died, and another required a respirator. Only 1 of the

9 participants receiving BCAAs became unable to walk during the study period. This study is too small to give conclusive evidence, but it does suggest that BCAAs might be helpful for this disease.

However, other studies found no effect, and one actually found a slight increase in deaths during the study period among those treated with BCAAs compared to placebo.

Muscular Dystrophy

One double-blind, placebo-controlled study found leucine (one of the amino acids in BCAAs) ineffective at the dose of 0.2 g per kilogram body weight (for example, 15 g daily for a 75-kilogram woman) in 96 individuals with muscular dystrophy. Over the course of 1 year, no differences were seen between the effects of leucine and placebo.

Safety Issues

BCAAs are believed to be safe; when taken in excess, they are simply converted into other amino acids. However, like other amino acids, BCAAs may interfere with medications for **Parkinson's disease**.

Interactions You Should Know About

If you are taking **medication for Parkinson's disease** (such as **levodopa**), BCAAs may reduce its effectiveness.

Bromelain

PRINCIPAL PROPOSED USES: *Athletic Injuries, Digestive Problems, Phlebitis, Sinusitis, Surgery*

OTHER PROPOSED USES: *Arthritis, Chronic Venous Insufficiency, Easy Bruising, Gout, Hemorrhoids, Dysmenorrhea, Ulcerative Colitis*

Bromelain is not actually a single substance, but rather a collection of protein-digesting enzymes (also called *proteolytic enzymes*) found in pineapple juice and in the stem of pineapple plants. It is primarily produced in Japan, Hawaii, and Taiwan, and much of the original research was performed in the first two of those locations. Subsequently, European researchers developed an interest and, by 1995, bromelain had become the thirteenth most common individual herbal product sold in Germany.

What Is Bromelain Used for Today?

Bromelain (often in combination with other proteolytic enzymes) is used in Europe to aid in recovery from **surgery** and **athletic injuries**, as well as to treat sinusitis and **phlebitis**.

Other proposed uses of bromelain include chronic venous insufficiency (closely related to **varicose veins**),

Bromelain

hemorrhoids, other diseases of the veins, **bruising**, osteoarthritis, **rheumatoid arthritis**, **gout**, **ulcerative colitis**, and **dysmenorrhea** (menstrual pain). However, there is little real evidence that bromelain is effective for these conditions.

Bromelain is definitely useful as a digestive enzyme. Unlike most digestive enzymes, bromelain is active both in the acid environment of the stomach and the alkaline environment of the small intestine. This may make it particularly effective as an oral digestive aid for those who do not digest food properly.

Bromelain may also increase the absorption of various drugs, particularly antibiotics such as amoxicillin and tetracycline. This could offer both risks and benefits.

Bromelain is widely available in groceries as a meat tenderizer.

What Is the Scientific Evidence for Bromelain?

While most large enzymes are broken down in the digestive tract, those found in bromelain appear to be absorbed whole to a certain extent. This finding makes it reasonable to suppose that bromelain can actually produce systemic (whole body) effects. Once in the blood, bromelain appears to reduce inflammation, "thin" the blood, and affect the immune system. These influences may be responsible for some of bromelain's therapeutic effects.

See also **Proteolytic Enzymes** for a discussion of combination products that often contain bromelain.

Injury and Surgery

The evidence for bromelain as a treatment for injuries and surgeries is mixed.

A double-blind, placebo-controlled study evaluated 160 women who received episiotomies (surgical cuts in the perineum) during childbirth. Participants given 40 mg of bromelain 4 times daily for 3 days, beginning 4 hours after delivery, showed a statistically significant decrease in edema, inflammation, and pain. Ninety percent of patients taking bromelain demonstrated excellent or good responses compared to 44% in the placebo group. However, another double-blind study of 158 women who received episiotomies failed to find significant benefit.

In a double-blind, controlled trial, 95 patients undergoing treatment for cataracts were given 40 mg of bromelain or placebo (along with other treatments) 4 times daily for 2 days prior to surgery and 5 days post-operatively.

Overall, less inflammation was noted in the bromelain-treated group compared to the placebo group.

Benefits were also seen in double-blind, placebo-controlled studies of dental, nasal, or foot surgery. However, a study of 154 people undergoing facial plastic surgery found no benefit.

A somewhat informal controlled study of 146 boxers suggested that bromelain helps bruises to heal more quickly. Another study—this one without any type of control group—found that bromelain reduced swelling, pain at rest, and tenderness among 59 patients with blunt trauma injuries, including bruising.

People who engage in intense exercise to which they are not accustomed may experience a set of symptoms called *delayed onset muscle soreness* (DOMS), consisting of pain, reduced flexibility, and weakness of the muscles involved. Bromelain has been proposed for this condition, but a small double-blind, placebo-controlled study failed to find it effective.

Sinusitis

In a double-blind trial, 48 patients with moderately severe to severe sinusitis received bromelain or placebo for 6 days. All patients were placed on standard therapy for sinusitis, which included antihistamines, analgesics, and antibiotics. Upon completion of the study, inflammation was reduced in 83% of those taking bromelain compared to 52% of the placebo group. Breathing difficulty was relieved in 78% of the bromelain group and 68% of the placebo group. Overall, good to excellent results were observed in 87% of patients treated with bromelain compared to 68% on placebo.

Benefits were also seen in two other studies enrolling a total of more than 100 individuals with sinusitis.

Dosage

Recommended dosages of bromelain vary with the form used. Due to the wide variation, we suggest following label instructions.

Safety Issues

Bromelain appears to be essentially nontoxic and it seldom causes side effects other than occasional mild gastrointestinal distress or allergic reactions.

However, because bromelain "thins" the blood to some extent, it shouldn't be combined with drugs such as Coumadin (warfarin) without a doctor's supervision.

According to one small animal study, bromelain might interact with sedative medications, increasing their effect. As noted above, it might also increase blood levels of various antibiotics, which could present risks in some cases. In addition, one trial suggests that doses of bromelain eight times higher than standard recommendations might increase heart rate (but not blood pressure).

Safety in young children, pregnant or nursing women, or those with liver or kidney disease has not been established.

Interactions You Should Know About

If you are taking medications that thin the blood, such as **Coumadin** (warfarin) or **heparin**, sedative drugs such as **benzodiazepines**, or **antibiotics**, bromelain might amplify their effect.

Buchu

Barosma betulina, Agathosma betulina, Agathosma crenultata

PRINCIPAL PROPOSED USES: *None*

NOT RECOMMENDED USES: *Urinary Tract Infections and Inflammation*

Buchu has a long tradition of use for the treatment of bladder and urinary tract problems, especially urinary tract infections. In South Africa, buchu and other plants similar to it are additionally used for stomach aches, joint pain, and colds and flus. The leaves are the part used medicinally.

What Is Buchu Used for Today?

Many herbalists use buchu as a part of herbal combinations designed for kidney and bladder problems. Buchu is said to have a *diuretic effect*, meaning that it increases the flow of urine. However, there is no meaningful scientific documentation of this or any other medicinal effect of buchu.

Buchu contains various bioflavonoids, including **diosmin**, **rutin**, and **quercetin**. Its **essential oil** contains a variety of aromatic substances, including limonene and menthone, along with the known liver toxin pulegone. While it is commonly said that the essential oil has antimicrobial effects, the only published study on the subject failed to find activity in this regard. This study did, however, find possible antispasmodic actions, which could potentially reduce the pain of bladder infections.

Dosage

Buchu is typically taken at a dose of 1 to 2 g of dried leaf 3 times daily, with meals. However, due to the toxicity of one of the constituents of buchu, we do not recommend using it at all.

Safety Issues

Because buchu contains the known liver toxin pulegone, the herb should be used only with great caution, if at all. It also frequently causes stomach upset. It definitely should not be used by young children, pregnant or nursing women, or people with liver or kidney disease.

In addition, if buchu does in fact have diuretic effects as claimed, people taking the medication lithium should use buchu only under the supervision of a physician, as dehydration can be a danger with this medication.

Interactions You Should Know About

If you are taking **lithium**, do not use buchu except under the supervision of a physician.

Bugleweed

Bugleweed

Lycopus virginicus

PRINCIPAL PROPOSED USES: *None*

OTHER PROPOSED USES: *Cyclic Mastalgia (Cyclic Breast Pain), Hyperthyroidism*

Bugleweed (*Lycopus virginicus*), from the mint family, is a native of North America. It is closely related to the European herb called *gypsywort* or *gypsyweed* (*L. europaeus*). For medicinal purposes, these two plants are often used interchangeably. The leaves of bugleweed are long and thin and grow in pairs from the stem. Small whitish flowers grow around the stem at the base of each pair of leaves.

The juice of bugleweed can be used as a fabric dye and it was reportedly used by gypsies to darken their skin, which may be the origin of the common names applied to the European species of *Lycopus*.

Bugleweed also has a long-standing reputation as a medicinal plant. Herbalists have traditionally used bugleweed as a sedative, to treat mild heart conditions, and to reduce fever and mucus production in flus and colds. More recently, bugleweed has been suggested as a treatment for hyperthyroidism and mastodynia (breast pain).

What Is Bugleweed Used for Today?

Several very preliminary studies suggest that bugleweed may be helpful for treating mild **hyperthyroidism**.

Hyperthyroidism is a condition in which the thyroid gland releases excessive amounts of thyroid hormone. Symptoms include weight loss, weakness, heart palpitations, and anxiety. Test tube and animal studies suggest that bugleweed may reduce thyroid hormone by decreasing levels of TSH (a hormone that stimulates the thyroid gland) and by impairing thyroid hormone synthesis. In addition, bugleweed may block the action of thyroid-stimulating antibodies found in Grave's disease.

Note: Self-treatment of hyperthyroidism can be dangerous. Physician supervision is necessary to determine why the thyroid is overactive to design a specific treatment plan.

Bugleweed may also reduce levels of the hormone prolactin, which is primarily responsible for the production of breast milk. Elevated levels of prolactin may also cause breast pain in women; based on this finding, bugleweed has been recommended as a treatment for **cyclic mastalgia** (breast tenderness that comes and goes with the menstrual cycle). However, due to its effects on thyroid hormone, we do not recommend that it be used for this purpose.

Dosage

The dosage of bugleweed must be adjusted by measuring thyroid hormone levels.

Safety Issues

The safety of bugleweed has not been established. Long-term or high-dose use of the herb may cause an enlarged thyroid. Bugleweed should not be used by individuals with hypothyroidism (low thyroid hormone) or an enlarged thyroid gland. Pregnant or nursing women should also avoid bugleweed because of potential effects on their children as well as on breast milk production.

Bugleweed should not be combined with thyroid medications. It may also interfere with diagnostic procedures that rely on radioactive isotopes to evaluate the thyroid.

Interactions You Should Know About

If you are taking **thyroid medications**, do not use bugleweed.

If you are undergoing tests of your thyroid function, do not use bugleweed except on physician advice.

Burdock

Arctium lappa

PRINCIPAL PROPOSED USES: *Acne, Eczema, Psoriasis*
OTHER PROPOSED USES: *Cancer, Rheumatoid Arthritis*

The common burdock, that well-known source of annoying burrs matted in dogs' fur, is also a medicinal herb of considerable reputation. Called *gobo* in Japan, burdock root is said to be a food that provides deep strengthening to the immune system. In ancient China and India, herbalists used it in the treatment of respiratory infections, abscesses, and joint pain. European physicians of the Middle Ages and later used it to treat cancerous tumors, skin conditions, venereal disease, and bladder and kidney problems.

Burdock was a primary ingredient in the famous (or infamous) Hoxsey cancer treatment. Harry Hoxsey was a former coal miner who parlayed a traditional family remedy for cancer into the largest privately owned cancer treatment center in the world, with branches in 17 states. (It was shut down in the 1950s by the FDA. Harry Hoxsey himself subsequently died of cancer.) Other herbs in his formula included red clover, poke, prickly ash, bloodroot, and barberry. Burdock is also found in the famous herbal cancer remedy Essiac.

Despite this historical enthusiasm, there is no significant evidence that burdock is an effective treatment for cancer or any other illness.

What Is Burdock Used for Today?

Burdock is widely recommended for the relief of dry, scaly skin conditions such as **eczema** and **psoriasis**. It is also used for treating **acne**. It can be taken internally as well as applied directly to the skin. Burdock is sometimes recommended for **rheumatoid arthritis**. Unfortunately, there is as yet no real scientific evidence for any of these uses.

Dosage

A typical dosage of burdock is 1 to 2 g of powdered dry root 3 times per day.

Safety Issues

As a food commonly eaten in Japan (it is often found in *sukiyaki*), burdock root is believed to be safe. However, in 1978, the *Journal of the American Medical Association* caused a brief scare by publishing a report of burdock poisoning. Subsequent investigation showed that the herbal product involved was actually contaminated with the poisonous chemical atropine from an unknown source. Safety in young children, pregnant or nursing women, or those with severe liver or kidney disease is not established.

Interactions You Should Know About

If you are taking **insulin** or **oral medications to reduce blood sugar**, it is possible that burdock will increase its effect.

Butcher's Broom

Ruscus aculeatus

PRINCIPAL PROPOSED USES: *Chronic Venous Insufficiency*

OTHER PROPOSED USES: *Hemorrhoids, Surgery Support (Lymphedema Following Breast Cancer Surgery)*

So named because its branches were a traditional source of broom straw used by butchers, this Mediterranean evergreen bush has a long history of traditional use in the treatment of urinary conditions. More recently, it has been studied as a treatment for vein-related conditions.

What Is Butcher's Broom Used for Today?

Butcher's broom has been approved by Germany's Commission E as supportive therapy for **chronic venous insufficiency**. Venous insufficiency, a condition closely related to varicose veins, involves pain, swelling and fatigue in the calves. Commission E also recommends butcher's broom for the treatment of **hemorrhoids**.

This recommendation was in place before any meaningful studies had been performed evaluating butcher's broom for either of these purposes. However, several studies performed subsequently now provide preliminary supporting evidence for its use in chronic venous insufficiency.

No substantial studies have evaluated butcher's broom for hemorrhoids, but because hemorrhoids are similar to varicose veins, it is a reasonable supposition that butcher's broom might be helpful.

Various treatments used for venous insufficiency have also shown promise for treating arm swelling (lymphedema) following **surgery** for **breast cancer**. One study suggests that butcher's broom may be helpful for this condition as well.

What Is the Scientific Evidence for Butcher's Broom?

Venous Insufficiency

A well-designed and reported double-blind trial evaluated the effectiveness of a standardized butcher's broom extract in 166 women with chronic venous insufficiency. For a period of 12 weeks, participants received either placebo or butcher's broom (one tablet twice daily containing 36.0 to 37.5 mg of a methanol dry extract concentrated at 15–20:1). The results showed that leg swelling (the primary measurement used) decreased significantly in the butcher's broom group as compared to the placebo group.

Similar results were seen in a 12-week, double-blind, placebo-controlled trial with 148 participants.

Another 12-week, double-blind, placebo-controlled trial with 141 participants used a combination of butcher's broom extract and the bioflavonoid trimethylhesperidin chalcone, and found benefits. Marginal benefits were seen in a much smaller study using this combination.

Lymphedema

In a double-blind study, 57 women with lymphedema received either placebo or butcher's broom combined with the modified citrus bioflavonoid trimethylhesperidin chalcone. The results indicated that use of the combination therapy resulted in significantly less swelling.

Dosage

A typical dose of butcher's broom is 36.0 to 37.5 mg twice daily of a methanol extract concentrated at a level of 15–20:1. This should supply about 7–11 mg ruscogenin (also called *ruscogenine*) daily.

For hemorrhoids, butcher's broom is sometimes applied as an ointment or in the form of a suppository.

Safety Issues

In clinical trials, use of butcher's broom has not been associated with any serious adverse effects. However, comprehensive safety studies have not been reported. Maximum safe doses in young children, pregnant or nursing women, or those with liver or kidney disease have not been established.

Butterbur

Petasites hybridus

PRINCIPAL PROPOSED USES: *Allergies, Migraine Headaches (Prevention)*
OTHER PROPOSED USES: *Asthma, Musculoskeletal Pain, Ulcer Protection*

Butterbur can be found growing along rivers, ditches, and marshy areas in northern Asia, Europe, and parts of North America. It sends up stalks of reddish flowers very early in spring, before producing very large heart-shaped leaves with a furry gray underside. Once the leaves appear, butterbur somewhat resembles rhubarb—one of its common names is bog rhubarb. It is also sometimes referred to as "umbrella leaves" due to the size of its foliage. Other more or less descriptive common names abound, including blatterdock, bogshorns, butter-dock, butterly dock, capdockin, flapperdock, and langwort.

Butterbur is often described as possessing an unpleasant smell, but being malodorous hasn't protected it from harvesting by humans. The plant has a long history of use as an anti-spasmodic, thought to be effective for such conditions as stomach cramps, whooping cough, and asthma.

Externally, butterbur has been applied as a poultice over wounds or skin ulcerations.

What Is Butterbur Used for Today?

A special toxin-free butterbur extract has been investigated for the treatment of a variety of illnesses. Two double-blind trials suggest that this butterbur extract may be useful for preventing **migraine headaches**. In addition, meaningful evidence indicates that this extract is helpful for **hay fever**.

There is some evidence that butterbur has anti-inflammatory and anti-spasmodic effects and, on this basis, it has been proposed as a treatment for a variety of **musculoskeletal pain** conditions; however, meaningful clinical trials have not been reported. Butterbur has also undergone highly preliminary investigation for treatment of **asthma** and for protecting the stomach lining from injury, thereby helping to prevent **ulcers**.

Preliminary evidence suggests that butterbur is *not* likely to be particularly effective for allergic skin diseases, such as **eczema**.

What Is the Scientific Evidence for Butterbur?

Migraines

Two double-blind, placebo-controlled studies suggest that butterbur extract may be helpful for preventing migraines, although the optimum dosage is not clear.

Butterbur extract was tested as a migraine preventive in a double-blind, placebo-controlled study involving 60 men and women who experienced at least three migraines per month. After 4 weeks without any conventional medications, participants were randomly assigned to take either 50 mg of butterbur extract or placebo twice daily for 3 months.

The results were positive: both the number of migraine attacks and the total number of days of migraine pain were significantly reduced in the treatment group as compared to the placebo group. Three out of four individuals taking butterbur reported improvement, as compared to only one out of four in the placebo group. No significant side effects were noted.

In another double-blind, placebo-controlled study performed by different researchers, 202 people with migraine headaches received either 50 mg twice daily of butterbur extract, 75 mg twice daily, or placebo. Over the 3 months of the study, the frequency of migraine attacks gradually decreased in all three groups. However, the group receiving the higher dose of butterbur extract showed significantly greater improvement than those in the placebo group. The lower dose of butterbur failed to prove significantly more effective than placebo.

Based on these two studies, it does appear that butterbur extract is helpful for preventing migraines, and that 75 mg twice daily is more effective than 50 mg twice daily. However, further research is necessary to establish this with certainty.

Hay Fever (Allergic Rhinitis)

Butterbur appears to affect the immune system in ways that suggest it should be helpful for hay fever (technically, "seasonal allergic rhinitis"). On this basis, it has been tested as an allergy treatment, with positive results in substantial studies.

In a 2-week, double-blind, placebo-controlled study of 186 people with intermittent allergic rhinitis, use of butterbur at a dose of three tablets daily, or only one tablet daily, reduced allergy symptoms as compared to placebo. Significantly greater benefits were seen in the higher-dose group. Such "dose dependency" is generally taken as a confirming sign that a treatment really works.

In another double-blind study, 330 people were given either butterbur extract (one tablet three times daily), the antihistamine fexofenadine (Allegra), or placebo. The results showed that butterbur and fexofenadine were equally effective and both were more effective than placebo.

A previous 2-week, double-blind study of 125 individuals with hay fever compared a standardized butterbur extract against the antihistamine drug certizine. According to ratings by both doctors and patients, the two treatments proved about equally effective. Unfortunately, this study did not use a placebo group.

Two much smaller studies produced inconsistent results.

Dosage

The usual dosage of butterbur is 50–75 mg twice daily of a standardized extract that has been processed to remove potentially dangerous chemicals called *pyrrolizidine alkaloids* (see Safety Issues below).

Warning: Use of any butterbur product that contains pyrrolizidine alkaloids is definitely not recommended.

Safety Issues

In studies involving adults and children, burping and other mild gastrointestinal complaints have been the main side effect of butterbur extract.

Butterbur contains liver-toxic and possibly carcinogenic components called *pyrrolizidine alkaloids*. Fortunately, it is possible to remove these compounds from butterbur products. In Germany, the maximum allowable content of pyrrolizidine alkaloids in butterbur products has been set at 1 mcg per daily recommended dose.

Butterbur should not be used by pregnant or nursing women, young children, or people with severe kidney or liver disease, until further safety testing has been performed.

Calcium

SUPPLEMENT FORMS/ALTERNATE NAMES: *Bonemeal, Calcium Aspartate, Calcium Carbonate, Calcium Chelate, Calcium Citrate, Calcium Citrate Malate, Calcium Gluconate, Calcium Lactate, Calcium Orotate, Dolomite, Oyster Shell Calcium, Tricalcium Phosphate*

PRINCIPAL PROPOSED USES: *Osteoporosis, Premenstrual Syndrome (PMS)*

OTHER PROPOSED USES: *Attention Deficit Disorder, Colon Polyps and Cancer Prevention, Dysmenorrhea (Menstrual Pain), High Cholesterol, Hypertension, Migraine Headaches, Periodontal Disease, Polycystic Ovary Syndrome, Preeclampsia, Weight Loss*

Calcium is the most abundant mineral in the body, making up nearly 2% of total body weight. More than 99% of the calcium in your body is found in your bones, but the other 1% is perhaps just as important for good health. Many enzymes depend on calcium in order to work properly, as do your nerves, heart, and blood-clotting mechanisms.

To build bone, you need to have enough calcium in your diet. But in spite of calcium-fortified orange juice and the best efforts of the dairy industry, most Americans are calcium deficient. Calcium supplements are a simple way to make sure you're getting enough of this important mineral.

One of the most important uses of calcium is to help prevent and treat osteoporosis, the progressive loss of bone mass to which postmenopausal women are especially vulnerable. Calcium works best when combined with vitamin D.

Other meaningful evidence suggests that calcium may have an additional important use: reducing PMS symptoms.

Requirements/Sources

Although there are some variations between recommendations issued by different groups, the official U.S. and Canadian recommendations for daily intake of calcium are as follows:

- Infants 0–6 months, 210 mg
  7–12 months, 270 mg
- Children 1–3 years, 500 mg
  4–8 years, 800 mg
- Males and females 9–18 years, 1,300 mg
  19–50 years, 1,000 mg
  51 years and older, 1,200 mg
- Pregnant women 1,000 mg (1,300 mg if under 19 years old)
- Nursing women 1,000 mg (1,300 mg if under 19 years old)

To absorb calcium, your body also needs an adequate level of vitamin D (for more information, see the article on **vitamin D**).

Various medications may impair calcium absorption or metabolism, either directly or through effects on vitamin D. People who use these may benefit by taking extra calcium and vitamin D. Implicated medications include corticosteroids, heparin, isoniazid, and anticonvulsants. **Note**: Calcium carbonate might interfere with the effects of anticonvulsant drugs, and for that reason should not be taken at the same time of day.

Milk, cheese, and other dairy products are excellent sources of calcium. Other good sources include orange juice or soy milk fortified with calcium, fish canned with its bones (such as sardines), dark green vegetables, nuts and seeds, and calcium-processed tofu.

Many forms of calcium supplements are available on the market, each with its own advantages and disadvantages.

Naturally Derived Forms of Calcium

These forms of calcium come from bone, shells, or the earth: bonemeal, oyster shell, and dolomite. Animals concentrate calcium in their shells and calcium is found in minerals in the earth. These forms of calcium are economical and you can get as much as 500 to 600 mg in one tablet. However, there are concerns that the natural forms of calcium supplements may contain significant amounts of lead. The level of contamination has decreased in recent years, but still may present a health risk. Calcium supplements rarely list the lead content of their source, although they should. The lead concentration should always be less than 2 parts per million.

Refined Calcium Carbonate

This is the most common commercial calcium supplement and it is also used as a common antacid. Calcium carbonate is one of the least expensive forms of calcium, but it can cause constipation and bloating, and it may not be well absorbed by people with reduced levels of stomach acid. Taking it with meals improves absorption because stomach acid is released to digest the food. (See next section, Chelated Calcium.)

Chelated Calcium

Chelated calcium is calcium bound to an organic acid (citrate, citrate malate, lactate, gluconate, aspartate, or orotate). The chelated forms of calcium offer some significant advantages and disadvantages compared with calcium carbonate.

Certain forms of chelated calcium (calcium citrate and calcium citrate malate) are widely thought to be significantly better absorbed and more effective for osteoporosis treatment than calcium carbonate. However, while some studies support this belief, others do not. The discrepancy may be due to the particular calcium carbonate products used; some calcium carbonate formulations may dissolve better than others.

One study found that calcium citrate malate in orange juice is markedly better absorbed than tricalcium phosphate/calcium lactate in orange juice.

A form of calcium called *active absorbable algal calcium* (AAACa) has also been promoted as superior to calcium carbonate, but the study upon which claims of benefit are founded actually used quite questionable statistical methods (technically, post-hoc subgroup analysis).

Chelated calcium is much more expensive and bulkier than calcium carbonate. In other words, you have to take larger pills, and more of them, to get enough calcium. It is not at all uncommon to need to take five or six large capsules daily to supply the necessary amount, a quantity some people may find troublesome.

Therapeutic Dosages

Unlike some supplements, calcium is not taken at extra high doses for special therapeutic benefit. Rather, for all its uses it should be taken in the amounts listed under Requirements/Sources, along with the recommended level of vitamin D.

Calcium absorption studies have found evidence that your body can't absorb more than 500 mg of calcium at one time. Therefore, it is most efficient to take your total daily calcium in two or more doses.

Use of **prebiotics** known as "inulin fructans" may improve calcium absorption.

It isn't possible to put all the calcium you need in a single **multivitamin/mineral** tablet, so this is one supplement that should be taken on its own. Furthermore, if taken at the same time, calcium may interfere with the absorption of chromium and manganese. This means that it is best to take your multivitamin and mineral pill at a separate time from your calcium supplement.

Although the calcium present in some antacids or supplements may alter the absorption of **magnesium**, this effect apparently has no significant influence on overall magnesium status. Calcium may also interfere with iron absorption, but the effect may be too slight to cause a problem. Some studies show that calcium may decrease zinc absorption when the two are taken together as supplements; however, studies have found that, in the presence of meals, zinc levels may be unaffected by increases of either dietary or supplemental calcium.

Therapeutic Uses

According to most, though not all, studies, use of calcium (especially in the form of calcium citrate) combined with vitamin D may modestly slow the bone loss that leads to **osteoporosis**.

A rather surprising potential use of calcium came to light when a large, well-designed study found that calcium is an effective treatment for **premenstrual syndrome** (PMS). Calcium supplementation reduced all major symptoms, including headache, food cravings, moodiness, and fluid retention. It is at least remotely possible that there may be a connection between these two uses of calcium: weak evidence hints that PMS might be an early sign of future osteoporosis.

One small but carefully conducted study suggests that getting enough calcium may help control symptoms of **menstrual pain**.

Evidence is inconsistent on whether getting enough calcium may reduce the risk of developing colon **cancer** or colon polyps (a precancerous condition).

Individuals who are deficient in calcium may be at greater risk of developing **high blood pressure**. Among individuals who already have hypertension, increased intake of calcium might slightly decrease blood pressure, according to some but not all studies.

Calcium supplements might slightly improve the **cholesterol** profile.

One preliminary study suggests that supplementation with calcium and vitamin D may be helpful for women with polycystic ovary syndrome.

Calcium supplementation has also been tried as a treatment to prevent **preeclampsia** in pregnant women. While the evidence from studies is conflicting, calcium supplementation might offer at least a minimal benefit.

The drug metformin, used for diabetes, interferes with the absorption of **vitamin B_{12}**. Interestingly, calcium supplements may reverse this, allowing the B_{12} to be absorbed normally.

Rapid **weight loss** in overweight postmenopausal women appears to accelerate osteoporosis slightly. For this reason, taking calcium and vitamin D supplements may be especially appropriate for women on a severe weight-loss diet.

It has been suggested that calcium supplements, or high-calcium diets, may slightly enhance weight loss, but current evidence is inconsistent and, overall, more negative than positive.

Finally, calcium is also sometimes recommended for **attention deficit disorder**, **migraine headaches**, and **periodontal disease**, but there is as yet no meaningful evidence that it is effective for these conditions.

What Is the Scientific Evidence for Calcium?

Osteoporosis

A number of double-blind, placebo-controlled studies indicate that calcium supplements (especially as calcium citrate, and taken with vitamin D) are slightly helpful in preventing and slowing down bone loss in postmenopausal women. However, the effect is relatively mild, and may not be strong enough to reduce the rate of osteoporotic fractures. Note that use of calcium and vitamin D must be continual. Any improvements in bone rapidly disappear once the supplements are stopped. Calcium carbonate may not be effective. One study found benefits for male seniors using a calcium and vitamin D–fortified milk product. (See, however, possible increased risk of prostate cancer discussed in Safety Issues below.)

Calcium and vitamin D supplementation may help bones heal that have become fractured due to bone thinning.

Calcium supplements may do a better job of strengthening bones when people have relatively high protein intake.

Calcium supplementation might be useful for young girls as a way to "put calcium in the bank"—building up a supply for the future in order to prevent later osteoporosis; however, again the benefits appear to be relatively modest at most and may only reach a point of significance when exercise is also increased.

One study found that in calcium-deficient pregnant women, calcium supplements can improve the bones of their unborn children.

Evidence suggests that the use of calcium combined with vitamin D can help protect against the bone loss caused by corticosteroid drugs, such as prednisone. A review of five studies covering a total of 274 participants reported that calcium and vitamin D supplementation significantly prevented bone loss in corticosteroid-treated individuals. For example, in a 2-year, double-blind, placebo-controlled study that followed 65 individuals with rheumatoid arthritis taking low-dose corticosteroids, daily supplementation with 1,000 mg of calcium and 500 IU of vitamin D reversed steroid-induced bone loss, causing a net bone gain.

There is some evidence that essential fatty acids may enhance the effectiveness of calcium. In one study, 65 postmenopausal women were given calcium along with either placebo or a combination of omega-6 fatty acids (from **evening primrose oil**) and omega-3 fatty acids (from **fish oil**) for a period of 18 months. At the end of the study period, the group receiving essential fatty acids had higher bone density and fewer fractures than the placebo group. However, a 12-month, double-blind trial of 42 postmenopausal women found no benefit. The explanation for the discrepancy may lie in the differences between the women studied. The first study involved women living in nursing homes, while the second studied healthier women living on their own. The latter group of women may have been better nourished and already received enough essential fatty acids in their diet.

Premenstrual Syndrome (PMS)

According to a large and well-designed study published in a 1998 issue of *American Journal of Obstetrics and Gynecology*, calcium supplements are a simple and effective treatment for a wide variety of PMS symptoms. In a double-blind, placebo-controlled study of 497 women, 1,200 mg daily of calcium as calcium carbonate reduced PMS symptoms by half over a period of three menstrual cycles. These symptoms included mood swings, headaches, food cravings, and bloating. These results corroborate earlier, smaller studies.

High Cholesterol

In a 12-month study of 223 postmenopausal women, use of calcium citrate at a dose of 1 g daily improved the ratio of HDL ("good") cholesterol levels to LDL ("bad") cholesterol levels. The extent of this improvement was statistically significant (as compared to the placebo group), but not very large in practical terms. Similarly modest benefits were seen in a previous, smaller double-blind, placebo-controlled study. A third double-blind, placebo-controlled study failed to find any statistically significant effects.

Colon Cancer

Evidence from observational studies that a high calcium intake is associated with a reduced incidence of colon cancer, but not all studies have found this association.

Some but not all evidence from intervention trials supports these findings.

A 4-year, double-blind, placebo-controlled study followed 832 individuals with a history of colon polyps. Participants received either 3 g daily of calcium carbonate or placebo. The calcium group experienced 24% fewer polyps overall than the placebo group. Since colon polyps are the precursor of most colon cancer, this finding strongly suggests benefit. Another, similar sized study found that calcium carbonate at a dose of 1,200 mg daily may have a more pronounced effect on dangerous polyps than on benign ones. However, a gigantic (36,282 participant), very long-term (average 7 years) study of post-menopausal women failed to find that calcium carbonate supplements at a dose of 1,000 mg daily had any effect on the incidence of colon cancer.

The reason for these discrepancies remains unclear.

It is possible that an inadequate dose of calcium was used in the large study just mentioned.

Safety Issues

In general, it's safe to take up to 2,500 mg of calcium daily, although this is more than you need. Greatly excessive intake of calcium can cause numerous side effects, including dangerous or painful deposits of calcium within the body.

Note: If you have cancer, hyperparathyroidism, or sarcoidosis, you should take calcium only under a physician's supervision.

Some evidence hints that use of calcium supplements might slightly increase **kidney stone** risk. However, increased intake of calcium from *food* does not seem to have this effect, and could even help prevent stones. One study found that if calcium supplements are taken with food, there is no increased risk. Calcium citrate supplements may be particularly safe regarding kidney stones because the citrate portion of this supplement is used to *treat* kidney stones.

Large observational studies have found that, in men, higher intakes of calcium are associated with an increased risk of **prostate cancer**. This seems to be the case whether the calcium comes from milk or from calcium supplements.

Calcium supplements combined with high doses of vitamin D might interfere with some of the effects of drugs in the calcium channel blocker family. It is very important that you consult your physician before trying this combination.

Concerns have been raised that the aluminum in some antacids may not be good for you. There is some evidence that calcium citrate supplements might increase the absorption of aluminum; for this reason, it might not be a good idea to take calcium citrate at the same time of day as aluminum-containing antacids. Another option is to use different forms of calcium or to avoid antacids containing aluminum.

When taken over the long term, thiazide diuretics tend to increase levels of calcium in the body by decreasing the amount excreted by the body. It's not likely that this will cause a problem. Nonetheless, if you are using thiazide diuretics, you should consult with your physician on the proper doses of calcium and vitamin D for you.

Finally, calcium may interfere with the absorption of antibiotics in the tetracycline and fluoroquinolone families as well as thyroid hormone. If you are taking any of these drugs, you should take your calcium supplements at least 2 hours before or after your medication dose.

Interactions You Should Know About

If you are taking:

- Corticosteroids, heparin, or isoniazid: You may need more calcium.
- Aluminum hydroxide: You should take calcium citrate at least 2 hours apart to avoid increasing aluminum absorption.
- The anticonvulsants phenytoin (Dilantin), carbamazepine, phenobarbital, or primidone: You may need more calcium; however, it may be advisable to take your dose of anticonvulsant and your calcium supplement at least 2 hours apart because each interferes with the other's absorption.
- Antibiotics in the tetracycline or fluoroquinolone (Cipro, Floxin, Noroxin) families or thyroid hormone: You should take your calcium supplement at least 2 hours before or after your dose of medication because calcium interferes with the absorption of these medications (and vice versa).
- Thiazide diuretics: Do not take extra calcium except on the advice of a physician.
- Calcium channel blockers: Do not take calcium together with high-dose vitamin D except on the advice of a physician.
- Calcium: You may need extra iron, manganese, zinc, and chromium. Ideally, you should take calcium at a different time of day from these other minerals because it may interfere with their absorption.
- Soy: A constituent of soy called *phytic acid* can interfere with the absorption of calcium, so it may be advisable to wait 2 hours after taking calcium supplements to eat soy (or vice versa).
- Metformin: Taking supplemental calcium may be helpful.

Calendula

PRINCIPAL PROPOSED USES: *Canker Sores, Eczema, Hemorrhoids, Minor Burns, Minor Wounds, Varicose Veins*

Calendula, well known as one of the ornamental marigolds, blooms month after month from early spring to first frost. Because *calend* means "month" in Latin, the plant's lengthy flowering season is believed to have given calendula its name. The herb has been used to heal wounds and treat inflamed skin since ancient times.

An active ingredient that might be responsible for calendula's traditional medicinal properties has not been discovered. One theory suggests that volatile oils in the plant act synergistically with other constituents called *xanthophylls.*

What Is Calendula Used for Today?

Experiments on rats and other animals suggest that calendula cream exerts wound-healing and anti-inflammatory effects, but double-blind, placebo-controlled studies have not yet been reported. The best study on calendula so far was a controlled trial comparing calendula to the standard treatment trolamine for the prevention of skin irritation caused by radiation therapy. Interestingly, the researchers used trolamine for comparison not because it has been proven effective but more as a kind of acceptable placebo (trolamine is not thought to do very much, even though it's widely used). The study found calendula more effective than trolamine. However, because this was not a double-blind study, the results mean little; mere expectation of benefit is likely to cause patients and experimenters to perceive benefit.

Creams made with calendula flower are a nearly ubiquitous item in the German medicine chest, used for everything from children's scrapes to **eczema**, burns, and poorly healing wounds. These same German products are widely available in the United States as well.

Calendula cream is also used to soothe **hemorrhoids** and **varicose veins**, and the tea reportedly reduces the discomfort of **canker sores**. However, as yet there is no scientific evidence for any of these uses.

Dosage

Calendula cream is generally applied 2 or 3 times daily to the affected area. For oral use as a mouthwash, pour boiling water over 1 to 2 teaspoons of calendula flowers and allow to steep for 10 to 15 minutes.

Safety Issues

Calendula is generally regarded as safe. Neither calendula cream nor calendula taken internally has been associated with any adverse effects other than occasional allergic reactions and animal studies have found no significant toxic effects. However, the same studies found that in high doses, calendula acts like a sedative and also reduces blood pressure. For this reason, it might not be safe to combine calendula with sedative or blood pressure medications.

Interactions You Should Know About

If you are taking:

> - **Sedative drugs: Calendula might increase the sedative effect.**
> - **Medications to reduce blood pressure: Internal use of calendula might amplify the blood pressure-lowering effect.**

Candytuft

Iberis amara

ALTERNATE NAMES/RELATED TERMS: *Clown's Mustard*
PRINCIPAL PROPOSED USES: *Dyspepsia (in Herbal Combinations)*
OTHER PROPOSED USES: *Gastrointestinal Side Effects Caused by Medications, Irritable Bowel Syndrome*

Candytuft, also known as *clown's mustard*, is a white flowering plant found originally in Spain. It's a member of the *Brassicaceae* family, making it a relative of cabbage and broccoli. Traditionally, it was used in the treatment of arthritis, gout, enlarged heart, and asthma. The seeds, stems, roots, and leaves have all been used medicinally.

What Is Candytuft Used for Today?

Candytuft is widely used in Germany for treatment of **dyspepsia**. This term indicates chronic digestive distress that occurs in the absence of any identifiable cause, such as an ulcer. Symptoms include stomach discomfort, gas, bloating, belching, appetite loss, and nausea.

Several studies, enrolling a total of hundreds of participants, have found benefits for dyspepsia with use of an herbal combination therapy containing candytuft as the primary ingredient.

The other herbs in the combination are **matricaria flower**, **peppermint leaves**, caraway, **licorice root**, and **lemon balm**. Some studies utilized an augmented preparation containing angelica root, celandine, and **milk thistle** as well. In the subsequent text, we shall refer to the first mixture as the *primary* candytuft combination and the augmented one as the *modified* preparation.

Besides dyspepsia, candytuft combinations have shown potential for decreasing the gastrointestinal side effects caused by a variety of medications and for reducing lower digestive tract symptoms of **irritable bowel syndrome**.

What Is the Scientific Evidence for Candytuft?

A double-blind, placebo-controlled trial of 120 people with dyspepsia evaluated the primary candytuft combination described above. The study design was somewhat complicated, but in essence it found that 4 weeks of treatment with candytuft was more effective than placebo in reducing dyspepsia symptoms.

In another double-blind study, this one enrolling 60 people with dyspepsia, use of either the primary or the modified candytuft herbal combination proved more effective than placebo.

Benefits with the primary mixture were also seen in two other double-blind, placebo-controlled studies enrolling a total of about 200 people. In addition, a double-blind comparative study found that both candytuft combinations were equally effective as the standard drug cisapride.

Dosage

A typical dosage of the tested candytuft preparation is 20 drops 3 times daily.

Safety Issues

In controlled clinical trials, use of the tested candytuft preparation has not resulted in any significant side effects. Note that the studied preparation is manufactured in Germany under conditions that are more closely regulated than herbal manufacturing in the U.S. Formulations made outside of Germany might present unrecognized safety risks. Even with the tested product, comprehensive safety studies have not been performed. Safety for pregnant or nursing women, young children, or individuals with severe liver or kidney disease has not been established.

Caraway
Carum carvi

PRINCIPAL PROPOSED USES: *Dyspepsia (Non-specific Indigestion), Intestinal Gas*

OTHER PROPOSED USES:

Oral: *Irritable Bowel Syndrome*

Topical: *Canker Sores, Periodontal Disease*

Caraway has a long history of use as a *carminative*, an herb said to relieve gas pain. Mentions of caraway for digestive problems can be found in Egyptian records, and the herb has been used in Europe for this purpose since at least the Middle Ages. The seeds or their **essential oil** are the part of the plant used medicinally.

What Is Caraway Used for Today?

Only double-blind, placebo-controlled studies can prove a treatment effective, and thus far such studies have not been performed on caraway alone. (For more information on why such studies are essential, see **Why Does This Book Rely on Double-blind Studies?**) However, a few double-blind studies have been reported on combination products containing caraway oil for the treatment of **dyspepsia** (non-specific stomach distress).

For example, a double-blind, placebo-controlled study of 39 people found that an enteric-coated **peppermint oil** and caraway oil combination taken 3 times daily by mouth for 4 weeks significantly reduced dyspepsia pain as compared to placebo. Of the treatment group, 63.2% of participants were pain-free after 4 weeks, compared to 25% of the placebo group. In other double-blind, placebo-controlled studies, a combination of caraway, **bitter candytuft**, **feverfew**, peppermint leaves, **licorice root**, and **lemon balm** also proved effective for dyspepsia.

Double-blind comparative studies have also been reported. One such study of 118 people found that the combination of peppermint and caraway oil was about as effective as the standard drug cisapride (a drug used for dyspepsia that is no longer available). After 4 weeks,

the herbal combination reduced dyspepsia pain by 69.7%, whereas the conventional treatment reduced pain by 70.2%. Finally, a preparation of peppermint, caraway, fennel, and wormwood oil was compared to the drug metoclopramide in a double-blind study enrolling 60 people. After 7 days, 43.3% of the treatment group was pain-free, compared to 13.3% of the metoclopramide group.

Far weaker evidence hints that caraway extracts may have **anti-cancer**, antibacterial, and **antidiabetic** actions. However, the evidence for these potential benefits is far too weak to rely on.

Caraway oil is said to be helpful for **irritable bowel syndrome**. Teas made from caraway are recommended for **periodontal disease** and **canker sores**. However, there is no meaningful supporting evidence for any of these uses.

Dosage

A typical dose of caraway is 0.05 to 0.2 ml of the essential oil taken 3 times daily.

Safety Issues

Caraway is generally regarded as safe when used in recommended doses. However, essential oils can be toxic to very young children, and excessive doses could be dangerous for adults as well. Maximum safe dosages in young children, pregnant or nursing women, or people with severe liver or kidney disease have not been established.

Carnitine

SUPPLEMENT FORMS/ALTERNATE NAMES: *Acetyl-L-Carnitine (ALC), L-Acetyl-Carnitine (LAC), L-Carnitine, Propionyl-L-Carnitine*

PRINCIPAL PROPOSED USES: *Angina, Chronic Obstructive Pulmonary Disease, Congestive Heart Failure, Diabetic Peripheral Neuropathy, Heart Attack, Hyperthyroidism, Intermittent Claudication, Male Infertility, Male Sexual Dysfunction, Peyronie's Disease*

OTHER PROPOSED USES: *Alzheimer's Disease, Chronic Fatigue Syndrome, Depression, Diabetes, Diabetic Cardiac Autonomic Neuropathy, High Cholesterol, HIV Support (Toxicity Caused by AZT), Hyperactivity in Fragile X Syndrome, Sports Performance Enhancement, Weight Loss*

Carnitine is an amino acid the body uses to turn fat into energy. It is not normally considered an essential nutrient because the body can manufacture all it needs. However, supplemental carnitine could in theory improve the ability of certain tissues to produce energy. This has led to the use of carnitine for various muscle diseases as well as heart conditions.

Sources

There is no dietary requirement for carnitine. However, a few individuals have a genetic defect that hinders the body's ability to make carnitine. In addition, diseases of the liver, kidneys, or brain may inhibit carnitine production. Certain medications, especially the antiseizure drugs valproic acid (Depakene) and phenytoin (Dilantin), may reduce carnitine levels; however, whether taking extra carnitine would be helpful has not been determined. Heart muscle tissue, because of its high energy requirements, is particularly vulnerable to carnitine deficiency.

The principal dietary sources of carnitine are meat and dairy products, but to obtain therapeutic dosages a supplement is necessary.

Therapeutic Dosages

Typical adult dosages for the diseases described here range from 500 to 1,000 mg three times daily. For children, one study used 50 mg/kg twice daily, up to a maximum of 4 g daily.

Carnitine is taken in three forms: L-carnitine (for heart and other conditions), propionyl-L-carnitine (for heart conditions), and acetyl-L-carnitine (for Alzheimer's disease). The dosage is the same for all three forms.

Therapeutic Uses

Carnitine is primarily used for heart-related conditions. Some evidence suggests that it can be used along with conventional treatment for **angina** to improve symptoms and reduce medication needs. When combined with conventional therapy, it may or may not help prevent medical complications or sudden cardiac death in the months following a **heart attack**.

Lesser evidence suggests that it may be helpful for a condition called *intermittent claudication* (pain in the legs after walking due to narrowing of the arteries), as well as for **congestive heart failure**. In addition, a few studies suggest that carnitine may be useful for **cardiomyopathy**.

Carnitine may also be helpful for improving exercise tolerance in people with **chronic pulmonary obstruction disease** (COPD), more commonly known as emphysema.

Warning: You should not attempt to self-treat any of these serious medical conditions, nor should you use carnitine as a substitute for standard drugs.

Growing, if not entirely consistent, evidence suggests that L-carnitine or acetyl-L-carnitine, or their combination, may be helpful for improving sperm function. If true, this would mean that carnitine could be helpful for some forms of **male infertility**.

Carnitine has also shown promise for improving **male sexual function** and improving mental and physical **fatigue** in seniors.

Two studies found evidence that carnitine is helpful for **Peyronie's disease**, a condition affecting the penis.

Some studies have found evidence that one particular form of carnitine, acetyl-L-carnitine, might be helpful in **Alzheimer's disease**, but the two most recent and largest studies found no benefit. One review evaluated published and unpublished double-blind, placebo-controlled trials and concluded that acetyl-L-carnitine may only be helpful for very mild Alzheimer's disease.

In preliminary trials, acetyl-L-carnitine has shown some promise for treatment of **depression** or dysthymia (a milder condition related to depression).

Some evidence suggests that carnitine may be useful for improving blood sugar control in people with type 2 (adult-onset) **diabetes.** Better evidence suggests benefit with acetyl-L-carnitine for a major complication of diabetes, **diabetic peripheral neuropathy** (injury to nerves of the extremities caused by diabetes). Acetyl-L-carnitine might help prevent diabetic cardiac autonomic neuropathy (injury to the nerves of the heart caused by diabetes). However, one study found that carnitine supplements had an adverse effect on **triglyceride levels** in people with diabetes.

Much weaker evidence suggests possible benefits for neuropathy caused by the chemotherapy drugs **cisplatin** and paclitaxel.

Some evidence suggests that carnitine may be able to improve **cholesterol profile**.

A genetic condition called *fragile X syndrome* can cause behavioral disturbances, such as hyperactivity, along with mental retardation, autism, and alterations in appearance. A preliminary study of 17 boys found that acetyl-L-carnitine might help to reduce hyperactive behavior associated with this condition. Ordinary carnitine has shown a bit of promise for **attention deficit and hyperactivity disorder** (ADHD).

Weak evidence hints that carnitine may help people with degeneration of the cerebellum (the structure of the brain responsible for voluntary muscular movement). One very small study suggests carnitine may be helpful for reducing symptoms of **chronic fatigue syndrome**. Another study suggests that carnitine may be of value for treating **hyperthyroidism** and severe liver disease.

Weak evidence also suggests that carnitine may be helpful for decreasing the toxicity of AZT (a drug used to treat **AIDS**).

One study failed to find carnitine effective for promoting **weight loss**, although another found that carnitine might lead to improvements in body composition (fat–muscle ratio).

Carnitine is widely touted as a physical **performance enhancer**, but there is no real evidence that it is effective, and some research indicates that it is not.

Little to no evidence supports other claimed benefits, such as treating irregular heartbeat, Down's syndrome, muscular dystrophy, and alcoholic fatty liver disease.

What Is the Scientific Evidence for Carnitine?

Angina

Carnitine might be a good addition to standard therapy for angina. In one controlled study, 200 individuals with angina (the exercise-induced variety) took either 2 g daily of L-carnitine or were left untreated. All the study participants continued to take their usual medication for angina. Those taking carnitine showed improvement in several measures of heart function, including a significantly greater ability to exercise without chest pain. They were also able to reduce the dosages of some of their heart medications (under medical supervision) as their symptoms decreased.

Unfortunately, the results of this study can't be fully trusted because researchers didn't use a double-blind protocol. (For more information on why double-blinding is so important, see **Why Does This Book Rely on Double-blind Studies?**.) Another trial that did use a double-blind, placebo-controlled design tested L-carnitine in 52 people with angina and found evidence of benefit.

In addition, several small studies (some of them double-blind) tested propionyl-L-carnitine for the treatment of angina and also found evidence of benefit.

Intermittent Claudication

People with advanced hardening of the arteries, or **atherosclerosis**, often have difficulty walking due to lack of blood flow to the legs, a condition called *intermittent claudication*. Pain may develop after walking less than half a block. Although carnitine does not increase blood flow, it appears to improve the muscle's ability to function under difficult circumstances. A 12-month, double-blind, placebo-controlled trial of 485 patients with intermittent claudication evaluated the potential benefits of propionyl-L-carnitine. Participants with relatively severe disease showed a 44% improvement in walking distance as compared to placebo. However, no improvement was seen in those with mild disease. Another double-blind study followed 245 people and also found benefit.

Similar results have been seen in most but not all other studies of L-carnitine or propionyl-L-carnitine. Propionyl-L-carnitine may be more effective for intermittent claudication than plain carnitine.

Congestive Heart Failure

Several small studies have found that carnitine, often in the form of propionyl-L-carnitine, can improve symptoms

Carnitine

of congestive heart failure. In one trial, benefits were maintained for 60 days after treatment with carnitine was stopped.

After a Heart Attack

L-carnitine has shown inconsistent promise for use after a heart attack.

A double-blind, placebo-controlled study that followed 101 people for 1 month after a heart attack found that use of L-carnitine, in addition to standard care, reduced the size of the infarct (dead heart tissue).

In the months following a severe heart attack, the left ventricle of the heart often enlarges and the pumping action of the heart becomes less efficient. Some evidence suggests that L-carnitine can help prevent heart enlargement, but that it does not improve heart function. In a 12-month, double-blind, placebo-controlled study of 472 individuals who had just undergone a heart attack, use of carnitine at a dose of 6 g/day significantly decreased the rate of heart enlargement. However, heart function was not significantly altered.

A 3-month, double-blind, placebo-controlled study of 60 individuals who had just undergone a heart attack also failed to find improvements in heart function. (Heart enlargement was not studied.)

Results consistent with those of the studies above were seen in a 6-month, double-blind, placebo-controlled study of 2,330 people who had just had a heart attack. Carnitine failed to produce significant reductions in mortality or heart failure (serious decline in heart function) over the 6-month period. However, the study did find reductions in early death. (Unfortunately, for statistical reasons, the meaningfulness of this last finding is questionable: reduction in early death was a secondary endpoint rather than a primary one.)

Note: Carnitine is used along with conventional treatment, not as a substitute for it.

Diabetic Neuropathy

High levels of blood sugar can damage the nerves leading to the extremities, causing pain and numbness. This condition is called *diabetic peripheral neuropathy*. Nerve damage may also develop in the heart, a condition called *cardiac autonomic neuropathy*. Acetyl-L-carnitine has shown considerable promise for diabetic peripheral neuropathy and some promise for cardiac autonomic neuropathy.

Two 52-week, double-blind, placebo-controlled studies, involving a total of 1,257 people with diabetic peripheral neuropathy, evaluated the potential benefits of ALC taken at 500 mg or 1,000 mg daily. The results showed that use of ALC, especially at the higher dose, improved sensory perception and decreased pain levels. In addition, the supplement appeared to promote nerve fiber regeneration.

A small study found some potential benefits for cardiac autonomic neuropathy.

Male Sexual Function

Carnitine has shown promise for improving male sexual function. One double-blind, placebo-controlled study of 120 subjects compared a combination of propionyl-L-carnitine (2 g per day) and acetyl-L-carnitine (2 g per day) against testosterone for the treatment of male aging symptoms (sexual dysfunction, depression, and fatigue). The results indicated that both testosterone and carnitine improved erectile function, mood, and fatigue, as compared to placebo. However, no improvements were seen in the placebo group. This is an unusual occurrence in studies of erectile dysfunction so it casts some doubt on the study results.

A double-blind study of 40 men evaluated propionyl-L-carnitine (2 g per day) in diabetic men with erectile dysfunction who had not responded well to Viagra. The results indicated that carnitine significantly enhanced the effectiveness of Viagra.

In another double-blind study, a combination of the propionyl and acetyl forms of carnitine enhanced the effectiveness of Viagra in men who suffered from erectile dysfunction caused by prostate surgery.

Male Infertility

Growing evidence suggests that L-carnitine or acetyl-L-carnitine or their combination may be helpful for improving sperm quality and function, thereby potentially aiding male fertility.

For example, in one double-blind, placebo-controlled study of 60 men, use of combined L-carnitine (2 g per day) and acetyl-L-carnitine (also at 2 g per day) significantly improved sperm quality.

Chronic Obstructive Pulmonary Disease (COPD)

Evidence from three double-blind, placebo-controlled studies enrolling a total of 49 people suggests that L-carnitine can improve exercise tolerance in COPD, presumably by improving muscular efficiency in the lungs and other muscles.

Alzheimer's Disease

Numerous double- or single-blind studies involving a total of more than 1,400 people have evaluated the potential benefits of acetyl-L-carnitine in the treatment of Alzheimer's disease and other forms of dementia. However, while early studies found evidence of modest benefit, two large and well-designed studies failed to find acetyl-L-carnitine effective at all.

The first of these was a double-blind, placebo-controlled trial that enrolled 431 participants for 1 year. Overall, acetyl-L-carnitine proved no better than placebo. However, because a close look at the data indicated that the supplement might help people who develop Alzheimer's disease at an unusually young age, researchers performed a follow-up trial. This 1-year, double-blind, placebo-controlled trial evaluated acetyl-L-carnitine in 229 patients with early onset Alzheimer's. Unfortunately, no benefits were seen here either.

One review of the literature concluded that acetyl-L-carnitine may be helpful for mild cases of Alzheimer's disease, but not more severe cases.

Mild Depression

A double-blind study of 60 seniors with dysthymia (a mild form of depression) found that treatment with 3 g of carnitine daily over a 2-month period significantly improved symptoms as compared to placebo. Positive results were seen in two other studies as well, one of depression and one of dysthymia.

Hyperthyroidism

Enlargement of the thyroid (goiter) can be due to many causes, including cancer and iodine deficiency. In some cases, thyroid enlargement occurs without any known cause, so-called benign goiter.

Treatment of benign goiter generally consists of taking thyroid hormone pills. This causes the thyroid gland to become less active and the goiter shrinks. However, there may be undesirable effects as well. Symptoms of hyperthyroidism (too much thyroid hormone) can develop, including heart palpitations, nervousness, weight loss, and bone breakdown.

A double-blind, placebo-controlled trial found evidence that use of L-carnitine could alleviate many of these symptoms. This 6-month study evaluated the effects of L-carnitine in 50 women who were taking thyroid hormone for benign goiter. The results showed that a dose of 2 or 4 g of carnitine daily protected participants' bones and reduced other symptoms of hyperthyroidism.

Carnitine is thought to affect thyroid hormone by blocking its action in cells. This suggests a potential concern: carnitine might be harmful for people who have low or borderline thyroid levels to begin with. This possibility has not been well explored as yet.

Peyronie's Disease

Peyronie's disease is an inflammatory condition of the penis that develops in stages. In the first stage, penile pain occurs with erection; next, the penis becomes curved; finally, erectile dysfunction may occur. Many medications have been tried for Peyronie's disease, with some success. One such drug is tamoxifen (better known as a treatment to prevent breast cancer recurrence). A 3-month double-blind study compared the effectiveness of acetyl-L-carnitine to the drug tamoxifen in 48 men with Peyronie's disease. Acetyl-L-carnitine (at a dose of 1 g daily) reduced penile curvature while tamoxifen did not; in addition, the supplement reduced pain and slowed disease progression to a greater extent than tamoxifen.

Safety Issues

L-carnitine in its three forms appears to be quite safe. However, individuals with low or borderline-low thyroid levels should avoid carnitine because it might impair the action of thyroid hormone.

Individuals on dialysis should not receive this (or any other supplement) without a physician's supervision.

The maximum safe dosages for young children, pregnant or nursing women, or those with severe liver or kidney disease have not been established.

Interactions You Should Know About

If you are taking:

➤ **Antiseizure medications, particularly valproic acid (Depakote, Depakene) but also phenytoin (Dilantin): You may need extra carnitine.**
➤ **Thyroid medication: Do not take carnitine except under a physician's supervision.**

Carnosine

SUPPLEMENT FORMS/ALTERNATE NAMES: *L-Carnosine*

PRINCIPAL PROPOSED USES: *Anti-aging Nutrient*

OTHER PROPOSED USES: *Alzheimer's Disease and Related Conditions, Autism, Cataracts*

L-carnosine, not to be confused with **L-carnitine**, is a substance manufactured in the human body, made by combining the amino acids alanine and histidine. The highest levels of carnosine are found in the brain and nervous system, the lens of the eye, and skeletal muscle tissue. Its exact function in the body is not known.

Requirements/Sources

The body manufactures carnosine from common dietary proteins and, for this reason, there is no daily requirement of this substance.

Therapeutic Dosages

Among advocates of carnosine, there is a controversy regarding whether the proper dose is 50 to 150 mg per day or nearer to 1,000 mg daily. However, until carnosine has actually been shown to have any medical benefits, this argument cannot be settled.

Therapeutic Uses

Carnosine is widely marketed as an anti-aging nutrient. However, while there are a large *number* of studies that hint carnosine might help slow various aspects of aging, the quality of these studies is as yet far too low to provide any reliable evidence for benefit.

There is some actual evidence that carnosine may be helpful for children with **autistic spectrum disorders**. In a double-blind, placebo-controlled trial, 31 children with autism were given either carnosine (400 mg twice daily) or placebo for a period of 8 weeks. The results showed that children given carnosine showed significant improvements compared to those given placebo. While this was too small a trial to allow definitive conclusions, it is definitely promising.

Like numerous other substances, carnosine has **antioxidant properties**, meaning that it neutralizes dangerous, naturally occurring substances called *free radicals*.

Free radicals are thought to play a role in many illnesses and, on this basis, many antioxidant substances have been studied for potential health-promoting properties. The best evaluated are **beta-carotene**, **vitamin E**, and **vitamin C**. However, despite massive amounts of research, these supplements have yet to live up to their apparent promise. Some websites claim that carnosine acts as an antioxidant in a unique way, fighting the "second wave" effects that follow attacks by free radicals. However, there is no meaningful evidence to support this theory or the hypothesis that such an effect, if it truly exists, would provide any health benefits.

Other weak evidence hints that oral carnosine might be helpful for **cataracts**, **wound healing**, **Alzheimer's disease** and other forms of dementia, and various forms of **heart disease**.

Safety Issues

The use of carnosine has not been associated with any significant side effects. However, the body deploys a range of enzymes, called *carnosinases*, to break down carnosine. There may be a reason for the presence of these enzymes, and overcoming them by providing large amounts of supplemental carnosine could conceivably cause harm in some as-yet unrecognized way. Maximum safe doses in young children, pregnant or nursing women, or people with severe liver or kidney disease have not been established.

Carob

Carob

ALTERNATE NAMES/RELATED TERMS: *Locust Bean Gum*
PRINCIPAL PROPOSED USES: *Diarrhea, High Cholesterol*
OTHER PROPOSED USES: *Esophageal Reflux in Infants*

Carob is a warm-climate tree that grows up to 50 feet in height. Its long, reddish pods contain seeds used as medicine and food. The seed consists of three different parts: the outer husk, the nutritive endosperm (analogous to the white edible portion of the coconut), and the inner seed, or germ. The endosperm is converted to locust bean gum, a thickening agent used in numerous prepared foods. The entire pod, when dried and ground, is called *carob powder*. Carob powder is used both as a chocolate-like flavoring and as a medicinal substance for treatment of diarrhea.

What Is Carob Used for Today?

Carob is rich in insoluble fiber. Like other sources of fiber, carob has shown some promise for improving **cholesterol** profile. In a small (58-participant), double-blind, placebo-controlled study, use of carob powder at a dose of 15 g daily significantly reduced levels of LDL ("bad") cholesterol as compared to placebo.

Carob also contains tannins, astringent substances found in many plants. Foods rich in tannins are often recommended for treatment of diarrhea. (Your mother may have recommended black tea when you came down with diarrhea, on the same principle.) A double-blind clinical trial of 41 infants with diarrhea found that carob powder (at a dose of 1 g per kilogram per day) significantly speeded resolution of diarrhea as compared to placebo.

The portion of carob that is made into locust bean gum contains soluble fiber in the galactomannan family. Like other forms of soluble fiber, it has shown potential (though it has not been proven) benefit for enhancing **weight loss** and controlling **blood sugar levels**.

Some infants have a tendency to regurgitate after eating. A small, double-blind, placebo-controlled study found that use of locust bean gum as a thickening agent in baby formula significantly reduced the amount and frequency of regurgitation.

Dosage

A typical dose of carob powder for the treatment of diarrhea or high cholesterol in adults is 15 to 20 g daily. The dose is reduced proportionately by weight for treating diarrhea in children. Like other fiber sources, carob should be taken with plenty of water. Note that severe diarrhea in children or infants requires professional medical care.

Safety Issues

Carob powder and locust bean gum, as widely consumed foods, are believed to have a high degree of safety. Locust bean gum has been extensively evaluated and found noncarcinogenic and nontoxic. There are no known risks in pregnant or nursing women.

Cartilage

SUPPLEMENT FORMS/ALTERNATE NAMES: *Bovine Cartilage, Shark Cartilage*

PRINCIPAL PROPOSED USES: *None*

OTHER PROPOSED USES: *Cancer Treatment, Minor Wounds, Osteoarthritis, Psoriasis*

Cartilage is a tough connective tissue found in many parts of the body. Your ears and nose are made from cartilage and so is the gliding surface in your joints.

One constituent of cartilage, **chondroitin**, is widely used in Europe to treat osteoarthritis. Cartilage itself has also been proposed as a treatment for osteoarthritis.

The most commonly used forms of cartilage come from cows (bovine cartilage) and sharks. Provocative evidence suggests that shark cartilage might have some value in the treatment of cancer. However, properly designed studies have not yet been completed to tell us whether it really works.

Sources

Unless your uncle works at a slaughterhouse or you're brave enough to prepare your own cartilage from whole sharks, the preferred source of cartilage is your health food store or pharmacy, where you can purchase this supplement in pill or powdered form.

Therapeutic Dosages

Various doses of cartilage have been used in different studies, ranging from 2.5 mg to 60 g daily.

Therapeutic Uses

Based on the belief that sharks don't get cancer, shark cartilage has been heavily marketed as a cure for **cancer**. While this justification is a myth (sharks do get cancer), shark cartilage has, in fact, shown some promise for cancer treatment. Shark cartilage (like other forms of cartilage) contains substances that tend to inhibit *angiogenesis* (the growth of new blood vessels). Since cancers must build new blood vessels to feed themselves, this effect might be beneficial. Double-blind, placebo-controlled studies on special formulations of shark cartilage for the treatment of cancer are now underway. It has also been suggested that the antiangiogenic properties of shark cartilage may make it helpful for **psoriasis**, but this hypothesis has not yet undergone proper study.

Shark cartilage also inhibits substances called *matrix metalloproteases* (MMPs). These little-understood enzymes affect the "extracellular matrix," the framework of substances that lie between cells in the body. MMPs are thought to play a role in diseases of the cornea, gums, skin, blood vessels, and joints, as well as cancer and illnesses that involve excessive fibrous tissue. On this basis, shark cartilage has been proposed for a wide variety of medical conditions, from **cataracts** to **scleroderma**; however, there are no meaningful studies as yet that can tell us whether it offers any benefit.

Cartilage in general has been proposed as a treatment for the common "wear and tear" type of arthritis known as **osteoarthritis**. The idea behind this is straightforward: because osteoarthritis is a disease of the joints and because cartilage is one of the elements that make up your joints, adding cartilage to the diet might help. This idea sounds a bit too simplistic to be believable, but it is the same principle behind the use of **glucosamine** and chondroitin (specific substances found in the joints) for osteoarthritis. Since well-designed studies have found those treatments effective, perhaps cartilage itself will ultimately be proven to work. However, such studies of cartilage have not yet been performed.

Finally, highly preliminary studies hint that cartilage may help heal **minor wounds**.

What Is the Scientific Evidence for Cartilage?

A number of test tube experiments have found that shark cartilage extracts prevent new blood vessels from forming in chick embryos and other test systems. As mentioned above, this effect could conceivably mean that shark cartilage might fight cancer. These findings have led to other test tube experiments, animal studies, and preliminary human trials to investigate the possible anticancer effects of shark cartilage. The results suggest that a particular liquid shark cartilage extract might be useful in the treatment of various cancers, including lung, prostate, and breast cancer. However, not all studies have been positive.

In any case, only double-blind, placebo-controlled trials can provide conclusive data. (For information on why such studies are essential, see **Why Does This Book Rely on Double-blind Studies?**) So far, the only reported study of this type on shark cartilage for cancer failed to find benefit.

Safety Issues

Because cartilage is just common, ordinary gristle, it is presumably safe to consume. However, for reasons that are not at all clear at this time, there is a report of an individual who developed liver inflammation after taking shark cartilage supplements. He recovered fully when the supplements were discontinued.

Catnip
Nepeta cataria

PRINCIPAL PROPOSED USES: *None*

OTHER PROPOSED USES: *Indigestion (especially when caused by stress), Insomnia*

Although catnip has a stimulating effect on virtually all felines, in humans it is traditionally used as a sleep aid. It has also been used for digestive and menstrual problems, as a uterine stimulant in childbirth, and as a symptomatic treatment for colds. Publications from the late 1960s suggested that the plant, when smoked, produced a psychedelic high not unlike marijuana, but it was later discovered that the researchers had, in fact, mixed up the two plants.

What Is Catnip Used for Today?

Catnip is primarily used by today's herbalists as a treatment for **insomnia**, as well as for mild stomach upset, especially when caused by stress. One ingredient of catnip, trans-cis-nepetalactone, is the active ingredient so far as cats are concerned. Most (but not all) cats respond to this substance with a complex reaction called the *catnip response* that can go on for about an hour.

Nepetalactone is similar to a class of substances called *valepotriates*, found in the sedative herb valerian. This has attracted some attention, as valerian also is used for insomnia and stomach discomfort.

However, as valepotriates are no longer considered to be the active ingredients in valerian, it is not clear that this relationship has any significance.

As yet, there is no real evidence that catnip produces any effect at all in humans. Tests conducted on chicks and rats have produced conflicting results, although high doses of essential oil of catnip have increased sleeping times in the latter.

Dosage

Catnip tea is most commonly made by mixing 1 to 2 teaspoons (1 to 2 g) of the dried herb, or half that amount of the liquid extract, per cup of water (240 ml) and can be consumed up to 3 times a day.

Safety Issues

Although comprehensive safety studies have not been performed, catnip tea is generally regarded as safe. However, due to its traditional use as a uterine stimulant, pregnant women should probably avoid catnip. Safety for young children or individuals with severe liver or kidney disease has not been established.

Cat's Claw

Uncaria tomentosa, Uncaria guianensis

PRINCIPAL PROPOSED USES: *Osteoarthritis, Rheumatoid Arthritis*

VARIOUS VIRAL DISEASES: *AIDS, Feline Leukemia Virus, Genital and Oral Herpes, Shingles (Herpes Zoster)*

OTHER PROPOSED USES: *Allergies, Ulcers*

Cat's claw is an herb popular among the indigenous people of Peru, where it is used to treat cancer, diabetes, ulcers, arthritis, and infections, as well as to assist in recovery from childbirth. It is also used as a contraceptive. There are two primary species of cat's claw used medicinally: *Uncaria tomentosa* and *Uncaria guianensis.*

What Is Cat's Claw Used for Today?

Cat's claw is most often marketed as a treatment for viral diseases, such as **herpes**, **shingles**, **AIDS**, and feline leukemia virus. However, the evidence for these uses is extremely preliminary.

The most meaningful study yet performed on cat's claw suggests that the *Uncaria guianensis* species might be helpful for an entirely different condition: **osteoarthritis.**

In addition, one double-blind trial indicates that a certain type of *Uncaria tomentosa* may be modestly helpful for people with **rheumatoid arthritis.**

Cat's claw has also been proposed as a treatment for **allergies** and **stomach ulcers**, but there is no meaningful evidence as yet that it is effective for these conditions.

What Is the Scientific Evidence for Cat's Claw?

Osteoarthritis

A 4-week, double-blind, placebo-controlled trial evaluated the potential benefits of cat's claw (*Uncaria guianensis* species) for the treatment of osteoarthritis. A total of 45 individuals with osteoarthritis were enrolled. Of these, 30 were treated with cat's claw extract and 15 were given placebo. Individuals in the treatment group showed reduced pain with activity as compared to those in the placebo group. However, no comparative im-provements were seen in knee pain at rest or at night, nor in knee circumference.

This pilot trial suggests that the *Uncaria guianensis* species of cat's claw may be a useful treatment for osteoarthritis. However, more research will be necessary to verify this potential use of the herb.

Rheumatoid Arthritis

In a double-blind, placebo-controlled trial of 40 individuals undergoing conventional treatment for rheumatoid arthritis, use of an extract made from *Uncaria tomentosa* modestly improved symptoms in individuals with rheumatoid arthritis, as compared to placebo. The researchers conducting this trial made use of recent information indicating that there are two different subtypes of *Uncaria tomentosa*, identifiable based on the chemicals found in them. For this trial, they used the form containing pentacyclic oxindole alkaloids, as opposed to tetracyclic oxindole alkaloids.

Dosage

Numerous widely varying forms of cat's claw are available commercially. The optimum dosage of each type is not known. In addition, the precise differences in action between the two species of cat's claw, *Uncaria tomentosa* and *Uncaria guianensis*, as well as the pentacyclic and tetracyclic forms of *Uncaria tomentosa* (see above) are not known.

Safety Issues

In general, use of cat's claw has not been associated with adverse effects more serious than occasional digestive upset or allergic reactions. However, full safety studies have not been completed and there has been one report of kidney failure apparently triggered by cat's claw.

Safety in young children, pregnant or nursing women, or those with severe liver or kidney disease has not been established.

Some evidence suggests that cat's claw might inter-act with various medications by affecting their metabolism in the liver, but the extent of this effect has not been fully determined.

Cayenne
Capsicum frutescens, Capsicum annuum

PRINCIPAL PROPOSED USES:

Topical Uses: *Diabetic Peripheral Neuropathy, Osteoarthritis, Post-Herpetic Neuralgia*

Oral Uses: *Dyspepsia*

OTHER PROPOSED USES:

Topical Uses: *Back Pain, Cluster Headaches, Fibromyalgia, Nerve Pain Following Surgery, Psoriasis*

Oral Uses: *Protecting the Stomach from Ulcers Caused by Anti-Inflammatory Drugs*

The capsicum family includes red peppers, bell peppers, pimento, and paprika, but the most famous medicinal member of this family is the common cayenne pepper.

Cayenne and related peppers have a long history of use as digestive aids in many parts of the world, but the herb's recent popularity has, surprisingly, come through conventional medicine.

What Is Cayenne Used for Today?

Many people think that hot peppers cause inflammation to tissues and that this is the source of the classic hot pepper sensation. However, hot peppers don't actually have any damaging effect; they merely *simulate* the sensations produced by damage. (Herbs like **garlic**, **ginger**, horseradish, and mustard actually can *cause* tissue damage.)

Here's how it works: all hot peppers contain a substance called *capsaicin*. When applied to tissues, capsaicin causes release of a chemical called *substance P.* Substance P is ordinarily released when tissues are damaged; it is part of the system the body uses to detect injury. When hot peppers artificially release substance P, they trick the nervous system into thinking that an injury has occurred. The result: A sensation of burning pain.

When capsaicin is applied regularly to a part of the body, substance P becomes depleted in that location. This is why individuals who consume a lot of hot peppers gradually build up a tolerance.

It's also the basis for a number of medical uses of capsaicin. When levels of substance P are reduced in an area, all pain in that area is somewhat reduced. Because of this effect, capsaicin cream is widely used for the treatment of various painful conditions.

Under the brand name Zostrix, a cream containing concentrated capsaicin has been approved by the FDA for the treatment of post-herpetic neuralgia, the pain that often lingers after an attack of **shingles**. There is also relatively good evidence that topical capsaicin can modestly decrease the pain of **diabetic peripheral neuropathy** and other forms of peripheral neuropathy nerve pain following cancer surgery and the pain of arthritis. Capsaicin cream may be helpful for other forms of pain as well, including **fibromyalgia**, **back pain**, and **cluster headaches**. However, the benefits seen with capsaicin are seldom dramatic; in many cases, other pain-relieving treatments are used simultaneously.

Besides pain-related conditions, some evidence indicates that topical capsaicin may be helpful for **psoriasis** and possibly other skin conditions as well (especially those that involve itching).

Cayenne can be taken internally as well. It appears that oral use of cayenne might reduce the pain of minor indigestion (**dyspepsia**). This may seem like an odd use of the herb; intuitively, it seems that hot peppers should be hard on the stomach. However, remember that hot peppers don't actually damage tissues—they merely produce sensations similar to those caused by actual damage. Apparently, by depleting substance P in the stomach they reduce sensations of discomfort. In fact, some evidence suggests that oral use of cayenne or capsaicin can actually protect the stomach against **ulcers** caused by anti-inflammatory drugs. However, contrary to some reports, cayenne does not appear to be able to kill *Helicobacter pylori*, the stomach bacteria implicated as a major cause of ulcers.

In addition, it appears that, contrary to long-standing belief, hot peppers do not cause increased pain in people with **hemorrhoids**.

What Is the Scientific Evidence for Cayenne?

Oral Uses of Cayenne

➤ *Dyspepsia*

In a double-blind, placebo-controlled study, 30 individuals with dyspepsia were given either 2.5 g daily of red pepper powder (divided up and taken prior to meals) or placebo for 5 weeks. By the third week of treatment, individuals taking red pepper were experiencing significant improvements in pain, bloating, and nausea as compared to placebo, and these relative improvements lasted through the end of the study.

A placebo-controlled crossover study failed to find benefit, but it only enrolled 11 participants, far too few to have much chance of identifying a treatment effect.

Topical Uses of Cayenne

All double-blind studies of topical capsaicin (or cayenne) suffer from one drawback: it isn't really possible to hide the burning sensation that occurs during initial use of the treatment. For this reason, such studies probably aren't truly double-blind. It has been suggested that instead of an inactive placebo, researchers should use some other substance (such as camphor) that causes at least mild burning. However, such treatments might also have therapeutic benefits; they have a long history of use for pain as well.

Because of these complications, the evidence for topical treatments cited below is less meaningful than it might at first appear.

➤ *Pain*

Capsaicin cream is well established as a modestly helpful pain-relieving treatment for post-herpetic neuropathy (the pain that lingers after an attack of shingles), peripheral neuropathy (nerve pain that occurs most commonly as a side effect of diabetes, but may occur with **HIV** as well as other conditions), nerve pain after **cancer surgery**, and **osteoarthritis**.

Weaker evidence supports the use of topical capsaicin for fibromyalgia.

Capsaicin instilled into the nose may be helpful for cluster headaches. (The fact that this has even been considered a viable treatment option shows how painful cluster headaches can be!)

Actual cayenne rather than capsaicin has been tested for pain as well. A 3-week, double-blind trial of 154 individuals with back pain found that cayenne applied topically as a "plaster" improved pain to a greater extent than placebo.

➤ *Skin Conditions*

A double-blind, placebo-controlled trial of nearly 200 individuals found that use of topical capsaicin can improve itching as well as overall severity of psoriasis. Benefits were also seen in a smaller double-blind study of topical capsaicin for psoriasis.

Topical capsaicin is thought to be helpful for various itchy skin conditions, such as prurigo nodularis, but double-blind studies are lacking.

Dosage

Capsaicin creams are approved over-the-counter drugs and should be used as directed. If the burning sensation that occurs with initial use is too severe, using weaker forms of the cream at first may be advisable.

For treatment of dyspepsia, cayenne may be taken at a dosage of 0.5 to 1 g 3 times daily (prior to meals).

Safety Issues

Capsaicin creams commonly cause an unpleasant burning sensation when they are first applied; this sensation disappears over subsequent days as treatment is continued.

As a commonly used food, cayenne is generally recognized as safe. Contrary to some reports, cayenne does not appear to aggravate stomach ulcers.

Interactions You Should Know About

If you are taking:

➤ **The asthma drug theophylline: Cayenne might increase the amount you absorb, possibly leading to toxic levels.**
➤ **Nonsteroidal anti-inflammatory drugs: Cayenne might protect your stomach from damage.**

Cetylated Fatty Acids

PRINCIPAL PROPOSED USES: *Osteoarthritis*

OTHER PROPOSED USES: *Psoriasis*

In 2004, a special mixture of fats called *cetylated fatty acids* began to be widely marketed as a treatment for osteoarthritis. Although the claims associated with this product appear to exceed what has actually been proven, it is fair to say that cetylated fatty acids have shown definite promise in preliminary trials.

Requirements/Sources

There is no dietary requirement for cetylated fatty acids.

Therapeutic Dosages

Cetylated fatty acids are used both orally and as a topical cream.

A typical oral dose of cetylated fatty acids is 1,000 to 2,000 mg daily. Cetylated fatty acid creams are applied 2 to 4 times daily to the affected area.

Therapeutic Uses

Three double-blind, placebo-controlled studies have found cetylated fatty acids helpful for **osteoarthritis**. Two involved a topical product and one used an oral formulation.

In one of the studies that used a cream preparation, 40 people with osteoarthritis of the knee applied either cetylated fatty acids or placebo to the affected joint. The results over 30 days showed greater improvements in range of motion and functional ability among people using the real cream than those using the placebo cream.

In another 30-day study, also enrolling 40 people with knee arthritis, use of cetylated fatty acid cream improved postural stability, presumably due to decreased pain levels.

In addition, a 68-day, double-blind, placebo-controlled study of 64 people with knee arthritis tested an oral cetylated fatty acid supplement (the supplement also contained lesser amounts of **lecithin** and **fish oil**). Participants in the treatment group experienced improvements in swelling, mobility, and pain level as compared to those in the placebo group. Inexplicably, the study report does not discuss whether or not side effects occurred.

While this is a promising body of research, it is far from definitive. Current advertising claims for cetylated fatty acids go far beyond the existing evidence. For example, a number of websites claim that cetylated fatty acids are more effective than **glucosamine** or **chondroitin**. However, no comparison studies have been performed upon which such a claim could be rationally based.

It's not known how cetylated fatty acids might help osteoarthritis. Proponents cite the known benefits of fish oil for **rheumatoid arthritis**, but since the fatty acids in fish oil are rather different from those in cetylated fatty acids and the origin of rheumatoid arthritis is quite unlike that of osteoarthritis, there is little relevance to these observations. Proponents also make multiple specific claims, including that cetylated fatty acids reduce inflammation, protect cartilage from damage, lubricate cell membranes, and increase fluid in joints. However, none of these explanations have more than speculative scientific support. At present, if in fact cetylated fatty acids help osteoarthritis, we do not know how they might do so.

Cetylated fatty acid creams have also been proposed for treatment of **psoriasis**.

Safety Issues

Cetylated fatty acids appear to have a low level of toxicity, according to safety studies conducted by the primary manufacturer. However, maximum safe doses in young children, pregnant or nursing women, or people with severe liver or kidney disease have not been established.

Chamomile

German (*Matricaria recutita*), Roman (*Chamaemelum nobile*)

PRINCIPAL PROPOSED USES: *Skin Inflammation (Eczema, Skin Inflammation Caused by Radiation Therapy)*

OTHER PROPOSED USES: *Digestive Upset, Mouth Sores Caused by Chemotherapy, Tension and Stress*

Two distinct plants are known as chamomile and are used interchangeably: German and Roman chamomile. Although distantly related botanically, they both look like miniature daisies and are traditionally thought to possess similar medicinal benefits.

Over a million cups of chamomile tea are drunk daily, testifying to its good taste, at least. Chamomile was used by early Egyptian physicians for fevers and by ancient Greeks, Romans, and Indians for headaches and disorders of the kidneys, liver, and bladder.

The modern use of chamomile dates back to 1921, when a German firm introduced a topical form. This cream became a popular treatment for a wide variety of skin disorders, including eczema, bedsores, skin inflammation caused by radiation therapy, and contact dermatitis (for example, poison ivy).

What Is Chamomile Used for Today?

Germany's Commission E authorizes the use of topical chamomile preparations for a variety of diseases of the skin and mouth.

Chamomile tea is also said to reduce mild tension and stress and to aid **indigestion**.

What Is the Scientific Evidence for Chamomile?

There is no reliable evidence that chamomile is effective for the treatment of any health condition.

Skin Diseases

A controlled study of 161 individuals found chamomile cream equally effective as 0.25% hydrocortisone cream for the treatment of **eczema**. However, this study did not use a placebo group and does not appear to have been double-blind. For this reason, the results are not reliable. (For information on why double-blind studies are so important, see **Why Does This Book Rely on Double-blind Studies?**.)

A study of 72 individuals with eczema found somewhat odd results: in this trial, chamomile was not significantly more effective than placebo, but both were better than 0.5% hydrocortisone cream. It is difficult to interpret what these paradoxical results actually mean, but they certainly cannot be taken as proof that chamomile cream is effective.

In a double-blind study, chamomile cream proved *less* effective for reducing inflammation of the skin than hydrocortisone cream or witch hazel cream.

Finally, in a single-blind trial, 50 women receiving **radiation therapy** for breast cancer were treated with either chamomile or placebo. Chamomile failed to prove superior to placebo for preventing skin inflammation caused by radiation therapy.

Mouth Sores

A double-blind, placebo-controlled trial of 164 individuals did not find chamomile mouthwash effective for treating the mouth sores caused by chemotherapy with the drug 5-FU.

Dosage

Chamomile cream is applied to the affected area 1 to 4 times daily.

Chamomile tea can be made by pouring boiling water over 2 to 3 heaping teaspoons of flowers and steeping for 10 minutes.

Chamomile tinctures and pills should be taken according to the directions on the label. Alcoholic tincture may be the most potent form for internal use.

Safety Issues

Chamomile is listed on the FDA's GRAS (generally recognized as safe) list.

Reports that chamomile can cause severe reactions in people allergic to ragweed have received significant media attention. However, when all the evidence is examined, it does not appear that chamomile is actually more allergenic than any other plant. The cause of these reports may be products contaminated with "dog chamomile," a highly allergenic and bad-tasting plant of similar appearance.

Chamomile also contains naturally occurring coumarin compounds that might act as "blood thinners" under certain circumstances. There is one case report in which it appears that use of chamomile combined with the anticoagulant warfarin led to excessive "blood thinning" resulting in internal bleeding. Some evidence suggests that chamomile might interact with other medications as well through effects on drug metabolism, but the extent of this effect has not been fully determined.

Safety in young children, pregnant or nursing women, or those with liver or kidney disease has not been established, although there have not been any credible reports of toxicity caused by this common beverage tea.

Interactions You Should Know About

If you are taking blood-thinning medications such as **warfarin** (Coumadin), **heparin**, **clopidogrel** (Plavix), **ticlopidine** (Ticlid), or **pentoxifylline** (Trental), you should avoid using chamomile as it might increase their effects. This could potentially cause problems.

Chasteberry

Vitex agnus-castus

PRINCIPAL PROPOSED USES: *Cyclic Breast Discomfort (Often Associated with PMS), Other PMS Symptoms*

OTHER PROPOSED USES: *Amenorrhea, Female Infertility, Irregular Menstruation, Menopausal Symptoms*

Chasteberry is frequently called by its Latin names: *vitex* or, alternatively, *agnus-castus*. A shrub in the verbena family, chasteberry is commonly found on riverbanks and nearby foothills in central Asia and around the Mediterranean Sea. After its violet flowers have bloomed, a dark brown, peppercorn-size fruit with a pleasant odor reminiscent of peppermint develops. This fruit is used medicinally.

As the name implies, for centuries chasteberry was thought to counter sexual desire. A drink prepared from the plant's seeds was used by the Romans to diminish libido, and in ancient Greece, young women celebrating the festival of Demeter wore chasteberry blossoms to show that they were remaining chaste in honor of the goddess. Monks in the Middle Ages used the fruit for similar purposes, yielding the common name "monk's pepper."

What Is Chasteberry Used for Today?

The modern use of chasteberry dates back to the 1950s, when the German pharmaceutical firm Madaus Company first produced a standardized extract. This herb

has become a standard European treatment for cyclic breast tenderness, a condition related to PMS that is sometimes called *cyclic mastitis*, **cyclic mastalgia**, *mastodynia*, or *fibrocystic breast disease*. Chasteberry also appears to be useful for general **PMS** symptoms.

Chasteberry is believed to work by suppressing the release of prolactin from the pituitary gland. Prolactin is a hormone that naturally rises during pregnancy to stimulate milk production. Inappropriately increased production of prolactin may be a factor in cyclic breast tenderness, as well as other symptoms of PMS.

Elevated prolactin levels can also cause a woman's period to become irregular and even stop. For this reason, chasteberry is sometimes tried when menstruation is irregular or stops altogether (amenorrhea). **Note:** We recommend that you do not attempt to self-treat significant menstrual irregularities without a full medical evaluation. There could be a serious medical condition causing the problem that you wouldn't want to miss.

High prolactin levels can also cause infertility in women. For this reason, chasteberry is sometimes tried as a fertility drug; however, the two double-blind studies

Chasteberry

performed to evaluate this possible use failed to return statistically significant results.

Finally, chasteberry is sometimes used for **menopausal symptoms**, but there is as yet no evidence that it is effective.

What Is the Scientific Evidence for Chasteberry?

There is a growing body of scientific research supporting the use of chasteberry.

Cyclic Mastalgia

A double-blind, placebo-controlled trial of 97 women with symptoms of cyclic mastalgia found that treatment with chasteberry extract significantly reduced pain intensity by the end of one menstrual cycle. The reduction continued to increase throughout the second menstrual cycle and, at the end of both the first and second cycle, women in the treated group were doing better than those receiving placebo.

However, something interesting happened in the third cycle. The benefits of chasteberry treatment reached a plateau, while the placebo group continued to improve. At the end of the third cycle, those receiving chasteberry were still doing better, but the difference was no longer statistically significant.

Another double-blind trial of 104 women compared placebo against two forms of chasteberry (liquid and tablet) for at least three menstrual cycles. The results showed statistically significant and comparable improvements in the treated groups as compared to placebo.

Benefits were also seen in a double-blind trial that enrolled 160 women with cyclic breast pain. The women were given either chasteberry, a drug related to progesterone, or placebo, and were followed for at least four menstrual cycles. Although there were many dropouts, the results again suggest that chasteberry is superior to placebo.

Premenstrual Syndrome (PMS)

A double-blind, placebo-controlled study of 178 women found that treatment with chasteberry over three menstrual cycles significantly reduced general PMS symptoms. The dose used was 1 tablet 3 times daily of a dry chasteberry extract. Women in the treatment group experienced significant improvements in symptoms, including irritability, depression, headache, and breast tenderness.

Unfortunately, there is little corroborating evidence as yet for this one well-designed study. A previous double-blind trial compared chasteberry to vitamin B_6 (pyridoxine) instead of a placebo. The two treatments proved equally effective. However, because vitamin B_6 itself has not been shown effective for PMS, these results mean little.

Two other studies are often cited in support of chasteberry as a treatment for PMS. These were rather informal reports of a total of about 3,000 women with PMS given chasteberry by their physicians. The physicians rated chasteberry as effective about 90% of the time, but in the absence of a control group, these reports are not very meaningful.

Irregular Menstruation

One double-blind trial followed 52 women with a form of irregular menstruation known as *luteal phase defect*. This condition is believed to be related to excessive prolactin release. After 3 months, the women who took chasteberry showed significant improvements.

Dosage

The typical dose of dry chasteberry extract is 20 mg taken 1 to 3 times daily. Chasteberry is also sold as a liquid extract to be taken at a dosage of 40 drops each morning. However, extracts that require lower or higher dosing are also available. We recommend following the label instructions.

Safety Issues

There haven't been any detailed studies of the safety of chasteberry. However, its widespread use in Germany has not led to any reports of significant adverse effects, other than a single case of excessive ovarian stimulation possibly caused by chasteberry.

Because it lowers prolactin levels, chasteberry is not an appropriate treatment for pregnant or nursing women. Safety in young children or those with severe liver or kidney disease has not been established.

There are no known drug interactions associated with chasteberry. However, it is quite conceivable that the herb could interfere with hormones or medications that affect the pituitary gland.

Interactions You Should Know About

If you are taking **hormones** or **drugs that affect the pituitary**, such as **bromocriptine**, it is possible that chasteberry might interfere with their action.

Chinese Skullcap

Scutellaria baicalensis

ALTERNATE NAMES/RELATED TERMS: *Baicalein, Baicalin*

PRINCIPAL PROPOSED USES: *None*

OTHER PROPOSED USES: *Anxiety, Cancer Treatment, Enhancing Antibiotic Activity, Hypertension, Liver Protection*

*S*cutellaria baicalensis, also called *Chinese skullcap*, is a member of the mint family and has long been used in traditional Chinese herbal medicine. Chinese skullcap has been incorporated in herbal formulas designed to treat such widely varying conditions as cancer, liver disease, allergies, skin conditions, and epilepsy. The root is the part used medicinally.

Note: Chinese skullcap is substantially different from **American skullcap** (*Scutellaria lateriflora*).

What Is Chinese Skullcap Used for Today?

The root of Chinese scullcap contains the flavonoids baicalin, wogonin, and baicalein, and most studies have involved these substances rather than the whole herb.

Highly preliminary evidence suggests that baicalin can enhance the activity of antibiotics against antibiotic-resistant staph bacteria. Other highly preliminary evidence suggests that baicalin, wogonin, and baicalein may have **anti-cancer**, anti-inflammatory, **liver-protective**, **anti-anxiety**, and **antihypertensive** effects. However, for none of these uses does the evidence approach the level necessary to truly establish a treatment as effective.

Research involving combination herbal therapies containing Chinese skullcap is discussed in the **Traditional Chinese Herbal Medicine** article.

Dosage

The optimum doses, if any, of baicalin, wogonin, and baicalein have not been established. Chinese skullcap is typically taken at a dose of 3 to 9 g daily as part of an herbal combination.

Safety Issues

Baicalin, wogogin, and baicalein appear to have a low order of toxicity, though comprehensive safety studies have not been performed. There have been case reports of liver injury associated with use of skullcap products, but these may have been due to adulteration by the herb germander.

One animal study found worrisome evidence that baicalin might markedly reduce the absorption of the drug cyclosporine, used to prevent organ transplant rejection.

Safety in young children, pregnant or nursing women, or people with severe liver or kidney disease has not been established.

Interactions You Should Know About

If you are taking the drug **cyclosporine**, do not use Chinese skullcap or its constituents.

Chitosan

SUPPLEMENT FORMS/ALTERNATE NAMES: *Chitin (Chitosan Is the Deacetylated Form)*

PRINCIPAL PROPOSED USES: *None*

OTHER PROPOSED USES: *Antimicrobial, High Blood Pressure, High Cholesterol, Kidney Failure, Wound Healing (Topical Chitosan)*

PROBABLY NOT EFFECTIVE USES: *Weight Loss*

Chitosan is a form of fiber chemically processed from crustacean shells. Like other forms of fiber, such as oat bran, chitosan is not well digested by the human body. As it passes through the digestive tract, it seems to have an ability to bond with ingested fat and carry it out in the stool. For this reason, it has been tried as an agent for lowering cholesterol and reducing weight. However, the results in studies have been more negative than positive.

In addition, chitosan has been tried as a treatment for kidney failure and as an aid in wound healing.

Note: We do not recommend the use of chitosan in children or pregnant women due to concerns about possible growth retardation (see Safety Issues below).

Requirements/Sources

Chitosan can be extracted from the shells of shrimp, crab, or lobster. It is also found in yeast and some fungi. Another inexpensive source of chitin is "squid pens," a byproduct of squid processing; these are small, plastic-like, inedible pieces of squid that are removed prior to eating.

Therapeutic Dosages

The standard dosage of chitosan is 3 to 6 g per day, to be taken with food.

Chitosan can deplete the body of certain minerals (see Safety Issues below). For this reason, when using chitosan, it may be helpful to take supplemental calcium, vitamin D, selenium, magnesium, and other minerals.

Also, according to a preliminary study in rats, taking **vitamin C** along with chitosan might provide additional benefit in lowering cholesterol.

Therapeutic Uses

On the basis of chitosan's supposed ability to bind fat in the intestines, it has been tried as a treatment for **high cholesterol**. However, the evidence regarding whether it really works is generally more negative than positive. At best, chitosan appears to offer no more than minimal benefit for high cholesterol.

Chitosan has also been proposed as a **weight loss** treatment on the same principle. However, the current balance of evidence suggests that chitosan does *not*, in fact, significantly aid weight loss.

Weak evidence hints that chitosan may be helpful in kidney failure. When used for this purpose, it is thought to work by binding with toxins in the digestive tract and causing them to be excreted.

Studies in dogs have found that topically applied chitosan can help heal **wounds**. This effect might be due to stimulation of new tissue growth; in addition, topical chitosan appears to kill bacteria such as *Streptococcus*, which may also contribute to wound healing. Chitosan may also have activity against *Candida albicans*, a form of yeast that causes **vaginal infections**.

Highly preliminary evidence suggests that oral chitosan may inhibit the expected rise in **blood pressure** after a high-salt meal. It has also been suggested that chitosan can **stimulate the immune system** and **prevent cancer**, but there is no reliable evidence as yet that it offers these benefits.

Animal studies suggest that some forms of chitosan may help to prevent bone loss; however, because chitosan also interferes with mineral absorption, the net effect in humans might actually be to increase bone loss (see Safety Issues below).

What Is the Scientific Evidence for Chitosan?

High Cholesterol

An 8-week, double-blind, placebo-controlled trial of 51 women found that use of chitosan at a dose of 1,200 mg twice daily slightly reduced LDL ("bad") cholesterol as compared to placebo, but it did not affect total or HDL ("good") cholesterol levels. Another 8-week trial, this one enrolling 84 people, also found modest benefits.

However, a 4-month, double-blind, placebo-controlled trial of 88 individuals found no improvement in cholesterol with 1,000 mg 3 times daily of a different chitosan product. A 7-month study of 84 men given placebo or 1,200 mg of chitosan daily also failed to find benefit. Furthermore, in a 10-month, double-blind, placebo-controlled study of 130 men and women, use of a special microcrystalline form of chitosan at a dose of 1,200 mg twice daily again failed to improve cholesterol profile.

These contradictory results suggest that if chitosan actually improves cholesterol profile at all, it does so to only a minimal extent.

Weight Loss

Chitosan has been widely advocated as a weight loss supplement, on the basis of its supposed ability to bind fat in the digestive tract. However, despite some positive results in a small preliminary study, by far the largest and best-designed trial failed to find benefit. In this 6-month, double-blind, placebo-controlled study of 250 overweight people, use of chitosan at a dose of 3 g daily failed to enhance weight loss to any meaningful extent as compared to placebo.

Other studies have also failed to find benefit. Overall, it appears that chitosan is not effective for weight loss.

Kidney Failure

People with kidney failure experience numerous health problems, including anemia, fatigue, and loss of appetite. In one open study, researchers tested chitosan supplements in 80 people with kidney failure receiving ongoing hemodialysis treatment. Half the participants were given 45 mg tablets for a total of about 1,500 mg of chitosan daily for 12 weeks; the other half were not given a supplement. Those in the treatment group showed a significant decrease in urea and creatinine levels. Further, they had a rise in hemoglobin levels and reported improved overall strength, appetite, and sleep, as well. However, these results must be taken with grain of salt, for only double-blind, placebo-controlled studies can prove a treatment effective. (For information on why this is so, see **Why Does This Book Rely on Double-blind Studies?**)

Safety Issues

There is significant evidence that long-term, high-dose chitosan supplementation can result in malabsorption of some crucial vitamins and minerals, including **calcium, magnesium, selenium,** and **vitamins A, D, E,** and **K**. In turn, this appears to lead to a risk of **osteoporosis** in adults and growth retardation in children. For this reason, adults taking chitosan should also take supplemental vitamins and minerals, making especially sure to get enough vitamin D, calcium, and magnesium.

Another possible risk of long-term ingestion of high doses of chitosan is that it could change the intestinal flora and allow the growth of unhealthful bacteria.

Finally, there has been a case report of arsenic poisoning caused by long-term use of chitosan supplements. Shellfish, it appears, can concentrate arsenic in their shells as part of their normal development; this in turn may lead to arsenic-laced chitosan supplements.

Pregnant or nursing women and young children should probably avoid chitosan altogether.

Choline

PRINCIPAL PROPOSED USES: *Alzheimer's Disease, Stroke*

OTHER PROPOSED USES: *Bipolar Disease, Cancer Prevention, Cirrhosis, Hepatitis, High Cholesterol, HIV Support*

Choline has only recently been recognized as an essential nutrient. Choline is part of the neurotransmitter acetylcholine, which plays a major role in the brain; for this reason, many studies have been designed to look at choline's role in brain function.

Choline functions as a part of a major biochemical process in the body called *methylation*; choline acts as a methyl donor. Until recently, it was thought that the body could use other substances to substitute for choline, such as **folate, vitamins B$_6$** and **B$_{12}$,** and the amino acid methionine. But recent evidence has finally shown that, for some people, adequate choline supplies cannot be maintained by other nutrients and must be obtained independently through diet or supplements.

Requirements/Sources

Choline is widespread in the foods we eat. The average diet provides about 500 to 1,000 mg of choline per day. Lecithin, a fatty constituent in foods, is a major source of choline; it is comprised mostly of a type of choline called *phosphatidylcholine* (PC). (Lecithin and PC have been studied separately as treatments for a variety of illnesses; for more information on these supplements, see the full article on **lecithin**.)

According to U.S. and Canadian guidelines, the recommended daily intake of choline is as follows:

> Infants 0–6 months, 125 mg
>   7–12 months, 150 mg
> Children 1–3 years, 200 mg
>   4–8 years, 250 mg
>   9–13 years, 375 mg
> Males 14 years and older, 550 mg
> Females 14–18 years, 400 mg
>   19 years and older, 425 mg
> Pregnant women, 450 mg
> Nursing women, 550 mg

Therapeutic Dosages

Most studies of choline as a treatment for diseases have used between 1 and 30 g of choline or choline-containing supplements per day. This wide range is due to the existence of several different types of choline supplements, all with varying amounts of the active ingredient.

Therapeutic Uses

A form of choline called *choline alfoscerate* has shown promise for Alzheimer's disease.

A substance related to choline called *CDP-choline* (or *citcholine*) may be slightly helpful for enhancing recovery from **strokes**.

Slight evidence hints that lecithin or pure choline may be helpful for people with **bipolar disorder**. Lecithin has failed to prove effective for **tardive dyskinesia**. Lecithin has also failed to prove effective for improving **cholesterol profile** levels.

Some evidence suggests that individuals with **HIV**

who are low in choline may experience more rapid disease progression. However, there is no direct evidence that choline supplements offer any benefit for people with HIV.

Numerous studies have found that diets very low in choline lead to impaired liver function. But these diets are contrived: one would have to work very hard to get so little choline in the diet! To what degree additional choline may benefit people with pre-existing liver damage is an area of ongoing research. In a double-blind study, use of phosphatidlycholine enhanced the effect of interferon in people with **chronic hepatitis C** but not those with chronic hepatitis B. Open studies have yielded mixed results.

Finally, there are theoretical reasons to believe that choline might have **cancer-preventive** properties. The notion stems from its function as a methyl donor. Methyl units are essential for RNA and DNA replication—a process ongoing in every cell of the body. The theory goes like this: Diets lacking sufficient methyl donors (such as choline) may cause an error in RNA or DNA synthesis, leading to a mutated gene and, hypothetically, to cancer initiation. Indeed, in rats fed diets very low in choline and other methyl donors, cancer rates increased. However, again, it is a long step from the effects of an artificially low-choline diet to taking choline supplements.

Choline as phosphatidylcholine may reduce homocysteine levels. This in turn might reduce heart disease risk, although the proposed homocysteine–heart disease connection remains far from proven. (See the **High Homocysteine** article for more information.)

What Is the Scientific Evidence for Choline?

Alzheimer's Disease

In a 6-month, double-blind, placebo-controlled trial, 261 people with mild to moderate Alzheimer's disease were given either placebo or choline alfoscerate (a special form of choline) at a dose of 400 mg 3 times daily. The results indicated that people receiving the supplement improved slightly over the course of the trial, while those given placebo worsened.

Weak evidence from highly preliminary studies hints that CDP-choline may improve mental function in Alzheimer's disease. Double-blind trials using lecithin as a source of choline failed to find benefit.

Strokes

Four double-blind, placebo-controlled studies enrolling a total of 1,372 people have evaluated the potential effectiveness of CDP choline in the treatment of strokes.

Overall, the evidence suggests that use of CDP-choline in the period immediately following a stroke slightly improves the chances of full recovery.

Safety Issues

The tolerable upper intake (the highest daily intake over a prolonged time known to pose no risks to most members of a healthy population) of choline has been set at 3.5 g daily for adults.

In higher dosages, minor but annoying side effects may occur, such as abdominal discomfort, diarrhea, and nausea. Maximum safe dosages for young children, pregnant or nursing women, or those with severe liver or kidney disease have not been determined.

Chondroitin

SUPPLEMENT FORMS/ALTERNATE NAMES: *Chondroitin Sulfate*

PRINCIPAL PROPOSED USES: *Osteoarthritis*

OTHER PROPOSED USES: *Atherosclerosis, High Cholesterol, Sports and Fitness Support:*
  Enhancing Recovery

Chondroitin sulfate is a naturally occurring substance in the body. It is a major constituent of cartilage—the tough, elastic connective tissue found in the joints.

Based on the evidence of preliminary double-blind studies, chondroitin is widely used as a treatment for **osteoarthritis**, the typical arthritis that many people suffer as they get older.

There is some evidence that chondroitin might go beyond treating symptoms and actually protect joints from damage. Current medical treatments for osteoarthritis, such as **nonsteroidal anti-inflammatory drugs** (NSAIDs), treat the symptoms but don't actually slow the disease's progression, and they may actually make it get worse faster. Chondroitin (along with **glucosamine**) may take the treatment of osteoarthritis to a new level. However, more research needs to be performed to prove definitively that this exciting possibility is real.

Sources

Chondroitin is not an essential nutrient. Animal cartilage is the only dietary source of chondroitin. (When it's on your plate, animal cartilage is called *gristle*.) Unless you enjoy chewing gristle, you'd do best to obtain chondroitin in pill form from a health food store or pharmacy.

Therapeutic Dosages

The usual dosage of chondroitin is 400 mg taken 3 times daily, indefinitely. Two studies (mentioned below) used an "on and off" schedule of chondroitin (taking it for 3 months, going off of it for 3 months, and then taking it again). Other studies involved taking chondroitin daily. Regardless of which way you use it, be patient! The results are thought to take weeks to develop.

In commercial products chondroitin is often combined with glucosamine. Preliminary information from one animal study suggests that this combination may be superior to either treatment alone.

There are large differences between chondroitin products based on their chemical structure. This can be expected to lead to significant differences in absorption and hence effectiveness. Most likely, chondroitin products with physically smaller molecules (fewer than 16,900 daltons) are better absorbed. In addition, a review conducted in 2003 by the respected testing organization Consumerlab.com found that some products sold as providing chondroitin actually contained far less chondroitin than stated on the label (or even contained none at all). It may be advisable to use the exact products that were tested in double-blind trials.

Therapeutic Uses

Numerous double-blind studies have found evidence that chondroitin can relieve the symptoms of osteoarthritis and possibly also slow the progression of the disease; however, the largest and generally best-designed study failed to find benefit.

Chondroitin has also been proposed as a treatment for other conditions, such as **atherosclerosis**, **interstitial cystitis**, and **high cholesterol**, but as yet the evidence that it might help is far too weak to rely upon at all.

One small double-blind study evaluated chondroitin for reducing **muscle soreness caused by intense exercise** but failed to find benefit.

What Is the Scientific Evidence for Chondroitin?

For years, experts stated that oral chondroitin couldn't possibly work because its molecules are so big that it seemed doubtful that they could be absorbed through the digestive tract. However, in 1995 researchers laid this objection to rest when they found evidence that up to 15% of chondroitin is absorbed intact.

Reducing Symptoms of Osteoarthritis

Most but not all double-blind, placebo-controlled studies indicate that chondroitin can relieve symptoms of osteoarthritis.

For example, one study enrolled 85 people with osteoarthritis of the knee and followed them for 6 months. Participants received either 400 mg of chondroitin sulfate twice daily or placebo. At the end of the trial, doctors rated the improvement as good or very good in 69% of those taking chondroitin sulfate but in only 32% of those taking placebo.

Another way of comparing the results is to look at maximum walking speed among participants. Whereas individuals in the chondroitin group were able to improve their walking speed gradually over the course of the trial, walking speed did not improve at all in the placebo group. Additionally, there were improvements in other measures of osteoarthritis, such as pain level, with benefits seen as early as 1 month. This suggests that chondroitin was able to stop the arthritis from gradually getting worse (see also Slowing the Progression of Osteoarthritis below).

Good results were seen in a 12-month, double-blind trial that compared chondroitin against placebo in 104 people, a 12-month trial of 42 people, and a 12-month study of 120 people.

In two of these studies, chondroitin was taken for two separate 3-month periods separated by 3 months of no treatment; in the others it was taken continuously. No comparison of these two ways of using chondroitin has been published.

Benefits were also seen in two other double-blind, placebo-controlled trials involving a total of more than 350 individuals.

Another double-blind study compared chondroitin to the anti-inflammatory drug dicoflenac and found equivalent benefits.

Additional studies combined glucosamine with chondroitin. A 6-month, double-blind, placebo-controlled study of 93 people with knee arthritis found that a combination of glucosamine and chondroitin (along with manganese) was more effective than placebo. Another double-blind, placebo-controlled study evaluated chondroitin/glucosamine for **temporomandibular joint disease** (TMJ) but found equivocal results.

However, a very large (1,583 participants) and well-designed study failed to find either chondroitin or glucosamine plus chondroitin more effective than placebo. It has been suggested that chondroitin, like glucosamine, may primarily show benefit in studies funded by manufacturers of chondroitin products.

Slowing the Progression of Osteoarthritis

Osteoarthritis tends to worsen with time. As mentioned earlier, no conventional treatment for osteoarthritis protects joints from progressive damage. Growing evidence tells us that chondroitin can do this, but it is too early to consider the matter settled.

One study examined the progression of osteoarthritis in 119 people for 3 years. In this double-blind, placebo-controlled trial, those who took 1,200 mg of chondroitin daily showed lower rates of severe joint damage. Only 8.8% of the chondroitin group developed severely damaged joints during the 3 years of the study, compared with almost 30% of the placebo group. This suggests that chondroitin was slowing the progression of osteoarthritis.

Protective effects were also seen in three 1-year studies enrolling a total of more than 200 people.

Animal studies provide some additional evidence for a joint-protecting benefit.

How Does Chondroitin Work for Osteoarthritis?

Scientists are unsure how chondroitin sulfate works, but one of several theories (or all of them) might explain its mode of action.

At its most basic level, chondroitin may help cartilage by providing it with the building blocks it needs to repair itself. Chondroitin is also believed to block enzymes that break down cartilage in the joints. Another theory holds that chondroitin increases the amount of hyaluronic acid in the joints. Hyaluronic acid is a protective fluid that keeps the joints lubricated. Finally, chondroitin may have a mild anti-inflammatory effect.

Safety Issues

Chondroitin generally does not cause much in the way of side effects, besides occasional mild digestive distress. However, there is one case report of an exacerbation of asthma caused by use of a glucosamine-chondroitin product. In addition, there are theoretical concerns that chondroitin might have a mild blood-thinning effect, based on its chemical similarity to the anticoagulant drug heparin. Reassuringly, there are no case reports of any problems relating to this, and studies suggest that chon-droitin has at most a mild anticoagulant effect. Nonetheless, prudence suggests that, based on these findings, chondroitin should not be combined with blood-thinning drugs such as warfarin (Coumadin), heparin, and aspirin, except under physician supervision. In addition, individuals with bleeding problems such as hemophilia or who are temporarily at risk for bleeding (for example, undergoing surgery or labor and delivery) should avoid chondroitin.

Interactions You Should Know About

If you are using drugs that impair blood coagulation, such as **warfarin** (Coumadin), **heparin**, **aspirin**, **clopidogrel** (Plavix), **ticlopidine** (Ticlid), or **pentoxifylline** (Trental), do not use chondroitin except under physician supervision.

Chromium

SUPPLEMENT FORMS/ALTERNATE NAMES: *Chromium Chloride, Chromium Picolinate, Chromium Polynicotinate, High-Chromium Brewer's Yeast*

PRINCIPAL PROPOSED USES: *Diabetes, Heart Disease Prevention, Insulin Resistance and Abnormal Glucose Tolerance*

OTHER PROPOSED USES: *Acne, Depression, Functional Hypoglycemia, High Cholesterol, Migraine Headaches, Psoriasis, Sports Performance Enhancement, Syndrome X, Weight Loss ("Fat Burning")*

Chromium is a mineral the body needs in very small amounts, but it plays a significant role in human nutrition. Chromium's most important function in the body is to help regulate the amount of glucose (sugar) in the blood. Insulin plays a starring role in this fundamental biological process by regulating the movement of glucose out of the blood and into cells. Scientists believe that insulin uses chromium as an assistant (technically, a *cofactor*) to "unlock the door" to the cell membrane, thus allowing glucose to enter the cell. In the past, it was believed that, to accomplish this, the body first converted chromium into a large chemical called *glucose tolerance factor* (GTF). Intact GTF was thought to be present in certain foods, such as Brewer's yeast, and for that reason such products were described as superior sources of chromium. However, subsequent investigation indicated that researchers were actually creating GTF inadvertently during the process of chemical analysis. Scientists now believe that there is no such thing as GTF. Rather, chromium appears to act in concert with a very small protein called *low molecular weight chromium-binding substance* (LMWCr) to assist insulin's action. LMWCr does not permanently bind chromium and is not a likely source of chromium in foods.

Based on chromium's close relationship with insulin, this trace mineral has been studied as a treatment for diabetes. The results have been somewhat positive: it seems fairly likely that chromium supplements can improve blood sugar control in people with diabetes. Chromium also might be helpful for milder abnormalities in blood sugar metabolism. One study suggests that chromium might aid in weight loss as well, but other studies failed to find this effect.

Requirements/Sources

The official U.S. recommendations for daily intake are as follows:

➤ **Infants 0–6 months, 0.2 mcg**
  7–12 months, 5.5 mcg
➤ **Children 1–3 years, 11 mcg**
  4–8 years, 15 mcg
➤ **Males 9–13 years, 25 mcg**
  14–50 years, 35 mcg
  50 years and older, 30 mcg
➤ **Females 9–13 years, 21 mcg**
  14–18 years, 24 mcg
  19–50 years, 25 mcg
  50 years and older, 20 mcg
➤ **Pregnant women, 30 mcg (29 mcg if 18 years or younger)**
➤ **Nursing women, 45 mcg (44 mcg if 18 years or younger)**

Some evidence suggests that chromium deficiency may be relatively common. However, this has not been proven, and the matter is greatly complicated by the fact that we lack a good test to identify chromium deficiency.

Severe chromium deficiency has only been seen in hospitalized individuals receiving nutrition intravenously. Symptoms include problems with blood sugar control that cannot be corrected by insulin alone.

Corticosteroid treatment may cause increased chromium loss in the urine. It is possible that this loss of chromium may contribute to corticosteroid-induced diabetes.

Chromium is found in drinking water, especially hard water, but concentrations vary widely. Many good sources of chromium, such as whole wheat, are depleted of this important mineral during processing. The most concentrated sources of chromium are brewer's yeast (not nutritional or torula yeast) and calf liver. Two ounces of brewer's yeast or 4 ounces of calf liver supply between 50 and 60 mcg of chromium. Other good sources of chromium are whole grains, beer, and cheese.

Calcium carbonate interferes with the absorption of chromium.

Therapeutic Dosages

The dosage of chromium used in studies ranges from 200 to 1,000 mcg daily. However, there may be potential risks in the higher dosages of chromium (see Safety Issues below).

Some products state that they contain "GTF chromium." Some of these products are manufactured from brewer's yeast, which was once thought to contain GTF. Others contain chromium as chromium nicotinate, which bears a faint resemblance to the proposed GTF molecule. However, since GTF is no longer believed to exist, this claim should be disregarded.

Therapeutic Uses

Chromium has principally been studied for its possible benefits in improving blood sugar control in people with **diabetes**. Several, but not all, studies suggest that people with adult-onset (type 2) diabetes may show some improvement when given appropriate dosages of chromium. One study suggests that chromium may also be useful for **diabetes that occurs during pregnancy**. In addition, nondiabetic individuals with mildly impaired blood sugar control might attain better control of blood sugar with chromium supplementation. Since mild impairment of blood sugar control is believed to increase risk of heart disease, chromium supplementation might help reduce **heart disease rates**.

Chromium has been sold as a "fat burner" and is also said to help build muscle tissue. While most studies evaluating chromium's ability to promote **weight loss** have not found benefits, the largest study did find some evidence that chromium can enhance fat loss.

Studies evaluating chromium as a **performance enhancer** or aid to bodybuilding have yielded almost entirely negative results.

Studies on whether chromium can improve **cholesterol** levels have returned mixed results. However, one study suggests that chromium combined with **grape seed extract** might have a beneficial effect. In addition, among individuals taking beta-blockers, chromium may raise levels of HDL ("good") cholesterol.

When depression is characterized by rapid mood changes, excessive sleeping and eating, a sense of leaden paralysis, and extreme sensitivity to negative life events, the condition is called *atypical depression*. A very small (15 participants) double-blind, placebo-controlled study found that chromium picolinate might be helpful for this form of **depression**; however, a much larger study failed to find statistically significant benefits.

According to some researchers, impaired blood sugar control, high cholesterol, weight gain, and high blood pressure are all part of a bigger picture, called *metabolic syndrome*, or *syndrome* X. Since chromium may be helpful for the first three of these conditions, chromium deficiency has been proposed as the cause of syndrome X. However, this has not been proven.

One study failed to find that chromium picolinate at 200 mcg/day can improve symptoms of polycystic ovaries (a common cause of **infertility**).

Chromium has also been proposed as a treatment for **acne**, **migraine headaches**, and **psoriasis**, but there is as yet no real evidence that it works.

What Is the Scientific Evidence for Chromium?

Diabetes

The evidence regarding use of chromium for type 2 (adult onset) diabetes, as well as other forms of diabetes, remains incomplete and inconsistent.

In a double-blind, placebo-controlled study, 180 people with type 2 diabetes were given placebo, 200 mcg of chromium picolinate, or 1,000 mcg of chromium picolinate daily. Individuals taking 1,000 mcg showed marked improvements in blood sugar levels. Lesser but still significant benefits were also seen in the 200-mcg group but not in the placebo group.

A double-blind trial of 78 individuals with type 2 diabetes compared two forms of chromium (brewer's yeast and chromium chloride) against placebo. This rather complex crossover study consisted of four 8-week intervals of treatment in random order. The results in the 67 participants who completed the study showed that both forms of chromium significantly improved blood sugar control.

Positive results were also seen in two other double-blind, placebo-controlled studies enrolling a total of more than 100 people with type 2 diabetes. One of these studies involved people with severe type 2 diabetes and found that though use of chromium did not allow a reduction in medication dosage, it did improve blood sugar control overall. However, several studies have failed to find benefit for people with type 2 diabetes. These contradictory findings suggest that the benefit, if any, is small.

One placebo-controlled study of 30 women with pregnancy-related diabetes found that supplementation with chromium (at a dosage of 4 or 8 mcg chromium picolinate for each kilogram of body weight) significantly improved blood sugar control.

Chromium has also shown some promise for treating diabetes caused by corticosteroid treatment.

Improved Blood Sugar Control in People Without Diabetes

Many people develop impaired responsiveness to insulin (insulin resistance) and mildly abnormal blood sugar levels. A few small, double-blind trials have found that chromium supplementation may be helpful, although two studies found no benefit. Another small double-blind trial found that chromium improved the body's response to insulin among overweight people at risk of developing diabetes. There is growing evidence that mildly impaired blood sugar control increases the risk of heart disease (see Heart Disease Prevention below), suggesting that chromium supplementation might be useful.

Weight Loss ("Fat Burning")

The evidence is mixed on whether chromium is an effective aid for reducing weight or improving body composition (improving the ratio of fatty tissue to lean tissue).

In one study, 219 people were given either placebo or 200 or 400 mcg of chromium picolinate daily. Participants were not advised to follow any particular diet. Over a period of 72 days, people taking chromium experienced significantly greater weight loss than those not taking chromium—more than 2½ pounds versus about ¼ pound. Interestingly, people taking chromium actually gained lean body mass, so the loss of fatty tissue was even more dramatic: more than 4 pounds versus less than ½ pound. However, a very high dropout rate makes the results of this study somewhat unreliable.

However, in another double-blind study by the same researcher, 130 moderately overweight people attempting to lose weight were given either placebo or 400 mcg of chromium daily. At the end of the trial, no statistically significant differences in weight or body composition were seen between groups. Researchers were able to show benefit only by resorting to fairly complicated statistical maneuvers.

In a third study, 44 overweight women were given either placebo or 400 mcg of chromium per day. All participants were placed on an exercise program. Over a period of 12 weeks, no differences were seen between the two groups in terms of body weight, waist circumference, or percentage body fat. A small double-blind trial of older women undergoing resistance training also failed to find evidence of benefit. Generally negative results were seen in other small double-blind trials as well.

When larger studies find positive results and smaller studies do not, it often indicates that the treatment under study is only weakly effective. This may be the case with chromium as a weight-loss treatment.

Heart Disease Prevention

Insulin resistance, as well as mildly elevated blood sugar levels, appears to increase risk of heart disease. Chromium supplementation might help by improving insulin responsiveness and normalizing blood sugar.

In support of this, an observational trial found associations between higher chromium intake and reduced risk of heart attack.

Safety Issues

Although the precise upper limit of safe chromium intake is not known, it is believed that chromium is safe when taken at a dosage of 50 to 200 mcg daily. Side effects appear to be rare.

However, chromium is a heavy metal and might conceivably build up and cause problems if taken to excess. There is one report of kidney, liver, and bone marrow damage in a person who took 1,200 to 2,400 mcg of chromium for several months; in another report, as little as 600 mcg for 6 weeks was enough to cause damage. Such problems appear to be quite rare and it is possible that these individuals already had health problems that predisposed them to such a reaction. The risk of chromium toxicity is believed to be higher in individuals who already have liver or kidney disease.

Nonetheless, based on these reports, it's possible that the dosage of chromium found most effective for individuals with type 2 diabetes—1,000 mcg daily—

might present some health risks. For example, there is some evidence that if chromium is taken in high enough amounts, it may be converted from its original safe form (chromium 3) into a known carcinogen, chromium 6. We advise seeking medical supervision before taking more than 200 mcg of chromium daily.

Also, keep in mind that if you have diabetes and chromium is effective, you may need to cut down your dosage of any medication you take for diabetes. Medical supervision is advised.

There are also several concerns about the picolinate form of chromium in particular. Picolinate can alter levels of neurotransmitters. This has led to concern among some experts that chromium picolinate might be harmful for individuals with **depression**, **bipolar disease**, or **schizophrenia**. There has also been one report of a severe skin reaction caused by chromium picolinate.

Finally, there are also concerns, still fairly theoretical and uncertain, that chromium picolinate could cause adverse effects on DNA.

The maximum safe dosage of chromium for women who are pregnant or nursing and for individuals with severe liver or kidney disease has not been established.

Interactions You Should Know About

If you are taking:

- Calcium carbonate supplements or antacids: You may need extra chromium. You should also separate your chromium supplement and your doses of these substances by at least 2 hours because they may interfere with chromium's absorption.
- Corticosteroids: You may need extra chromium.
- Oral diabetes medications or insulin: Seek medical supervision before taking chromium because you may need to reduce your dose of these medications.
- Beta-blockers: Chromium supplementation may improve levels of HDL ("good") cholesterol.

Cinnamon

Cinnamomum zeylanicum

PRINCIPAL PROPOSED USES: *Diabetes, High Cholesterol*

OTHER PROPOSED USES: *Antimicrobial, Improving Appetite, Indigestion, Ulcers*

Most Americans consider cinnamon a simple flavoring, but in traditional Chinese medicine, it's one of the oldest remedies, prescribed for everything from diarrhea and chills to influenza and parasitic worms. Cinnamon comes from the bark of a small Southeast Asian evergreen tree and is available as an oil, extract, or dried powder. It's closely related to cassia (*C. cassia*) and contains many of the same components, but the bark and oils from *C. zeylanicum* are thought to have a better flavor.

What Is Cinnamon Used for Today?

Based on the results of one preliminary double-blind, placebo-controlled study, cinnamon has been widely advertised as an effective treatment for type 2 **diabetes** as well as **high cholesterol**. However, as described below, this conclusion was premature.

Germany's Commission E approves cinnamon for **improving appetite** and relieving **indigestion**; however, these uses are not backed by reliable scientific evidence.

Two animal studies weakly suggest that an extract of cinnamon bark taken orally may help prevent **stomach ulcers**.

Preliminary results from test tube and animal studies suggest that cinnamon oil and cinnamon extract have antifungal, antibacterial, and antiparasitic properties. For example, cinnamon has been found to be active against *Candida albicans*, the fungus responsible for vaginal **yeast infections** and thrush (oral yeast infection), *Helicobacter pylori* (the bacteria that causes stomach ulcers), and even head lice. However, it's a long way from studies of this type to actual proof of effectiveness. Until cinnamon is tested in double-blind human trials, we can't conclude that it can successfully treat these or any other infections. (For information on why double-blind studies are so important, see **Why Does This Book Rely on Double-blind Studies?**)

What Is the Scientific Evidence for Cinnamon?

Based on previous animal studies that had suggested potential benefits of cinnamon for diabetes, researchers in Pakistan performed a double-blind, placebo-controlled trial in people. In this 40-day study, 60 people with type 2 diabetes were given cinnamon at a dose of 1, 3, or 6 g daily. The results reportedly indicated that use of cinnamon improved blood sugar levels by 18–29%, total cholesterol by 12–26%, LDL ("bad") cholesterol by 7–27%, and triglycerides by 23–30%. These results were said to be statistically significant as compared to the beginning of the study and to the placebo group.

However, this study has some odd features. The most important is that it found no significant difference in benefit between the various doses of cinnamon. This is called lack of a *dose-related effect* and it generally casts doubt on the results of a study. The researchers counter that perhaps even 1 g of cinnamon is sufficient to produce the maximum cholesterol-lowering effect and, therefore, higher doses simply didn't add any further benefit. There is another problem with this study as well: no improvements were seen in the placebo group. This, too, is unusual, and it also casts doubt on the results.

In an attempt to replicate these results, a group of Dutch researchers performed a carefully designed 6-week, double-blind, placebo-controlled study of 25 people with diabetes. All participants were given 1.5 g of cinnamon daily. The results failed to show *any* detectible effect on blood sugar, insulin sensitivity, or cholesterol profile. Although this second study was smaller than the first because it had fewer groups ("arms"), overall, its statistical power is similar.

Another study, this one involving 79 people given 3 g of cinnamon daily for 4 months, found marginal benefits at most.

At present, therefore, it would be premature to consider cinnamon an evidence-based treatment for diabetes or high cholesterol.

Dosage

Typical recommended dosages of ground cinnamon bark are 1 to 4 g daily. Cinnamon oil is generally used at a dose of 0.05 to 0.2 g daily.

Safety Issues

As a widely used food spice, ground cinnamon bark is believed to be safe. However, cinnamon's **essential oil** is much more concentrated than the powdered bark commonly used for baking. There is some evidence that high doses of cinnamon oil might depress the central nervous system. Germany's Commission E recommends that pregnant women avoid taking cinnamon oil or high doses of the bark. Maximum safe doses in young children, nursing women, or individuals with severe liver or kidney disease have not been determined.

When used topically, cinnamon bark oil may cause flushing and a burning sensation. Some people have reported strong burning sensations or mouth ulcers after chewing cinnamon-flavored gum or candy. However, these reactions disappeared within days of discontinuing the gum.

Citrulline

ALTERNATE NAME/RELATED TERM: *L-Citrulline Malate*
PRINCIPAL PROPOSED USES: *Enhancing Sports Performance*
OTHER PROPOSED USES: *Alzheimer's Disease, Fatigue, Impotence*

Citrulline is a non-essential amino acid, meaning that the body can manufacture it from other nutrients. Within the body, citrulline is converted to the amino acid **L-arginine**. Some of the proposed uses of citrulline supplements are based on raising levels of arginine. Citrulline also plays a role in a physiological process called *the urea cycle*, in which toxic ammonia is converted to urea.

Requirements/Sources

The body manufactures citrulline from the essential amino acid glutamine. Deficiency of citrulline is unlikely to occur.

Therapeutic Dosages

A typical dose of citrulline is 6 to 18 g daily. It is commonly sold in the form of citrulline malate.

Therapeutic Uses

There is little scientific support for any use of citrulline supplements.

Citrulline is most commonly marketed today as a supplement for **enhancing sports performance**. Based on exceedingly speculative reasoning, it is often described as an aerobic complement to the supplement **creatine**. Supposedly, citrulline enhances aerobic exercise capacity (relatively low-intensity exercise), while creatine enhances anaerobic exercise capacity (high-intensity exercise). However, while there have been numerous double-blind studies on creatine, available evidence on citrulline as a sports supplement is so scant that no conclusions whatsoever can be based on it. The only meaningful study reported thus far found that citrulline *reduced* rather than enhanced exercise capacity. Current enthusiasm for the supplement is therefore based entirely on testimonials. Since placebos increase sense of energy and well-being, and since they may even enhance performance, enthusiastic testimonials about a new and exciting supplement should be received with considerable caution.

Other proposed uses of citrulline are based on the fact that the body converts citrulline to the amino acid arginine. It is claimed by some that citrulline supplements are actually more effective at raising arginine levels than arginine supplements. However, this has not been established in any scientific sense. Furthermore, arginine itself is not a proven treatment for any condition. For example, citrulline is marketed as a treatment for **impotence** based on the assumption that arginine is effective for impotence. However, current evidence supporting arginine as an impotence treatment is weak at best and citrulline itself has not been studied for this use in any meaningful way. Again, numerous testimonials are offered, but they mean little: placebos are very effective for impotence.

Very preliminary studies conducted in France in the late 1970s hint that citrulline may improve mental func-tion in people with **Alzheimer's disease** and also reduce general **fatigue**. However, these studies were not conducted at the level of modern scientific standards and have not been followed up.

Safety Issues

As a naturally occurring amino acid, citrulline is believed to be safe. However, maximum safe doses in young children, pregnant or nursing women, or people with severe liver or kidney disease have not been established.

Citrus aurantium

ALTERNATE NAMES/RELATED TERMS: *Bitter Orange, Seville Orange, Sour Orange*
PRINCIPAL PROPOSED USES: *Weight Loss*
OTHER PROPOSED USES: *Anxiety, Cancer Prevention, Depression, Viral Infections*

Citrus aurantium is the Latin name for a fruit called *Seville orange* or *bitter orange*. The juice, peel, and essential oil have all been used medicinally. Traditional uses include digestive problems, epilepsy, fatigue, insomnia, infections, respiratory problems, skin problems, and many other uses. As a flavoring, essence of bitter orange is found in the drinks Triple Sec and Cointreau.

What Is *Citrus aurantium* Used for Today?

Citrus aurantium juice and peel contain the stimulant chemical synephrine as well as related stimulants such as octopamine, tyramine, N-methyltyramine, and horde-line. On this basis, *Citrus aurantium* has been widely marketed as a **weight-loss product**. However, there is no reliable evidence that *Citrus aurantium* is effective, and there is considerable reason to worry that it may cause harm (see Safety Issues below). The reassuring statement made by some manufacturers that *Citrus aurantium* offers the "benefits of ephedra without the risks" is not supported by scientific evidence.

The only published double-blind, placebo-controlled trial on *Citrus aurantium* juice did not test the herb alone, but rather evaluated a combination product that also contained caffeine and **St. John's wort**. While the results were somewhat positive, overall the study was too preliminary to reach reliable conclusions. An even less reliable study evaluated the synephrine constituent of *Citrus aurantium* and found possible "fat burning" actions. In view of the weakness of the evidence in favor of *Citrus aurantium* and the considerable evidence that it presents health risks, we recommend against using it for weight loss.

Other evidence, far too weak to rely upon at all, hints that synephrine-rich *Citrus aurantium* extracts might have **antidepressant effects**.

Besides synephrine and other stimulants, whole *Citrus aurantium* peel contains citral, limonene, and several **citrus bioflavonoids**, including hesperidin, neo-hesperidin, naringin, and rutin. Weak evidence hints that these substances might have **cancer-preventive** and antiviral actions.

The **essential oil** of *Citrus aurantium* contains linalool and the fragrant substance limonene and might have antianxiety and sedative effects. However, neither of these proposed uses has more than extremely preliminary supporting evidence.

Dosage

Many *Citrus aurantium* products are made from the juice and/or concentrated extracts of the peel and are said to contain a fixed percentage of synephrine or total amines. A typical recommended dosage of such products ranges from 100 to 150 mg 2 to 3 times daily. However, these doses may be unsafe.

Safety Issues

Most of the safety concerns regarding *Citrus aurantium* relate to its stimulant constituents.

The drug synephrine is known to produce many unpleasant and possibly dangerous side effects, including headache, agitation, rapid heart rate, and heart palpitations. In some people, it can cause **angina pectoris**, kidney damage, increased pressure in the eye, and reduced blood circulation to the heart and the extremities. The other stimulant amines in *Citrus aurantium* may increase such effects. There is one case report of a heart attack that appears possibly related to use of a *Citrus aurantium* supplement, and another that links the herb to stroke. *Citrus aurantium* juice or concentrated extracts can raise blood pressure and increase heart rate and, therefore, should not be used by individuals with **cardiovascular disease** or **high blood pressure**. The herb should also be avoided by people with **glaucoma**.

Synephrine can also interact with numerous medications and other drugs, including stimulants (for example, ephedrine, pseudoephedrine [Sudafed], Ritalin, and even caffeine) and anesthetics. The tyramine constituent of *Citrus aurantium* can cause deadly side effects when combined with drugs in the MAO inhibitor family.

The peel and essential oil of *Citrus aurantium* may cause photosensitivity (increased tendency to react to sun exposure). For this reason, combination treatment with drugs that cause the same side effect (such as sulfa antibiotics) is not recommended.

Finally, *Citrus aurantium* juice can alter the way that the liver processes various medications, potentially raising or lowering their levels.

In particular, the drugs cyclosporine and felodipine (a calcium channel blocker) are thought to be affected by *Citrus aurantium* juice, but numerous other drugs may interact with it as well. For this reason, we recommend that if you are taking any medication that is critical to your health, you should not take *Citrus aurantium* juice.

Safety in young children, pregnant or nursing women, or people with severe liver or kidney disease has not been established.

Interactions You Should Know About

If you are taking:

➤ **Drugs in the MAO inhibitor family: Do not use *Citrus aurantium* at all.**
➤ **Ephedrine, pseudoephedrine (Sudafed), Ritalin, cyclosporine, calcium channel blockers, drugs that cause photosensitivity (such as sulfa antibiotics), or any medication that is critical to your health: Do not use *Citrus aurantium* without consulting a physician.**

Citrus Bioflavonoids

SUPPLEMENT FORMS/ALTERNATE NAMES: *Bioflavonoid, Diosmetin, Diosmin, Hesperidin, Naringin, Narirutin, Neohesperidin, Nobiletin, Rutin, Tangeretin*

PRINCIPAL PROPOSED USES: *Hemorrhoids, Chronic Venous Insufficiency*

OTHER PROPOSED USES: *Easy Bruising, Hypertension, Leg Ulcers, Lymphedema Following Breast Cancer Surgery, Nosebleeds*

Citrus fruits are well known for providing ample amounts of **vitamin C**. But they also supply bioflavonoids, substances that are not required for life but that may improve health. The major bioflavonoids found in citrus fruits are diosmin, hesperidin, rutin, naringin, tangeretin, diosmetin, narirutin, neohesperidin, nobiletin, and quercetin.

This article addresses the first five bioflavonoids listed above. Please see the article on **quercetin** for information on this supplement. A modified form of rutin, **oxerutin**, is also discussed in its own article.

Citrus bioflavonoids and related substances are widely used in Europe to treat diseases of the blood vessels and lymph system, including hemorrhoids, chronic venous insufficiency, leg ulcers, easy bruising, nosebleeds, and lymphedema following breast cancer surgery. These compounds are thought to work by strengthening the walls of blood vessels.

Requirements/Sources

Citrus fruits contain citrus bioflavonoids in varying proportions. Even different brands of citrus juice may vary widely in their bioflavonoid concentrations and composition. For use as a supplement, bioflavonoids are extracted either from citrus fruits or other plant sources, such as buckwheat.

Therapeutic Dosages

A typical dosage of citrus bioflavonoids is 500 mg twice daily. The most studied citrus bioflavonoid treatment is a special micronized (finely ground) combination of diosmin (90%) and hesperidin (10%).

Therapeutic Uses

Double-blind trials suggest that a micronized combination preparation of diosmin and hesperidin may be helpful for **hemorrhoids**.

Diosmin and hesperidin, as well as the bioflavonoid rutin, may also be helpful for **chronic venous insufficiency**, a condition in which the veins in the legs begin to weaken.

At least one good double-blind trial also found diosmin and hesperidin to be helpful for individuals who develop **bruises** or **nosebleeds** easily.

Citrus bioflavonoids have also been tried, with some success, for treating lymphedema (arm swelling) following **breast cancer surgery**.

Note: Do not use bioflavonoid combinations containing tangeretin if you are taking tamoxifen for breast cancer.

In addition, highly preliminary evidence suggests that citrus bioflavonoids may help reduce **cholesterol** levels, control inflammation, benefit people with **diabetes**, reduce **allergic reactions**, and **prevent cancer.**

"Sweetie fruit," a bioflavonoid-rich hybrid of grapefruit and pummelo, has shown a bit of promise for treatment of **high blood pressure**.

What Is the Scientific Evidence for Citrus Bioflavonoids?

Hemorrhoids

A 2-month, double-blind, placebo-controlled trial of 120 individuals with recurrent hemorrhoid flare-ups found that treatment with combined diosmin and hesperidin significantly reduced the frequency and severity of hemorrhoid attacks. Another double-blind, placebo-controlled trial of 100 individuals had positive results with the same bioflavonoids in relieving symptoms once a flare-up of hemorrhoid pain had begun. A 90-day, double-blind trial of 100 individuals with bleeding hemorrhoids also found significant benefits for both treatment of acute attacks and prevention of new ones. Finally, this bioflavonoid combination was found to compare favorably with surgical treatment of hemorrhoids. However, less-impressive results were seen in a double-blind, placebo-controlled study in which all participants were given a fiber laxative with either combined diosmin and hesperidin or placebo.

Two studies claimed to find that diosmin/hesperidin reduces pain after hemorrhoid surgery. In fact, these studies show little to nothing, as the researchers failed to use a placebo group and simply compared treated participants to untreated participants. (For information on why this matters, see **Why Does This Book Rely on Double-blind Studies?.**)

Chronic Venous Insufficiency

A 2-month, double-blind, placebo-controlled trial of 200 people with relatively severe chronic venous insufficiency found that treatment with diosmin/hesperidin significantly improved symptoms as compared to placebo.

Another double-blind, placebo-controlled trial of diosmin/hesperidin enrolled 101 people with relatively *mild* chronic venous insufficiency. The results showed little difference between the two groups; the authors theorize that diosmin/hesperidin might be more effective in *severe* chronic venous insufficiency.

A 2-month, double-blind, placebo-controlled trial evaluated the effects of diosmin/hesperidin in 107 people with nonhealing leg ulcers (sores) caused by venous insufficiency or other conditions. The results indicated that treatment significantly improved the rate of healing.

Also, a 3-month, double-blind, placebo-controlled trial of 67 individuals evaluated buckwheat tea (a good source of rutin) for chronic venous insufficiency. The results showed less leg swelling in the treated group.

One study supposedly showed that the supplement oxyrutin is more effective than diosmin/hesperidin for chronic venous insufficiency, but the study was too poorly designed to provide meaningful results.

Easy Bruising

Some people bruise particularly easily due to fragile capillaries. A 6-week, double-blind, placebo-controlled study of 96 people with this condition found that combined diosmin and hesperidin decreased symptoms of capillary fragility, such as bruising and nosebleeds.

Two rather poorly designed studies from the 1960s found benefits with a combination of vitamin C and citrus bioflavonoids for decreasing bruising in collegiate athletes.

Lymphedema

Breast cancer surgery sometimes causes persistent swelling of the arm (lymphedema) caused by damage to lymph vessels. Citrus bioflavonoids as well as other natural supplements have shown promise for this condition. In a 3-month, double-blind study, 57 women with lymphedema received either placebo or combination therapy consisting of the modified citrus bioflavonoid trimethylhesperidin chalcone plus the bioflavonoid-rich herb **butcher's broom**. The results indicated that use of the bioflavonoid combination resulted in significantly less swelling.

Safety Issues

Extensive investigations of diosmin and hesperidin have found them to be essentially nontoxic and free of drug interactions. The combination has been given to 50 pregnant women in a research study, without apparent harm to mothers or babies.

However, the citrus bioflavonoid tangeretin may interfere with the action of tamoxifen, a drug used to treat breast cancer.

One highly preliminary study suggests that some citrus bioflavonoids in the diet of pregnant women might increase the risk of infant leukemia; hesperidin did not produce this effect and diosmin was not tested.

Interactions You Should Know About

If you are taking **tamoxifen** for breast cancer, you should avoid citrus fruits and juices and the citrus bioflavonoid tangeretin.

Cleavers

Galium aparine

PRINCIPAL PROPOSED USES: *None*

OTHER PROPOSED USES: *Bladder Infections, Fluid Retention, Swollen Glands*

The leaves of the cleavers plant (*Galium aparine*) have small hooked hairs that cause it to "cleave" to the fingers when touched, hence the name. The whole leaf has been used as a flavoring in soups and stews. Roasted seeds are used as a coffee substitute. The leaves and flowers are used medicinally. Cleavers is primarily used for urinary problems and fluid retention, on the basis of its apparent diuretic (urine-stimulating) effects. It has also been recommended for enlarged lymph nodes, tonsillitis, hepatitis, and snake bites.

What Is Cleavers Used for Today?

Cleavers is often included in herbal mixtures offered for the treatment of kidney and bladder problems, including **bladder infections**, **kidney stones**, and **prostatitis**. It is also said to help "cleanse" the lymph system. However, there has not been any meaningful scientific evaluation of the herb. Even animal and test-tube studies are essentially lacking.

Dosage

A typical recommended dose of cleavers is 1 cup of tea 3 times daily, made by steeping 10 to 15 g of the herb in a cup of hot water.

Safety Issues

Cleavers has not undergone any meaningful safety testing. Safety in young children, pregnant or nursing women, or people with severe liver or kidney disease has not been established.

In case cleavers does, in fact, have diuretic effects as claimed, people taking the medication lithium should use cleavers only under the supervision of a physician, as dehydration can be dangerous with this medication.

Interactions You Should Know About

If you are taking **lithium**, do not use cleavers except under the supervision of a physician.

Coenzyme Q₁₀

SUPPLEMENT FORMS/ALTERNATE NAMES: *CoQ₁₀, Ubiquinone*
PRINCIPAL PROPOSED USES: *Cardiomyopathy, Congestive Heart Failure, Heart Attack Recovery, Hypertension, Nutrient Depletion/Interference Caused by Various Medications*
OTHER PROPOSED USES: *Amyotrophic Lateral Sclerosis (Lou Gehrig's Disease), Diabetes, Kidney Failure, Migraine Headaches, Parkinson's Disease, Periodontal Disease, Sports Performance Enhancement*

Coenzyme Q₁₀ (CoQ₁₀), also known as ubiquinone, is a major part of the body's mechanism for producing energy. The name of this supplement comes from the word *ubiquitous*, which means "found everywhere." Indeed, CoQ₁₀ is found in every cell in the body. It plays a fundamental role in the mitochondria, the parts of the cell that produce energy from glucose and fatty acids.

Japanese scientists first reported therapeutic properties of CoQ₁₀ in the 1960s. Some evidence suggests that CoQ₁₀ might assist the heart during times of stress on the heart muscle, perhaps by helping it use energy more efficiently.

CoQ₁₀'s best-established use is for congestive heart failure, but the evidence that it works is not entirely consistent. Ongoing research suggests that it may also be useful for other types of heart problems, Parkinson's disease, and several additional illnesses. It is generally used in addition to, rather than instead of, standard therapies.

CoQ₁₀ supplementation might also be of value for counteracting side effects of certain prescription medications.

Sources

Every cell in your body needs CoQ₁₀, but there is no dietary requirement as the body can manufacture CoQ₁₀ from scratch.

Therapeutic Dosages

The typical recommended dosage of CoQ₁₀ is 30 to 300 mg daily, often divided into 2 or 3 doses; higher daily intakes have been used in some studies. CoQ₁₀ is fat-soluble and may be better absorbed when taken in an oil-based soft gel form rather than in a dry form, such as tablets and capsules.

Therapeutic Uses

Although not all studies have been positive, the best-documented use of CoQ₁₀ is for treating **congestive heart failure**. Keep in mind that CoQ₁₀ is taken *along with* conventional medications, not as a replacement for them.

Weaker evidence suggests that this supplement may be useful for **heart attack** recovery, **cardiomyopathy**, **hypertension**, **diabetes**, strengthening the heart prior to heart surgery, **migraine headaches**, and **Parkinson's disease**.

CoQ₁₀ has shown the potential to prevent heart damage and other side effects caused by certain types of **cancer chemotherapy**. This evidence is weak, however, and as yet it cannot be stated with any certainty that CoQ₁₀ is actually helpful.

CoQ₁₀ has shown some preliminary promise as an aid to the treatment of kidney failure.

Note: People with severe illnesses, such as heart disease, cancer, or kidney failure, should not use CoQ₁₀, or any supplement, except under physician supervision.

Highly preliminary studies suggest CoQ₁₀ might be helpful for **amyotrophic lateral sclerosis**. CoQ₁₀ has been tried but not found effective for the treatment of Huntington's disease.

Certain medications may interfere with the body's production of CoQ$_{10}$ or partially block its function. The best evidence regards cholesterol-lowering drugs in the statin family, such as lovastatin (Mevacor), simvastatin (Zocor), and pravastatin (Pravachol); these medications impair CoQ$_{10}$ synthesis as an inevitable side effect of their mechanism of action. Since these drugs are used to protect the heart and since CoQ$_{10}$ deficiency could in theory impair heart function, it has been suggested that this side effect may work against the intended purpose of taking statins. (Note also that the supplement red yeast rice contains statin drugs, and people who use this supplement might benefit from CoQ$_{10}$ on the same principles.) However, there is only weak and inconsistent evidence to indicate CoQ$_{10}$ supplements offer any specific benefit to people taking statins. For several other categories of drugs, the evidence that they interfere with CoQ$_{10}$ is provocative but less than solid. These include oral diabetes drugs (especially glyburide, phenformin, and tolazamide), beta-blockers (specifically propranolol, metoprolol, and alprenolol), antipsychotic drugs in the phenothiazine family, tricyclic antidepressants, methyldopa, hydrochlorothiazide, clonidine, and hydralazine.

CoQ$_{10}$ has also been suggested as a **performance enhancer** for athletes. However, while one double-blind study of 25 highly trained cross-country skiers found some benefit, most studies evaluating potential sports supplement uses of CoQ$_{10}$ have returned negative rather than positive results.

CoQ$_{10}$ is also sometimes claimed to be an effective treatment for **periodontal disease**. However, the studies on which this idea is based are too flawed to be taken as meaningful.

One preliminary study of CoQ$_{10}$ for people undergoing treatment for **HIV** found conflicting results; the supplement appeared to improve general well-being, but it did not protect mitochondria (as the researchers had hoped it would) and actually seemed to worsen symptoms of nerve-related pain (peripheral neuropathy).

CoQ$_{10}$ has additionally been proposed as a treatment for a wide variety of other conditions, including **angina**, **cancer**, **male infertility**, muscular dystrophy, and **obesity**, but there is, as yet, no evidence that it is effective.

What Is the Scientific Evidence for Coenzyme Q$_{10}$?

Congestive Heart Failure

Most but not all studies tell us that CoQ$_{10}$ can be helpful for people with congestive heart failure (CHF). In this serious condition, the heart muscles become weakened, resulting in poor circulation and shortness of breath.

People with CHF have significantly lower levels of CoQ$_{10}$ in heart muscle cells than do healthy people. This fact alone does not prove that CoQ$_{10}$ supplements will help CHF; however, it prompted medical researchers to try using CoQ$_{10}$ as a treatment for heart failure.

The largest study was a 1-year, double-blind, placebo-controlled trial of 641 people with moderate to severe congestive heart failure. Half were given 2 mg per kilogram body weight of CoQ$_{10}$ daily; the rest were given placebo. Standard therapy was continued in both groups. The participants treated with CoQ$_{10}$ experienced a significant reduction in the severity of their symptoms. No such improvement was seen in the placebo group. The people who took CoQ$_{10}$ also had significantly fewer hospitalizations for heart failure.

Similarly positive results were also seen in other double-blind studies involving a total of more than 250 participants. One double-blind study found that in people with heart failure so severe they were waiting for a heart transplant, use of CoQ$_{10}$ improved subjective symptoms.

However, two very well-designed, double-blind studies published in 1999 and 2000 enrolling a total of about 85 people with congestive heart failure failed to find any evidence of benefit. The reason for this discrepancy is not clear.

Cardiomyopathy

Cardiomyopathy is the general name given to conditions in which the heart muscle gradually becomes diseased. Several small studies suggest that CoQ$_{10}$ supplements are helpful for some forms of cardiomyopathy.

Hypertension

An 8-week, double-blind, placebo-controlled study of 59 men already taking medications for high blood pressure found that 120 mg daily of CoQ$_{10}$ reduced blood pressure by about 9% as compared to placebo.

A 12-week, double-blind, placebo-controlled study of 83 people with isolated systolic hypertension (a type of high blood pressure in which only the "top" number is high) found that use of CoQ$_{10}$ at a dose of 60 mg daily improved blood pressure measurements to a similar extent.

Similarly, in a 12-week, double-blind, placebo-controlled trial of 74 people with diabetes, use of CoQ$_{10}$ at a dose of 100 mg twice daily significantly reduced blood pressure as compared to placebo.

Anti-hypertensive effects were also seen in previous smaller trials, most of which were not double-blind.

Heart Attack Recovery

In a double-blind trial, 144 people who had recently experienced a heart attack were given either placebo or 120 mg of CoQ_{10} daily for 1 year, along with conventional treatment. The results showed that participants receiving CoQ_{10} experienced significantly fewer heart-related problems, such as episodes of angina pectoris or arrhythmia or recurrent heart attacks.

A double-blind study of 49 people who had suffered a full cardiac arrest requiring cardiopulmonary resuscitation (CPR) found that use of CoQ_{10} along with mild hypothermia (chilling of the body) was more effective than mild hypothermia plus placebo.

Note: Individuals recovering from a heart attack should not take any herbs or supplements except under the supervision of a physician.

Parkinson's Disease

In a double-blind trial, 28 people with Parkinson's disease were given either placebo or 360 mg of CoQ_{10} daily, along with conventional care. The results indicated that use of the supplement produced a mild improvement in symptoms.

In a previous study, CoQ_{10} showed some promise for slowing the progression of Parkinson's disease. In this 16-month, double-blind, placebo-controlled trial, 80 people with Parkinson's disease were given either CoQ_{10} (at a dose of 300, 600, or 1,200 mg daily) or placebo. Participants in this trial had early stages of the disease and did not yet need medication. The results suggested that CoQ_{10}, especially at the highest dose, might have slowed disease progression. However, various statistical technicalities made the results inconclusive.

Further trials will be necessary to confirm (or deny) these encouraging results.

Diabetes

In the 12-week, double-blind, placebo-controlled trial of 74 people with diabetes mentioned above, use of CoQ_{10} at a dose of 100 mg twice daily significantly improved blood sugar control as compared to placebo. Similar benefits were seen in the 8-week, double-blind, placebo-controlled study of 59 men also described above. However, a third study failed to find any effect on blood sugar control.

Safety Issues

In general, CoQ_{10} appears to be extremely safe. No significant side effects have been found, even in studies

that lasted a year. However, people with severe heart disease should not take CoQ_{10} (or any other supplement) except under a doctor's supervision.

As noted above, two studies suggest that CoQ_{10} might reduce blood sugar levels in people with diabetes. While this could potentially be helpful for treatment of diabetes, it might present a risk as well; people with diabetes who are using CoQ_{10} might inadvertently push their blood sugar levels dangerously low. However, another trial in people with diabetes found no effect on blood sugar control. The bottom line: If you have diabetes, make sure to track your blood sugar closely if you start taking CoQ_{10} (or, indeed, any herb or supplement).

CoQ_{10} chemically resembles **vitamin K**. Since vitamin K counters the anticoagulant effects of warfarin (Coumadin), it has been suggested that CoQ_{10} may have the same effect. However, a small double-blind study found no interaction between CoQ_{10} and warfarin. Nonetheless, in view of warfarin's low margin of safety, prudence indicates physician supervision before combining CoQ_{10} with warfarin.

CoQ_{10} might also interact with reverse transcriptase inhibitors used for treatment of HIV (for example, lamivudine and zidovudine). These medications can cause damage to the mitochondria, the energy-producing subunits of cells, leading in turn to a variety of side effects, including lactic acidosis (a dangerous metabolic derangement), peripheral neuropathy (injury to nerves in the extremities), and lipodystrophy (cosmetically undesirable rearrangement of fat in the body). The supplement CoQ_{10} has been tried for minimizing these side effects, but unexpected results occurred. In a double-blind, placebo-controlled study, use of CoQ_{10} improved general sense of well-being in people with HIV infection using reverse transcriptase inhibitors; however, for reasons that are unclear, it actually worsened symptoms of peripheral neuropathy. For this reason, people with HIV who have peripheral neuropathy symptoms should use CoQ_{10} only with caution.

The maximum safe dosages of CoQ_{10} for young children, pregnant or nursing women, or those with severe liver or kidney disease have not been determined.

Interactions You Should Know About

If you are taking:

> ► **Cholesterol-lowering drugs in the statin family, red yeast rice, beta-blockers (specifically propranolol, metoprolol, and alprenolol), antipsychotic drugs in**

the phenothiazine family, tricyclic antidepressants, methyldopa, hydrochlorothiazide, clonidine, hydralazine, or *oral diabetes drugs* (especially glyburide, phenformin, and tolazamide): You may need more CoQ_{10}.

➤ Warfarin (Coumadin): You should not take CoQ_{10} except on a physician's advice.
➤ Reverse transcriptase inhibitors (for HIV infection): CoQ_{10} might improve general sense of well-being, but worsen peripheral neuropathy symptoms.

Cola Nut

Cola acuminata and *Cola nitida*

PRINCIPAL PROPOSED USES: *Fatigue*

Indigenous to Western Africa, the cola tree is cultivated today in many tropical climates, including Central and South America, the West Indies, Sri Lanka, and Malaysia. Cola nuts are actually seeds removed from their seed coats. Traditionally, they are chewed raw or taken in pulverized or liquid extract form. Of the various species of cola nuts, the two most commonly edible kinds are *Cola acuminata* and *Cola nitida.*

Cola contains caffeine and related chemicals and, for this reason, is a stimulant. For thousands of years, people in Africa have chewed the seeds to enhance mental alertness and fight fatigue. Centuries ago, Arabs traded gold dust for cola nuts before starting out on long treks across the Sahara.

Cola nut has been used in folk medicine as an aphrodisiac and an appetite suppressant, and to treat morning sickness, migraine headache, and indigestion. It has also been applied directly to the skin to treat wounds and inflammation. The tree's bitter twig has been used as well to clean the teeth and gums.

What Is Cola Nut Used for Today?

Based on the cola nut's caffeine content, Germany's Commission E has approved its use for the treatment of **fatigue**.

Cola is ingested daily by millions as one of the main ingredients in cola soft drinks. It is also used in diet and "high-energy" products such as food bars and as a flavoring in alcoholic beverages, frozen dairy desserts, candy, baked goods, gelatins, and puddings. However, the caffeine-containing cola nut, used in original recipes for Coca-Cola, should not be confused with **gotu kola**.

Because of its caffeine content, cola nut would be expected to increase urination, stimulate the heart and lungs, and help analgesics, such as aspirin, to function more effectively.

Dosage

Germany's Commission E recommends the following daily dosage of cola: 2 to 6 g of cola nut, 0.25 to 0.75 g of cola extract, 2.5 to 7.5 g of cola liquid extract, 10 to 30 g of cola tincture, or 60 to 180 g of cola wine.

Safety Issues

Although comprehensive safety studies have not been performed, moderate amounts of cola nut are generally regarded as safe. The Council of Europe and the U.S. Food and Drug Administration have approved it as a food additive. The typical side effects associated with cola nut are those of caffeine, including nervousness, heart irregularities, headaches, and sleeplessness.

Cola is not advised for individuals with stomach **ulcers** due to both its caffeine and its tannin content. Tannins, found in many plants, are substances that can irritate the stomach.

Coleus forskohlii

PRINCIPAL PROPOSED USES: *Allergies, Asthma, Bladder Infections (for Pain Relief), Eczema, Glaucoma, Hypertension, Irritable Bowel Syndrome, Menstrual Cramps, Weight Loss*

OTHER PROPOSED USES: *Psoriasis*

A member of the mint family, *Coleus forskohlii* grows wild on the mountain slopes of Nepal, India, and Thailand. In traditional Asian systems of medicine, it was used for a variety of purposes, including treating skin rashes, asthma, bronchitis, insomnia, epilepsy, and angina. But modern interest is based almost entirely on the work of a drug company, Hoechst Pharmaceuticals.

Like other drug manufacturers, Hoechst regularly screens medicinal plants in hopes of discovering new medications. In 1974, work performed in collaboration with the Indian Central Drug Research Institute found that the rootstock of *Coleus forskohlii* could lower blood pressure and decrease muscle spasms. Intensive study identified a substance named forskolin that appeared to be responsible for much of this effect.

Like certain drugs used for asthma, forskolin increases the levels of a fundamental natural compound known as *cyclic AMP*. Cyclic AMP plays a major role in many cellular functions, and some drugs that affect it relax the muscles around the bronchial tubes.

What Is *Coleus forskohlii* Used for Today?

Herb manufacturers have begun to offer extracts of *Coleus forskohlii* that have been specially manufactured to contain high levels of forskolin.

Forskolin has been found to stabilize the cells that release histamine and other inflammatory compounds. This suggests that *Coleus forskohlii* may be a useful treatment for **asthma**, **eczema**, and other allergic conditions.

Studies have also found that forskolin relaxes smooth muscle tissue. For this reason, *Coleus forskohlii* has been suggested as a treatment for **dysmenorrhea** (menstrual cramps), **angina**, **irritable bowel syndrome** (spastic colon), crampy bladder pain (as in **bladder infections**), and **hypertension** (high blood pressure). Smooth muscle relaxation also suggests another possible way the herb might benefit asthma.

Coleus forskohlii has also been proposed as a treat-
ment for **psoriasis**, because that disease appears to be at least partly related to low levels of cyclic AMP in skin cells.

What Is the Scientific Evidence for *Coleus forskohlii*?

The scientific evidence for the herb *Coleus forskohlii* as a treatment for any disease is weak. What is known relates to the substance forskolin rather than the whole herb.

One small double-blind study indicates that a concentrated forskolin extract might increase the rate of "fat burning," thereby potentially enhancing **weight loss**. Another small double-blind study hints that forskolin taken by inhalation may be as effective as standard asthma inhalers. In addition, forskolin eyedrops have shown promise in improving **glaucoma**. Animal studies and open studies in humans suggest that forskolin can reduce blood pressure and dilate the bronchial tubes in the lungs.

Dosage

A common dosage recommendation is 50 mg 2 or 3 times a day of an extract standardized to contain 18% forskolin.

However, because such an extract provides significant levels of forskolin, a drug with wide-ranging properties, we recommend that *Coleus forskohlii* extracts be taken only with a doctor's supervision.

Safety Issues

The safety of *Coleus forskohlii* and forskolin has not been fully evaluated, although few significant risks have been noted in studies performed thus far. Caution should be exercised when combining this herb with blood-pressure medications and "blood thinners."

In 2005 in Italy, several cases of acute poisoning were reported, apparently caused by accidental contamination of *Coleus forskohlii* products with similar-appearing plants in the deadly nightshade family. Safety in young children, pregnant or nursing women, or those with severe liver or kidney disease has not been established.

Interactions You Should Know About

If you are taking blood pressure medications, such as **beta-blockers**, **clonidine**, or **hydralazine**, or blood-thinning drugs, such as **warfarin** (Coumadin), **heparin**, **clopidogrel** (Plavix), **ticlopidine** (Ticlid), or **pentoxifylline** (Trental), then *Coleus forskohlii* should only be used under the supervision of a physician.

Colostrum

PRINCIPAL PROPOSED USES: *Prevention and Treatment of Infectious Diarrhea*

OTHER PROPOSED USES: *Lichen Planus, Sjogren's Syndrome, Sore Throat and Other Upper Respiratory Infections, Sports Supplement, Ulcer Prevention*

Colostrum is the fluid that new mothers' breasts produce during the first day or two after birth. It gives newborn infants a rich mixture of antibodies and growth factors that help them get a good start.

Although colostrum has been available since the first mammals walked the earth, it is relatively new as a nutritional supplement. The resurgence of breastfeeding in the 1970s sparked a revival of interest in colostrum for both infants and adults.

However, most commercial colostrum preparations come from cows, not humans. The antibodies a mother cow gives to her calf are designed to fend off bacteria that are dangerous to cows; these may be very different from those that pose risks to humans. Nonetheless, colostrum also contains substances that might offer general benefits, such as growth factors (which stimulate the growth and development of cells in the digestive tract and perhaps elsewhere) and transfer factor (which may have general immune-activating properties). In addition, some researchers have used a special form of colostrum called *hyperimmune colostrum*, created by inoculating cows with bacteria and viruses that affect humans. The cow in turn makes antibodies to them and secretes those antibodies into its colostrum. Hyperimmune colostrum has shown considerable promise as an infection-fighting agent.

Hyperimmune colostrum, however, is not available over the counter as a dietary supplement. Non-hyperimmune colostrum might have some value too, but the evidence is much weaker.

Requirements/Sources

Breastfeeding is the healthiest way to nourish a newborn, and a mother's colostrum is undoubtedly good for a baby. But don't believe claims (by at least one manufacturer) that most babies would die without colostrum. Colostrum is good for health, but it's not essential for life.

Colostrum has just become available in capsules that contain its immune proteins in dry form.

Therapeutic Dosages

The usual recommended dosage of colostrum is 10 g daily. In studies of colostrum as a sports supplement for athletes, the much higher dose of 60 g a day was used.

Note: Most of the studies of colostrum for infectious conditions used colostrum prepared by immunizing cows against specific diseases (hyperimmune colostrum). This form is not generally available as a dietary supplement.

Therapeutic Uses

Many, but not all, studies have found that hyperimmune colostrum might be able to help prevent or treat various forms of infectious **diarrhea**.

Colostrum has also shown some promise as a **sports supplement**, presumably because it contains growth factors, but study results are inconsistent.

For years, people with **ulcers** were advised to eat a bland diet and drink lots of milk. Although this treatment was eventually found to be ineffective, according to one study in rats and a small human trial, ordinary colostrum (although not milk) might help protect the stomach from damage caused by anti-inflammatory drugs. It has been hypothesized that colostrum's growth factors help stimulate the stomach to regenerate.

Weak evidence suggests that oral hygiene products containing ordinary colostrum might have beneficial effects in a disease of the mouth called *lichen planus*, as well as in the condition known as **Sjogren's syndrome** (which also affects the mouth, by reducing salivary flow). One study found that colostrinin, a substance extracted from colostrum, might be helpful for **Alzheimer's disease**.

Ordinary colostrum has been suggested as a treatment for short bowel syndrome (a condition following digestive tract surgery), chemotherapy-induced mouth ulcers, and inflammatory bowel disease (**Crohn's disease** and **ulcerative colitis**), but as yet there is no real evidence that it is effective.

A study cited by some colostrum manufacturers as showing that colostrum can prevent or treat upper respiratory infections (such as colds) was actually far too preliminary to do more than hint at benefits. A proper double-blind, placebo-controlled study of 148 adults failed to find colostrum helpful for shortening the duration of a sore throat.

What Is the Scientific Evidence for Colostrum?

Infectious Diarrhea

Preliminary evidence suggests that hyperimmune colostrum might help prevent or possibly treat infectious diarrhea.

For example, a double-blind, placebo-controlled trial of 80 children with rotavirus diarrhea found that hyperimmune colostrum (prepared by immunizing cows with rotavirus) reduced symptoms and shortened recovery time. Similar results were seen in another double-blind trial of about the same size. However, colostrum prepared by immunizing cows with a monkey form of rotavirus was not found effective for treating rotavirus in a double-blind trial of 135 children. The difference between these results may lie in the level and type of antibodies found in the particular colostrums used.

Both hyperimmune and normal colostrum have been tried for prevention or treatment of *Cryptosporidium* infection in people with AIDS, but the evidence that it works is weak at best.

Other studies suggest that hyperimmune colostrum might help prevent infection with shigella, as well as *E. coli* (a common cause of traveler's diarrhea). However, studies have not found it effective for treating the diarrhea resulting from shigella or *E. coli* infection once it takes hold.

A study of Bangladeshi children infected with *Helicobacter pylori* (the organism that causes digestive ulcers) found no benefits with hyperimmune colostrum.

Sports Performance

Colostrum contains the growth factor IGF-1, which may help build muscle, and on this basis colostrum has been proposed as a sports supplement. However, results are conflicting on whether it really works.

In a double-blind, placebo-controlled study, use of colostrum over an 8-week training period did not improve performance on an exercise-to-exhaustion test; however, it did improve performance on a repeat bout 20 minutes later. This suggests potential benefits for enhancing recovery of energy following heavy exercise.

Another 8-week double-blind study found that use of colostrum enhanced sprinting performance but not endurance exercise in elite hockey players. Previous double-blind studies found improvements in rowing performance and vertical jump.

A small double-blind study found that colostrum, as compared to whey protein, increased lean mass in healthy men and women undergoing aerobic and resistance training. However, no improvements in performance were seen in this trial.

Interestingly, it appears that the IGF-1 in colostrum is not directly absorbed into the body. Nonetheless, consumption of colostrum does appear to increase IGF-1 levels in the blood. The explanation for this is unclear.

Safety Issues

Colostrum does not seem to cause any significant side effects. However, comprehensive safety studies have not been performed. Safety in young children or women who are pregnant or nursing has not been established.

Coltsfoot

Tussilago farfara

PRINCIPAL PROPOSED USES: *We recommend against the medicinal use of coltsfoot for any purpose.*

The herb coltsfoot has a long history of use in the herbal medicine of Europe and Asia as a treatment for coughs and sore throats. It does not appear that traditional herbalists recognized that this treatment, which they often recommended for use by children, may cause liver damage.

What Is Coltsfoot Used for Today?

Germany's Commission E, the scientific body assigned to approving the use of herbal treatments in Germany, once approved coltsfoot for the treatment of sore throat. However, coltsfoot was subsequently banned due to its content of potentially liver-toxic substances called *pyrrolizidine alkaloids* (see Safety Issues below).

Safety aside, there is no meaningful evidence that coltsfoot has any medicinal effects. Only double-blind, placebo-controlled trials can prove a treatment effective, and none have been reported for coltsfoot. (For information on why this type of study is essential, see **Why Does This Book Rely on Double-blind Studies?**) Interestingly, much the same situation prevails for conventional cough syrups, none of which have been proven effective. However, they at least appear to be safe.

Dosage

Horticulturists have developed a form of coltsfoot that does not carry toxic pyrrolizidine alkaloids. Products of this type, when available, should be safer. Nonetheless, since we don't know whether coltsfoot offers any benefit, it's not possible to state an effective dosage.

Safety Issues

The pyrrolizidine alkaloids found in coltsfoot are known to have potential liver-toxic and cancer-promoting effects. One case report indicates that use of a coltsfoot tea caused severe liver problems in an infant that gradually disappeared when the tea was stopped. In another case, an infant developed liver disease and died because the mother drank tea containing coltsfoot during her pregnancy. Similar pyrrolizidine alkaloids are found in the herb comfrey, which has been associated with additional cases of liver injury.

Supporters of herbal therapy have defended the use of coltsfoot on the grounds that it was used for many thousands of years without harm. Unfortunately, there is a flaw in this reasoning. Traditional herbalists would be expected to notice immediate, dramatic reactions to herbal formulas, and one can assume with some confidence that treatments used for thousands of years are unlikely to cause such immediate problems in very many people who take them. However, certain types of harm could be expected to elude the detection of traditional herbalists. These include safety problems that are delayed, occur relatively rarely, or are difficult to detect without scientific instruments. How would a traditional herbalist ever know, for example, if a treatment caused liver failure in 1 out of 100,000 people who used it, especially if such failure took 2 or more years to develop? If such a death did occur in the herbalist's patient population, it would probably be attributed to hepatitis or some other common cause. These factors may explain why **traditional Chinese herbal medicine** uses treatments that are now recognized as dangerous, such as mercury, arsenic, lead, and the kidney-toxic herbs in the *Aristolochia* family.

Coltsfoot appears to fall into the same category. Most people can probably take coltsfoot for a short time and suffer no injury. A few people (especially infants), however, may have greater sensitivity and suffer harm. Many more people may experience harm if they use coltsfoot for a prolonged period of time.

For all these reasons, we strongly recommend against using coltsfoot.

Comfrey

Symphytum officinale

PRINCIPAL PROPOSED USES:

Topical Uses: *Back Pain, Sports Injuries (Sprains and Strains)*

Oral Uses: *Oral use of comfrey should be avoided under all circumstances.*

OTHER PROPOSED USES:

Topical Uses: *Back Pain, Broken Bones, Bruises, Sports Injures (Sprains and Strains), Varicose Veins*

NOT RECOMMEND USES: *Wound Healing (Broken Skin)*

Comfrey is a high-yielding leafy green plant that has been used for centuries as a feed crop for animals and a medicine for humans. However, in 2001, it was removed as an oral dietary supplement from the U.S. market and, soon afterwards, as a commercial animal food source. These actions were taken because comfrey contains dangerous levels of toxic pyrrolizidine alkaloids and its use has led to severe liver injury and death.

Traditionally, oral or topical use of comfrey was said to help bones heal more rapidly, and this is the origin of its Latin name *Symphytum* (meaning "drawing together"). It was also used orally for the treatment of digestive and lung problems. Topical comfrey creams have been used to treat minor wounds, bruises, sprains, and varicose veins.

What Is Comfrey Used for Today?

Comfrey is commonly included in salves and creams that also contain such herbs as **aloe**, **goldenseal**, **calendula**, and **vitamin E**. Such preparations are marketed for treatment of **minor wounds**. However, for safety reasons, comfrey should not be applied to broken skin. Therefore, it should not be used for the treatment of lacerations or abrasions (cuts and scrapes).

Topical comfrey appears to be safe when used for contusions and bruises. Furthermore, there is some evidence that topical comfrey might be useful in the treatment of ankle sprains. In a double-blind, placebo-controlled study of 142 people with acute ankle sprain, use of comfrey cream for 8 days significantly enhanced rate of recovery. Comfrey proved more effective than placebo in measurements of pain, swelling, and mobility. More modest benefits were seen in an-

other double-blind trial, this one enrolling 203 people with ankle sprain and comparing a high-comfrey to a low-comfrey product.

Another double-blind, placebo-controlled study, this one enrolling 215 people, found comfrey cream helpful for treatment of **back pain**.

Additional studies, generally of lower quality, suggest possible benefit for shoulder tendonitis and knee injuries.

The active ingredients in comfrey are not known, but may include rosmaric acid, choline, and allantoin.

Dosage

The tested form of topical comfrey contains 10% of a 2.5:1 juice extract made from fresh pressed plant sap; in other words, every 100 g of cream contains the equivalent of 25 g of comfrey sap.

Note: The toxic pyrrolizidine alkaloids in comfrey can be absorbed through the skin. For this reason, it has been recommended that when using comfrey preparations, the daily amount of pyrrolizidine alkaloids should not exceed 100 mcg. Unfortunately, few products are labeled to indicate their pyrrolizidine alkaloid content. Furthermore, the common analytic methods used for testing pyrrolizidine alkaloid content may fail to measure a certain chemical form of these toxins (the N-oxide form), leading to results that are too low by a factor of 10 or more. For all these reasons, it may be prudent to avoid topical comfrey products entirely. If you nonetheless wish to use comfrey as a topical treatment, we recommend the following general guidelines:

➤ **Do not apply comfrey for more than 4 to 6 weeks per year.**

Conjugated Linoleic Acid

➢ **Do not use for more than 10 days in a row.**
➢ **Do not apply to broken skin.**
➢ **Do not use in children.**

Safety Issues

Comfrey contains substances called *pyrrolizidine alkaloids* that are both toxic to the liver and carcinogenic.

The main form of liver disease seen with comfrey is a blockage of small veins that can lead to liver cirrhosis and eventually liver failure (hepato-occlusive disease). Liver transplantation may be required. Oral use of comfrey for as brief a time as 5 to 7 days in a child and 19 to 45 days in adults has resulted in severe liver disease and death. Long-term use of very low dosages may also cause harm.

In general, the root of the plant contains more pyrrolizidine alkaloids than the leaves. Related species of comfrey, such as *Symphytum uplandicum* and *Symphytum asperum*, contain even higher levels of these toxins and may be mistakenly sold as ordinary comfrey.

Pyrrolizidine alkaloids can be absorbed through the skin, though to what extent is unclear. For this reason, even topical comfrey should be used only with caution. Use of comfrey should be avoided entirely by young children, pregnant or nursing women, and people with liver disease.

Conjugated Linoleic Acid

SUPPLEMENT FORMS/ALTERNATE NAMES: *CLA*

PRINCIPAL PROPOSED USES: *Improving Body Composition*

OTHER PROPOSED USES: *Cancer Prevention, Diabetes, High Cholesterol*

Conjugated linoleic acid (CLA) is a mixture of different isomers, or chemical forms, of linoleic acid. Linoleic acid is an essential fatty acid—a type of fat that your body needs for optimum health.

Based on preliminary evidence, CLA has been promoted as a "fat-burning" supplement and as a treatment for diabetes. However, there is little evidence that it works, and growing evidence that CLA might actually *worsen* blood sugar control in people who are overweight.

Requirements/Sources

Although linoleic acid itself is an important nutritional source of essential fatty acids, there is no evidence that you need to get *conjugated* linoleic acid in your diet. CLA does occur in food, but it would be very difficult to get the recommended dose that way. Supplements are the only practical source.

Therapeutic Dosages

The typical dosage of CLA ranges from 3 to 5 g daily. As with all supplements taken at this high a dosage, it is important to purchase a reputable brand, as even very small amounts of a toxic contaminant could quickly add up.

Therapeutic Uses

While CLA is often called a **weight-loss** supplement, studies have generally failed to confirm this proposed benefit. A meta-analysis (systematic statistical review) of all the data found minimal benefits at most, whether for weight or body composition (ratio of muscle to fat).

Note: Contrary to early reports, CLA does *not* appear to be a useful supplement for people with diabetes and might, in fact, contribute to diabetes in overweight people. In addition, it might increase cardiovascular risk in another manner. See Safety Issues below.

Some animal and test-tube studies suggest that CLA might help prevent cancer, but the evidence is preliminary and inconsistent.

A small, double-blind trial found weak evidence that CLA might be useful for **high cholesterol**.

One study failed to find that CLA can enhance immune function.

Safety Issues

CLA appears to be a generally safe nutritional substance. However, there are some concerns with its use.

During the course of investigations into its effect on fat, CLA was found to act somewhat similarly to some oral medications used for diabetes. This led to research into the possible usefulness of CLA as a treatment for diabetes. In one study, CLA reduced blood sugar levels in diabetic rats as effectively as a standard diabetes treatment. The same researchers also performed a small, double-blind, placebo-controlled trial in humans. The results indicated that CLA improved insulin responsiveness in people with type 2 (adult onset) diabetes. However, several subsequent studies found opposite and rather alarming results: Use of CLA by people with diabetes may *worsen* blood sugar control; in overweight people without diabetes, CLA might decrease insulin sensitivity, creating a pre-diabetic state. At present, therefore, individuals with diabetes or who are at risk for it should not use CLA except under physician supervision.

One study found that CLA impairs endothelial function, suggesting that it might increase cardiovascular risk.

Concerns have also been raised regarding use of CLA by nursing mothers. A double-blind, placebo-controlled study indicates that use of CLA reduces the fat content of human breast milk. Since infants depend on the fat in breast milk to provide adequate calories and on certain fats to aid proper growth and development, it is probably prudent for nursing mothers to avoid CLA supplements.

Maximum safe dosages of CLA for young children, pregnant women, or those with severe liver or kidney disease have not been determined.

Copper

SUPPLEMENT FORMS/ALTERNATE NAMES: *Copper Complexes of Various Amino Acids, Copper Gluconate, Copper Picolinate, Copper Sulfate*

PRINCIPAL PROPOSED USES: *To Balance High Zinc Intake*

OTHER PROPOSED USES: *Heart Disease, High Cholesterol, Osteoarthritis, Osteoporosis, Rheumatoid Arthritis*

The human body contains only 70 to 80 mg of copper in total, but it's an essential part of many important enzymes. Copper's possible role in treating disease is based on the fact that these enzymes can't do their jobs without it. However, there is little direct evidence that taking extra copper can treat any disease.

Requirements/Sources

The official U.S. recommendations for daily intake of copper are as follows:

- Infants 0–6 months, 200 mcg
  7–12 months, 220 mcg
- Children 1–3 years, 340 mcg
  4–8 years, 440 mcg
- Males and females 9–13 years, 700 mcg
  14–18 years, 890 mcg
  19 years and older, 900 mcg
- Pregnant women, 1,000 mcg
- Nursing women, 1,300 mcg

High zinc intake reduces copper stores in the body; for this reason, if you are taking zinc in doses above nutritional levels (as, for example, in the treatment of **macular degeneration**), you will need extra copper.

In addition, if you are taking iron or large doses of vitamin C, you may need extra copper. Ideally, you should take copper at least 2 hours apart from these two nutrients, so that they don't interfere with each other's absorption.

Oysters, nuts, legumes, whole grains, sweet potatoes, and dark greens are good sources of copper. Drinking water that passes through copper plumbing is a good source of this mineral and sometimes it may even provide too much.

Therapeutic Dosages

For the various therapeutic uses described in the next section, copper is often recommended at a high (but still safe) dose of 1 to 3 mg (1,000 to 3,000 mcg) daily.

Therapeutic Uses

Copper has been proposed as a treatment for **osteoporosis**, based primarily on studies that found benefit using combinations of various trace minerals, including copper. However, one study found that copper supplements taken alone may not be helpful.

One researcher, L. M. Klevay, has claimed in more than a dozen papers that copper deficiencies increase the risk of **high cholesterol** and heart disease, but he has failed to supply any real evidence that this idea is true. A small, double-blind, placebo-controlled study of copper supplements for reducing heart disease risk factors, such as cholesterol profile, found no benefit.

Copper has long been mentioned as a possible treatment for **osteoarthritis** and **rheumatoid arthritis**, but there is as yet no real evidence that it works.

Safety Issues

The following daily doses of copper should not be exceeded:

- ➤ **Children 1–3 years, 1,000 mcg**
  4–8 years, 3,000 mcg
  9–13 years, 5,000 mcg
- ➤ **Males and females 14–18 years, 8,000 mcg**
  19 years and older, 10,000 mcg
- ➤ **Pregnant or nursing women, 10,000 mcg (8,000 mcg if 18 years old or younger)**

Maximum safe dosages of copper for individuals with severe liver or kidney disease have not been determined.

Interactions You Should Know About

If you are taking:

- ➤ **Zinc: You need to make sure to get enough copper.**
- ➤ **Iron, supplements, or high doses of *vitamin C*: You may need extra copper. If you do take a copper supplement, it might be ideal to take it either 2 hours before or after these other substances.**

Cordyceps

Cordyceps sinensis

PRINCIPAL PROPOSED USES: *None*

OTHER PROPOSED USES: *Cancer Prevention, Diabetes, Fatigue, High Blood Pressure, High Cholesterol, Immune Support, Kidney Protection, Liver Support, Lupus, Male Sexual Dysfunction, Sports Performance, Viral Hepatitis*

Although *Cordyceps sinensis* is often described as an herb, it's actually a combination of a parasitic fungus and the larvae of a moth (a caterpillar). The fungus attacks the caterpillar and destroys it from within. The remaining structures of the caterpillar, along with the fungus, are dried and sold as cordyceps.

Cordyceps has a long history of use in China as a *tonic*, a substance said to generally strengthen the body, particularly following illness. It was also used to treat bronchitis, kidney failure, and tuberculosis.

What Is Cordyceps Used for Today?

Cordyceps is widely marketed today as treatment for a great many conditions. However, there is no reliable scientific evidence that it actually provides any medical benefits.

Most research on cordyceps was done in China and is not up to modern scientific standards. In general, double-blind, placebo-controlled studies are the most reliable form of evidence. (For information on the reasons why, see **Why Does This Book Rely on Double-blind Studies?**.) However, such studies have to be performed and reported according to certain standards. Although several double-blind studies have been reported on cordyceps, they all fall considerably short of the level necessary for scientific validity. These somewhat dubious double-blind trials hint that cordyceps might be helpful for reducing **high cholesterol** and improving **male sexual function**.

Evidence is more negative than positive regarding whether cordyceps is helpful for **enhancing sports performance**.

Weak evidence hints that cordyceps may modulate the immune system, which means that it stimulates some aspects of the immune system while suppressing others.

On this basis, it has been tried in China as an aid in organ transplant surgery and for the treatment of **viral hepatitis** and **lupus**.

Highly preliminary test-tube and animal studies hint that cordyceps may help fight **stress**, control blood sugar levels (potentially making it useful in **diabetes**), **reduce cancer risk**, **lower high blood pressure**, and help protect the kidney against damage caused by the drugs **cyclosporin** and **gentamycin**.

Other test-tube studies hint that cordyceps may stimulate production of hormones such as cortisone and testosterone. However, contrary to what some websites say, these studies are far too preliminary to indicate any therapeutic hormonal effect.

Dosage

Typical traditional recommended doses of cordyceps range from 5 to 10 g per day. Concentrated extracts are also available, taken at a lower dosage.

Safety Issues

Use of cordyceps does not generally cause apparent side effects. However, comprehenseive safety studies have not been reported. In addition, there are two case reports in which cordyceps products contained enough lead to cause lead poisoning. Safety in young children, pregnant or nursing women, or people with severe liver or kidney disease has not been established.

Coriolus versicolor

Trametes versicolor

ALTERNATE NAMES/RELATED TERMS: *Kawaratake, Turkey Tail, Yun Zhi*
PRINCIPAL PROPOSED USES: *Cancer Treatment Support*
OTHER PROPOSED USES: *Cancer Prevention*

Coriolus versicolor is a common tree fungus, often seen by hikers as a stiff, rounded, horizontal protuberance from tree trunks, with concentric lines of varying color. In **traditional Chinese herbal medicine**, this fungus is used to strengthen overall vitality and treat lung and liver problems as well as other conditions.

What is *Coriolus versicolor* Used for Today?

Currently, extracts of *Coriolus versicolor* called *polysaccharide-K* (PSK) and *polysaccharopeptide* (PSP) are under study as immune stimulants for use alongside

Corydalis

chemotherapy in the treatment of cancer. These two related substances, made from slightly different strains of the fungus, are thought to act as *biological response modifiers*, meaning that they affect the body's response to cancer.

According to most but not all reported trials, most of which were performed in Asia, both PSK and PSP can enhance the effects of various forms of standard cancer treatment.

For example, in a 28-day, double-blind, placebo-controlled study of 34 people with advanced non–small-cell lung cancer, use of *Coriolus* extracts along with conventional treatment significantly slowed the progression of the disease.

It is thought that *Coriolus* extracts work by stimulating the body's own cancer-fighting cells. PSK and PSP may also have **cancer-preventive** effects.

In addition, very weak evidence hints that extracts of *Coriolus versicolor* might be helpful for **HIV infection**.

Dosage

A typical dosage of PSK or PSP as an adjunct to standard cancer treatment is 2 to 6 g daily. For prevention of cancer, some experts recommend 500 mg daily, but there is no real scientific basis for this recommendation.

Safety Issues

According to Chinese studies, PSP and PSK appear to be relatively nontoxic, both in the short and long term.

Few side effects have been reported in clinical trials. However, safety in young children, pregnant or nursing women, or people with severe liver or kidney disease has not been established.

Corydalis

Corydalis turtschaninovii, Corydalis yanhusuo

ALTERNATE NAMES/RELATED TERMS: *Yan Hu So*
PRINCIPAL PROPOSED USES: *Pain (Many Types, Including Peripheral Neuropathy, Painful Menstruation, and Pain Caused by Soft-Tissue Injuries)*
OTHER PROPOSED USES: *Cataracts, Heart Arrhythmias, Preventing Blood Clots*
Note: *We recommend against using this herb at all.*

Widely used in Chinese herbal medicine, the herb corydalis is said to alleviate pain by "moving Qi" and "stimulating the blood." These expressions refer to traditional concepts included within the complex theories of **traditional Chinese herbal medicine**. In terms of Western diagnostic categories, corydalis may be recommended for **soft-tissue injuries**, **menstrual discomfort**, and abdominal pain.

The part of the plant used medicinally is the rhizome (underground stalk).

What Is Corydalis Used for Today?

There is no reliable evidence that corydalis or its constituents offer any medicinal benefits. Corydalis contains a number of active and potentially dangerous chemicals in the alkaloid family, including tetrahydropalmatine (THP), corydaline, protopine, tetrahydrocoptisine, tetrahydrocolumbamine, and corybulbine. Of these, THP may be the most active, as well as the most toxic (see Safety Issues below).

Only double-blind, placebo-controlled studies can actually show that a treatment works, and there is only one such study that is relevant to corydalis. This trial tested THP as a treatment for a type of heart rhythm abnormality called *supraventricular arrhythmia*. Reportedly, use of THP produced significant benefits as compared to placebo. However, this study was conducted in China, and there is considerable skepticism about the validity of Chinese medical trials. (For information on why double-blind studies are essential, see **Why Does This Book Rely on Double-blind Trials?**)

Much weaker evidence from animal and test-tube studies hints that THP or corydalis extracts might have pain-relieving, sedative, and anti-inflammatory effects. Corydalis constituents may also affect neurotransmitters in the brain, including dopamine and GABA. Equally weak evidence hints at benefits for preventing or treating **cataracts**, reducing blood coagulation, and **lowering blood pressure**. However, none of this research remotely approaches the level of evidence that can prove a treatment effective.

Dosage

Corydalis is usually taken at a dose of 5 to 10 g daily or equivalent quantities of an extract.

Safety Issues

Corydalis has not undergone any meaningful safety testing. The herb is known to produce immediate side effects, including nausea and fatigue, in some people. In addition, there are serious safety concerns related to its alkaloid constituent, THP. Use of products containing THP has repeatedly been associated with severe and potentially fatal liver injury.

In addition, there are three reports that use of THP by young children has led to life-threatening suppression of the central nervous system.

For these reasons, we strongly recommend against the use of corydalis, especially by young children, pregnant or nursing women, or people with liver disease.

Cranberry

Vaccinium macrocarpon

PRINCIPAL PROPOSED USES: *Prevention and Possibly Treatment: Bladder Infections*

OTHER PROPOSED USES:

Prevention and Treatment: *Periodontal Disease, Ulcers*

Prevention Only: *Cancer, Heart Disease*

The cranberry plant is a close relative of the common blueberry. Native Americans used it both as food and for the treatment of bladder and kidney diseases. The Pilgrims learned about cranberry from local tribes and quickly adopted it for their own use. Subsequent physicians used it for bladder infections, for "bladder gravel" (small bladder stones), and to remove "blood toxins."

In the 1920s, researchers observed that drinking cranberry juice makes the urine more acidic. Since common urinary tract–infection bacteria such as *E. coli* dislike acidic surroundings, physicians concluded that they had discovered a scientific explanation for the traditional uses of cranberry. This discovery led to widespread medical use of cranberry juice for treating bladder infections. Cranberry fell out of favor with physicians after World War II, but it became popular again during the 1960s—as a self-treatment.

What Is Cranberry Used for Today?

Cranberry is widely used today to prevent **bladder infections**, although as yet the evidence to support this use remains limited. Contrary to the research from the 1920s, it now appears that cranberry's acidification of the urine is not likely to play an important role in the treatment of bladder infections; current study has focused instead on cranberry's apparent ability to block bacteria from adhering to the bladder wall. If the bacteria can't hold on, they will be washed out with the stream of urine. Interestingly, studies have found that in women who frequently develop bladder infections, bacteria seem to have a particularly easy time holding on to the bladder wall. This suggests that cranberry juice can actually get to the root of their problem.

Just as cranberry seems to prevent adhesion of

Cranberry

bacteria to the bladder, preliminary evidence suggests that it might also help prevent the adhesion of the ulcer-causing bacteria *Helicobacter pylori* to the stomach wall. One double-blind, placebo-controlled trial performed in China reported that use of cranberry reduced levels of helicobacter infection in infected individuals. Theoretically, this could reduce the risk of **ulcers**.

Other preliminary evidence suggests that the same actions of cranberry juice might make it useful for treating or preventing **cavities** or **gum disease**. However, there is one kink to work out before cranberry could be practical for this purpose: the sweeteners added to cranberry juice aren't good for your teeth, but without them cranberry juice is very bitter.

Cranberry has also been investigated as a possible aid in reducing the risk of **heart disease** and **cancer**, and as a treatment for **diabetes**, but there is no meaningful evidence as yet that it is actually helpful for these conditions.

One study failed to find cranberry significantly effective for **enhancing mental function**.

What Is the Scientific Evidence for Cranberry?

The only reliable evidence for the use of cranberry juice for preventing bladder infections comes from a 1-year, double-blind, placebo-controlled study of 150 sexually active women that compared placebo against both cranberry juice (8 ounces 3 times daily) and cranberry tablets. The results showed that both forms of cranberry significantly reduced the number of episodes of bladder infections; cranberry tablets were more cost-effective.

A double-blind study of 376 hospitalized seniors attempted to determine whether a low dose of cranberry juice (as cranberry juice cocktail, 10 ounces daily—a very low dose compared to the previous study) would help prevent acute infections. It failed to find benefit, perhaps in part due to the dosage of cranberry as well as the low number of infections that developed overall.

Another double-blind study evaluated cranberry juice cocktail for the *treatment* of chronic bladder infections. This trial followed 153 women with an average age of 78.5 years for a period of 6 months. Many women of this age group have what are called *chronic asymptomatic bladder infections*: signs of bacteria in the urine without any symptoms. Half of the participants were given 10 ounces a day of a standard commercial cranberry cocktail drink, the other a placebo drink prepared to look and taste the same. Both treatments contained the same amount of **vitamin C** to eliminate the possible antibacterial influence of that supplement. Despite the weak preparation of cranberry used, the results showed a 58% decrease in the incidence of bacteria and white blood cells in the urine.

Three other double-blind, placebo-controlled studies evaluated the effectiveness of cranberry extract for eliminating bacteria in the urine of people with bladder paralysis (neurogenic bladder). The results showed no benefit.

Finally, a year-long open trial of 150 women found that regular use of a cranberry juice/lingonberry combination reduced the rate of urinary tract infection as compared to a probiotic drink or no treatment. However, because this study was not double-blind, the results are unreliable. (For information on why double-blind studies are so important, see **Why Does This Book Rely on Double-blind Studies?**.)

Dosage

The usual dosage of dry cranberry juice extract is 300 to 400 mg twice daily. For people who prefer juice, 8 to 16 ounces daily should suffice. Pure cranberry juice, not sugary cranberry juice cocktail with its low percentage of cranberry, should be used for best effect.

Safety Issues

As a food, cranberry is thought to have a good safety profile.

Five case reports suggest that cranberry could interact with the drug warfarin (Coumadin), potentially leading to internal bleeding. However, a formal study failed to find evidence of such an interaction. This study was somewhat indirect, however, in that it did not evaluate the effects of cranberry on warfarin action, but rather on another drug that is metabolized similarly in the body. Prudence would therefore suggest continued caution at this time.

Cranberry juice might allow the kidneys to excrete weakly alkaline drugs more rapidly, thereby reducing their effectiveness. These include many antidepressants and prescription painkillers.

Indirect evidence suggests that regular use of cranberry concentrate tablets might increase risk of **kidney stones**.

Interactions You Should Know About

If you are taking:

➤ Warfarin (Coumadin): Use of cranberry might lead to excessive bleeding.

➤ Weakly alkaline drugs, which include many antidepressants and prescription painkillers: Cranberry might decrease their effectiveness.

Creatine

SUPPLEMENT FORMS/ALTERNATE NAMES: *Creatine Monohydrate*

PRINCIPAL PROPOSED USES: *Sports Performance Enhancement*

OTHER PROPOSED USES: *Amyotrophic Lateral Sclerosis (ALS), Cancer Treatment Support, Chronic Obstructive Pulmonary Disease (COPD), Congestive Heart Failure, Disuse Atrophy Following Injury, Enhancing Mental Function (Following Sleep Deprivation), High Triglycerides, Huntington's Disease, Improved Ratio of Body Fat to Muscle, McArdle's Disease, Mitochondrial Illnesses, Muscular Dystrophy, Myotonic Dystrophy, Weight Loss*

Creatine is a naturally occurring substance that plays an important role in the production of energy in the body. The body converts it to phosphocreatine, a form of stored energy used by muscles.

Although the evidence for creatine is not definitive, it has the most evidence behind it among all the sports supplements. Numerous small double-blind studies suggest that it can increase athletic performance in sports that involve intense but short bursts of activity.

The theory behind its use is that supplemental creatine can build up a reserve of phosphocreatine in the muscles, to help them perform on demand. Supplemental creatine may also help the body make new phosphocreatine faster when it has been used up by intense activity.

Sources

Although some creatine exists in the daily diet, it is not an essential nutrient because your body can make it from the amino acids **L-arginine**, glycine, and **L-methionine**. Provided you eat enough animal protein (the principal source of these amino acids), your body will make all the creatine you need for good health.

Meat (including chicken and fish) is the most important dietary source of creatine and its amino acid building blocks. For this reason, vegetarian athletes may potentially benefit most from creatine supplementation.

Therapeutic Dosages

For bodybuilding and exercise enhancement, a typical dosage schedule starts with a "loading dose" of 15 to 30 g daily (divided into 2 or 3 separate doses) for 3 to 4 days, followed by 2 to 5 g daily. Some authorities recommend skipping the loading dose. (By comparison, we typically get only about 1 g of creatine in the daily diet.)

Creatine's ability to enter muscle cells can be increased by combining it with glucose, fructose, or other simple carbohydrates; in addition, prior use of creatine might enhance the sports benefits of carbohydrate-loading.

Caffeine may block the effects of creatine.

Therapeutic Uses

Creatine is one of the best-selling and best-documented supplements for enhancing **athletic performance**, but the scientific evidence that it works is far from complete. The best evidence we have points to potential benefits in forms of exercise that require repeated short-term bursts of high-intensity exercise; this has been seen more in artificial laboratory studies, however, rather than in studies involving athletes carrying out normal sports. It might also be helpful for resistance exercise (weight training), although not all studies have found benefit.

Creatine has also been proposed as an aid to promote **weight loss** and to reduce the proportion of fat to muscle in the body, but there is little evidence that it is effective for this purpose.

Preliminary evidence suggests that creatine supplements may be able to reduce levels of **triglycerides** in the blood. (Triglycerides are fats related to cholesterol that also increase risk of heart disease when elevated in the body.)

Creatine supplements might also help counter the loss of muscle strength that occurs when a limb is immobilized, such as following **injury** or **surgery**; however, not all results have been positive.

Preliminary studies, including small double-blind trials, suggest (somewhat inconsistently) that creatine might be helpful for reducing fatigue and increasing strength in various illnesses where muscle weakness occurs, including **congestive heart failure**, **chronic obstructive pulmonary disease** (COPD), Huntington's disease, McArdle's disease, mitochondrial illnesses, myotonic dystrophy, and muscular dystrophy.

Evidence from animal and open human trials suggested that creatine improved strength and slowed the progression of **amyotrophic lateral sclerosis** (ALS), and for this reason, many people with ALS have tried it. However, these hopes were dashed in 2003 when the results of a 10-month, double-blind, placebo-controlled trial of 175 people with ALS were announced. Use of creatine at a dose of 10 g daily failed to provide any benefit at all in terms of symptoms or disease progression. Negative results were also seen in a subsequent, slightly smaller study. Creatine also does not appear to strengthen muscles in people with wrist weakness due to nerve injury.

Long-term use of corticosteroid drugs can slow a child's growth. One animal study suggests that use of supplemental creatine may help prevent this side effect.

Creatine has also shown some promise for **improving mental function**, particularly after sleep deprivation.

One study failed to find creatine helpful for maintaining muscle mass during treatment for colon **cancer**.

What Is the Scientific Evidence for Creatine?

Exercise Performance

Several small double-blind studies suggest that creatine can improve performance in exercises that involve repeated short bursts of high-intensity activity.

For example, a double-blind study investigated creatine and swimming performance in 18 men and 14 women. Men taking the supplement had significant increases in speed when doing 6 bouts of 50-meter swims starting at 3-minute intervals, as compared with men taking placebo. However, their speed did not improve when swimming 10 sets of 25-yard lengths started at 1-minute intervals. It may be that the shorter rest time between laps was not enough for the swimmers' bodies to resynthesize phosphocreatine.

Interestingly, none of the women enrolled in the study showed any improvement with the creatine supplement. The authors of this study noted that women normally have more creatine in their muscle tissue than men do, so perhaps creatine supplementation (at least at this level) is not of benefit to women as it appears to be for men. Further research is needed to fully understand this gender difference in response to creatine.

In another double-blind study, 16 physical education students exercised 10 times for 6 seconds on a stationary cycle, alternating with a 30-second rest period. The results showed that individuals who took 20 g of creatine for 6 days were better able to maintain cycle speed. Similar results were seen in many other studies of repeated high-intensity exercise, although generally benefits are minimal in studies involving athletes engaged in normal sports rather than contrived laboratory tests.

Isometric exercise capacity (pushing against a fixed resistance) also may improve with creatine, according to some, but not all, studies.

In addition, two double-blind, placebo-controlled studies, each lasting 28 days, provide some evidence that creatine and creatine plus HMB (beta hydroxymethyl butyrate) can increase lean muscle and bone mass. The first study enrolled 52 college football players during off-season training and the other followed 40 athletes engaged in weight training.

However, studies of endurance or nonrepeated exercise have *not* shown benefits. Therefore, creatine probably won't help you for marathon running or single sprints.

High Triglycerides

A 56-day, double-blind, placebo-controlled study of 34 men and women found that creatine supplementation can reduce levels of triglycerides in the blood by about 25%. Effects on other blood lipids such as total cholesterol were insignificant.

Congestive Heart Failure

Easy fatigability is one unpleasant symptom of congestive heart failure. Creatine supplementation has been tried as a treatment for this symptom, with some positive results.

A double-blind study examined 17 men with congestive heart failure who were given 20 g of creatine daily for 10 days. Exercise capacity and muscle strength increased in the creatine-treated group. Similarly, muscle endurance improved in a double-blind, placebo-controlled crossover study of 20 men with chronic heart failure. Treatment with 20 g of creatine for 5 days increased the amount of exercise they could complete before they reached exhaustion.

These results are promising, but further study is needed.

Safety Issues

Creatine appears to be relatively safe. No significant side effects have been found with the regimen of several days of a high dosage (15 to 30 g daily) followed by 6 weeks of a lower dosage (2 to 3 g daily). A study of 100 football players found no adverse consequences during 10 months to 5 years of creatine supplementation. Creatine does not appear to adversely affect the body's ability to exercise under hot conditions.

However, there are some potential concerns with creatine. Because it is metabolized by the kidneys, fears have been expressed that creatine supplements could cause kidney injury, and there are two worrisome case reports. However, evidence suggests that creatine is safe for people whose kidneys are healthy to begin with and who don't take excessive doses. Furthermore, a 1-year, double-blind study of 175 people with amyotrophic lateral sclerosis found that use of 10 g of creatine daily did not adversely affect kidney function. Nonetheless, individuals with kidney disease, especially those on dialysis, should avoid creatine.

Another concern revolves around the fact that creatine is metabolized in the body to the toxic substance formaldehyde. However, it is not clear whether the amount of formaldehyde produced in this way will cause any harm. Three deaths have been reported in individuals taking creatine, but other causes were most likely responsible.

It has also been suggested that use of oral creatine would increase urine levels of the carcinogen N-nitrososarcosine, but this does not seem to be the case.

A few reports suggest that creatine could, at times, cause **heart arrhythmias**.

As with all supplements taken in very high doses, it is important to purchase a high-quality form of creatine, as contaminants present even in very low concentrations could conceivably build up and cause problems.

Damiana

Turnera diffusa

PRINCIPAL PROPOSED USES: *Male Sexual Capacity*

OTHER PROPOSED USES: *Asthma, Depression, Difficulty Achieving Orgasm in Women, Digestive Problems, Impotence in Men, Menstrual Disorders, Respiratory Diseases*

The herb damiana has been used in Mexico for some time as a male aphrodisiac. Classic herbal literature of the nineteenth century describes it as a "tonic," or general body strengthener.

What Is Damiana Used for Today?

Damiana continues to be a popular aphrodisiac for males. However, if it works at all, the effect appears to be rather mild. No scientific trials have been reported.

Damiana is also sometimes said to be helpful for treating **asthma** and other respiratory diseases, depression, digestive problems, menstrual disorders, and various forms of sexual dysfunction—for example, **impotence** in men and inability to achieve orgasm in women. However, again there is no real evidence that it works for any of these conditions.

Like the herb **uva ursi**, damiana contains arbutin, although at a concentration about 10 times lower. Arbutin is a urinary antiseptic, but the levels present in damiana are probably too small to make this herb a useful treatment for bladder infections.

Dosage

The proper dosage of damiana is 2 to 4 g taken 2 to 3 times daily or as directed on the label.

Safety Issues

Damiana appears to be safe at the recommended dosages. It appears on the FDA's GRAS (generally recognized as safe) list and is widely used as a food flavoring. The only common side effect of damiana is occasional mild gastrointestinal distress. However, because damiana contains low levels of cyanide-like compounds, excessive doses may be dangerous. Safety in young children, pregnant or nursing women, or those with severe liver or kidney disease is not established.

Dandelion

Taraxacum officinale

PRINCIPAL PROPOSED USES: *None*

OTHER PROPOSED USES:

Leaves: *Fluid Retention, Nutritional Supplement*
Root: *Constipation, Detoxification, Liver Support*

The common dandelion, enemy of suburban lawns, is an unusually nutritious food. Its leaves contain substantial levels of vitamins A, C, D, and B complex, as well as iron, magnesium, zinc, potassium, manganese, copper, choline, calcium, boron, and silicon.

Worldwide, the root of the dandelion has been used for the treatment of a variety of liver and gallbladder problems. Other historical uses of the root and leaves include the treatment of breast diseases, water retention, digestive problems, joint pain, fever, and skin diseases.

The most active constituents in dandelion appear to be eudesmanolide and germacranolide, substances unique to this herb. Other ingredients include taraxol, taraxerol, and taraxasterol, along with stigmasterol, beta-sitosterol, caffeic acid, and p-hydroxyphenylacetic acid.

What Is Dandelion Used for Today?

Dandelion leaves are widely recommended as a food supplement for **pregnant women** because of the many nutrients they contain. The scientific basis for any other potential use of dandelion is scanty.

Dandelion leaves have been found to produce a mild diuretic effect, which has led to its proposed use for people who suffer from mild fluid retention, such as may occur in **premenstrual syndrome** (PMS). However, no double-blind, placebo-controlled studies have been reported on the effectiveness of dandelion for this purpose.

In the folk medicine of many countries, dandelion root is regarded as a "**liver tonic**," a substance believed to support the liver in an unspecified way. This led to its use for many illnesses traditionally believed to be caused by a "sluggish" or "congested" liver, including constipation, headaches, eye problems, gout, skin problems, fatigue, and boils. Building on this traditional thinking, some modern naturopathic physicians believe that dandelion can help detoxify, or clean out, the liver and gallbladder. This concept has led to the additional suggestion that dandelion can reduce the side effects of medications processed by the liver, as well as relieve symptoms of diseases in which impaired liver function plays a role. However, while preliminary studies do suggest that dandelion root stimulates the flow of bile, there is as yet no meaningful scientific evidence that this observed effect leads to any of the benefits described above.

Dandelion root is also used like other bitter herbs to improve appetite and treat **minor digestive disorders**. When dried and roasted, it is sometimes used as a coffee substitute. Finally, dandelion root is sometimes recommended for mild **constipation**.

Dosage

A typical dosage of dandelion root is 2 to 8 g 3 times daily of dried root; 250 mg 3 to 4 times daily of a 5:1 extract; or 5 to 10 ml 3 times daily of a 1:5 tincture in 45% alcohol. The leaves may be eaten in salad or cooked.

Safety Issues

Dandelion root and leaves are believed to be quite safe, with no side effects or likely risks other than rare allergic reactions. Dandelion is on the FDA's GRAS (generally recognized as safe) list and approved for use as a food flavoring by the Council of Europe.

However, based on dandelion root's effect on bile secretion, Germany's Commission E has recommended that it not be used at all by individuals with obstruction of the bile ducts or other serious diseases of the gallbladder, and that it be used only under physician supervision by those with **gallstones**.

Some references state that dandelion root can cause hyperacidity and thereby increase **ulcer** pain, but this concern has been disputed.

Because the leaves contain so much **potassium**, they probably resupply any potassium lost due to dandelion's mild diuretic effect, although this has not been proven.

People with known allergies to related plants, such as **chamomile** and **yarrow**, should use dandelion with caution.

There are no known drug interactions with dandelion. However, based on what we know about dandelion root's effects, there might be some risk when combining it with pharmaceutical diuretics or drugs that reduce blood sugar levels. In addition, individuals taking the medication lithium should use herbal diuretics such as dandelion leaf only under the supervision of a physician, as being dehydrated can be dangerous when using this medication.

Safety in young children, pregnant or nursing women, or those with severe liver or kidney disease has not been established.

Interactions You Should Know About

If you are taking *diuretic drugs, lithium, insulin* or *oral medications that reduce blood sugar levels*, use dandelion only under doctor's supervision.

Deer Velvet

SUPPLEMENT FORMS/ALTERNATE NAMES: *Deer Antler, Velvet Antler*

PRINCIPAL PROPOSED USES: *Male Sexual Dysfunction*

OTHER PROPOSED USES: *Adaptogen, Cancer Prevention, Drug Addiction Support, Immune Support, Liver Protection, Osteoarthritis, Osteoporosis Treatment, Pain Control, Sports Performance and Bodybuilding Enhancement*

Deer velvet is the common name of a product made from the growing antlers of deer, during a stage when they are covered in soft velvety hair. New Zealand is a major exporter of deer velvet, shipping tens of millions of dollars worth to Asia and the U.S. each year.

According to Asian tradition, deer velvet has *tonic* properties, meaning that it tends to enhance energy and vitality. More recently, it has been called an *adaptogen*. This term, invented by early Soviet scientists, refers to a hypothetical treatment that can be described as follows: An adaptogen should help the body adapt to stresses of various kinds, whether heat, cold, exertion, trauma, sleep deprivation, toxic exposure, radiation, infection, or psychological stress. Furthermore, an adaptogen should cause no side effects, be effective in treating a wide variety of illnesses, and help return an organism toward balance no matter what may have gone wrong.

The only indisputable example of an adaptogen is a healthful lifestyle. By eating right, exercising regularly, and generally living a life of balance and moderation, you will increase your physical fitness and ability to resist illnesses of all types. The herb **ginseng** is widely said to have adaptogenic properties. However, there is no reliable evidence that any herb or supplement actually has adaptogenic properties, and the term is not accepted by conventional medicine.

What Is Deer Velvet Used for Today?

In the 1960s, an injectible form of deer velvet was used by Japanese physicians to treat **male sexual dysfunction**. Deer velvet first began to become popular in the U.S. beginning in the late 1990s. Today, numerous books and websites claim that deer velvet can enhance sexual performance by increasing levels of male hormones. However, these claims are based on extremely preliminary research. Only double-blind, placebo-controlled studies can actually prove a treatment effective, and the one study of this type reported for deer velvet failed to find evidence of benefit. (For information on why double-blind studies are essential, see **Why Does This Book Rely on Double-blind Studies?**.)

In this study, 32 healthy men ages 45 to 60 were given either deer velvet (1 g daily) or placebo for 12 weeks. The results showed no significant change in sexual function or male hormone levels in the treated group as compared to the placebo group.

Deer velvet also contains **cartilage**. On this basis, as well as one study in dogs, it has been promoted as a treatment for **osteoarthritis**; however, cartilage is not a proven treatment for this condition. Numerous other proposed benefits of deer velvet are based on test-tube studies or other forms of evidence that are too preliminary to rely upon at all. These include **cancer prevention**, **drug addiction support**, **immune support**, **liver protection**, **osteoporosis treatment**, pain control, **sports performance**, and bodybuilding enhancement.

Dosage

A typical dosage of deer velvet is 1 g daily, taken all at once or divided throughout the day.

Safety Issues

Other than occasional allergic reactions, deer velvet does not appear to cause many obvious, immediate side effects. However, there are concerns based on contamination with the tranquilizers and anesthetics used during the process of removing the horn from the deer. One of these substances used, xylazine, is carcinogenic, and studies have found that low but potentially dangerous levels of xylazine are contained in deer velvet product.

Another set of risks derives from the proposed effects of deer velvet: raising male hormone levels. If deer velvet does in fact increase male hormones as it is advertised to do, this could lead to a range of potential problems; however, as noted above, there is no real evidence that deer velvet actually does raise such hormones.

Safety in young children, pregnant or nursing women, or people with severe liver or kidney disease has not been established.

Dehydroepiandrosterone

SUPPLEMENT FORMS/ALTERNATE NAMES: *DHEA, DHEA Sulfate*

PRINCIPAL PROPOSED USES: *Lupus*

OTHER PROPOSED USES: *Adrenal Failure, Alzheimer's Disease, Chronic Fatigue Syndrome, Depression, Fibromyalgia, HIV Support, Immune Support, Impotence, Menopause, Osteoporosis, Preventing Heart Disease, Schizophrenia, Sexual Dysfunction in Women, Sports Performance Enhancement*

PROBABLY NOT EFFECTIVE USES: *Enhancing General Well-being in Seniors*

Dehydroepiandrosterone (DHEA), a hormone produced by the adrenal glands, is the most abundant hormone in the *steroid* family found in the bloodstream. Your body uses DHEA as the starting material for making the sex hormones testosterone and estrogen.

A meaningful body of evidence indicates that DHEA might be helpful for the autoimmune disease lupus, at least in women. DHEA may also help prevent osteoporosis (again, in women). Additionally, DHEA appears to be beneficial when taken along with standard treatment for women with adrenal failure.

Other uses with some evidence include improving sexual function in men and women and alleviating depression. DHEA does *not* appear to be effective for improving general well-being in seniors. Keep in mind that DHEA is not a natural supplement. The DHEA you can buy at the store is made by a synthetic chemical process and it is a hormone, not a nutrient. Although DHEA appears to be safe to use in the short term, its safety when taken for prolonged periods is unknown.

Sources

The body makes its own DHEA; we get very little in our diets. DHEA production peaks early in life and begins to decline as we reach adulthood. By age 60, our bodies produce just 5 to 15% as much as when we were 20. It's not clear whether this decline in DHEA is a bad thing, but some believe that it may contribute to the aging process.

For use as a dietary supplement, DHEA is manufactured synthetically from substances found in soybeans. Contrary to popular belief, there is no DHEA in **wild yam**.

Therapeutic Dosages

A typical therapeutic dosage of DHEA is 50 to 200 mg daily, although some studies used dosages above and below this range. A cream containing 10% DHEA may also be used; it is typically applied to the skin at a dosage of 3 to 5 g daily.

Physicians sometimes check DHEA levels and adjust the daily dose to achieve blood levels of 20 to 30 nmol/L.

Therapeutic Uses

Much of the evidence of benefits with DHEA involves results seen in women.

A meaningful body of evidence indicates that DHEA may help reduce symptoms in women with **lupus**.

Some evidence hints that DHEA may be helpful for preventing or treating **osteoporosis** in postmenopausal women over age 70 and perhaps in other demographics as well.

Two double-blind studies of seniors found that ongoing use of DHEA could improve **female sexual function**. In one double-blind study, however, younger women did not benefit from a one-time dose of DHEA. DHEA has also shown some promise for improving **erectile dysfunction** in men who have low DHEA blood levels to begin with.

Three double-blind studies hint that DHEA might be helpful for **depression**.

DHEA might also be helpful for people with adrenal failure, according to some but not all studies. **Note:** The term "adrenal failure" refers to total loss of function of the adrenal glands, caused by surgery or infection. The term "adrenal weakness" as used by practitioners of naturopathy refers to something more subtle and vague.

One double-blind, placebo-controlled study indicates that DHEA might enhance the effects of drug treatment of **schizophrenia**. DHEA might also reduce Parkinson's disease–like side effects caused by antipsychotic drugs in the **phenothiazine** family.

A small double-blind trial suggests that DHEA may improve subjective feelings of well-being in people

Dehydroepiandrosterone

with **HIV**. However, another small trial failed to find benefits.

Highly preliminary evidence suggests that DHEA might help improve symptoms of chronic fatigue syndrome, improve **immune response** to vaccinations, and strengthen immunity following burns. Weak evidence also suggests that DHEA supplements might reduce the risk of **heart disease**, especially in men.

One small double-blind study found evidence that DHEA at a dose of 25 mg daily might reduce **menopausal symptoms**; however, in this study, use of DHEA led to altered levels of numerous other hormones, suggesting a potential for hazardous side-effects.

For several other proposed uses of DHEA, study results are more negative than positive.

Primarily because DHEA naturally decreases with age, this hormone has been widely hyped as a kind of fountain of youth. However, eight studies have found that DHEA supplementation does not improve mood, mental function, or **general well-being** in older people, and three studies found that use of DHEA does not increase muscle mass in seniors.

One study did find potential memory-enhancing benefits in younger people.

Athletes have used DHEA on the controversial assumption that it limits the body's response to cortisol and thereby causes an increase in muscle tissue growth. However, current evidence remains inconsistent at best on whether DHEA will aid muscle building or enhance **sports performance** ability.

In a 6-month, double-blind, placebo-controlled trial of 58 people with **Alzheimer's disease**, use of DHEA at 50 mg twice daily did not improve symptoms.

One small study failed to find DHEA helpful for **Sjogren's syndrome**. Another study failed to find DHEA helpful for **fibromyalgia**.

DHEA has been proposed as an aid to **weight loss**, but the little evidence that is available suggests that it does not work. A supplement related to DHEA, 3-acetyl-7-oxo-dehydroepiandrosterone (also called 7-oxy or 7-keto-DHEA), has also been advocated for enhancing weight loss, and there is at least a small amount of supporting evidence.

What Is the Scientific Evidence for Dehydroepiandrosterone?

Lupus

A 12-month, double-blind, placebo-controlled trial of 381 women with mild or moderate lupus (systemic lupus erythematosus, or SLE) evaluated the effects of DHEA at a dose of 200 mg daily. While participants in both treatment and placebo groups improved (the power of placebo is amazing!), DHEA was more effective, reducing many symptoms of the disease. However, DHEA was found to adversely affect cholesterol levels (specifically, the ratio of total cholesterol to HDL cholesterol) and raise levels of testosterone. For this reason, study authors recommend the monitoring of serum cholesterol and keeping watch for adverse effects caused by increased testosterone.

Similarly, in a double-blind, placebo-controlled study of 120 women with SLE, use of DHEA at a dose of 200 mg daily significantly decreased symptoms and reduced the frequency of disease flare-ups.

A smaller study found equivocal evidence that a lower dose of DHEA (30 mg daily for women over 45, and 20 mg daily for women under 45) might also work.

Positive results were also seen in earlier small studies.

Even if DHEA is not strong enough to completely control symptoms of SLE on its own, it might allow a reduction in dosage of the more dangerous standard medications. In addition, it might directly help offset some of the side effects of corticosteroid treatment, such as accelerated osteoporosis, although the evidence for this benefit remains weak and inconsistent.

Osteoporosis

DHEA appears to be helpful for osteoporosis in older women. A double-blind, placebo-controlled trial of 280 men and women ranging in age from 60 to 79 years evaluated the effects of 50 mg of DHEA daily for 1 year. The results suggest that DHEA can fight osteoporosis in women over 70. However, younger women did not respond to treatment with DHEA.

Additional evidence that DHEA might help osteoporosis in older women comes from other clinical trials as well as observational studies.

DHEA might also be helpful for preventing osteoporosis in women with **anorexia**. Women with this condition often experience bone loss, at least in part due to decreases in estrogen levels. In a 1-year, double-blind study, women with anorexia were randomly assigned to receive either DHEA at a dose of 50 mg per day or standard hormone replacement therapy. The results showed equivalent bone preservation in both groups. However, because there is considerable doubt whether hormone replacement therapy is helpful for preventing bone loss caused by anorexia, these results mean relatively little.

DHEA does not appear to affect men's bones to any significant extent.

Adrenal Insufficiency

Two double-blind trials support adding DHEA to the usual hormone regimen for adrenal failure. One double-blind, placebo-controlled crossover trial evaluated the effects of DHEA in 24 women with this condition. The results showed that DHEA at a dose of 50 mg daily improved sexual function, feelings of overall well-being, and cholesterol levels during a 4-month treatment period. Another double-blind crossover trial enrolled 39 men and women and found improvements in general feelings of well-being, mood, and energy level over a 3-month treatment period. However, another double-blind study failed to find benefit with a dose of 25 mg daily.

Improving Libido and Sexual Function in Women

Some evidence suggests that DHEA may be helpful for improving sexual function in older women, but not in younger women.

The 1-year, double-blind, placebo-controlled trial of 280 men and women previously described in the Osteoporosis section (above) also looked for effects on sexual function. The results indicate that for women over 70, daily use of DHEA at 50 mg improves libido. Neither men nor younger women responded. Two other studies did not find benefit, but they enrolled many fewer people and also ran for a shorter time.

Two small, double-blind, placebo-controlled studies tested whether a one-time dose of DHEA at 300 mg could increase sexual arousability in pre- or postmenopausal women respectively. The results again indicate that DHEA is effective for older women but not for younger women.

Improving Sexual Function in Men

A double-blind, placebo-controlled study enrolled 40 men with erectile dysfunction who also had low measured levels of DHEA. The results showed that DHEA at a dose of 50 mg daily significantly improved sexual performance; however, the authors failed to provide a statistical analysis of the results, making the meaningfulness of this study impossible to determine.

Sports Performance Enhancement

A small double-blind study found no performance enhancement with DHEA at a dose of 150 mg per day for men undergoing weight training. In addition, a 12-week, double-blind study of 40 trained male athletes given either DHEA or androstenedione at 100 mg daily found no improvement in lean body mass or strength, or change in testosterone levels.

A 12-month, double-blind, placebo-controlled crossover trial of 16 people aged 50 to 65 found some evidence of fat loss and strength improvement in the male participants during the period in which they received 100 mg of DHEA daily. No improvement was seen in female participants.

Safety Issues

DHEA appears to be safe when taken in therapeutic doses, at least in the short term. One study found no significant side effects in 50 women who took up to 200 mg daily for up to 1 year.

However, DHEA, even at the low dose of 25 mg per day, may decrease levels of HDL ("good") cholesterol. In addition, in women DHEA may increase levels of male sex hormones along with estrogens and progesterone. This could lead to acne and growth of facial and body hair. Effects on hormones in men may be less significant, although one study in HIV-infected men found that DHEA supplements increase level of testosterone, dihydrotestosterone, androstenedione, and estrone.

Concerns have been raised by one study in rats and another in trout that linked DHEA to liver cancer. However, at least four other animal studies suggest that DHEA may have some anticancer effects.

A 15-year human observational trial looking for a connection between naturally occurring DHEA levels and breast cancer found no relationship, either positive or negative. However, another study found a relationship between higher levels of DHEA and ovarian cancer. Overall, the long-term safety of DHEA supplements remains unknown. This is the case with many supplements, but because there are animal studies suggesting that DHEA might increase the risk of liver cancer, caution is warranted. Estrogen is one example of a hormone that increases the risk for certain forms of cancer, and it took years for researchers to discover that risk. Keep in mind also that the body converts DHEA into other hormones, including estrogen and testosterone. This could be dangerous for women with hormone-influenced diseases, such as breast cancer.

We also don't know whether DHEA interacts with other hormone treatments, such as estrogen, although it certainly stands to reason that it might. The safety of DHEA in young children, pregnant or nursing women, and people with severe liver or kidney disease has not been established.

Devil's Claw

Harpagophytum procumbens

PRINCIPAL PROPOSED USES:

Pain and Inflammation: *Back Pain, Gout, Muscle Pain, Osteoarthritis, Rheumatoid Arthritis*
Digestive Problems: *Loss of Appetite, Mild Stomach Upset*

Devil's claw is a native of South Africa, so named because of its rather peculiar appearance. Its large tuberous roots are used medicinally after being chopped up and dried in the sun for 3 days.

Native South Africans used the herb to reduce pain and fever and stimulate digestion. European colonists brought devil's claw back home, where it became a popular treatment for arthritis.

What Is Devil's Claw Used for Today?

In modern Europe, devil's claw is used to treat all types of joint pain, including **osteoarthritis**, **rheumatoid arthritis**, and **gout**. Devil's claw is also used for soft-tissue (muscle-related or tendon-related) pain.

Like other bitter herbs (and this is one of the bitterest!), devil's claw is said to improve appetite and relieve mild stomach upset.

What Is the Scientific Evidence for Devil's Claw?

The evidence for devil's claw is fairly preliminary, with the largest and most well-designed studies showing marginal benefits at best. Most studies have evaluated it for treatment of arthritis.

A double-blind study compared devil's claw to the European drug diacerhein. Diacerhein is a member of a drug category not recognized in the United States: the so-called slow-acting drugs for osteoarthritis (SADOAs). Unlike anti-inflammatory drugs, such as ibuprofen, SADOAs don't give immediate relief, but rather act over a period of weeks to gradually reduce arthritis pain. The supplements **glucosamine** and **chondroitin** have been proposed as natural SADOAs.

In this trial, 122 individuals with osteoarthritis of the hip and/or knee were given either devil's claw or diacerhein for a period of 4 months. The results showed that devil's claw was as effective as diacerhein, as measured by pain levels, mobility, and need for pain-relief medications (such as acetaminophen or ibuprofen). While this might seem impressive, diacerhein itself is only slightly effective, and in such cases, comparative studies must use a placebo group to achieve reliable results.

Another double-blind study followed 89 individuals with rheumatoid arthritis for a 2-month period. The group given devil's claw showed a significant decrease in pain intensity and improved mobility. A third double-blind study of 50 people with various types of arthritis found that 10 days of treatment with devil's claw provided significant pain relief. A fourth study compared devil's claw against Vioxx, an anti-inflammatory drug (currently off the market). While widely reported as showing that devil's claw was equally effective as the drug, in fact it was too small to produce statistically meaningful results.

Other studies have evaluated devil's claw for treatment of muscular tension and discomfort. One of these was a 4-week, double-blind, placebo-controlled trial that evaluated 63 patients with muscular tension or pain in the back, shoulder, and neck. The results showed significant pain reduction in the treatment group as compared to the placebo group. However, a double-blind study of 197 individuals with **back pain** found devil's claw marginally effective at best. Similarly unimpressive results were seen in a previous double-blind study of 118 people with back pain.

We don't know how devil's claw might work. Some studies have found an anti-inflammatory effect but others have not. Apparently, the herb doesn't produce the same changes in prostaglandins as standard anti-inflammatory drugs.

Dosage

A typical dosage of devil's claw is 750 mg 3 times daily of a preparation standardized to contain 3% iridoid glycosides.

Safety Issues

Devil's claw appears to be quite safe, with no evidence of toxicity at doses many times higher than recommended. A 6-month open study of 630 people with arthritis showed no side effects other than occasional mild gastrointestinal distress. Devil's claw is not recommended for people with ulcers. According to one case report, the herb devil's claw might increase the potential for bleeding while taking warfarin. Safety in young children, pregnant or nursing women, or those with severe liver or kidney disease has not been established.

Interactions You Should Know About

If you are taking blood-thinning medications such as **warfarin** (Coumadin) or **heparin**, devil's claw might enhance their effects, possibly producing a risk of bleeding.

Diindolylmethane

SUPPLEMENT FORMS/ALTERNATE NAMES: *DIM*

PRINCIPAL PROPOSED USES: *Reducing Cancer Risk*

OTHER PROPOSED USES: *"Balancing" Hormone Levels, Cervical Dysplasia, Female Sexual Function, Male Sexual Function*

Diindolylmethane (DIM) is produced when the substance **indole-3-carbinol** (I3C) is digested. Indole-3-carbinol, found in broccoli and other vegetables, has shown considerable promise for **cancer prevention**. Some of its benefits in this regard may occur after it is converted by the body to DIM.

DIM also has complex interactions with the hormone estrogen, which could lead to either positive or negative effects on cancer risk.

Requirements/Sources

There is no dietary requirement for DIM. Good natural sources include broccoli, Brussels sprouts, cabbage, and cauliflower.

Therapeutic Dosages

Manufacturers selling DIM products typically recommend about 500 to 1,000 mg daily. The optimal dose (if there is any) is not known.

Therapeutic Uses

Numerous test-tube and animal studies hint that DIM might help prevent various types of **cancer**, especially breast, cervical, prostate, and uterine cancer.

However, this evidence is far too preliminary to serve as the basis for recommending that anyone use DIM. As with many proposed cancer-preventing substances, there are also circumstances in which DIM might actually *increase* the risk of cancer.

Some of DIM's apparent anticancer benefits appear to derive from its complex interactions with estrogen.

DIM appears to alter liver function in such a manner that an increased amount of estrogen becomes metabolized into inactive forms. In addition, DIM blocks certain effects of estrogen on cells; however, it may enhance other effects of estrogen. The overall effect is far too complex and poorly understood to be described as "balancing estrogen in the body," which is what many websites say about DIM.

DMAE

DIM also appears to have an anti-testosterone effect, which could make it helpful for preventing or treating breast cancer. Again, on some websites this effect has been over-optimistically termed "balancing testosterone levels."

Highly preliminary evidence hints that DIM may offer benefit for diseases caused by human papilloma virus (HPV). These include **cervical dysplasia** and respiratory papillomatosis.

According to some manufacturers, DIM can enhance **sexual function in men** or **women** and also **enhance sports performance**. However, there is no evidence that it actually works.

Safety Issues

DIM is thought to be a relatively nontoxic substance. However, comprehensive safety studies have not been completed. Due to DIM's complex interactions with estrogen and testosterone, it has the potential for causing hormonal disturbances. Safety in young children, pregnant or nursing women, or people with severe liver or kidney disease has not been established.

Although there are no known drug interactions with DIM, the substance has shown considerable potential for interacting with many medications.

For this reason, we recommend that if you use any medication that is critical for your health, do not use DIM except under a physician's supervision.

DMAE

SUPPLEMENT FORMS/ALTERNATE NAMES: *2-Dimethylaminoethanol, Deanol*
PRINCIPAL PROPOSED USES: *Attention Deficit Hyperactivity Disorder*
OTHER PROPOSED USES: *Alzheimer's Disease, Huntington's Chorea, Tardive Dyskinesia*

DMAE (2-dimethylaminoethanol) is a chemical that has been used to treat a number of conditions affecting the brain and central nervous system. Like other such treatments, it is thought to work by increasing production of the neurotransmitter acetylcholine, although this has not been proven.

Requirements/Sources

DMAE is sold in pharmacies and health food stores, as well as on the Internet, as a nutritional supplement.

Therapeutic Dosages

Manufacturers' recommended dosages and those used in clinical studies vary between 400 and 1,800 mg daily.

Therapeutic Uses

Preliminary evidence suggests that DMAE may be helpful for **attention deficit hyperactivity disorder** (ADHD).

More widely marketed today as a memory and mood enhancer, DMAE is said to improve intellectual functioning; however, there are no clinical studies that support its use for these purposes. The basis for such claims probably stems from its purported ability to increase levels of a neurotransmitter called *acetylcholine*. Drugs and supplements called *cholinergics* that increase acetylcholine have been used to treat **Alzheimer's disease**, **tardive dyskinesia**, and Huntington's chorea. Because DMAE was believed to be a cholinergic, it has been tried for all of these disorders. However, well-designed, double-blind, placebo-controlled studies have yielded almost entirely negative results. In addition, there is some controversy over whether DMAE really increases acetylcholine at all.

What Is the Scientific Evidence for DMAE?

Attention Deficit Hyperactivity Disorder

There is some evidence that DMAE may be helpful for attention deficit hyperactivity disorder (ADHD), according to studies performed in the 1970s. Two such studies were reported in a review article on DMAE. Fifty children aged 6 to 12 years who had been diagnosed with hyperkinesia (their diagnosis today would likely be ADHD) participated in a double-blind study comparing DMAE to placebo. The dose was increased from 300 mg daily to 500 mg daily by the third week, and continued for 10 weeks. Evaluations revealed statistically significant test score improvements in the treatment group compared to the placebo group.

Another double-blind study compared DMAE with both methylphenidate (Ritalin) and placebo in 74 children described as having unspecified "learning disabilities" (also probably what we would call ADHD today). The study found significant test score improvement for both treatment groups over a 10-week period. Positive results were also seen in a small open study.

Alzheimer's Disease

Most people over the age of 40 experience some memory loss, but Alzheimer's disease is much more serious, leading to severe mental deterioration (dementia) in the elderly. Microscopic examination shows that in the areas of the brain involved in higher thought processes, nerve cells have died and disappeared, particularly cells that release the chemical acetylcholine. Drugs such as tacrine and danazol and supplements such as **huperzine A** are used for Alzheimer's based on their ability to increase acetylcholine levels. Because DMAE is also thought to increase acetylcholine, trials have been performed to test its effectiveness for the same purpose. However, there is no real evidence as yet that it works.

A double-blind, placebo-controlled study involving 27 patients with Alzheimer's disease tested DMAE as a treatment. Thirteen participants were placed in the group receiving DMAE; however, 6 of them had to drop out of the study because of side effects, such as drowsiness, increased confusion, and elevated blood pressure. In those completing the trial, no differences were seen between the treatment group and those taking placebo.

An open trial enrolling 14 patients found no improvement in either memory or cognitive function. The researchers did note improvements in symptoms of depression, but in the absence of a placebo group this observation means little.

Tardive Dyskinesia

Tardive dyskinesia (TD) is a potentially permanent side effect of drugs used to control **schizophrenia**. This late-developing (tardy, or tardive) complication consists of annoying, uncontrollable movements (dyskinesias), particularly in the face.

Based on its supposed cholinergic effect, DMAE has been proposed as a treatment for TD. Although some case reports and open studies seemed to suggest that DMAE might be useful for this purpose, properly designed studies using double-blind methods and placebo control groups have not borne this out. Of 12 double-blind studies reviewed, only one found DMAE to be significantly effective when compared with placebo. A meta-analysis of proposed treatments for TD found DMAE to be no more effective than placebo. It seems likely, though not entirely certain, that the benefits seen in open studies and individual cases were the result of a placebo effect. However, it is also possible that some particular individuals respond well to DMAE, even if most don't.

Huntington's Chorea

Huntington's chorea is a genetically inherited disease that results in personality changes and, somewhat similarly to TD, uncontrolled spastic movements. It doesn't usually become symptomatic until a person's age reaches the late thirties or older, although about 10% of people with Huntington's will begin to show signs of the disorder in childhood or adolescence.

DMAE was not found to be an effective treatment for Huntington's chorea in double-blind, placebo-controlled trials, although mixed results have been obtained using DMAE in open trials.

Safety Issues

Although most clinical investigations using DMAE report that the participants experienced no side effects, enough researchers have found adverse reactions to suggest that some caution is appropriate in using this supplement. One study, as noted above, reports increased confusion, drowsiness, and elevated blood pressure; another reports headache and muscle tension as possible adverse effects; and another paper suggests that weight loss and insomnia may accompany use of DMAE. There is also one case report of a woman who developed severe TD after taking DMAE for 10 years for a hand tremor. Besides this, a number of manufacturers warn against the use of DMAE by people with epilepsy or a history of convulsions.

Maximum safe dosages for young children, pregnant or nursing women, or people with severe liver or kidney disease have not been established.

Dong Quai

Angelica sinensis

ALTERNATE NAMES/RELATED TERMS: *Dang Kwai, Dong Kwai, Dang Quai, Tang Quai*

PRINCIPAL PROPOSED USES: *Dysmenorrhea, Menstrual Disorders in General, Premenstrual Syndrome (PMS)*

PROBABLY INEFFECTIVE USES: *Menopausal Symptoms*

One of the major herbs used in **traditional Chinese herbal medicine**, *Angelica sinensis* is closely related to European *Angelica archangelica*, a common garden herb and the flavoring in Benedictine and Chartreuse liqueurs. The carrot-like roots of this fragrant plant are harvested in the fall after about 3 years of cultivation and stored in airtight containers prior to processing.

Traditionally, dong quai is said to be one of the most important herbs for strengthening the *xue*. The Chinese term *xue* is often translated as "blood," but it actually refers to a complex concept in traditional Chinese medicine, of which the Western notion of blood is only a part. In the late 1800s, an extract of dong quai known as Eumenol became popular in Europe as a "female tonic," and this is how most people consider it in the West.

What Is Dong Quai Used for Today?

Dong quai is often recommended as a treatment for menstrual cramps, **premenstrual syndrome** (PMS), and other problems related to menstruation, as well as hot flashes and other **menopausal symptoms**. However, the scientific evidence supporting these uses is very weak, consisting primarily of test-tube and animal studies, as well as a few open studies of humans. Only double-blind, placebo-controlled studies can actually show a treatment effective, and a 24-week study that compared the effects of dong quai against a placebo in 71 postmenopausal women found no benefit.

Dosage

We recommend using dong quai under the supervision of an herbalist qualified in traditional Chinese herbal medicine, not because the herb is dangerous, but because it is difficult to self-prescribe Chinese herbal formulas.

If you wish to self-treat with dong quai, a typical dosage is 10 to 40 drops of dong quai tincture 1 to 3 times daily or 1 standard 00 gelatin capsule 3 times daily.

Safety Issues

Dong quai is generally believed to be nontoxic. According to Chinese studies, which may not have been up to current scientific standards, very large amounts have been given to rats without causing harm. Side effects are rare and primarily consist of mild gastrointestinal distress and occasional allergic reactions (such as rash).

Contrary to popular belief, dong quai does not appear to have estrogen-like actions. However, according to an article in the *Singapore Medical Journal*, a 35-year-old man who used a prepared herbal formula called *Dong Quai pills* developed enlargement of his breasts. Such enlargement would typically result if a man used estrogen. The authors of the article blamed the dong quai itself. However, a more likely explanation is that the prepared herbal formula was spiked with synthetic estrogen. There are numerous reports of prepackaged Asian herb products containing unlabeled constituents, including conventional medications designed to enhance their effects.

Interestingly, in a test-tube study, dong quai was again found to be non-estrogenic, and yet it nonetheless stimulated the growth of breast cancer cells. Although the mechanism of this effect is not known, the results suggest that women who have had breast cancer should avoid using dong quai.

Dong quai may interact with the blood-thinning drug Coumadin (warfarin), increasing the risk of bleeding, according to one case report. Dong quai might also conceivably interact with other blood-thinning drugs, such as heparin, aspirin, Plavix (clopidogrel), Ticlid (ticlopidine), or Trental (pentoxifylline).

Certain constituents of dong quai can cause **photosensitivity** (increased sensitivity to the sun), but this has not been observed to occur in people using the whole herb.

Safety in young children, pregnant or nursing women, or those with severe liver or kidney disease has not been established. One case report suggests that dong quai usage by a nursing mother caused elevated blood pressure in both the mother and child.

Interactions You Should Know About

If you are taking blood-thinning drugs such as **warfarin** (Coumadin), **heparin**, **clopidogrel** (Plavix), **ticlopidine** (Ticlid), **pentoxifylline** (Trental), or **aspirin**, dong quai might interact and increase the risk of bleeding.

Echinacea

Echinacea purpurea, E. angustifolia, E. pallida

PRINCIPAL PROPOSED USES: *Colds and Flus (Treatment, not Prevention)*

OTHER PROPOSED USES: *Chronic Bronchitis (Acute Flare-ups), Genital Herpes*

PROBABLY NOT EFFECTIVE USES: *Colds and Flus (Prevention), General Immune Support*

The decorative plant *Echinacea purpurea*, or purple coneflower, has been one of the most popular herbal medications in both the United States and Europe for over a century.

Native Americans used the related species *Echinacea angustifolia* for a wide variety of problems, including respiratory infections and snakebite. Herbal physicians among the European colonists quickly added the herb to their repertoire. Echinacea became tremendously popular toward the end of the nineteenth century, when a businessman named H.C.F. Meyer promoted an herbal concoction containing *E. angustifolia*. The garish, exaggerated, and poorly written nature of his labeling helped define the characteristics of a "snake oil" remedy.

However, serious manufacturers developed an interest in echinacea as well. By 1920, the respected Lloyd Brothers Pharmaceutical Company of Cincinnati, Ohio, counted echinacea as its largest-selling product. In Europe, physicians took up the American interest in *E. angustifolia* with enthusiasm. Demand soon outstripped the supply coming from America and, in an attempt to rapidly plant echinacea locally, the German firm Madeus and Company mistakenly purchased a quantity of *Echinacea purpurea* seeds. This historical accident is the reason why most echinacea today belongs to the *purpurea* species instead of *angustifolia*. Another family member, *Echinacea pallida*, is also used.

Echinacea was the number one cold and flu remedy in the United States until it was displaced by sulfa anti-

biotics. Ironically, antibiotics are not effective for colds, while echinacea appears to offer some real help. Echinacea remains the primary remedy for minor respiratory infections in Germany, where over 1.3 million prescriptions are issued each year.

What Is Echinacea Used for Today?

In Europe, and increasingly in the U.S. as well, echinacea products are widely used to treat colds and flus.

The best scientific evidence about echinacea concerns its ability to help you recover from **colds and minor flus** more quickly. The old saying goes that "a cold lasts 7 days, but if you treat it, it will be over in a week." However, good, if not entirely consistent, evidence tells us that echinacea can actually help you get over colds much faster. It also appears to significantly reduce symptoms while you are sick. Echinacea may also be able to "abort" a cold, if taken at the first sign of symptoms. However, taking echinacea regularly throughout cold season is probably not a great idea. Evidence suggests that it does *not* help prevent colds.

Until recently, it was believed that echinacea acted by stimulating the immune system. Test-tube and animal studies had found that various constituents of echinacea can increase antibody production, raise white blood cell counts, and stimulate the activity of key white blood cells. However, most recent studies have tended to cast doubt on this theory. The fact that regular use of echinacea does not appear to help prevent colds (or genital herpes) also somewhat argues against an immune-strengthening effect. Thus, at present, it can only be said that we don't understand the means by which echinacea affects cold symptoms.

Echinacea has been proposed for the treatment and/or prevention of other acute infections as well. One small double-blind study found that use of an herbal combination containing echinacea enhanced the effectiveness of antibiotic treatment for acute flare-ups of **chronic bronchitis**. However, another study failed to find benefit for **ear infections** in children.

Finally, echinacea is frequently proposed for **general immune support**. However, as discussed above, there is some reason to think that it is not effective for this purpose.

What Is the Scientific Evidence for Echinacea?

Reducing the Symptoms and Duration of Colds

Double-blind, placebo-controlled studies enrolling a total of more than 1,000 individuals have found that various forms and species of echinacea can reduce cold symptoms and help you get over a cold faster. The best evidence regards products that include the aboveground portion of *E. purpurea*.

For example, in one double-blind, placebo-controlled trial, 80 individuals with early cold symptoms were given either an aboveground *E. purpurea* extract or placebo. The results showed that individuals who were given echinacea recovered significantly more quickly: just 6 days in the echinacea group versus 9 days in the placebo group.

Another study found evidence that aboveground *E. purpurea* can reduce the severity of cold symptoms, but that *E. purpurea* root may not be effective. In this double-blind trial, 246 individuals with recent onset of a respiratory infection were given either placebo or one of three *E. purpurea* preparations: two formulations of a product made of 95% aboveground herb (leaves, stems, and flowers) and 5% root, and one made only from the roots of the plant. The results showed significant improvements in symptoms, such as runny nose, sore throat, sneezing, and fatigue, with the aboveground preparations, but the root preparation was not effective.

Symptom reduction with a whole plant formulation of *E. purpurea* was seen in a double-blind, placebo-controlled study of 282 people.

However, another double-blind, placebo-controlled study of aboveground *E. purpurea*, enrolling 120 people, failed to find benefits as compared to placebo treatment. An even larger trial (407 participants) failed to find a widely used aboveground *E. purpurea* extract helpful for treating children with respiratory infections. The reasons for these negative outcomes are unclear.

In other studies, benefits were seen with a preparation of *E. pallida* root and an herbal beverage tea containing aboveground portions of *E. purpurea* and *E. angustifolia* (as well as some *E. purpurea* root extract).

A double-blind, placebo-controlled study failed to find benefit with a dry herb product consisting largely of *E. purpurea* root and *E. angustifolia* root. Another study failed to find benefit with *E. angustifolia* root extract.

The bottom line: At present, the best supporting evidence for echinacea involves the aboveground portion or whole plant extract of *E. purpurea*, but even here the results are less than fully consistent.

"Aborting" a Cold

A double-blind study suggests that echinacea can not only make colds shorter and less severe, it might also be able to stop a cold that is just starting. In this study, 120 people were given *E. purpurea* or a placebo as soon as they started showing signs of getting a cold.

Participants took either echinacea or placebo at a dosage of 20 drops every 2 hours for 1 day, then 20 drops 3 times a day for a total of up to 10 days of treatment. The results were promising. Fewer people in the echinacea group felt that their initial symptoms actually developed into "real" colds (40% of those taking echinacea versus 60% taking the placebo actually became ill). Also, among those who did come down with "real" colds, improvement in the symptoms started sooner in the echinacea group (4 days instead of 8 days). Both of these results were statistically significant.

Preventing Colds

Several studies have attempted to discover whether the daily use of echinacea can prevent colds from even starting, but the results have not been promising.

In one double-blind, placebo-controlled trial, 302 healthy volunteers were given an alcohol tincture containing either *E. purpurea* root, *E. angustifolia* root, or placebo for 12 weeks. The results showed that *E. purpurea* was associated with perhaps a 20% decrease in the number of people who got sick and *E. angustifolia* with a 10% decrease. However, the difference was not statistically significant. This means that the benefit, if any, was so small that it could have been due to chance alone.

Another double-blind, placebo-controlled study enrolled 109 individuals with a history of four or more colds during the previous year and gave them either *E. purpurea* juice or placebo for a period of 8 weeks. No benefits were seen in the frequency, duration, or severity of colds. (**Note:** This paper is actually a more detailed look at a 1992 study widely misreported as providing evidence of benefit.)

Similar results were seen in three other studies as well, enrolling a total of more than 300 individuals.

A study often cited as evidence that echinacea can prevent colds actually found no benefit in the 609 participants taken as a whole. Only by looking at subgroups of participants (a statistically questionable procedure) could researchers find any evidence of benefit, and it was still slight.

However, a recent study using a combination product containing echinacea, **propolis**, and **vitamin C** did find preventive benefits. In this double-blind, placebo-controlled study, 430 children age 1 to 5 years were given either the combination or placebo for 3 months during the winter. The results showed a statistically significant reduction in frequency of respiratory infections. It is not clear which components of this mixture were responsible for the apparent benefits seen.

Dosage

Echinacea is usually taken at the first sign of a cold and continued for 7 to 14 days. Longer-term use of echinacea is not recommended. The best (though not entirely consistent) evidence supports the use of products made from the aboveground portions of *E. purpurea* (specifically, flowers, leaves, and stems); *E. pallida* root has also shown promise, but *E. purpurea* root appears to be ineffective.

The typical dosage of echinacea powdered extract is 300 mg 3 times a day. Alcohol tincture (1:5) is usually taken at a dosage of 3 to 4 ml 3 times daily, echinacea juice at a dosage of 2 to 3 ml 3 times daily, and whole dried root at 1 to 2 g 3 times daily. There is no broad agreement on what ingredients should be standardized in echinacea tinctures and solid extracts.

Note: A survey of available echinacea products found many problems. In this 2003 analysis, about 10% had no echinacea at all; about half were mislabeled as to the species of echinacea present; more than half the standardized preparations did not contain the labeled amount of standardized constituents; and the total milligrams of echinacea stated on the label generally had little to do with the actual milligrams of herb present. A subsequent analysis performed in 2004 by the respected testing organization, ConsumerLab.com, also found many problems.

Many herbalists feel that liquid forms of echinacea are more effective than tablets or capsules, because they think that part of echinacea's benefit is due to activation of the tonsils through direct contact. However, there is no real evidence to support this contention.

Finally, **goldenseal** is frequently combined with echinacea in cold preparations. However, there is not a shred of evidence that oral goldenseal stimulates immunity, nor did traditional herbalists use it for this purpose.

Safety Issues

Echinacea appears to be generally safe. Even when taken in very high doses, it has not been found to cause any toxic effects.

Reported side effects are also uncommon and usually limited to minor gastrointestinal symptoms, increased urination, and mild allergic reactions. However, severe allergic reactions have occurred occasionally, some of them life-threatening. In Australia, one survey found that 20% of allergy-prone individuals were allergic to echinacea.

Other concerns relate to echinacea's possible immune-stimulating properties. Immunity is a two-edged sword that the body keeps under careful control; excessively strong immune reactions can be dangerous. Based on this concern, echinacea should be used only with caution (if at all) by individuals with autoimmune disorders, such as multiple sclerosis, lupus, and rheumatoid arthritis.

Furthermore, a recent case report strongly suggests that use of echinacea can trigger episodes of erythema nodosum (EN). EN is an inflammatory condition that involves tender nodules under the skin. These nodules often arise after cold-like symptoms. In this report, a 41-year-old man took echinacea on four separate occasions when he thought he was developing a cold, and each time he developed EN instead. When he stopped using echinacea for this purpose, he remained free of EN outbreaks for a full year of follow-up. The cause of EN is not known, but it involves increased activity of certain immune cells; echinacea has been observed to cause similar effects in the same immune cells, suggesting that the relationship is not coincidental.

One study raised questions about possible anti-fertility effects of echinacea. When high concentrations of echinacea were placed in a test tube with hamster sperm and ova, the sperm were less able to penetrate the ova. However, since we have no idea whether this much echinacea can actually come in contact with sperm and ova when they are in the body rather than a test tube, these results may not be meaningful in real life.

Animal studies of echinacea are supportive of safety in pregnancy. One human study found a bit of evidence that use of echinacea during pregnancy does not increase risk of birth defects, but this evidence is not strong enough to absolutely rely on.

Furthermore, studies dating back to the 1950s suggest that echinacea is safe in children. Nonetheless, the safety of echinacea in young children or pregnant or nursing women cannot be regarded as established. In addition, safety in those with severe liver or kidney disease has also not been established.

Two studies suggest that echinacea might interact with various medications by affecting their metabolism in the liver, but the significance of these largely theoretical findings remains unclear.

Elderberry

Sambucus nigra

PRINCIPAL PROPOSED USES: *Colds and Flus*

OTHER PROPOSED USES: *Herpes, High Cholesterol, HIV Support*

Native Americans used tea made from elderberry flowers to treat respiratory infections. They also used the leaves and flowers in poultices applied to wounds, and the bark, suitably aged, as a laxative. The berries are frequently made into beverages, pies, and preserves, but they have also been used to treat arthritis.

What Is Elderberry Used for Today?

A product containing elderberry, as well as small amounts of **echinacea** and **bee propolis**, has been widely marketed as a **cold and flu** remedy. Weak evidence suggests that this mixture may stimulate the immune system and also inhibit viral growth. In a preliminary double-blind study, this mixture was found to reduce symptoms and speed recovery from influenza A, the type of influenza for which flu shots are given. A few of the participants in this study had influenza B (a milder form of influenza), and the elderberry mixture appeared to be helpful for them as well. Another preliminary double-blind study evaluated people with influenza B and also found benefit.

Elderberry has also shown some preliminary promise for use in other viral infections, including HIV and **herpes**.

Based on promising results in an uncontrolled study, researchers performed a small, double-blind, placebo-controlled study on the potential benefits of elderberry for improving cholesterol levels. Unfortunately, at the dose used, no benefits were evident.

Dosage

Elderberry-flower tea is made by steeping 3 to 5 g of dried flowers in 1 cup of boiling water for 10 to 15 minutes. A typical dosage is 1 cup 3 times daily. Standardized extracts should be taken according to the directions on the product's label.

Safety Issues

Elderberry flowers are generally regarded as safe. Side effects are rare and consist primarily of occasional mild gastrointestinal distress or allergic reactions. Nonetheless, safety in young children, pregnant or nursing women, or those with severe liver or kidney disease has not been established.

Elecampane

Inula helenium

PRINCIPAL PROPOSED USES: *Asthma, Chronic Respiratory Diseases, Poor Digestion*

The Latin name of elecampane comes from Helen of Troy, who was supposed to have carried elecampane with her while being abducted from Sparta. Revered by the ancient Greeks and Romans, this herb was recommended for treating such diverse problems as indigestion, melancholy, sciatica, bronchitis, and asthma.

What Is Elecampane Used for Today?

Some modern herbalists regard elecampane as a long-term treatment for respiratory diseases such as **asthma** and bronchitis, especially when excessive mucus is a notable feature. However, there is no real evidence that it is effective for this purpose.

Elecampane is also sometimes recommended as a daily supplement to improve general digestion.

One of elecampane's constituents, alantolactone, has been used in concentrated form as a treatment for intestinal parasites, but it isn't clear whether the whole herb is particularly effective for this purpose.

Dosage

A typical dosage of elecampane root is 1.5 to 4 g 3 times daily, either in capsule form or boiled in water as tea.

Safety Issues

The only reported adverse effects of elecampane are occasional allergic reactions. However, safety in young children, pregnant or nursing women, or those with severe liver or kidney disease has not been established.

Eleutherococcus senticosus

ALTERNATE NAMES/RELATED TERMS: *Eleuthero; Ginseng, Russian; Ginseng, Siberian; Russian ginseng; Siberian ginseng*

PRINCIPAL PROPOSED USES: *Adaptogen, Stress*

OTHER PROPOSED USES: *Chronic Fatigue Syndrome, Herpes, Sports Performance*

Eleutherococcus senticosus is only distantly related to the true ginseng species (**Panax ginseng** and **P. quinquefolius**) and possesses entirely different, unrelated chemical constituents. However, it is popularly called *Russian* or *Siberian ginseng*. The origin of this misnomer lies in the work of a Soviet scientist, I. I. Brekhman, who believed that *Eleutherococcus* has the same properties as ginseng and popularized it as a less-expensive alternative herb.

According to Brekhman, *Eleutherococcus* and ginseng are both **adaptogens**. This term refers to a hypothetical treatment defined as follows: An adaptogen should help the body adapt to stresses of various kinds, whether heat, cold, exertion, trauma, sleep deprivation, toxic exposure, radiation, infection, or psychological stress. Furthermore, an adaptogen should cause no side effects, be effective in treating a wide variety of illnesses, and help return an organism toward balance no matter what may have gone wrong.

Perhaps the only indisputable example of an adaptogen is a healthful lifestyle. By eating right, exercising regularly, and generally living a life of balance and moderation, you will increase your physical fitness and ability to resist illnesses of all types. Brekhman felt certain that both *Eleutherococcus* and ginseng produced similarly universal benefits. However, there is little to no meaningful evidence supporting this theory.

Herbs sold under the name ciwuja are most likely *Eleutherococcus* as well.

What Is *Eleutherococcus senticosus* Used for Today?

If Brekhman is right, ginseng (whether *Eleutherococcus* or *Panax*) should be the right treatment for most of us. Modern life is tremendously stressful, and if an herb could help us withstand **stress**, it would be a useful herb indeed. *Eleutherococus* is widely used for this purpose in Russia and Eastern Europe, and is popular elsewhere as well. However, there is little meaningful evidence to support this theory. Existing evidence on the supposed adaptogenic properties of *Eleutherococcus* falls far beneath current scientific standards.

Better-quality studies have evaluated the potential usefulness of *Eleutherococcus* for specific conditions. Most, however, have failed to find benefit.

In the one unquestionably positive study, a 6-month, double-blind, placebo-controlled trial of 93 men and women with recurrent herpes infections, treatment with *Eleutherococcus* (2 g daily) reduced the frequency of outbreaks by approximately 50%.

Although *Eleutherococcus* is widely used as a **sports supplement**, evidence from studies is largely negative. For example, a double-blind, placebo-controlled study of 20 athletes over an 8-week period found no improvement in physical performance. In addition, a small, double-blind, crossover trial found *Eleutherococcus* ineffective for improving performance in endurance exercise (specifically, prolonged cycling). Finally, in a small, double-blind, placebo-controlled trial of endurance athletes, use of *Eleutherococcus* actually *increased* physiological signs of stress during intensive training.

One study failed to find *Eleutherococcus* helpful for **chronic fatigue syndrome**.

Several double-blind studies enrolling a total of about 500 people have evaluated a combination therapy (Kan Jang) containing *Eleutherococcus* and the herb andrographis for the treatment of **upper respiratory infections** and found benefit. In general, these studies have found that use of the combination therapy may decrease both severity and duration of upper respiratory infections. However, it is not clear whether the presence of the *Eleutherococcus* adds any benefit beyond that of the andrographis constituent, which when taken alone has shown efficacy in clinical trials. For more information, see the **Andrographis** article.

Dosage

The typical recommended daily dosage of *Eleutherococcus* is 2 to 3 g whole herb or 300 to 400 mg of extract daily.

Safety Issues

According to studies performed primarily in the former Soviet Union, *Eleutherococcus* appears to present a low order of toxicity in both the short and long term. Human trials have not resulted in any significant side effects. Safety in pregnant or nursing women, young children, or people with severe liver or kidney disease is not known.

One report suggests that *Eleutherococcus* may alter the results of a test for digoxin. However, it is not clear whether it was the *Eleutherococcus* or a contaminant (for example, digoxin mixed with the herb) that caused these problems.

Interactions You Should Know About

If you are taking **digoxin**, *Eleutheroccocus* may interfere with blood tests designed to measure digoxin level.

Ephedra

Ephedra sinica

ALTERNATE NAMES/RELATED TERMS: *Ma Huang*

PRINCIPAL PROPOSED USES: *Asthma*

QUESTIONABLE USES: *Sexual Dysfunction in Women, Weight-loss Aid*

On Dec. 30, 2003, the U.S. Food and Drug Administration (FDA) issued a consumer alert regarding the safety of dietary supplements containing ephedra. The FDA determined that consuming these supplements poses an unnecessary risk of illness or injury and that consumers should stop buying and using ephedra products immediately. The FDA also notified manufacturers and marketers of these dietary supplements that effective 60 days (March 2004) after the publication of its final ruling, the sale of all products containing ephedra in the United States would be banned. However, this ruling was overturned in April of 2005 based on provisions of the law governing supplement sales and marketing (Dietary Supplementation and Health Education Act, or DSHEA). With medications, the manufacturer is required to prove safety, but with supplements the situation is reversed: the burden of proof is on the FDA to prove lack of safety. The judge ruled that the FDA had failed to prove ephedra dangerous when used according to label instructions. However, the FDA in general lacks the resources to prove that supplements are unsafe. It is fair to say at present that ephedra's safety is unproven and there are clearly possible risks.

The Chinese herb ma huang is a member of a primitive family of plants that look like thin, branching, connected straws. A related species, *Ephedra nevadensis*, grows wild in the American Southwest and is widely called *Mormon tea*. However, only the Asian species of ephedra contains the active compounds ephedrine and pseudoephedrine.

Ma huang was traditionally used by Chinese herbalists during the early stages of respiratory infections and also for the short-term treatment of certain kinds of asthma, eczema, hay fever, narcolepsy, and edema.

Japanese chemists isolated ephedrine from ma huang at the turn of the century and it soon became a primary treatment for asthma in the United States and abroad. Ephedra's other major ingredient, pseudoephedrine, became the decongestant Sudafed.

What Is Ephedra Used for Today?

Although it can still be found in a few over-the-counter drugs for **asthma**, physicians seldom prescribe ephedrine anymore. The problem is that ephedrine mimics the effects of adrenaline and causes symptoms such as rapid heartbeat, high blood pressure, agitation, insomnia, nausea, and loss of appetite. The newer asthma drugs are much safer and easier to tolerate.

Meaningful evidence suggests ephedrine/caffeine combinations can assist in **weight loss**. **Note:** Due to safety risks, we strongly recommend that you seek a physician's supervision before attempting to lose weight with ephedrine/caffeine combination therapy. We do not recommend using herbal sources of ephedrine for weight loss at all (see Safety Issues below).

One highly preliminary study has been used to claim that ephedrine is helpful for women with **sexual dysfunction**. However, this trial was very small, enrolled women without sexual problems, and only examined sexual responsiveness to visual stimuli; at this time, we do not recommend that women with sexual dysfunction use ephedra. Another study examined the possible benefits of ephedrine for treatment of female sexual dysfunction caused by antidepressants in the **SSRI** family (such as Prozac). Ephedrine failed to prove more effective than placebo.

There is no meaningful evidence that ephedra enhances **sports performance**.

Note: Individuals taking ephedra or ephedrine may test positive for methamphetamine (speed) on drug screening.

What Is the Scientific Evidence for Ephedra?

Evidence suggests that ephedrine/caffeine combinations can aid weight loss and help keep the weight off for up to 6 months. However, the benefits are modest.

For example, in a double-blind, placebo-controlled

trial, 180 overweight individuals were placed on a weight-loss diet and given either ephedrine/caffeine (20 mg/200 mg), ephedrine alone (20 mg), caffeine alone (200 mg), or placebo 3 times daily for 24 weeks. The results showed that the ephedrine/caffeine treatment significantly enhanced weight loss, resulting in a loss of more than 36 pounds as compared to only 29 pounds in the placebo group, a 7-pound difference. Neither ephedrine nor caffeine alone produced any benefit. Contrary to some reports, participants did not develop tolerance to the treatment. For the whole 6 months of the trial, the treatment group maintained the same relative weight-loss advantage over the placebo group.

A few side effects were seen in this study, primarily insomnia, dizziness, and tremor, but they tended to fade away after a few weeks. Keep in mind that participants were screened prior to the study and were eliminated if they had high blood pressure or any other serious disease, or if they used medications or illegal drugs that might interact with stimulants.

Another study compared ephedrine/caffeine with the no-longer-available drug dexfenfluramine (Redux), related to fenfluramine of fen-phen fame. A total of 103 overweight individuals were enrolled in this 15-week, double-blind trial. All were placed on a weight-loss diet. Half were given ephedrine/caffeine at the usual dose, while the others were given 15 mg of dexfenfluramine. The results showed comparable weight loss in both groups.

Finally, a double-blind, placebo-controlled trial enrolled 225 heavy smokers who wanted to quit but were afraid of gaining weight. At 12 weeks after quitting smoking, individuals taking ephedrine and caffeine had gained significantly less weight. At that point, the dosage was gradually reduced and the difference between the groups declined. (Contrary to the hopes of the experimenters, ephedrine/caffeine use did not help individuals quit smoking.)

Benefits have also been seen in smaller studies using herbal sources of ephedrine.

We don't know exactly how ephedrine/caffeine works. However, caffeine has actions that cause fat breakdown and enhance metabolism. Ephedrine suppresses appetite and increases energy expenditure. The combination appears to produce synergistic effects, with appetite suppression probably the most important overall factor.

Dosage

The dosage of ephedra should be adjusted according to the amount of the ephedrine it provides. For adults, no more than 25 mg should be taken at one time and a total daily intake of 100 mg should not be exceeded. However, a survey of ephedra-containing dietary supplements found that ephedrine content as listed on the label was frequently incorrect. In addition, other chemicals were often present that could increase safety risks (see Safety Issues below). For this reason, we do not recommend using herbal ephedra at all.

Safety Issues

While ephedra is an herb with a long history of use in Chinese herbal medicine, Chinese tradition attaches numerous warnings: it should only be used by very robust people, for certain specific purposes, and only for a short period of time. These ancient warnings seem to have been disregarded in the transition of ephedra use from Asia to the United States, where it is now often sold for continuous use by overweight, relatively unhealthy people. Herbal products containing ephedra cause the majority (64%) of reported adverse effects from herbs in the U.S. This proportion is particularly impressive given that less than 1% of all herbal products sold in the U.S. contain ephedra. On a per-use basis, for example, ephedra has 720 times the risk of causing harm as ginkgo biloba.

There are many reasons for this high rate of risk. While it is possible for healthy individuals under physician supervision to use ephedrine or ephedrine/caffeine combinations safely, in individuals with heart disease, and even occasionally in those with no known heart conditions, ephedrine can cause serious disturbances of the heart rhythm and possibly sudden death; strokes have also occurred. Use of herbal ephedra, as opposed to ephedrine, may present additional dangers. As noted above, there is no ready way to be sure of the dose of the *drug* ephedrine you are getting when you purchase the *herb* ephedra, creating potential risk of overdosage. In addition, some ephedra products contain potentially more toxic chemicals related to ephedrine, such as (+)-norpseudoephedrine.

Besides heart problems and strokes, use of ephedra has been associated with severe inflammation of the liver (in at least one case requiring a liver transplant) and of the heart. In these cases, it appears likely that ephedra (or an unidentified contaminant in the herb) triggered an autoimmune reaction.

In addition, people taking ephedra or ephedrine may develop an unusual form of kidney stones that actually contain ephedrine. Temporary psychosis has also been linked to use of ephedra.

Finally, there are indications that certain preparations of ephedra may be toxic to the nervous system.

Based on the known risks of ephedrine, as well as the evidence described above, ephedra should definitely not be taken by a person with:

- Cardiovascular disease, including:
  - Angina
  - Abnormalities of heart rhythm
  - Hardening of the arteries
  - High blood pressure
  - High cholesterol
  - Intermittent claudication
  - History of stroke
- Enlargement of the prostate
- Diabetes
- Hepatitis
- Myocarditis
- Vasculitis
- Diseases of the nervous system
- Glaucoma
- Hyperthyroidism

Ephedra may be particularly risky for:

- Young children
- Pregnant or nursing women
- People with kidney disease
- People with liver disease

Furthermore, one should never combine ephedra with monoamine-oxidase inhibitors (MAO inhibitors), such as Nardil (phenelzine), or fatal reactions may develop.

Interactions You Should Know About

If you are taking:

- MAO inhibitors: Do not take ephedra.
- any stimulant drugs (including caffeine): Do not take ephedra except under physician supervision.

Essential Oil Monoterpenes

PRINCIPAL PROPOSED USES: *Acute Bronchitis, Chronic Bronchitis, Sinus Infections*
OTHER PROPOSED USES: *Colds and Flus*

Eucalyptus oil is a standard ingredient in cough drops and cough syrups, as well as oils added to humidifiers. A standardized combination of eucalyptus oil plus two other **essential oils** has been studied for effectiveness in a variety of respiratory conditions. This combination therapy contains cineole from eucalyptus, d-limonene from citrus fruit, and alpha-pinene from pine. Because these oils are all in a chemical family called *monoterpenes*, the treatment is called *essential oil monoterpenes*.

Therapeutic Uses of Essential Oil Monoterpenes

Most, though not all, studies indicate that oral use of essential oil monoterpenes can help acute bronchitis, chronic bronchitis, and sinus infections.

For example, a double-blind, placebo-controlled trial of 676 people with **acute bronchitis** found that 2 weeks' treatment with essential oil monoterpenes was more effective than placebo and equally effective as antibiotic treatment for reducing symptoms and aiding recovery. Also, a 3-month, double-blind, placebo-controlled trial of 246 people with chronic bronchitis found that regular use of essential oil monoterpenes helped prevent the typical worsening of **chronic bronchitis** that occurs during the winter.

Additionally, in a double-blind, placebo-controlled study of about 300 people, use of essential oil monoterpenes improved symptoms of acute sinusitis.

One study weakly indicates that essential oil monoterpenes may be helpful for colds in children.

Essential oil monoterpenes are thought to work by thinning mucus.

Dosage

In studies, this essential oil combination was taken at a dose of 300 mg 3 to 4 times daily.

Safety Issues

Other than minor gastrointestinal complaints, no side effects have been reported with this essential oil combination. However, be advised that essential oils can be toxic if taken in excess. Maximum safe doses in young children, women who are pregnant or nursing, and individuals with severe liver or kidney disease have not been established.

Estriol

SUPPLEMENT FORMS/ALTERNATE NAMES: *Oestriol, Tri-Estrogen*
PRINCIPAL PROPOSED USES: *Menopausal Symptoms, Osteoporosis*

Several forms of estrogen occur naturally in a woman's body. The ovary produces a form named estradiol, which is converted into another important estrogen called *estrone*. Estriol is yet another form of estrogen metabolized from estradiol, weaker than the other two, but still active.

The estrogen tablets prescribed for menopausal symptoms usually contain estradiol, estrone, or a combination of the two. Some alternative medicine physicians have popularized the use of estriol as an alternative, and there is no doubt that estriol is also effective for symptoms of menopause. However, despite claims that it is safer than other forms of estrogen, the balance of evidence suggests that, in fact, estriol presents precisely the same risks (see Safety Issues below).

Requirements/Sources

Estriol is manufactured in the body from estrone, estradiol, and **androstenedione**. When taken as a drug, it is manufactured synthetically or extracted from animal products.

Therapeutic Dosages

The usual dose of estriol is 2 to 8 mg taken once daily. Estriol is also commonly sold in combination with other forms of estrogen.

Therapeutic Uses

Like more common forms of estrogen, estriol is used for the treatment of **menopausal symptoms**. Double-blind, placebo-controlled studies and other controlled trials have found oral or vaginal estriol effective for symptoms of menopause, including hot flashes, night sweats, insomnia, vaginal dryness, and recurrent urinary tract infections; estriol may also help prevent **osteoporosis**.

Estriol might cause less vaginal bleeding as a side effect than other forms of estrogen, although this has not been definitively established.

Some alternative practitioners claim that estriol actually fights cancer, as opposed to estrogen, which increases risk of some cancers. However, this claim is based on exaggerated interpretations of very weak studies. It is more likely that estriol increases cancer risk in much the same way as other forms of estrogen (see Safety Issues below).

Safety Issues

Like other forms of estrogen, oral estriol stimulates the growth of uterine tissue. This leads to risk of uterine cancer. In a placebo-controlled study of 1,110 women, uterine tissue stimulation was seen among women given estriol orally (1 to 2 mg daily) as compared to those given placebo. Another large study found that oral estriol increased the risk of uterine cancer. In a third study of

48 women, estriol (1 mg twice daily) caused uterine tissue stimulation. In contrast, a 12-month, double-blind trial of oral estriol (2 mg daily) in 68 Japanese women found no effect on the uterus. It may be that the high levels of soy in the Japanese diet altered the results.

For this reason, to protect the uterus, estriol, like other forms of estrogen, needs to be balanced with progesterone. Additionally, one study suggests that estriol is less likely to affect the uterus when taken in a once-daily dose rather than in multiple daily doses.

However, the uterus isn't the only organ at risk of cancer. Test-tube studies suggest that estriol is just as likely to cause breast cancer as any other form of estrogen. While this preliminary evidence doesn't constitute proof, it does raise alarm bells. Until proven otherwise, estriol must be regarded as increasing breast cancer risk.

As with other forms of estrogen, vaginal estriol preparations are safer than oral preparations.

Eucalyptus
Eucalyptus globulus

PRINCIPAL PROPOSED USES: *Common Cold (Oral, Lozenge, Inhaled)*
OTHER PROPOSED USES: *Asthma (Inhaled or Oral), Cough (Lozenge or Inhaled), Insect Repellant (Topical), Sore Throat (Lozenge)*

The eucalyptus tree originated in Australia and Tasmania, but has now been spread to all other inhabited continents. There are many different varieties of eucalyptus, with somewhat differing constituents. The most common type used medicinally is eucalyptus globules. Its essential oil contains eucalyptol (cineol or cineole).

Eucalyptus oil has a long history of use as a topical antiseptic. It has also been used as a lozenge or inhalation therapy for asthma, cough, sore throat, and other respiratory conditions.

What Is Eucalyptus Used for Today?

A standardized combination of cineol from eucalyptus, d-limonene from citrus fruit, and alpha-pinene from pine has been studied for effectiveness in a variety of respiratory conditions. These oils are all in a chemical family called *monoterpenes* and, for this reason, the combined treatment is called ***essential oil monoterpenes***. This combination is discussed in a separate article of that name. Other combination therapies containing eucalyptus oil are discussed in the article titled **Aromatherapy**.

Eucalyptus oil or its constituents taken alone have undergone only limited study. It appears to be most promising as a treatment for the comment cold. However, concerns about safety have limited its use.

In a double-blind, placebo-controlled study of 152 people, use of cineol at a dose of 200 mg 3 times daily markedly improved symptoms of the **common cold**. Benefits were seen in such symptoms as nasal congestion, headache, and overall malaise. Few significant side effects were seen in this study, but the product used was of pharmaceutical grade and not all dietary supplements of eucalyptus oil may be equally safe.

In another study, 32 people on steroids to control severe **asthma** (steroid-dependent asthma) were given either placebo or cineole (200 mg 3 times daily) for 12 weeks. The results showed that people using cineole were able to gradually reduce their steroid dosage to a greater extent than those taking placebo. **Note:** Reduction of steroid dosage should be done only under the supervision of a physician.

Cineole or eucalyptus oil applied topically has also shown some potential value for repelling **mosquito bites**.

Dosage

The studied dosage of cineole is 200 mg 3 times daily for adults. Internal use of cineole or eucalyptus oil should be avoided in children.

For use as an insect repellent, 25 to 50 ml of the oil is added to 500 ml of water. Do not use in children under age 12.

As an inhalant, a few drops of eucalyptus oil are added to a vaporizer.

Safety Issues

Internal use of eucalyptus oil at appropriate doses by healthy people can cause nausea, heartburn, vomiting, diarrhea, and skin rash. Excessive dosages can be fatal, especially to children. Inhalation of the oil can exacerbate asthma in some people. Application of cineole to the entire body resulted in severe nervous system poisoning in a 6-year-old child. In general, eucalyptus oil should not be used by young children, pregnant or nursing women, or people with severe liver or kidney disease.

Although no drug interactions of eucalyptus are firmly documented, there are theoretical reasons to believe it could interact with a number of medications, either raising or lowering their levels. Therefore, people taking any oral or injected medication that is critical to their health or well-being should avoid internal use of eucalyptus until more is known.

Eyebright

Euphrasia officinale L.

PRINCIPAL PROPOSED USES: *None*

NOT RECOMMENDED USES: *Conjunctivitis or Other Diseases of the Eye*

The herb eyebright has been used since the Middle Ages as an eyewash for infection or inflammation of the eye. However, as much as one would like to believe that all traditions are wise, eyebright appears to have been selected for treating eye diseases not because it works particularly well, but because its petals look bloodshot. This follows from the classic medieval philosophic attitude known as the *Doctrine of Signatures*, which states that herbs show their proper use by their appearance.

What Is Eyebright Used for Today?

Like many herbs, eyebright contains astringent substances and volatile oils that are probably at least slightly antibacterial. But there's no evidence that eyebright is particularly effective for treating conjunctivitis (pink eye) or any other eye disease; Germany's Commission E recommends against using it. Warm compresses consisting of nothing but water (or ordinary black tea) are probably equally effective under the same conditions.

Eyebright tea is also sometimes taken internally to treat jaundice, respiratory infections, and memory loss. However, there is no evidence that it is effective for any of these conditions.

Dosage

Traditionally, eyebright tea is made by boiling 1 tablespoon of the herb in a cup of water. This is then used as an eyewash or taken internally up to 3 times daily.

Safety Issues

Eyebright can cause tearing of the eyes, itching, redness, and many other symptoms, probably due to direct irritation. It appears to be safe when taken internally, but not many studies have been performed. Safety in young children, pregnant or nursing women, or those with severe liver or kidney disease has not been established.

False Unicorn

Chamaelirium luteum

PRINCIPAL PROPOSED USES: *Dysmenorrhea (Painful Menstruation)*

OTHER PROPOSED USES: *Infertility, Pelvic Inflammatory Disease, Premenstrual Syndrome (PMS)*

NOT RECOMMENDED USES: *Morning Sickness, Pregnancy Support (Preventing Miscarriages)*

The herb false unicorn is native to North America east of the Mississippi River. It is similar in appearance but unrelated to "true" unicorn, *Aletris farinose.*

The root is the portion used medicinally. Native Americans and subsequently European physicians believed that false unicorn stimulates the uterus, promoting menstruation. It was used for dysmenorrhea (painful menstruation), amenorrhoea (absent menstruation), and irregular menstruation, as well as infections of the female genital tract.

What Is False Unicorn Used for Today?

Some contemporary herbalists claim that false unicorn can help "balance" the female reproductive system, normalizing hormone levels and optimizing ovarian action. On this basis, they recommend it for preventing miscarriages and treating **infertility, dysmenorrhea**, **premenstrual syndrome** (PMS), pelvic inflammatory disease, and **morning sickness**. However, there is no meaningful evidence to support any of these uses. (For more information on why scientific studies are essential to determine whether folk uses of an herb are valid, see **Why Does This Book Rely on Double-blind Studies?**.)

Some herbalists support these proposed effects by referring to the presence of the hormone-like substance diosgenin in false unicorn. They claim that diosgenin either has hormonal properties or that the body can use it to create hormones. This concept, however, is based on a widespread misconception. It is true that diosgenin is used by industrial chemists as a raw material from which to economically synthesize sex hormones. This fact has been sufficient to lead to an association in people's minds between diosgenin and hormones. However, diosgenin itself does *not* have any hormonal properties, and while chemists can convert diosgenin into female hormones, the body does not do so.

Dosage

A typical dose of false unicorn is 1 to 2 g 3 times daily or an equivalent amount in tincture form.

Safety Issues

False unicorn has not undergone any meaningful safety evaluation. Even though it is traditionally recommended for use during pregnancy, its reputation as a uterine stimulant would seem to suggest it shouldn't be taken by pregnant women.

Safety in young children, nursing women, or people with severe liver or kidney disease has not been established.

Fennel

Foeniculum vulgare

PRINCIPAL PROPOSED USES: *Infantile Colic*

OTHER PROPOSED USES: *Dyspepsia (Indigestion), Intestinal Gas, Menstrual Pain*

The herb fennel has a long history of use as both food and medicine. Traditionally, it is said to act as a *carminative*, a term that means that it helps the body expel gas. Other traditional uses include increasing breast-milk production, easing childbirth, soothing cough, promoting menstrual flow, soothing indigestion, and enhancing libido. Fennel is also a common ingredient in "gripe water," a traditional (and highly alcoholic) preparation used for treating infant colic.

What Is Fennel Used for Today?

Animal and test-tube studies hint at a number of potential medicinal effects of fennel or its constituents, such as relaxing smooth muscles, stimulating the flow of bile, and reducing pain. However, only double-blind, placebo-controlled studies in humans can actually show a treatment effective. Only one such study of this type has been performed for fennel.

This trial enrolled 125 infants with **colic** who received either placebo or fennel seed oil at a dose of 12 mg daily per kg of body weight. The results were promising. About 40% of the infants receiving fennel showed relief of colic symptoms, as compared to only 14% in the placebo group, a significant difference. Another way to view the results involves looking at hours of inconsolable crying. In the treated group, infants cried about 9 hours per week, compared to 12 hours in the placebo group. While these are promising results, confirmation by an independent research group is necessary before the treatment can be accepted as effective.

Previously, a small, double-blind, placebo-controlled study found similar benefits with a tea containing fennel as well as other herbs (**chamomile**, vervain, **licorice**, and **lemon balm**).

No other proposed uses of fennel have undergone study in double-blind trials. One study commonly cited as evidence that fennel is helpful for **menstrual pain** actually proved nothing at all. This was an open trial that compared fennel to the drug mefenamic acid. Because participants and researchers were aware of which treatment was which, the power of suggestion had free play, making the results almost meaningless. (For more information, see **Why Does This Book Rely on Double-blind Studies?**)

At one time it was thought that fennel had estrogen-like effects, making it a **phytoestrogen**. However, subsequent research has tended to indicate that fennel does not have significant phytoestrogen activity.

Dosage

A typical dose of fennel is 1 to 1½ teaspoons of seeds per day, either in capsules or as tea.

Safety Issues

As a widely consumed food spice, fennel is thought to have a high safety factor. However, according to one placebo-controlled study with rats, fennel impairs the absorption of the antibiotic ciprofloxacin (Cipro). Fennel might be expected to interfere similarly with other drugs in the ciprofloxacin family, the fluoroquinolone drugs. Allowing 2 hours between taking ciprofloxacin and fennel should reduce the potential for an interaction, but may not eliminate it. For this reason, it may be advisable to avoid taking fennel during therapy with ciprofloxacin or other antibiotics in this family.

Maximum safe doses of fennel in young children, pregnant or nursing women, or people with severe liver or kidney disease have not been established.

Interactions You Should Know About

If you are taking drugs in the **fluoroquinolone** family such as ciprofloxacin (Cipro), do not use fennel.

Fenugreek

Trigonella foenumgraecum

PRINCIPAL PROPOSED USES: *Constipation, Diabetes, High Cholesterol*

For millennia, fenugreek has been used both as a medicine and as a food spice in Egypt, India, and the Middle East. It was traditionally recommended for increasing milk production in nursing women and for the treatment of wounds, bronchitis, digestive problems, arthritis, kidney problems, and male reproductive conditions.

What Is Fenugreek Used for Today?

Present interest in fenugreek focuses on its potential benefits for people with **diabetes** or **high cholesterol**. Numerous animal studies and preliminary trials in humans have found that fenugreek can reduce blood sugar and serum cholesterol levels in people with diabetes. Like other high-fiber foods, it may also be helpful for **constipation**.

What Is the Scientific Evidence for Fenugreek?

In a 2-month, double-blind study of 25 individuals with type 2 diabetes, use of fenugreek (1 g per day of a standardized extract) significantly improved some measures of blood sugar control and insulin response as compared to placebo. Triglyceride levels decreased and HDL ("good") cholesterol levels increased, presumably due to the enhanced insulin sensitivity.

Similar benefits have been seen in animal studies and open human trials, as well.

Dosage

Because the seeds of fenugreek are somewhat bitter, they are best taken in capsule form. The typical dosage is 5 to 30 g of defatted fenugreek taken 3 times a day with meals. The one double-blind study of fenugreek used 1 g per day of a water/alcohol fenugreek extract.

Safety Issues

As a commonly eaten food, fenugreek is generally regarded as safe. The only common side effect is mild gastrointestinal distress when it is taken in high doses.

Animal studies have found fenugreek essentially non-toxic and no serious adverse effects have been seen in a 2-year follow-up of human trials.

However, extracts made from fenugreek have been shown to stimulate uterine contractions in guinea pigs. For this reason, pregnant women should not take fenugreek in dosages higher than is commonly used as a spice, perhaps 5 g daily. Besides concerns about pregnant women, safety in young children, nursing women, or those with severe liver or kidney disease has also not been established.

Because fenugreek can lower blood sugar levels, it is advisable to seek medical supervision before combining it with diabetes medications.

Interactions You Should Know About

If you are taking diabetes medications such as **insulin** or **oral hypoglycemic drugs**, fenugreek may enhance their effects. This may cause excessively low blood sugar and you may need to reduce your dose of medication.

Feverfew

Tanacetum parthenium

PRINCIPAL PROPOSED USES: *Migraine Headaches*

OTHER PROPOSED USES: *Osteoarthritis, Rheumatoid Arthritis*

Originally native to the Balkans, this relative of the common daisy was spread by deliberate planting throughout Europe and the Americas. Feverfew's feathery and aromatic leaves have long been used medicinally to improve childbirth, promote menstruation, induce abortions, relieve rheumatic pain, and treat severe headaches.

Contrary to popular belief, feverfew is not used for lowering fevers. Actually, according to one source, "feverfew" is a corruption of the name "featherfoil." Featherfoil became featherfew and ultimately feverfew. In a weird historical reversal, this name then led to a widespread belief among herbalists that feverfew could lower fevers. After a while they noticed that it didn't work and then angrily rejected feverfew as a useless herb! Feverfew remained out of fashion until a serendipitous event occurred in the late 1970s.

At that time, the wife of the chief medical officer of the National Coal Board in England suffered from serious migraine headaches. When workers in the industry learned of this fact, a sympathetic miner suggested she try a folk treatment he had used. She followed his advice and chewed feverfew leaves. The results were dramatic: her migraines disappeared almost completely.

Her husband was impressed, too. He used his high office to gain the ear of a physician who specialized in migraine headaches, Dr. E. Stewart Johnson of the London Migraine Clinic. Johnson subsequently experimented with feverfew in his practice and seemed to observe good results. This led to the studies described below.

What Is Feverfew Used for Today?

Feverfew is primarily used for the *prevention* of **migraine headaches**. For this purpose, it is taken daily. There has been no formal investigation of feverfew as a *treatment* for migraines that have already started, although one double-blind study evaluating feverfew as a preventive agent did find hints of possible symptom-reducing benefits.

It is important to remember that serious diseases may occasionally first present themselves as migraine-type headaches. For this reason, proper medical diagnosis is essential if you suddenly start having migraines without a previous history or if the pattern of your migraines changes significantly.

Feverfew is sometimes recommended for **osteoarthritis** or **rheumatoid arthritis**, but there is no evidence at all that it works.

What Is the Scientific Evidence for Feverfew?

Five meaningful double-blind, placebo-controlled studies have been performed to evaluate feverfew's effectiveness as a preventive treatment for migraines. The best of the positive trials used a feverfew extract made by extracting the herb with liquid carbon dioxide. Two other trials that used whole feverfew leaf also found it effective; however, two studies that used feverfew extracts did not find benefit.

In a well-conducted 16-week, double-blind, placebo-controlled study of 170 people with migraines, use of a feverfew extract at a dose of 6.25 mg 3 times daily resulted in a significant decrease in headache frequency as compared to the effect of the placebo treatment. In the treatment group, headache frequency decreased by 1.9 headaches per month, as compared to a reduction of 1.3 headaches per month in the placebo group. The average number of headaches per month prior to treatment was 4.76 headaches. The extract used in this study was made utilizing liquid carbon dioxide.

A previous study using the same extract had failed to find benefit, but it primarily enrolled people with less frequent migraines.

Two other studies used whole feverfew leaf and found benefit. The first followed 59 people for 8 months. For 4 months, half received a daily capsule of powdered feverfew leaf; the other half took placebo. The groups were then switched and followed for an additional 4 months. Treatment with feverfew produced a 24% reduction in the number of migraines and a significant decrease in nausea and vomiting during the headaches. A subsequent double-blind study of 57 people with migraines found that use of feverfew leaf could decrease the severity of migraine headaches. Unfortunately, this trial did not report whether there was any change in the frequency of migraines; it is possible, therefore, that this study actually showed a symptom-reducing effect rather than a preventive benefit.

One study using an alcohol extract failed to find benefit.

Dosage

The tested liquid-carbon-dioxide feverfew extract is taken at a dose of 6.25 mg 3 times daily. To replicate the dosage of feverfew used in the two positive studies of whole leaf described above, take 80 to 100 mg of powdered whole feverfew leaf daily.

Safety Issues

Animal studies suggest that feverfew is essentially nontoxic. In one 8-month study, there were no significant differences in side effects between the treated and control groups. There were also no changes in measurements on blood tests and urinalysis.

In a survey involving 300 people, 11.3% reported mouth sores from chewing feverfew leaf, occasionally accompanied by general inflammation of tissues in the mouth. A smaller percentage reported mild gastrointestinal distress. However, mouth sores do not seem to occur in people who use encapsulated feverfew leaf powder, the usual form.

In view of its use as a folk remedy to promote abortions, feverfew should probably not be taken during pregnancy.

Because feverfew might slightly inhibit the activity of blood-clotting cells known as platelets, it should not be combined with strong anticoagulants, such as Coumadin (warfarin) or heparin, except on medical advice. Feverfew might also increase the risk of stomach problems if combined with anti-inflammatory drugs such as aspirin.

Safety in young children, pregnant or nursing women, or those with severe kidney or liver disease has not been established.

Interactions You Should Know About

If you are taking **warfarin** (Coumadin), **heparin**, **aspirin** or other **nonsteroidal anti-inflammatory drugs**: Do not use feverfew except on medical advice.

Fish Oil

SUPPLEMENT FORMS/ALTERNATE NAMES: *Docosahexaenoic Acid (DHA), Eicosapentaenoic Acid (EPA), Omega-3 Fatty Acids, Omega-3 Oil(s)*

PRINCIPAL PROPOSED USES: *Heart Disease Prevention, Rheumatoid Arthritis*

OTHER PROPOSED USES: *Allergies, Angina, Asthma, Attention Deficit and Hyperactivity Disorder (ADHD), Bipolar Disorder, Borderline Personality Disorder, Cancer Treatment Support, Chronic Fatigue Syndrome, Crohn's Disease, Depression, Diabetic Neuropathy, Dysmenorrhea (Menstrual Pain), Eczema (Prevention), Epilepsy, Gout, HIV Support, Hypertension, Kidney Stones, Lupus, Male Infertility, Migraine Headaches, Multiple Sclerosis, Osteoporosis, Pregnancy Support, Prevention of Premature Birth, Prostate Cancer (Prevention), Psoriasis, Raynaud's Phenomenon, Retinitis Pigmentosa, Schizophrenia, Sickle-cell Anemia, Strokes (Prevention), Ulcerative Colitis, Undesired Weight Loss Caused by Cancer*

Fish oil contains omega-3 fatty acids, one of the two main classes of essential fatty acids. (**Omega-6 fatty acids** are the other main type.) Essential fatty acids are special fats that the body needs for optimum health.

Interest in the potential therapeutic benefits of omega-

Fish Oil

3 fatty acids began when studies of the Inuit (Eskimo) people found that, although their diets contain an enormous amount of fat from fish, seals, and whales, they seldom suffer heart attacks. This is presumably because those sources of fat are very high in omega-3 fatty acids.

Subsequent investigation found that the omega-3 fatty acids found in fish oil have various effects that tend to reduce risk of heart disease and strokes. However, research into whether use of fish oil actually prevents these diseases, while somewhat positive, remains incomplete and somewhat inconsistent. In recognition of this, the FDA has allowed supplements containing fish oil or its constituents to carry a label that states: "Supportive but not conclusive research shows that consumption of EPA and DHA omega-3 fatty acids may reduce the risk of coronary heart disease."

Fish oil has also shown promise as an anti-inflammatory treatment for conditions such as rheumatoid arthritis, menstrual pain, and lupus. In addition, it may be helpful for various psychiatric conditions.

Requirements/Sources

There is no daily requirement for fish oil. However, a healthy diet should provide at least 5 g of essential fatty acids daily.

Many grains, fruits, vegetables, sea vegetables, and vegetable oils contain significant amounts of essential omega-6 and/or omega-3 fatty acids, but oil from cold-water fish is the richest natural source of omega-3 fats. It is commonly stated that people require a certain optimum ratio of omega-3 to omega-6 fatty acids in the diet, but there is no real evidence for this belief.

Therapeutic Dosages

Typical dosages of fish oil are 3 to 9 g daily, but this is not the upper limit. In one study, participants ingested 60 g daily.

The most important omega-3 fatty acids found in fish oil are called *eicosapentaenoic acid* (EPA) and *docosahexaenoic acid* (DHA). In order to match the dosage used in several major studies, you should take enough fish oil to supply about 2 to 3 g of EPA (2,000 to 3,500 mg) and about 1 to 2.5 g of DHA daily (1,000 to 2,500 mg). Far higher doses have been used in some studies, however.

DHA and EPA are not identical and might not have identical effects. For example, DHA may be more effective than EPA for thinning the blood and reducing blood

pressure, while the reverse may be true for reducing triglyceride levels.

Some manufacturers add vitamin E to fish oil capsules to keep the oil from becoming rancid. Another method is to remove all the oxygen from the capsule.

If possible, purchase fish oil products certified as free of significant levels of mercury, toxic organochlorines, and PCBs (see Safety Issues below).

Flaxseed oil also contains omega-3 fatty acids, although of a different kind. It has been suggested as a less smelly substitute for fish oil. However, it is far from clear whether flaxseed oil is therapeutically equivalent to fish oil.

Therapeutic Uses

Consumption of fish oil alters the body's production of certain substances in the class of chemicals called *prostaglandins*. Some prostaglandins increase inflammation while others decrease it. The prostaglandins whose production is enhanced by fish oil fall into the anti-inflammatory category. Based on this, fish oil has been tried as a treatment for early stages of **rheumatoid arthritis**, with positive results. It is thought to significantly reduce symptoms without causing side effects and may magnify the benefits of standard arthritis drugs. However, while some standard medications can slow the progression of the disease, there is no evidence that fish oil can do this.

Fish oil's anti-inflammatory properties are the likely explanation for its apparent benefit in **dysmenorrhea** (menstrual pain), as seen in two studies. Similarly, fish oil may be helpful for the autoimmune disease **lupus**. (However, two studies failed to find fish oil helpful for kidney disease caused by lupus.) Evidence is mixed regarding whether fish oil is beneficial for **Crohn's disease** or **ulcerative colitis**, conditions in which parts of the digestive tract are highly inflamed.

Incomplete evidence hints but does not prove that fish or fish oil might help prevent death caused by **heart disease**. This effect, if it exists, seems to result from several separate actions, including (most predominately) reducing **high triglyceride levels**, as well as raising HDL ("good") cholesterol levels, "thinning" the blood, lowering levels of **homocysteine**, preventing dangerous heart arrhythmias, slowing heart rate, improving blood vessel tone, and decreasing **blood pressure**. These effects also support findings that fish oil may help prevent **strokes**. However, results are conflicting on whether people with **angina** should take fish oil or increase intake of fatty fish;

one large study actually found that fish oil *increased* risk of sudden death.

For reasons that are almost entirely unclear, fish oil might have positive effects on various psychiatric disorders. According to one small double-blind study, high doses of fish oil may produce benefits in **bipolar disorder** (more commonly known as manic-depressive illness), reducing risk of relapse and improving emotional state. It might also offer benefits in **depression, schizophrenia**, and borderline personality disorder. In one study, DHA failed to augment the effectiveness of standard therapy for **attention deficit disorder**. However, two studies that evaluated the potential benefits of fish oil combined with omega-6 fatty acids found some evidence of benefit.

Small studies also suggest that fish oil may be helpful in **Raynaud's phenomenon** (a condition in which a person's hands and feet show abnormal sensitivity to cold temperatures), **sickle-cell anemia**, and a form of kidney disease called *IgA nephropathy*.

According to some, but not all, studies, fish oil may help treat the **undesired weight loss** often experienced by people with cancer. In addition, highly preliminary evidence hints that DHA might enhance the effects of the **cancer chemotherapy** drug doxorubicin and decrease side effects of the chemotherapy drug irinotecan.

Use of fish oil by **pregnant women** might help prevent premature birth, although evidence is inconsistent. In addition, use of fish oil by pregnant women may support healthy brain function and help prevent eczema and allergies in offspring.

Intriguing but not yet at all reliable evidence hints that fish oil or its constituents might be helpful for treating **kidney stones**, alleviating the symptoms of **chronic fatigue syndrome**, reducing the risk of prostate **cancer**, decreasing seizure frequency in people with **epilepsy**, and, when taken with **vitamin A**, slowing the progression of a retinitis pigmentosa (a condition in which the retina gradually degenerates).

Fish oil has also been proposed as a treatment for many other conditions, including **diabetic neuropathy, allergies**, and **gout**, but there has been little real scientific investigation of these uses.

Some, but not all, studies suggest that fish oil combined with omega-6 essential fatty acids may augment the effectiveness of calcium in the treatment of **osteoporosis**. One promising, but highly preliminary, double-blind, placebo-controlled study suggests that the same combination therapy may improve symptoms of the severe neurological illness called *Huntington's disease*.

For several other conditions, the current balance of the evidence suggests that fish oil is *not* effective.

For example, despite widely publicized claims that fish oil helps **asthma**, most preliminary studies have failed to provide evidence that it is effective, and one study found that fish oil can actually worsen aspirin-related asthma. However, there is some evidence that use of fish oil could help prevent exercise-induced asthma in athletes.

Similarly, a 16-week, double-blind, placebo-controlled study of 167 individuals with recurrent **migraine headaches** found that fish oil did not significantly reduce headache frequency or severity. Conflicting results have been seen in other, much smaller trials of fish oil for migraines.

One study found weak evidence that use of fish oil might decrease aggressive behavior in young girls (but, in this study, not in young boys). Another study found benefit in developmental coordination disorder (a condition in which children suffer from lack of physical coordination as well as problems with learning and behavior).

Fish oil is also sometimes recommended for enhancing immunity in **HIV** infection. However, one 6-month, double-blind study found that a combination of the omega-3 fatty acids in fish oil plus the amino acid arginine was no more effective than placebo in improving immune function in people with HIV. Fish oil, however, might help individuals with HIV gain weight.

There is no evidence, as yet, that use of fish oil reduces cancer risk.

Preliminary studies have suggested that fish oil could help symptoms of **multiple sclerosis**; however, the largest double-blind study on the subject found no difference between people taking fish oil and those taking olive oil (used as a placebo).

Although one study found fish oil somewhat helpful in **psoriasis**, a much larger study found no benefit.

DHA has been evaluated as a possible treatment for **male infertility**, but a double-blind trial of 28 men with impaired sperm activity found no benefit.

Combination therapy with GLA and fish oil has failed to prove effective for **cyclic breast pain**.

One study failed to find fish oil more effective than placebo for treating **stress**.

What Is the Scientific Evidence for Fish Oil?

Heart Disease Prevention

Studies on fish or fish oil for preventing cardiovascular disease, slowing the progression of cardiovascular disease, and preventing heart-related death have returned somewhat contradictory results. One review (technically a meta-analysis) of many studies on the subject published in 2002 concluded that when all the evidence is put together, it appears that fish or fish oil can reduce overall mortality, heart disease mortality, and sudden cardiac death. However, another review published in 2004 failed to find trustworthy evidence of benefit, and an even more recent study found that use of fish oil *increases* risk of sudden death in people with stable heart disease. These contradictory results suggest that fish oil's benefit to heart disease, if any, is slight.

As noted earlier, fish oil is hypothesized to exert several separate effects that act together to help protect the heart. The most important action of fish oil may be its apparent ability to reduce high triglyceride levels. Like cholesterol, triglycerides are a type of fat in the blood that tends to damage the arteries, leading to heart disease. According to most, though not all, studies, fish oil supplements can reduce triglycerides by about 25 to 30%. A slightly modified form of fish oil (ethyl-omega-3 fatty acids) has been approved by the FDA as a treatment for elevated triglycerides. However, in some studies, use of fish oil has markedly raised LDL ("bad") cholesterol, which might offset some of the benefit.

Fish oil has been specifically studied for reducing triglyceride levels in people with diabetes, and it appears to do so safely and effectively. It also seems to remain effective in individuals who are already using statin drugs to control lipid levels (both people with and without diabetes). However, one study found that the standard drug **gemfibrozil** is more effective than fish oil for reducing triglycerides.

Some but not all studies suggest that fish, fish oil, or EPA or DHA separately may additionally raise the level of HDL ("good") cholesterol and possibly improve other aspects of cholesterol profile as well. This too should help prevent heart disease.

Additionally, fish oil may help the heart by "thinning" the blood and by reducing blood levels of homocysteine, although not all studies have found a positive effect.

Studies contradict one another on whether fish oil can lower blood pressure, but on balance the supplement does seem to exert a modest positive effect. A 6-week, double-blind, placebo-controlled study of 59 overweight men suggests that the DHA in fish oil, but not the EPA, is responsible for this benefit.

Evidence is conflicting on whether fish oil helps prevent heart arrhythmias.

Fish oil may slightly reduce heart *rate*. This effect could contribute to preventing heart attacks and other heart problems.

Rheumatoid Arthritis

The results of numerous small double-blind trials indicate that omega-3 fatty acids in fish oil can help reduce the symptoms of rheumatoid arthritis. The benefits of the fish oil effect may be enhanced by a vegetarian diet. Simultaneous supplementation with olive oil (about two teaspoons daily) may further increase the benefits. However, unlike some conventional treatments, fish oil probably does not slow the progression of rheumatoid arthritis.

Menstrual Pain

Regular use of fish oil may reduce the pain of menstrual cramps.

In a 4-month study of 42 young women aged 15 to 18, half the participants received a daily dose of 6 g of fish oil, providing 1,080 mg of EPA and 720 mg of DHA daily. After 2 months, they were switched to placebo for another 2 months. The other group received the same treatments in reverse order. The results showed that these young women experienced significantly less menstrual pain while they were taking fish oil.

Another double-blind study followed 78 women, who received either fish oil, seal oil, fish oil with vitamin B_{12} (7.5 mcg daily), or placebo for three full menstrual periods. Significant improvements were seen in all treatment groups, but the fish oil plus vitamin B_{12} proved most effective and its benefits continued for the longest time after treatment was stopped (3 months). The researchers offered no explanation why vitamin B_{12} should be helpful.

Bipolar Disorder

A 4-month, double-blind, placebo-controlled study of 30 individuals suggests that fish oil can enhance the effects of standard treatments for bipolar disorder, reducing risk of relapse and improving emotional state. Eleven of the 14 individuals who took fish oil improved or remained well during the course of the study, while only 6 out of the 16 given placebo responded similarly.

Another small study found that ethyl-EPA (a modified form of EPA) is helpful for the depressive phase of bipolar disease.

Depression

A 4-week, double-blind, placebo-controlled trial evaluated the potential benefits of fish oil in 20 individuals with depression. All but one participant were also taking standard antidepressants and had been taking them for at least 3 months. By week 3, the level of depression had improved to a significantly greater extent in the fish oil group than in placebo group. Six of 10 participants given fish oil, but only one of 10 given placebo, showed at least a 50% reduction in depression scores by the end of the trial. (A reduction of this magnitude is considered a "cure.")

A double-blind, placebo-controlled study of 70 people who were still depressed despite standard therapy found that additional treatment with ethyl-EPA (a modified form of EPA) improved symptoms. Similar add-on benefits were also seen in other double-blind studies of ethyl-EPA or mixed essential fatty acids. However, one study failed to find benefit with fish oil as an add-on treatment. Another double-blind study failed to find DHA alone helpful for depression.

Schizophrenia

Five double-blind, placebo-controlled studies have been performed on EPA for the treatment of schizophrenia, with benefits seen in four out of the five.

Raynaud's Phenomenon

In small, double-blind studies, fish oil has been found to reduce the severe finger and toe responses to cold temperatures that occur in Raynaud's phenomenon. However, these studies suggest that a higher than usual dosage must be used to get results, perhaps 12 g daily.

Osteoporosis

There is some evidence that essential fatty acids may enhance the effectiveness of calcium in osteoporosis. In one study, 65 postmenopausal women were given calcium along with either placebo or a combination of omega-6 fatty acids (from evening primrose oil) and omega-3 fatty acids (from fish oil) for a period of 18 months. At the end of the study period, the group receiving essential fatty acids had higher bone density and fewer fractures than the placebo group.

However, a 12-month, double-blind trial of 42 postmenopausal women found no benefit.

The explanation for the discrepancy may lie in the differences between the women studied. The first study involved women living in nursing homes, while the second studied healthier women living on their own. The latter group of women may have been better nourished and already received enough essential fatty acids in their diet.

Lupus

Lupus is a serious autoimmune disease that can cause numerous problems, including fatigue, joint pain, and kidney disease. One small, 34-week, double-blind, placebo-controlled crossover study compared placebo against daily doses of EPA (20 g) from fish oil. A total of 17 individuals completed the trial. Of these, 14 showed improvement when taking EPA, while only 4 did so when treated with placebo. Another small study found similar benefits with fish oil over a 24-week period. However, two small studies failed to find fish oil helpful for lupus nephritis (kidney damage caused by lupus).

Attention Deficit and Hyperactivity Disorder (ADHD)

Based on evidence that essential fatty acids are necessary for the proper development of brain function in growing children, EFAs have been tried for the treatment of ADHD and related conditions.

A preliminary double-blind, placebo-controlled trial found some evidence that a supplement containing fish oil and **evening primrose oil** might improve ADHD symptoms. However, a high dropout rate makes the results of this trial somewhat unreliable. Another small study examined fish oil in children with ADHD who had thirst and skin problems. Benefits were seen with fish oil, but they occurred with placebo as well, and to about the same extent.

In a double-blind, placebo-controlled trial of children already using stimulant therapy, addition of DHA for 4 months failed to further improve symptoms.

Safety Issues

Fish oil appears to be generally safe. The most common problem is fishy burps. However, there are some safety concerns to consider.

For example, it has been suggested that some fish oil products contain excessive levels of toxic substances such as organochlorines and PCBs. If possible, try to purchase fish oil products certified not to contain significant levels of these contaminants. **Note:** Various types of fish contain mercury, but this has not been a problem with fish oil supplements, according to reports on Consumerlab.com.

Fish oil has a mild blood-thinning effect, and in one case report it increased the effect of the blood-thinning medication Coumadin (warfarin). Fish oil does not seem to cause bleeding problems when it is taken by itself or with aspirin. Nonetheless, people who are at risk of bleeding complications for any reason should probably consult a physician before taking fish oil.

Fish oil does not appear to raise blood sugar levels in people with diabetes. Nonetheless, if you have diabetes, you should not take any supplement except on the advice of a physician.

Fish oil may also raise the level of LDL ("bad") cholesterol; it is possible, however, that this effect may be short-lived and that levels return to normal with continued use.

If you decide to use cod liver oil as your fish oil supplement, make sure you do not exceed the safe maximum intake of vitamin A and **vitamin D**. These vitamins are fat-soluble, which means that excess amounts tend to build up in your body, possibly reaching toxic levels. The official maximum daily intake of vitamin A is 3,000 mcg for pregnant women as well as other adults. Look at the bottle label to determine how much vitamin A you are receiving. (It is less likely that you will get enough vitamin D to produce toxic effects.)

Interactions You Should Know About

If you are taking **warfarin** (Coumadin) or **heparin**, do not take fish oil except on the advice of a physician.

Flaxseed

ALTERNATE NAMES/RELATED TERMS: *Linseed*

PRINCIPAL PROPOSED USES: *Constipation, Heart Disease (Prevention), High Cholesterol*

OTHER PROPOSED USES: *Cancer Prevention, Diverticulitis, Dyspepsia, High Cholesterol, Irritable Bowel Syndrome, Lupus Nephritis, Menopausal Symptoms, Skin Inflammation (Topical Use of the Herb)*

Flaxseeds are the hard, tiny seeds of *Linum usitatissimum*, the flax plant, which has been widely used for thousands of years as a source of food and clothing. There are at least three flaxseed components with potential health benefits. The first is fiber, valuable in treating **constipation**. Flaxseed also contains alpha-linolenic acid, a type of **omega-3 fatty acid** similar to the omega-3 fatty acids found in fish oil in some ways, but significantly different in others, and perhaps offering some of the same benefits. Finally, substances called *lignans* in flaxseed have **phytoestrogenic** properties, making them somewhat similar to the **isoflavones** in soy.

The oil made from flaxseed has no appreciable amounts of lignans, but it does contain alpha-linolenic acid. See the **Flaxseed Oil** and **Lignans** articles for more information on these substances.

What Is Flaxseed Used for Today?

The fiber in flaxseed binds with water, swelling to form a gel which, like other forms of fiber, helps soften the stool and move it along in the intestines. One study found that flaxseed can help with chronic constipation in irritable bowel disease. Germany's Commission E authorizes the use of flaxseed for various digestive problems, such as chronic constipation, **irritable bowel syndrome**, **diverticulitis**, and general **stomach discomfort**.

Flaxseed may be slightly helpful for improving **cholesterol profile**, according to some, but not all, studies. Purified alpha linolenic acid or lignans alone have not consistently shown benefits. It may be the generic fiber and not the other specific ingredients in flaxseed that benefit cholesterol levels.

Flaxseed, its lignans, and its oil have undergone a small amount of investigation for potential **cancer prevention** or cancer treatment possibilities.

Flaxseed has shown some promise for treating kidney disease associated with **lupus** (lupus nephritis).

Because it is believed to have soothing properties, flaxseed is sometimes used for symptomatic relief of stomach distress and applied externally for inflammation of the skin. However, research on these potential uses is essentially non-existent.

Although flaxseed is often advocated for the treatment of symptoms related to **menopause**, a sizable 12-month study failed to find it more helpful than wheat germ placebo. Besides failing to improve immediate symptoms, such as hot flashes, flaxseed did not appear to provide any protection against loss of bone density. A previous, much smaller study by the same researchers found it equally effective for menopausal symptoms as hormone replacement therapy, but due to the absence of a placebo group and the high rate of placebo response in menopausal symptoms, these results cannot be taken as indicating much.

Another study failed to find that flaxseed has any effect on **blood pressure**.

What Is the Scientific Evidence for Flaxseed?

Constipation

In a double-blind study, 55 people with chronic constipation caused by irritable bowel syndrome received either ground flaxseed or psyllium seed (a well-known treatment for constipation) daily for 3 months. Those taking flaxseed had significantly fewer problems with constipation, abdominal pain, and bloating than those taking psyllium. The flaxseed group had even further improvements in constipation and bloating while continuing their treatment in the 3 months after the double-blind part of the study ended. The researcher concluded that flaxseed relieved constipation more effectively than psyllium.

Cholesterol and Atherosclerosis

Some but not all human studies have found that flaxseed improves cholesterol profile. However, the benefits, if they do exist, are very modest. For example, in a double-blind study of about 200 post-menopausal women, use of flaxseed at a dose of 40 g daily produced measurable improvements in cholesterol profile, but the improvements were so small that the researchers considered them "clinically insignificant."

It has been claimed that flaxseed might also have a direct effect in helping to prevent **atherosclerosis**, based on its lignan ingredients, but the evidence upon which these claims are based is limited to studies in rabbits.

Cancer

Some evidence hints that flaxseed or its lignan components might have cancer-preventive properties. Observational studies and other forms of highly preliminary evidence suggest that people who eat more lignan-containing foods have a lower incidence of breast and perhaps colon cancer.

The lignans in flaxseed are phytoestrogens, plant chemicals mimicking the effects of estrogen in the body: phytoestrogens hook onto the same spots on cells where estrogen attaches. If there is little estrogen in the body, for example after menopause, lignans may act like weak estrogen. However, when natural estrogen is abundant, lignans may reduce the hormone's effects by displacing it from cells; displacing estrogen in this manner might help prevent those cancers that depend on estrogen, such as breast cancer, from starting and developing. (This is also, in part, how soy is believed to work in breast cancer prevention, although the phytoestrogens in soy are isoflavones.)

Some preliminary research indicates that these lignans may also fight cancer in other ways, perhaps by acting as **antioxidants**.

Animal studies using flaxseed and its lignans offer supporting evidence for a potential cancer-preventive or even cancer-treatment effect; several found that one or the other inhibited breast and colon cancer in animals and reduced metastases from melanoma (a type of skin cancer) in mice. Test-tube studies have found that flaxseed or one of its lignans inhibited the growth of human breast cancer cells and that the lignans enterolactone and enterodiol inhibited the growth of human colon tumor cells.

This preliminary research is promising, but much more is needed before we can draw any conclusions.

Although much of this anticancer work has focused on the lignans in flaxseed, one study also found that flaxseed oil—which contains no appreciable amounts of lignans—slowed the growth of malignant breast tumors in rats.

Therapeutic Dosages

According to the European Scientific Cooperative on Phytotherapy (ESCOP), the usual dose of flaxseed for constipation is 5 g of whole, cracked, or freshly crushed seeds soaked in water and taken with a glassful of liquid 3 times a day. Expect effects to begin 18 to 24 hours later. Because of this time delay, it's recommended that flaxseed be taken for a minimum of 2 to 3 days. Children aged 6 to 12 should be given half the adult dose, while children younger than 6 should be treated only under the guidance of a physician.

In one study, people received 6 to 24 g per day of flaxseed for 6 months for constipation caused by irritable bowel syndrome.

To soothe an upset stomach, soak 5 to 10 g of whole flaxseed in a half cup of water, strain after 20 to 30 minutes, then drink. For painful skin inflammations, the recommended dose is 30 to 50 g of crushed or powdered seed applied externally as a warm poultice or compress.

Like other sources of fiber, flaxseed should be taken with plenty of fluids or it may actually worsen constipation. Also, it's best to start with smaller doses and then increase.

Safety Issues

Flaxseed is generally believed to be safe. However, there are some potential risks to consider.

As with many substances, there have been reports of life-threatening allergic reactions to flaxseed.

Because of its potential effects on estrogen, pregnant or breast-feeding women should probably avoid flaxseed. One study found that pregnant rats who ate large amounts of flaxseed (5% or 10% of their diet) or one of its lignans gave birth to offspring with altered reproductive organs and functions—in humans, eating 25 g of flaxseed per day amounts to about 5% of the diet. Lignans were also found to be transferred to baby rats during nursing. Additionally, a study of postmenopausal women found that use of flaxseed reduced estrogen levels and increased levels of prolactin. This suggests hormonal effects that could be problematic in pregnancy.

Flaxseed may not be safe for women with a history of estrogen-sensitive cancer, such as breast or uterine cancer. A few test-tube studies suggest that certain cancer cells can be stimulated by lignans such as those present in flaxseed. Other studies found that lignans inhibit cancer cell growth. As with estrogen, lignans' positive or negative effects on cancer cells may depend on dose, type of cancer cell, and levels of hormones in the body. If you have a history of cancer, particularly breast cancer, talk with your doctor before consuming large amounts of flaxseeds.

If you have diabetes, flaxseed (like other high-fiber foods) may delay glucose absorption. This may lead to better blood sugar control but it also may increase the risk of hypoglycemic reactions. Talk with your doctor about appropriate use.

Finally, flaxseeds contain tiny amounts of cyanide-containing substances, which can be a problem among livestock eating large amounts of flax. While normal cooking and baking of whole flaxseeds or flour eliminates any detectable amounts of cyanide, it is at least theoretically possible that eating huge amounts of raw or unprocessed flaxseeds or flaxseed meal could pose a problem. However, most authorities do not think this presents much of a risk in real life.

Flaxseed Oil

SUPPLEMENT FORMS/ALTERNATE NAMES: ALA, *Alpha-linolenic Acid, Linseed Oil*

PRINCIPAL PROPOSED USES: *None*

OTHER PROPOSED USES: *Bipolar Disorder, Cancer Prevention, Heart Disease Prevention, High Blood Pressure, High Cholesterol, Pregnancy Support, Rheumatoid Arthritis*

Flaxseed oil is derived from the hard, tiny seeds of the flax plant. It has been proposed as a less smelly alternative to fish oil. Like fish oil, flaxseed oil contains omega-3 fatty acids, a type of fat your body needs as much as it needs vitamins.

However, it's important to realize that the omega-3 fatty acids in flaxseed oil aren't identical to what you get from fish oil. Flaxseed oil contains alpha-linolenic acid (ALA), while fish oil contains eicosapentaenoic acid (EPA) and docosahexaenoic acid (DHA). The effects and potential benefits may not be the same.

Whole flaxseeds contain another important group of chemicals known as *lignans*. Lignans are being stud-ied for use in preventing cancer. However, flaxseed *oil* contains no lignans.

Requirements/Sources

Flaxseed oil contains both omega-3 and omega-6 fatty acids, which are essential to health. Although the exact daily requirement of these essential fatty acids is not known, deficiencies are believed to be fairly common. Flaxseed oil may be an economical way to ensure that you get enough essential fatty acids in your diet.

The essential fatty acids in flax can be damaged by

exposure to heat, light, and oxygen (essentially, they become rancid). For this reason, you shouldn't cook with flaxseed oil. A good product should be sold in an opaque container and the manufacturing process should keep the temperature below 100 degrees Fahrenheit. Some manufacturers combine the product with vitamin E because it helps prevent rancidity.

Therapeutic Dosages

A typical dosage is 1 to 2 tablespoons of flaxseed oil daily. It can be taken in capsule form or made into salad dressing. Some people find the taste pleasant, although others would politely disagree.

For whole flaxseed, a typical dose is 1 tablespoon of the seed (not ground) with plenty of liquid 2 to 3 times daily.

Therapeutic Uses

The best use of flaxseed oil is as a general nutritional supplement to provide essential fatty acids. There is little evidence that it is effective for any specific therapeutic purpose.

Flaxseed oil has been proposed as a less smelly alternative to fish oil for the prevention of **heart disease**. Although fish oil is much better studied, there is some evidence that flaxseed oil or whole flaxseed may reduce LDL ("bad") **cholesterol**, perhaps slightly reduce

high blood pressure, and, overall, slow down **atherosclerosis**.

In addition, one study found that a diet high in ALA (from sources other than flaxseed oil) was associated with a reduced risk of heart disease. However, there were so many other factors involved that it is hard to say what caused what.

One very preliminary study hints that flaxseed oil may enhance the effects of conventional treatments for **bipolar disorder** when combined with conventional medications.

It has been suggested that flaxseed oil may have **anticancer** effects due to its ALA and lignan content. However, the supporting evidence for this belief is incomplete and somewhat contradictory (some studies actually found weak evidence of increased cancer risk with higher ALA intake). Although fish oil appears to be effective for reducing symptoms of **rheumatoid arthritis**, one study failed to find flaxseed oil helpful for this purpose. One study failed to find flaxseed oil helpful for **preventing premature birth**.

Safety Issues

Flaxseed oil appears to be a safe, nutritional supplement when used as recommended. However, due to the contradictory evidence regarding its effects on cancer (as described above), it should not be taken by people at high risk of cancer except on physician's advice.

Folate

SUPPLEMENT FORMS/ALTERNATE NAMES: *Folic Acid, Folacin*

PRINCIPAL PROPOSED USES: *Cancer Prevention, Depression, Heart Disease Prevention, Prevention of Birth Defects, Reduction of Methotrexate Side Effects*

OTHER PROPOSED USES: *Bipolar Disorder, Gout, Improving Action of Drugs in the Nitroglycerin Family, Migraine Headaches, Nutritional Support for Cigarette Smokers, Osteoarthritis, Osteoporosis, Periodontal Disease, Restless Legs Syndrome, Rheumatoid Arthritis, Seborrheic Dermatitis, Vitiligo*

Folate, a B vitamin, plays a critical role in many biological processes. It participates in the crucial biological process known as methylation and plays an important role in cell division: without sufficient

amounts of folate, cells cannot divide properly. Adequate folate intake can reduce the risk of heart disease and prevent serious birth defects, and it may lessen the risk of developing certain forms of cancer.

Requirements/Sources

Folate requirements rise with age. The official U.S. and Canadian recommendations for daily intake are as follows:

- Infants 0–6 months, 65 mcg
  7–12 months, 80 mcg
- Children 1–3 years, 150 mcg
  4–8 years, 200 mcg
- Males 9–13 years, 300 mcg
  14 years and older, 400 mcg
- Females 9–13 years, 300 mcg
  14 years and older, 400 mcg
- Pregnant women, 600 mcg
- Nursing women, 500 mcg

Until recently, folate deficiency was fairly common in the developed world, causing thousands of children to be born with preventable birth defects. However, in 1998, widespread fortification of cereal products began in the U.S. and Canada. As a result, the prevalence of folate deficiency has begun to decrease in these countries. Deficiency appears to be most common today among individuals who are African-American, Hispanic, or of Asian/Pacific Islander race/ethnicity, as well as younger people and those who are overweight.

Various drugs may impair your body's ability to absorb or utilize folate, including antacids, bile acid sequestrants (such as cholestyramine and colestipol), H_2 blockers, methotrexate, oral medications used for diabetes, various antiseizure medications (carbamazepine, phenobarbital, phenytoin, primidone, and valproate), sulfasalazine and possibly certain other NSAID-type drugs, high-dose triamterene, nitrous oxide, and the antibiotic **trimethoprim-sulfamethoxazole**. In addition, some of these drugs might put pregnant women at higher risk of giving birth to children with various kinds of birth defects; taking folate supplements may help reduce this risk. Oral contraceptives may also affect folate slightly, but there doesn't appear to be a need for supplementation.

Good sources of folate include dark green leafy vegetables, oranges, other fruits, rice, brewer's yeast, beef liver, beans, asparagus, kelp, soybeans, and soy flour.

Therapeutic Dosages

For most uses, folate should be taken at nutritional doses, about 400 mcg daily for adults. However, higher dosages—up to 10 mg daily—have been used to treat specific diseases. Before taking more than 400 mcg daily, it is important to make sure that you don't have a vitamin B_{12} deficiency (see Safety Issues below).

A particular kind of digestive enzyme taken as a supplement, pancreatin, may interfere with the absorption of folate. You can get around this by taking the two supplements at different times of day.

Therapeutic Uses

The use of folate supplements by **pregnant women** dramatically decreases the risk that their children will be born with a serious birth defect called *neural tube defect*. This congenital problem consists of problems with the brain or spinal cord.

Folate supplements may also help prevent other types of birth defects, such as defects of the heart, palate, and urinary tract; conversely, drugs that impair folate action may increase risk of birth defects. (See Requirements/Sources above for a list of the drugs involved.) An observational study suggests that folate supplements may reduce this risk in pregnant women taking such drugs.

Folate also lowers blood levels of **homocysteine**, which in turn has been hypothesized to reduce risk of heart disease and other conditions. Studies conflict on the optimum dose of folate for this purpose, but 100 to 400 mcg appears to produce significant homocysteine-lowering effects and 800 mcg daily may produce maximum effects. However, there is as yet no meaningful evidence that reducing homocysteine is beneficial, and considerable evidence that it is not.

Based on very preliminary evidence, folate has been suggested as a treatment for **depression**. One double-blind, placebo-controlled trial found that folate supplements at a dose of 500 mcg daily may help antidepressants work more effectively in women, but perhaps not in men.

Studies hint that a deficiency in folate might predispose people to develop **cancer** of the cervix, colon, lung, breast, pancreas, and mouth. Large observational studies suggest that folate supplements may help prevent colon cancer, especially when taken for many years; this may be especially true in people with **ulcerative colitis**. High-dose folate (10 mg daily) might be helpful for normalizing abnormalities in the appearance of the cervix (as seen under a microscope) in women taking oral contraceptives, but it does not appear to reverse actual **cervical dysplasia**.

Folate deficiency may also increase the risk of **Alzheimer's disease**, although this has not yet been proven.

Folate supplements may reduce drug side effects in individuals taking the drug methotrexate for certain conditions. Folate may also reduce side effects of the anti-seizure drug carbamazepine.

Folate supplements may help medications in the nitroglycerin family remain effective.

Very high dosages of folate may be helpful for **gout**, although some authorities suggest that it was actually a contaminant of folate that caused the benefit seen in some studies. Furthermore, other studies have found no benefit at all.

Based on intriguing but not yet definitive evidence, folate in various dosages has been suggested as a treatment for **bipolar disorder**, **osteoarthritis** (in combination with vitamin B_{12}), **osteoporosis**, **restless legs syndrome**, **rheumatoid arthritis**, **seborrheic dermatitis**, and **vitiligo** (splotchy loss of skin pigmentation). Other conditions for which it has been suggested include **migraine headaches** and **periodontal disease**.

Folate does *not* appear to be helpful for **enhancing mental function** in seniors.

What Is the Scientific Evidence for Folate?

Birth Defects

Very strong evidence tells us that regular use of folate by pregnant women can reduce the risk of neural tube defect by 50 to 80%. Less direct evidence suggests that folate can help prevent other kinds of birth defects, especially among women using medications that interfere with folate.

Depression

One study found that people with depression who do not respond well to antidepressants are likely to be low in folate.

A 10-week, double-blind, placebo-controlled trial of 127 individuals with severe major depression found that folate supplements at a dose of 500 mcg daily significantly improved the effectiveness of fluoxetine (Prozac) in female participants. Improvement in male participants was not significant, but blood tests taken during the study suggested that higher intake of folate might be necessary for men.

Methotrexate Side Effects

Methotrexate is used in cancer chemotherapy as well as for treating inflammatory diseases such as rheumatoid arthritis and **psoriasis**. While often highly effective, it can produce a number of severe side effects. These include liver toxicity as well as gastrointestinal distress. In addition, use of methotrexate is thought to raise levels of homocysteine, potentially increasing risk of heart disease.

Supplementation with folate may help. Methotrexate is called a *folate antagonist* because it prevents the body from converting folate to its active form. In fact, this inactivation of folate plays a role in methotrexate's therapeutic effects. This leads to an interesting Catch-22: methotrexate use can lead to folate deficiency, but taking extra folate could theoretically prevent methotrexate from working properly.

However, evidence suggests that individuals who take methotrexate for rheumatoid arthritis, juvenile rheumatoid arthritis, or psoriasis can safely use folate supplements. Not only does the methotrexate continue to work properly, but its usual side effects may decrease as well.

For example, in a 48-week, double-blind, placebo-controlled trial of 434 individuals with active rheumatoid arthritis, use of folate helped prevent liver inflammation caused by methotrexate. This effect allowed more participants to continue methotrexate therapy; the development of liver inflammation often requires people to stop using the drug. A slightly higher dose of methotrexate was needed to reach the same level of benefit as taking methotrexate alone, but researchers felt this was worth it.

In the study just described, folate supplements did not reduce the incidence of mouth sores and nausea. However, in other studies folate supplements did reduce these side effects, both in individuals receiving methotrexate for rheumatoid arthritis and in those with psoriasis.

In addition, two studies of individuals with rheumatoid arthritis found that use of folate supplements corrected the methotrexate-induced rise in homocysteine without affecting disease control.

Note: Folate supplements have been found safe only as supportive treatment in the specific conditions noted above. It is not known, for example, whether folate supplements are safe for use by individuals taking methotrexate for cancer treatment.

Safety Issues

Folate at nutritional doses is extremely safe. The only serious potential problem is that folate supplementation can mask the early symptoms of vitamin B_{12} deficiency (a special type of anemia), potentially allowing more irreversible symptoms of nerve damage to develop. For this reason, when taking more than 400 mcg daily, it is

[488]

COLLINS ALTERNATIVE HEALTH GUIDE

Fructo-Oligosaccharides

important to get your B_{12} level checked. See the article on **vitamin B_{12}** for more information.

Very high dosages of folate, greater than 5 mg (5,000 mcg) daily, can cause digestive upset. The maximum recommended dosage of folate for pregnant or nursing women is 1,000 mcg daily (800 mcg if under 19 years old).

Media reports that use of folate by pregnant women may increase their risk of breast cancer are based on a single study of highly questionable validity. At present, this is not considered a significant concern, but further research will follow.

As mentioned previously, the antiseizure drug phenytoin may interfere with folate absorption. However, folate may reduce the effectiveness of phenytoin. If you are taking phenytoin, you should consult with a physician about the proper dosage of folate for you.

Also as noted above, individuals who are taking the drug methotrexate for rheumatoid arthritis, juvenile rheumatoid arthritis, or psoriasis can safely take folate supplements at the same time. However, if you are taking methotrexate for any other purpose, do not take folate except on the advice of a physician.

Interactions You Should Know About

If you are taking:

➤ Aspirin and other anti-inflammatory medications, drugs that reduce stomach acid (such as antacids, H_2 blockers, and proton pump inhibitors), bile acid sequestrants (such as cholestyramine and colestipol), carbamazepine, estrogen-replacement therapy, nitrous oxide, oral contraceptives, oral hypoglycemic drugs, phenobarbital, primidone, sulfa antibiotics, triamterene, valproic acid, or the antibiotic trimethoprim-sulfamethoxazole: You may need to take extra folate.

➤ Phenytoin: You may need more folate. However, too much folate can interfere with this medication and cause seizures! Physician supervision is essential.

➤ Drugs in the nitroglycerin family: Folate may help them remain effective.

➤ Pancreatin (a proteolytic enzyme): It may be advisable to separate your dose of pancreatin from your dose of folate by at least 2 hours in order to avoid absorption problems.

➤ Methotrexate for rheumatoid arthritis, juvenile rheumatoid arthritis, or psoriasis: Evidence suggests that folate supplements may reduce side effects of the drug without decreasing its benefits. Nonetheless, physician supervision is highly recommended. Note: If you are taking methotrexate for other conditions, folate might decrease the drug's effectiveness.

Fructo-Oligosaccharides

ALTERNATE NAMES/RELATED TERMS: *FOS, Galacto-oligosaccharides, GOS, Inulin, Prebiotics*

PRINCIPAL PROPOSED USES: *None*

OTHER PROPOSED USES: *Diabetes (Blood Sugar Control), High Cholesterol, Irritable Bowel Syndrome, Traveler's Diarrhea*

Fructo-oligosaccharides (FOS) are starches that the human body cannot fully digest. Inulin and galacto-oligosaccharides (GOS) are similar substances also discussed in this article.

When a person consumes FOS, the undigested portions provide nourishment for bacteria in the digestive tract. "Friendly" bacteria (**probiotics**) may respond particularly well to this nourishment. Because FOS feed probiotics, they are sometimes called *prebiotics*.

Low doses of FOS are often provided, along with probiotic supplements, to aid probiotic growth. High doses of FOS (and related substances) have been advocated for a variety of health conditions. However, currently, the available scientific evidence for benefit remains more negative than positive.

Requirements/Sources

There is no daily requirement for FOS. FOS and related substances are found in asparagus, Jerusalem artichoke, leeks, onions, and soybeans, among other foods.

Therapeutic Dosages

When taken simply for promoting healthy bacteria, FOS are often taken at a dose of 4 to 6 g daily. When used for therapeutic purposes, the typical dose of FOS is 10 to 20 g daily, divided into 3 doses and taken with meals. Side effects are common at a daily intake 15 g or more (see Safety Issues below).

Therapeutic Uses

Animal studies hint that FOS, GOS, and inulin can significantly improve **cholesterol** profile; however, study outcomes in humans have been inconsistent at best.

At most, it appears that FOS might improve cholesterol profiles by 5%, an amount too small to make much of a difference in most circumstances. These relatively poor results might be due to that fact that humans cannot tolerate doses of FOS much above 15 g daily without developing gastrointestinal side effects.

FOS has also been suggested for preventing **traveler's diarrhea**. However, in a large (244-participant) double-blind study, FOS at a dose of 10 g daily again offered only minimal benefits. Probiotics themselves might be a better bet.

According to most studies, FOS at 10 to 20 g daily do not improve blood sugar control in people with type 2 **diabetes**.

FOS have been advocated as a treatment for **irritable bowel syndrome**. However, in a 12-week, double-blind, placebo-controlled study of 98 people, treatment at a dose of 20 g daily slightly worsened symptoms initially, then produced no effect.

Small double-blind studies found that FOS at a dose of 10 g daily may improve **magnesium** absorption in postmenopausal women. Whether this is beneficial remains unclear, since magnesium deficiency is not believed to be a widespread problem. FOS may also slightly increase **copper** absorption, but they do not appear to affect absorption of **calcium**, **zinc**, or **selenium**.

Safety Issues

FOS appear to be generally safe. However, they can cause bloating, flatulence, and intestinal discomfort at daily doses of 15 g or higher. People with lactose intolerance may particularly suffer from these side effects.

Gamma-Linolenic Acid

SUPPLEMENT FORMS/ALTERNATE NAMES: *GLA, Omega-6 Fatty Acids; Omega-6 Oil(s); Sources of GLA include Black Currant Seed Oil, Borage Oil, Evening Primrose Oil*

PRINCIPAL PROPOSED USES: *Diabetic Neuropathy*

OTHER PROPOSED USES:

GLA Alone: *Attention Deficit and Hyperactivity Disorder (ADHD), Cyclic Mastalgia, Kidney Stones, Premenstrual Syndrome (PMS), Raynaud's Phenomenon, Rheumatoid Arthritis, Ulcerative Colitis, Weight Loss*

In Combination with Fish Oil: *Attention Deficit and Hyperactivity Disorder (ADHD), Huntington's Disease, Osteoporosis*

PROBABLY NOT EFFECTIVE USES: *Eczema*

GLA (gamma-linolenic acid) is one of the two main types of *essential fatty acids*. These are "good" fats that are as necessary for your health as vitamins. Specifically, GLA is an omega-6 fatty acid. (For more information on the other major category of essential fatty acids, omega-3, see the article on **fish oil**.)

Gamma-Linolenic Acid

The body uses essential fatty acids to make various prostaglandins and leukotrienes. These substances influence inflammation and pain; some of them increase symptoms, while others decrease them. Taking GLA may swing the balance over to the more favorable prostaglandins and leukotrienes, making it helpful for diseases that involve inflammation.

There is some evidence that GLA may be helpful for diabetic neuropathy. It is widely used in the U.K. and other parts of Europe to treat **eczema** and **cyclic mastalgia** (a condition marked by breast pain associated with the menstrual cycle). Current evidence, however, suggests that it may not help. There are many other proposed uses of GLA based on fairly weak evidence.

Requirements/Sources

The body ordinarily makes all the GLA it needs from linoleic acid, an omega-6 essential fatty acid found in many foods. In certain circumstances, however, the body may not be able to convert linoleic acid to GLA efficiently. These include advanced age, diabetes, high alcohol intake, eczema, cyclic mastitis, viral infections, excessive saturated fat intake, elevated cholesterol levels, and deficiencies of vitamin B_6, zinc, magnesium, biotin, or calcium. In such cases, taking GLA supplements may make up for a genuine deficiency.

Very little GLA is found in the diet. Borage oil is the richest supplemental source (17 to 25% GLA), followed by black currant oil (15 to 20%) and evening primrose oil (7 to 10%). Borage and evening primrose are the most common sources used in studies.

Therapeutic Dosages

The typical dosage of GLA when it is used in hopes of alleviating cyclic mastalgia or eczema is about 200 to 400 mg daily (about 2 to 4 g of evening primrose oil or 1 to 2 g borage oil). Diabetic neuropathy is typically treated with about 400 to 600 mg daily (about 4 to 6 g of evening primrose or 2 to 3 g of borage oil), and in rheumatoid arthritis doses as high as 2,000 to 3,000 mg have been tried. (Doses this high can only be obtained from purified GLA, as one would need impractically high doses of evening primrose oil or borage oil to get enough.)

GLA should be taken with food. Full benefits (if there are any) may take more than 6 months to develop.

Therapeutic Uses

GLA has shown some promise for the treatment of **diabetic neuropathy**, a complication of diabetes. This condition consists of pain and/or numbness due to progressive nerve damage. However, supporting evidence that GLA is effective for this use is quite limited.

Perhaps the most common use of GLA has been as a treatment for eczema. It was once widely dispensed for this purpose by the British health-care system, but the balance of the evidence indicates that for eczema, GLA is just a placebo treatment.

GLA is also a popular treatment for cyclic mastalgia (breast pain that cycles with the menstrual period), but the evidence regarding its effectiveness is more negative than positive. GLA is additionally said to be useful for general **premenstrual syndrome** (PMS) symptoms, but the supporting evidence for this use is very weak.

Despite many positive anecdotes, GLA has failed to prove effective for **attention deficit and hyperactivity disorder** (ADHD). One study that used GLA plus fish oil did find weak evidence of benefits. Extremely weak evidence hints that evening primrose oil might be more effective for ADHD if combined with zinc, but this is more of an untested hypothesis than a conclusion.

GLA has been studied for numerous other conditions, such as **rheumatoid arthritis, Raynaud's phenomenon** (a condition in which the fingers and toes react to cold in an exaggerated way), **weight loss, ulcerative colitis, kidney stones, multiple sclerosis,** and increasing the effectiveness of the drug tamoxifen in the treatment of breast **cancer. Note:** Individuals undergoing treatment for cancer should not take GLA (or any other supplement) except under physician supervision.

Other studies have investigated the potential benefits of combination treatment using GLA and fish oil. Conditions studied include **osteoporosis, chronic fatigue syndrome, periodontitis** (gum disease), and Huntington's disease. In these trials, some promising (but far from definitive) results have been seen. However, this combination therapy has failed to prove effective for cyclic mastalgia.

GLA is sometimes suggested as a treatment for **tardive dyskinesia**, but two double-blind studies have failed to find it helpful for this disorder. GLA has also failed to prove effective for the itching caused by kidney dialysis.

Thus far, we've mentioned only a fraction of the conditions for which GLA has been proposed as a treatment. Others include **asthma, allergies, bursitis, endo-**

metriosis, **heart disease**, **irritable bowel syndrome**, prostate cancer, **benign prostatic hyperplasia** (BPH), and Sjogren's disease. However, none of these potential uses has as yet been scientifically evaluated to any significant extent.

What Is the Scientific Evidence for Gamma-Linolenic Acid?

Diabetic Neuropathy

Diabetic neuropathy is a gradual degeneration of nerves caused by diabetes. There is some evidence that GLA can be helpful, if you give it long enough to work. In one double-blind, placebo-controlled study, 111 people with mild diabetic neuropathy received either 480 mg daily of GLA or placebo. After 12 months, the group taking GLA was doing significantly better than the placebo group. Good results were seen in a smaller study as well. However, these promising findings lack further research validation.

There is some preliminary evidence that GLA may be more effective for diabetic neuropathy when it is combined with **lipoic acid**.

Eczema

Despite the fact that GLA (usually as evening primrose oil) is widely used in Europe to treat eczema, it appears most likely that the treatment is not truly effective. The anecdotes of cure that abound are, most likely, simply testimonials to the placebo effect (as well as a strong marketing campaign by one evening primrose oil supplier).

A 1989 review of the literature found significant benefit in the nine double-blind controlled studies performed to that date, all involving evening primrose oil. This study led to widespread sales of one evening primrose oil product. However, this review has been sharply criticized for including poorly designed studies and possibly misinterpreting study results.

Improvements in symptoms were also seen in a later double-blind study of 48 children with eczema.

However, more recent and better conducted research has failed to find any benefit. For example, a 16-week, double-blind study involving 58 children with eczema found no difference between the effects of evening primrose oil and placebo (substantial improvements were seen, but to the same extent for placebo and evening primrose oil). Lack of specific benefit was also seen with evening primrose oil or evening primrose oil plus fish oil in a 16-week, double-blind, placebo-controlled study of 102 individuals with eczema. Finally, a double-blind trial followed 39 people with hand dermatitis for 24 weeks and again found no greater benefits than those produced by placebo.

GLA from borage oil has also failed to prove effective. In a 24-week, double-blind study of 160 adults with eczema, the treatment provided no greater benefits than placebo. The same was seen in a 12-week, double-blind, placebo-controlled study of 151 adults and children with eczema.

Finally, in a double-blind, placebo-controlled study of 118 infants at high risk for developing eczema in the future, a GLA supplement made from borage oil failed to provide a significant protective effect.

Cyclic Mastalgia

Cyclic mastalgia, also known as fibrocystic breast disease, cyclic mastitis, and mastodynia, is a condition in which a woman's breasts become painful during the week or two before her menstrual period. The discomfort is accompanied by swelling, inflammation, and sometimes actual cysts that form in the breasts. It is often associated with other symptoms of premenstrual syndrome (PMS).

We do not know the cause of cyclic mastalgia, but some researchers believe that it is associated with an imbalance of fatty acids in the body. On this basis, evening primrose oil became a popular treatment for cyclic mastalgia. However, there are considerable doubts regarding whether it is actually effective.

The main supporting evidence comes from three controlled studies that appeared to find benefit. Unfortunately, all of these suffered from significant limitations in study design and reporting, and cannot be taken as reliable. A much better quality study found that evening primrose oil, by itself or with fish oil, is not more effective than placebo for cyclic breast pain. (As with eczema, placebo treatment itself was found to be quite effective.) Other studies have found evening primrose oil ineffective for established breast cysts.

Other Premenstrual Symptoms

Although several small studies suggest that GLA as evening primrose oil is helpful in reducing overall PMS symptoms, all of these studies suffer from serious flaws that make the results difficult to trust.

Rheumatoid Arthritis

According to many studies, fish oil, a source of omega-3 essential fatty acids, improves symptoms of rheumatoid arthritis. A few studies suggest that GLA may also help. One double-blind study followed 56 people with rheumatoid arthritis for 6 months. Participants received either 2.8 g daily of purified GLA or placebo. The group taking GLA experienced significantly fewer symptoms than the placebo group, and the improvements grew over time.

Other small studies have found similar results. The overall conclusion appears to be that purified GLA might offer some benefit for rheumatoid arthritis, especially when used along with standard treatment for rheumatoid arthritis, but the evidence is weak.

Raynaud's Phenomenon

High dosages of evening primrose oil may be useful for Raynaud's phenomenon, a condition in which a person's hands and feet show abnormal sensitivity to cold temperature. A small double-blind study found that GLA produced significantly better results than placebo. Similar results have been obtained with the omega-3 fatty acids found in fish oil. However, larger studies would be necessary to actually establish effectiveness.

Osteoporosis

There is some evidence that essential fatty acids may enhance the effectiveness of calcium for the treatment or prevention of osteoporosis. In one study, 65 postmenopausal women were given calcium along with either placebo or a combination of omega-6 fatty acids (from evening primrose oil) and omega-3 fatty acids (from fish oil) for a period of 18 months. At the end of the study period, the group receiving essential fatty acids had higher bone density and fewer fractures than the placebo group.

However, a 12-month, double-blind trial of 42 postmenopausal women found no benefit.

The explanation for the discrepancy may lie in the differences between the women studied. The first study involved women living in nursing homes, while the second studied healthier women living on their own. The latter group of women may have been better nourished and already received enough essential fatty acids in their diet.

Attention Deficit and Hyperactivity Disorder (ADHD)

Based on evidence that essential fatty acids are necessary for the proper development of brain function in growing children, essential fatty acids have been tried for the treatment of ADHD and related conditions. A prelimi-

nary double-blind, placebo-controlled trial found some evidence that a supplement containing fish oil and evening primrose oil might improve ADHD symptoms. However, a high rate of dropouts makes the results of this study less than reliable. A repeat study found this combination no better than placebo.

Evening primrose oil by itself was found no better than placebo in a double-blind, placebo-controlled trial. In another small, placebo-controlled, comparative trial, evening primrose oil proved less effective than standard medical treatment.

Weight Loss

A 12-week, double-blind study that enrolled 100 significantly overweight women compared the effectiveness of evening primrose oil to placebo. No difference was seen between the groups. However, there was a high dropout rate in this trial (over 25%), which somewhat decreases the meaningfulness of the results. In addition, many participants were known to have "refractory obesity," meaning that they had already failed to respond to other forms of treatment.

Another double-blind trial tested the unusual hypothesis that evening primrose might only work in individuals with a family history of obesity. A total of 47 people with a family history of obesity were enrolled in this study. The results showed that use of evening primrose oil produced a small but significant loss of weight. Interestingly, participants whose parents were both obese showed even better response.

Considering the contradictory nature of this evidence, more research is necessary to determine whether evening primrose oil is really useful for weight loss.

Safety Issues

Most of the safety information we have regarding GLA comes from experience with evening primrose oil.

Animal studies suggest that evening primrose oil is completely nontoxic and noncarcinogenic. More than 4,000 people have taken GLA or evening primrose oil in scientific studies, and no significant adverse effects have ever been noted.

Early reports suggested the possibility that GLA might worsen temporal lobe epilepsy, but there has been no later confirmation.

The maximum safe dosage of GLA for young children, pregnant or nursing women, or those with severe liver or kidney disease has not been established.

Gamma Oryzanol

PRINCIPAL PROPOSED USES: *High Cholesterol*

OTHER PROPOSED USES: *Heart Disease Prevention, Menopausal Symptoms, Sports Performance and Bodybuilding, Ulcers (Protection)*

Gamma oryzanol is a mixture of substances derived from rice bran oil, including sterols and ferulic acid. It has been approved in Japan for several conditions, including menopausal symptoms, mild anxiety, stomach upset, and high cholesterol. In the U.S., it is widely used as a sports supplement, as well as for reducing cholesterol. However, there is no more than preliminary evidence that gamma oryzanol is effective for any purpose.

Sources

There is no daily requirement for gamma oryzanol.

Rice bran oil is the principal source of gamma oryzanol, but it is also found in the bran of wheat and other grains, as well as various fruits, vegetables, and herbs. However, to get enough gamma oryzanol to reach typical therapeutic dosages, you will need to take supplements.

Therapeutic Dosages

A typical dosage of gamma oryzanol is 500 mg daily.

Therapeutic Uses

Like many other vegetable oils, rice bran oil appears to improve cholesterol profile. Preliminary evidence, including small double-blind, placebo-controlled trials, suggests that the gamma oryzanol portion of rice bran oil may contribute an additional cholesterol-lowering benefit beyond the effects of the fatty acids. Gamma oryzanol is thought to work by impairing cholesterol absorption in the digestive tract.

Additionally, gamma oryzanol has **antioxidant** properties. It has been hypothesized that antioxidants can help protect against heart disease, cancer, and other illnesses; however, it must be kept in mind that gigantic studies looking for such benefits with the antioxidants **vitamin E** and **beta-carotene** have returned negative results.

Gamma oryzanol is used by some athletes based on early reports that suggested gamma oryzanol enhances muscle growth and sports performance. According to numerous websites, gamma oryzanol produces these benefits by increasing levels of testosterone, growth hormone, and other anabolic (muscle-building) hormones. However, there is no real evidence that gamma oryzanol either affects these hormones or enhances performance, and some evidence that it does not: a double-blind, placebo-controlled study found that 9 weeks' consumption of gamma oryzanol at a dose of 500 mg daily affected neither anabolic hormone levels nor performance.

Evidence from animal studies suggests that gamma oryzanol may help prevent **ulcers**, but meaningful human trials are lacking.

Gamma oryzanol has also been advocated as a treatment for **menopausal symptoms**, but the basis of this potential use consists of evidence far too weak to be relied upon at all. In one study, gamma oryzanol injected into rats altered levels of circulation luteinizing hormone (LH). This in turn *might* conceivably help menopausal symptoms, but it is a long way from theoretical benefits in rats to proof of effectiveness in humans. One open study sometimes touted as direct evidence for benefit in menopause lacked a control group and therefore means nothing.

Safety Issues

In the late 1970s, a batch of rice bran oil was contaminated by PCBs (polychlorobiphenyls), resulting in the poisoning of more than 2,000 people. This led to studies on the safety of gamma oryzanol products. On balance, the results of these investigations suggest that gamma oryzanol, when taken at normal doses, is non-toxic and non-carcinogenic. However, the maximum safe dosages for young children, pregnant or nursing women, or those with severe liver or kidney disease have not been established.

Garlic

Allium sativum

PRINCIPAL PROPOSED USES: *Common Cold (Prevention), Heart Disease (Prevention), Insect Repellent*

OTHER PROPOSED USES: *Athlete's Foot, "Blood Thinning," Cancer Prevention, Candida, Diabetes, Hypertension, Immune Support, Middle Ear Infections (Reducing Pain), Topical Antibiotic, Vaginal Infections, Yeast Hypersensitivity*

PROBABLY NOT EFFECTIVE USES: *High Cholesterol, Oral Antibiotic, Ulcers*

The story of garlic's role in human history could fill a book, as indeed it has, many times. Its species name, *sativum*, means "cultivated," indicating that garlic does not grow in the wild. So fond have humans been of this herb that garlic can be found almost everywhere in the world, from Polynesia to Siberia.

From Roman antiquity through World War I, garlic poultices were used to prevent **wound** infections. The famous microbiologist Louis Pasteur performed some of the original work showing that garlic could kill bacteria. In 1916, the British government issued a general plea for the public to supply it with garlic in order to meet wartime needs. Garlic was called *Russian penicillin* during World War II because, after running out of antibiotics, the Russian government turned to this ancient treatment for its soldiers.

After World War II, Sandoz Pharmaceuticals manufactured a garlic compound for intestinal spasms and the Van Patten Company produced another for lowering blood pressure.

What Is Garlic Used for Today?

Garlic is widely used as an all-around treatment for preventing or slowing the progression of **atherosclerosis** (the cause of most **heart attacks** and **strokes**). However, there is actually relatively little in the way of meaningful evidence that it works for this purpose. The balance of the evidence suggests that garlic is not very effective (if at all) for treating **high cholesterol,** and there is only minimal evidence that it offers any benefits for people with **high blood pressure.** Garlic does appear to have some blood-thinning effects, but whether this translates into any medical benefit remains unclear.

Garlic has a long folkloric history as a treatment for colds and is commonly stated to strengthen the im-

mune system. However, up until 2001, there was no supporting evidence for this use. Since then, however, evidence including a well-designed double-blind study does suggest that regular use of garlic extract can help prevent **colds**.

In addition, folklore suggesting that garlic ingestion can ward off **insect bites** may have some truth to it, at least when garlic is taken regularly for several weeks.

When applied topically, garlic can kill fungi, and there is preliminary evidence suggesting that ajoene, a compound derived from garlic, might help treat **athlete's foot**. Topical garlic can also kill bacteria on contact; however, if you take garlic by mouth, it will not work like an antibiotic throughout your system. Furthermore, oral garlic has failed to prove effective for killing *Helicobacter pylori*, the stomach bacteria implicated as a major cause of **ulcers**.

Traditionally, garlic was often combined with the herb mullein in oil products designed to reduce the pain of middle ear infections (**otitis media**, not external ear infections known commonly as swimmer's ear), and two double-blind studies support this use. **Note:** While these products may reduce pain, it is very unlikely that they have any actual effect on the infection because the eardrum prevents them from reaching the site of infection.

Highly preliminary evidence suggests that regular intake of garlic as food may reduce **cancer** risk.

Based on extremely weak evidence, garlic has been proposed as a treatment for problems related to the yeast *Candida albicans*, such as **vaginal yeast infections**, oral yeast infections (thrush), and the purported condition discussed in some alternative medicine circles as **yeast hypersensitivity syndrome**. Garlic has also been proposed as a treatment for **asthma** and **diabetes**, but there is no supporting evidence for these uses.

What Is the Scientific Evidence for Garlic?

Atherosclerosis

Scant evidence hints that garlic might help prevent atherosclerosis, the most common cause of heart attacks and strokes.

Garlic preparations have been found to slow hardening of the arteries in animal studies.

In a double-blind, placebo-controlled study that followed 152 people for 4 years, standardized garlic powder at a dosage of 900 mg daily significantly slowed the development of atherosclerosis as measured by ultrasound. Unfortunately, this study suffered from some statistical problems that make its results less than fully reliable.

An observational study of 200 people measured the flexibility of the aorta, the main artery exiting the heart. Participants who took garlic showed more flexibility, indicating less atherosclerosis. However, because this was not a double-blind trial, its results prove little.

Heart Attack Prevention

In one study, 432 people who had suffered a heart attack were given either garlic oil extract or no treatment over a period of 3 years. The results showed a significant reduction of second heart attacks and about a 50% reduction in death rate among those taking garlic.

High Cholesterol

A number of studies published in the 1980s and early 1990s found evidence that garlic preparations can reduce high cholesterol. However, virtually all subsequent studies have failed to find any significant benefit. The accumulating impact of these repeated negative results indicates that garlic is not, in fact, effective for improving cholesterol profile.

Hypertension (High Blood Pressure)

Numerous studies have found weak evidence that garlic lowers blood pressure slightly, perhaps in the neighborhood of 5 to 10% more than placebo. However, all of these studies suffered from significant flaws, and most were performed on people who did not have high blood pressure. At present, it is not clear whether garlic actually has any effects on blood pressure.

One study followed 47 subjects with an average starting blood pressure of 171/101. Over a period of 12 weeks, half were treated with 600 mg of garlic powder daily, standardized to 1.3% alliin, while the other half were given placebo. The results showed a statistically significant drop of 11% in the systolic blood pressure and 13% in the diastolic pressure. In comparison, blood pressure fell in the placebo group by 5% and 4%, respectively. However, this study suffers from a significant problem: the average starting blood pressure of the placebo and the treated groups were quite different, making comparisons unreliable.

Cold Prevention

The herb garlic has a long history of use for treating or preventing colds. However, up until 2001, there was no scientific evidence that it actually works for this purpose. A U.S. study reported in that year does provide meaningful preliminary evidence that garlic might possess cold-fighting powers. In this 12-week, double-blind, placebo-controlled trial, 146 people received either placebo or a garlic extract between November and February.

The results showed that participants receiving garlic were almost two-thirds less likely to catch colds than those receiving placebo. Furthermore, participants who did catch colds recovered about one day faster in the garlic group as compared to the placebo group.

A study performed in Russia also reported benefits.

Thus, regular use of garlic might help prevent colds. However, there is no evidence as yet that if you take garlic at the onset of a cold you will recover more quickly.

Insect Repellent

A 20-week, double-blind, placebo-controlled crossover trial followed 80 Swedish soldiers and measured the number of tick bites received during the garlic and the placebo treatments. The results showed a modest but statistically significant reduction in tick bites when soldiers consumed 1,200 mg of garlic daily for 8 to 10 weeks. Unfortunately, the type of garlic used in this study was not stated.

However, another study failed to find one-time use of garlic helpful for repelling mosquitoes.

Cancer Prevention

Evidence from observational studies suggests that garlic may help prevent cancer, particularly cancer of the stomach and colon. In one of the best of these trials, the Iowa Women's Study, a group of 41,837 women were questioned as to their lifestyle habits in 1986 and then followed continuously in subsequent years. At the 4-year follow-up, questionnaires showed that women whose diets included significant quantities of garlic were approximately 30% less likely to develop colon cancer.

The interpretations of studies like this one are always a bit controversial. For example, it's possible that the women who ate a lot of garlic also made other healthful lifestyle choices. While researchers looked at this possibility very carefully and concluded that garlic was a common factor, it is not clear that they are right. What is really needed to settle the question is an intervention trial, where some people are given garlic and others are given a placebo. However, none has yet been performed that evaluated garlic for cancer prevention.

Antimicrobial

There is no question that raw garlic can kill a wide variety of microorganisms by direct contact, including fungi, bacteria, viruses, and protozoa. A double-blind study reported in 1999 found that a cream made from the garlic constituent ajoene was just as effective for fungal skin infections as the standard drug terbinafine. These findings may explain why garlic was traditionally applied directly to wounds in order to prevent infection (but keep in mind that it can burn the skin). Nevertheless, there is no real evidence that taking garlic orally can kill organisms throughout the body. Thus, it's not an antibiotic in the usual sense. It's more of an antiseptic.

Oral garlic could theoretically offer benefits against organisms in the stomach or intestines, because it can come into direct contact with them. However, there is only the scantiest evidence as yet that it works for any specific infection of this type. For example, despite test-tube evidence that garlic can kill *Helicobacter pylori* (the cause of ulcers), studies in people have not been promising.

Dosage

A typical dosage of garlic is 900 mg daily of a garlic powder extract standardized to contain 1.3% alliin, providing about 12,000 mcg of alliin daily. However, a great deal of controversy exists over the proper dosage and form of garlic. Most everyone agrees that 1 or 2 raw garlic cloves per day are adequate for most purposes, but virtual trade wars have taken place over the potency and effectiveness of various dried, aged, or deodorized garlic preparations. The problem has to do with the way garlic is naturally constructed.

A relatively odorless substance, alliin, is one of the most important compounds in garlic. When garlic is crushed or cut, an enzyme called *allinase* is brought in contact with alliin, turning it into allicin. The allicin itself then rapidly breaks down into entirely different compounds. Allicin is most responsible for garlic's strong odor. It can also blister the skin and kill bacteria, viruses, and fungi. Presumably the garlic plant uses allicin as a form of protection from pests and parasites. Allicin also may provide much of the medicinal benefits of garlic.

When you powder garlic to put it in a capsule, it acts like cutting the bulb. The chain reaction starts: alliin contacts allinase, yielding allicin, which then breaks down. Unless something is done to prevent this process, garlic powder won't have any alliin or allicin left by the time you buy it.

Some garlic producers declare that alliin and allicin have nothing to do with garlic's effectiveness and simply sell products without it. This is particularly true of aged powdered garlic and garlic oil. But others feel certain that allicin is absolutely essential. However, in order to make garlic relatively odorless, they must prevent the alliin from turning into allicin until the product is consumed. To accomplish this feat, they engage in marvelously complex manufacturing processes, each unique and proprietary. How well each of these methods work is a matter of finger-pointing controversy.

The best that can be said at this point is that in most of the clinical studies of garlic, the daily dosage supplied at least 10 mg of alliin. This is sometimes stated in terms of how much allicin will be created from that alliin. The number you should look for is 4 to 5 mg of "allicin potential."

Alliin-free aged garlic also appears to be effective when taken at a dose of 1 to 7.2 g daily.

Note: Do not confuse essential oil of garlic with garlic oils. The term "garlic oil" refers to garlic extracted by means of oil. Garlic essential oil is the pure oily component of the herb, and, like other **essential oils**, it is potentially toxic.

Safety Issues

As a commonly used food, garlic is on the FDA's GRAS (generally recognized as safe) list. Rats have been fed gigantic doses of aged garlic (2,000 mg per kilogram body weight) for 6 months without any signs of negative effects. Long-term treatment with standardized garlic powder at a dose equivalent to three times the usual dose, along with fish oil, produced no toxic effects in rats.

The only common side effect of garlic is unpleasant breath odor. Even "odorless garlic" produces an offensive smell in up to 50% of those who use it.

Other side effects occur only rarely. For example, a study that followed 1,997 people who were given a normal dose of deodorized garlic daily over a 16-week period showed a 6% incidence of nausea, a 1.3% incidence of dizziness on standing (perhaps a sign of low blood pressure), and a 1.1% incidence of allergic reactions. There were also a few reports of bloating, headaches, sweating, and dizziness.

When raw garlic is taken in excessive doses, it can cause numerous symptoms, such as stomach upset, heartburn, nausea, vomiting, diarrhea, flatulence, facial flushing, rapid pulse, and insomnia.

Topical garlic can cause skin irritation, blistering, and even third-degree burns, so be very careful about applying garlic directly to the skin.

Since garlic "thins" the blood, it is not a good idea to take high-potency garlic pills immediately prior to or after surgery or labor and delivery, because of the risk of excessive bleeding. Similarly, garlic should not be combined with blood-thinning drugs such as Coumadin (warfarin), heparin, aspirin, Plavix (clopidogrel), Ticlid

(ticlopidine), or Trental (pentoxifylline). In addition, garlic could conceivably interact with natural products with blood-thinning properties, such as ginkgo, policosanol, or high-dose vitamin E.

Garlic may also combine poorly with certain HIV medications. Two people with HIV experienced severe gastrointestinal toxicity from the HIV drug ritonavir after taking garlic supplements. Garlic might also reduce the effectiveness of some drugs used for HIV.

Garlic is presumed to be safe for pregnant women (except just before and immediately after delivery) and nursing mothers, although this has not been proven.

Interactions You Should Know About

If you are taking:

➤ **Blood-thinning drugs such as warfarin (Coumadin), heparin, aspirin, clopidogrel (Plavix), ticlopidine (Ticlid), or pentoxifylline (Trental): Do not use garlic except on medical advice.**

➤ **Ginkgo, policosanol, or high-dose vitamin E: Taking garlic at the same time might conceivably cause a risk of bleeding problems.**

➤ **Medications for HIV: Do not use garlic.**

Genistein

PRINCIPAL PROPOSED USES: *None*

OTHER PROPOSED USES:

    Prevention: *Cancer, Osteoporosis*

    Treatment: *Amyotrophic Lateral Sclerosis (ALS), High Cholesterol, Menopausal Symptoms, Osteoporosis*

G enistein, a naturally occurring chemical present in soy, has attracted scientific interest for its possible benefits in cancer and heart disease prevention. Genistein is a type of chemical called a *phytoestrogen*—an estrogen-like substance present in some plants. There are two main types of phytoestrogens: **isoflavones** and **lignans**. Soy is the most abundant source of isoflavones, with genistein the most abundant isoflavone in soy. Red clover is also a good course of genistein.

Like other phytoestrogens, genistein can work in two ways: either by increasing or decreasing the effects of estrogen. This happens because genistein binds to special sites on cells called *estrogen receptors*. Genistein stimulates these receptors, but not as strongly as real estrogen; at the same time, it blocks estrogen itself from attaching. The net result is that when there is a lot of estrogen in the body, such as before menopause, genistein may partly block its effects. Since estrogen appears to increase the risk of various forms of cancer, regular use of genistein by premenopausal women might help reduce this risk. On the other hand, if there is little human estrogen present, such as after menopause, genistein can partly make up for it. This is one rationale for using genistein to prevent osteoporosis.

Genistein might also be helpful for reducing heart disease risk.

Requirements/Sources

Genistein is found in high quantities in soy and in negligible quantities in a few other foods. Most soy foods contain about 1 to 2 mg of genistein per gram of protein.

Therapeutic Dosages

The optimum dosage of genistein is unknown. In Asia, population groups who eat soy foods daily containing 20 to 80 mg of genistein have lower rates of breast and prostate cancer than do groups in the West with less genistein in their diets. However, we don't know whether genistein (or even soy isoflavones generally) are responsible for this effect.

Therapeutic Uses

Double-blind, placebo-controlled studies have found that genistein may be helpful for preventing **heart disease** and preventing or treating **osteoporosis**. Weaker evidence suggests potential benefits in **cancer prevention, cancer treatment**, and **amyotrophic lateral sclerosis** (ALS).

Isoflavone mixtures containing genistein have undergone considerably more study than genistein alone. Mixed isoflavones have shown promise for most of the conditions just mentioned, as well as **menopausal symptoms** and **cyclic mastalgia**.

What Is the Scientific Evidence for Genistein?

Osteoporosis

Estrogen has a powerful protective effect on bone. In women, osteoporosis most often occurs after menopause when the ovaries stop producing estrogen. Animal studies as well as a double-blind, placebo-controlled trial in humans suggest that genistein can help restore bone protection.

In one 12-month study, 90 women aged 47 to 57 were given genistein, standard hormone replacement therapy (HRT), or placebo. The results showed that genistein increased bone density to approximately the same extent as HRT. No adverse effects on the uterus or breast were seen.

Interestingly, unlike estrogen, which primarily helps prevent the destruction of bone, evidence suggests that genistein may also assist in creating new bone.

However, in one animal study, while a small dose of genistein helped protect the rats' bones, a larger dose of genistein seemed to have the opposite effect—causing increasing bone destruction. Studies in humans are needed to determine whether genistein is truly effective and to find the optimum dose.

Other studies have evaluated the effects of soy products containing other constituents besides genistein.

Cancer

Genistein may help reduce risk of various forms of cancer. In one study, newborn female rats treated with genistein had less breast cancer later in life than those treated with placebo. However, other studies suggest that genistein or other isoflavones could promote breast cancer under certain conditions. (See Safety Issues below.)

In the test tube, genistein has been found to suppress the growth of a wide range of cancer cells, including forms of cancer that are not affected by estrogen. For example, genistein has been found to inhibit skin cancer when it was applied to the skin of mice or fed to rats. Furthermore, in test-tube studies, genistein has been found to enhance the effects of chemotherapy drugs.

Heart Disease

One double-blind, placebo-controlled study found that use of genistein helped relax the artery wall (the endothelium), an effect that would be expected to help prevent heart disease. In addition, test-tube studies suggest that genistein may help keep cholesterol in the blood from depositing in blood vessel walls. Finally, very early test-tube research suggests that genistein may also inhibit the formation of blood clots, which are a major cause of heart attacks.

Safety Issues

Most safety studies that have implications for genistein involved mixed isoflavones from soy or red clover.

Additionally, some evidence suggests that the genistein in particular might impair immunity. One study in mice found that injected genistein has negative effects on the thymus gland (an organ that is important for immunity) and also causes changes in the prevalence of various white blood cells consistent with impaired immunity. Although the genistein was injected rather than administered orally, the blood levels of genistein that these injections produced were not excessively high; they were comparable to (or even lower than) what occurs in children fed soy milk formula. In addition, there are several reports of impaired immune responses in infants fed soy formula. While it is too early to conclude that genistein impairs immunity, these findings are a potential cause for concern.

Gentian

Gentiana lutea

PRINCIPAL PROPOSED USES: *Poor Appetite, Poor Digestion*

For reasons that aren't entirely clear, bitter plants have the capacity to stimulate appetite, and gentian ranks high on the scale of bitterness. Two of its constituents, gentiopicrin and amarogentin, taste bitter even when diluted by a factor of 50,000!

In traditional European herbology, gentian and other bitter herbs are believed to strengthen the digestive system when taken over a period of time. However, in Chinese medicine, gentian is regarded as a rather intense herb that should seldom be taken over the long term. We are not sure which view is right, although we tend to lean toward the Chinese viewpoint and recommend gentian only for short-term use.

What Is Gentian Used for Today?

Gentian extracts are widely sold in liquor stores under the name "bitters," for the purpose of increasing appetite. Tinctures are also sold medicinally for the same purpose.

Dosage

A typical dosage of gentian is 20 drops of tincture 15 minutes before meals. To make the intensely bitter taste more tolerable, you can mix the tincture in juice or water.

Safety Issues

Gentian is somewhat mutagenic, meaning that it can cause changes in the DNA of bacteria. For this reason, gentian should not be taken during pregnancy. Safety in young children, nursing women, or those with severe liver or kidney disease is also not established.

In the short term, gentian rarely causes any side effects, except for occasional worsening of ulcer pain and heartburn. (For some people, it relieves stomach problems.)

Germander

Teucrium chamaedrys

PRINCIPAL PROPOSED USES: *This toxic herb should not be used for treatment of any condition.*

The herb germander is a dramatic counterexample to the widely held belief that if a treatment has been used for thousands of years, it must be safe. Germander grows wild in the Mediterranean region, especially in Greece and Syria. It has a long tradition of use for **gout**, as well as febrile illnesses, **asthma**, coughs, **depression**, and **congestive heart failure**. It was also said to improve digestion and increase appetite. What traditional herbalists appear to have missed is that germander is toxic to the liver.

In the 1980s, germander became a popular treatment for weight control in France. A small epidemic of hepatitis was the result. Subsequent research demonstrated conclusively that the herb is toxic to the liver, but has not precisely identified the constituents at fault. Problems have also occurred when products labelled as containing **American skullcap** have turned out to contain germander instead.

Germander was subsequently banned in France and many other countries. Unfortunately, numerous websites continue to promote the use of this herb. We recommend avoiding germander entirely.

Ginger

Zingiber officinale

PRINCIPAL PROPOSED USES: *Motion Sickness, Morning Sickness in Pregnancy, Post-surgical Nausea*
OTHER PROPOSED USES: *Atherosclerosis, Migraine Headaches, Osteoarthritis, Rheumatoid Arthritis*

Native to southern Asia, ginger is a 2- to 4-foot-long perennial that produces grass-like leaves up to a foot long and almost an inch wide. Although it's called *ginger root* in the grocery store, the part of the herb used is actually the rhizome, the underground stem of the plant, with its bark-like outer covering scraped off.

Ginger has been used as food and medicine for millennia. Arabian traders carried ginger root from China and India to be used as a food spice in ancient Greece and Rome, and tax records from the second century A.D. show that ginger was a delightful source of revenue to the Roman treasury.

Chinese medical texts from the fourth century B.C. suggest that ginger is effective in treating nausea, diarrhea, stomachaches, cholera, toothaches, bleeding, and rheumatism. Ginger was later used by Chinese herbalists to treat a variety of respiratory conditions, including coughs and the early stages of colds.

Ginger's modern use dates back to the early 1980s, when a scientist named D. Mowrey noticed that ginger-filled capsules reduced his nausea during an episode of flu. Inspired by this, he performed the first double-blind study of ginger. Germany's Commission E subsequently approved ginger as a treatment for indigestion and motion sickness.

One of the most prevalent ingredients in fresh ginger is the pungent substance gingerol. However, when ginger is dried and stored, its gingerol rapidly converts to the substances shogaol and zingerone. Which, if any, of these substances, has medicinal effects remains unknown.

What Is Ginger Used for Today?

Some evidence suggests that ginger may be at least slightly helpful for the prevention and treatment of various forms of nausea, including motion sickness, the **nausea and vomiting of pregnancy** (morning sickness), and **post-surgical nausea**.

Note: If you are pregnant or undergoing surgery, do not self-treat with ginger except under physician supervision.

Scant preliminary evidence suggests that ginger might be helpful for **osteoarthritis**.

Ginger has been suggested as a treatment for numerous other conditions, including **atherosclerosis, migraine headaches, rheumatoid arthritis, high cholesterol, ulcers, depression,** and **impotence**. However, there is negligible evidence for these uses.

In traditional Chinese medicine, hot ginger tea taken at the first sign of a **cold** is believed to offer the possibility of averting the infection. However, once more there is no scientific evidence for this use.

What Is the Scientific Evidence for Ginger?

Nausea

The evidence for ginger's effectiveness in various forms of nausea remains mixed. It has been suggested that, in some negative studies, poor-quality ginger powder might have been used.

In general, while most antinausea drugs influence the brain and the inner ear, ginger appears to act directly on the stomach.

⮞ *Motion Sickness*

Ginger has shown inconsistent promise for treatment of motion sickness. A double-blind, placebo-controlled study of 79 Swedish naval cadets at sea found that 1 g of ginger could decrease vomiting and cold sweating but without significantly decreasing nausea and vertigo. Benefits were also seen in a double-blind study of 36 individuals given ginger, dimenhydrinate, or placebo.

However, a 1984 study funded by NASA using intentionally stimulated motion sickness found that ginger was not any more effective than placebo. Two other small studies have also failed to find any benefit. The reason for the discrepancy may lie in the type of ginger used or the severity of the stimulant used to bring on motion sickness.

⮞ *Nausea and Vomiting of Pregnancy*

Four double-blind, placebo-controlled studies enrolling a total of 246 women found ginger more effective than placebo for treatment of morning sickness. For example, a double-blind, placebo-controlled trial of 70 pregnant women evaluated the effectiveness of ginger for morning sickness. Participants received either placebo or 250 mg of powdered ginger 3 times daily for a period of 4 days. The results showed that ginger significantly reduced nausea and vomiting. No significant side effects occurred. Other studies have compared ginger to **vitamin B$_6$** and found equal benefits, but since vitamin B$_6$ itself is not a solidly established treatment for morning sickness—the evidence for its effectiveness rests largely on one study—this finding doesn't say much.

Note: Despite its use in these studies, ginger has not been proven safe for pregnant women.

⮞ *Post-surgical Nausea*

Although there have been some positive studies, on balance, the evidence regarding ginger for reducing nausea and vomiting following surgery is discouraging.

A double-blind British study compared the effects of ginger, placebo, and metoclopramide (Reglan) in the treatment of nausea following gynecological surgery. The results in 60 women indicated that both treatments produced similar benefits as compared to placebo.

A similar British study followed 120 women receiving elective laparoscopic gynecological surgery. Whereas nausea and vomiting developed in 41% of the participants given placebo, in the groups treated with ginger or metoclopramide these symptoms developed in only 21% and 27%, respectively. Benefits were also seen in a double-blind study of 80 people.

However, a double-blind study of 108 people undergoing similar surgery found no benefit with ginger as compared to placebo. Negative results were also seen in another recent study of 120 women and another of 180 women.

The Bottom Line: If ginger is effective for post-surgical nausea at all, the effect must be very slight.

⮞ *Other Forms of Nausea*

One study failed to find ginger helpful for reducing nausea caused by the **cancer chemotherapy** drug **cisplatin**.

Osteoarthritis

A large double-blind study (more than 250 participants) found that a combination of ginger and another Asian spice called *galanga* (*Alpinia galanga*) can significantly improve arthritis symptoms. This study was widely publicized as proving that ginger is effective for osteoarthritis. However, the study design makes it impossible to draw any conclusions on the effectiveness of the ginger component of the mixture. Ginger alone has only been

Ginkgo

tested in two very small double-blind studies, and they had contradictory results.

Dosage

For most purposes, the standard dosage of powdered ginger is 1 to 4 g daily, divided into 2 to 4 doses per day.

To prevent motion sickness, it may be best to begin treatment 1 or 2 days before a trip and continue it throughout the period of travel.

Safety Issues

Ginger is on the FDA's GRAS (generally recognized as safe) list as a food, and the treatment dosages of ginger are comparable to dietary usages. No significant side effects have been observed.

Like onions and **garlic**, extracts of ginger inhibit blood coagulation in test-tube experiments. European studies with actual oral ginger taken alone in normal quantities have not found any significant effect on blood coagulation, but it is still theoretically possible that a very weak anticoagulant could amplify the effects of drugs that have a similar effect, such as Coumadin (warfarin), heparin, Plavix (clopidogrel), Ticlid (ticlopidine), Trental (pentoxifylline), and aspirin. One fairly solid case report appears to substantiate these theoretical concerns: use of a ginger product markedly (and dangerously) increased the effect of an anticoagulant drug closely related to Coumadin. However, a double-blind study failed to find any interaction between ginger and Coumadin, leaving the truth regarding this potential risk unclear.

The maximum safe doses of ginger for pregnant or nursing women, young children, or individuals with severe liver or kidney disease have not been established.

Interactions You Should Know About

If you are taking strong blood-thinning drugs such as **warfarin** (Coumadin), **heparin**, **clopidogrel** (Plavix), **ticlopidine** (Ticlid), **pentoxifylline** (Trental), or even **aspirin**: Ginger might possibly increase the risk of bleeding problems.

Ginkgo
Ginkgo biloba

PRINCIPAL PROPOSED USES: *Alzheimer's Disease, Enhancing Memory and Mental Function in Healthy People, Intermittent Claudication, Non-Alzheimer's Dementia*

OTHER PROPOSED USES: *Antipsychotic Medications (Increasing Efficacy and Reducing Side Effects of Phenothiazines and Atypical Antipsychotics), Complications of Diabetes, Depression, Glaucoma, Macular Degeneration, Multiple Sclerosis, Premenstrual System (PMS), Raynaud's Phenomenon, Vertigo, Vitiligo*

PROBABLY NOT EFFECTIVE USES: *Altitude Sickness, Sexual Dysfunction in Women or Men Caused by Antidepressant Drugs, Tinnitus*

Traceable back 300 million years, the ginkgo is the oldest surviving species of tree. Although it died out in Europe during the Ice Age, ginkgo survived in China, Japan, and other parts of East Asia. It has been cultivated extensively for both ceremonial and medical purposes, and some particularly revered trees have been lovingly tended for more than 1,000 years.

In traditional Chinese herbology, tea made from ginkgo seeds has been used for numerous problems, most particularly asthma and other respiratory illnesses. The leaf was not used. But in the 1950s, German researchers started to investigate the medical possibilities of ginkgo leaf extracts rather than remedies using the seeds. Thus, modern ginkgo preparations are not the same as the traditional Chinese herb, and the comparisons often drawn are incorrect.

What Is Ginkgo Used for Today?

Presently, ginkgo is the most widely prescribed herb in Germany, reaching a total prescription count of more than 6 million in 1995. German physicians consider it to be as effective as any drug treatment for **Alzheimer's disease** and other severe forms of memory and mental function decline.

Inconsistent evidence hints that ginkgo might also be helpful for **enhancing memory** and mental function in seniors without severe memory loss. Weak evidence hints that ginkgo (alone or in combination with **ginseng** or **vinpocetine**) may be helpful for enhancing memory or alertness in younger people.

In addition, ginkgo appears to be effective for the treatment of restricted circulation in the legs due to hardening of the arteries known as **intermittent claudication**.

Weak evidence from preliminary double-blind trials hints that ginkgo may also be helpful for **glaucoma**, **macular degeneration**, **multiple sclerosis**, **premenstrual system** (PMS), **Raynaud's phenomenon**, **sudden hearing loss**, **vertigo**, and **vitiligo**.

Although study results conflict, on balance the evidence suggests that ginkgo is *not* helpful for **tinnitus** (ringing in the ear).

Two small, preliminary double-blind trials found that ginkgo biloba can help prevent **altitude sickness**. Based on these encouraging results, researchers conducted a large-scale, double-blind study enrolling *ten times* more people than the total number enrolled in the other two trials combined. Unfortunately, in this definitive trial, gingko failed to prove more effective than placebo. (The drug acetazolamide, however, did produce significant benefits.)

Numerous case reports and uncontrolled studies raised hopes that ginkgo might be an effective treatment for **impotence** or **difficulty achieving orgasm in women** that can be caused by certain antidepressant drugs. However, as always, double-blind, placebo-controlled studies are necessary to truly establish efficacy (see **Why Does This Book Rely on Double-blind Studies?**). When these studies were finally performed, the results indicated that ginkgo does not actually provide this benefit.

One small study failed to find ginkgo helpful for the treatment of **cocaine dependence**.

Chinese research suggests that ginkgo might enhance the effects of drugs used for **schizophrenia** (both phenothiazines as well as atypical antipsychotic drugs).

An open study evaluated combination therapy with ginkgo extract and the chemotherapy drug 5FU for the treatment of pancreatic cancer, on the theory that ginkgo might enhance blood flow to the tumor and thereby help 5FU penetrate better. The results were promising, but much better research must be performed before ginkgo can be recommended for this use.

Ginkgo has also been proposed as a treatment for **depression** and **diabetic retinopathy**, but there is little evidence that it is effective for these conditions. **Note:** There are some theoretical safety concerns regarding ginkgo and **diabetes**. See Safety Issues below for more information.

What Is the Scientific Evidence for Ginkgo?

Alzheimer's Disease and Non-Alzheimer's Dementia

In the past, European physicians believed that the cause of mental deterioration with age (senile dementia) was reduced circulation in the brain due to atherosclerosis. Since ginkgo is thought to improve circulation, they assumed that ginkgo was simply getting more blood to brain cells and thereby making them work better.

However, the contemporary understanding of age-related memory loss and mental impairment no longer considers chronically restricted circulation the primary issue. Ginkgo (and other drugs used for dementia) may instead function by directly stimulating nerve-cell activity and protecting nerve cells from further injury, although improvement in circulatory capacity may also play a role.

According to a 1992 article published in *Lancet*, more than 40 double-blind, controlled trials had at that time evaluated the benefits of ginkgo in treating various forms of dementia. Of these, eight were rated of good quality, involving a total of about 1,000 people and producing positive results in all but one study. The authors of the *Lancet* article felt that the evidence was strong enough to conclude that ginkgo extract is an effective treatment for this condition.

Most studies reported since 1992 have supported this conclusion, including a large U.S. study published in the *Journal of the American Medical Association*. The U.S. trial enrolled more than 300 people with Alzheimer's disease or non-Alzheimer's dementia. Participants

Ginkgo

were given either 40 mg of *Ginkgo biloba* extract or placebo 3 times daily. The results showed significant (but not dramatic) improvements in the treated group.

One fairly large study of ginkgo extract found no benefit. This 24-week, double-blind, placebo-controlled study of 214 people with either mild to moderate dementia or ordinary age-associated memory loss found no effect with ginkgo extract at a dose of 240 or 160 mg daily. However, this study has been sharply criticized for a number of serious flaws in its design.

Enhancing Mental Function in Healthy People

Ginkgo has shown less consistent promise for enhancing mental function in people who experience the relatively slight decline in cognitive function that typically accompanies increased age.

For example, in a double-blind, placebo-controlled trial, 241 seniors complaining of mildly impaired memory were given either placebo or ginkgo for 24 weeks. The results showed that ginkgo produced modest improvements in certain types of memory.

Another double-blind, placebo-controlled trial examined the effects of ginkgo extract in 40 men and women (ages 55 to 86) who did not suffer from any mental impairment. Over a 6-week period, the results showed improvements in measurements of mental function.

Possible benefits were seen in six other trials as well, involving a total of about 250 people.

Set against these positive findings is the 24-week study mentioned above, which found no benefit in ordinary age-related memory loss. The reason for this negative outcome may be flaws in this trial's design, as noted above. However, three other studies enrolling a total of about 400 seniors also failed to find significant benefit with daily use of ginkgo. Another double-blind, placebo-controlled study used a one-time dose of ginkgo and again found no benefits.

Several other studies enrolling a total of about 250 people have examined the effects of ginkgo on memory and mental function in younger people, but the largest of these failed to find benefit. According to one study, benefits may be present early on and then decline after several weeks.

Besides ginkgo alone, several double-blind, placebo-controlled studies evaluated combined treatment with ginseng and ginkgo or vinpocetine and ginkgo for enhancing mental function in young people, and most found some evidence of benefit. In two studies, ginkgo

combined with the **Ayurvedic** herb brahmi failed to improve mental function.

The bottom line: It's not clear whether ginkgo actually enhances memory and mental function in healthy people. Benefits, if they do exist, are probably slight.

Intermittent Claudication

In intermittent claudication, impaired circulation can cause a severe, cramp-like pain in one's legs after walking only a short distance. According to nine double-blind, placebo-controlled trials, ginkgo can significantly increase pain-free walking distance.

One double-blind study enrolled 111 people for 24 weeks. Subjects were measured for pain-free walking distance by walking up a 12% slope on a treadmill at 3 kilometers per hour (about 2 miles per hour). At the beginning of treatment, both the placebo and ginkgo (120 mg daily) groups were able to walk about 350 feet without pain. By the end of the trial, both groups had improved (the power of placebo is amazing!), although the ginkgo group improved significantly more: participants taking ginkgo showed about a 40% increase in pain-free walking distance as compared to only a 20% improvement in the placebo group.

Similar improvements were also seen in a double-blind, placebo-controlled trial of 60 people who had achieved maximum benefit from physical therapy.

A 24-week, double-blind, placebo-controlled study of 74 people with intermittent claudication found that ginkgo at a dose of 240 mg per day was more effective than at 120 mg per day.

Premenstrual Symptoms

One double-blind, placebo-controlled study evaluated the benefits of ginkgo extract for women with PMS symptoms. This trial enrolled 143 women, 18 to 45 years of age, and followed them for two menstrual cycles. Each woman received either the ginkgo extract (80 mg twice daily) or placebo on day 16 of the first cycle. Treatment was continued until day 5 of the next cycle and resumed again on day 16 of that cycle.

As compared to placebo, ginkgo significantly relieved major symptoms of PMS, especially breast pain and emotional disturbance.

Macular Degeneration

Macular degeneration, one of the most common causes of vision loss in seniors, may respond to ginkgo.

In a 6-month, double-blind, placebo-controlled study

of 20 people with macular degeneration, use of ginkgo at a dose of 160 mg daily resulted in improved visual acuity.

A 24-week, double-blind study of 99 people with macular degeneration compared ginkgo extract at a dose of 240 mg per day with ginkgo at a dose of 60 mg daily. The results showed that vision improved in both groups, but to a greater extent with the higher dose.

Vertigo

A 3-month, double-blind trial of 70 people with a variety of vertiginous syndromes found that ginkgo extract given at a dose of 160 mg twice daily produced results superior to placebo. By the end of the trial, 47% of the people given ginkgo had significantly recovered versus only 18% in the placebo group.

Glaucoma

A small, double-blind, placebo-controlled trial found that use of ginkgo extract at a dose of 120 mg daily for 8 weeks significantly improved the visual field in people with glaucoma.

Tinnitus

Studies of *Ginkgo biloba* extract for treating tinnitus have yielded conflicting results. While some small studies found benefit, the largest and best-designed of these trials failed to find ginkgo effective. In a 12-week, double-blind trial, 1,121 people with tinnitus were given either placebo or standardized ginkgo at a dose of 50 mg 3 times daily. The results showed no difference between the treated and the placebo groups.

Dosage

The standard dosage of ginkgo is 40 to 80 mg 3 times daily of a 50:1 extract standardized to contain 24% ginkgo-flavone glycosides. Levels of toxic ginkgolic acid and related alkylphenol constituents should be kept under 5 parts per million.

In an analysis performed in 2006 by the respected testing organization ConsumerLab.com, some tested ginkgo products were found to be contaminated with lead.

Safety Issues

Ginkgo appears to be relatively safe. Extremely high doses have been given to animals for long periods of time without serious consequences, and results from human trials are also generally reassuring. Safety in young children, pregnant or nursing women, or those with severe liver or kidney disease, however, has not been established.

In all the clinical trials of ginkgo up through 1991 combined, involving a total of almost 10,000 participants, the incidence of side effects produced by ginkgo extract was extremely small. There were 21 cases of gastrointestinal discomfort and even fewer cases of headaches, dizziness, and allergic skin reactions.

However, there are a few potential problems. Perhaps the most serious have been the numerous case reports of internal bleeding associated with use of ginkgo (spontaneous as well as following surgery). Based on these reports, as well as previous evidence that ginkgo inhibits platelet function, studies have been performed to determine whether ginkgo significantly affects bleeding time or other measures of blood coagulation, with somewhat inconsistent results. Prudence suggests that ginkgo should not be used by anyone during the periods before or after surgery or labor and delivery, or by those with bleeding problems such as hemophilia.

It also seems reasonable to hypothesize that ginkgo might also interact with blood-thinning drugs, amplifying their effects on coagulation. However, two studies found no interaction between ginkgo and warfarin (Coumadin). While these findings are reassuring, prudence indicates physician supervision before combining ginkgo with blood-thinning drugs.

One study found that when high concentrations of ginkgo were placed in a test tube with hamster sperm and ova, the sperm were less able to penetrate the ova. However, since we have no idea whether this much ginkgo can actually come into contact with sperm and ova when they are in the body rather than a test tube, these results may not be meaningful in real life.

The ginkgo extracts approved for use in Germany are processed to remove alkylphenols, including ginkgolic acids, which have been found to be toxic. The same ginkgo extracts are available in the United States. However, other ginkgo extracts and whole ginkgo leaf might contain appreciable levels of these dangerous constituents.

Seizures have also been reported with the use of ginkgo leaf extract in people with previously well-controlled epilepsy; in one case, the seizures were fatal. It has been suggested that ginkgo might interfere with the effectiveness of some anti-seizure medications, specifically **phenytoin** and **valproic acid**. Another possible explanation is contamination of ginkgo leaf products with ginkgo seeds, the seeds of the ginkgo plant contain a neurotoxic substance called *4-methoxypyridoxine* (MPN). Finally, the drug tacrine (also used to improve memory) has been associated with seizures, and ginkgo may affect the brain in ways similar to tacrine. Regardless of the explanation, prudence suggests that people with **epilepsy** should avoid ginkgo.

According to a study in rats, ginkgo extract may cause the body to metabolize the drug nicardipine (a calcium channel blocker) more rapidly, thereby decreasing its effects. In addition, this finding also suggests potential interactions with numerous other drugs, although more research is needed to know for sure which ones might be affected.

Antibiotics in the aminoglycoside family can cause hearing loss by damaging the nerve carrying hearing sensation from the ear. One animal study evaluated the potential benefits of ginkgo for preventing hearing loss and found instead that the herb increased damage to the nerve. Based on this finding, individuals using aminoglycosides should avoid ginkgo.

It has been suggested that ginkgo might cause problems for people with type 2 diabetes, both by altering blood levels of medications as well as by directly affecting the blood sugar regulating system of the body. However, the most recent and best-designed studies have failed to find any such actions. Nonetheless, until this situation is clarified, people with diabetes should use ginkgo only under physician supervision.

Interactions You Should Know About

If you are taking:

➤ **Blood-thinning drugs such as warfarin (Coumadin), heparin, aspirin, clopidogrel (Plavix), ticlopidine (Ticlid), or pentoxifylline (Trental): Simultaneous use of ginkgo could theoretically cause bleeding problems and should not be undertaken without physician supervision.**

➤ **Calcium channel blockers: Ginkgo might reduce their effectiveness.**

➤ **Antipsychotic medications in the phenothiazine family, as well as atypical antipsychotic drugs (such as clozapine and olanzapene): Ginkgo might help them work better, with fewer side effects.**

➤ **Aminoglycoside antibiotics: Use of ginkgo might increase risk of hearing loss.**

➤ **Medications to prevent seizures: Ginkgo might interfere with their effectiveness.**

Ginseng

Panax ginseng, Panax quinquefolius

PRINCIPAL PROPOSED USES: *Colds and Flus, Diabetes, Enhancing Mental Function, Immune Support, Improving General Well-being, Stress*

OTHER PROPOSED USES: *Cancer Prevention, Male Sexual Function, Sports Performance*

PROBABLY INEFFECTIVE USES: *Menopause*

There are three different herbs commonly called *ginseng*: Asian or Korean ginseng (*Panax ginseng*), American ginseng (*Panax quinquefolius*), and Siberian "ginseng" (**Eleutherococcus senticosus**). The latter herb is actually not ginseng at all and is discussed in a separate article.

Asian ginseng is a perennial herb with a taproot resembling the shape of the human body. It grows in northern China, Korea, and Russia; its close relative, *Panax quinquefolius*, is cultivated in the United States. Because ginseng must be grown for 5 years before it is harvested, it commands a high price, with top-quality roots easily selling for more than $10,000. Dried, unprocessed ginseng root is called *white ginseng* and steamed, heat-dried root is *red ginseng*. Chinese herbalists believe that each form has its own particular benefits.

Ginseng is widely regarded by the public as a stimulant, but according to everyone who uses it seriously, that isn't the right description. In traditional Chinese herbology, *Panax ginseng* was used to strengthen the digestion and the lungs, calm the spirit, and increase overall energy. When the Russian scientist Israel I. Brekhman became interested in the herb prior to World War II, he came up with a new idea about ginseng: he decided that it was an **adaptogen**.

The term adaptogen refers to a hypothetical treatment described as follows: an adaptogen should help the body adapt to stresses of various kinds, whether heat, cold, exertion, trauma, sleep deprivation, toxic exposure, radiation, infection, or psychological stress. Furthermore, an adaptogen should cause no side effects, be effective in treating a wide variety of illnesses, and help return an organism toward balance no matter what may have gone wrong.

Perhaps the only indisputable example of an adaptogen is a healthful lifestyle. By eating right, exercising regularly, and generally living a life of balance and moderation, you will increase your physical fitness and ability to resist illnesses of all types. Whether there are any substances that can do as much remains unclear. However, Brekhman felt certain that ginseng produced similarly universal benefits.

Interestingly, traditional Chinese medicine (where ginseng comes from) does not entirely agree. There is no one-size-fits-all in Chinese medical theory. Like any other herb, ginseng is said to be helpful for those people who need its particular effects, and neutral or harmful for others. But in Europe, Brekhman's concept has taken hold and ginseng is widely believed to be a universal adaptogen.

What Is Ginseng Used for Today?

If Brekhman is right, ginseng should be the right treatment for most of us. Modern life is tremendously stressful, and if an herb could help us withstand it, it would be a useful herb indeed. Ginseng is widely used for this purpose in Russia and Eastern Europe. However, the scientific basis for this use is largely limited to animal studies and human trials of unacceptably low quality.

There have been a few better-quality studies of vari-

ous forms of ginseng for certain more specific purposes—strengthening immunity against **colds and flus** and other infections (including **herpes**), helping to control **diabetes**, **stimulating the mind**, **increasing a general sense of well-being**, and **improving physical performance capacity**—and some of these have found positive results. (See **What Is the Scientific Evidence for Ginseng?** below.)

The active ingredients in ginseng are believed to be substances known as ginsenosides. Ginseng low in ginsenosides may not be effective. However, different ginsenosides appear to have differing actions, and the exact mixture of the ginsenosides in a given ginseng product may play a large role in its efficacy.

Two preliminary studies suggest that Korean red ginseng may have some benefits for **impotence** (erectile dysfunction).

A poorly designed study using an untreated control group found indications that *Panax ginseng* might improve sperm count and motility, thereby enhancing **male fertility**.

Highly preliminary evidence suggests that *Panax quinquefolius* might help breast cancer **chemotherapy** drugs work better. *Panax ginseng* is also said to help prevent **cancer** and fight chemical dependency, but the scientific evidence for these uses is minimal at best.

One study failed to find *Panax ginseng* helpful for **menopausal symptoms**.

What Is the Scientific Evidence for Ginseng?

Adaptogenic Effects

Numerous studies have evaluated the effects of oral *Panax ginseng* on animals under conditions of extreme **stress**. The results suggest that ginseng increases physical endurance and causes physiological changes that may help the body adapt to adverse conditions. In addition, studies in mice found that consuming *Panax ginseng* before exposure to a virus significantly increased the survival rate and the number of antibodies produced. However, most of these studies fall far beneath modern scientific standards.

Cold and Flus

A double-blind, placebo-controlled study of 323 people found meaningful evidence that an extract of American ginseng taken at 400 mg daily may help prevent the common cold. Participants who used the extract over 4 months experienced a reduced number of colds as compared to those taking the placebo. Comparative benefits were also seen regarding the percentage of participants who developed two or more colds, and the severity and duration of cold symptoms that did develop. Similar benefits were also seen in a study of 43 people.

In addition, two double-blind, placebo-controlled studies indicate that *Panax quinquefolius* may be able to prevent flu-like illness in seniors.

A double-blind, placebo-controlled study suggests that *Panax ginseng* can also help prevent flu-like illnesses. This trial enrolled 227 participants at three medical offices in Milan, Italy. Half were given ginseng at a dosage of 100 mg daily, the other half placebo. Four weeks into the study, all participants received influenza vaccine. The results showed a significant decline in the frequency of colds and flus in the treated group compared to the placebo group (15 versus 42 cases). Also, antibody measurements in response to the vaccination rose higher in the treated group than in the placebo group.

On a much more theoretical level, two other studies found evidence that *Panax ginseng* increases the number of immune cells in the blood, while a third study did not find this effect. (In any case, measuring changes in the number of immune cells is not a reliable method of demonstrating immune-enhancement.)

A nonblinded pilot study provides weak evidence that *Panax ginseng* might be helpful in **chronic bronchitis**.

Diabetes

In preliminary double-blind studies performed by a single research group, use of American ginseng (*Panax quinquefolius*) appeared to improve blood sugar control.

The same researchers reported potential benefit with Korean red ginseng as well.

A different research group tested ordinary *Panax ginseng* and claimed to find it effective. However, this study was somewhat substandard in both its design and reporting. In other studies (conducted by the research group mentioned in the previous paragraph), ordinary *Panax ginseng* seemed to *worsen* blood sugar control rather than improve it. It appears possible that certain ginsenosides (found in high concentrations in some American ginseng products) may lower blood sugar while others (found in high concentration in some *Panax ginseng* products) may raise it. It has been suggested that since the actions of these various constituents are not well defined at this

time, ginseng should *not* be used to treat diabetes until more is known.

Mental Function

Several studies have found indications that *Panax ginseng* might enhance mental function. However, the specific benefits seen have varied considerably from trial to trial, tending to make the actual cognitive effects of ginseng (if there are any) difficult to discern. A double-blind, placebo-controlled study found that *Panax ginseng* can improve some aspects of mental function. Over a period of 2 months, 112 healthy, middle-aged adults were given either ginseng or placebo. The results showed that ginseng improved abstract thinking ability. However, there was no significant change in reaction time, memory, concentration, or overall subjective experience between the two groups.

Another double-blind, placebo-controlled study of 50 men found that 8-week treatment with a *Panax ginseng* extract improved ability in completion of a detail-oriented editing task. Also, a double-blind trial of 16 healthy males found favorable changes in ability to perform mental arithmetic in those given *Panax ginseng* for 12 weeks.

A double-blind, placebo-controlled trial of 60 elderly people found that 50 or 100 days of treatment with *Panax ginseng* produced improvements in numerous measures of mental function, including memory, attention, concentration, and ability to cope. Benefits were still evident at the 50-day follow-up. However, virtually no improvement was seen in the placebo group, a result that is highly unusual and raises doubts about the accuracy of the study.

In addition, three double-blind, placebo-controlled studies evaluated combined treatment with *Panax ginseng* and ginkgo and found some evidence of improved mental function.

Sports Performance

The evidence for *Panax ginseng* as a sports supplement is mixed at best. An 8-week, double-blind, placebo-controlled trial evaluated the effects of *Panax ginseng* with and without exercise in 41 individuals. The participants were given either ginseng or placebo and then underwent exercise training or remained untrained throughout the study. The results showed that ginseng improved aerobic capacity in individuals who did not exercise, but offered no benefit in those who did exercise. In a 9-week, double-blind, placebo-controlled trial of 30 highly trained athletes, treatment with *Panax ginseng* alone or in combination with **vitamin E** produced significant improvements in aerobic capacity. Another double-blind, placebo-controlled trial of 37 individuals also found some benefit.

A double-blind, placebo-controlled study of 120 people found that *Panax ginseng* gradually improved reaction time and lung function over a 12-week treatment period among those 40 to 60 years old. No benefits were seen in younger individuals.

However, numerous studies have failed to find *Panax ginseng* effective. For example, an 8-week double-blind trial that followed 31 healthy men in their 20s found no evidence of ergogenic benefit. Many other small trials of *Panax ginseng* also failed to find evidence of benefit.

General Well-being

A double-blind study compared the effects of a nutritional supplement with and without *Panax ginseng* extract on the feeling of well-being in 625 people whose average age was just under 40 years old. Quality of life was measured by a set of 11 questions. People taking the ginseng-containing supplement reported significant improvement compared to those taking the non-ginseng supplement (the control group). Similar findings were reported in a double-blind, placebo-controlled study of 36 people newly diagnosed with diabetes. After 8 weeks, participants who had been taking 200 mg of ginseng daily reported improvements in mood, well-being, vigor, and psychophysical performance that were significant compared to the reports of control participants.

A 12-week, double-blind, placebo-controlled study of 120 people found improvement in general well-being among women aged 30 to 60 years and men aged 40 to 60 years, but not among men aged 30 to 39 years.

However, a double-blind, placebo-controlled trial of 30 young people found marginal benefits at 4 weeks and no significant benefits at 8 weeks. Similarly, a 60-day, double-blind, placebo-controlled trial of 83 adults in their mid-20s found no effect on mood or psychological well-being.

Impotence (Erectile Dysfunction)

Two double-blind, placebo-controlled trials, involving a total of about 135 people, have found evidence that Korean red ginseng may improve erectile function.

In the better of the two trials, 45 participants received either placebo or Korean red ginseng at a dose of 900 mg 3 times daily for 8 weeks.

The results indicate that while using Korean red ginseng, men experienced significantly better sexual function than while they were taking placebo.

Preventing Cancer

An observational study on ginseng and cancer prevention has been widely publicized, but a close look at the data arouses serious suspicions. This study was performed in South Korea and followed a total of 4,587 men and women aged 39 years and older from 1987 to 1991. People who regularly consumed *Panax ginseng* were compared with otherwise similar individuals (matched in sex, age, alcohol use, smoking, and education and economic status) who did not.

The reported results were impressive. Those who used ginseng showed a 60% decrease in risk of death from cancer. Lung cancer and gastric cancer were particularly reduced. The more ginseng consumed, the greater the effect.

However, there is something a bit fishy about this study. Use of ginseng fewer than 3 times per year caused a 54% reduction in risk. It is difficult to believe that so occasional a use of ginseng could reduce cancer mortality by more than half!

Menopause

A double-blind, placebo-controlled study of 384 women experiencing menopausal symptoms found no significant benefit with *Panax ginseng* and no evidence of hormonal effects.

Dosage

The typical recommended daily dosage of *Panax ginseng* is 1 to 2 g of raw herb or 200 mg daily of an extract standardized to contain 4 to 7% ginsenosides. In one study of American ginseng (*Panax quinquefolius*) for diabetes, the dose used was 3 g daily.

Note: There are dozens of ginsenosides in ginseng. Because different ginsenosides have different effects, two different ginseng products with similar *total* ginsenoside content will not necessarily have similar efficacy. Unfortunately, current scientific knowledge does not allow us at present to make informed recommendations on which specific ginsenosides are useful for which conditions.

Ginseng

Ordinarily, a 2- to 3-week period of using ginseng is recommended, followed by a 1- to 2-week "rest" period. Russian tradition suggests that ginseng should not be used by those under 40. However, there is no scientific evidence to support these recommendations.

Safety Issues

Ginseng appears to be nontoxic, both in the short and long term, according to the results of studies in mice, rats, chickens, and dwarf pigs.

Reported side effects are rare. There are a few case reports of breast tenderness, postmenopausal vaginal bleeding, and menstrual abnormalities associated with *Panax ginseng* use. Such side effects suggest that it has estrogenic properties. However, a large double-blind trial of *Panax ginseng* found no estrogen-like effects. Another double-blind trial found no effects on estrogen or testosterone, and a carefully designed test-tube study showed that ginseng is not estrogenic. Therefore, it is possible that these apparent side effects were coincidental; another possibility is that adulterants in the ginseng product used caused the problem. Ginseng and other Asian herbal products have often been found to contain unlisted herbs and pharmaceuticals.

Estrogen itself stimulates the growth of breast cancer cells. Interestingly, in a test-tube study, *Panax ginseng* was again found to be non-estrogenic, and yet it nonetheless stimulated the growth of breast cancer cells. Although the mechanism of this effect is not known, the results suggest that women who have had breast cancer should avoid using ginseng.

Unconfirmed reports suggest that highly excessive doses of *Panax ginseng* can cause insomnia, raise blood pressure, increase heart rate, and possibly cause other significant effects. Whether some of these cases were actually caused by caffeine mixed in with ginseng remains unclear. One double-blind study failed to find any effect on blood pressure.

One case report and one double-blind trial suggest that *Panax ginseng* can reduce the anticoagulant effects of Coumadin (warfarin), but another trial failed to find such an interaction. The reason for this discrepancy is not clear, but prudence would nonetheless suggest not combining ginseng and warfarin.

Two reports indicate that combination treatment with *Panax ginseng* and antidepressant drugs may result in a manic episode.

There are also theoretical concerns regarding use of ginseng by people with diabetes. If it is true, as the preliminary studies discussed above suggest, that ginseng can in fact reduce blood sugar levels, people with diabetes who take ginseng might need to reduce their dose of medication. On the other hand, if certain types of ginseng have the opposite effect (as researchers hypothesize), this could necessitate an increase in medication. The bottom line: People with diabetes should only use ginseng under physician supervision.

In 1979, an article was published in the *Journal of the American Medical Association* claiming that people can become addicted to *Panax ginseng* and develop blood pressure elevations, nervousness, sleeplessness, diarrhea, and hypersexuality. However, this report has since been thoroughly discredited and should no longer be taken seriously.

Chinese tradition suggests that *Panax ginseng* should not be used by pregnant or nursing mothers, and one animal study hints that ginseng use by a pregnant mother could cause birth defects. Safety in young children or people with severe liver or kidney disease has not been established.

Interactions You Should Know About

If you are taking:

➢ **Antidepressants:** *Panax ginseng* **might cause manic episodes.**
➢ **Insulin or oral hypoglycemics: Various forms of ginseng may unpredictably alter your dosage need.**
➢ **Warfarin (Coumadin):** *Panax ginseng* **might possibly decrease its effect.**
➢ **Influenza vaccine: Panax ginseng might help it work better.**

Glucomannan

PRINCIPAL PROPOSED USES: *High Cholesterol*

OTHER PROPOSED USES: *Constipation, Diabetes, High Blood Pressure, Weight Loss*

Glucomannan is a dietary fiber derived from the tubers of *Amorphophallus konjac*. Konjac flour (made from these tubers) is used to make a jelly called *konyaku*, a common food product in Japan.

Fiber-containing foods, such as oats, are known to help reduce cholesterol and improve constipation, and may also help regulate blood sugar and assist in weight reduction by creating a feeling of fullness. However, many people have a hard time consuming enough fiber from food, so turn to fiber supplements, such as guar gum and pectin, to help fulfill their daily requirements. Glucomannan offers one advantage over these forms of fiber: much smaller doses are necessary. When glucomannan is placed in water, it can swell up to 17 times its original volume. These qualities make it potentially quite convenient as a fiber supplement.

Requirements/Sources

Although glucomannan can be derived from other sources such as yeast, most studies have used glucomannan purified from the konjac root.

Therapeutic Dosages

Most of the studies described here used 3 to 5 g per day in divided doses before meals. However, there are concerns regarding the form of glucomannan used (see Safety Issues below).

Therapeutic Uses

Several small controlled studies have found glucomannan to be effective for improving the **cholesterol** profile. Glucomannan appears to reduce LDL ("bad") cholesterol and, according to some studies, increase HDL ("good") cholesterol. In addition, it may improve **blood pressure**.

By expanding in the stomach, glucomannan might be useful for people trying to lose weight. Many people report a feeling of fullness after taking glucomannan, and some studies found a significant **weight loss** among those taking glucomannan compared to those

on placebo. However, not all studies of glucomannan for weight loss have had positive results.

Glucomannan may also help the body to regulate blood sugar levels and, therefore, could be helpful in treating diabetes. Additionally, glucomannan might be helpful for individuals who experience episodes of low blood sugar following stomach surgery.

Like other dietary fibers, glucomannan may help treat **constipation**.

What Is the Scientific Evidence for Glucomannan?

High Cholesterol and High Blood Pressure

In a double-blind study, 63 people were given either 3.9 g per day of glucomannan or placebo for 4 weeks and then switched to the other treatment. While taking glucomannan, participants showed significant reductions in total cholesterol, LDL cholesterol, and triglycerides, as compared to placebo. In addition, their systolic blood pressure (the upper number in the blood pressure reading) was also reduced. However, there was no significant increase in HDL cholesterol and no improvement in the ratio of LDL to HDL cholesterol.

Participants in another study were given either 3 g per day of glucomannan or placebo over an 8-week period. The glucomannan group showed improvements in total and HDL cholesterol as well as a reduction in systolic blood pressure. Those taking glucomannan also lost weight, whereas the placebo group gained weight over the length of the trial.

Several other controlled studies have found similar results.

Weight Loss

A few small double-blind studies suggest that glucomannan may be helpful for people trying to lose weight; however, in other studies, no such benefit was seen.

One double-blind, placebo-controlled trial of 20 women who were more than 20% over their ideal weight found glucomannan to be more effective than placebo at promoting weight loss. All participants were instructed not to change their eating or exercise habits while on the treatment. Those in the treatment group took 1 g of glucomannan 3 times a day for 8 weeks and lost an average of 5.5 pounds during that period; in comparison, those in the placebo group gained an average of 1.5 pounds, a significant difference. The glucomannan group also had a reduction of total and LDL cholesterol as well as triglyceride levels.

Benefits were also seen in a double-blind, placebo-controlled trial of 28 overweight people who had just experienced a heart attack.

However, another double-blind trial of 60 obese children did not find a significant difference in weight loss between the glucomannan and the placebo groups. In this study, the children received either 1 g of glucomannan or placebo twice a day for 8 weeks.

Diabetes

A study of individuals with diabetes tested the effectiveness of glucomannan fiber-enriched biscuits against wheat bran biscuits for blood sugar control. While using the glucomannan biscuits, people experienced a significant improvement in glucose control as compared to the wheat bran biscuits.

Other studies have also found evidence that glucomannan can improve blood sugar control as well as cholesterol profile.

Safety Issues

In Japan, food products containing glucomannan have a long history of use and are believed to be safe. However, there are some concerns about taking glucomannan as a supplement.

Some people taking glucomannan complain of excess gas, stomach distension, or mild diarrhea. These symptoms usually abate within a couple of days of treatment or with a reduction of the dosage.

In a few cases, glucomannan tablets have caused obstruction of the esophagus when they expanded before reaching the stomach. In response to these reports, tablets of this type have been banned. Capsules, however, do not seem to pose the same risk because their casing prevents the glucomannan from contacting water until it reaches the stomach. The dramatic expansion of glucomannan has also raised some concerns that it could cause an obstruction in the intestines; nonetheless, as of yet, there have been no reports of this actually happening.

One option to offset all expansion risk is to mix glucomannan powder in water so that it expands before it is ingested; however, this strategy defeats the convenience of this form of fiber.

Glucosamine

SUPPLEMENT FORMS/ALTERNATE NAMES: *Glucosamine Hydrochloride, Glucosamine Sulfate, N-Acetyl Glucosamine*

PRINCIPAL PROPOSED USES: *Osteoarthritis (Relieving Symptoms and Possibly Slowing the Course of the Disease)*

OTHER PROPOSED USES: *Muscle Injury Prevention, Osteochondritis, Tendinitis*

Glucosamine, most commonly used in the form glucosamine sulfate, is a simple molecule derived from glucose, the principal sugar found in blood. In glucosamine, one oxygen atom in glucose is replaced by a nitrogen atom. The chemical term for this modified form of glucose is *amino sugar.*

Glucosamine is produced naturally in the body, where it is a key building block for making cartilage.

Some, but not all, studies suggest that glucosamine supplements can relieve pain and improve mobility in **osteoarthritis**, a disease in which cartilage in joints becomes stiffer and may wear away. Besides possibly relieving symptoms, there is some evidence that glucosamine might actually slow the progression of the disease.

Sources

There is no U.S. Dietary Reference Intake (formerly known as the Recommended Dietary Allowance) for glucosamine. Your body makes all the glucosamine it needs from building blocks found in foods.

Glucosamine is not usually obtained directly from food. Glucosamine supplements are derived from chitin, a substance found in the shells of shrimp, lobsters, and crabs.

Therapeutic Dosages

For osteoarthritis, a typical dosage of glucosamine is 500 mg 3 times daily. A 1,500-mg dose taken once daily may also be effective. Be patient: Results take weeks to develop.

Glucosamine is available in three forms: glucosamine sulfate, glucosamine hydrochloride, and N-acetyl glucosamine. All three forms are sold as tablets or capsules. There is some dispute over which form is best. One study provides some evidence that glucosamine hydrochloride and glucosamine sulfate are equally effective.

Glucosamine is often sold in combination with chondroitin. It is not known whether this combination treatment is better than glucosamine alone, although animal studies suggest that this may be the case.

Therapeutic Uses

Glucosamine is widely accepted as a treatment for osteoarthritis. However, the current evidence from double-blind studies is highly inconsistent, with many of the most recent and best-designed studies failing to find significant benefit. According to the positive studies, glucosamine acts more slowly than conventional treatments, such as ibuprofen, but eventually produces approximately equivalent benefits. Unlike conventional treatments, glucosamine might also help prevent progressive joint damage, thereby slowing the course of the disease.

Glucosamine has also shown some promise for osteochondritis of the knee, a cartilage disease related to osteoarthritis.

Some athletes use glucosamine, in the (unproved) belief that it can prevent **muscle and tendon injuries**. It has also been suggested as a treatment for **tendinitis**. However, there is no meaningful scientific evidence to support these potential uses.

What Is the Scientific Evidence for Glucosamine?

Osteoarthritis

⇒ *Symptom Relief*

Inconsistent evidence suggests that glucosamine supplements might relieve pain and other symptoms of osteoarthritis. Two types of studies have been performed, those that compared glucosamine against placebo and those that compared it against standard medications.

In the placebo-controlled category, one of the best trials was a 3-year, double-blind study of 212 people with osteoarthritis of the knee. Participants receiving glucosamine showed reduced symptoms as compared to those receiving placebo.

Benefits were also seen in other double-blind, placebo-controlled studies, enrolling a total of more than 800 people and ranging in length from 4 weeks to 3 years.

Other double-blind studies enrolling a total of more than 400 people compared glucosamine against ibuprofen and found glucosamine equally effective as the drug. Furthermore, one of the placebo-controlled trials noted above (unfortunately, only reported in abstract form) also included people given the drug piroxicam and again found equivalent benefits.

However, more recent studies have been less promising. In four studies involving a total of about 500 people, use of glucosamine failed to provide any meaningful improvement in symptoms. A fifth study evaluated the effects of *stopping* glucosamine after taking it for 6 months. In this double-blind study of 137 people with osteoarthritis of the knee, participants who stopped using glucosamine (and, unbeknownst to them, took placebo instead) did no worse than people who stayed on glucosamine. In addition, a very large (1,583-participant) study failed to find either glucosamine (as glucosamine hydrochloride) or glucosamine plus chondroitin more effective than placebo. It appears that most of the positive studies were funded by manufacturers of glucosamine products and most of the studies performed by neutral researchers failed to find benefit.

⇒ *Slowing the Course of the Disease*

Conventional treatments for osteoarthritis reduce the symptoms but don't slow the actual progress of the disease; in fact, nonsteroidal anti-inflammatory drugs,

Glutamine

such as indomethacin, may actually speed the progression of osteoarthritis by interfering with cartilage repair and promoting cartilage destruction. Glucosamine appears to be more helpful in this regard.

A 3-year, double-blind, placebo-controlled study of 212 people found indications that glucosamine may protect joints from further damage. Over the course of the study, individuals given glucosamine showed some actual improvement in pain and mobility, while those given placebo worsened steadily. Perhaps even more importantly, x-rays showed that glucosamine treatment prevented progressive damage to the knee joint.

A separate 3-year study enrolling 202 people confirmed these results.

Knee Pain Due to Osteochondritis

A 12-week, double-blind, placebo-controlled study examined the effectiveness of glucosamine at 2,000 mg daily of 50 people with continuing knee pain, mostly caused by osteochondritis (damage to the articular cartilage of the knee) rather than osteoarthritis. The results were somewhat equivocal, but appeared to indicate that glucosamine could improve symptoms. Some participants may have had osteoarthritis too, however, so the results of this study are a bit difficult to interpret.

Safety Issues

Glucosamine appears to be a generally safe treatment, and has not been associated with significant side effects. A few case reports and animal studies raised concerns that glucosamine might be harmful for individuals with diabetes, but subsequent studies have tended to lay these concerns to rest.

There is one case report of an allergic reaction to a glucosamine/chondroitin product, causing exacerbation of asthma.

Glutamine

SUPPLEMENT FORMS/ALTERNATE NAMES: *L-Glutamine*

PRINCIPAL PROPOSED USES: *None*

OTHER PROPOSED USES: *Angina, Attention Deficit Disorder, Crohn's Disease, Enhancing Mental Function, Food Allergies, HIV Support, Irritable Bowel Syndrome, Overtraining Syndrome, Post-exercise Colds, Ulcerative Colitis, Ulcers, Undesired Weight Loss*

Glutamine, or L-glutamine, is an amino acid derived from another amino acid, glutamic acid. Glutamine plays a role in the health of the immune system, digestive tract, and muscle cells, as well as other bodily functions. It appears to serve as a fuel for the cells that line the intestines. Heavy exercise, infection, surgery, and trauma can deplete the body's glutamine reserves, particularly in muscle cells.

The fact that glutamine does so many good things in the body has led people to try glutamine supplements as a treatment for various conditions, including preventing the infections that often follow endurance exercise, reducing symptoms of overtraining syndrome, improving nutrition in critical illness, alleviating allergies, and treating digestive problems.

Sources

There is no daily requirement for glutamine, because the body can make its own supply. As mentioned earlier, various severe stresses may result in a temporary glutamine deficiency.

High-protein foods such as meat, fish, beans, and dairy products are excellent sources of glutamine. Typical daily intake from food ranges from approximately 1 to 6 g.

Therapeutic Dosages

Typical therapeutic dosages of glutamine used in studies range from 3 to 30 g daily, divided into several separate doses.

Therapeutic Uses

Endurance athletes frequently catch **colds** after completing a marathon or similar forms of exercise. Preliminary evidence, including one small, double-blind, placebo-controlled trial, suggests that glutamine supplements might help prevent such infections.

Another small, double-blind, placebo-controlled trial suggests that glutamine might support standard therapy for **angina**. **Note:** Angina is too dangerous a disease for self-treatment. If you have angina, do not take glutamine (or any other supplement) except on the advice of a physician.

Because, as noted above, cells of the intestine use glutamine for fuel, the supplement has been tried as a supportive treatment for various digestive conditions, with mixed results. Tested uses include reducing diarrhea caused by the drug nelfinavir (used for treatment of **HIV**), digestive distress caused by **cancer** chemotherapy, and symptoms of **inflammatory bowel disease**.

Glutamine appears to help reduce leakage through the intestinal wall. On this basis, glutamine has also been suggested as a treatment for **food allergies**, according to the idea that, in some people, whole proteins leak through the wall of the digestive tract and enter the blood, causing allergic reactions (so-called leaky gut syndrome). However, as yet there is no reliable evidence that glutamine actually provides any benefits for food allergies.

Preliminary evidence suggests glutamine combined with **antioxidants** or other nutrients may help people with HIV to **gain weight**. Glutamine (often combined with other nutrients) also appears to be useful as a nutritional supplement for people undergoing recovery from major surgery or critical illness.

Glutamine has been tried as an ergogenic aid for bodybuilders, but two small trials failed to find any evidence of benefit.

Based on glutamine's role in muscle, it has been suggested that glutamine might be useful for athletes experiencing overtraining syndrome. As the name suggests, this syndrome is the cumulative effect of a training regimen that allows too little rest and recovery between workouts. Symptoms include depression, fatigue, reduced performance, and physiological signs of stress. Glutamine supplements have additionally been proposed as treatment for **attention deficit disorder**, **ulcers**, and as a "brain booster." However, there is little to no scientific evidence for any of these uses.

What Is the Scientific Evidence for Glutamine?

Infections in Athletes

Endurance exercise temporarily reduces immunity to infection. This effect may be due in part to reduction of glutamine in the body, although not all studies agree.

A double-blind, placebo-controlled study evaluated the benefits of supplemental glutamine (5 g) taken at the end of exercise in 151 endurance athletes. The results showed a significant decrease in infections among treated athletes. Only 19% of the athletes taking glutamine got sick, as compared to 51% of those on placebo.

Recovery from Critical Illness

One small double-blind study found that glutamine supplements might have significant nutritional benefits for seriously ill people. In this study, 84 critically ill hospital patients were divided into two groups. All the patients were being fed through a feeding tube. One group received a normal feeding-tube diet, whereas the other group received this diet plus supplemental glutamine. After 6 months, 14 of the 42 patients receiving glutamine had died, compared with 24 of the control group. The glutamine group also left both the intensive care ward and the hospital significantly sooner than the patients who did not receive glutamine. Benefits have been seen in other controlled trials as well.

HIV Support

One double-blind, placebo-controlled study of 25 people found that use of glutamine at 30 g daily for 7 days reduced diarrhea caused by the protease inhibitor nelfinavir.

In addition, combination supplements containing glutamine may help reverse HIV-related weight loss. For example, a double-blind, placebo-controlled study found that a combination of glutamine and antioxidants (**vitamins C** and **E, beta-carotene, selenium,** and **N-acetyl cysteine**) led to significant weight gain in people with HIV who had lost weight. Another small double-blind trial found that combination treatment with glutamine, **arginine**, and **beta-hydroxy beta-methylbutyrate**

Glutamine

(HMB) could increase muscle mass and possibly improve immune status.

Cancer Chemotherapy

There is mixed evidence regarding whether glutamine can reduce the side effects of cancer chemotherapy. A double-blind, placebo-controlled trial of 70 people undergoing chemotherapy with the drug 5-FU for colorectal cancer found that glutamine at a dose of 18 g daily improved intestinal function and structure, and reduced the need for anti-diarrhea drugs. However, a double-blind trial of 65 women undergoing various forms of chemotherapy for advanced breast cancer failed to find glutamine at 30 g per day helpful for reducing diarrhea.

Angina

Researchers conducted investigations in rats, and found that glutamine could protect the heart from damage caused by loss of oxygen. Based on these findings, they went on to evaluate the effects of glutamine in ten people with chronic angina who were also taking standard medication. In this double-blind, placebo-controlled trial, each participant received a single oral dose of glutamine (80 mg per kg of body weight) or placebo 40 minutes before a treadmill test. A week later, each participant received the opposite treatment. The results showed that use of glutamine significantly enhanced the ability of participants to exercise without showing signs of heart stress. Based on the results in rats, researchers suggest that a higher dose of glutamine would be worth trying.

Crohn's Disease

Because glutamine is the major fuel source for cells of the small intestine, glutamine has been proposed as a treatment for Crohn's disease, a disease of the small intestine. However, two double-blind trials enrolling a total of 30 people found no benefit.

Sports Performance

A double-blind, placebo-controlled trial of 31 people ranging from 18 to 24 years of age evaluated the potential benefits of glutamine as a sports supplement for improving response to resistance training (weight lifting). Participants received either placebo or glutamine at a dose of 0.9 g per kg of lean tissue mass. After 6 weeks of resistance training, participants taking glutamine showed no relative improvement in performance, composition, or muscle protein degradation.

Similarly, negative results were seen in a small, double-blind, placebo-controlled trial of weightlifters using a dose of 0.3 g per kg of total body weight.

Safety Issues

As a naturally occurring amino acid, glutamine is thought to be a safe supplement when taken at recommended dosages. However, those who are hypersensitive to monosodium glutamate (MSG) should use glutamine with caution, as the body metabolizes glutamine into glutamate. Also, because many anti-epilepsy drugs work by blocking glutamate stimulation in the brain, high dosages of glutamine might conceivably overwhelm these drugs and pose a risk to people with **epilepsy**.

Finally, in one case report, high doses of the supplement L-glutamine (more than 2 g per day) may have triggered episodes of mania in two people not previously known to have **bipolar disorder**.

Maximum safe dosages for young children, pregnant or nursing women, or those with severe liver or kidney disease have not been determined.

Interactions You Should Know About

If you are taking:

- Antiseizure medications, including carbamazepine, phenobarbital, phenytoin (Dilantin), primidone (Mysoline), and valproic acid (Depakene): Use glutamine only under medical supervision.
- Nelfinavir or other protease inhibitors for HIV, or cancer chemotherapy drugs: Use of glutamine may reduce intestinal side effects.

Glutathione

PRINCIPAL PROPOSED USES: *None*

OTHER PROPOSED USES: *Antioxidant*

In the body, dangerous naturally occurring substances called *free radicals* pose a risk of harm to many tissues. The body deploys an "antioxidant defense system" to hold them in check. Glutathione, a protein made from the amino acids cysteine, glutamic acid, and glycine, is one of the most important elements of this system.

Glutathione does much of its work in the liver, although it is also found elsewhere in the body. Besides fighting free radicals, it helps keep various essential biological molecules in a chemical state called *reduced* (as opposed to *oxidized*). In addition, glutathione can act on toxins, such as pesticides, lead, and dry-cleaning solvents, transforming them in such a way that the body can excrete them more easily.

Nutrients such as **vitamin C** and **vitamin E** also help neutralize free radicals. In the 1990s, such **antioxidant** supplements were widely promoted for preventing a variety of diseases, including cancer and heart disease. (Unfortunately, this hope has largely floundered as the results of large, reliable studies have come in.) During this period, oral glutathione became popular as an additional antioxidant supplement. Unfortunately, glutathione is not absorbed when taken by mouth, so such supplements are almost certainly useless. It may be possible, however, to raise glutathione levels in the body by taking other supplements, such as vitamin C, cysteine, **lipoic acid**, and **N-acetylcysteine.** Whether doing so would offer any health benefits remains unclear.

Requirements/Sources

There is no dietary requirement for glutathione. The body makes it from scratch, utilizing vitamins and common amino acids found in food.

Glutathione levels in the body are reduced by cigarette smoking. Various diseases are associated with reduced levels of glutathione, including cancer, **cataracts**, **diabetes**, and **HIV infection.**

Therapeutic Dosages

A typical recommended dose of oral glutathione is 50 mg twice daily. However, as noted above, when glutathione is taken by mouth it is destroyed. Therefore, no matter what the dose, it won't make any difference.

It is possible that some glutathione may be absorbed if it is held in the mouth and allowed to dissolve, but this has not been well studied.

A more promising method for raising glutathione levels in the body involves taking supplemental cysteine or antioxidant supplements. Evidence suggests that cysteine (often supplied in the form of whey protein, which is high in cysteine) can raise glutathione levels in people with **cancer**, **hepatitis**, or HIV.

In addition, because vitamin C has overlapping functions with glutathione, vitamin C supplements may spare some of the body's glutathione from being used up, thereby increasing its levels in the body. The antioxidant supplement lipoic acid appears to raise glutathione levels as well.

Other supplements that might raise glutathione levels include N-acetylcysteine, **glutamine**, **methionine**, and **S-adenosyl methionine** (SAMe).

Therapeutic Uses

Various websites promote glutathione for a wide variety of health problems, from preventing aging to enhancing sports performance. However, oral glutathione supplements are almost certainly useless for any condition since they are not absorbed.

There is a bit of evidence that injected glutathione might offer a few heath benefits, such as preventing blood clots during surgery, reducing the side effects and increasing the effectiveness of cancer chemotherapy drugs such as **cisplatin**, treating **male infertility**, and alleviating symptoms of early **Parkinson's disease.** Although oral glutathione is not likely to provide the same benefits, it is at least theoretically possible that taking the nutrients described in the previous section (and

Glycine

thereby raising glutathione levels indirectly) could offer similar benefits. However, there is no direct evidence to indicate that this hypothesis is true.

Safety Issues

Oral glutathione should be entirely safe, since it is not absorbed.

Glycine

PRINCIPAL PROPOSED USES: *Schizophrenia*

OTHER PROPOSED USES: *Cancer Prevention, Diabetes, Enhancing Memory and Mental Function, Epilepsy, Immune Support, Kidney Protection, Liver Protection, Prostate Enlargement (BPH), Sports Performance, Strokes*

Glycine is the simplest of the 20 different amino acids used as building blocks to make proteins for your body. It works in concert with glutamine, a substance that plays a major role in brain function. Glycine has shown some promise as an aid in the treatment of **schizophrenia**, and may have other uses related to the brain as well, such as **enhancing mental function**.

Requirements/Sources

Your body is able to make glycine using another amino acid, serine. Because you can manufacture glycine, you don't really have to consume any, so it's called a *nonessential amino acid*. Most of us get about 2 g of glycine a day from the foods we regularly eat anyway. This dietary glycine comes mostly from high-protein foods like meat, fish, dairy products, and legumes. For treating certain disease conditions, however, much larger amounts than are normally consumed have been advocated; such high doses can only be obtained by taking supplements.

Therapeutic Dosages

Dosages of oral glycine used in clinical trials for therapeutic purposes range from 2 g to 60 g daily.

Therapeutic Uses

Several studies have evaluated glycine as a supportive treatment for schizophrenia. Preliminary evidence suggests that high doses of glycine (from 15 to 60 g daily) can augment the effectiveness of most medications used for this disease. The one notable exception is clozapine (Clozaril); one study suggests that glycine may actually *decrease* the effectiveness of this drug (see Safety Issues below).

One large double-blind study suggests that low doses of glycine may be helpful for limiting the spreading brain damage that occurs during **stroke**. However, there are also theoretical concerns that glycine could increase such damage (see Safety Issues below), so you should not try this treatment except under physician supervision.

A small double-blind study found evidence that glycine may help improve long-term blood sugar control in people with type 2 diabetes.

One small study weakly suggests that glycine may enhance memory and mental function.

Glycine alone and in combination with other amino acids has shown a bit of promise for enhancing wound healing.

Animal studies suggest that dietary glycine may protect against chemically induced damage to the liver or kidneys.

Other studies in laboratory animals suggest that dietary glycine may prevent tumor formation and growth in the livers of mice and rats. However, it is too early to say whether glycine has **cancer preventive** effects in humans.

Manufacturers advertising glycine supplements have made a number of additional claims for it, including prevention of **epileptic seizures**, reducing acid in the stomach, **multiple sclerosis, boosting the immune system,** and calming the mind. It is also proposed as a **sports supplement,** said to work in this capacity by increasing release of human growth hormone (HGH). As yet, there is no real scientific evidence that glycine works for any of these purposes.

Because it has a sweet taste, glycine has also been recommended as a sugar substitute for people with diabetes.

What Is the Scientific Evidence for Glycine?

Schizophrenia

Glycine may enhance the effectiveness of drugs used for schizophrenia, especially those in the older **phenothiazine** category. It has also shown promise for the newer drugs risperidone and olanzapine. However, it may not be helpful for people using clozapine.

Phenothiazine drugs are most effective for the "positive" symptoms of schizophrenia, such as hallucinations and delusions. (Such symptoms are called *positive* because they indicate the presence of abnormal mental functions, rather than the absence of normal mental functions.) In general, however, these medications are less helpful for the "negative" symptoms of schizophrenia, such as apathy, depression, and social withdrawal. Glycine might be of benefit here.

A double-blind, placebo-controlled trial enrolled 22 participants who continued to experience negative symptoms of schizophrenia despite standard therapy. The results showed that the use of glycine significantly improved negative symptoms. As a bonus, glycine also appeared to reduce some of the side effects caused by the prescription drugs. No changes were seen in positive symptoms (for instance, hallucinations), but it isn't possible to tell whether that is because these symptoms were already being controlled by prescription medications or if glycine simply has no effect on those particular symptoms of schizophrenia.

Three earlier double-blind, placebo-controlled clinical trials of glycine together with standard drugs for schizophrenia also found it to be helpful for negative symptoms. All of these studies used very small groups (from 12 to 18 people), so much larger trials are still needed to verify glycine's effectiveness.

The trials just discussed were conducted before the newer antipsychotic drugs, known as atypical antipsychotics, were widely available. These drugs cause fewer side effects, and also provide benefits for the negative symptoms of schizophrenia along with the positive. One study found that glycine augmented the effectiveness of two of these drugs: olanzapine and risperidone. However, another study suggests that adding glycine to the atypical antipsychotic clozapine may not be a good idea. In this study, glycine was found to reduce the benefits of clozapine. Two other double-blind, placebo-controlled trials of glycine and clozapine simply failed to find benefit.

Stroke

Glycine's potential usefulness for treating individuals who have undergone strokes was investigated in a double-blind, placebo-controlled study with 200 participants. The results suggest that glycine can protect against the spreading damage to the brain that usually follows a stroke. Participants were given either 1 to 2 g of glycine sublingually (dissolved under the tongue) or placebo treatment for a period of 5 days. The results suggest that glycine can prevent neural damage. This appears to be an impressive result, but further research is necessary.

Although other researchers using glycine for brain disorders have reported that such small doses of glycine would not be sufficient to cross the blood–brain barrier, measurements of amino acids in the cerebrospinal fluid during the above study suggest that it did enter the brain. However, there are potential concerns that high-dose glycine could *increase* stroke damage (see Safety Issues below).

Safety Issues

No serious adverse effects from using glycine have been reported, even at doses as high as 60 g per day. One participant in the 22-person trial described above developed stomach upset and vomiting, but it ceased when the glycine was discontinued.

In contradiction to the study on strokes mentioned above, theoretical concerns have been raised that suggest glycine might actually increase brain injury in strokes. In fact, drugs that block glycine have been investigated as treatments to limit stroke damage. However, the authors of the study on strokes described above make an argument that suggests the overall effect of glycine is protective. Until this controversy is settled, prudence suggests not using glycine following a stroke, except on the advice of a physician.

In addition, as noted above, it is possible that use of glycine could reduce the benefits of clozapine.

Maximum safe doses for young children, pregnant or nursing women, or people with liver or kidney disease are not known.

Interactions You Should Know About

If you are taking **clozapine**: Do not take glycine except on the advice of a physician.

Goldenrod

Solidago spp.

PRINCIPAL PROPOSED USES: *Bladder Infections, Bladder/Kidney Stones*

Goldenrod is often falsely accused of being an intensely allergenic plant, because of its unfortunate tendency to bloom brightly at the same time and often in locations quite near to the truly allergenic ragweed. However, actual allergic reactions to this gorgeous herb are unusual.

There are numerous species of goldenrod (27 have been collected in Indiana alone), but all seem to possess similar medicinal properties, and various species are used interchangeably in Europe.

What Is Goldenrod Used for Today?

In Germany, goldenrod is used as a supportive treatment for bladder infections, irritation of the urinary tract, and bladder/kidney stones. Goldenrod is said to wash out bacteria and **kidney stones** by increasing the flow of urine and, also, to soothe inflamed tissues and calm muscle spasms in the urinary tract. It isn't used as a cure in itself, but rather as an adjunct to other, more definitive treatments such as (in the case of bladder infections) antibiotics.

However, we don't know whether goldenrod actually helps. Several studies have found that goldenrod does in fact increase urine flow, but there is no direct evidence that this in turn leads to any other medical benefits.

Warning: Urinary conditions such as kidney stones are potentially serious. For this reason, medical advice is recommended.

Dosage

A typical dosage is 3 to 4 g of dried herb 2 to 3 times daily. Make sure to drink plenty of water while taking goldenrod, to help it do its job.

Safety Issues

The safety of goldenrod hasn't been fully evaluated. However, no significant reactions or side effects have been reported. Safety in young children, pregnant and nursing women, or those with severe liver or kidney disease has not been established. Individuals taking the medication lithium should use herbal diuretics such as goldenrod only under the supervision of a physician, as dehydration can be dangerous with this medication.

Interactions You Should Know About

If you are taking **lithium**: Do not use goldenrod except under the supervision of a physician.

Goldenseal

Hydrastis canadensis

PRINCIPAL PROPOSED USES: *None*

OTHER PROPOSED USES:

Topical Uses: *Athlete's Foot and Other Fungal Infections, Minor Wounds, Vaginal Yeast Infections*

Oral Uses: *Congestive Heart Failure, Dyspepsia, Heart Arrhythmias, High Blood Pressure, High Cholesterol, Infectious Diarrhea, Irritable Bowel Syndrome, Urinary Tract Infections*

INCORRECT USES: *Common Cold, Immune Support, Masking Positive Findings on Drug Screens*

Although goldenseal root is one of the most popular herbs sold today, it is taken almost entirely for the wrong reasons. Originally, it was used by Native Americans both as a dye and as a treatment for skin disorders, digestive problems, liver disease, diarrhea, and eye irritations. European settlers learned of the herb from the Iroquois and other tribes and quickly adopted goldenseal as a part of early colonial medical care.

In the early 1800s, an herbalist named Samuel Thompson created a wildly popular system of medicine (some would say personality cult) that swept the country. Thompson spoke of goldenseal as a nearly magical cure for many conditions. His evangelism led to a dramatic upsurge in demand, followed by over-collection and decimation of the wild plant. Prices skyrocketed and then collapsed when Thompsonianism faded away.

Goldenseal has passed through several more booms and busts. Today, it is again in great demand, but now it is under intentional cultivation.

What Is Goldenseal Used for Today?

Goldenseal contains a substance called *berberine* that has been found to inhibit or kill many microorganisms, including fungi, protozoa, and bacteria. On this basis, contemporary herbalists often use goldenseal as a topical antibiotic for skin wounds, as well as to treat viral **mouth sores** and superficial fungal infections, such as **athlete's foot**. However, there is no direct scientific evidence that goldenseal is effective for any of these purposes.

Note that goldenseal probably is not likely to work as an oral antibiotic because the blood levels of berberine that can be achieved by taking goldenseal orally are far too low to matter. However, goldenseal could theoretically be beneficial in treating sore throats and diseases of the digestive tract (such as **infectious diarrhea**) because it can contact the affected area directly. Similarly, since berberine is concentrated in the bladder, goldenseal could be useful for bladder infections. Nonetheless, again there is as yet no direct evidence that goldenseal is effective for any of these uses.

Extremely weak evidence (far too weak to rely upon at all) suggests that goldenseal or berberine may have actions that could lead it to be helpful for various heart-related conditions, including **arrhythmias**, **congestive heart failure**, **high cholesterol**, and **high blood pressure**. Similarly, infinitesimal evidence hints that goldenseal could be helpful for conditions in which spasms of smooth muscle play a role, such as **dyspepsia** (nonspecific stomach distress) and **irritable bowel syndrome**, as well as various forms of pain caused by inflammation.

Ironically, goldenseal's most common uses are entirely inappropriate. Goldenseal is frequently combined with the herb **echinacea** to be taken as a "traditional immune booster" and "antibiotic" for the prevention and treatment of colds. However, as the noted herbalist Paul Bergner has pointed out, there are three things wrong with this packaging: (1) there is no credible evidence that goldenseal increases immunity (only one study even hints at an immune-strengthening effect, and it hints weakly), (2) colds are caused by viruses and don't respond to antibiotics, even if goldenseal were an effect systemic (whole body) antibiotic, which it almost certainly isn't, and (3) goldenseal was never used traditionally for the common cold.

The other myth that has helped drive the sales of goldenseal is the widespread street belief that it can block a positive drug screen. The origin of this false idea dates back to a work of fiction published in 1900 by a pharmacist and author named John Uri Lloyd. In *Stringtown on the Pike*, Lloyd's most successful novel, a dead man is found to have traces of goldenseal in his stomach. In fact, he had taken goldenseal regularly as a digestive aid, but a toxicology expert mistakes the goldenseal for strychnine and deduces intentional murder.

This work of fiction sufficed to create a folkloric connection between goldenseal and drug testing. Although the goldenseal in the story actually made a drug test come out falsely positive, this has been turned around to become a belief that goldenseal can make urine drug screens come out negative. A word to the wise: it doesn't work.

Dosage

When used as a topical treatment for **minor skin wounds**, a sufficient quantity of goldenseal cream, ointment, or powder should be applied to cover the wound. Make sure to clean the wound at least once a day to prevent goldenseal particles from being trapped in the healing tissues.

For mouth sores and sore throats, goldenseal tincture is swished or gargled. Goldenseal may also be used as strong tea for this purpose, made by boiling 0.5 to 1 g in a cup of water. Warning: it tastes very bitter! Goldenseal tea is also used as a douche for **vaginal yeast infections**.

Safety Issues

Although there are no reports of severe adverse effects attributable to use of goldenseal, this herb has not undergone much safety testing.

One study suggests that topical use of goldenseal could cause photosensitivity (an increased tendency to react to sun exposure).

Goldenseal should not be used by pregnant women, for at least three reasons: goldenseal has been reported to cause uterine contractions, and berberine may increase levels of bilirubin and cause genetic damage. The last of these effects indicates that individuals with elevated bilirubin levels (jaundice) should also avoid use of goldenseal. Safety in young children, nursing women, or those with severe liver or kidney disease is also not established.

Just as there are incorrect rumors regarding the benefits of goldenseal, there are popular but incorrect beliefs regarding its health risks. For example, it is often said that goldenseal can disrupt the normal bacteria of the intestines. However, there is no scientific evidence that this occurs. Another fallacy is that small overdoses of goldenseal are toxic, causing ulcerations of the stomach and other mucous membranes. This idea is based on a misunderstanding of old literature.

Some evidence suggests that goldenseal might interact with various medications by altering the way they are metabolized in the liver. One study found that berberine impairs metabolism of the drug **cyclosporine**, thereby raising its levels. This could potentially cause toxicity.

Gotu Kola

Centella asiatica

PRINCIPAL PROPOSED NATURAL USES: *Venous Insufficiency/Varicose Veins*

OTHER PROPOSED NATURAL USES: *Anal Fissures, Anxiety, Burn Healing, Cellulite, Hemorrhoids, Improving Mental Performance, Keloid Scars, Liver Cirrhosis, Periodontal Disease, Scleroderma, Wound Healing*

Gotu kola is a creeping plant native to subtropical and tropical climates. Gotu kola has a long history of use in Ayurvedic medicine (the traditional medicine of India) to promote wound healing and slow the progress of leprosy. It was also reputed to prolong life, increase energy, and enhance sexual potency. Other uses of gotu kola included treating skin diseases, anxiety, diarrhea, menstrual disorders, vaginal discharge, and venereal disease.

Based on these many traditional indications, gotu kola was accepted as a drug in France in the 1880s. British physicians in Africa used a special extract to treat leprosy.

What Is Gotu Kola Used for Today?

The best-documented use of gotu kola is to treat **chronic venous insufficiency**, a condition closely related to varicose veins. In these conditions, blood pools in the legs, causing aching, pain, heaviness, swelling, fatigue, and unsightly visible veins. Preliminary double-blind, placebo-controlled studies indicate that gotu kola extract provides improvement in major venous insufficiency symptoms, reducing swelling, pain, fatigue, sensation of heaviness, and fluid leakage from the veins. However, no studies have evaluated whether regular use of gotu kola can make visible varicose veins disappear, or prevent new ones from developing.

Gotu kola has also been suggested as a treatment for **hemorrhoids** because they are a type of varicose vein, but there is no direct evidence that it is helpful for this purpose.

Like other herbs used for the treatment of varicose veins, gotu kola is thought to work by strengthening connective tissues. This has led to trials of gotu kola extracts for preventing or treating keloid scars, and treating anal fissures, bladder ulcers, **burns**, cellulite, dermatitis, **liver cirrhosis**, **periodontal disease**, **scleroderma**, and **wounds**. However, again there is no real evidence as yet that gotu kola is effective for any of these conditions.

One study provides weak evidence that gotu kola might be helpful for **anxiety**.

Gotu kola has a reputation for improving memory, and the positive results from a study in rats performed in 1992 produced a temporary rush of public interest in gotu kola as a "brain booster." However, benefits in humans have not been demonstrated.

Gotu kola should not be confused with the caffeine-containing kola nut, used in original recipes for Coca-Cola.

What Is the Scientific Evidence for Gotu Kola?

Venous Insufficiency/Varicose Veins

There is significant but not definitive scientific evidence for the effectiveness of gotu kola for the treatment of **varicose veins/venous insufficiency**.

For example, a 2-month, double-blind, placebo-controlled study of 94 people with venous insufficiency of the lower limb compared the benefits of gotu kola extract at 120 mg daily and 60 mg daily against a placebo. The results showed a significant dose-related improvement in the treated groups in symptoms such as subjective heaviness, discomfort, and edema.

Another 2-month study of double-blind design enrolled 90 people with varicose veins and compared the benefits of gotu kola at 60 mg and 30 mg daily against placebo. Again, the results showed improvements in both treated groups, but greater improvement at the higher dose.

In one study of people with venous insufficiency, 2 weeks of treatment with gotu kola extracts was shown to reduce the time necessary for the swelling to disappear.

Another study of double-blind design followed 87 people with varicose veins and compared the benefits of gotu kola at 60 mg and 30 mg daily against placebo. Again, the results showed improvements in both treated groups, but greater improvement at the higher dose.

Anxiety

Gotu kola has been used in traditional Ayurvedic medicine to treat anxiety. Because evidence suggests that easy startling is related to anxiety, researchers have attempted to test this use by measuring the acoustic startle response. In this double-blind, placebo-controlled trial, 40 study participants were given either gotu kola or placebo and then subjected to sudden loud noises. Researchers measured eye blinks and found a significantly reduced startle response in those treated with gotu kola. This suggests, but doesn't prove, that gotu kola may be helpful for anxiety.

Dosage

The usual dosage of gotu kola is 20 to 60 mg 3 times daily of an extract standardized to contain 40% asiaticoside, 29 to 30% asiatic acid, 29 to 30% madecassic acid, and 1 to 2% madecassoside. When using it for venous insufficiency, gotu kola takes at least 4 weeks to work.

For the prevention of keloid scars (a purpose for which gotu kola has *not* been proven effective), the herb is typically taken for 3 months prior to surgery and for another 3 months afterwards.

Safety Issues

When taken orally, gotu kola seldom causes any side effects other than the occasional allergic skin rash, and safety studies suggest that it is essentially non-toxic. However, one animal study hints that gotu kola might have carcinogenic effects if applied topically to the skin.

Although gotu kola has not been proven safe for pregnant or nursing women, studies in rabbits suggest that it does not harm fetal development, and Italian physicians have given it to pregnant women. Safety in young children and those with severe liver or kidney disease has not been established.

Grass Pollen Extract

PRINCIPAL PROPOSED USES: *Prostate Enlargement (BPH)*

OTHER PROPOSED USES: *High Cholesterol, Menopausal Symptoms, Premenstrual Syndrome (PMS), Prostate Cancer, Prostatitis*

Like the more famous saw palmetto, extracts of grass pollen are used to treat prostate enlargement. The grass mixture utilized to make this preparation consists of 92% rye, 5% timothy, and 3% corn. Grass pollen has also been investigated for its potential to treat prostatitis, prostate cancer, symptoms of menopause and PMS, and for reducing cholesterol.

Related grass pollen extracts are used for allergy shots. The grass pollen extracts described here have their allergenic component removed, and so can't possibly work to treat hay fever (see Safety Issues below). Grass pollen is also an entirely different product than **bee pollen**.

Sources

Grass pollen extract tablets for prostate disease are available in pharmacies and health food stores or can be ordered from a number of sources on the Internet.

Therapeutic Dosages

The recommended dosage for grass pollen extract tablets is between 80 and 120 mg per day.

Therapeutic Uses

Two double-blind, placebo-controlled studies found that grass pollen extract can help reduce symptoms of **be-**

nign prostate enlargement (technically called *benign prostatic hyperplasia*, or BPH).

One small, double-blind study found evidence that a product containing grass pollen, the pistils (seed-bearing parts) of grass, and royal jelly (a product made by bees) may be helpful for **premenstrual syndrome (PMS)**. Another small double-blind study found benefit with the same combination for treatment of **menopausal symptoms**.

Grass pollen extract has also shown promise for treating **prostatitis**. In a 6-month, double-blind study of 60 men with non-bacterial prostatitis, use of the grass pollen extract was more effective than placebo in relieving symptoms.

Grass pollen has additionally been investigated for its usefulness in treating prostate cancer and **high cholesterol**. Animal studies also suggest that it may **protect the liver** from damage by some types of poisons. However, the scientific evidence for all of these other proposed uses remains very weak.

What Is the Scientific Evidence for Grass Pollen Extract?

Two double-blind, placebo-controlled studies found that grass pollen extract can improve symptoms of BPH.

In the first double-blind, placebo-controlled study, 103 people with BPH were assigned to take either placebo or

2 capsules of a standardized grass pollen extract 3 times daily for a period of 12 weeks. At the end of the study, 69% of the participants who had been taking the grass pollen had reduced the number of trips they had to make to the bathroom at night. In the placebo group, only 37% reported improvement in this symptom. The amount of urine remaining in the bladder following urination was reduced in the treatment group by 24 ml and by 4 ml for the placebo group. Both of these were statistically significant improvements for those taking grass pollen.

The second double-blind, placebo-controlled study lasted longer but enrolled fewer participants. Fifty-seven men with prostate enlargement were enrolled in the study, with 31 taking 92 mg of the grass pollen extract daily for 6 months and the remaining 26 taking placebo. As with the previous study, statistically significant improvements in nighttime frequency of urination and emptying of the bladder were found with use of grass pollen extract. Additionally, 69% of the participants receiving treatment reported overall improvement, while only 29% of the group taking the placebo felt they had improved—another statistically significant difference.

An important finding in this study was that, according to ultrasound measurements, prostate size decreased in men taking grass pollen. Not all treatments for BPH can reduce prostate size. It may be that treatments that shrink the prostate can reduce the need for surgery—such is the case, at least, with the prescription drug finasteride. Whether grass pollen offers this same potential benefit is not yet known.

Two additional studies compared grass pollen to other alternative treatments for prostate enlargement, rather than to placebo. An open study pitted grass pollen against **pygeum**. Although pygeum is considered a more established treatment for prostate enlargement, grass pollen appeared to work better. The pollen extract was found to be significantly more effective in improving the flow of urine, emptying of the bladder, and the participants' perceptions of relief. Those in the grass pollen group also had a significant reduction in prostate size while there was no reduction of size in the pygeum group. It appears from this that grass pollen is a more effective treatment than pygeum, but since the study was not blinded, the results are somewhat questionable. (For more information on why double-blind studies are so important, see **Why Does This Book Rely on Double-blind Studies?**.)

A double-blind comparative study pitted grass pollen against an amino acid preparation and found no significant difference between the two. Unfortunately, since we don't know how well the amino acid medication works, the result has little meaning.

No one is certain how the grass pollen extract might cause the beneficial results seen in the studies. One theory is that it inhibits the body's manufacturing of prostaglandins and leukotrienes, which might relieve congestion and act as an anti-inflammatory. This, however, probably would not explain the reduction in prostate size, meaning that there may be more than one mechanism at work.

Safety Issues

No serious side effects have been reported with the use of grass pollen extract. No adverse reactions were observed in any of the clinical trials discussed above, although one review author mentioned rare reports of stomach upset and skin rash.

Although many people are allergic to grass pollen, the grass pollen products discussed in this article are processed to remove allergenic proteins. For this reason, it is unlikely that grass-allergic individuals will have an allergic reaction.

Maximum safe doses for young children, pregnant or nursing women, or those with liver or kidney disease are not known.

Greater Celandine

Chelidonium majus

PRINCIPAL PROPOSED USES: *None*

OTHER PROPOSED USES: *Dyspepsia, Warts (Topical Use)*

Note: *Greater celandine contains toxic constituents and we recommend against using it.*

The herb greater celandine (*Chelidonium majus*), a relative of the poppy, contains an orange-colored juice that has been used medicinally for thousands of years. It has been applied topically for eye and skin problems and taken internally for bronchitis, jaundice, indigestion, cancer, and whooping cough. However, traditional herbalists appear to have missed one major problem with this herb: it can damage the liver.

What Is Greater Celandine Used for Today?

Test-tube and animal studies provide weak evidence that greater celandine may both stimulate and relax the gallbladder.

In Europe, it is commonly believed that minor gallbladder problems are a cause of indigestion. On this basis, celandine was approved in 1985 by Germany's Commission E as a treatment for what we would call **dyspepsia**, or non-specific digestive distress. While there is some supporting evidence for this use, in view of the safety risks associated with celandine (see Safety Issues below), we do not recommend using it for this purpose (or any other).

Very preliminary evidence suggests that constituents of celandine may also have cancer preventive and antimicrobial properties.

Celandine has also traditionally been advocated as a topical treatment for **warts**. However, there is no reliable evidence that it is effective for this purpose.

Dosage

A typical dosage of greater celandine extract is standardized to supply 4 mg of the substance chelidonine 3 times daily. However, we suggest that you do not use it at all. (See Safety Issues.)

For the treatment of warts, greater celandine is applied directly to the wart and allowed to dry there.

Safety Issues

Numerous case reports indicate that use of celandine can lead to severe, potentially fatal liver injury.

It should be noted that most people who use greater celandine do not develop liver problems. It may be that certain individuals have an especially high level of susceptibility. However, since it is not possible to determine in advance who would be at risk, we recommend that, until more is known, the internal use of greater celandine should be avoided entirely.

Green-Lipped Mussel

Perna canaliculus

PRINCIPAL PROPOSED USES: *Osteoarthritis*

OTHER PROPOSED USES: *Asthma, Rheumatoid Arthritis*

The green-lipped mussel, a common appetizer in sushi restaurants, contains healthy fats in the omega-3 family. Like **fish oil**, another source of omega-3 fatty acids, green-lipped mussel has shown some promise for reducing inflammation. Inflammation is the cause of symptoms in numerous illnesses, ranging from arthritis to asthma. On this basis, green-lipped mussel has been promoted as a treatment for these conditions. However, the evidence that it provides any meaningful benefits remains highly preliminary.

Therapeutic Uses

There are two major forms of arthritis: **osteoarthritis** and **rheumatoid arthritis**. Rheumatoid arthritis is primarily a disease of inflammation, and the anti-inflammatory omega-3 fatty acids found in fish oil have been successfully used to treat it. Inflammation plays a relatively less important role in osteoarthritis. However, green-lipped mussel has been tried for both conditions, with, at present, inconclusive results.

Unlike standard **nonsteroidal anti-inflammatory drugs** (NSAIDs), which harm the stomach wall, green-lipped mussel might actually help prevent **ulcers**.

Green-lipped mussel has also shown some promise for **asthma**.

What Is the Scientific Evidence for Green-Lipped Mussel?

Arthritis

The evidence regarding use of green-lipped mussel for arthritis remains weak and inconsistent.

Several animal studies performed by a single research group have reported that green-lipped mussel reduces symptoms of osteoarthritis. However, the results from human studies remain inconsistent. There are five reported controlled studies of green-lipped mussel for osteoarthritis, and, of these, only two found benefit.

Asthma

In an 8-week, double-blind, placebo-controlled trial of 46 people with allergic asthma, those who received a green-lipped mussel extract showed some improvement in wheezing and peak flow of air.

Therapeutic Dosages

A typical dose of green-lipped mussel is about 200 mg per day of the lipid extract or 1,000 mg per day of the freeze-dried powder.

Safety Issues

In studies, green-lipped mussel has not caused much in the way of side effects other than occasional mild digestive distress. People with shellfish allergies, however, should avoid green-lipped mussel.

Unlike oysters, green-lipped mussel does not appear to contain heavy metals.

Green Tea

Camellia sinensis

PRINCIPAL PROPOSED USES: *Cancer Prevention, Gingivitis*
OTHER PROPOSED USES: *Heart Disease Prevention, High Cholesterol, Liver Disease Prevention, Rosacea, Sun Damage Protection, Weight Loss*

People have been drinking tea for thousands of years, but in the last couple of decades a number of potential health benefits have been attributed to this ancient beverage. Black tea and green tea are made from the same plant, but a higher level of the original substances endure in the less-processed green form.

What Is Green Tea Used for Today?

Green tea contains high levels of substances called *catechin polyphenols*, known to possess strong antioxidant, anticarcinogenic, antitumorigenic, and even antibiotic properties. Based on these findings, as well as observational studies, green tea has become popular as a daily drink for preventing **cancer** and **heart disease**. However, some observational trials failed to find indications of benefit with green tea. Furthermore, only double-blind, placebo-controlled studies can prove a treatment effective, and there is little direct evidence of this type regarding green tea and cancer or heart disease prevention. (For more information on why double-blind studies are so important, see **Why Does this Book Rely on Double-blind Studies?**.) One such study found that green teas produced short-term improvements in cholesterol profile, but they disappeared after 4 weeks. More positive results were seen in a study that evaluated a form of green tea enriched with the substance theaflavin, found in black tea. In this fairly large (more than 200 participants), 3-month study, use of the tea product resulted in significant, ongoing reductions in LDL ("bad") cholesterol as compared to placebo.

Preliminary studies suggest that certain green tea polyphenols may help prevent skin cancer if they are applied directly to the skin. In addition, there is some evidence that green tea constituents might help protect the skin from **sun damage**. Unlike normal sunscreen preparations, green tea does not physically block ultraviolet light. Rather, it seems to protect cells from some of the damage caused by ultraviolet light. Because it works by such a different mechanism of action, green tea might offer synergistic benefits if combined with standard sunscreens. However, in an 8-week, double-blind, placebo-controlled study of 40 women who *already* had symptoms of aging skin, combined use of oral green tea and a topical green tea cream failed to prove more effective than placebo. Some possible benefits were seen in microscopic evaluation of skin condition.

Topical green tea extracts have also shown a bit of promise for the treatment of **cervical dysplasia**, while oral green tea extracts might reduce risk of prostate cancer, according to a small pilot study.

A small, double-blind, placebo-controlled trial found weak evidence that green tea chew candy might reduce gum inflammation in individuals with **periodontal disease** (gingivitis).

Green tea has been proposed as means of preventing **liver disease**, but the evidence for this use remains unconvincing.

Green tea is sometimes recommended for **weight loss** on the basis of rather theoretical evidence that it speeds up metabolism. However, there is little direct scientific backing for this use. Other evidence indicates that if green tea increases metabolism at all, the effect is extremely small. A study using oolong tea enriched with green tea catechins found some apparent weight-loss benefit; however, another study failed to find green tea itself helpful for preventing weight regain after weight loss. In yet another study, use of green tea failed to produce significant weight loss in overweight women with polycystic ovary syndrome.

One preliminary study, available only in abstract form, found some evidence that green tea cream may be helpful for **rosacea**. The results of another study weakly hint that green tea extracts taken orally might reduce symptoms of **benign prostatic hyperplasia**.

One study found that inhaled tea catechins could reduce levels of resistant staph carried in the sputum of disabled seniors. **Note:** Do not attempt to inhale green tea products.

Dosage

Studies weakly suggest that 3 cups of green tea daily might provide protection against cancer. However, because not everyone wants to take the time to drink green tea, manufacturers have offered extracts that can be taken in pill form. A typical dosage is 100 to 150 mg 3 times daily of a green tea extract standardized to contain 80% total polyphenols and 50% epigallocatechin gallate. Whether these extracts offer any benefit remains unknown. Furthermore, there are serious concerns about liver toxicity with use of green tea extracts (see Safety Issues below).

Warning: In an analysis performed in 2006 by the respected testing organization ConsumerLabs.com, some tested green tea products were found to be contaminated with lead.

Safety Issues

As a widely consumed beverage, green tea is generally regarded as safe. It does contain caffeine, at perhaps a slightly lower level than black tea, and can therefore cause insomnia, nervousness, and the other well-known symptoms of excess caffeine intake.

Green tea extracts, however, may not be safe. There are several case reports in which use of a concentrated green tea extract was associated with liver inflamma-

tion. In most cases, liver problems disappeared after the extract was discontinued, but in one case, permanent liver failure ensued, requiring liver transplantation. While it is not certain that the green tea extract *caused* the liver problems, nor how it might do so, these reports do raise significant concerns about use of green tea extracts.

Green tea should not be given to infants and young children. There are theoretical concerns that high dosages of EGCG might be unsafe for pregnant women.

Dried green tea leaf contains significant levels of vitamin K on a per-weight basis. On this basis, it has been stated that people using blood thinners in the warfarin (Coumadin) family should avoid green tea, because vitamin K antagonizes the effect of those drugs. However, green tea taken as a *beverage* provides such small amounts of the vitamin that the risk seems minimal for normal consumption. There is one case report of problems that developed in a person on warfarin who consumed as much as a gallon of green tea daily.

Interactions You Should Know About

If you are taking:

➤ **MAO inhibitors: The caffeine in green tea could cause serious problems.**
➤ **Warfarin (Coumadin): Avoid drinking large quantities of green tea.**

Guarana
Paullinia cupana

PRINCIPAL PROPOSED USES: *Enhancing Mental Function, Fatigue*
OTHER PROPOSED USES: *Sports Performance Enhancement, Weight Loss*

Guarana, an herb from the Amazon rain forest, has a long history of use as a stimulant beverage. It has also been used to treat arthritis, diarrhea, and headaches.

What Is Guarana Used for Today?

Like tea, coffee, and chocolate, guarana contains alkaloids in the caffeine family, such as theobromine and theophylline. Caffeine is known to reduce pain, treat **mi-**

graine headaches, and, of course, fight fatigue. In addition, it may, under certain circumstances, **enhance sports performance, improve mental function**, and modestly aid **weight loss**.

Most of the proposed uses of guarana fall into line with these effects of caffeine. For example, in one double-blind, placebo-controlled study, use of guarana alone or guarana plus **ginseng** appeared to significantly improve mental function. Interestingly, the amount of caffeine in the guarana preparation used was very small and would not seem to account for the apparent benefits. However, this study was small and had some problems in its design. In two other studies, no benefits were seen.

Another double-blind, placebo-controlled study tested the effects of guarana plus ephedra for weight loss. In this trial, a total of 67 overweight people were given either placebo or a combination of guarana and ephedra for a period of 8 weeks. The results showed significantly greater weight loss in the treated group than in the placebo group. However, ephedra is an unsafe substance. (See the **Ephedra** article for more information.)

Dosage

A typical dose of guarana supplies 50 mg of caffeine, about half the amount in a cup of strong coffee. However, a 1998 analysis of products on the market indicated that many guarana products contain less than the advertised amount of guarana.

Safety Issues

The side effects of guarana would be expected to be similar to those of tea or coffee, such as heartburn, gastritis, insomnia, anxiety, and heart arrhythmias (benign palpitations or more serious disturbances of heart rhythm). Combination products containing guarana and ephedra would be expected to present additional risk. Finally, all drug interactions that can occur with caffeine would be expected to occur with guarana as well (see Interactions You Should Know About).

Young children, pregnant or nursing women, or people with heart disease should not use guarana.

Interactions You Should Know About

If you are taking:

> - **MAO inhibitors:** The caffeine in guarana could cause dangerous drug interactions.
> - **Stimulant drugs such as Ritalin:** The stimulant effects of guarana might be amplified.
> - **Drugs to prevent heart arrhythmias or treat insomnia or anxiety:** Guarana might interfere with their actions.

Guggul
Commiphora mukul

PRINCIPAL PROPOSED USES: *High Cholesterol*
OTHER PROPOSED USES: *Acne, Diabetes, Weight Loss*

Guggul, the sticky gum resin from the mukul myrrh tree, plays a major role in **Ayurveda**, the traditional herbal medicine of India. It was traditionally combined with other herbs for the treatment of arthritis, skin diseases, pains in the nervous system, obesity, digestive problems, infections in the mouth, and menstrual problems.

What Is Guggul Used for Today?

Based on preliminary studies, guggul has become a popular herbal treatment for **high cholesterol**. However, the best-designed trial failed to find benefit.

Other potential uses of guggul have no more than minimal supporting evidence. One small study hints that guggul might be helpful for **acne**. In addition, a study in mice found potential **antidiabetic** effects.

Recently, guggul has been promoted as a **weight-loss** agent. Supposedly, it works by enhancing thyroid function. However, there is little evidence that guggul actually affects the thyroid, and one small, double-blind, placebo-controlled trial failed to find it effective for weight loss.

What Is the Scientific Evidence for Guggul?

High Cholesterol

Three double-blind studies performed in India found evidence that guggul can reduce cholesterol levels. However, the largest placebo-controlled study failed to find benefit.

One of the positive placebo-controlled studies enrolled 61 individuals and followed them for 24 weeks. After 12 weeks of following a healthy diet, half the participants received placebo and the other half received guggul at a dose providing 100 mg of guggulsterones daily. The results after 24 weeks of treatment showed that the treated group experienced an 11.7% decrease in total cholesterol, along with a 12.7% decrease in LDL ("bad" cholesterol), a 12% decrease in triglycerides, and an 11.1% decrease in the total cholesterol/HDL ("good" cholesterol) ratio. These improvements were significantly greater than what was seen in the placebo group.

Similar results were seen in a double-blind, placebo-controlled trial of 40 individuals.

A double-blind study of 228 individuals given either guggul or the standard drug clofibrate found approximately equal efficacy between the two treatments. However, the absence of a placebo group makes these results less than reliable.

In contrast to these results, a double-blind, placebo-controlled study of 103 people failed to find guggul effective at a dose of 75 mg or 150 mg of guggulsterones daily. In fact, the herb seemed to worsen levels of LDL ("bad") cholesterol. The reason for this discrepancy is not clear.

Acne

A small controlled trial compared oral gugulipid (50 mg of guggulsterones twice daily) against tetracycline for the treatment of acne and reported equivalent results. Unfortunately, the study report does not state whether this trial was double-blind, and it also lacked a placebo group. (For information on why this matters, see **Why Does This Book Rely on Double-blind Studies?**.)

Dosage

Guggul is manufactured in a standardized form that provides a fixed amount of guggulsterones, the presumed active ingredients in guggul. The typical daily dose should provide 100 mg of guggulsterones.

Safety Issues

In clinical trials of standardized guggul extract, no significant side effects other than occasional mild gastrointestinal distress or allergic skin rashes have been seen. Laboratory tests conducted in the course of these trials did not reveal any alterations in liver or kidney function, blood cell numbers and appearance, heart function, or blood chemistry.

Drugs in the **statin family** used to reduce cholesterol can cause a potentially serious condition called *rhabdomyolysis*, in which muscle fibers break down. One case report hints that this could occur with guggul as well.

Safety in young children, pregnant or nursing women, or those with severe liver or kidney disease has not been established.

Gymnema

Gymnema sylvestre

PRINCIPAL PROPOSED USES: *Diabetes*

Native to the forests of India, *Gymnema sylvestre* (also called *gumar*) has a coincidental double relationship to sugar: when placed on the tongue, it blocks the sensation of sweetness, and when taken internally, it might help control blood sugar levels in people with diabetes. (There doesn't seem to be any connection between these two uses.)

Practitioners of **Ayurveda** (the traditional medicine of

India) first used gymnema to treat diabetes almost 2,000 years ago. In the 1920s, preliminary scientific studies found some evidence that gymnema leaves can reduce blood sugar levels, but nothing much came of this observation for decades. Research in India picked up again in the 1980s and 90s, leading to the publication of promising preliminary studies in people.

What Is Gymnema Used for Today?

Gymnema has become increasingly popular in the United States as a supportive treatment for diabetes. However, the evidence that it works remains weak. Only double-blind, placebo-controlled studies can prove a treatment effective, and none have yet been reported for gymnema. Current evidence is limited to a few animal studies and human open trials.

Warning: This herb is advocated as a support to standard treatment, not as a replacement for it. Gymnema definitely cannot be used as a substitute for insulin treatment and has not been proven strong enough for use in lieu of oral diabetes medications. However, there are also potential risks involved in adding gymnema to an existing treatment regimen. See Safety Issues below.

Dosage

Gymnema is usually taken at a dosage of 400 to 600 mg daily of an extract standardized to contain 24% gymnemic acid.

Safety Issues

When used in appropriate dosages, gymnema appears to be fairly safe, although extensive studies have not been performed. One obvious risk is that if gymnema is successful, it may lower blood sugar levels too far, causing a dangerous hypoglycemic reaction. For this reason, medical supervision is essential.

Safety in young children, pregnant or nursing women, or those with severe kidney or liver disease has not been established.

Interactions You Should Know About

If you are taking **insulin** or **oral medications to reduce blood sugar levels**: Gymnema might cause them to work even better, potentially causing hypoglycemia. Therefore, you may need to reduce your dose of medication.

Hawthorn
Crataegus oxyacantha

PRINCIPAL PROPOSED USES: *Congestive Heart Failure*

OTHER PROPOSED USES: *Benign Heart Palpitations, High Blood Pressure, Orthostatic Hypotension (in Combination with Camphor)*

The name "hawthorn" is derived from "hedgethorn," reflecting this spiny tree's use as a living fence in much of Europe. Besides protecting estates from trespassers, hawthorn has also been used medicinally since ancient times. Roman physicians used hawthorn as a heart drug in the first century A.D., but most of the literature from that period focuses on its symbolic use for religious rites and political ceremonies.

During the Middle Ages, hawthorn was used for the treatment of dropsy, a condition we now call congestive heart failure. It was also used for treating other heart ailments, as well as for sore throat.

What Is Hawthorn Used for Today?

Meaningful evidence indicates that hawthorn is a safe and effective treatment for **congestive heart failure** (CHF). Like other treatments used for CHF, hawthorn improves the heart's pumping ability. However, it may offer some important advantages over certain conventional drugs used for this condition.

Digoxin, as well as other medications that increase the power of the heart, also make the heart more susceptible to dangerous irregularities of rhythm (arrhythmias). In contrast, preliminary evidence indicates that hawthorn may have the unusual property of both strengthening the heart and stabilizing it against arrhythmias.

It is thought to do so by lengthening what is called the *refractory period*. This term refers to the short period following a heartbeat during which the heart cannot beat again. Many irregularities of heart rhythm begin with an early beat. Digoxin shortens the refractory period, making such a premature beat more likely, while hawthorn protects against such potentially dangerous breaks in the heart's even rhythm.

Another advantage of hawthorn is its lower toxicity. With digoxin, the difference between the proper dosage and the toxic dosage is dangerously small. Hawthorn has an enormous range of safe dosing.

However, keep in mind that digoxin is itself an outdated drug. There are many newer drugs for CHF (such as ACE inhibitors) that are much more effective and have been proven to save lives. Hawthorn has not been shown to provide the same benefit. And it is not clear whether one can safely combine hawthorn with other drugs that affect the heart. Furthermore, CHF is simply too dangerous a condition to rely solely on self-treatment.

The bottom line: If you have CHF, do not use hawthorn except under close physician supervision.

In addition to CHF, hawthorn is sometimes used as a treatment for annoying heart palpitations that have been thoroughly evaluated and found to be harmless. Common symptoms include occasional thumping as well as episodes of racing heartbeat. These may occur without any identifiable cause and may not require any medical treatment, except for purposes of comfort. However, there is no evidence that hawthorn is effective for this purpose. Furthermore, because there are many dangerous kinds of heart palpitations, it is absolutely necessary to get a thorough checkup first. It is only worth considering hawthorn as a treatment for palpitations if a doctor tells you that you have no medically significant heart problems.

Hawthorn is sometimes recommended for the treatment of **high blood pressure**, but its effects appear to be marginal at best. Furthermore, there is some evidence that a combination herbal treatment made from haw-

thorn and camphor can help prevent the sudden fall in blood pressure that may occur on standing up from a sitting or lying position (orthosatic hypotension). In these studies, hawthorn acted to *increase* blood pressure.

Hawthorn has also been tried for other heart-related conditions, such as **angina** and **atherosclerosis** in general, but there is no reliable evidence to support these uses.

What Is the Scientific Evidence for Hawthorn?

At least nine reasonable-quality, double-blind, placebo-controlled trials, involving a total of more than 750 participants, have found hawthorn effective for the treatment of mild to moderate congestive heart failure.

In one of the best of these studies, 209 people with relatively advanced congestive heart failure (technically, New York Heart Association [NYHA] class III) were given either 1,800 mg or 900 mg of standardized hawthorn extract or matching placebo. The results after 16 weeks of therapy showed significant improvements in the hawthorn groups as compared to the placebo groups. Benefits in the high-dose hawthorn group included a reduction in subjective symptoms as well as an increase in exercise capacity. Subjective symptoms improved to a similar degree in the lower-dose hawthorn group, but there was no improvement in exercise capacity.

A comparative study suggests that hawthorn extract (900 mg) is about as effective as a low dose of the conventional drug captopril. However, while captopril and other standard drugs in the same family have been shown to help reduce hospitalizations and mortality associated with CHF, there is no similar evidence for hawthorn.

Dosage

The usual dosage of hawthorn is 300 to 600 mg 3 times daily of an extract standardized to contain about 2 to 3% flavonoids or 18 to 20% procyanidins. Studies indicate that full effects may take up to 6 months to develop, although some improvement should be apparent much sooner.

Safety Issues

Hawthorn appears to be safe. Germany's Commission E lists no known risks, contraindications, or drug interactions with hawthorn, and mice and rats have been given very large doses without showing significant toxicity. In clinical trials, reported side effects were rare, consisting primarily of mild stomach upset and occasional allergic reactions (skin rash).

Perhaps the biggest risk with hawthorn is that using it instead of conventional treatment might increase risk of death or other complications of CHF. In addition, it is not known whether hawthorn can be safely combined with other drugs that affect the heart. Therefore (to reit-erate), do not self-treat CHF with hawthorn! A physician's supervision is essential.

Safety in young children, pregnant or nursing women, or those with severe liver, heart, or kidney disease has not been established.

Interactions You Should Know About

If you are taking any medications that affect the heart: It is possible that taking hawthorn could cause problems.

He Shou Wu
Polygonum multiflorum

ALTERNATE NAMES/RELATED TERMS: *Fo Ti*

PRINCIPAL PROPOSED USES: *None*

OTHER PROPOSED USES: *Aging in General, Constipation, Enhancing Mental Function, Graying Hair, Heart Disease Prevention, High Cholesterol, Immune Support, Insomnia*

The name of this herb literally means "Black-haired Mr. He," in reference to an ancient story of a Mr. He who restored his vitality, sexual potency, and youthful appearance by taking the herb now named after him. He shou wu is widely used in China for the traditional purpose of restoring black hair and other signs of youth.

Traditional Chinese herbal medicine ordinarily recommends the use of herbs in complex formulas, but He shou wu is also often taken as a single herb. He shou wu is often called *fo ti*; pure, unprocessed root is named white *fo ti*, while herb boiled in black-bean liquid according to a traditional process is called red *fo ti*. The two forms are said to have somewhat different properties.

What Is He Shou Wu Used for Today?

He shou wu is widely marketed today as a general anti-aging herb, said to reduce **cholesterol**, prevent heart disease, prevent age-related loss of mental function, improve sleep, and extend life span. However, the evidence supporting these uses is far too preliminary to meaningfully indicate effectiveness for any of these proposed uses.

He shou wu is reputed to strengthen immunity; however, one constituent of the herb, emodin, has shown some promise as an immune system suppressant!

Finally, He shou wu has a traditional reputation as a mild laxative. In support of this, it has been pointed out that emodin belongs to a family of chemicals called *anthraquinones*; other members of this family act as laxatives. However, animal research has failed to find any evidence that emodin itself has a laxative effect.

Dosage

A typical dose of He shou wu is 3 g of the raw herb 3 times daily, or according to the label for processed extracts. For most purposes, the processed or "red" *fo ti* is said to be superior. However, the raw herb is said to be more effective for constipation.

Safety Issues

Detailed modern safety studies have not been performed on this herb. Immediate side effects are infrequent, primarily limited to mild diarrhea and the rare allergic reaction. Safety for young children, pregnant or nursing women, or those with severe kidney or liver disease has not been established.

Case reports relate use of a popular He shou wu product to liver inflammation. However, it is not clear whether He shou wu herb itself was responsible; Asian herbal preparations of this type have frequently been found to contain unlisted toxic ingredients, either due to poor quality control or deliberate adulteration.

Hibiscus

Hibiscus sabdariffa

ALTERNATE NAMES/RELATED TERMS: *Roselle*
PRINCIPAL PROPOSED USES: *High Blood Pressure*
OTHER PROPOSED USES: *Cancer Prevention, High Cholesterol, Liver Protection*

The red-flowered hibiscus shrub is a widely cultivated ornamental and, because of its pleasant, tangy taste, it is a common constituent of herbal beverage teas. Medicinally, hibiscus has been taken internally for the treatment of various forms of digestive upset, along with scurvy, anxiety, and fevers. It is said to have an antiseptic and astringent effect when used topically.

What is Hibiscus Used for Today?

Animal studies have suggested that hibiscus might have a **blood pressure–lowering effect**. Based on this, preliminary human studies were conducted, with somewhat promising results.

In one study, 54 people with hypertension were given either hibiscus tea or no extra treatment for 2 weeks. By the end of the study, people in the hibiscus group had significantly improved blood pressure as compared to those in the group receiving no extra treatment. Unfortunately, these results aren't as impressive as they may sound; for a variety of reasons, people who are enrolled in a study and given a treatment tend to improve, regardless of whether the treatment itself actually works. In order to actually show that a treatment works, it must be compared against a placebo.

Another flawed study enrolled 90 people with hypertension and compared the effectiveness of hibiscus (10 g dried hibiscus calyx in water daily) against the standard drug captopril (25 mg twice daily). The results showed equal benefit. Unfortunately, once more the study is less meaningful than it sounds. This study also failed to use a placebo group and it, too, was not double-blind. (For detailed information on why double-blind, placebo-controlled studies are essential, see **Why Does This Book Rely on Double-blind Studies?**)

Hibiscus contains substances called *anthocyanins*, **antioxidants** similar to those found in **bilberry**, **cranberry**, and red wine. Very weak evidence, too weak to be relied upon at all, hints that hibiscus or its anthocyanin constituents may have **anti-cancer** and **liver-protective** effects, and might also improve **cholesterol** profile.

Dosage

A typical daily adult dosage of hibiscus is 10 g of dried calyx (part of the flower).

Safety Issues

As a widely used beverage tea, hibiscus is presumed to have a high degree of safety. However, comprehensive safety testing has not been performed. Maximum safe doses in pregnant or nursing women, young children, or individuals with severe liver or kidney disease have not been established.

Some evidence suggests that hibiscus might slightly alter the metabolism of the drug **acetaminophen**, though the effect is probably not large enough to be very important.

Histidine

SUPPLEMENT FORMS/ALTERNATE NAMES: *L-Histidine*

PRINCIPAL PROPOSED USES: *None*

OTHER PROPOSED USES: *Rheumatoid Arthritis*

Histidine is a semi-essential amino acid, which means your body normally makes as much as it needs. Like most other amino acids, histidine is used to make proteins and enzymes. The body also uses histidine to make histamine, the culprit behind the swelling and itching you feel in an allergic reaction.

It appears that people with rheumatoid arthritis may have low levels of histidine in their blood. This has led to some speculation that histidine supplements might be a good treatment for this kind of arthritis, but so far no studies have confirmed this.

Sources

Although histidine is not required in the diet, histidine deficiencies can occur during periods of very rapid growth. Dairy products, meat, poultry, fish, and other protein-rich foods are good sources of histidine.

Therapeutic Dosages

A typical therapeutic dosage of histidine is 4 to 5 g daily.

Therapeutic Uses

Although individuals with **rheumatoid arthritis** appear to have reduced levels of histidine in the blood, this by itself doesn't prove that taking histidine will help. One study designed to evaluate this question directly found no significant benefit.

Safety Issues

As a necessary nutrient, histidine is believed to be safe. However, maximum safe dosages of histidine have not been determined for young children, pregnant or nursing women, or those with severe liver or kidney disease. As with other supplements taken in large doses, it is important to purchase a quality product, as contaminants present even in very small percentages could conceivably add up and become toxic.

Hops

Humulus lupulus

PRINCIPAL PROPOSED USES: *None*

OTHER PROPOSED USES: *Anxiety, Breast Enhancement, Digestive Problems, Insomnia, Menopausal Symptoms*

Hops (the fruiting bodies of the hop plant) is most famous as the source of beer's bitter flavor, but it has a long history of use in herbal medicine as well. In Greece and Rome, hops was used as a remedy for poor digestion and intestinal disturbances. The Chinese used the herb for these purposes as well as to treat leprosy and tuberculosis.

As cultivation of hops for beer spread through Europe, it gradually became obvious that workers in hop fields tended to fall asleep on the job, more so than could be explained by the tedium of the work. This observation led to enthusiasm for using hops as a sedative. However, subsequent investigation suggests that much of the sedative effect seen in hop fields is due to an oil that evaporates quickly in storage.

Despite the absence of this oil, dried hop preparations do appear to be somewhat calming. While the exact reason is not clear, it seems that a sedating substance known as methylbutenol develops in the dried herb over a period of time. It may also be manufactured in the body from other constituents of dried hops.

What Is Hops Used for Today?

Germany's Commission E authorizes the use of hops for "discomfort due to restlessness or anxiety and sleep disturbances." However, scientists have had difficulty proving that hops causes sedation. Because its sedative effect is mild at most, the herb is often combined with other natural treatments for **anxiety** and **insomnia**, such as **valerian**.

Hops has fairly strong estrogen-like properties, making it a phytoestrogen. The basis for this activity is a constituent called *8-prenyl naringenin*. Like soy (another phytoestrogen), hops has been proposed as a treatment for **menopausal symptoms**. It is also marketed as a **breast enhancement** product. However, there is no direct evidence as yet that it works for either of these purposes.

Like other bitter plants, hops is also used to improve appetite.

Dosage

The standard dosage of hops is 0.5 g taken 1 to 3 times daily.

Safety Issues

Hops is believed to be nontoxic. However, as with all herbs, some people are allergic to it. Interestingly, some species of dogs, greyhounds in particular, appear to be sensitive to hops, with reports of deaths occurring. The mechanism of this toxicity is not yet known. Those taken with the popular hobby of brewing beer at home are advised to keep pets away from the relatively large quantity of hops used in this process.

As noted above, hops has estrogen-like effects. Like estrogen itself, hops might stimulate the growth of breast cancer cells. On this basis, women who have had breast cancer, or who are at high risk for it, should probably avoid hops until more is known. (Beer does not appear to contain enough of the active phytoestrogen in hops, 8-prenyl naringenin, to matter.) Children should also probably abstain from hops, to avoid producing unwanted estrogen-like effects. Safety in pregnant or nursing women or people with severe liver or kidney disease has not been established.

One animal study suggests that hops might increase the effect of sedative drugs, so do not take hops with other medications for insomnia or anxiety except under a physician's supervision.

Interactions You Should Know About

If you are taking **sedative drugs**: Do not take hops except under a physician's supervision.

Horehound

Marrubium vulgare

PRINCIPAL PROPOSED USES: *Cough*

OTHER PROPOSED USES: *Asthma, Loss of Appetite, Sore Throat*

The herb horehound has been used since Roman times as a treatment for coughs and other respiratory problems, as well as rabies. It was popular among Native North Americans as well. Teas and syrups of horehound continued to be used through the nineteenth century for coughs and lung complaints, as well as for menstrual problems. Although the herb itself has a strong bitter taste, horehound candy is considered pleasant by some and it is still available in traditional candy stores.

What Is Horehound Used for Today?

Horehound is recommended by some current herbalists as a treatment for **cough, asthma,** and **sore throat.** In addition, like other bitter herbs, horehound is thought to enhance appetite, and Germany's Commission E has approved it for this use. However, there is no reliable scientific evidence to support these uses. Only double-blind, placebo-controlled studies can prove a treatment effective, and none have been performed on horehound. (For information on why such studies are essential, see **Why Does This Book Rely on Double-blind Studies?**)

It is commonly stated that horehound loosens bronchial mucous, but there is no meaningful evidence to support this claim. Very weak evidence (far too weak to be relied upon at all), hints that horehound or its constituents, marrubenol and marrubiin, might have smooth-muscle relaxant, **antidiabetic, blood pressure–lowering,** and non-narcotic pain-reducing effects.

Dosage

A typical dose of horehound is 1.5 g 3 times daily of the dry herb or 2 to 6 tablespoons daily of the pressed juice.

Safety Issues

Horehound is thought to be relatively nontoxic, but it has not undergone any meaningful safety study. Horehound is traditionally not recommended for use by pregnant women. Safety in young children, nursing women, or people with severe liver or kidney disease has not been evaluated.

Horny Goat Weed

Epimedium grandiflorum, Epimedium sagittatum

PRINCIPAL PROPOSED USES: *Female Sexual Dysfunction, Male Sexual Dysfunction*

OTHER PROPOSED USES: *Menopausal Symptoms*

Horny goat weed is an ornamental plant that also has a long history of traditional use in Asian herbal medicine. Its whimsical name is said to derive from folk observations that goats who grazed on the herb became unusually sexually active. Horny goat weed is said to "tonify the kidney yang"; this is an expression whose meaning cannot be fully explained without entering into the theoretical framework of **traditional Chinese medicine,** but in a loose sense it signifies warming and invigorating the core energy of the body. Traditional uses of the herb (generally in formulas involving several other herbs as well) include treatment of male sexual dysfunction, prostate and urinary problems, low back pain, knee pain, poor memory, emotional timidity, and general symptoms of aging. The aboveground portion of the plant is used medicinally.

What Is Horny Goat Weed Used for Today?

Horny goat weed is currently marketed as a **sexual stimulant for both men** and **women**, and also as a treatment for **menopausal symptoms**. However, there is no meaningful scientific evidence to support these proposed uses. Statements on multiple websites claim that it increases testosterone levels, inhibits acetylcholinesterase (a chemical important in the function of the nervous system), and has been shown to act as an aphrodisiac in mice. However, the references cited on these sites do not support these statements. What limited scientific evidence is available is at best far too preliminary to prove anything at all.

According to test-tube studies, a different species in the same family, *Epimedium brevicornum*, may have estrogenic activity, but even if this were to apply to horny goat weed as well, it wouldn't indicate effectiveness for menopausal symptoms. Many herbs with estrogenic effects in the test tube do not appear to help menopausal symptoms (and the one herb that most reliably appears to affect menopausal symptoms, **black cohosh**, does not have estrogenic effects in the test tube).

A study of yet another distinct species, *Epimedium koreanum*, seems to be the source of the widespread claim that horny goat weed affects acetylcholinesterase.

In fact, only double-blind, placebo-controlled studies can begin to prove a treatment effective, and none have been performed on horny goat weed taken by itself. The only study of this type tested a combination of horny goat weed, **maca**, *Lepidium meyenii*, *Mucuna pruriens*, and *Polypodium vulgare*. It supposedly found benefit, but its design and reporting were markedly inadequate and the results are unreliable.

Dosage

A typical dose of horny goat weed is 250 to 1,000 mg daily.

Safety Issues

The safety of horny goat weed is unknown. There is one case report in which use of a horny goat weed product caused rapid heart rate and manic-like mood changes in a 66-year-old man. It is not clear whether the herb itself caused the symptoms, as it is possible the product used by this individual might have been adulterated or contaminated with an unlisted active substance.

Safety in young children, pregnant or nursing women, or people with severe liver or kidney disease has definitely not been established.

Horse Chestnut

Aesculus hippocastanum

PRINCIPAL PROPOSED USES: *Venous Insufficiency (Related to Varicose Veins)*
OTHER PROPOSED USES: *Hemorrhoids, Minor Injuries, Phlebitis*

The horse chestnut tree is widely cultivated for its bright white, yellow, or red flower clusters. Closely related to the Ohio buckeye, this tree produces large seeds known as horse chestnuts. A superstition in many parts of Europe suggests that carrying these seeds in your pocket will ward off rheumatism. More serious medical uses date back to nineteenth-century France, where extracts were used to treat hemorrhoids.

What Is Horse Chestnut Used for Today?

Serious German research of this herb began in the 1960s and ultimately led to the approval of a horse chestnut extract for vein diseases of the legs. Horse chestnut is the third most common single-herb product sold in Germany, after ginkgo and St. John's wort. In Japan, an injectable form of horse chestnut is widely used to reduce inflammation after surgery or injury; however, it is not available in the United States and it may present safety risks.

The active ingredients in horse chestnut appear to be a group of chemicals called *saponins*, of which aescin is considered the most important. Aescin appears to reduce swelling and inflammation. It's not exactly clear how aescin might work, but theories include "sealing" leaking capillaries, improving the elastic strength of veins, preventing the release of enzymes (known as glycosaminoglycan hydrolases) that break down collagen and open holes in capillary walls, decreasing inflammation, and blocking other various physiological events that lead to vein damage.

Horse chestnut is most often used as a treatment for **venous insufficiency**. This is a condition associated with varicose veins, when the blood pools in the veins of the leg and causes aching, swelling, and a sense of heaviness. While horse chestnut appears to reduce these symptoms, no studies have evaluated whether it can make visible varicose veins disappear or prevent new ones from developing.

Because **hemorrhoids** are actually a form of varicose veins, horse chestnut is used for them as well, and one double-blind, placebo-controlled study suggests that it may be effective.

Another double-blind study found that a topically applied gel made from horse chestnut may be helpful for bruises. Oral horse chestnut has also been proposed for minor injuries and **surgery**, but published studies on this potential use were not double-blind, and hence mean little. (For the reasons why double-blind studies are important, see **Why Does This Book Rely on Double-blind Studies?**.)

Finally, horse chestnut is sometimes used along with conventional treatment in cases where the veins of the lower legs become seriously inflamed (**phlebitis**). **Note:** Phlebitis is potentially dangerous and requires a doctor's supervision.

What Is the Scientific Evidence for Horse Chestnut?

Venous Insufficiency

More than 800 individuals have been involved in double-blind, placebo-controlled studies of horse chestnut for treating venous insufficiency.

One of the largest of these trials followed 212 people over a period of 40 days. It was what is called a *crossover study* because the participants initially received horse chestnut or placebo, and then were crossed over to the other treatment (without their knowledge) after 20 days. The results showed that horse chestnut produced significant improvement in leg edema, pain, and sensation of heaviness. However, the design of this study was not quite up to modern standards.

A better-designed double-blind study of 74 individuals also found benefit.

Good results were also seen in a partially double-blind, placebo-controlled study, which compared the effectiveness of horse chestnut to that of compression stockings, a standard treatment. This study followed 240 people over a course of 12 weeks. Compression stockings worked faster at reducing swelling, but by the end of the study the results were equivalent and both treatments were better than placebo.

However, a small double-blind trial suggests that **oligomeric proanthocyanidins** (OPCs) from pine bark are more effective than horse chestnut for the treatment of venous insufficiency.

Hemorrhoids

A double-blind, placebo-controlled study of 80 people with symptomatic hemorrhoids evaluated the use of a horse chestnut product providing 40 mg of aescin 3 times daily. The results indicated that use of horse chestnut produced noticeable subjective improvements in pain, bleeding, and swelling within a week; within 2 weeks, the benefits were visible by objective examination.

Bruises

A double-blind study of 70 people found that about 10 g of 2% aescin gel, applied externally to bruises in a single dose 5 minutes after they were induced, reduced bruise tenderness.

Dosage

The most common dosage of horse chestnut is 300 mg twice daily, standardized to contain 50 mg aescin per dose, for a total daily dose of 100 mg aescin.

Horse chestnut preparations should certify that a toxic constituent called *esculin* has been removed (see Safety Issues). Also, a delayed-release formulation must be used to prevent gastrointestinal upset.

Safety Issues

Whole horse chestnut is classified as an unsafe herb by the FDA. Eating the nuts or drinking a tea made from the leaves can cause horse chestnut poisoning, the symptoms of which include nausea, vomiting, diarrhea, salivation, headache, breakdown of red blood cells, convulsions, and circulatory and respiratory failure possibly leading to death. However, manufacturers of the typical European standardized extract formulations remove the most toxic constituent (esculin) and standardize the quantity of aescin. To prevent stomach irritation caused by another ingredient of horse chestnut, the extract is supplied in a controlled-release product, which reduces the incidence of irritation to below 1%, even at higher doses.

Properly prepared horse chestnut products appear to be quite safe. After decades of wide usage in Germany, there have been no reports of serious harmful effects, and even mild reported reactions have been few in number.

In animal studies, horse chestnut and its principal ingredient aescin have shown a low degree of toxicity, producing no measurable effects when taken at dosages seven times higher than normal. Dogs and rats have been treated for 34 weeks with this herb without harmful effects.

Individuals with severe kidney problems should avoid horse chestnut. In addition, injectable forms of horse chestnut can be toxic to the liver. The safety of horse chestnut in young children and pregnant or nursing women has not been established. However, 13 pregnant women were given horse chestnut in a controlled study without noticeable harm. Furthermore, studies in pregnant rats and rabbits found no injury to embryos at doses up to 10 times the human dose and changes of questionable significance at 30 times the dose.

Horse chestnut should not be combined with anticoagulant, or blood-thinning, drugs, as it may amplify their effect.

Interactions You Should Know About

If you are taking **aspirin**, **clopidogrel** (Plavix), **ticlopidine** (Ticlid), **pentoxifylline** (Trental), or anticoagulant drugs, such as **warfarin** (Coumadin) or **heparin**: Do not use horse chestnut except under medical supervision.

Horsetail

Equisetum arvense

PRINCIPAL PROPOSED USES: *Brittle Nails, Osteoporosis, Rheumatoid Arthritis*

Horsetail is a living fossil, the sole descendent of primitive plants that served as dinosaur snacks 100 million years ago. Horsetail contains unusually high levels of the element silicon, making the herb so abrasive that it can be used for polishing. In addition, the plant can incorporate dissolved gold and other minerals into its structure.

Medicinally, horsetail has been used for treating urinary disorders, wounds, gonorrhea, nosebleeds, digestive disorders, gout, and many other conditions.

What Is Horsetail Used for Today?

Silicon plays a role in bone health and, for this reason, horsetail has been recommended to prevent or treat **osteoporosis**, and to strengthen **brittle nails.** The famous German herbalist Rudolf Weiss also suggests that horsetail can relieve symptoms of **rheumatoid arthritis.** However, there is no real scientific evidence for these proposed uses.

Dosage

The standard dosage of horsetail is 1 g in capsule or tea form up to 3 times daily, as needed. Medicinal horsetail should *not* be confused with its highly toxic relative, the marsh horsetail (*Equisetum palustre*).

Safety Issues

Noticeable side effects from standard dosages of horsetail tea are rare. However, horsetail contains an enzyme that damages vitamin B_1 (thiamin) and has caused severe illness and even death in livestock that consumed too much of it. In Canada, horsetail products are required to undergo heating or other forms of processing to inactivate this harmful constituent.

Also, perhaps because horsetail contains low levels of nicotine, children have been known to become seriously ill from using the branches as blow guns. This plant can also concentrate toxic metals present in its environment.

For all of the above reasons, horsetail is not recommended for young children, pregnant or nursing women, or those with severe kidney or liver disease.

Individuals taking the medication lithium should use herbal diuretics such as horsetail only under the supervision of a physician, as becoming dehydrated while taking this medication can be dangerous.

Horsetail may also cause loss of potassium, which may be dangerous for people taking drugs in the digitalis family.

Interactions You Should Know About

If you are taking:

- ➤ **Drugs in the digitalis family: Use horsetail only under medical supervision.**
- ➤ **Lithium: Do not use horsetail except under the supervision of a physician.**

Huperzine A

PRINCIPAL PROPOSED USES: *Alzheimer's Disease and Other Forms of Dementia, Ordinary Age-related Memory Loss*

Huperzine A is a potent chemical derived from a particular type of club moss (*Huperzia serrata*). Like caffeine and cocaine, huperzine A is a medicinally active, plant-derived chemical that belongs to the class known as alkaloids. It was first isolated in 1948 by Chinese scientists. This substance is really more a drug than an herb, but it is sold over the counter as a dietary supplement for memory loss and mental impairment.

Studies in animals suggested that it could improve memory skills. These findings led to human trials (described below) and the subsequent marketing of the huperzine A as a treatment for Alzheimer's disease and related conditions. It is also sold as a "brain booster" for enhancing memory and mental function in people without Alzheimer's disease.

Huperzine A inhibits the enzyme acetylcholinesterase. This enzyme breaks down acetylcholine, a substance that plays an important role in mental function. When the enzyme that breaks it down is inhibited, acetylcholine levels in the brain tend to rise. Drugs that inhibit acetylcholinesterase (such as tacrine and donepezil) improve memory and mental functioning in people with Alzheimer's and other severe conditions. The research on huperzine A indicates that it works in much the same way. The chemical action of huperzine A is very precise and specific. It "fits" into a niche on the enzyme where acetylcholine is supposed to attach. Because huperzine A is in the way, the enzyme can't grab and destroy acetylcholine. This mechanism has been demonstrated by considerable

scientific work, including sophisticated computer modeling of the shape of the molecule. Huperzine A may also help protect nerve cells from damage.

Note that while huperzine A is sold as a dietary supplement, in all essential ways it is simply a typical drug. Huperzine A is highly purified in a laboratory and is just a single chemical. It is simply not much like an herb. Herbs contain hundreds or thousands of chemicals. Huperzine A resembles drugs such as digoxin, codeine, Sudafed, and vincristine (a chemotherapy drug), which are also highly purified chemicals taken from plants. If we wish to call huperzine A natural treatment, we need to call these (and dozens of other standard drugs) natural as well.

What Is the Scientific Evidence for Huperzine A?

All clinical trials of huperzine A to date were performed in China and reported in Chinese.

A double-blind, placebo-controlled study evaluated 103 people with **Alzheimer's disease** who received either huperzine A or placebo twice daily for 8 weeks. About 60% of the treated participants showed improvements in memory, thinking, and behavioral functions compared to 36% of the placebo-treated group, and the difference was significant.

Benefits were also seen in an earlier double-blind trial using injected huperzine A in 160 individuals with dementia or other memory disorders.

However, not all studies have been positive. Another double-blind trial of 60 individuals with Alzheimer's disease found no significant difference in symptoms between the treated and the placebo groups. Such contradictory results are common when a treatment is only modestly effective, as may be the case here.

Huperzine A is also promoted for improving memory in healthy individuals, but the supporting evidence for this claim appears to be limited to one small, poorly designed trial.

Dosage

Huperzine A is a highly potent compound with a recommended dose of only 100 to 200 mcg twice a day for age-related memory loss. We recommend using it only under a doctor's supervision.

Safety Issues

Perhaps because it works so specifically, huperzine A appears to have few side effects. However, children, pregnant or nursing women, or those with high blood pressure or severe liver or kidney disease should not take huperzine A except on a doctor's recommendation. We also don't know for sure whether huperzine A interacts adversely with any drugs; however, it seems likely that huperzine might interact with drugs that function in a similar fashion (such as standard drugs for Alzheimer's disease).

Hydroxycitric Acid

SUPPLEMENT FORMS/ALTERNATE NAMES: *Garcinia cambogia, Gorikapuli, HCA, Hydroxycitrate, Malabar Tamarind*

PRINCIPAL PROPOSED USES: *None*

OTHER PROPOSED USES: *Weight Loss*

Hydroxycitric acid (HCA), a derivative of citric acid, is found primarily in a small, sweet, purple fruit called the *Malabar tamarind*, or, as it is most commonly called, *Garcinia cambogia*. Test-tube and animal research suggests that HCA may be helpful in weight loss because of its effects on metabolism. However, studies in humans have found mixed results.

Sources

HCA is not an essential nutrient. The Malabar tamarind is the only practical source of this supplement.

Therapeutic Dosages

A typical dosage of HCA is 250 to 1,000 mg 3 times daily. Supplements are available in many forms, including tablets, capsules, powders, and even snack bars. Products are often labeled *Garcinia cambogia* and standardized to contain a fixed percentage of HCA.

Therapeutic Uses

Although animal and test-tube studies, as well as one human trial, suggest that HCA might encourage **weight loss**, other studies have found no benefit.

What Is the Scientific Evidence for Hydroxycitric Acid?

It remains unclear whether HCA offers any weight-loss benefits.

In an 8-week double-blind, placebo-controlled trial of 60 overweight individuals, use of HCA at a dose of 440 mg 3 times daily produced significant weight loss as compared to placebo.

In contrast, a 12-week, double-blind, placebo-controlled trial of 135 overweight individuals, who were given either placebo or 500 mg of HCA (as *Garcinia cambogia* extract standardized to contain 50% HCA) 3 times daily, found no effect on body weight or fat mass. However, this study has been criticized for using a high-fiber diet, which is thought to impair HCA absorption.

A 12-week, double-blind trial of 89 individuals found that HCA had no effect on appetite. Another study tested HCA to see if it could cause weight loss by altering metabolism, but no effects on metabolism were found.

Safety Issues

The Malabar tamarind (from which HCA is extracted) is a traditional food and flavoring in Southeast Asia. No serious side effects have been reported from animal or human studies involving either fruit extracts or the concentrated chemical. However, formal safety studies have not been performed, and therefore, its safety remains unknown.

Hydroxymethyl Butyrate

SUPPLEMENT FORMS/ALTERNATE NAMES: *Beta-Hydroxy Beta-Methylbutyric Acid, HMB*
PRINCIPAL PROPOSED USES: *Muscle Building for Strength Athletes and Bodybuilders*
OTHER PROPOSED USES: *Enhancing Recovery from Heavy Exercise*

Technically "beta-hydroxy beta-methylbutyric acid," HMB is a chemical that occurs naturally in the body when the amino acid leucine breaks down.

Leucine is found in particularly high concentrations in muscles. During athletic training, damage to the muscles leads to the breakdown of leucine as well as increased HMB levels. Evidence suggests that taking HMB supplements might signal the body to slow down the destruction of muscle tissue. However, while promising, the research record at present is contradictory and marked by an absence of large studies.

Sources

HMB is not an essential nutrient, so there is no established requirement. HMB is found in small amounts in citrus fruit and catfish. To get a therapeutic dosage, however, you need to take a supplement in powder or pill form.

Therapeutic Dosages

A typical therapeutic dosage of HMB is 3 g daily.

Be careful not to confuse HMB with gamma hy-

droxybutyrate (GHB), a similar supplement. GHB can cause severe sedation, especially when combined with other sedating substances, such as alcohol or anti-anxiety drugs.

Therapeutic Uses

According to some but not all of the small double-blind trials performed thus far, HMB may improve response to weight training. One small, double-blind, placebo-controlled trial found hints that HMB might help prevent muscle damage during prolonged exercise, thereby potentially **enhancing recovery during athletic training**; however, a follow-up study failed to find this benefit.

Very weak evidence suggests that HMB might improve **blood pressure** and **cholesterol levels**.

What Is the Scientific Evidence for Hydroxymethyl Butyrate?

In a controlled study, 41 male volunteers age 19 to 29 years old were given either 0, 1.5, or 3 g of HMB daily for 3 weeks. The participants also lifted weights 3 days a week for 90 minutes. The results suggest that HMB can enhance strength and muscle mass in direct proportion to intake.

In another controlled study reported in the same article, 32 male volunteers took either 3 g of HMB daily or placebo and then lifted weights for 2 or 3 hours daily, 6 days a week for 7 weeks. The HMB group saw a significantly greater increase in its bench-press strength than the placebo group. However, there was no significant difference in body weight or fat mass by the end of the study.

Similarly, a double-blind, placebo-controlled trial of 39 men and 36 women found that over a period of 4 weeks, HMB supplementation improved response to weight training.

Two placebo-controlled studies in women found that 3 g of HMB had no effect on lean body mass and strength in sedentary women, but it did provide an additional benefit when combined with weight training. In addition, a double-blind study of 31 men and women, 70 years old, undergoing resistance training, found significant improvements in fat-free mass attributable to the use of HMB (3 g daily).

However, other small studies have found marginal or no benefits with HMB for enhancing body composition or strength.

When the results of small studies contradict one another, it often means that the studied treatment produces minimal benefits at most, and this may be the case with HMB. Larger trials will be necessary to truly determine the extent of its effect.

Safety Issues

HMB seems to be safe when taken at standard doses. Clinical trials have not found any significant adverse effects with short-term HMB use. Short- and long-term toxicological studies in animals have also found no evidence of harm. However, full safety studies have not been performed, so HMB should not be used by young children, pregnant or nursing women, or those with severe liver or kidney disease, except on the advice of a physician.

As with all supplements taken in very large doses, it is important to purchase a quality product, as an impurity present even in very small percentages could add up to a real problem.

Hyssop
Hyssop officinalis

PRINCIPAL PROPOSED USES: *None*
OTHER PROPOSED USES: *Asthma, Common Cold, Cough, Sore Throat*

The herb hyssop (*Hyssop officinalis*) has a long history of use in both religion and medicine. The biblical phrase "purge me with Hyssop, and I shall be clean" echoes the ancient Greek use of this herb for cleansing sacred sites. Various preparations of hyssop have been used medicinally for respiratory problems, including cough, chest congestion, sore throat, and bronchitis. Hyssop has also been used to treat a variety of digestive problems, including stomach pain and intestinal gas. The fragrant essential oil of hyssop is an ingredient in the liqueur Chartreuse.

What Is Hyssop Used for Today?

The **essential oil** of hyssop is still recommended by herbalists today for treatment of respiratory and digestive problems, such as the **common cold**, **asthma**, **acute bronchitis**, and **cough**, stomach upset, and **intestinal gas**. Hyssop tea is recommended as a gargle for sore throat. However, there is no meaningful evidence that it is effective for any of these purposes.

Very preliminary evidence, too weak to rely upon at all, hints that extracts of hyssop might have **anti-HIV**

activity. Other preliminary evidence weakly suggests that constituents in hyssop might reduce absorption of carbohydrates from the digestive tract. This has led to statements that hyssop is helpful for treating **diabetes** and aiding **weight loss**, but in reality the current evidence is far too weak to draw any such conclusion.

Dosage

A typical dose of hyssop essential oil is 1 to 2 drops daily. Hyssop tea is made by steeping 2 to 3 teaspoons of herb in a cup of hot water and may be taken 2 to 3 times daily for sore throat.

Safety Issues

Hyssop has undergone no more than minimal evaluation for safety. Hyssop tea is thought to be relatively benign, but hyssop essential oil (like most essential oils) is toxic in excessive doses. Some of its constituents might increase risk of seizures. For this reason, hyssop essential oil should not be used by people with **epilepsy**. It should also not be used by young children, pregnant or nursing women, or people with severe liver or kidney disease.

Indigo

Indigofera tinctoria, Indigofera oblongifolia

PRINCIPAL PROPOSED USES: *None*

OTHER PROPOSED USES: *Antiseptic, Liver Protection*

The leaves and branches of the indigo plant yield an exquisite blue dye; people around the globe have used it to color textiles and clothing for centuries. Before the development of synthetic blue dyes, indigo was cultivated for this pigment rather than for medicinal use.

In the traditional medicine of India and China, indigo was used in the treatment of conditions we would now call epilepsy, bronchitis, liver disease, and psychiatric illness. However, there is no real scientific evidence for any of these uses.

Warning: Several species of indigo are poisonous. See Safety Issues below for more information.

What Is Indigo Used for Today?

Based on its traditional use for liver problems, researchers have investigated whether indigo might protect the liver against chemically induced injury. Animal studies do suggest that extracts of the indigo species *Indigofera tinctoria* protect the liver from damage by toxic chemicals. No human trials, however, have been performed to examine indigo's effects on the liver.

The species *Indigofera oblongifolia* has been tested for its antibacterial and antifungal activity. In a test-tube

trial, this plant showed significant activity against certain types of bacteria and fungi. This research is still in its preliminary stages, so it is too early to tell whether *Indigofera oblongifolia* will prove useful for the treatment of any infectious diseases.

Note: A different plant called *wild indigo* (*Baptisia tinctoria*), in combination with **echinacea** and white cedar, has been studied as a possible immune stimulant. However, wild indigo is not part of the *Indigofera* family of plants and is not discussed here.

Dosage

No standard dosage of indigo has been established.

Safety Issues

The indigo species *Indigofera tinctoria* has a history of use in traditional medical systems and is regarded by herbalists as safe, other than the occasional allergic reactions that have been reported. However, comprehensive safety tests have not been performed. For this reason, indigo should not be used by pregnant or nursing women, young children, or individuals with severe liver or kidney disease. Safety in other individuals is unknown.

The species *Indigofera spicata* (formerly *Indigofera endecaphylla*), however, is poisonous: it has killed cattle and other animals and has caused birth defects in rats. Other indigo species have also been found to be lethal.

For this reason, it is important to avoid ingesting indigo internally unless you are absolutely certain that it has been harvested and processed by expert, reliable individuals.

Indole-3-Carbinol

SUPPLEMENT FORMS/ALTERNATE NAMES: *I3C*

PRINCIPAL PROPOSED USES: *Cancer Prevention*

OTHER PROPOSED USES: *Liver Protection, Respiratory Papillomatosis*

Indole-3-carbinol (I3C), a chemical found in vegetables of the broccoli family, is thought to possess cancer-preventive properties.

Indole-3-carbinol appears to work in several ways: (1) it facilitates the conversion of estrogen to a less cancer-promoting form, (2) it partially blocks the effects of estrogen on cells, (3) it directly kills or inhibits cancer cells, and (4) it reduces levels of free radicals that can promote cancer by damaging DNA.

Sources

I3C is found in cruciferous vegetables (*Brassica* plants), such as cabbage, broccoli, brussels sprouts, cauliflower, kale, kohlrabi, and turnips. A typical Japanese diet provides the equivalent of about 112 mg of I3C daily; intake in Western diets is lower.

Therapeutic Dosages

A 4-week, double-blind, placebo-controlled trial of 57 women found that a minimum dose of 300 mg of I3C daily may be necessary to reduce risk of estrogen-promoted cancers. Another study found benefits with 400 mg of I3C per day. However, until the overall effects of I3C are better understood, we recommend obtaining this substance through consumption of broccoli-family vegetables rather than taking it as a supplement (see Safety Issues below).

Therapeutic Uses

I3C is being studied as a chemopreventive agent: a substance that helps prevent **cancer**. Numerous animal studies suggest that I3C might help reduce the risk of estrogen-sensitive cancers as well as other types of cancer. One double-blind, placebo-controlled study in humans suggests that it can help reverse **cervical dysplasia**, a precancerous condition. Weaker evidence hints at benefits for vulvar intraepithelial neoplasia, a precancerous condition of the vulva. **Note:** Do not attempt to treat cervical dysplasia or any other precancerous or cancerous condition without physician supervision.

Some evidence indicates that I3C might also help prevent recurrences of a rare condition called *respiratory papillomatosis*. This disease involves benign tumors in the lungs, mouth, and vocal chords.

I3C has additionally been investigated as a **liver protectant**.

Further evidence suggests that I3C must be exposed to stomach acid to exert its full effects. For this reason, individuals with low stomach acid, such as those taking **H$_2$ blockers** (such as Zantac/ranitidine) or **proton pump inhibitors** (such as Prilosec/omeprazole), may not benefit as much from I3C.

What Is the Scientific Evidence for Indole-3-Carbinol?

A 12-week, placebo-controlled trial of 30 women with stage II or III cervical dysplasia found that treatment with I3C at a daily dose of 200 or 400mg significantly improved the rate at which the cervix spontaneously returned to normal.

Safety Issues

Studies in rats, chickens, guinea pigs, mice, and dogs suggest that I3C is safe at recommended doses.

Human trials have found no significant side effects with I3C.

However, one study of rats found increased abnormalities in male offspring, specifically related to their fertility. For this reason, I3C supplements should not be used by pregnant women.

There are other concerns with I3C as well. For example, despite its overall anticancer effects, there is some evidence that I3C has tumor-promoting properties under certain circumstances. For this reason, long-term use of concentrated I3C supplements may not be safe. In addition, individuals who have already had cancer shouldn't use I3C (or any other supplement) except under physician supervision. (But you don't need physician supervision to increase your broccoli intake!)

In addition, because it facilitates the inactivation of estrogen, it is possible that I3C might tend to promote **osteoporosis** in postmenopausal women and could interfere with estrogen therapies (such as birth control pills and hormone replacement therapy). However, this concern is purely theoretical at this time.

Interactions You Should Know About

If you are taking any medication that contains **estrogen** (including **birth control pills**): I3C might interfere with its action.

Inosine

PRINCIPAL PROPOSED USES: *None*

OTHER PROPOSED USES: *Heart Attack Recovery, Irregular Heartbeat, Sports Performance Enhancement, Tourette's Syndrome*

Inosine is an important chemical found throughout the body. It plays many roles, one of which is helping to make ATP (adenosine triphosphate), the body's main form of usable energy. Based primarily on this fact, inosine supplements have been proposed as an energy-booster for athletes, as well as a treatment for various heart conditions.

Sources

Inosine is not an essential nutrient. However, brewer's yeast and organ meats, such as liver and kidney, contain considerable amounts. Inosine is also available in purified form.

Therapeutic Dosages

When used as a sports supplement, a typical dosage of inosine is 5 to 6 g daily (see Safety Issues below).

Therapeutic Uses

Inosine has been proposed as a treatment for various forms of heart disease, from irregular heartbeat to recovery from **heart attacks**. However, the evidence that it offers any benefit to the heart remains far too preliminary to rely upon at all.

Inosine is better known as a performance enhancer for athletes, although most of the available evidence suggests that it *doesn't* work for this purpose.

Inosine has also been suggested as a possible treatment for Tourette's syndrome, a neurological disorder.

Safety Issues

Although no side effects have been reported with the use of inosine, long-term use should be avoided. A very preliminary double-blind crossover study that enrolled 7 participants suggests that high doses of inosine (5,000 to 10,000 mg per day for 5 to 10 days) may increase the risk of uric acid–related problems, such as gout or kidney stones.

The safety of inosine for young children, pregnant or nursing women, or those with serious liver or kidney disease has not been established.

As with all supplements taken in multigram doses, it is important to purchase a reputable product, because a contaminant present even in small percentages could add up to a real problem.

Inositol

SUPPLEMENT FORMS/ALTERNATE NAMES: *Inositol Hexaphosphate, IP6, Myoinositol, Phytic Acid, Vitamin B$_8$*

PRINCIPAL PROPOSED USES: *Depression, Panic Disorder*

OTHER PROPOSED USES: *Alzheimer's Disease, Attention Deficit Disorder, Bipolar Disorder, Bulimia, Cancer Prevention, Diabetic Neuropathy, Obsessive-Compulsive Disorder, Polycystic Ovarian Syndrome, Premenstrual Syndrome (PMS), Psoriasis Caused by Treatment with Lithium*

Inositol, unofficially referred to as "vitamin B$_8$," is present in all animal tissues, with the highest levels in the heart and brain. It is part of the membranes (outer coverings) of all cells and plays a role in helping the liver process fats, as well as contributing to the function of muscles and nerves.

Inositol may also be involved in depression. People who are depressed may have lower than normal levels of inositol in their spinal fluid. In addition, inositol participates in the action of *serotonin*, a neurotransmitter known to be a factor in depression. (Neurotransmitters are chemicals that transmit messages between nerve cells.) For these two reasons, inositol has been proposed as a treatment for depression, and preliminary evidence suggests that it may be helpful.

Inositol has also been tried for other psychological and nerve-related conditions.

Sources

Inositol is not known to be an essential nutrient. However, nuts, seeds, beans, whole grains, cantaloupe, and citrus fruits supply a substance called *phytic acid* (inositol hexaphosphate, or IP6), which releases inositol when acted on by bacteria in the digestive tract. The typical American diet provides an estimated 1,000 mg daily.

Therapeutic Dosages

Experimentally, inositol dosages of up to 18 g daily have been tried for various conditions.

Therapeutic Uses

Some but not all studies suggest that high-dose inositol may be useful for **depression**.

Inositol has also been studied for **bipolar disorder**, panic disorder, bulimia, and **obsessive-compulsive disorder**, but the evidence remains far from conclusive. Other potential uses include **Alzheimer's disease** and **attention deficit disorder**.

One small double-blind study found indications that inositol might be helpful for women with polycystic ovarian syndrome.

Another very small double-blind study found that inositol supplements could help reduce symptoms of **psoriasis** triggered or made worse by use of the drug **lithium**.

A small double-blind study failed to find inositol helpful for premenstrual dysphoric disorder, a severe form of **premenstrual syndrome** (PMS).

Inositol is sometimes proposed as a treatment for diabetic neuropathy, but there have been no double-blind, placebo-controlled studies on this subject, and two uncontrolled studies had mixed results.

Inositol has also been investigated for potential cancer-preventive properties.

What Is the Scientific Evidence for Inositol?

Depression

Small double-blind studies have found inositol helpful for depression. In one such trial, 28 depressed individuals were given a daily dose of 12 g of inositol for 4 weeks. By the fourth week, the group receiving inositol showed significant improvement compared to the placebo group.

However, a double-blind study of 42 people with severe depression that was not responding to standard antidepressant treatment found no improvement when inositol was added.

Panic Disorder

People with panic disorder frequently develop panic attacks, often with no warning. The racing heartbeat, chest pressure, sweating, and other physical symptoms can be so intense that they are mistaken for a heart attack. A small double-blind study (21 participants) found that people given 12 g of inositol daily had fewer and less severe panic attacks as compared to the placebo group.

A double-blind, crossover study of 20 individuals compared inositol to the antidepressant drug fluvoxamine (Luvox), a medication related to Prozac. The results over 4 weeks of treatment showed that the supplement was at least as effective as the drug.

Bipolar Disorder

In a 6-week, double-blind study, 24 individuals with bipolar disorder received either placebo or inositol (2 g 3 times daily for a week, then increased to 4 g 3 times daily) in addition to their regular medical treatment. The results of this small study failed to show statistically significant benefits; however, promising trends were seen that suggest a larger study is warranted.

Safety Issues

No serious ill effects have been reported for inositol, even with a therapeutic dosage that equals about 18 times the average dietary intake. However, no long-term safety studies have been performed.

Although inositol has sometimes been recommended for bipolar disorder, there is evidence to suggest inositol may trigger manic episodes in people with this condition. If you have bipolar disorder, you should not take inositol unless under a doctor's supervision.

Safety has not been established in young children, women who are pregnant or nursing, and those with severe liver and kidney disease. As with all supplements used in very large doses, it is important to purchase a reputable product, because a contaminant present even in small percentages could add up to a real problem.

Iodine

SUPPLEMENT FORMS/ALTERNATE NAMES: *Elemental Iodine, Iodide*

PRINCIPAL PROPOSED USES: *Correcting Nutritional Deficiency*

OTHER PROPOSED USES: *Cyclic Mastalgia*

Your thyroid gland, located just above the middle of your collarbone, needs iodine to make thyroid hormone, which maintains normal metabolism in all cells of the body. Principally found in seawater, dietary iodine can be scarce in many inland areas, and deficiencies were common before iodine was added to table salt. Iodine deficiency causes enlargement of the thyroid, a condition known as goiter. However, if you are not deficient in iodine, taking extra iodine will not help your thyroid work better, and it might even cause problems.

For reasons that are not clear, supplementary iodine might also be helpful for **cyclic mastalgia**.

Requirements/Sources

The official U.S. recommendations for daily intake of iodine are as follows:

> Infants 0–6 months, 110 mcg
> 7–12 months, 130 mcg
> Children 1–8 years, 90 mcg
> Males and females 9–13 years, 120 mcg
> 14 years and older, 150 mcg
> Pregnant women, 220 mcg
> Nursing women, 290 mcg

Iodine deficiency is rare in developed countries today because of the use of iodized salt.

Seafood and **kelp** contain very high levels of iodine, as do salty processed foods that use iodized salt.

Most iodine is in the form of iodide, but a few studies suggest that a special form of iodine called *molecular iodine* may be better than iodide (see What Is the Scientific Evidence for Iodine? below).

Therapeutic Dosages

A typical therapeutic dosage of iodide or iodine is 200 mcg daily.

Therapeutic Uses

Iodine supplements have been proposed as a treatment for **cyclic mastalgia** (breast pain and lumpiness that usually cycles in relation to the menstrual period, also called *cyclic mastitis* or *fibrocystic breast disease*).

What Is the Scientific Evidence for Iodine?

Three clinical studies provide weak evidence that supplements providing iodine may be helpful in treating cyclic mastalgia. These studies suggest that either iodide or iodine (the pure molecular form) might be useful. In the one double-blind, placebo-controlled trial among this group, a study that enrolled 56 individuals, molecular iodine was found superior to placebo in relieving pain and reducing the number of cysts.

Another of these studies compared molecular iodine to iodide. Molecular iodine was no more effective than iodide, but was deemed superior because it induced fewer side effects and did not affect the thyroid.

Safety Issues

When taken at the recommended dosage (see Requirements/Sources above), iodine and iodide are safe nutritional supplements. However, excessive doses of iodide can actually cause thyroid problems, including both **hypothyroidism** and **hyperthyroidism**! There is also a speculative link between excessive iodide intake and thyroid cancer. For these reasons, iodide intake above nutritional recommendations is not advised except under physician supervision.

Ipriflavone

PRINCIPAL PROPOSED USES: *Preventing and Treating Osteoporosis*
OTHER PROPOSED USES: *Bodybuilding*

Isoflavones are water-soluble chemicals found in many plants. Ipriflavone is a semisynthetic version of an isoflavone found in **soy**.

Soy isoflavones have effects in the body somewhat similar to those of estrogen. This should be beneficial, but it is possible that soy could present some of the risks of estrogen as well. In 1969, a research project was initiated to manufacture a type of isoflavone that would possess the bone-stimulating effects of estrogen without any estrogen-like activity elsewhere in the body. Such a product would help prevent osteoporosis but cause no other health risks.

Ipriflavone was the result. After 7 successful years of experiments with animals, human research was started in 1981. Today, ipriflavone is available in over 22 countries and in most drugstores in the United States as a nonprescription dietary supplement. It is an accepted treatment for osteoporosis in Italy, Turkey, and Japan.

According to all but one study, ipriflavone combined with calcium can slow and perhaps slightly reverse bone breakdown. It also seems to help reduce the pain of fractures caused by osteoporosis. However, since it does not appear to have any estrogenic effects anywhere else in the body, it shouldn't increase the risk of breast or uterine cancer. On the other hand, it won't reduce the hot flashes, night sweats, mood changes, or vaginal dryness of menopause, nor prevent heart disease.

Note: A recent, large study found that ipriflavone might reduce white blood cell count in some individuals. See Safety Issues below for more information.

Sources

Ipriflavone is not an essential nutrient and is not found in food. It must be taken as a supplement.

Therapeutic Dosages

The proper dosage of ipriflavone is 200 mg 3 times daily or 300 mg twice daily. A calcium supplement providing 1,000 mg of calcium daily should be taken as well.

Therapeutic Uses

Ipriflavone appears to be able to slow down and perhaps slightly reverse **osteoporosis**. It may be helpful for this purpose in ordinary postmenopausal osteoporosis, as well as in osteoporosis caused by medications. Ipriflavone also seems to ease the pain of fractures caused by osteoporosis.

Ipriflavone has also been proposed as a bodybuilding aid, but there is no meaningful evidence that it is helpful for this purpose.

What Is the Scientific Evidence for Ipriflavone?

Numerous double-blind, placebo-controlled studies involving a total of over 1,700 participants have examined the effects of ipriflavone on various forms of osteoporosis. Overall, it appears that ipriflavone can slow the progression of osteoporosis and perhaps reverse it to some extent. For example, a 2-year, double-blind study followed 198 postmenopausal women who showed evidence of bone loss. At the end of the study, there was a gain in bone density of 1% in the ipriflavone group and a loss of 0.7% in the placebo group. These numbers may sound small, but they can add up to a lot of bone over time.

However, the largest and longest study of ipriflavone found no benefit. In this 3-year trial of 474 postmenopausal women, no differences in the extent of osteoporosis were seen between the ipriflavone and placebo groups. How can this failure be accounted for, in view of all the successful trials that came before? Perhaps because the researchers in this study gave women only 500 mg of calcium daily. All other major studies of ipriflavone gave participants 1,000 mg of calcium daily. It's possible that ipriflavone requires the higher dose of calcium in order to work properly. Ipriflavone, like estrogen, probably works by fighting bone breakdown. However, there is some evidence that it may also increase new bone formation.

Combining ipriflavone with estrogen may enhance anti-osteoporosis benefits. However, we do not know for sure whether such combinations increase or reduce the other risks (or benefits) of estrogen.

Ipriflavone may also be helpful for preventing osteoporosis in women who are taking Lupron or **corticosteroids**, medications that accelerate bone loss. However, the combined use of ipriflavone and drugs that suppress the immune system, such as corticosteroids, presents potential risks.

Finally, for reasons that are not at all clear, ipriflavone appears to be able to reduce pain in osteoporosis-related fractures that have already occurred.

Safety Issues

About 3,000 people have used ipriflavone in clinical studies and, in all but two, no significant adverse effects were seen. However, these trials (a 3-year, double-blind trial of almost 500 women, as well as a small study) found worrisome evidence that ipriflavone can reduce levels of white blood cells called *lymphocytes*. For this reason, anyone taking ipriflavone for the long term should have periodic measurements taken of white blood cell count. In addition, ipriflavone should not be used by anyone with immune deficiencies, such as HIV, or by those who take drugs that suppress the immune system, except under physician supervision. There are other potential risks as well. Because ipriflavone is metabolized by the kidneys, individuals with severe kidney disease should have their ipriflavone dosage monitored by a physician. Individuals with ulcers should also avoid ipriflavone.

Also, although ipriflavone itself does not affect tissues outside of bone, some evidence suggests that if it is combined with estrogen, estrogen's effects on the uterus are increased. This might mean that the risk of uterine cancer would be elevated over taking estrogen alone. It should be possible to overcome this risk by taking progesterone along with estrogen, which is standard medical practice in any case. However, this finding does make one wonder whether ipriflavone–estrogen combinations raise the risk of breast cancer too, an estrogen side effect that has no easy solution. At present, there is no available information on this important subject.

Additionally, ipriflavone may interfere with certain drugs by affecting the way they are processed in the liver. For example, it may raise blood levels of the older asthma drug theophylline. It could also raise levels of caffeine, meaning that if you drink coffee while taking ipriflavone you might stay up longer than you expect! Ipriflavone could also interact with tolbutamide (a drug for diabetes), phenytoin (used for epilepsy), and Coumadin (a blood thinner). Such interactions are potentially dangerous, especially since phenytoin and Coumadin cause osteoporosis and some people might be tempted to try taking ipriflavone at the same time.

Iron

Interactions You Should Know About

If you are taking:

> Theophylline, tolbutamide, phenytoin (Dilantin), warfarin (Coumadin), or any other drug metabolized in the liver: Ipriflavone might change the levels of that drug in your body.

> Estrogen: Ipriflavone might help it strengthen your bones even more. However, it might also increase the risk of uterine cancer.
> Drugs that suppress the immune system, such as corticosteroids, methotrexate, or cyclosporine: Do not use ipriflavone except under medical supervision.

Iron

SUPPLEMENT FORMS/ALTERNATE NAMES: *Chelated Iron, Iron Sulfate*

PRINCIPAL PROPOSED USES: *Correction of Iron Deficiency, Sports Performance Enhancement*

OTHER PROPOSED USES: *Attention Deficit Disorder, Fatigue, HIV Support, Menorrhagia (Heavy Menstruation), Reduction of ACE Inhibitor Side Effects, Restless Legs Syndrome*

The element iron is essential to human life. As part of hemoglobin, the oxygen-carrying protein found in red blood cells, iron plays an integral role in nourishing every cell in the body with oxygen. It also functions as a part of myoglobin, which helps muscle cells store oxygen. Without iron, your body could not make ATP (adenosine triphosphate, the body's primary energy source), produce DNA, or carry out many other critical processes.

Iron deficiency can lead to anemia, learning disabilities, impaired immune function, fatigue, and depression. However, you shouldn't take iron supplements unless lab tests show that you are genuinely deficient.

Requirements/Sources

The official U.S. recommendations for daily intake of iron are as follows:

> Infants 0–6 months, 0.27 mg
> 7–12 months, 11 mg
> Children 1–3 years, 7 mg
> 4–8 years, 10 mg
> Males 9–13 years, 8 mg
> 14–18 years, 11 mg
> 19 years and older, 8 mg
> Females 9–13 years, 8 mg
> 14–18 years, 15 mg

> 19–50 years, 18 mg
> 50 years and older, 8 mg
> Pregnant women, 27 mg
> Nursing women 9 mg, (10 mg if 18 years old or younger)

Iron deficiency is the most common nutrient deficiency in the world; worldwide, at least 700 million individuals have iron-deficiency anemia. While iron deficiency is widespread in the developing world, it is also prevalent in developed countries. Groups at high risk are children, teenage girls, menstruating women (especially those with excessively heavy menstruation, known as menorrhagia), pregnant women, and the elderly.

There are two major forms of iron: *heme* iron and *nonheme* iron. Heme iron is bound to the proteins hemoglobin or myoglobin, whereas nonheme iron is an inorganic compound. (In chemistry, "organic" has a very precise meaning that has nothing to do with farming. An organic compound contains carbon atoms. Thus "inorganic iron" is an iron compound containing no carbon.) Heme iron, obtained from red meats and fish, is easily absorbed by the body. Nonheme iron, usually derived from plants, is less easily absorbed.

Rich sources of heme iron include oysters, meat, poultry, and fish. The main sources of nonheme iron are dried fruits, molasses, whole grains, legumes, leafy green

Iron

vegetables, nuts, seeds, and **kelp**. Acidic foods, such as fruit preserves and tomatoes, are a good source of iron when they've been cooked in iron or stainless steel cookware (some of the iron leaches into the food).

Iron absorption may be affected by the following substances: antibiotics in the quinolone (Floxin, Cipro) or tetracycline families, levodopa, methyldopa, carbidopa, penicillamine, thyroid hormone, captopril (and possibly other ACE inhibitors), calcium, soy, zinc, copper, or manganese, or multivitamin/multimineral tablets. Conversely, iron may inhibit their absorption, too.

In addition, drugs in the H_2 blocker or proton pump inhibitor families may impair iron absorption.

Therapeutic Dosages

The typical short-term therapeutic dosage to correct iron deficiency is 100 to 200 mg daily. Once your body's iron stores reach normal levels, however, this dose should be reduced to the lowest level that can maintain iron balance.

Therapeutic Uses

The most obvious use of iron supplements is to treat iron deficiency. Severe iron deficiency causes anemia, which in turn causes many symptoms. Iron deficiency too slight to cause anemia may impair health as well. Several, though not all, double-blind trials suggest that mild iron deficiency might impair **sports performance**. In addition, a double-blind, placebo-controlled study of 144 women with unexplained **fatigue** who also had low or borderline-low levels of ferritin (a measure of stored iron) found that iron supplement enhanced energy and well-being. However, don't take iron just because you feel tired. Make sure to get tested to see whether you are indeed deficient. With iron, more is definitely *not* better (see Safety Issues below).

Excessively heavy menstruation (menorrhagia) can certainly cause iron loss, and thereby may warrant iron supplements. Interestingly, a small double-blind trial found evidence that iron supplements might actually help reduce menstrual bleeding in women with menorrhagia who are also iron deficient.

A study of 71 **HIV-positive** children noted a high rate of iron deficiency. One observational study of 296 men with HIV infection linked high intake of iron to a decreased risk of AIDS 6 years later.

Individuals taking ACE inhibitors frequently develop a dry cough as a side effect. One study suggests that iron supplementation can alleviate this symptom. (However, iron can interfere with ACE inhibitor absorption, so it should be taken at a different time of day.)

Iron has also been tried as a treatment for **attention deficit disorder**, but there is as yet no real evidence that it works.

Preliminary studies have linked low iron levels to **restless legs syndrome**. However, a small double-blind study found no benefit with iron supplements among individuals who were not iron deficient.

What Is the Scientific Evidence for Iron?

Sports Performance

A double-blind, placebo-controlled trial of 42 non-anemic women with evidence of slightly low iron reserves found that iron supplements significantly enhanced sports performance. Participants were put on a daily aerobic training program for the latter 4 weeks of this 6-week trial. At the end of the trial, those receiving iron showed significantly greater gains in speed and endurance as compared to those given placebo.

In addition, a double-blind, placebo-controlled study of 40 non-anemic elite athletes with mildly low iron stores found that 12 weeks of iron supplementation enhanced aerobic performance.

Benefits with iron supplementation were also observed in other double-blind trials involving mildly low iron stores. However, other studies failed to find significant improvements, suggesting that the benefits of iron supplements for non-anemic, iron-deficient athletes is small at most.

Menorrhagia

One small double-blind study found good results using iron supplements to treat heavy menstruation. This study, which was performed in 1964, saw an improvement in 75% of the women who took iron (compared to 32.5% of those who took placebo). Women who began with higher iron levels did not respond to treatment. This suggests once more that supplementing with iron is only a good idea if you are deficient in it.

Safety Issues

At the recommended dosage, iron is quite safe. Excessive dosages, however, can be toxic—damaging the intestines and liver and possibly resulting in death. Iron poisoning in children is a surprisingly common problem, so make sure to keep your iron supplements out of their reach.

Mildly excessive levels of iron may be unhealthy for another reason: it acts as an oxidant (the opposite of an antioxidant), perhaps increasing the risk of cancer and heart disease, although this theory is controversial. Elevated levels of iron may also play a role in brain injury caused by **stroke**. In addition, excess iron appears to increase complications of **pregnancy**, and, if **breastfed** infants who are not iron-deficient are given iron supplements, the effects may be negative rather than positive.

Note: Simultaneous use of iron supplements and high-dose **vitamin C** can greatly increase iron absorption, possibly leading to excessive iron levels in the body.

One study found that iron does *not* impair absorption of the drug **methotrexate**.

Interactions You Should Know About

If you are taking:

➢ Antibiotics in the tetracycline or quinolone (Floxin, Cipro) families, levodopa, methyldopa, carbidopa, penicillamine, thyroid hormone, calcium, soy, zinc, copper, or manganese: To avoid absorption problems, wait at least 2 hours following your dose of medication or supplement before taking iron.
➢ Drugs that reduce stomach acid such as antacids, H2 blockers, and proton pump inhibitors: You may need extra iron.
➢ High doses of vitamin C: You may absorb too much iron.
➢ ACE inhibitors: Iron may reduce coughing side effect; however, to avoid absorption problems, you should wait at least 2 hours following your dose of medication before taking iron.

Isoflavones

SUPPLEMENT FORMS/ALTERNATE NAMES: *Red Clover Isoflavones, Soy Isoflavones*

PRINCIPAL PROPOSED USES: *High Cholesterol, Menopausal Symptoms*

OTHER PROPOSED USES: *Cancer Prevention, Cyclic Mastalgia, Enhancing Mental Function, Female Infertility, Osteoporosis, Premenstrual Syndrome (PMS)*

Isoflavones are water-soluble chemicals found in many plants. In this article, we will discuss a group of isoflavones that are *phytoestrogens*, meaning that they cause effects in the body somewhat similar to those of estrogen. The most investigated phytoestrogen isoflavones, **genistein** and daidzein, are found both in **soy** products and the herb **red clover**. Soy additionally contains glycitein, an isoflavone that is more estrogenic than genistein and daidzein but is usually present in relatively low amounts. Red clover also contains two other isoflavones: biochanin (which can be turned into genistein) and formonenetin (which can be turned into daidzein).

Certain cells in the body have *estrogen receptors,* special sites that allow estrogen to attach. When estrogen attaches to a cell's estrogen receptor, estrogenic effects occur in the cell. Isoflavones latch on to estrogen

receptors too, but produce weaker estrogenic effects. This leads to an interesting two-part action. When there is not enough estrogen in the body, isoflavones can stimulate cells with estrogen receptors and partly make up for the deficit. However, when there is plenty of estrogen, isoflavones may tend to block real estrogen from attaching to estrogen receptors, thereby reducing the net estrogenic effect. This may reduce some of the risks of excess estrogen (for example, breast and uterine cancer) while still providing some of estrogen's benefits (such as preventing osteoporosis).

Isoflavones also appear to directly reduce estrogen levels in the body, perhaps by fooling the body into thinking that it has plenty of estrogen.

Isoflavones are widely thought to be the active ingredients in soy products. However, growing evidence suggests that there are other active ingredients as well, such as proteins, fiber, and phospholipids.

Sources

Although isoflavones are not essential nutrients, they may help reduce the incidence of several diseases. Thus, isoflavones may be useful for optimum health, even if they are not necessary for life like a classic vitamin.

Roasted soybeans have the highest isoflavone content: about 167 mg for a 3.5-ounce serving. Tempeh (a cake of fermented soybeans) is next, with 60 mg, followed by soy flour with 44 mg. Processed soy products, such as soy protein and soy milk, contain about 20 mg per serving. The same isoflavones found in soy are also contained in certain red clover products.

Therapeutic Dosages

When purified isoflavones from red clover or soy are used, the dose generally ranges from about 40 to 80 mg daily. This is considerably higher than the average isoflavone intake in Japan, which is about 28 mg daily. (Postmenopausal Japanese women may consume closer to 50 mg daily.)

Therapeutic Uses

Soy products are known to improve **cholesterol** profile, but isoflavones may not be the active cholesterol-lowering ingredient in soy. Isoflavones may, however, improve other measures linked to cardiovascular risk, such as levels of blood sugar, insulin, and fibrinogen.

According to some but not all studies, soy protein or concentrated isoflavones from soy or red clover may reduce **menopausal symptoms** such as hot flashes and vaginal dryness.

However, isoflavones have failed to prove effective for the hot flashes that often occur in breast cancer survivors.

There is conflicting evidence regarding whether soy or isoflavones may be helpful for preventing **osteoporosis**, but on balance the evidence suggests a modest beneficial effect.

A small and poorly reported double-blind, placebo-controlled study provides weak evidence that red clover isoflavones might be helpful for **cyclic mastalgia**.

A combination product containing soy isoflavones, black cohosh, and dong quai has shown some promise for menstrual **migraines**.

One study found that use of soy isoflavones improved the effectiveness rate of in vitro fertilization (used for **female infertility**).

In a small double-blind trial, use of soy isoflavones appeared to reduce some symptoms of **premenstrual syndrome** (PMS).

Observational studies hint that soy may help prevent breast and uterine cancer in women. If this connection is real and not a statistical accident (observational studies are notorious for falling prey to statistical accidents), the explanation may lie in the estrogen-like action of soy isoflavones. As noted above, isoflavones decrease the action of regular estrogen by blocking estrogen receptor sites and may also reduce levels of circulating estrogen. Since estrogen promotes breast and uterine cancer, these effects could help prevent breast cancer. Soy also appears to lengthen the menstrual cycle by a few days, and this, too, would be expected to reduce breast cancer risk. However, only a large, long-term intervention trial could actually show that soy or isoflavones reduce breast and uterine cancer risk, and one has not been performed.

Observational studies also hint that soy might help prevent prostate cancer in men. Men have very low levels of circulating estrogen, so the net effect of increased soy consumption might be to increase estrogen-like activity in the body. Since real estrogen is used as a treatment to suppress prostate cancer, perhaps the mild estrogen-like activity of isoflavones has a similar effect. Isoflavones might also decrease testosterone levels, which would again be expected to provide benefit. In one double-blind study, men with early prostate cancer were given either isoflavones or placebo, and their PSA levels were monitored. (PSA is a marker for prostate cancer, with higher values generally showing increased numbers of cancer cells.) The results did show that use of isoflavones (60 mg daily) slightly reduced PSA levels. Whether this meant that soy actually slowed the progression of the cancer or simply lowered PSA directly is not clear from this study alone. However, in another study of apparently healthy men (not known to have prostate cancer), soy isoflavones at a dose of 83 mg per day did not alter PSA levels. Taken together, these two studies provide some direct evidence that soy isoflavones may be helpful for treating or preventing prostate cancer, but the case nonetheless remains highly preliminary.

According to most but not all studies, soy isoflavones are ineffective for **improving mental function**.

One study failed to find that soy protein with isoflavones improved general quality of life (health status, depression, and life satisfaction) in post-menopausal women. Soy isoflavones have also failed to prove effective for reducing levels of **homocysteine**.

What Is the Scientific Evidence for Isoflavones?

High Cholesterol

Numerous studies have found that soy can reduce blood cholesterol levels and improve the ratio of LDL ("bad") versus HDL ("good") cholesterol.

Although it was once thought that isoflavones are the ingredients in soy responsible for improving cholesterol profile, on balance current evidence suggests otherwise. Non-isoflavone constituents of soy, such as proteins, fiber, and phospholipids, may be equally or perhaps even more important than the isoflavones in soy.

It is also possible that the exact types of isoflavones in a particular product made a difference. One study of red clover isoflavones found evidence that biochanin—but not formononetin—can reduce LDL cholesterol.

Another study found that soy products may at times have an unusual isoflavone profile, containing high levels of the isoflavone glycitein rather than the more usual genistein and daidzein. Glycitein could be inactive regarding cholesterol reduction.

Finally, an interesting study suggests that the isoflavone daidzein may only be effective for reducing cholesterol when it is converted by intestinal bacteria into a substance called *equol*. It appears that only about one-third of people have the right intestinal bacteria to make equol.

Menopausal Symptoms

Although study results are not entirely consistent, the balance of the evidence suggests that isoflavones from soy may be helpful for symptoms of menopause, especially "hot flashes."

Improvements in hot flashes, as well as other symptoms, such as vaginal dryness, were seen in many studies of soy, mixed soy isoflavones, or genistein alone. One study found that people who are equol producers (see previous section) may experience greater benefits.

However, several other studies have failed to find benefit with whole soy or concentrated soy isoflavones. Another study failed to find benefit with a mixture of soy isoflavones and **black cohosh**.

Isoflavones from red clover have also shown inconsistent benefit, with the largest and most recent trial failing to find any reduction in hot-flash symptoms.

Furthermore, in double-blind, placebo-controlled trials, soy or purified isoflavones failed to reduce hot flashes among survivors of breast cancer.

What can one make of this mixed evidence? The problem here is that placebo treatment has a strong effect on menopausal symptoms. In such circumstances, statistical noise can easily drown out the real benefits of a treatment under study. Estrogen is so powerful for hot flashes and other menopausal symptoms that its benefits are almost always clear in studies; most likely, soy or concentrated isoflavones have a more modest effect, not always seen above the background.

Osteoporosis

Estrogen has a powerfully protective effect on bone. Study results on whether isoflavones have the same effect have produced inconsistent results. On balance, it is probably fair to summarize current evidence as indicating that isoflavones (either as soy, genistein, mixed isoflavones, or tofu extract) may have a modestly beneficial effect on bone density.

Interestingly, one small but long-term study suggests that **progesterone cream** (another treatment proposed for use in preventing or treating osteoporosis) may decrease the bone-sparing effect of soy isoflavones.

Bone is always subject to two influences: bone building and bone breakdown. Estrogen primarily works by reducing the bone breakdown part of the equation, thereby leading to a net result of increased bone growth. Some evidence suggests that isoflavones may act on both sides of this equation, directly stimulating new bone creation along with slowing bone breakdown.

Again, isoflavones may be more effective in equol producers.

Menstrual Migraines

In a 24-week, double-blind study, 49 women with menstrual migraines (migraine headaches associated with the menstrual cycle) received either placebo or a combination supplement containing soy isoflavones and extracts of **dong quai** and black cohosh. Beginning at the twentieth week, use of the herbal supplement resulted in decreased severity and frequency of headaches as compared to placebo. However, it is not clear which of the ingredients in the combination was helpful. The authors of the study apparently considered black cohosh and dong quai as phytoestrogens, but the current consensus is that they do not belong in that category.

Safety Issues

Studies in animals have found soy isoflavones essentially nontoxic. The long history of the use of soy as food in Asia would tend to suggest safety as well. However, as noted under the Therapeutic Dosages section above, typical recommended consumption of soy isoflavones exceeds the normal Asian consumption, so absolute safety cannot be assumed from historical consumption of soy as food. Concerns have been raised about estrogenic and other potential side effects of excessive soy isoflavone intake. In Japan, the maximum safe intake level of soy isoflavones has been set at a total of 70 to 75 mg daily (food plus supplement sources).

Overall, the estrogenic effect of soy isoflavones in women appears to be fairly minimal. Nonetheless, it is not zero: according to most but not all studies, use of soy has enough of an estrogen-like effect to slightly alter the menstrual cycle and change levels of sex hormones in young women. Thus, some of the risks of estrogen could in theory apply to isoflavones as well.

For example, because estrogen can stimulate breast cancer cells, there are theoretical concerns that isoflavones may not be safe for women who have already had breast cancer. While isoflavones in general should have an anti-estrogenic effect by blocking real estrogen, some studies in animals have found evidence that under certain circumstances soy isoflavones might stimulate breast cancer cells. Studies directly examining the effects of isoflavones on human breast tissue have produced contradictory results. Taking all this evidence together, prudence suggests that women who have had breast cancer, or are at high risk for it, should consult a physician before taking any isoflavone product.

Estrogen also stimulates uterine cells, leading to an increased risk of uterine cancer. Most studies have found that isoflavones do not stimulate uterine cells. However, one fairly large (365 participants) and long-term (5 years) study did find uterine stimulation in 3.37% of women on isoflavones and 0% of those on placebo. This could indicate an increased risk of uterine cancer with high-dose isoflavone use.

Similarly, preliminary studies and reports have raised concerns that intensive use of soy products or isoflavones by pregnant women could exert a hormonal effect that impacts unborn fetuses. Use of soy formula by infants is also of concern along these lines, as an infant subsisting on soy formula has a relatively enormous isoflavone intake; on a per-weight basis it may exceed the average Asian adult isoflavone intake by a factor of ten.

The drug tamoxifen blocks estrogen and is used to help prevent breast cancer recurrence in women who have had breast cancer. One animal study found that soy isoflavones might remove the benefit of tamoxifen treatment.

One double-blind study of post-menopausal women found the use of red clover isoflavones at a dose of 80 mg daily for 90 days resulted in increased levels of testosterone. The potential significance of this is unclear. In men, isoflavones might decrease testosterone levels, but the effect appears to be slight at most.

Other concerns relate to soy's potential effects involving the thyroid gland. When given to individuals with **impaired thyroid function**, soy products have been observed to reduce absorption of thyroid medication. In addition, some evidence hints that soy isoflavones may directly inhibit the function of the thyroid gland (though perhaps only in people who are iodine deficient). To make matters more confusing, studies of healthy humans and animals given soy isoflavones or other soy products have generally found that soy either had no effect on thyroid hormone levels or actually *increased* levels. The bottom line: In view of soy's complex effects regarding the thyroid, individuals with impaired thyroid function should not take large amounts of soy products except under the supervision of a physician.

While fears have been expressed by some experts that soy isoflavones might interfere with the action of oral contraceptives, one study of 36 women found reassuring results.

Some evidence suggests that the isoflavone genistein might impair immunity. One study in mice found that injected genistein has negative effects on the thymus gland (an organ that is important for immunity) and also causes changes in the prevalence of various white blood cells consistent with impaired immunity. Although the genistein was injected rather than administered orally, the blood levels of genistein that these injections produced were not excessively high; they were comparable to (or even lower than) what occurs in children fed soy milk formula. In addition, there are several reports of impaired immune responses in infants fed soy formula. While it is too early to conclude that genistein impairs immunity, these findings are a potential cause for concern.

One observational study raised concerns that soy

might impair mental function in adults. However, observational studies are far less reliable than clinical trials. Direct studies designed to test the potential effects of isoflavones on brain function, and lasting up to 12 months, have found either no effect or a slightly positive effect on brain function. While this does not rule out a harmful long-term effect on cognition, it is reassuring.

There exists one case report in which soy isoflavone supplements caused migraine headaches in a man who had never experienced migraines before; presumably this was a highly individual reaction, such as an allergy. Similarly, there is also a well-documented case report in which use of high-dose soy isoflavones caused extreme elevation in blood pressure in a woman participating in a scientific study (of soy isoflavones).

Ivy Leaf
Hedera helix

PRINCIPAL PROPOSED USES: *Asthma*

OTHER PROPOSED USES: *Acute Bronchitis, Chronic Bronchitis, Colds and Flus*

The climbing ivy that adorns the sides of buildings has a long history of traditional medicinal use. Herbalists used ivy for such disparate conditions as arthritis, bronchitis, dysentery, and whooping cough. Topical applications of the herb were used for skin problems such as lice, eczema, and sunburn.

What Is Ivy Leaf Used for Today?

Ivy leaf is one of many herbs used in Europe as an expectorant, a substance said to thin mucous and thereby loosen coughs. (In the United States, the herbal product guaifenesin takes this role in almost all over-the-counter cough formulas.) Germany's Commission E has approved ivy leaf for treatment of mucous in the respiratory passages. On this basis, it is often recommended for **asthma**, **acute bronchitis**, **chronic bronchitis**, **colds and flus**, and other respiratory problems. Unfortunately, there is almost no evidence that ivy leaf (or, indeed, any other expectorant) actually offers meaningful benefits.

Only one double-blind, placebo-controlled study of ivy leaf has been reported. (For information on why double-blind, placebo-controlled studies are essential to prove a treatment effective, see **Why Does This Book Rely on Double-blind Studies?**.) In this study, a total of 24 children with asthma received either placebo or ivy

leaf extract twice a day for a period of 3 days. The results showed modest improvement in asthma symptoms as measured by formal testing.

Other studies on ivy leaf compared various forms of the product to each other and thereby do not prove anything about efficacy. One double-blind study found ivy leaf equally effective as the expectorant drug ambroxol for chronic bronchitis; however, because ambroxol itself has not been proven effective, this study proves little.

Dosage

A typical dose of standardized ivy leaf extract is 25 drops twice per day in children, or 50 or more drops twice per day in adults.

Safety Issues

Fairly extensive monitoring indicates that ivy leaf rarely causes any noticeable side effects. Nausea and vomiting are possible with excessive doses or in very susceptible people. Ivy leaf is not recommended during pregnancy due to its emetine content.

Safety in nursing women, young children, or people with severe liver or kidney disease has not been established.

Juniper Berry

Juniper Berry
Juniperus communis

PRINCIPAL PROPOSED USES: *None*

OTHER PROPOSED USES: *Diuretic, Often Used for Bladder Infections, Osteoarthritis*

In Dutch, juniper is called *geniver*, from which came the English name *gin*. But juniper is not only good for making martinis. Its berries (actually not berries at all, but a portion of the cone) were used by the Zuni Indians to assist in childbirth, by British herbalists to treat congestive heart failure and stimulate menstruation, and by American nineteenth-century herbalists to treat congestive heart failure, gonorrhea, and urinary tract infections.

What Is Juniper Berry Used for Today?

Contemporary herbalists primarily use juniper as a diuretic ("water pill") component of herbal formulas designed to treat bladder infections. A typical combination might include **goldenrod**, dandelion, **uva ursi**, **parsley**, **cleavers**, and buchu. The volatile oils of juniper reportedly increase the rate of kidney filtration, thereby increasing urine flow and perhaps helping to "wash out" offending bacteria. However, there is no direct scientific evidence that juniper is effective, for bladder infections. Only a double-blind, placebo-controlled study can prove a treatment effective, and none have been reported with juniper.

Recently, gin-soaked raisins have been touted as an **arthritis** treatment. This is probably just a fad, but some weak evidence suggests that juniper may possess anti-inflammatory properties. Also, in test-tube studies, certain constituents of juniper have been found to inhibit the herpes virus. However, it is a long way from such studies to the conclusion that juniper is helpful for herpes infections.

Dosage

You can make juniper tea by adding 1 cup of boiling water to 1 tablespoon of juniper berries, covering, and allowing the berries to steep for 20 minutes. The usual dosage is 1 cup twice a day. However, juniper is said to work better as a treatment for bladder infections when combined with other herbs. Combination products should be taken according to label instructions.

Warning: Bladder infections can go on to become kidney infections. For this reason, seek medical supervision if your symptoms don't resolve in a few days or if you develop intense low back pain, fever, chills, or other signs of serious infection.

Safety Issues

Although juniper is regarded as safe and is widely used in foods, we don't recommend taking it during pregnancy. (We also recommend not drinking gin.) Remember, juniper was used historically to stimulate menstruation and childbirth. It has also been shown to cause miscarriages in rats.

Individuals taking the medication lithium should use herbal diuretics such as juniper only under the supervision of a physician, as being dehydrated when taking this medication can be dangerous.

Some texts warn that juniper oil may be a kidney irritant, but there is no real evidence that this is the case. Nonetheless, people with serious kidney disease probably shouldn't take juniper. Safety for young children, nursing women, or those with severe liver disease has also not been established.

Interactions You Should Know About

If you are taking **lithium**: Do not use juniper except under the supervision of a physician.

Kava

Piper methysticum

PRINCIPAL PROPOSED USES: *Anxiety*

OTHER PROPOSED USES: *Alcohol Withdrawal, Insomnia, Tension Headaches*

Kava is a member of the pepper family that has long been cultivated by Pacific Islanders for use as a social and ceremonial drink. The first description of kava came to the West from Captain James Cook on his celebrated voyages through the South Seas. Cook reported that on occasions when village elders and chieftains gathered together for significant meetings, they would hold an elaborate kava ceremony at the beginning to break the ice (not that there's much ice out there). Typically, each participant would drink two or three bowls of chewed-up kava mixed with coconut milk. Kava was also drunk in less-formal social settings as a mild intoxicant.

When they learned about kava's effects, European scientists set to work trying to isolate its active ingredients. However, it wasn't until 1966 that substances named kavalactones were isolated and found to be effective sedatives. One of the most active of these is dihydrokavain, which has been found to produce a sedative, painkilling, and anticonvulsant effect. Other named kavalactones include kavain, methysticin, and dihydromethysticin.

High doses of kava extracts are thought to cause muscle relaxation and even paralysis (without loss of consciousness) at very high doses. Kava also has local anesthetic properties, producing peculiar numbing sensations when held in the mouth.

The method of action of kava is not fully understood. Conventional tranquilizers in the Valium family interact with special binding sites in the brain called *GABA receptors*. Early studies of kava suggested that the herb does not affect these receptors. However, more recent studies have found an interaction. The early researchers may have missed the connection because kava appears to affect somewhat unusual parts of the brain.

Note: An accumulation of case reports suggests that kava products may rarely cause severe liver injury, and this has led to a banning of kava by many countries. See Safety Issues below for more information.

What Is Kava Used for Today?

In 1990, Germany's Commission E authorized the use of kava for relieving "states of nervous anxiety, tension, and agitation," based on evidence from several double-blind studies. However, case reports of liver damage later led Germany and other countries to ban the sale of kava.

Like other anxiety-reducing drugs, kava could be useful for **insomnia**, but most of the supporting evidence for this use remains highly preliminary. One small double-blind study found that daily use of kava reduced sleep disturbances linked to anxiety. However, a larger study failed to find benefits in people with both insomnia and anxiety.

One animal study suggests that kava may also have value as an aid to **alcohol withdrawal**. (However, individuals who abuse alcohol are probably at increased risk of harm from kava. See Safety Issues.) Kava has been additionally proposed as a treatment for **tension headaches**, but it has not been evaluated for this purpose.

What Is the Scientific Evidence for Kava?

There have been at least 11 placebo-controlled studies of kava, involving a total of more than 700 people. Most found kava helpful for anxiety symptoms.

One of the best of these was a 6-month, double-blind study that tested kava's effectiveness in 100 people with various forms of anxiety. Over the course of the trial, they were evaluated with a list of questions called the *Hamilton Anxiety Scale* (HAM-A). The HAM-A assigns a total score based on such symptoms as restlessness, nervousness, heart palpitations, stomach discomfort, dizziness, and chest pain. Lower scores indicate reduced anxiety. Participants who were given kava showed significantly improved scores beginning at 8 weeks and continuing throughout the duration of the treatment.

This study is notable for the long delay before kava was effective. Previous studies had shown a good response in 1 week. The reason for this discrepancy is unclear.

Several double-blind, placebo-controlled studies have specifically tested kava for the treatment of the anxiety that often occurs during **menopause**. In the most recent one, 40 women were given either kava plus standard hormone therapy or hormone therapy alone for a period of 6 months. The results showed that women given kava experienced greater improvement in symptoms than those given hormone therapy alone.

However, not all studies have been positive. One double-blind, placebo-controlled study failed to find kava effective for people with generalized anxiety disorder (GAD). Another study failed to find kava more effective than placebo for people with both anxiety and insomnia.

Besides these placebo-controlled studies, one 6-month, double-blind study compared kava against two standard anxiety drugs (oxazepam and bromazepam) in 174 people with anxiety symptoms. Improvement in HAM-A scores was about the same in all groups. Another study found kava equally effective as the drugs buspirone and opipramol.

A 5-week, double-blind, placebo-controlled trial studied 40 people who had been taking standard antianxiety drugs (benzodiazepines) for an average duration of 20 months. Participants were gradually tapered off their medications and switched to kava or placebo. Individuals taking kava showed some improvement in anxiety symptoms. This would appear to indicate that kava can successfully substitute for benzodiazepine drugs. However, participants who were switched from benzodiazepines to placebo showed little to no increase in anxiety, suggesting perhaps that they didn't really need medication after all! Thus, the results of this study are hard to interpret.

Note: This trial involved close medical supervision and very gradual tapering of benzodiazepine dosages. Do not discontinue antianxiety medications without such supervision, as withdrawal symptoms can be life-threatening!

One study purported to find evidence that kava helps reduce reactions to **stressful situations**, but because it lacked a placebo group, the results mean little.

Dosage

A typical dosage of kava when used for treatment of anxiety is 300 mg/day of a product standardized to contain 70% kavalactones. A lower dose of 150 mg/day has also been tested, but may be less effective.

The typical dosage for insomnia is 210 mg of kavalactones 1 hour before bedtime.

Safety Issues

Until recently, kava had been considered a safe herb. Animal studies have shown that kava dosages of up to 4 times the normal amount cause no health problems, and 13 times the normal dosage causes only mild problems in rats. A study of 4,049 people who took a rather low dose of kava (70 mg of kavalactones daily) for 7 weeks found side effects in 1.5% of cases. These were mostly mild gastrointestinal complaints and allergic rashes. A 4-week study of 3,029 people given 240 mg of kavalactones daily showed a 2.3% incidence of basically the same side effects. One review of the literature concluded that "the data support the safety of kava in treating anxiety at 280 mg kava lactones/day for 4 weeks."

However, a growing number of case reports have raised serious concerns about kava's safety. These reports suggest that, occasionally, even normal doses of kava can cause severe liver injury. Based on these reports, regulatory agencies have taken action in numerous countries banning or restricting sale of kava. However, case reports are notorious for failing to show cause and effect, and some well-regarded experts who have reviewed the literature feel that kava has not been shown unsafe. At present, if you wish to use this herb, we recommend that you seek physician supervision to monitor for liver inflammation. People with liver problems, who drink alcohol excessively, or who take medications that can harm the liver are probably at increased risk of harm by kava.

There are other safety concerns as well. For example, kava should not be used by individuals who have had "acute dystonic reactions." These consist of spasms in the muscles of the neck and movements of the eyes, and are believed related to effects on dopamine. They are typically caused by antipsychotic drugs, which affect dopamine. Kava might trigger such reactions too.

At ordinary doses, kava does not appear to produce mental cloudiness. However, high doses cause inebriation and can lead to charges of driving under the influence of drugs.

One study suggests that kava does not amplify the effects of alcohol. However, there is a case report indicating that kava can increase the effects of certain sedative drugs. For this reason, kava probably should not be combined with any drugs that depress mental function. Kava should also not be combined with antipsychotic drugs or drugs used for **Parkinson's disease**, due to the potential for increased problems with movement.

The German Commission E monograph warns against the use of kava during pregnancy and nursing. Safety in young children and individuals with kidney disease has not been established.

Interactions You Should Know About

If you are taking:

> - **Medications for insomnia or anxiety, such as benzo-diazepines: Do not take kava in addition to them.**

> - **Antipsychotic drugs: Kava might increase the risk of a particular side effect consisting of sudden abnormal movements, called a *dystonic reaction*.**
> - **Levodopa for Parkinson's disease: Kava might reduce its effectiveness.**
> - **Medications that can irritate the liver: Avoid kava. (Numerous medications have this potential. Ask your physician to see if this concern applies to you.)**

Kelp

SUPPLEMENT FORMS/ALTERNATE NAMES: *Kombu*

PRINCIPAL PROPOSED USES: *Nutrient-rich Food*

OTHER PROPOSED USES: *Cancer Prevention, Colds and Flus, Herpes, High Blood Pressure, HIV Support, Weight Loss*

Kelp refers to several species of large, brown algae that can grow to enormous sizes far out in the depths of the ocean. Kelp is a type of seaweed, but not all seaweed is kelp: "seaweed" loosely describes any type of vegetation growing in the ocean, including many other types of algae and plants.

Kelp is a regular part of a normal human diet in many parts of the world, such as Japan, Alaska, and Hawaii. It is also incorporated into some vitamin and mineral supplements because of its nutrient value. Kelp is a good source of folic acid (a B vitamin), as well as many other vitamins and minerals—especially **iodine**; but iodine is also a potential source of side effects (see Safety Issues below).

Requirements/Sources

Supplements containing kelp can be purchased at most pharmacies and health food stores. Kelp used in food preparation is available at groceries that stock specialties for Asian cooking.

Therapeutic Dosages

There is no appropriate "therapeutic" dosage of kelp, as it is not yet known whether kelp is truly therapeutic for any conditions. However, because of its high iodine content, it is important not to overdo your use of kelp. The iodine content in 17 different kelp supplements studied by one group of researchers varied from 45 to 57,000 mcg per tablet or capsule. The recommended daily intake for iodine is 150 mcg per day for people over the age of 4, and taking a great deal more than this can cause thyroid problems (see Safety Issues below).

Therapeutic Uses

Kelp is used primarily as a nutrient-rich food supplement.

The results of highly preliminary test-tube and animal studies have suggested other potential uses for kelp. For example, there is some evidence that elements in kelp might help to prevent infection with several kinds of viruses, including **influenza**, herpes simplex, and **HIV**. Similarly weak evidence hints that kelp possesses cancer preventive effects, and may lower **blood pressure**. However, far more research, including double-blind, placebo-controlled studies, would be necessary to know whether kelp is actually helpful for any of these health problems.

Additionally, kelp has been marketed as a weight-loss product, but there are no meaningful scientific studies to indicate that it is effective for this purpose.

Another common claim regarding kelp is that, because of its high iodine content, it can help all kinds of thyroid problems. This claim, however, is misleading and even dangerous. It is true that if you are deficient in iodine, kelp is probably good for you, but iodine deficiency is rare, and taking extra iodine when you don't need it can *cause* dysfunction of the thyroid (see Safety Issues below).

Safety Issues

Taking excessive kelp can overload the body with iodine and cause either **hypothyroidism** or **hyperthyroidism**—conditions in which the thyroid gland either produces too little or too much thyroid hormone. This is a potentially dangerous side effect and is definitely cause for caution. If your thyroid gland is already functioning incorrectly, you should avoid high doses of kelp except on a physician's advice.

Additionally, published reports describe two cases of **acne** apparently caused or worsened by taking large doses of kelp. This effect is also believed to be due to the large amounts of iodine in the supplement.

Finally, some kelp supplements have been found to contain levels of arsenic high enough to be toxic. Seawater contains highly diluted arsenic, but kelp (like other ocean life) can concentrate arsenic in its tissues, and there are reports of two people with symptoms of arsenic poisoning who had been consuming kelp.

Kombucha Tea

ALTERNATE NAMES/RELATED TERMS: *Kargasoki Mushroom, Kargasoki Tea, Kargasok Tea, Kombucha Mushroom, Manchurian Mushroom*

PRINCIPAL PROPOSED USES: *None*

OTHER PROPOSED USES: *Numerous Exaggerated Claims*

Just like friends can pass along sourdough starter, a small, round, flat, gray, gelatinous object has become a popular gift among those interested in natural medicine. You insert this object in sweetened black tea and let it ferment for 7 days. By the end of the week, you have a strong-tasting drink and a big, flat, gray, gelatinous object you can cut up and pass on to your friends.

Described variously as Manchurian mushroom, Kombucha tea, or just Kombucha, this tea is said to have been used for centuries to cure a wide variety of illnesses. The earliest known scientific analysis of Kombucha occurred in Germany in the 1930s, and subsequent studies have provided accurate information about this dubious product.

The word *kombucha* literally means "tea made from kombu seaweed." However, what is called *Kombucha tea* today has no seaweed in it. Furthermore, despite the name Manchurian mushroom, Kombucha is not a mushroom either. The gelatinous mass is a colony of numerous species of fungi and bacteria living together, and the same microorganisms permeate the tea. The precise composition of any sample of Kombucha depends to a great extent on what was floating around in your kitchen when you grew it.

The most common microorganisms found in Kombucha tea include species of *Brettanomyces*, *Zygosaccharomyces*, *Saccharomyces*, *Candida*, *Torula*, *Acetobacter*, and *Pichia*. However, some analyzed specimens have been found to contain completely different organisms, and there is no guarantee that they will be harmless.

What Is Kombucha Tea Used for Today?

Kombucha tea is widely supposed to have miraculous medicinal properties, ranging from curing cancer to restoring gray hair to its original color. Other reputed effects include normalizing weight, improving blood pressure, increasing energy, decreasing arthritis pain, restoring normal bowel movements, removing wrinkles, curing acne, strengthening bones, improving memory, and generally solving every health problem that exists.

However, there is no evidence that Kombucha tea is effective for these or any other uses.

Dosage

The *Collins Alternative Health Guide* does not recommend the use of homemade Kombucha tea. Commercially produced Kombucha should be safer, but it has no known medicinal effects.

Safety Issues

In a set of animal studies, researchers prepared a batch of Kombucha and found that it was essentially non-toxic when taken at appropriate doses. However, because Kombucha is a complex and variable mixture of microorganisms, it isn't clear that any other batch of the tea would be equally safe. In fact, there are case reports that suggest that Kombucha preparations can cause such problems as nausea, jaundice, shortness of breath, throat tightness, headache, dizziness, liver inflammation, and even unconsciousness. It isn't clear whether the cause of these symptoms is an unusual reaction to a generally nontoxic substance or a response to unusual toxins that developed in a particular batch of Kombucha.

In addition, there is one case report of severe lead poisoning caused by regular use of Kombucha brewed in a ceramic pot. When brewed or stored in some ceramics, the risk of lead poisoning results because Kombucha tea is acidic. Many ceramic glazes contain a low level of lead that would not make the pottery dangerous for ordinary use; but if an acidic solution like Kombucha is steeped in them for a long time, a dangerous amount of lead may leech into the solution.

There is also one report of Kombucha becoming infected with anthrax and passing along the infection to an individual who rubbed it on his skin to alleviate pain. Apparently, anthrax from nearby cows got into the Kombucha mixture and grew luxuriantly.

Krill Oil

PRINCIPAL PROPOSED USES: *Dysmenorrhea, High Cholesterol, Premenstrual Syndrome (PMS)*
OTHER PROPOSED USES: See *All Uses of* Fish Oil

Krill are tiny, shrimp-like crustaceans that flourish in the Antarctic Ocean and provide food for numerous aquatic animals. Oil made from krill has come on the market as an alternative to fish oil. Like fish oil, krill oil contains the omega-3 fatty acids eicosapentaenoic acid (EPA) and docosahexaenoic acid (DHA). Krill also contains **omega-6 fatty acids**, an antioxidant in the **carotenoid** family called *astaxanthin*, and substances called *phosopholipids*.

Requirements/Sources

Many grains, fruits, vegetables, sea vegetables, and vegetable oils contain significant amounts of essential fatty acids, but krill oil is an especially rich source.

Carotenoids are also found in many foods, especially yellow/orange and dark green fruits and vegetables. They are not essential nutrients (except insofar as some can be converted to **vitamin A**), but they might offer some health benefits.

Phospholipids are utilized in the body for numerous purposes, but they are not essential nutrients.

Dosage

A typical recommended dose of krill oil is 1 to 3 g daily.

Therapeutic Uses

Based on its omega-3 fatty acid content, krill oil would be expected to have many of the same effects as fish oil. See the full **Fish Oil** article for a detailed discussion of these potential benefits.

A few studies have evaluated krill oil specifically. In one double-blind, placebo-controlled study, 120 people with **high cholesterol** were given krill oil, fish oil, or placebo. The results over 3 months showed that krill oil (taken by student participants at a dose ranging from 1 to 3 g daily depending on body mass and which of two groups they were in) improved all aspects of cholesterol profile as compared to placebo and was more effective than fish oil (taken at the fixed dose of 3 g daily). Krill oil also reduced blood sugar levels.

Though these results need to be confirmed by independent trials, they are certainly promising.

Another double-blind study compared krill oil against fish oil for treatment of symptoms of **premenstrual syndrome** (PMS) and **dysmenorrhea** (menstrual cramps). This study suffered from many problems in design and reporting, but appeared to show that krill oil was more effective than fish oil for treating both of these conditions.

Safety Issues

Based on its known constituents, krill oil would be expected to have little to no toxicity. Side effects seen in studies are limited to occasional digestive distress and allergic reactions. The only known potential concerns relate to possible blood-thinning effects: Fish oil is known to decrease blood coagulation, and in one case report it increased the effect of the blood-thinning medication **warfarin** (Coumadin). People who are at risk of bleeding complications for any reason should therefore consult a physician before taking krill oil. Maximum safe doses in young children, pregnant or nursing women, or people with severe liver disease have not been established.

Kudzu

Pueraria lobata

PRINCIPAL PROPOSED USES: *None*

OTHER PROPOSED USES: *Alcoholism, Common Cold, Menopausal Symptoms*

Kudzu is cooked as food in China and also is used as an herb in **traditional Chinese medicine**. However, in the United States, kudzu has become an invasive pest. It was deliberately planted earlier this century for use as animal fodder and to control soil erosion. It turned out to be incredibly prolific and soon spread throughout the South like an alien invader. The problem is that kudzu can grow a foot a day during the summer, and as much as 60 feet a year, giving it the folk name "mile-a-minute vine." It swallows telephone poles, chokes trees, and takes over yards.

What Is Kudzu Used for Today?

Besides cooking with it, feeding it to animals, and weaving baskets out of its rubbery vines, kudzu may also be useful in treating **alcoholism**. In Chinese folk medicine, a tea brewed from kudzu root is believed to be useful in sobering up people who are intoxicated by alcohol. Taking the hint, a 1993 study evaluated the effects of kudzu in a species of hamsters known to enjoy drinking alcohol to intoxication. Ordinarily, if given a choice, the Syrian golden hamster will prefer alcohol to water, but administration of kudzu reversed that preference.

This animal study, along with another one involving rats, led to widespread speculation that kudzu may be useful in the treatment of human alcoholism. However, the results of the two small reported human trials are conflicting.

In academic Chinese herbology (as opposed to Chinese folk medicine), kudzu has different applications. One classic herbal formula containing kudzu is used for the treatment of **colds** accompanied by pain in the neck. However, there is no scientific evidence that it is effective for this condition.

Kudzu contains **isoflavones** similar to those found in **soy**. These substances are known to have an estrogen-like effect. On this basis, kudzu has been proposed as a treatment for **menopausal symptoms**. However, the one published double-blind trial failed to find benefit.

Dosage

The standard dosage of kudzu ranges from 9 to 15 g daily, in tea or tablets.

Safety Issues

Based on its extensive food use, kudzu is believed to be reasonably safe. However, safety in young children, pregnant or nursing women, or those with severe kidney or liver disease has not been established.

Lady's Slipper Orchid
Cypripedium species

PRINCIPAL PROPOSED USES: *None*

OTHER PROPOSED USES:

    Oral Uses: *Anxiety, Insomnia*

    Topical Uses: *Musculoskeletal Pain*

The common name "lady's slipper" refers to the distinctive shape of these beautiful orchids, members of the genus *Cypripedium* that are native to North America and Europe, as well as the *Paphiopedilum* species native to Southeast Asia. Other "slipper" orchid species are native to South America. Typically, the yellow lady's slipper *Cypripedium calceolus var. pubescens* (now called *Cypripedium parviflorum var. pubescens*) is used medicinally in Europe and North America. *Cypripedium montanum*, the rare mountain lady's slipper native to North America, is also *wildcrafted* (collected in the wild).

Many of the *Cypripedium* lady's slipper species are endangered and have proven very difficult to cultivate; even just collecting the flower alone may be enough to kill the plant, and transplantation from the wild is rarely successful. Alternatively, some herbalists recommend using the roots of another species called *stream orchid* or *helleborine* (*Epipactis helleborine*), which has the same purported effects, is more widespread, and is relatively easy to cultivate.

Traditionally, lady's slipper root was classified as a *nervine*, indicating its purported healing and calming effect on the nerves. This term, however, is no longer used in medicine today.

What Is Lady's Slipper Orchid Used for Today?

Despite a complete absence of scientific evidence that it is effective, lady's slipper is sometimes used today either alone or as a component of formulas intended to treat **anxiety** or **insomnia**.

Lady's slipper is also sometimes used topically as a

Lapacho

poultice or plaster for relief of muscular pain, but again there is no evidence that it is effective.

Dosage

The optimum oral dosage of lady's slipper is not known. A typical recommendation for *Cypripedium* species is 3 to 9g of root or 2 to 6ml of a tincture of fresh or dried root.

For muscle-pain relief, a topical application of fresh

or dried roots mashed into a poultice or plaster is sometimes used.

Safety Issues

The safety of any medicinal application of these orchid species has not been established. Contact with the small hairs on some species can cause skin irritation.

Lapacho

Tabebuia impestiginosa, T. avellanedae

ALTERNATE NAMES/RELATED TERMS: *Pau d'Arco, Taheebo*

PRINCIPAL PROPOSED USES: *None*

OTHER PROPOSED USES: *Bladder Infections, Cancer, Colds and Flus, Diarrhea, Pain in General, Psoriasis, Ulcers, Vaginal Infections, Yeast Hypersensitivity Syndrome ("Chronic Candida")*

The inner bark of the lapacho tree plays a central role in the herbal medicine of several South American indigenous peoples. They use it to treat cancer as well as a great variety of infectious diseases.

There has been very little scientific investigation of lapacho as a whole herb. However, an enormous amount of scientific interest has focused on three constituents of lapacho: lapachol, lapachone, and isolapachone. The relevance of these findings to the use of lapacho itself remains unclear.

What Is Lapacho Used for Today?

Based on its traditional uses, lapacho is sometimes recommended by herbalists as a treatment for **cancer**. However, there is no reliable scientific evidence that the herb is effective. Test-tube studies have found that lapachone can kill cancer cells by inhibiting an enzyme called *topoisomerase*, and there are hopes that effective anti-cancer drugs may eventually be produced through chemical modification of lapachone. Nonetheless, this does not indicate that lapacho is effective against cancer in humans; it would be difficult to take

enough of the herb to provide active levels of lapachone.

Similarly, test-tube studies have found that constituents of lapacho (especially lapachone, isolapachone, and lapachol) may be able to kill various microorganisms, including various fungi and the parasites that cause schistosomiasis, malaria, and sleeping sickness. These findings have led to the widespread belief that lapacho is useful against the yeast *Candida Albicans*, a common cause of vaginitis, as well as the purported condition colloquially known as chronic Candida; unfortunately, the supporting research remains far too preliminary to meaningfully show clinical benefits.

Similarly, these studies have been twisted to support claims that lapacho is useful for many infections, including **colds and flus** and bladder infections. However, there are at least two problems with this reasoning. First, lapacho has been tested primarily against fungi and parasites; there is little evidence that it can kill viruses (the cause of colds) or bacteria (the cause of most bladder infections). Furthermore, even if lapacho can kill these microorganisms on direct contact, this does not imply that it would be effective if taken by mouth. Consider this analogy: wine easily kills the cold virus on direct contact, but if you drink wine when you have a cold you're not likely to get well faster. Similarly, hundreds of herbal products kill microorganisms in the test tube but fail to prove effective as systemic antibiotics. A substance taken by mouth has to survive the digestive tract and passage through the liver and reach sufficient concentrations in the bloodstream to produce a meaningful effect. Few substances can do this without simultaneously proving toxic to the body; that's why antibiotics were not invented until the twentieth century and remain difficult to invent even today. Until lapacho's potential effects as an oral antibiotic are examined directly, it is not reasonable to assume that the herb is likely to help systemic infections.

Lapacho and its constituents have also been investigated for potential use in the treatment of pain, **psoriasis**, and **ulcers**; however, the evidence for benefit is as yet too preliminary to rely upon at all.

Dosage

Lapacho contains many components that don't dissolve in water, so making tea from the herb is not the best idea. It's better to take capsulized powdered bark; a typical dose is 300 to 500 mg 3 times daily. The inner bark of the lapacho tree is said to be the most effective part of the plant.

Safety Issues

When taken in normal dosages, lapacho has not been found to cause any obvious side effects. However, full safety studies have not been performed. Furthermore, the anti-cancer actions of lapachone raise serious concerns about the safety of lapacho for pregnant women, because like cancer cells, cells of a developing fetus rapidly divide. Also, a study in animals found that lapachol caused fetal death. For all these reasons, pregnant or nursing women should not use lapacho. Safety in young children or those with severe liver or kidney disease has also not been established.

Larch Arabinogalactan
Hypericum perforatum

PRINCIPAL PROPOSED USES: *Immune Support*
OTHER PROPOSED USES: *Cancer Treatment, Ear Infections*

Arabinogalactins, substances found in many plants, are long molecules made of the sugars galactose and arabinose linked together in a chain. Arabinogalactan extracted from the Western larch tree (larch arabinogalactan, or LA) has been proposed as an immune stimulant.

Therapeutic Uses

Test-tube and animal studies suggest that LA has several potentially positive effects on the immune system. It appears to activate a type of white blood cell called a *natural killer*, or NK cell, and perhaps other white blood cells as well; it may also possibly alter levels of immune-related substances such as interleukins, interferon, and properdin.

On the basis of these findings, LA has been advocated as a supplement for **general immune support**. However, this recommendation is premature. It is a very, very long way from basic science of this type to evidence that a treatment has real effectiveness. Many plant substances appear to activate the immune system; this may be merely because the immune system regards them as "the enemy" and mobilizes to fight them. It takes double-blind, placebo-controlled trials to determine whether theoretical effects translate into real-life benefits and, thus far, only one such study has been performed on LA as an immune stimulant. Unfortunately, this single meaningful trial was not designed to determine the actual medical benefits (if any) of LA. Rather, it primarily continued the theoretical investigation of LA's effects on components of the immune system.

In this trial, 48 healthy women were assigned to receive one of four treatments: LA, echinacea, LA plus echinacea, or placebo. Researchers evaluated various laboratory measurements of immune function. The results failed to show that LA by itself had any effect on immunity.

Other extremely preliminary research hints that LA might enhance the effectiveness of drugs used in **cancer treatment**, help antibiotics fight **ear infections** and other infections, and enhance the immune system in people with conditions such as **chronic viral hepatitis**, **HIV**, and **chronic fatigue syndrome**. However, all these suggestions are highly speculative and lack reliable supporting evidence.

There is no doubt, however, that LA is a good dietary fiber source. Like less expensive forms of fiber, it appears to have beneficial effects in the colon.

A 6-month study failed to find LA helpful for improving **cholesterol profile**.

Dosage

A typical dose of powdered LA is 3 to 9 g daily.

Safety Issues

Based on animal studies and limited evidence in humans, LA appears to be essentially nontoxic. However,

like other sources of dietary fiber, LA might lead to colonic problems like bloating and flatulence.

One additional set of potential risks derives from its supposed benefits: If LA does in fact meaningfully stimulate the immune system, it might be dangerous. The immune system is balanced on a knife's edge. An immune system that is too relaxed fails to defend us from infections; an immune system that is too active attacks healthy tissues, causing autoimmune diseases. If LA truly boosts immunity, it might cause or worsen such conditions as **lupus**, **Crohn's disease**, **asthma**, **Graves' disease**, **Hashimoto's thyroiditis**, **multiple sclerosis**, or **rheumatoid arthritis**, among other problems. In addition, people who take immune suppressant drugs for organ transplants would be at risk of organ rejection. However, there is no actual evidence that it causes problems.

Maximum safe doses in young children, pregnant or nursing women, or people with severe liver or kidney disease have not been established.

Interactions You Should Know About

If you are taking an immunosuppressant drug such as **cyclosporine**, **methotrexate**, or **corticosteroids**, use of LA could conceivably decrease the drug's effectiveness by stimulating your immune system.

Lecithin

SUPPLEMENT FORMS/ALTERNATE NAMES: *Egg Lecithin, Phosphatidylcholine in Lecithin, Soy Lecithin*

PRINCIPAL PROPOSED USES: *None*

OTHER PROPOSED USES: *Alzheimer's Disease, Bipolar Disorder, High Cholesterol, Liver Disease, Parkinson's Disease, Tardive Dyskinesia, Tourette's Syndrome*

For decades, lecithin has been a popular treatment for high cholesterol (although there is surprisingly little evidence that it works). More recently, lecithin has been proposed as a remedy for various psychological and neurological diseases, such as Tourette's syn-

drome, Alzheimer's disease, and bipolar disorder (also known as manic depression).

Lecithin contains a substance called *phosphatidylcholine* (PC) that is presumed to be responsible for its medicinal effects. Phosphatidylcholine is a major part of

Lecithin

the membranes surrounding our cells. However, when you consume phosphatidylcholine, it is broken down into the nutrient *choline* rather than being carried directly to cell membranes. Choline acts like folate, TMG (trimethylglycine), and SAMe (S-adenosylmethionine) to promote methylation (see the article on **TMG** for further discussion of this subject). It is also used to make *acetylcholine* a nerve chemical essential for proper brain function.

This article discusses lecithin and phosphatidylcholine. For more information on the effects and possible benefits of **choline** alone, see the full article.

Sources

Neither lecithin nor its ingredient, phosphatidylcholine, is an essential nutrient; however, choline has recently been recognized as essential. For use as a supplement or a food additive, lecithin is often manufactured from soy.

Therapeutic Dosages

Ordinary lecithin contains about 10 to 20% phosphatidylcholine. However, European research has tended to use products concentrated to contain 90% phosphatidylcholine in lecithin, and the following dosages are based on that type of product. For psychological and neurological conditions, doses as high as 5 to 10 g taken 3 times daily have been used in studies. For liver disease, a typical dose is 350 to 500 mg taken 3 times daily; and for high cholesterol, 500 to 900 mg taken 3 times daily has been tried.

Therapeutic Uses

For a while, lecithin/phosphatidylcholine was one of the most commonly recommended natural treatments for **high cholesterol**. However, this idea appears to rest entirely on studies of unacceptably low quality. The best-designed studies have failed to find any evidence of benefit. In Europe, phosphatidylcholine is also used to treat **liver diseases**, such as alcoholic fatty liver, **alcoholic hepatitis**, **liver cirrhosis**, and **viral hepatitis**. However, research into these potential uses remains preliminary and has yielded contradictory results.

Some evidence hints that phosphatidylcholine may reduce **homocysteine levels**, which in turn might potentially reduce heart disease risk.

Because phosphatidylcholine plays a role in nerve function, it has also been suggested as a treatment for various psychological and neurological disorders, such as **Alzheimer's disease**, **bipolar disorder**, **Parkinson's disease**, Tourette's syndrome, and **tardive dyskinesia** (a late-developing side effect of drugs used for psychosis). However, the evidence that it works is limited to small studies with conflicting results.

Safety Issues

Lecithin is believed to be generally safe. However, some people taking high dosages (several grams daily) experience minor but annoying side effects, such as abdominal discomfort, diarrhea, and nausea. Maximum safe dosages for young children, pregnant or nursing women, or those with severe liver or kidney disease have not been determined.

Lemon Balm
Melissa officinalis

ALTERNATE NAMES/RELATED TERMS: *Melissa*

PRINCIPAL PROPOSED USES:

Topical Lemon Balm: *Oral and Genital Herpes*

Oral Lemon Balm: *Sedative (Insomnia, Anxiety, Nervous Stomach)*

Inhaled Essential Oil of Lemon Balm (Aromatherapy): *Reducing Agitation in Dementia*

Commonly called by its Latin first name, *Melissa*, lemon balm is a native of southern Europe, often planted in gardens to attract bees. Its leaves give off a delicate lemon odor when bruised.

Medical authorities of ancient Greece and Rome mentioned topical lemon balm as a treatment for wounds. The herb was later used orally as a treatment for influenza, insomnia, anxiety, depression, and nervous stomach.

What Is Melissa Used for Today?

Topical lemon balm is most popular today as a treatment for genital or oral **herpes**. It appears to make flare-ups less intense and last for a shorter period of time, but it doesn't completely eliminate them. Regular use of lemon balm might help prevent flare-ups, but this potential use hasn't been properly studied.

Note: While conventional treatments can reduce infectivity and thereby help prevent the spread of herpes, there is no evidence as yet that lemon balm offers this benefit. Keep in mind also that common sense methods of avoiding passing on herpes are not entirely effective: many people are infectious even when they do not have obvious symptoms and use of a condom does not entirely prevent the spread of the virus. Therefore, if you are sexually active with a non-infected partner who wishes to remain that way, we strongly recommend that you use suppressive drug therapy.

There is some evidence that oral use of lemon balm has sedative effects and it is currently used for **insomnia**, **anxiety**, and nervous stomach. Inhaled essential oil of lemon balm may also have calming effects.

What Is the Scientific Evidence for Lemon Balm?

Herpes Infection

Numerous test-tube studies have found that extracts of lemon balm possess antiviral properties. We don't really know how it works, but the predominant theory is that the herb blocks viruses from attaching to cells.

One double-blind, placebo-controlled study followed 66 individuals who were just starting to develop a cold sore (oral herpes). Treatment with melissa cream produced significant benefits on day 2, reducing intensity of discomfort, number of blisters, and the size of the lesion. (The researchers specifically looked at day 2 because, according to them, that is when symptoms are most pronounced.)

Another double-blind study followed 116 individuals with oral or genital herpes. Participants used either melissa cream or placebo cream for up to 10 days. The results showed that use of the herb resulted in a significantly better rate of recovery than those given placebo.

Relatively informal observations suggest that regular use of lemon balm cream may help reduce the frequency of herpes flare-ups.

Sedative Effect

Lemon balm extracts have been found to produce a sedative effect in mice. Based on this, human trials have been performed.

In a 4-month, double-blind, placebo-controlled study of 42 people with **Alzheimer's disease**, use of an oral lemon balm extract significantly decreased their tendency to become agitated.

In another study, lemon balm essential oil applied to the skin in the form of a cream also reduced agitation in

71 people with Alzheimer's disease. The researchers considered this a form of **aromatherapy**, a treatment in which the odor of a substance is said to produce the benefit. However, one of the first things to disappear in Alzheimer's disease is the sense of smell; it is more likely, therefore, that the lemon balm worked via absorption through the skin.

Lemon balm has also shown sedative and anti-anxiety effects in two small studies of healthy people.

In other studies, combination therapies containing lemon balm plus **valerian** have shown modest promise as sedatives for the treatment of insomnia.

Dosage

For treatment of an active flare-up of herpes, the proper dosage is 4 thick applications daily of a standardized lemon balm (70:1) cream. The dosage may be reduced to twice daily for preventive purposes.

The best lemon balm extracts are standardized by their capacity to inhibit the growth of herpes virus in a petri dish. To make sure the extract has been properly prepared, manufacturers place cells in such a growing medium and then add herpes virus. Normally, the virus will gradually destroy all the cells. But when little disks containing lemon balm are added, cells in the immediate vicinity are protected. Although manufacturers use this method as a form of quality control, it also provides evidence that lemon balm really works.

When taken orally for its calming effect, the standard dosage of lemon balm is 1.5 to 4.5 g of dried herb daily; extracts and tinctures should be taken according to label instructions.

Safety Issues

Topical lemon balm is not associated with any significant side effects, although allergic reactions are always possible. Oral lemon balm is on the FDA's GRAS (generally recognized as safe) list. However, according to one study cited above, lemon balm reduces alertness and impairs mental function; for this reason, individuals engaging in activities that require alertness, such as operating a motor vehicle, should avoid using lemon balm beforehand.

In addition, one animal study suggests that if lemon balm is taken at the same time as standard sedative drugs, excessive sedation might occur.

Interactions You Should Know About

If you are taking sedative medications, use of oral lemon balm might amplify the effect, potentially leading to excessive sedation.

Licorice

Glycyrrhiza glabra

PRINCIPAL PROPOSED USES: *None*

OTHER PROPOSED USES:

   Oral Uses (DGL Form): *Heartburn (Esophageal Reflux), Mouth Sores, Ulcers*
   Topical Uses (Whole Herb): *Eczema, Herpes, Psoriasis*
   Oral Uses (Whole Herb): *Asthma, Chronic Fatigue Syndrome, Cough*

A member of the pea family, licorice root has been used since ancient times both as food and as medicine. In Chinese herbology, licorice is an ingredient in nearly all herbal formulas for the traditional purpose of "harmonizing" the separate herbs involved.

The herb licorice contains a substance called *glycyrrhizin*. When taken in high enough amounts, glycyrrhizin produces effects similar to those of the natural hormone aldosterone, causing fluid retention, increased blood pressure, and loss of potassium. To prevent this, manufacturers have found a way to remove glycyrrhizin from licorice, producing the safer product deglycyrrhizinated licorice (DGL).

What Is Licorice Used for Today?

DGL has shown some promise for the treatment of **ulcers**. Weak evidence hints that it might also help prevent ulcers caused by **anti-inflammatory drugs**.

DGL is also sometimes recommended for relieving the discomfort of canker sores and other mouth sores, but this potential use has not been studied scientifically.

Creams containing whole licorice (often combined with **chamomile** extract) are advocated for a variety of skin diseases, including **eczema**, **psoriasis**, and **herpes**, but as yet there is only supporting evidence for the first of these uses.

Whole licorice, not DGL, is used as an expectorant for respiratory problems such as **coughs** and **asthma**.

Licorice has been suggested as a treatment for **chronic fatigue syndrome (CFS)**, based on the observation that people with CFS appear to suffer from low levels of certain adrenal hormones. The glycyrrhizin portion of licorice may relieve symptoms by mimicking the effects of these hormones. However, this is a fairly dangerous approach to treatment that should be tried only under medical supervision. In addition, studies of drugs that even more closely imitate adrenal hormones have not found benefit.

What Is the Scientific Evidence for Licorice?

Eczema

Creams containing whole licorice (often combined with extract of chamomile) are in wide use as "natural hydrocortisone creams." However, there is only preliminary supporting evidence for this use. In one double-blind, placebo-controlled trial of 30 people, licorice gel at 2% was more effective than placebo or 1% gel for reducing symptoms of eczema.

Licorice has constituents that increase the activity of naturally occurring (or artificially supplied) corticosteroids and this might explain some of the benefits seen. In addition, licorice contains licochalcone A, a substance hypothesized to have anti-inflammatory effects.

Ulcer Treatment

Two controlled studies suggest that regular use of DGL in a combination product also containing antac-

ids can heal ulcers as effectively as drugs in the Zantac family. Unfortunately, these studies do not prove that DGL was effective; antacids themselves can help heal ulcers and, in any case, the studies were not double-blind. (For information on why this matters, see **Why Does This Book Rely on Double-blind Studies?**.)

Furthermore, if it does work, DGL would have to be taken continuously to avoid ulcer recurrence. In some cases, drug treatment can prevent the recurrence of ulcers permanently by eradicating the bacteria *Helicobacter pylori*. There is no evidence as yet that DGL can do the same.

Ulcer Prevention

A very preliminary study suggests that DGL might help prevent ulcers caused by aspirin and related medications (such as ibuprofen).

Dosage

For supportive treatment of ulcer pain along with conventional medical care, the standard dose is two to four 380-mg tablets of DGL taken before meals and at bedtime. The same tablets can be allowed to slowly dissolve in the mouth for possible relief of mouth sore pain.

A typical dose of whole licorice is 5 to 15 g daily. However, we do not recommend the use of doses this high for more than a few weeks. For long-term consumption, about 0.3 g of licorice root daily should be safe for most adults. (See Safety Issues below.) Individuals who wish to take a higher dose should do so only under the supervision of a physician.

For the treatment of eczema, psoriasis, or herpes, 2% licorice gel or cream is applied twice daily to the affected area.

Safety Issues

Use of whole licorice has not been associated with significant adverse effects in the short term. However, 2 or more weeks of use may cause high blood pressure, fluid retention, and symptoms related to loss of potassium. Such effects are especially dangerous for people who take the drug digoxin or medications that deplete the body of potassium (such as thiazide and loop diuretics) or who have high blood pressure, heart disease, diabetes, or kidney disease.

Current evidence indicates that individuals who wish to take whole licorice on a long-term basis without any risk of these side effects should not consume more than 0.2 mg of glycyrrhizin per kilogram of body weight daily. For a person who weighs 130 pounds, this works out to 12 mg of glycyrrhizin daily. Based on a typical 4% glycyrrhizin content, this is the equivalent of 0.3 grams of licorice root.

Whole licorice may have other side effects as well. For example, it appears to reduce testosterone levels in men. For this reason, men with **impotence, infertility,** or decreased libido may wish to avoid this herb. Licorice may also increase both the positive and negative effects of corticosteroids, such as prednisone and hydrocortisone cream. In addition, some evidence suggests that licorice might affect the liver's ability to metabolize other medications as well, but the extent of this effect has not been fully determined.

Whole licorice possesses significant estrogenic activity and some evidence indicates that licorice increases risk of premature birth. For these reasons, it shouldn't be taken by pregnant or nursing women or women who have had breast cancer.

Maximum safe doses for young children, nursing women, or those with severe liver or kidney disease have not been established.

It is believed, but not proven, that most or all of the major side effects of licorice are due to glycyrrhizin. For this reason, DGL has been described as entirely safe. However, comprehensive safety studies on DGL have not been reported.

Interactions You Should Know About

If you are taking:

- ➤ **Digoxin:** Long-term use of licorice can be dangerous.
- ➤ **Thiazide or loop diuretics:** Use of licorice might lead to excessive potassium loss.
- ➤ **Corticosteroid treatment:** Licorice could increase both its negative and positive effects. Do not take licorice internally if using corticosteroids.
- ➤ **Aspirin or other anti-inflammatory drugs:** Regular use of DGL might help lower the risk of ulcers.

Lignans

PRINCIPAL PROPOSED USES: *None*

OTHER PROPOSED USES: *Cancer Prevention, Elevated Cholesterol, Kidney Disease, Menopausal Symptoms*

Lignans are naturally occurring chemicals widespread within the plant and animal kingdoms. Several lignans—with intimidating names such as secoisolariciresinol—are considered to be *phytoestrogens*, plant chemicals that mimic the hormone estrogen. These are especially abundant in **flaxseeds** and sesame seeds. Bacteria in our intestines convert the naturally occurring phytoestrogens from flaxseed into two other lignans, enterolactone and enterodiol, which also have estrogen-like effects. In this article, the term *lignans* refers to these two specific lignans as well as the phytoestrogen kind, but not to the wide variety of other lignans.

Lignans are being studied for possible use in cancer prevention, particularly breast cancer. Like other phytoestrogens (such as **soy isoflavones**), they hook onto the same spots on cells where estrogen attaches. If there is little estrogen in the body (after menopause, for example), lignans may act like weak estrogen; but when natural estrogen is abundant in the body, lignans may instead reduce estrogen's effects by displacing it from cells. This displacement of the hormone may help prevent those cancers, such as breast cancer, that depend on estrogen to start and develop. In addition, at least one test-tube study suggests that lignans may help prevent cancer in ways that are unrelated to estrogen.

Requirements/Sources

The richest source of lignans is flaxseed (sometimes called *linseed*), containing more than 100 times the amount found in other foods! **Flaxseed oil,** however, does not contain appreciable amounts of lignans. Sesame seed is an equally rich source. Other food sources are pumpkin seeds, whole grains, cranberries, and black or green tea.

Therapeutic Dosages

Effective dosages of purified lignans have not been determined. In studies of flaxseed as a source of lignans, flaxseed has been taken at a dose of 5 to 38 g daily.

Cooking flaxseed apparently does not decrease the amount of lignans absorbed by the body.

Therapeutic Uses

A number of preliminary human and animal studies suggest that lignans may be helpful for **cancer prevention**, particularly of breast and colon cancer, as well as reduction of cholesterol. Other highly preliminary research suggests that flaxseeds or lignans may decrease menopausal symptoms and improve kidney function in various types of kidney disease (specifically, lupus nephritis and polycystic kidney disease).

Warning: Flaxseed or other treatments for kidney disease should be taken only under a doctor's supervision due to the serious nature of these disorders.

Despite positive preliminary results in animal studies, a small double-blind, placebo-controlled study in humans failed to find lignans helpful for improving **cholesterol profile**.

What Is the Scientific Evidence for Lignans?

The most promising use for lignans is in cancer prevention. According to observational studies, people who eat more lignan-containing foods have a lower incidence of breast and, perhaps, colon cancer. This, however, does not prove that lignans are the cause of the benefit, for other factors in these foods, or in the characteristics of the people who consume these foods, may have been responsible. Double-blind, placebo-controlled studies are necessary to prove that a medical treatment provides benefits and none have yet been reported for lignans. (For information on why this type of study is so important, see **Why Does This Book Rely on Double-blind Studies?**)

Nonetheless, animal studies offer additional support for a potential cancer-preventive or even cancer-treatment effect. Several studies showed that lignan-rich foods or lignans found in flax inhibited breast and colon cancer in animals and reduced metastases from melanoma (a type of skin cancer) in mice. Test-tube studies have found that flaxseed or one of its lignans inhibited the growth of human breast cancer cells and that the lignans enterolactone and enterodiol inhibited the growth of human colon tumor cells.

In many of these studies it isn't clear whether lignans are responsible for the benefit seen, as flaxseeds contain many other substances. Animal and human studies have begun to examine specific lignans and results seem to confirm that at least some of the positive effects probably come from the lignans themselves; still, until more and better designed trials are done, we will not know lignans' precise effects on the human body or the precise dose needed to prevent cancer.

Safety Issues

Women who are pregnant or breast-feeding should avoid high intake of flaxseed or purified lignans. One study found that pregnant rats who ate large amounts of flaxseed (5 or 10% of their diet) or a purified lignan present in flaxseed gave birth to offspring with altered reproductive organs and functions and that lignans were also transferred to the baby rats during nursing. In humans, eating 25 g of flaxseed per day amounts to about 5% of the diet.

High intake of lignans may not be safe for women with a history of estrogen-sensitive cancer, such as breast cancer or uterine cancer. A few test-tube studies suggest that certain cancer cells can be stimulated by lignans such as those present in flaxseed. Other studies found that lignans inhibit cancer cell growth. As with estrogen, lignans' positive or negative effects on cancer cells may depend on dose, type of cancer cell, and levels of hormones in the body. If you have a history of cancer, particularly breast cancer, talk with your doctor before consuming large amounts of flaxseeds.

Other potential concerns are discussed in the safety section of the **flaxseed** article.

Ligustrum

Ligustrum lucidum

ALTERNATE NAMES/RELATED TERMS: *Glossy Privet Tree*

PRINCIPAL PROPOSED USES: *Immune Support*

OTHER PROPOSED USES: *Cancer Prevention, Cancer Treatment Support, HIV Support, Liver Protection*

The berries of the glossy privet tree, *Ligustrum lucidum*, have a long history of use in **traditional Chinese herbal medicine** as an herb that helps "tonify the yin." This expression cannot be fully explained without entering into the theoretical framework of traditional Chinese medicine, but it may be said loosely to indicate a strengthening effect on some of the functions of the body. As part of herbal combinations (traditional Chinese herbal medicine seldom uses single-herb preparations), ligustrum is used for such purposes as turning gray hair black, alleviating ringing in the ear, and treating vertigo.

One of the most famous combination therapies containing ligustrum is named *Erzhi Wan,* or "Two-Solstices Pill." It consists of ligustrum berries harvested at the winter solstice, combined with another herb (*Eclipta alba*) harvested at the summer solstice. The combined treatment is thought of as providing a balance of two opposite "energies."

What Is Ligustrum Used for Today?

Ligustrum is currently marketed as a treatment for strengthening the immune system and, on this basis, is often recommended for use by people undergoing treatment for **cancer** or **HIV**. However, there is no meaningful scientific evidence that ligustrum provides any benefit for these, or any other, conditions.

Very weak evidence from test-tube and animal studies hints that ligustrum might have anti-parasitic, anti-viral, **liver-protective**, immunomodulatory (this means "altering" immune function, rather than, as commonly misunderstood, "strengthening" it), and **cancer-preventive** effects. However, this evidence is too preliminary to rely upon at all. Only double-blind, placebo-controlled studies can prove a treatment effective and none have been performed on ligustrum. (For information on why such studies are essential, see **Why Does This Book Rely on Double-blind Studies?**.)

Dosage

A typical dose of ligustrum berries is 5 mg taken 2 or 3 times daily.

Safety Issues

Although use of ligustrum appears to be well tolerated in general, the herb has not undergone any meaningful safety evaluation at the level of modern scientific standards. Safety in young children, pregnant or nursing women, or people with severe liver or kidney disease is definitely not established.

Linden

Tilia cordata, Tilia platyphyllos, and other *Tilia* spp.

PRINCIPAL PROPOSED USES: *Common Cold*

OTHER PROPOSED USES: *Anxiety, Dyspepsia, Insomnia, Liver Protection, Viral Hepatitis*

Linden flowers have a pleasant, tangy taste and, for this reason, the tree is sometimes called *lime flower*. Besides use in beverages and liqueurs, linden flower has a long history of medicinal use for such conditions as colds and flus, digestive distress, anxiety, migraine headaches, and insomnia. The wood of the linden tree has been used for liver problems, kidney stones, and gout.

What Is Linden Used for Today?

Linden flower has been approved by Germany's Commission E for the treatment of **cold symptoms**. Unfortunately, there is no meaningful evidence that it is helpful for this purpose. Linden is said to promote sweating and this, in turn, has long been presumed to be helpful for people with colds; however, there is no meaningful evidence that sweating helps colds, or that linden promotes sweating.

Other proposed uses of linden also lack scientific support. Two exceedingly preliminary studies that evaluated linden flower for potential **sedative** or **anti-anxiety** effects returned contradictory results. Very weak evidence hints that linden flower might help reduce symptoms of digestive upset and **protect the liver** from toxins. One highly preliminary study found possible anti-inflammatory and pain-relieving effects with linden leaf. However, none of this research approaches the level of meaningful evidence. Only

double-blind, placebo-controlled studies can show a treatment effective and none have been performed on linden. (For information on why such studies are essential, see **Why Does This Book Rely on Double-blind Studies?**.)

Other proposed benefits of linden that lack any meaningful supporting evidence include the claims that linden flower reduces **blood pressure**, prevents blood clots, and decreases risk of **stroke** or **heart attack**, and that linden bark can treat **viral hepatitis**.

Dosage

Linden flower is usually taken at a dose of 2 to 4 g daily, often as tea. A daily dose of linden wood is prepared by boiling 15 to 40 g in water for several hours.

Safety Issues

Linden is widely believed to be a safe herb, but it has not undergone comprehensive safety testing. Numerous texts state that when taken in high doses linden can be toxic to the heart, but this appears to have been a case of authors quoting one another for decades in succession; the original source of this concern is unclear. Safety in young children, pregnant or nursing women, or people with severe liver or kidney disease has not been established.

Lipoic Acid

SUPPLEMENT FORMS/ALTERNATE NAMES: *Alpha-lipoic Acid, Thioctic Acid*

PRINCIPAL PROPOSED USES:

Neuropathic Conditions: *Burning Mouth Syndrome, Diabetic Neuropathy (Peripheral Neuropathy and Cardiac Autonomic Neuropathy)*

OTHER PROPOSED USES: *Cancer Prevention, Cataract Prevention, Diabetes (Blood Sugar Control), Glaucoma, Heart Disease Prevention, Liver Disease, Sun-damaged Skin*

Lipoic acid, also known as alpha-lipoic acid, is a sulfur-containing fatty acid. It is found inside every cell of the body, where it helps generate the energy that keeps us alive and functioning. Lipoic acid is a key part of the metabolic machinery that turns glucose (blood sugar) into energy for the body's needs.

Lipoic acid is an **antioxidant**, which means that it neutralizes naturally occurring but harmful chemicals known as *free radicals*. Unlike other antioxidants, which work only in water or fatty tissues, lipoic acid is unusual in that it functions in both water and fat. By comparison, vitamin E works only in fat and vitamin C works only in water. This gives lipoic acid an unusually broad spectrum of antioxidant action.

Antioxidants are a bit like kamikaze pilots, sacrificing themselves to knock out free radicals. One of the more interesting findings about lipoic acid is that it may help regenerate other antioxidants that have been used up. In addition, lipoic acid may be able to do the work of other antioxidants when the body is deficient in them.

It is thought that certain nerve diseases are at least partially caused by free radical damage. Thanks to its combined fat and water solubility, lipoic acid can get into all the parts of a nerve cell and potentially protect it against such damage. This is the rationale for studies on the potential benefits of lipoic acid for diabetic neuropathy.

Sources

A healthy body makes enough lipoic acid to supply its requirements; external sources are not necessary. However, several medical conditions appear to be accompanied by low levels of lipoic acid—specifically **diabetes**, **liver cirrhosis**, and **atherosclerosis**—which suggests

(but definitely does not prove) that supplementation would be helpful.

Liver and yeast contain some lipoic acid. Nonetheless, supplements are necessary to obtain therapeutic dosages.

Therapeutic Dosages

The typical dosage of oral lipoic acid for treating complications of diabetes is 100 to 200 mg 3 times daily. In studies that found benefits, several weeks of treatment were often necessary for full effects to develop.

For use as a general antioxidant, a lower dosage of 20 to 50 mg daily is commonly recommended, although there is no evidence that taking lipoic acid in this way offers any health benefit.

Therapeutic Uses

Lipoic acid has been widely used for decades in Germany to treat diabetic peripheral neuropathy. This is a condition caused by **diabetes** in which nerves leading to the arms and legs become damaged, resulting in numbness, pain, and other symptoms. Free radicals are hypothesized to play a role in neuropathy, and on this basis lipoic acid has been tried as a treatment. However, the evidence for benefit is largely limited to studies that used the intravenous form of this supplement.

Another set of nerves may become damaged in diabetes as well: the *autonomic nerves* that control internal organs. When this occurs in the heart (*cardiac autonomic neuropathy*) it leads to irregularities of heart rhythm. There is some evidence that lipoic acid supplements may be helpful for this condition.

Preliminary and sometimes contradictory evidence suggests that lipoic acid may improve other aspects of diabetes, including blood sugar control and the development of long-term complications, such as diseases of the heart, kidneys, and small blood vessels.

In addition, lipoic acid may be helpful for **burning mouth syndrome** (BMS), a condition characterized by unexplained scalding sensations in the mouth.

A cream containing 5% lipoic acid has shown promise for the treatment of sun-damaged skin.

One animal study suggests that lipoic acid might help prevent age-related hearing loss. Similarly weak evidence hints that lipoic acid might be helpful for glaucoma. Other uses for which lipoic acid has been proposed include preventing **cancer** and **heart disease**, and treating or preventing **cataracts**.

What Is the Scientific Evidence for Lipoic Acid?

Diabetic Peripheral Neuropathy

There is some evidence that intravenous lipoic acid can reduce symptoms of diabetic peripheral neuropathy, at least in the short term. However, the evidence for oral lipoic acid remains weak and contradictory.

A double-blind, placebo-controlled study of 500 people with diabetic neuropathy found that intravenous lipoic acid helped reduce symptoms over a 3-week period; however, long-term oral supplementation did not prove effective.

A previous double-blind, placebo-controlled study also found benefit with intravenous lipoic acid.

A few studies found oral lipoic acid effective; however, they were too small or too poorly designed to mean much.

There is some preliminary evidence that lipoic acid may be more effective if it is combined with **gamma-linolenic acid** (GLA), another supplement used for diabetic peripheral neuropathy.

Diabetic Autonomic Neuropathy

There is better evidence for *oral* lipoic acid in a form of diabetic neuropathy affecting the nerves that supply the heart: autonomic neuropathy.

Not only does diabetes damage the nerves in the arms and legs, but it can also affect deep nerves that control organs such as the heart and digestive tract. The DEKAN (Deutsche Kardiale Autonome Neuropathie) study followed 73 people with diabetes who had symptoms caused by nerve damage affecting the heart. Treatment with 800 mg daily of oral lipoic acid showed statistically significant improvement compared to placebo and caused no significant side effects.

Burning Mouth Syndrome (BMS)

Individuals with BMS feel chronic scalding pain in the mouth, as if they had consumed an excessively hot drink. Although the cause of BMS is not known, the symptoms resemble those of neuropathy and for that reason researchers have investigated the potential benefits of lipoic acid.

In a 2-month, double-blind trial involving 60 people with BMS, use of lipoic acid significantly reduced symptoms as compared to placebo.

Safety Issues

Lipoic acid appears to have no significant side effects at dosages up to 1,800 mg daily.

Safety for young children, women who are pregnant or nursing, or those with severe liver or kidney disease has not been established.

Lobelia

Lobelia inflata

PRINCIPAL PROPOSED USES: *Cigarette Addiction*

OTHER PROPOSED USES: *Asthma, Chemical Dependency, Depression, Enhancing Memory, Insomnia, Pain Reduction*

The herb lobelia was originally used by Native Americans in the New England region. It was subsequently popularized by Samuel Thomson, the founder of an idiosyncratic form of medicine called *Thomsonianism*. The enduring popularity of lobelia is one of the legacies of this nineteenth-century enthusiasm. (**Goldenseal** is another herb popularized by Thomson.) The traditional names of the herb capture its traditional uses: wild tobacco, asthma weed, gagroot, and pukeweed. Dried lobelia tastes and smells somewhat like tobacco and, for this reason, it was sold as a tobacco substitute. Lobelia was also used to treat asthma and stimulate vomiting.

The Thomsonians additionally claimed that lobelia could relax muscles and nerves. On this basis, they used it for anxiety, epilepsy, kidney stones, insomnia, menstrual cramps, muscle spasms, spastic colon, and tetanus.

What Is Lobelia Used for Today?

The major active ingredient of lobelia is a substance called *lobeline*. It is widely stated that lobeline is chemically similar to nicotine and, on this basis, it has been marketed as a **treatment to help quit smoking**. However, this belief appears to be a type of urban legend; lobeline is not in fact chemically similar to nicotine.

Interestingly, chemists investigating the lobeline–nicotine myth found that lobeline may diminish certain effects of nicotine in the body, specifically nicotine-induced release of the substance dopamine. Since dopamine is believed to play a significant role in drug addiction, these findings can be taken as hinting that lobeline might be useful for **treating drug addiction**. Potential benefits have been found for addiction to amphetamines.

Dopamine also plays a role in cigarette addiction. For this reason, despite lobeline's lack of similarity to nicotine, it is at least possible that lobelia could be helpful for people who wish to stop smoking. Unfortunately, despite its widespread marketing for this purpose, there has never been any meaningful evidence that it works.

Other proposed uses of lobelia also lack supporting evidence. For example, while studies in horses have found that injected lobeline causes the animals to breathe more deeply, it is a long way from a finding like this to the widespread claims that lobelia is helpful for **asthma**. Similarly, animal studies hint that lobeline might **enhance memory** and reduce pain, and, in addition, that beta-amyrin palmitate, another constituent of lobelia, might have antidepressant and sedative properties.

However, there have not yet been any human studies on these potential benefits of the herb.

Dosage

Lobelia is generally sold in the form of a vinegar tincture. The typical dose of this tincture is 20 to 60 drops taken 3 times daily.

Safety Issues

It is widely stated that lobelia is a dangerously toxic herb. However, herbalist Paul Bergner undertook a review of published literature and discovered that each author who described lobelia as toxic was merely quoting another author, in a kind of game of telephone going back nearly 200 years. The original published reference upon which this sequence of hearsay reporting appears to have been based is a note in the *American New Dispensatory* of 1810, in which an "eminent physician" is quoted as stating that if a person consumes lobelia and doesn't vomit, death will follow. The ultimate origin of this claim may have been the claims made by the prosecution in a widely publicized trial of Samuel Thomson in which he was accused of committing murder through use of lobelia.

In fact, there are no reported cases of death caused by *Lobelia inflata* in animals or humans. Considering how widely lobelia was used under the Thomsonians, the concern that it reliably causes death appears to be a significant overstatement. Lobelia may present health risks, but if so, they have not been documented.

Short-term side effects that have been reported in association with lobelia include stomach pain, heartburn, nausea, vomiting, and dizziness. Lobeline also appears to trigger coughing and a sense of choking, for reasons that are unclear.

The fact that lobeline restricts dopamine release suggests at least a possibility that lobelia could worsen symptoms of **Parkinson's disease** (in which dopamine levels are low) and possibly interfere with the action of drugs used for **schizophrenia** or **attention deficit disorder** (which also act on dopamine). These concerns are, however, purely theoretical at this time.

Safety in young children, pregnant or nursing women, or people with severe liver or kidney disease has not been established.

Lomatium

Lomatium dissectum

PRINCIPAL PROPOSED USES: *Anti-Viral*

OTHER PROPOSED USES: *Acute Bronchitis, Colds and Flus, Herpes, HIV, Sinusitis, Viral Hepatitis*

An herb of bright yellow, umbrella-shaped flowers, lomatium was widely used among native peoples of North America as a treatment for a variety of infections, especially those involving the lungs. Reportedly, use of this herb protected the Washoe Indian tribe of Nevada from suffering any deaths during the 1917–18 worldwide pandemic of influenza. It was also said to be useful for pneumonia and tuberculosis.

What Is Lomatium Used for Today?

Lomatium is currently regarded by some herbalists as an effective treatment for many types of viral infection, including **HIV**, **viral hepatitis**, **colds and flus**, **acute bronchitis**, sinusitis, and **herpes**. However, there is no meaningful scientific evidence that lomatium is helpful for these conditions, or indeed that it has any antiviral effects at all. The story mentioned above about the great influenza pandemic of 1917–18 cannot be taken as meaningful evidence of benefit; like all other great plagues, the influenza pandemic gave rise to innumerable rumors of cures, none of which have held up to scientific testing.

At most, there is exceedingly weak evidence from a small number of test-tube studies hinting hint that *Lo-matium* species might have antiviral properties. However, tens or hundreds of thousands of substances have shown antiviral effects in the test tube; very seldom do benefits hypothesized from preliminary test-tube studies hold up when human studies are performed. Only double-blind, placebo-controlled studies can show a treatment effective and no studies of this type have been performed on lomatium. (For information on why such studies are essential, see **Why Does This Book Rely on Double-blind Studies?**)

Dosage

Lomatium is typically used in the form of a resin-free extract, taken at a dose of 1 to 3 ml daily.

Safety Issues

Lomatium has not undergone any modern safety testing. Reportedly, lomatium resin frequently causes allergic reactions leading to a whole-body rash; this is why resin-free products are sold. In addition, lomatium may cause digestive distress. Safety in young children, pregnant or nursing women, or people with severe liver or kidney disease has not been evaluated.

Lutein

PRINCIPAL PROPOSED USES: *None*

OTHER PROPOSED USES: *Atherosclerosis, Cataracts, Macular Degeneration, Retinitis Pigmentosa*

Lutein, a chemical found in green vegetables, is a member of a family of substances known as **carotenoids**. **Beta-carotene** is the most famous nutrient in this class. Like beta-carotene, lutein is an **antioxidant** that protects our cells against damage caused by dangerous, naturally occurring chemicals known as *free radicals*.

Recent evidence has found that lutein may play an important role in protecting our eyes and eyesight. It may work in two ways: by acting directly as a kind of natural sunblock and also by neutralizing free radicals that can damage the eye.

Sources

Lutein is not an essential nutrient. However, it is possible that it may be useful for optimal health.

Green vegetables are the best source of lutein, especially spinach, kale, collard greens, romaine lettuce, leeks, and peas. Unlike beta-carotene, lutein is *not* found in high concentrations in yellow and orange vegetables such as carrots.

Therapeutic Dosages

We don't know how much lutein is necessary for a therapeutic effect, but estimates range from 5 to 30 mg daily.

Therapeutic Uses

According to theoretical findings and two preliminary double-blind studies, it appears that use of lutein supplements might help prevent or slow the development of **age-related macular degeneration** (ARMD) and possibly **cataracts**, the two most common causes of vision loss in seniors.

Lutein has also shown a hint of promise for treatment of retinitis pigmentosa, an inherited form of eye disease that causes progressive vision loss.

Very weak evidence hints that lutein might help prevent **atherosclerosis**.

What Is the Scientific Evidence for Lutein?

Most but not all observational studies suggest that people who eat foods containing lutein are less likely to develop cataracts and perhaps macular degeneration as well, the two most common causes of vision loss in adults. Furthermore, there are good theoretical reasons to believe that lutein may play an important role in protecting the eyes.

Lutein is the main *pigment* (coloring chemical) in the center of the retina, the region of maximum visual sensitivity known as the *macula*. Macular degeneration consists of injury to the macula and leads to a severe loss in vision. One of the main causes of macular degeneration appears to be sun damage to the sensitive tissue. Lutein appears to act as a natural eyeshade, protecting the retina against too much light. It is also an antioxidant, meaning that it fights dangerous, naturally occurring substances called *free radicals*. Free radicals may play a role in macular degeneration.

Based on this information, researchers conducted a double-blind, placebo-controlled trial of lutein. The study enrolled 90 people with dry-type macular degeneration and followed them for 12 months. The participants received either lutein (10 mg), lutein plus other antioxidants, and a multivitamin/mineral supplement, or placebo. At the end of the study period, participants who had taken lutein alone or lutein plus the other nutrients showed improvements in vision, while no change in vision was seen in the placebo group.

While these are promising findings, further study will be necessary to establish the apparent benefit of lutein for ARMD.

Besides protecting the macula, lutein may also shield the lens of the eye from light damage, slowing the development of cataracts. One small 2-year, double-blind, placebo-controlled trial found some evidence that lutein may improve vision in people who already have cataracts.

Safety Issues

Although lutein is a normal part of the diet, there has not been a formal evaluation of lutein's safety when taken as a concentrated supplement. Maximum safe dosages for young children, pregnant or nursing women, or those with severe liver or kidney disease have not been established.

Lycopene

PRINCIPAL PROPOSED USES: *None*

OTHER PROPOSED USES:

> Prevention: *Cancer Prevention, Cataracts, Exercise-induced Asthma, Heart Disease, High Blood Pressure, Intrauterine Growth Retardation, Leukoplakia, Macular Degeneration, Preeclampsia*
> Treatment: *Cancer Treatment, Male Infertility*

Lycopene is a powerful **antioxidant** found in tomatoes and pink grapefruit. Like the better-known supplement **beta-carotene**, lycopene belongs to the family of chemicals known as *carotenoids*. As an antioxidant, it is about twice as powerful as beta-carotene.

There is some evidence that lycopene may help prevent cancer and other diseases, but conclusive proof is lacking. Thus far, the best evidence for lycopene has to do with preventing complications during pregnancy.

Sources

Lycopene is not a necessary nutrient. However, like other substances found in fruits and vegetables, it may be very important for optimal health.

Tomatoes are the best source of lycopene. Happily, cooking doesn't destroy lycopene, so pizza sauce is just as good as a fresh tomato. In fact, some studies indicate that cooking tomatoes in oil may provide lycopene in a way that the body can use better, although not all studies agree. Lycopene is also found in watermelon, guava, and pink grapefruit. Synthetic lycopene is also available, and appears to be as well absorbed as natural-source lycopene.

Therapeutic Dosages

The optimum dosage for lycopene has not been established, but the amount found helpful in studies generally fell in the range of 4 to 8 mg daily.

It has been suggested the lycopene is better absorbed when it is taken with fats such as olive oil, but one study failed to find any meaningful change in absorption.

Therapeutic Uses

Some but not all observational studies suggest that foods containing lycopene may help prevent **macular degeneration**, **cataracts**, cardiovascular disease, and **cancer**. However, observational studies are highly unreliable means of determining the effectiveness of medical treatments; only double-blind studies can do so, and few have yet been performed that relate to these potential uses of lycopene. (For more information on why double-blind trials are so important, see **Why Does This Book Rely on Double-blind Studies?**.)

The best study of lycopene thus far evaluated its possible benefits for pregnant women. The results of this preliminary double-blind trial hint that lycopene supplements may help prevent **preeclampsia** (a dangerous complication of pregnancy) as well as intrauterine growth retardation (inadequate growth of the fetus).

Preliminary controlled trials have found suggestive evidence that lycopene or a standardized tomato extract containing lycopene might be helpful for the prevention or treatment of **prostate cancer**. Tomato extract has also shown some promise for **high blood pressure**.

Leukoplakia is a precancerous condition of the mouth. A small double-blind, placebo-controlled study found that lycopene supplements might help reverse this condition.

One highly preliminary study weakly suggests that tomato extracts containing lycopene might be helpful in the treatment of **breast cancer**, while lycopene alone is not. Very weak evidence hints that lycopene might help prevent testicular damage caused by the **cancer chemotherapy** drug adriamycin.

Very weak evidence also suggests that the same tomato-based lycopene supplements might be helpful for treating **male infertility** and for preventing **heart disease**.

Results of studies have been inconsistent regarding the effects of lycopene and exercise-induced **asthma**.

One observational study failed to find that high consumption of lycopene reduced risk of developing **diabetes**.

High intake of tomato paste may offer weak protection against **sunburn**.

What Is the Scientific Evidence for Lycopene?

A double-blind study of 251 women evaluated the potential benefits of lycopene during pregnancy. Participants in this study received either placebo or 2 mg of lycopene twice daily. For reasons that are not at all clear, use of lycopene appeared to reduce risk of preeclampsia as well as inadequate growth of the fetus.

While these results are promising, researchers are cautious about drawing conclusions: several other nutritional substances have shown promise for preventing preeclampsia in preliminary trials, only to fail when larger and more definitive studies were done.

Safety Issues

Lycopene is believed to be a safe supplement, as evidenced by the fact that researchers felt comfortable giving it to pregnant women. However, maximum safe dosages are not known.

Note: We suggest that pregnant women should consult with a physician before taking any herbs or supplements.

Lysine

SUPPLEMENT FORMS/ALTERNATE NAMES: *L-Lysine, Lysine Hydrochloride*
PRINCIPAL PROPOSED USES: *Herpes Simplex Prevention (Cold Sores, Genital Herpes)*

Lysine is an essential amino acid, one that you need to get from food. Some evidence suggests that supplemental lysine may be able to help prevent **herpes infections** (cold sores and genital herpes).

Requirements/Sources

Most people need about 1 g of lysine per day. The requirement may be greater for athletes and people recovering from major injuries, especially burns. The richest sources of lysine are animal proteins, such as meat and poultry, but it is also found in dairy products, eggs, and beans.

Therapeutic Dosages

A typical therapeutic dosage of lysine for herpes infections is 1 g 3 times daily. You can take this as a regular part of your diet in hopes of preventing herpes flare-ups or, perhaps, at the first sign of an attack. Although the evidence isn't strong, there may be some advantage to restricting your intake of foods that contain a lot of arginine, such as chocolate, peanuts, other nuts and seeds, and, to a lesser extent, wheat.

Therapeutic Uses

Some small studies suggest that *regular* use of lysine supplements can help prevent flare-ups of cold sores and genital herpes, although other studies have not found benefit. Lysine has also been proposed as a treatment to take at the *onset* of a flare-up, but at least one study failed to find it effective for this purpose.

Both cold sores and genital herpes are caused by a virus called *herpes simplex*. After you are first infected, this virus hides in certain nerve cells, and reemerges under times of **stress**. Test tube research suggests that lysine fights this virus by blocking arginine, an amino acid the virus needs in order to replicate. For this reason, lysine might be most effective when used in conjunction with a low-arginine diet. However, this widely stated claim has not been proven. (Note that if this is true, it would be essential to avoid taking arginine supplements if you have herpes.)

What Is the Scientific Evidence for Lysine?

When taken in sufficient doses, it appears that regular use of lysine supplements might be able to reduce the number and intensity of herpes flare-ups.

One double-blind, placebo-controlled study followed 52 participants with a history of herpes flare-ups. While receiving 3 g of L-lysine every day for 6 months, the treatment group experienced an average of 2.4 fewer herpes flare-ups than the placebo group—a significant difference. The lysine group's flare-ups were also significantly less severe and healed faster.

Another double-blind, placebo-controlled crossover study on 41 subjects also found improvements in the frequency of attacks. Interestingly, this study found that 1,250 mg of lysine daily worked, but 624 mg did not.

Other studies, including one that followed 65 individuals, found no benefit, but they used lower dosages of lysine.

Although some are promising, none of these studies are large enough to give conclusive answers. At this point, more evidence is needed to determine whether lysine is effective for preventing herpes simplex.

Many people use lysine in a different way: they take it at the onset of a herpes attack. However, a double-blind, placebo-controlled study evaluating this method found no benefit. (Consider using the herb **lemon balm** instead.)

Safety Issues

Although lysine is an essential part of the diet, the safety of concentrated lysine supplements has not been well studied. In animal studies, high dosages have caused gallstones and elevated cholesterol levels, so you may want to use caution when using lysine if you have either of these problems. Maximum safe dosages for young children, pregnant or nursing women, or those with severe liver or kidney disease have not been established.

Interactions You Should Know About

If you are taking lysine to treat herpes: **Arginine** might counteract the potential benefit.

Maca
Lepidium meyenii

PRINCIPAL PROPOSED USES: *Male Sexual Dysfunction*

OTHER PROPOSED USES: *Adaptogen (Fighting Stress), Benign Prostate Enlargement (BPH), Diabetes, Fatigue, Female Infertility, Female Sexual Dysfunction, Hypertension, Male Infertility*

Maca is a Peruvian root vegetable used both as food and medicine. It is sometimes called *Peruvian ginseng*, not because the plants have any botanical relationship, but because their traditional uses are somewhat similar. Traditionally, maca has been said to increase energy and stamina and to enhance both fertility and sex drive in men and women.

What Is Maca Used for Today?

Maca is widely marketed for improving **male sexual function**, **female sexual function**, and both **male fertility** and **female fertility**. However, at present there is no reliable evidence that it actually provides any benefits at all.

Much of the evidence for maca comes from animal studies. In one study in rats, use of maca enhanced male sexual function. Animal studies have had mixed results regarding male and female fertility.

There are two published human trials on maca, performed by a single research group.

In one small 12-week, double-blind, placebo-controlled study, use of maca at 1,500 mg or 3,000 mg increased male libido. While this was an interesting finding, the study did not report benefits in male sexual *function*, just *desire*. Since loss of sexual function (specifically, impotence) is a more common problem in men than loss of sexual desire, these results do not justify the widespread claim that maca has been shown to act like a kind of herbal Viagra.

Another small study found that 4 months of maca use increased sperm count and sperm function. Unfortunately, this study failed to use a control group and, for this reason, its results are essentially meaningless. (For more information on why studies must use a control group, see **Why Does This Book Rely on Double-blind Studies?**.)

There are no human trials on maca for female fertility or female sexual function.

Contrary to widespread reporting, maca does not appear to increase testosterone levels or, in fact, affect any male hormones.

Other animal studies hint that maca might offer benefits for **prostate enlargement**, **stress**, **diabetes**, and **high blood pressure**. However, this evidence is as yet too weak to justify any claims regarding maca and these conditions.

Dosage

The usual dose of maca is 500 to 1,000 mg 3 times a day.

Safety Issues

In the two reported human clinical trials, use of maca has not led to any serious adverse effects. However, this herb has not undergone comprehensive safety testing. Safety in young children, pregnant or nursing women, or people with severe liver or kidney disease has not been established.

Magnesium

SUPPLEMENT FORMS/ALTERNATE NAMES: *Magnesium Chloride, Magnesium Citrate, Magnesium Fumarate, Magnesium Gluconate, Magnesium Malate, Magnesium Oxide, Magnesium Sulfate*

PRINCIPAL PROPOSED USES: *Diabetes, Hypertension, Kidney Stones, Migraine Headaches, Noise-related Hearing Loss*

OTHER PROPOSED USES: *Angina, Asthma, Atherosclerosis, Autism, Congestive Heart Failure, Coronary Artery Disease, Dysmenorrhea (Painful Menstruation, Premenstrual Syndrome (PMS), Fatigue, Fibromyalgia, Glaucoma, Low HDL ("Good") Cholesterol, Mitral Valve Prolapse, Osteoporosis, Preeclampsia, Pregnancy-induced Leg Cramps, Restless Legs Syndrome, Stroke*

NOT RECOMMENDED USES: *Following a Heart Attack*

Magnesium is an essential nutrient, meaning that your body needs it for healthy functioning. It is found in significant quantities throughout the body and used for numerous purposes, including muscle relaxation, blood clotting, and the manufacture of ATP (adenosine triphosphate, the body's main energy molecule).

It has been called *nature's calcium channel blocker*. The idea refers to magnesium's ability to block calcium

Magnesium

from entering muscle and heart cells. A group of prescription heart medications work in a similar way, although much more powerfully. This may be the basis for some of magnesium's effects when it is taken as a supplement in fairly high doses.

Requirements/Sources

Requirements for magnesium increase as we grow and age. The official U.S. and Canadian recommendations for daily intake are as follows:

- ➤ Infants 0–6 months, 30 mg
  7–12 months, 75 mg
- ➤ Children 1–3 years, 80 mg
  4–8 years, 130 mg
- ➤ Males 9–13 years, 240 mg
  14–18 years, 410 mg
  19–30 years, 400 mg
  31 years and older, 420 mg
- ➤ Females 9–13 years, 240 mg
  14–18 years, 360 mg
  19–30 years, 310 mg
  31 years and older, 320 mg
- ➤ Pregnant women 18 years and younger, 400 mg
  19–30 years, 350 mg
  31–50 years, 360 mg
- ➤ Nursing women 18 years and younger, 360 mg
  19–30 years, 310 mg
  31–50 years, 320 mg

Note: These recommendations refer to total intake from food plus supplements. The average diet provides a daily intake of magnesium very close to these amounts.

In the United States, the average dietary intake of magnesium is lower than the recommended daily allowance; however, it is unclear whether this truly indicates deficiency or if the recommended allowance is too high. Alcohol abuse, **surgery**, diabetes, **zinc** supplements, certain types of diuretics (thiazide and loop diuretics, but not potassium-sparing diuretics), estrogen and oral contraceptives, and the medications cisplatin and cyclosporin have been reported to reduce your body's level of magnesium or increase magnesium requirements. If you are taking potassium supplements, you may receive greater benefit from them if you take extra magnesium as well.

While it is sometimes said that **calcium** interferes with magnesium absorption, this effect is apparently too small to have a significant effect on overall magnesium status.

Kelp is very high in magnesium, as are wheat bran, wheat germ, almonds, and cashews. Other good sources include blackstrap molasses, brewer's yeast (not to be confused with nutritional yeast), buckwheat, nuts, and whole grains. You can also get appreciable amounts of magnesium from collard greens, dandelion greens, avocado, sweet corn, cheddar cheese, sunflower seeds, shrimp, dried fruit (figs, apricots, and prunes), and many other common fruits and vegetables.

Therapeutic Dosages

A typical supplemental dosage of magnesium ranges from the nutritional needs described above to as high as 600 mg daily. For premenstrual syndrome (PMS) and dysmenorrhea (painful menstruation), an alternative approach is to start taking 500 to 1,000 mg daily, beginning on day 15 of the menstrual cycle and continuing until menstruation begins.

Magnesium citrate may be slightly more absorbable than other forms of magnesium.

Therapeutic Uses

Preliminary double-blind studies suggest that regular use of magnesium supplements may help prevent **migraine headaches**, **hearing loss** caused by exposure to loud noises, and **kidney stones**, and help treat **high blood pressure**, **angina**, **dysmenorrhea** (menstrual cramps), pregnancy-induced leg cramps, and **premenstrual syndrome** (PMS) (including menstrual migraines).

People with **diabetes** are often deficient in magnesium and, according to some (but not all) studies, magnesium supplementation may enhance blood sugar control and insulin sensitivity in people with diabetes or prediabetic conditions.

One study found that magnesium supplements might be helpful for people with **mitral valve prolapse** who also have low levels of magnesium in the blood.

There is some evidence that magnesium may decrease the **atherosclerosis** risk caused by hydrogenated oils, the margarine-like fats found in many "junk" foods.

Studies on magnesium supplements for improving sports performance have returned contradictory results.

Magnesium supplements do not appear to be very helpful, if at all, for preventing **preeclampsia**.

(Magnesium, taken by injection rather than orally, however, is probably helpful for *treating* preeclampsia that already exists.)

Magnesium is sometimes said to decrease symptoms of **restless legs syndrome**, but the evidence that it works consists solely of open trials without a placebo group and such studies are not trustworthy. Very weak evidence hints at possible benefits for **insomnia**.

Magnesium has also been suggested as a treatment for **Alzheimer's disease**, **attention deficit disorder**, **fatigue**, **fibromyalgia**, low HDL ("good") **cholesterol**, **osteoporosis**, **periodontal disease**, **rheumatoid arthritis**, and **stroke**. However, there is virtually no evidence at all that it is effective for any of these conditions.

Magnesium is sometimes suggested for stabilizing the heart after a **heart attack**, but one study actually found that use of magnesium slightly increased risk of sudden death, repeat heart attack, or need for bypass surgery in the year following the initial heart attack. However, magnesium may be helpful in **congestive heart failure** (CHF).

Despite some early enthusiasm, combination therapy with **vitamin B$_6$** and magnesium has not been found helpful in **autism**.

Alternative medical literature frequently mentions magnesium as a treatment for **asthma**. However, this idea seems to be based entirely on the use of intravenous magnesium as an emergency treatment for asthma. When you take something by mouth, it's a very different matter from having it injected into your veins. There is no real evidence that oral magnesium helps asthma and even some evidence that it does not help.

Although magnesium is sometimes mentioned as a treatment to help keep the heart beating normally, a 6-month, double-blind trial of 170 people did not find it effective for preventing a particular heart rhythm abnormality called *atrial fibrillation*. However, a small double-blind, placebo-controlled trial found that magnesium supplements reduced episodes of arrhythmia in individuals with congestive heart failure. One possible explanation: People with congestive heart failure often take drugs (loop diuretics) that deplete magnesium. The combination of magnesium deficiency with digoxin (another drug given for CHF) may cause arrhythmias. Thus, it is possible that the benefits seen here were caused by correction of that depletion.

One double-blind, placebo-controlled study failed to find magnesium helpful in **glaucoma**.

What Is the Scientific Evidence for Magnesium?

Migraine Headaches

A double-blind study found that regular use of magnesium helps prevent migraine headaches. In this 12-week trial, 81 people with recurrent migraines were given either 600 mg of magnesium daily or placebo. By the last 3 weeks of the study, the treated group's migraines had been reduced by 41.6%, compared to a reduction of 15.8% in the placebo group. The only side effects observed were diarrhea (in about one-fifth of the participants) and, less often, digestive irritation.

Similar results have been seen in other smaller double-blind studies. One study found no benefit, but it has been criticized on many significant points, including using an excessively strict definition of what constituted benefit.

Noise-related Hearing Loss

One double-blind, placebo-controlled study on 300 military recruits suggests that 167 mg of magnesium daily can prevent hearing loss due to exposure to high-volume noise.

Kidney Stones

Magnesium inhibits the growth of calcium oxalate stones in the test tube and decreases stone formation in rats. However, human studies have had mixed results. In one 2-year open study, 56 people taking magnesium hydroxide had fewer recurrences of kidney stones than 34 people not given magnesium. In contrast, a double-blind (and, hence, more reliable) study of 124 people found that magnesium hydroxide was essentially no more effective than placebo.

Hypertension

Magnesium works with calcium and potassium to regulate blood pressure. Several studies suggest that magnesium supplements can reduce blood pressure in people with hypertension, although some have not.

Angina

In a double-blind, placebo-controlled trial of 187 people with angina, 6 months of treatment with magnesium at a dose of 730 mg daily improved exercise tolerance and enhanced overall quality of life. Benefits were also seen in a similar, smaller double-blind trial.

After a Heart Attack

In a 1-year, double-blind, placebo-controlled trial of 468 individuals who had just experienced a heart attack, use of a magnesium supplement at a dose of 360 mg daily failed to prevent heart-related events (defined as heart attack, sudden cardiac death, or need for cardiac bypass), and actually may have increased the risk slightly.

Dysmenorrhea

A 6-month, double-blind, placebo-controlled study of 50 women with menstrual pain found that treatment with magnesium significantly improved symptoms. The researchers reported evidence of reduced levels of prostaglandin F_2 alpha, a hormone-like substance involved in pain and inflammation.

Similarly positive results were seen in a double-blind, placebo-controlled study of 21 women.

Premenstrual Syndrome Symptoms

A double-blind, placebo-controlled study of 32 women found that magnesium taken from day 15 of the menstrual cycle to the onset of menstrual flow could significantly improve PMS symptoms, specifically mood changes.

Another small double-blind preliminary study found that regular use of magnesium could reduce symptoms of PMS-related fluid retention. In this study, 38 women were given magnesium or placebo for 2 months. The results showed no effect after one cycle, but by the end of two cycles, magnesium significantly reduced weight gain, swelling of extremities, breast tenderness, and abdominal bloating.

In addition, one small double-blind study (20 participants) found that magnesium supplementation can help prevent menstrual migraines.

Preliminary evidence suggests that the combination of magnesium and vitamin B_6 might be more effective than either treatment alone.

Pregnancy-induced Leg Cramps

Pregnant women frequently experience painful leg cramping. One double-blind trial of 73 pregnant women found that 3 weeks of magnesium supplements significantly reduced leg cramps as compared to placebo.

Safety Issues

The U.S. government has set the following upper limits for use of magnesium supplements:

- Children 1–3 years, 65 mg
  4–8 years, 110 mg
- Adults, 350 mg
- Pregnant or nursing women, 350 mg

In general, magnesium appears to be quite safe when taken at or below recommended dosages. The most common complaint is loose stools. However, people with severe kidney or heart disease should not take magnesium (or any other supplement) except on the advice of a physician. Maximum safe dosages have not been established for young children. There has been one case of death caused by excessive use of magnesium supplements in a developmentally and physically disabled child. Pregnant or nursing women should not exceed the nutritional dosages presented under Requirements/Sources.

If taken at the same time, magnesium can interfere with the absorption of antibiotics in the tetracycline family and, possibly, the drug nitrofurantoin. Also, when combined with oral diabetes drugs in the sulfonylurea family, magnesium may cause blood sugar levels to fall more than expected.

Interactions You Should Know About

If you are taking:

- Potassium supplements, manganese, loop diuretics and thiazide diuretics, oral contraceptives, estrogen-replacement therapy, cisplatin, cyclosporin, digoxin, or medications that reduce stomach acid: You may need extra magnesium.
- Antibiotics in the tetracycline family or nitrofurantoin (Macrodantin): You should separate your magnesium dose from doses of these medications by at least 2 hours to avoid absorption problems.
- Oral diabetes medications in the sulfonylurea family (Tolinase, Micronase, Orinase, Glucotrol, Diabinese, DiaBeta): Work closely with your physician when taking magnesium to avoid hypoglycemia.
- Amiloride: Do not take magnesium supplements except on medical advice.

Maitake

Grifola frondosa

PRINCIPAL PROPOSED USES: *Adaptogen (Improve Resistance to Stress), Strengthen Immunity*
OTHER PROPOSED USES: *Cancer Treatment, Diabetes, HIV Support, High Cholesterol, Hypertension*

Maitake is a medicinal mushroom used in Japan as a general promoter of robust health. Like the similarly described **reishi** fungus, innumerable healing powers have been attributed to maitake, ranging from curing cancer to preventing heart disease. Unfortunately, there hasn't been enough reliable research yet to determine whether any of these ancient beliefs are really true.

What Is Maitake Used for Today?

Contemporary herbalists classify maitake as an *adaptogen*, a substance said to help the body adapt to **stress** and resist infection (see the article on **ginseng** for further explanation about adaptogens). However, we lack definitive scientific evidence to show us that maitake (or any other purported adaptogen) really functions in this way.

Most investigation has focused on the polysaccharide constituents of maitake. This family of substances is known to affect the human immune system in complex ways and one in particular, beta-D-glucan, has been studied for its potential benefit in treating **cancer** and **HIV**. Highly preliminary studies also suggest that maitake may be useful in treating diabetes, **hypertension** (high blood pressure), and **high cholesterol**. However, there is no real evidence as yet that maitake is effective for these or any other illnesses.

Dosage

Maitake is an edible mushroom that can be eaten as food or made into tea. A typical dosage of dried maitake in capsule or tablet form is 3 to 7 g daily.

Safety Issues

Maitake is widely believed to be safe, although formal safety studies have not been performed. Safety in young children, pregnant or nursing women, or those with severe liver or kidney disease has not been established.

Malic Acid

SUPPLEMENT FORMS/ALTERNATE NAMES: *Apple Acid*
PRINCIPAL PROPOSED USES: *None*
OTHER PROPOSED USES: *Fibromyalgia*

The body synthesizes malic acid during the process of converting carbohydrates to energy. Extremely preliminary evidence suggests that individuals with the disease **fibromyalgia** (a disorder that involves fatigue and pain in the muscles) might have difficulty creating or utilizing malic acid. Such a deficiency could interfere with normal muscle function.

Based on this supposition, products containing malic acid and other nutrients were widely offered for sale to people with fibromyalgia. However, there is as yet no evidence that these products are in fact helpful.

Sources

The body produces its own malic acid. Many fruits and vegetables also supply malic acid, most notably apples.

Therapeutic Dosages

In studies and commercial products, the usual dose of malic acid for fibromyalgia is 1,200 to 2,800 mg per day, generally combined with **magnesium** and other nutrients.

Therapeutic Uses

Malic acid is a major ingredient in combination treatments used for fibromyalgia. However, there is no meaningful evidence that it works.

What Is the Scientific Evidence for Malic Acid?

In a double-blind, placebo-controlled trial, 24 individuals with fibromyalgia were given either placebo or malic acid (1,200 mg per day) combined with magnesium (300 mg daily). After 4 weeks of treatment, there was no significant difference between the placebo and malic acid groups.

The researchers then gave all participants the malic acid combination and increased the dose over a 6-month period. A significant improvement in fibromyalgia symptoms was found after the dose reached about 1,600 mg of malic acid with 400 mg of magnesium. However, because this part of the trial was not blinded or controlled, the results may be entirely due to the placebo effect. Only a properly designed double-blind, placebo-controlled trial of the higher malic acid dose could demonstrate that it really works and, as yet, none have been reported.

Safety Issues

Malic acid appears to be safe at recommended dosages. A few people reported loose stools at the higher doses in the above studies, possibly due to the magnesium in the combination.

Safety in pregnant or nursing women, children, or individuals with severe liver or kidney disease has not been established.

Manganese

SUPPLEMENT FORMS/ALTERNATE NAMES: *Manganese Chloride, Manganese Gluconate, Manganese Picolinate, Manganese Sulfate*

PRINCIPAL PROPOSED USES: *Dysmenorrhea (Menstrual Pain), Osteoporosis (In Combination with Other Minerals)*

OTHER PROPOSED USES: *Diabetes, Epilepsy, Muscle Sprains/Strains, Rheumatoid Arthritis, Tardive Dyskinesia*

Our bodies contain only a very small amount of manganese, but this metal is important as a constituent of many key enzymes. The chemical structure of these enzymes is interesting: large protein molecules cluster around a tiny atom of metal.

Manganese plays a particularly important role as part of the natural antioxidant enzyme superoxide dismutase (SOD), which helps fight damaging free radicals. It also helps energy metabolism, thyroid function, blood sugar control, and normal skeletal growth.

Requirements/Sources

The official U.S. recommendations for daily intake of manganese are as follows:

- Infants 0–6 months, 0.003 mg
  7–12 months, 0.6 mg
- Children 1–3 years, 1.2 mg
  4–8 years, 1.5 mg

➣ Males 9–13 years, 1.9 mg
  14–18 years, 2.2 mg
  19 years and older, 2.3 mg
➣ Females 9–18 years, 1.6 mg
  19 years and older, 1.8 mg
➣ Pregnant women, 2 mg
➣ Nursing women, 2.6 mg

The absorption of manganese may be impaired by simultaneous intake of antacids or calcium or iron supplements.

The best sources of dietary manganese are whole grains, legumes, avocados, grape juice, chocolate, seaweed, egg yolks, nuts, seeds, boysenberries, blueberries, pineapples, spinach, collard greens, peas, and green vegetables.

Therapeutic Dosages

A typical dosage used in studies on manganese is 3 to 6 mg daily. It is sometimes recommended at a much higher dose of 50 to 200 mg daily for 2 weeks following a muscle sprain or strain, but this dosage exceeds recommended safe intake levels (see Safety Issues below).

Therapeutic Uses

Because manganese plays a role in bone metabolism, it has been suggested as a treatment for **osteoporosis**, a condition in which bone mass deteriorates with age. However, we have no direct evidence that manganese is helpful, except perhaps in combination with other minerals.

One small but rigorous study suggests that making sure to get enough manganese may help control symptoms of **dysmenorrhea** (menstrual pain).

Manganese has also been suggested for the treatment of muscle strains and sprains, **rheumatoid arthritis**, and **tardive dyskinesia**, but there is no reliable evidence as yet to indicate that it actually helps.

People with **epilepsy** or **diabetes** have lower-than-normal levels of manganese in their blood. This suggests (but definitely doesn't prove) that manganese supplements might be useful for these conditions. Un-

fortunately, the studies that could prove or disprove this idea haven't been performed.

What Is the Scientific Evidence for Manganese?

Osteoporosis

Although manganese is known to play a role in bone metabolism, there is no direct evidence that manganese supplements can help prevent osteoporosis. However, one double-blind, placebo-controlled study suggests that a combination of minerals including manganese may be helpful. Fifty-nine women took either placebo, calcium (1,000 mg daily), or calcium plus a daily mineral supplement consisting of 5 mg of manganese, 15 mg of zinc, and 2.5 mg of copper. After 2 years, the group receiving calcium plus minerals showed better bone density than the group receiving calcium alone. But this study doesn't tell us whether it was the manganese or the other minerals that made the difference.

Dysmenorrhea (Menstrual Pain)

One very small but well-designed and carefully conducted double-blind study suggested that 5.6 mg of manganese daily might ease menstrual discomfort. In the same study, a lower dosage of 1 mg daily *wasn't* effective.

Safety Issues

Manganese is thought to be safe when taken by adults at a dose of 11 mg daily or less. The maximum safe dosage of manganese for pregnant or nursing women has also been established as 11 mg daily, or 9 mg if 18 years old or younger.

Very high exposure to manganese (due either to environmental pollution or manganese mining) has resulted in a serious psychiatric disorder known as "manganese madness."

Interactions You Should Know About

If you are taking:

➣ **Iron, copper, zinc, magnesium, or calcium: You may need extra manganese, and vice versa.**
➣ **Antacids: You may also need extra manganese.**

Marshmallow

Althaea officinalis

PRINCIPAL PROPOSED USES: *Asthma, Colds, Cough, Crohn's Disease, Skin Inflammation, Sore Throat, Ulcers*

The similarity in name between the herb marshmallow and the sweet treat is more than a coincidence, although the modern sugar puff ball no longer bears much relationship to the old-fashioned candy flavored with marshmallow herb.

Besides inspiring makers of campfire food, the marshmallow has also been used medicinally since ancient Greece. Hippocrates spoke of it as a treatment for bruises and blood loss, and subsequent Roman physicians recommended marshmallow for toothaches, insect bites, chilblains, and irritated skin. In medieval Europe, herbalists used marshmallow to soothe toothaches, coughs, sore throats, chapped skin, indigestion, and diarrhea.

What Is Marshmallow Used for Today?

Marshmallow contains large sugar molecules called *mucilage*, which are thought to exert a soothing effect on mucous membranes and this is the basis of most proposed uses of the herb. However, only double-blind, placebo-controlled studies can prove a treatment effective and no such studies of marshmallow have been reported at this time.

On the basis of its supposed soothing properties, tea or lozenges containing marshmallow tea are often recommended for **asthma**, **cough**, **colds**, and sore throat. Marshmallow taken as tea or in capsules is sometimes recommended for **Crohn's disease** or **ulcers** on the theory that mucilage might sooth the lining of the digestive tract. Finally, marshmallow ointment is sometimes recommended for irritated skin.

Dosage

Marshmallow can be made into a soothing tea by steeping roots overnight in water and diluting to taste. This tea can be drunk as desired for symptomatic relief. Alternatively, you can take marshmallow in capsules (5 to 6 g daily) or in tincture according to label directions.

Marshmallow ointments can be applied directly to soothe inflamed or irritated skin.

Safety Issues

Marshmallow is believed to be entirely safe. It is approved for use in foods and its chemical makeup does not suggest any but benign effects. However, detailed safety studies have not been performed. One study suggests that marshmallow can slightly lower blood sugar levels. For this reason, people with diabetes should use caution when taking marshmallow. Safety in young children, pregnant or nursing women, or those with severe liver or kidney disease has not been established.

Maté

Ilex paraguariensis

ALTERNATE NAMES/RELATED TERMS: *Yerba mate*

PRINCIPAL PROPOSED USES: *Enhancing Mental Function (Due to Caffeine Content), Enhancing Sports Performance (Due to Caffeine Content)*

OTHER PROPOSED USES: *Cancer Prevention, Weight Loss*

Maté is an evergreen tree native to Argentina, Brazil, Paraguay, and Uruguay. The leaves and small stems of the tree are used to make a tea-like caffeinated beverage. Maté has traditionally been used to enhance alertness and mental function and also to treat digestive problems.

What Is Maté Used for Today?

Maté is widely advertised as a healthful beverage, said to provide all the presumed benefits of green tea, such as preventing cancer and heart disease. However, the basis for this claim is largely theoretical. Maté does contain **antioxidant** polyphenols similar to those in tea, but this by itself does not demonstrate that maté is health-promoting; numerous substances with strong antioxidant properties have failed to prove beneficial in double-blind, placebo-controlled studies. Even **green tea** itself has not yet been proven to offer any health benefits.

In the test tube, maté has shown effects that suggest possible value for reducing cancer risk. However, these findings are far too preliminary to rely upon; in fact, there is stronger evidence that maté could, under certain circumstances, *increase* risk of cancer (see Safety Issues below).

Other proposed benefits of maté also largely lack foundation. One study found that an extract of maté could help slow glycation, a metabolic side effect of diabetes. These findings have been used to claim that maté is healthful for people with **diabetes**. However, this study did not involve people with diabetes; it involved chemicals in a test tube. Tens of thousands of substances show benefits in the test tube that fail to translate into real life; it is greatly premature to claim that maté is helpful for people with diabetes based on these exceedingly preliminary findings.

Similarly weak evidence hints that maté might increase fat metabolism and, on this basis, maté has been proposed as a **weight-loss agent**. However, there are no published human studies of maté that show any weight loss benefit. One small double-blind, placebo-controlled study evaluated an herbal preparation containing maté combined with **guarana** and **damiana**. The herbal mixture appeared to cause participants to feel full more quickly during a meal and to continue to feel full for longer after the meal; this led to modest, short-term weight loss. However, it is not clear to what extent the maté in this product played a role.

Another study found that maté might increase bile flow and speed the action of the intestines; these reported effects, even if real, do not indicate any particular health benefit.

Although some maté proponents attempted for many years to maintain that maté does not contain caffeine (supposedly it contained a chemical called *mateine*, which, in fact, does not exist), maté *does* contain caffeine. Depending on how it is brewed, maté tea contains somewhat more caffeine than black tea and slightly less caffeine than coffee. Based on this caffeine content, maté would be expected to **enhance mental function** and **improve sports performance**.

Dosage

A typical dose of maté is 3 to 10 g dried herb per cup. Concentrated extracts are also available. These should be taken according to label instructions.

Safety Issues

As a widely consumed beverage maté is generally assumed to be entirely safe. However, this may be an incorrect assumption. Numerous studies have found associations between high consumption of maté in South America and increased rates cancer of the esophagus, mouth, throat, and larynx. It is widely stated that this

Medium-Chain Triglycerides

increased risk is entirely due to the practice of drinking maté at very high temperatures. However, the underlying evidence is not so clear-cut. The data actually suggest that at least some of this increased risk is due to the maté itself, rather than the temperature at which it is consumed. In addition, maté consumption has also been associated with increased risk of kidney and lung cancer, which would not be expected to be influenced by beverage temperature. Finally, there is some direct evidence that maté has carcinogenic effects. Putting all this information together, it does appear that maté is at the very least slightly carcinogenic. However, so is charred hamburger; moderate use of maté is not likely to significantly increase cancer risk.

Other potential problems with maté relate to its caffeine content. Potential side effects of caffeine include heartburn, gastritis, insomnia, anxiety, and heart arrythmias (benign palpitations or more serious disturbances of heart rhythm). All drug interactions that can occur with caffeine would be expected to occur with maté as well (see next section).

Maximum safe doses have not been established in pregnant or nursing women, young children, or people with severe liver or kidney disease.

Interactions You Should Know About

If you are taking:

➤ **MAO inhibitors: The caffeine in maté could cause dangerous drug interactions.**
➤ **Stimulant drugs such as Ritalin: The stimulant effects of maté might be amplified.**
➤ **Drugs to prevent heart arrythmias or treat insomnia, heartburn, ulcers, or anxiety: The caffeine in maté might interfere with their action.**

Medium-Chain Triglycerides

SUPPLEMENT FORMS/ALTERNATE NAMES: *MCTs*
PRINCIPAL PROPOSED USES: *Undesired Weight Loss (Especially in AIDS)*
OTHER PROPOSED USES: *Performance Enhancement, Weight Loss (Enhancing Body Composition)*

Medium-chain triglycerides (MCTs) are fats with an unusual chemical structure that allows the body to digest them easily. Most fats are broken down in the intestine and remade into a special form that can be transported in the blood. But MCTs are absorbed intact and taken to the liver, where they are used directly for energy. In this sense, they are processed very similarly to carbohydrates.

MCTs are different enough from other fats that they can be used as fat substitutes by people (especially those with AIDS) who need calories but are unable to absorb or metabolize normal fats.

MCTs have also shown a bit of promise for improving body composition and enhancing athletic performance.

Sources

There is no dietary requirement for MCTs. Coconut oil, palm oil, and butter contain up to 15% MCTs (plus a lot of other fats). You can also buy MCTs as purified supplements.

Therapeutic Dosages

MCTs can be eaten as salad oil or used in cooking. When taken as an athletic supplement, dosages in the neighborhood of 85 mg daily are common.

Therapeutic Uses

Preliminary evidence suggests that MCTs are a useful fat substitute for those who have difficulty digesting fat. This makes MCTs potentially helpful for people with **AIDS**, who need to find a way to **gain weight** but cannot digest fat easily. MCTs might theoretically be helpful for those who have trouble digesting fatty foods because they lack the proper enzymes (pancreatic insufficiency), but taking digestive enzymes appears to be more effective.

Although this may sound paradoxical given the above, some evidence suggests that MCT consumption might also enhance the body's natural tendency to burn fat. On this basis, the supplement has been proposed as a **weight loss** aid. Unfortunately, the results of studies have generally failed to find any weight loss benefits. Some studies have, however, found that use of MCTs might produce improvements in body composition (ratio of fat to lean tissue). A related supplement called *structured medium- and long-chain triacylglycerols* (SMLCT) has been created to provide the same potential benefits as MCTs, but in a form that can be used as cooking oil. In a preliminary double-blind trial, SMLCT has also shown some promise for enhancing body composition.

Athletes often sip carbohydrate-loaded drinks during exercise. MCTs may provide an alternative. Like other fats, they provide more energy per ounce than carbohydrates; but unlike normal fats, this energy can be released rapidly. A number of double-blind trials using MCTs for improving high-intensity or endurance **exercise performance** have been conducted, but the results have been thoroughly inconsistent. This is not surprising, as none of these studies enrolled enough participants to provide trustworthy results.

Larger studies are necessary to discover whether MCTs are really as useful for athletes as the supplement's proponents claim.

What Is the Scientific Evidence for Medium-Chain Triglycerides?

A double-blind, placebo-controlled study on 24 men and women with AIDS suggests that MCTs can help improve AIDS-related fat malabsorption. In this disorder, fat is not digested; it passes unchanged through the intestines and the body is deprived of calories as well as fat-soluble vitamins.

The study participants were split into two groups: one received a liquid diet containing normal fats, whereas the other group received mostly MCTs. After 12 days, the participants on the MCT formula showed significantly less fat in their stool and better fat absorption than the other group.

Another double-blind study found similar results in 24 men with AIDS-related fat malabsorption.

The body depends on enzymes from the pancreas to digest fat. In one study, individuals with inadequate pancreatic function due to chronic pancreatitis appeared to be better able to absorb MCTs than ordinary fatty acids. However, this didn't turn out to mean much on a practical basis, because without taking extra digestive enzymes they could only just barely absorb the MCTs; whereas, if they took digestive enzymes, they absorbed ordinary fats as well as MCTs without difficulty.

Safety Issues

Studies in animals and humans tell us that MCTs are quite safe when consumed at a level of up to 50% of total dietary fat. However, some people who consume MCTs, especially on an empty stomach, experience annoying (but not severe) abdominal cramps and bloating.

The maximum safe dosage of MCTs in young children, pregnant or nursing women, or people with serious kidney or liver disease has not been established.

Melatonin

PRINCIPAL PROPOSED USES: *Insomnia, Jet Lag and Other Sleep Disorders*

OTHER PROPOSED USES:

Oral Uses: *Attention Deficit Disorder, Cancer (as an Addition to Conventional Therapy), Cluster Headaches, Epilepsy in Children, Fibromyalgia, Fighting Aging in General, Immune Support, Irritable Bowel Syndrome, Preventing Heart Disease, Quitting Smoking, Reducing Anxiety Before Surgery, Seasonal Affective Disorder, Tardive Dyskinesia*

Topical Uses: *Thinning Hair in Women*

Melatonin is a natural hormone that regulates sleep. During daylight, the pineal gland in the brain produces an important neurotransmitter called *serotonin*. (A *neurotransmitter* is a chemical that relays messages between nerve cells.) But at night, the pineal gland stops producing serotonin and instead makes melatonin. This melatonin release helps trigger sleep.

The production of melatonin varies according to the amount of light you're exposed to; for example, your body produces more melatonin in a completely dark room than in a dimly lit one.

Melatonin supplements appear to be helpful for people whose natural sleep cycle has been disturbed, such as travelers suffering from jet lag. Melatonin may also be helpful in various other sleep disorders.

Based on early reports that melatonin levels decline with age, the hormone was briefly marketed as a kind of fountain of youth. However, newer evidence suggests that melatonin levels do not decline with age after all.

Other potential benefits of melatonin remain largely speculative.

Sources

Melatonin is not a nutrient. However, travelers and workers on rotating or late shifts can experience sleep disturbances that seem to be caused by changing melatonin levels.

You can boost your melatonin production naturally by getting thicker blinds for the bedroom windows or wearing a night mask. You can also take melatonin tablets.

Therapeutic Dosages

Melatonin is typically taken half an hour before bedtime for the first 4 days after traveling.

For ordinary insomnia, melatonin is usually taken about 30 minutes to 1 hour before bedtime. To fall asleep on Sunday night after staying up late Friday and Saturday, one study suggests using melatonin 5.5 hours before the desired bedtime.

The optimum dose of melatonin is not clear, but it is probably in the 1 to 5 mg range.

Melatonin is available in two forms: immediate-release (just plain melatonin, also called *quick-release*) and slow-release (a special preparation, also called *controlled-release*, designed to spread melatonin absorption over many hours). It seems reasonable to suppose that quick-release melatonin helps in falling asleep, while slow-release melatonin helps in staying asleep, but study results are inconsistent on this issue.

Therapeutic Uses

Reasonably good evidence tells us that melatonin can help people with **jet lag** adjust to a new schedule. Although it probably works in part by resetting the biological clock, it also appears to decrease or block wakefulness-promoting circuits in the nervous system and may have other direct sedative effects. Based on this, melatonin has been tried for **insomnia** of various types, but results have been inconsistent.

In addition, two double-blind studies found that melatonin was useful for reducing **anxiety** prior to surgery, again presumably due to its sedative effects.

Two small double-blind, placebo-controlled studies found evidence that taken at 2.5 to 3 mg before bedtime may slightly reduce nighttime **blood pressure**.

Two preliminary double-blind trials hint that use of melatonin at a dose of 10 mg/day may reduce symptoms of **tardive dyskinesia**.

A preliminary double-blind study suggests that melatonin may improve quality of life in children with epilepsy, perhaps by improving sleep and reducing medication side effects.

One surprising double-blind study suggests that topical application of melatonin may increase hair growth in women with thinning hair, for reasons that are entirely unclear.

Oral melatonin has shown some potential for treating, **seasonal affective disorder, cluster headaches** and **irritable bowel syndrome**. Benefits were also seen in another small study, again unrelated to improvements in sleep.

Highly preliminary studies, including unblinded controlled trials, suggest that melatonin may enhance the effectiveness of standard therapy for breast cancer, prostate cancer, brain glioblastomas, non–small-cell lung cancer, and other forms of cancer. (For information on why such studies are unreliable, see **Why Does This Book Rely on Double-blind Studies?**.) Melatonin may also help decrease cancer chemotherapy side effects (see below).

Weak evidence supports a role for melatonin in reducing nicotine withdrawal symptoms.

On the basis of one uncontrolled trial, melatonin has been promoted as a treatment for **fibromyalgia**.

Based on theoretical reasoning and scant evidence, it has been suggested that melatonin can **boost the immune system**, prevent **heart disease**, and fight **aging** in general.

Some evidence suggests that melatonin is *not* helpful for **menopausal symptoms** or **chronic fatigue syndrome**.

What Is the Scientific Evidence for Melatonin?

Sleep Disorders

Melatonin appears to produce sedation comparable to that of conventional pharmaceuticals used for inducing sleep without impairing mental function. Melatonin has shown promise as a treatment for a variety of sleep disorders, of which the best studied is jet lag.

➢ Jet Lag

There is good evidence that melatonin can help you fall asleep when your bedtime rhythm has been disturbed by travel (jet lag).

For example, one double-blind, placebo-controlled study enrolled 320 people and followed them for 4 days after a long plane trip. The participants were divided

into four groups and given a daily dose of 5 mg of standard melatonin, 5 mg of slow-release melatonin, 0.5 mg of standard melatonin, or placebo. The group that received 5 mg of standard melatonin slept better, took less time to fall asleep, and felt more energetic and awake during the day than the other three groups.

Another small double-blind trial found that airplane crews experienced improved rest when using melatonin (10 mg) as compared to placebo, and equivalent benefits as compared to the drug zopiclone. Neither group experienced any impairment in mental function the following morning.

According to one review of the literature, melatonin treatment for jet lag is most effective for those who have crossed a significant number of time zones, perhaps eight.

➢ Shift Work

Studies of melatonin for the treatment of insomnia related to shift work have yielded relatively unimpressive results. Researchers have been surprised by these findings, but suggest that perhaps working at night upsets the biological rhythm even more profoundly than traveling over many time zones, too profoundly for melatonin to help.

➢ Sleep in the Elderly

Mixed results have been seen with the use of melatonin for treating insomnia in the elderly. Not only have many studies failed to find melatonin helpful, those studies with positive results found widely varying benefits; for example, some studies found a decreased time to falling asleep, but no change in sleep throughout the night, while others found the reverse. These differences have not followed dose or type of melatonin in any obvious way, making them somewhat suspect.

➢ General Insomnia

One small study failed to find benefit for general insomnia in healthy people.

➢ Sleep Problems in Children

A 4-week, double-blind trial evaluated the benefits of melatonin for children with difficulty falling asleep. A total of 40 children who had experienced this type of sleep problem for at least 1 year were given either placebo or melatonin at a dose of 5 mg. The results showed that use of melatonin significantly helped participants fall asleep more easily. Similar results were seen in a double-blind, placebo-controlled study of 62 children and in a study of 20 developmentally disabled children with sleep problems.

⇒ Delayed Weekend Sleep Pattern (Monday Morning Fatigue)

Many individuals stay up late on Friday and Saturday nights, and then find it difficult to get to sleep at a reasonable hour on Sunday. A small double-blind, placebo-controlled study found evidence that taking melatonin 5.5 hours before the desired Sunday bedtime improved the ability of participants to fall asleep.

⇒ Sleep in Hospitalized Patients

Benefits were seen in a small double-blind trial of patients in a pulmonary intensive care unit. It is famously difficult to sleep in an ICU and the resulting sleep deprivation is not helpful for those recovering from disease or surgery. In this study of 8 hospitalized individuals, 3 mg of controlled-release melatonin "dramatically improved" sleep quality and duration.

⇒ Other Sleep Problems and Sleep Problems Among People with Specific Medical Problems

Small double-blind trials have found benefits for improving sleep in people with diabetes, asthma (however, see Safety Issues below), head injury, schizophrenia, Alzheimer's disease, attention deficit disorder, and Parkinson's disease.

Blind people often have trouble sleeping on any particular schedule, because there are no "light cues" available to help them get tired at night. A small double-blind, placebo-controlled, crossover trial found that the use of melatonin at a dose of 10 mg per day was able to resynchronize participants' sleep schedules.

Some individuals find it impossible to fall asleep until early morning, a condition called *delayed sleep phase syndrome* (DSPS). Melatonin may be beneficial for this syndrome.

Individuals trying to quit using sleeping pills in the benzodiazepine family may find melatonin helpful. A double-blind, placebo-controlled study of 34 individuals who regularly used such medications found that melatonin at a dose of 2 mg nightly (controlled-release formulation) could help them discontinue the use of the drugs. Interestingly, another study failed to find melatonin helpful for reducing benzodiazepine use among people taking drugs in that family for anxiety.

Note: There can be risks in discontinuing benzodiazepine drugs. Consult your physician for advice.

Anxiety Prior to Surgery

Relaxing sedative medications are often used prior to surgery to help reduce the anxiety that often occurs while waiting for surgery to begin. A double-blind, placebo-controlled study of 75 women waiting for surgery compared melatonin against the standard drug midazolam. Although midazolam was more effective, melatonin was definitely superior to placebo and patients appeared to like each one equally. One advantage of melatonin was that it did not cause amnesia.

Benefits were also seen in a subsequent double-blind trial of 84 women and in a study of 105 children undergoing surgery. All of these studies on melatonin for reducing anxiety related to surgery were conducted by a single research group.

Cancer Treatment

Melatonin has been used with conventional anticancer therapy in more than a dozen clinical studies. Results have been surprisingly good, although this research must be considered preliminary. For example, a double-blind study on 30 people with advanced brain tumors suggested that melatonin might prolong life and also improve the quality of life. Participants received standard radiation treatment with or without 20 mg daily of melatonin. After 1 year, 6 of 14 individuals in the melatonin group were still alive, compared with just 1 of 16 from the control group. The melatonin group also had fewer side effects due to the radiation treatment—a notable improvement in their quality of life.

Improvements in symptoms and a possible reduction of mortality were also seen in other studies. Melatonin appears to work by increasing levels of the body's own tumor-fighting proteins, known as *cytokines*.

Cluster Headaches

Some evidence suggests that individuals with cluster headaches have lower than average levels of the hormone melatonin. In a double-blind, placebo-controlled study of 20 individuals with cluster headaches, use of melatonin (10 mg daily) for 14 days appeared to reduce headache severity and/or frequency in about half the participants. Overall, use of melatonin produced better effects than placebo.

Seasonal Affective Disorder

One study found that people with seasonal affective disorder (SAD) have higher levels of melatonin than those without the condition. On this basis, it would seem that supplemental melatonin should worsen SAD symptoms. However, the evidence for such an effect is inconsistent. Some researchers have proposed that interaction between SAD and melatonin might be more complex than merely high or low levels and that, when taken at certain times of day, melatonin might help the condition. A very small study found that when melatonin was given in the afternoon, it produced some benefit for people with SAD. However, a study of melatonin used in the early morning or the late evening failed to find any benefit.

Melatonin has shown equivocal effects for two conditions related to SAD: subsyndromal seasonal affective disorder (S-SAD) and weather associated syndrome (WAS). According to the one reported study, use of melatonin improved some symptoms but worsened others.

Safety Issues

A safety study found that melatonin at a dose of 10 mg daily produced no toxic effects when given to 40 healthy males for a period of 28 days. However, this does not prove that melatonin is safe when taken on a regular basis over the long term. Keep in mind that melatonin is not truly a food supplement but a hormone. As we know from other hormones used in medicine, such as estrogen and cortisone, harmful effects can take years to appear. Hormones are powerful substances that have many subtle effects in the body and we're far from understanding them fully. While in one small study, use of melatonin over an 8-day period by healthy men did not affect natural release of melatonin or levels of pituitary or sex hormones, another study found effects on testosterone and estrogen metabolism in men and possible impairment of sperm function, and a small study in women found possible effects on the important female hormone luteinizing hormone (LH).

Melatonin appears to cause drowsiness and decreased mental attention for about 2 to 6 hours after using it and may also impair balance. For this reason, you should not drive or operate machinery for several hours after taking melatonin. However, there doesn't appear to be any "hangover" the following day.

Based on theoretical ideas of how melatonin works, some authorities specifically recommend against using it in people with depression, schizophrenia, autoimmune diseases, and other serious illnesses. One study in postmenopausal women found evidence that melatonin might impair insulin action and glucose tolerance, suggesting that people with diabetes should not use it.

However, another study found melatonin safe and effective for people with diabetes. Because of these contradictions, we suggest that individuals with diabetes seek physician supervision before using melatonin.

Two exceedingly preliminary studies reported by one research group have led to publicized concerns that use of the supplement melatonin might increase night-time asthma. However, one double-blind study of melatonin in people with asthma found evidence of improved sleep without worsening of symptoms. Again, at the current state of knowledge caution must be advised for people with night-time asthma who wish to try melatonin.

Maximum safe dosages for young children, pregnant or nursing women, or those with serious liver or kidney disease have not been established.

Mesoglycan

SUPPLEMENT FORMS/ALTERNATE NAMES: *Aortic GAGs, Aortic Glycosaminoglycans, Chondroitin Polysulphate, Chondroitin Sulfate A, CSA, GAGs, Glycosaminoglycans, Mucopolysaccharide*
PRINCIPAL PROPOSED USES: *Atherosclerosis, Intermittent Claudication, Varicose Veins/Venous Insufficiency*
OTHER PROPOSED USES: *Hemorrhoids, High Cholesterol, Kidney Stones, Osteoarthritis, Phlebitis*

Mesoglycan is a type of substance found in many tissues in the body, including the joints, intestines, and the lining of blood vessels. Chemically, mesoglycan is related to the blood-thinning drug heparin and the supplement **chondroitin**. Unlike chondroitin, mesoglycan is primarily used to treat diseases of blood vessels. Preliminary evidence suggests that mesoglycan may be helpful for atherosclerosis, varicose veins, phlebitis, and hemorrhoids.

Sources

Mesoglycan is not an essential nutrient because the body usually manufactures it from scratch. For supplement purposes, mesoglycan is commercially extracted from the intestines of pigs. Very similar substances can be produced from cartilage, bone, and the lining of large blood vessels, and are often used interchangeably.

Therapeutic Dosages

The usual dosage of mesoglycan is 100 mg daily.

Therapeutic Uses

Most proposed uses of mesoglycan involve diseases of blood vessels. For example, evidence suggests that mesoglycan may slow the development of **hardening of the arteries**, perhaps by lowering **cholesterol levels**, "thinning" the blood, or through other effects.

People with severe hardening of the arteries sometimes develop blockage in the arteries of the legs, a condition called *intermittent claudication*. This condition limits the ability to walk by causing intense, crampy pain after walking a relatively short distance. There is some evidence that mesoglycan may help.

The conditions just discussed involve arteries. Mesoglycan may also be useful for various diseases of the veins, including **varicose veins/venous insufficiency**, **hemorrhoids**, and **phlebitis**.

One study suggests that a substance related to mesoglycan, hyaluronic acid, might be helpful for **asthma** when taken by inhalation.

Warning: Do not self-treat phlebitis. It is a potentially deadly disease.

Preliminary evidence suggests mesoglycan may additionally be useful in treating **kidney stones**.

The substance chondroitin is used for the treatment of **osteoarthritis**. Based on the chemical similarities between chondroitin and mesoglycan, researchers conducted a large (almost 400-participant) 5-year, double-blind, placebo-controlled study of injected mesoglycan for slowing the progression of osteoarthritis. Unfortunately, no benefits were seen.

What Is the Scientific Evidence for Mesoglycan?

Intermittent Claudication

A 20-week, double-blind, placebo-controlled trial that enrolled 242 people evaluated the effects of mesoglycan (100 mg a day orally, after a short course of injected treatment) for treating intermittent claudication. Significantly more participants in the mesoglycan group responded to treatment (defined as a greater than 50% improvement in walking distance) than in the placebo group.

Atherosclerosis in General

In a double-blind, comparative study, men with atherosclerosis in the arteries of the heart (coronary artery disease) were given either 200 mg daily of mesoglycan or no extra treatment. After 18 months, the layering of the vessel lining was 7.5 times greater in the untreated group than in the mesoglycan group, a significant difference. However, because this was not a double-blind, placebo-controlled trial, the results can't be taken as truly reliable. (For information on why double-blind studies are essential for proving a treatment effective, see **Why Does This Book Depend on Double-blind Studies?**.)

Additional preliminary evidence that mesoglycan might help atherosclerosis comes from other studies in animals and people.

We don't know for certain how mesoglycan might help atherosclerosis. There is some evidence that it can reduce cholesterol levels and also "thin" the blood.

Vein Diseases

Several studies suggest that mesoglycan may be helpful in the treatment of vein problems, such as varicose veins/venous insufficiency, phlebitis, and hemorrhoids. For example, in a double-blind, placebo-controlled trial, 183 individuals with leg ulcers caused by poor vein function were treated with either placebo or mesoglycan (first by injection and then orally) for 24 weeks. The results of this double-blind study suggest that mesoglycan significantly improved the rate at which the leg ulcers healed.

Safety Issues

Mesoglycan is essentially ground-up pig intestines and is believed to be safe, even if taken in large quantities. However, because mesoglycan appears to decrease blood clotting, it should not be combined with prescription blood thinners such as warfarin (Coumadin), clopidogrel (Plavix), ticlopidine (Ticlid), pentoxifylline (Trental), or heparin, or drugs in the aspirin family. Maximum safe dosages for young children, pregnant or nursing women, or those with severe liver or kidney disease have not been determined.

Interactions You Should Know About

If you are taking drugs that decrease blood clotting, such as **warfarin** (Coumadin), **heparin**, **clopidogrel** (Plavix), **ticlopidine** (Ticlid), **pentoxifylline** (Trental), or **aspirin**, do not use mesoglycan except under physician supervision.

Methionine

SUPPLEMENT FORMS/ALTERNATE NAMES: *L-Methionine*

PRINCIPAL PROPOSED USES: *None*

OTHER PROPOSED USES: *"Liver Support," Parkinson's Disease, Urinary Tract Infections*

Methionine is an essential amino acid—one of the building blocks of proteins and peptides that your body cannot manufacture from other chemicals. The body uses methionine to manufacture **creatine** and uses the sulfur in methionine for normal metabolism and growth.

One preliminary study suggests that methionine can prevent bacteria from sticking to urinary tract cells, which may make it useful for preventing **bladder infections**. (**Cranberry** juice is thought to help reduce the incidence of bladder infections in a similar fashion.)

Requirements/Sources

Depending on your body weight, you need between 800 and 1,000 mg of methionine daily for normal health.

Deficiency is unlikely, because enough methionine is generally available from the diet.

Meat, fish, dairy products, and other high-protein foods are good sources of methionine.

Therapeutic Dosages

A proper therapeutic dosage of methionine has not been determined. One study relating to urinary tract infections used a dosage of 500 mg 3 times daily.

Therapeutic Uses

Because it seems to discourage bacteria from sticking to the wall of the bladder, methionine has been suggested as a treatment for recurrent bladder infections.

However, the evidence that it works is limited to one small trial without a placebo control. (For information on why placebo-controlled trials are essential to prove a treatment effective, see **Why Does This Book Depend on Double-blind Studies?**.)

One study on rats suggests that methionine might protect the liver against the damaging effects of acetaminophen (Tylenol) poisoning. On this slim basis, methionine has been proposed as a general liver protectant. However, in this particular study the action of methionine was more to fight acetaminophen specifically than to protect the liver in general.

Very preliminary evidence suggests methionine might be helpful in treating **Parkinson's disease** (however, this should not be attempted except under physician supervision; see Safety Issues).

Safety Issues

Methionine is thought to be generally safe. However, the maximum safe dosages for young children, pregnant or nursing women, or those with serious liver or kidney disease have not been established.

Like other amino acids, methionine may interfere with the absorption or action of the drug levodopa, which is used for Parkinson's disease.

Interactions You Should Know About

If you are taking:

> **Methionine:** Make sure to get enough folate, vitamin B_6, and vitamin B_{12}.
> **Levodopa:** Methionine might interfere with its action.

Methyl Sulfonyl Methane

SUPPLEMENT FORMS/ALTERNATE NAMES: *MSM*

RELATED TERMS: *Dimethyl Sulfone (DMSO$_2$)*

PRINCIPAL PROPOSED USES: *Osteoarthritis*

OTHER PROPOSED USES: *Improving Growth of Nails and Hair, Interstitial Cystitis, Rheumatoid Arthritis, Snoring, Sports Injuries*

MSM (methyl sulfonyl methane) is a sulfur-containing compound normally found in many of the foods we eat. It is chemically related to DMSO (dimethyl sulfoxide), a popular (although unproven) treatment for arthritis. When DMSO is applied on the skin or taken orally, about 15% of it breaks down in the body to form MSM.

Some researchers have suggested that the resulting MSM could be responsible for the benefits attributed to DMSO. If so, MSM might be preferable as a treatment, because it does not cause some of the unpleasant side effects associated with DMSO treatment, such as body odor and bad breath. In addition, as a natural substance found in food, MSM would be expected to have a good safety profile. However, there is as yet no more than preliminary evidence that MSM is useful for any medical condition.

Requirements/Sources

There is no dietary requirement for MSM. However, it occurs naturally in cow's milk, meat, seafood, vegetables, fruits, and even coffee, tea, and chocolate. MSM supplements are sold in health-food stores and some pharmacies. Although creams and lotions containing MSM are also available, it is hard to see the purpose of these topical products since MSM, unlike DMSO, is not absorbed through the skin.

MSM supplies sulfur. Some advertisements for MSM claim that sulfur deficiency is widespread and that for this reason alone MSM will improve the health of almost everybody who takes it. However, there are numerous other dietary sources of sulfur, including, most prominently, many forms of ordinary protein.

Therapeutic Dosages

Dosages of oral MSM used for therapeutic purposes range from 1,500 mg to 10,000 mg daily, usually divided up into 3 daily doses.

Therapeutic Uses

Two small double-blind, placebo-controlled studies indicate that MSM may be helpful for **osteoarthritis**.

Small, unpublished trials have been used to claim that MSM is effective for the treatment of snoring, aiding the growth of nails and hair, and assisting in recovery from **sports injuries**. However, the design of each of these studies was substandard and the results were not subjected to any proper statistical analysis; therefore, they cannot be taken as meaningful evidence of efficacy.

One study in mice found positive effects of MSM in the treatment of **rheumatoid arthritis**. Other animal studies hint that MSM might have **cancer preventive** properties. Human studies on these potential uses of MSM have not been reported.

MSM has also been proposed as a treatment for **interstitial cystitis**, an inflammation in the wall of the bladder that causes frequent and painful urination. When prescribed for this condition, MSM is usually instilled directly into the bladder, although oral use has also been suggested. However, no clinical studies on this use have been performed: the only evidence for this treatment comes from case studies and anecdotal reports. Since interstitial cystitis is known to respond very positively to placebo, these reports mean little.

MSM has also been advocated for **allergies** (including drug allergies), **scleroderma**, **excess stomach acid**, and **constipation**, but there is no meaningful evidence whatsoever to support these proposed uses.

What Is the Scientific Evidence for Methyl Sulfonyl Methane?

In a double-blind, placebo-controlled study of 118 people with osteoarthritis of the knee, participants were given one of the following four treatments: glucosamine (500 mg 3 times daily), MSM (500 mg 3 times daily), a combination of glucosamine and MSM, or placebo. The study ran for 12 weeks. The results showed that both MSM and glucosamine improved arthritis symptoms as compared to placebo and that the combination of MSM and glucosamine was more effective than either one alone.

Benefits were also seen in a 12-week, double-blind, placebo-controlled trial of 50 people with osteoarthritis, utilizing MSM at a dose of 3 g twice daily.

Safety Issues

MSM is a natural component of the foods we normally eat and is not believed to be toxic. A laboratory study examining doses up to 8 g per kilogram of body weight per day (about 250 times the highest dose normally used by humans) reported that no toxic effects were seen.

Maximum safe doses for young children, pregnant or nursing women, or people with liver or kidney disease are not known. Possible drug interactions are also not known.

Methyl Sulfonyl Methane

Milk Thistle

Silybum marianum

PRINCIPAL PROPOSED USES: *Alcoholic Hepatitis, Liver Cirrhosis, Mushroom Poisoning (Special Intravenous Form Only), Protection from Liver-toxic Medications, Viral Hepatitis*

The milk thistle plant commonly grows from 2 to 7 feet in height, with spiny leaves and reddish-purple, thistle-shaped flowers. It has also been called *wild artichoke, holy thistle,* and *Mary thistle.* Native to Europe, milk thistle has a long history of use as both a food and a medicine. At the turn of the twentieth century, English gardeners grew milk thistle to use its leaves like lettuce (after cutting off the spines), the stalks like asparagus, the roasted seeds like coffee, and the roots (soaked overnight) like oyster plant. The seeds and leaves of milk thistle were used for medicinal purposes as well, such as treating jaundice and increasing breast milk production.

German researchers in the 1960s were sufficiently impressed with the history and clinical effectiveness of milk thistle to begin examining it for active constituents. In 1986, Germany's Commission E approved an oral extract of milk thistle standardized to 70% crude silymarin content as a treatment for liver disease. However, the evidence that it really works remains incomplete and inconsistent.

What Is Milk Thistle Used for Today?

Based on the extensive folk use of milk thistle in cases of jaundice, European medical researchers began to investigate its medicinal effects. It is currently used to treat **alcoholic hepatitis, liver cirrhosis,** liver poisoning, and **viral hepatitis,** as well as to **protect the liver in general** from the effects of liver-toxic medications. However, despite this wide usage, there is no definitive evidence that it is effective.

The active ingredients in milk thistle are assumed to be four substances known collectively as *silymarin,* of which apparently the most potent is named silibinin. When injected intravenously, silibinin is thought to act as an antidote to poisoning by the deathcap mushroom, *Amanita phalloides.* Animal studies suggest that milk thistle extracts can also protect against many other poisonous substances, from toluene to the drug acetaminophen. One animal study suggests that milk thistle can also protect against fetal damage caused by alcohol.

Silymarin is hypothesized to function by displacing toxins trying to bind to the liver as well as by causing the liver to regenerate more quickly. It may also act as an **antioxidant** and also stabilize liver cell membranes.

In Europe, milk thistle is often added as extra protection when patients are given medications known to cause liver problems. However, milk thistle failed to prove effective for preventing liver inflammation caused by the Alzheimer's drug Cognex (tacrine).

Milk thistle is also used in a vague condition known as minor hepatic insufficiency or "sluggish liver." This term is mostly used by European physicians and American naturopathic practitioners—conventional physicians in the U.S. don't recognize it. Symptoms are supposed to include aching under the ribs, fatigue, unhealthy skin appearance, general malaise, constipation, premenstrual syndrome, chemical sensitivities, and allergies.

Milk thistle may also offer some protection to the kidney.

Highly preliminary evidence hints that milk thistle might help reduce breast **cancer** risk. Milk thistle is sometimes recommended for **gallstones** and **psoriasis,** but there is little to no evidence as yet that it really helps these conditions.

What Is the Scientific Evidence for Milk Thistle?

As noted above, there is considerable evidence from studies in animals that milk thistle can protect the liver from numerous toxins. However, human studies of people suffering from various liver diseases have often yielded mixed results.

Acute Viral Hepatitis

A 21-day, double-blind, placebo-controlled study of 57 people with acute viral hepatitis found significant improvements in the group receiving milk thistle. A 35-day study of 151 individuals thought to have acute hepatitis found no benefit with milk thistle, but this study has been criticized for failing to document that the partici-pants actually had acute hepatitis.

Chronic Viral Hepatitis

While some studies have found milk thistle helpful for symptoms of chronic viral hepatitis B or C, the most re-cent and in some ways best-designed study failed to find benefit for hepatitis C.

Alcoholic Hepatitis

A double-blind, placebo-controlled study performed in 1981 followed 106 Finnish soldiers with alcoholic liver disease over a period of 4 weeks. The treated group showed a significant decrease in elevated liver enzymes and im-provement in liver histology (the microscopic structure of liver tissue), as evaluated by biopsy in 29 subjects.

Two similar studies provided essentially equivalent results. However, a 3-month, randomized, double-blind study of 116 people showed little to no additional benefit, perhaps because most participants reduced their alcohol consumption and almost half stopped drinking entirely. It is undoubtedly more effective for people with alcoholism to quit drinking than to continue drinking and take milk thistle! Another study found no benefit in 72 patients fol-lowed for 15 months.

Liver Cirrhosis

A double-blind, placebo-controlled study of 170 people with alcoholic or non-alcoholic cirrhosis found that in the group treated with milk thistle the 4-year survival rate was 58% as compared to only 38% in the placebo group. This difference was statistically significant.

A double-blind, placebo-controlled trial that en-rolled 172 people with cirrhosis for 4 years also found reductions in mortality, but they just missed the con-ventional cutoff for statistical significance. And a 2-year, double-blind, placebo-controlled study of 200 individuals with alcoholic cirrhosis found no reduction in mortality attributable to the use of milk thistle.

Other double-blind studies of people with various forms of cirrhosis have looked at changes in tests of liver function rather than mortality. Some found benefit while others did not.

Protection from Medications That Damage the Liver

Numerous medications can injure or inflame the liver. Preliminary evidence suggests that milk thistle might protect against liver toxicity caused by drugs such as acetaminophen, phenytoin (Dilantin), alcohol, and phenothiazines. However, according to a 12-week, double-blind study of 222 people, milk thistle does not seem to prevent the liver inflammation caused by the Alzheimer's drug tacrine (Cognex).

Dosage

The standard dosage of milk thistle is 200 mg 2 to 3 times a day of an extract standardized to contain 70% silymarin.

There is some evidence that silymarin bound to phos-phatidylcholine may be better absorbed. This form should be taken at a dosage of 100 to 200 mg twice a day.

Warning: Considering the severe nature of liver dis-ease, a doctor's supervision is essential. Also, do not inject milk thistle preparations that are designed for oral use!

Safety Issues

Milk thistle is believed to possess very little toxicity. Ani-mal studies have not shown any negative effects even when high doses were administered over a long period of time.

A study of 2,637 participants reported in 1992 showed a low incidence of side effects, limited mainly to mild gastrointestinal disturbance. However, on rare occasions severe abdominal discomfort may occur.

On the basis of its extensive use as a food, milk this-tle is believed to be safe for pregnant or nursing women and researchers have enrolled pregnant women in stud-ies. However, safety in young children, pregnant or nurs-ing women, and individuals with severe renal disease has not been formally established.

No drug interactions are known. However, one re-port has noted that silibinin (a constituent of silymarin) can inhibit a bacterial enzyme called *beta-glucuronidase*, which plays a role in the activity of certain drugs, such as oral contraceptives. This could theoretically reduce their effectiveness.

Interactions You Should Know About

If you are taking:

➤ Medications that could damage the liver, such as acetaminophen, phenytoin (Dilantin), alcohol, and phenothiazines: Milk thistle might be protec-tive for some of these drugs.

➤ Oral contraceptives: Milk thistle might reduce their effectiveness.

Mistletoe

Mistletoe

Viscum album

ALTERNATE NAMES/RELATED TERMS: *European Mistletoe*

PRINCIPAL PROPOSED USES: *Cancer Treatment Support (Injectible Form)*

OTHER PROPOSED USES: *Colds and Flus, Diabetes, Hypertension*

European mistletoe, famous during the Christmas season, is a semiparasitic plant that grows on trees in Europe and Asia. Its young leafy twigs and flowers were used as an "all-heal" or *panacea*, said to be helpful for virtually all diseases. The herb is also said to have played a role in Celtic religious celebrations.

Note: American mistletoe, Phoradendron leucarpum, is related to European mistletoe, but it is thought to be more toxic and has not been well studied.

What Is Mistletoe Used for Today?

In the twentieth century, mistletoe became popular in Germany through the advocacy of a mystic and philosopher named Rudolf Steiner. The school of medicine he founded, anthroposophical medicine, recommended injectible forms of mistletoe as a treatment for cancer. The initial basis for this use was Steiner's "clairvoyant" insight. Scientific tests were subsequently conducted with somewhat positive results, but current evidence is far from definitive.

Mistletoe extracts show anticancer effects in the test tube. However, test-tube studies cannot show a treatment effective; only controlled clinical trials can do that. A 2003 review of human trials found 10 human trials of injected mistletoe for cancer that met at least minimal scientific standards. Unfortunately, even these studies generally suffered from significant weaknesses in design. The review authors noted that the better-designed studies failed to find evidence of benefit, in terms of lengthened remission, improved quality of life, or chance of survival. Subsequent human trials have

also failed to reach adequate levels of scientific rigor and have therefore failed to clarify matters.

Oral uses of mistletoe have not undergone significant study. Very weak evidence, too weak to rely upon at all, hints that constituents of mistletoe might potentially offer benefit in diabetes and **colds and flus**. It is commonly stated that oral mistletoe products reduce blood pressure, but there is no scientific evidence to support this belief.

Dosage

Injectible mistletoe extracts should only be used under the supervision of a physician.

Mistletoe tea can be made by soaking 10 to 20 g of chopped leaves in 2 cups of water for 8 hours. A typical dose is 1 to 3 cups daily.

Safety Issues

In large clinical trials, use of injected pharmaceutical-grade mistletoe products has not been associated with serious adverse effects, although pain at the injection site and mild flu-like symptoms are common. Severe allergic reactions may occur rarely.

Oral use of a mistletoe product has been associated with hepatitis. Mistletoe berries and perhaps the leaves can cause severe toxicity, especially in children. American mistletoe may be more toxic than European mistletoe.

Mistletoe is not recommended for use in young children, pregnant or nursing women, or people with severe liver or kidney disease.

Molybdenum

PRINCIPAL PROPOSED USES: *None*

OTHER PROPOSED USES: *Female Sexual Dysfunction, General Well-Being, Insomnia, Male Sexual Dysfunction, Tooth Decay Prevention, Weight Loss*

Molybdenum is an essential trace mineral. Deficiency of molybdenum is rare, but may occur in certain parts of the world. Current marketing of molybdenum products for the treatment of medical conditions is not founded on any meaningful scientific evidence.

Requirements/Sources

Molybdenum is found in a variety of foods, including dark green leafy vegetables, legumes, and whole grains. Mineral water or "hard" tap water may aslo supply significant amounts of molybdenum.

Deficiency of molybdenum is believed to be rare. Although accurate Recommended Daily Intake levels for molybdenum have not been determined, less precise Safe and Adequate Intake levels have been set in the U.S. as follows:

> **Birth to 3 years of age: 15–50 mcg**
> **4–6 years of age: 30–75 mcg**
> **7–10 years of age: 50–150 mcg**
> **11 or older: 75–250 mcg**

Therapeutic Doses

There are no known uses of molybdenum that would suggest doses other than the Safe and Adequate Intake levels noted in the previous section.

Molybdenum is marketed both as a tablet and as a liquid supplement containing the mineral in dissolved form. Despite widespread claims, there is no evidence that one form of molybdenum is absorbed to a markedly superior extent than any other.

Therapeutic Uses

Websites that advocate molybdenum products make numerous health claims that lack scientific foundation. Some of these unsupported claims include the following:

> **Regulates the body's pH**
> **Enhances the body's ability to burn fat**
> **Eliminates toxins**
> **Promotes general well-being**
> **Prevents tooth decay**
> **Aids sleep**
> **Reduces allergic reaction to chemicals, such as MSG or sulfites**
> **Increases male and female libido**

None of these claims have any scientific support, and some (such as "regulating the body's pH") make no sense from a scientific point of view.

Additionally, it is often stated by some manufacturers of molybdenum products that a variety of disease are commonly caused or worsened by molybdenum deficiency. These include **acne, allergies, asthma, athlete's foot, Bell's palsy, bladder infection, candidiasis, canker sores, depression, diabetes, eczema,** Gulf War syndrome, **viral hepatitis,** *Herpes simplex,* **liver cirrhosis, lupus,** Lyme disease, **multiple sclerosis,** and **prostatitis.** However, again, all of these claims lack even the bare minimum of foundation.

In certain areas of China, molybdenum deficiency may occur relatively commonly. There are higher rates of some forms of cancer in these regions; however, when molybdenum supplementation was tried, it failed to make a difference, perhaps because other unidentified deficiencies were involved as well.

Safety Issues

When taken at recommended dosages, molybdenum should be safe. Excessive intake of molybdenum could in theory lead to copper deficiency. People with serious kidney disease should also avoid taking molybdenum (or any other supplement) except on the advice of a physician. One isolated report hints that excessive molybdenum intake can cause symptoms of psychosis.

Molybdenum

Motherwort

Motherwort

Leonurus cardiaca, Leonurus artemisia

PRINCIPAL PROPOSED USES: *None*

OTHER PROPOSED USES: *Irregular or Rapid Heartbeat, Uterine Stimulant*

NOT RECOMMENDED USES: *Pregnancy Support*

As its Latin name *cardiaca* suggests, motherwort has traditionally been used to treat heart conditions. The ancient Greeks and Romans employed motherwort to treat heart palpitations as well as depression, which they considered a problem of the heart. Centuries later, Europeans would believe motherwort helpful for "infirmities of the heart" but also considered the herb to have strengthening and stimulating effects on the uterus, using it to bring on a delayed menstrual period, as an aid during labor, and to relax a woman's womb after childbirth.

These uses of motherwort correspond well with those in traditional Chinese medicine, which employs the Asian variety, *Leonurus artemisia*, to treat menstrual disorders or to help a woman expel a dead fetus and placenta from her womb. In eastern China, women still drink a syrup made from motherwort to promote the recovery of the uterus after childbirth; the herb has a strong bitter taste, so visitors to a recovering mother often bring along sugar as a gift.

What Is Motherwort Used for Today?

Germany's Commission E has authorized motherwort for the treatment of rapid or irregular heartbeat caused by **anxiety** and **stress**, as well as part of an overall treatment plan for an overactive thyroid (**hyperthyroidism**, a condition that also causes irregular heartbeat).

However, as yet there is no real evidence to support these uses of the herb. The best that can be said is that in one test-tube study motherwort slowed the beating of normal rat heart cells and inhibited the effects of substances that usually speed up heart cell contractions.

Two other test-tube studies suggest that leonurine, a compound found in some species of motherwort, may affect the uterus. One of these studies found that low concentrations of leonurine induced uterine contractions, but that higher concentrations inhibited con-

tractions. These opposing effects might explain how motherwort could induce both labor and menstruation and yet could also relax the uterus after childbirth (as it is traditionally said to do). However, until properly designed human studies are performed, we won't have any clear idea whether motherwort is actually safe or effective for these traditional uses.

One poorly designed study suggests that motherwort might improve blood circulation. Another study of equally low quality hints that motherwort might protect brain tissue in people who have had a **stroke**.

One component of motherwort, ursolic acid, has been found to possess possible antiviral and antitumor properties; however, this extremely preliminary information should not be taken to mean that motherwort can fight viral infections or help treat cancer.

Dosage

The Commission E recommends a dose of 4.5 g of dried herb daily, or the equivalent.

Note: Irregular or rapid heartbeat can be a sign of serious medical illness. Do not self-treat these conditions with motherwort except under medical supervision. Also, do not combine motherwort with other heart medications, as they might interact unpredictably.

Safety Issues

The safety of motherwort has not been well studied; however, obvious side effects appear to be rare, except for occasional allergic reactions and gastrointestinal distress.

Because of the herb's traditional use for uterine stimulation and the corroborating results of some test-tube studies, motherwort should not be used by pregnant women until further scientific investigation has been performed.

In addition, preliminary animal evidence suggests that women with a history of breast cancer, or those at high risk for developing it, should avoid motherwort.

Safety in young children, nursing women, or people with severe liver or kidney disease has not been established.

Muira Puama

Ptychopetalum olacoides, P. uncinatum, P. guyanna

ALTERNATE NAMES/RELATED TERMS: *Potency wood*
PRINCIPAL PROPOSED USES: *Male Sexual Dysfunction*
OTHER PROPOSED USES: *Enhancing Mental Function*

Muira puama is a bush native to the Brazilian Amazon rain forest. Its bark and roots have been used traditionally for a variety of medicinal purposes, including impotence in men, loss of libido in women, nerve problems (including paralysis and tremor), anxiety, digestive problems, and arthritis.

What Is Muira Puama Used for Today?

Explorers brought muira puama to Europe, where it became popular primarily as a treatment for **impotence**. However, there has been no reliable scientific evaluation of the effectiveness of this herb.

One study is commonly cited as showing that muira puama is more effective for impotence than the drug yohimbine (from the herb **yohimbe**). However, this study actually shows nothing at all. It was an open trial, in which all participants took muira puama. The researchers simply compared the benefits seen in this trial to the benefits seen in other trials in which people took yohimbine. From a scientific perspective, this is not permissible. The placebo effect is strong and varies from study to study. One can assume without even performing the experiment that if men with sexual dysfunction are given a treatment that they believe might help them, they will be helped. To determine whether muira puama is helpful for impotence would require a double-blind, placebo-controlled study. To determine

whether it's more effective than yohimbine would require a double-blind study in which some people took muira puama and some took yohimbine. Since no double-blind studies of muira puama have been reported at all, use of this herb has to be regarded as entirely speculative. (For more information on why double-blind studies are essential, see **Why Does This Book Rely on Double-blind Studies?**.)

Weak evidence hints that muira puama may be helpful for **enhancing mental function** by increasing brain levels of acetylcholine, but this evidence is far too preliminary to indicate effectiveness.

Dosage

Muira puama is generally taken in the form of a liquid alcohol extract. Follow label instructions for dosage.

Safety Issues

From what limited evidence that is available, it does not appear that use of muira puama commonly causes significant side effects. However, a comprehensive formal safety evaluation has not been conducted. For this reason, muira puama should not be used by pregnant or nursing women, young children, or individuals with severe liver or kidney disease.

Mullein

Verbascum thapsus

PRINCIPAL PROPOSED USES: *None*

OTHER PROPOSED USES: *Asthma, Colds, Cough, Ear Infections (Topical, in Combination with Other Herbs), Sore Throat*

Also called *grandmother's flannel* for its thick, soft leaves, mullein is a common wildflower that can grow almost anywhere. It reaches several feet tall and puts up a spike of densely packed tiny yellow flowers. Mullein has served many purposes over the centuries, from making candlewicks to casting out evil spirits, but as medicine it was primarily used to treat diarrhea, respiratory diseases, and hemorrhoids.

What Is Mullein Used for Today?

Mullein contains a high proportion of *mucilage* (large sugar molecules); mucilage is generally thought to have a soothing effect. Mullein also contains saponins that may help loosen mucus. On this basis, mullein has been suggested as a treatment for asthma, **colds**, coughs, and sore throats. However, as yet there is no meaningful evidence that it is useful for any of these conditions.

Mullein is traditionally combined with other herbs in oil preparations to soothe the pain of **ear infections** (otitis media, or middle ear infection, but not "swimmer's ear," an external ear infection) and one study provides preliminary support for this use (see next section).

As with many herbs, test-tube studies have found that mullein can kill viruses on contact. In addition, an interesting but highly preliminary study suggests that mullein might help certain medications used for **influenza** work better. These findings, however, are far too scant to show that internal use of mullein will fight viral infections.

Oral mullein is said to be most effective when combined with other herbs of similar qualities, such as **yerba santa**, **marshmallow**, cherry bark, and **elecampane**, but there is no evidence to support this belief.

What Is the Scientific Evidence for Mullein?

Two double-blind trials enrolling a total of more than 250 children with eardrum pain caused by middle ear infection compared the effectiveness of an herbal preparation containing **garlic**, **St. John's wort**, and **calendula** against a standard anesthetic ear drop product (ametocaine and phenazone). The results indicated that the two treatments reduced pain to an equivalent extent. However, due to the strong placebo response in pain conditions, this study would have needed a placebo group to provide truly dependable evidence that the herb is effective.

Note: While herbal ear products may reduce pain, it is somewhat unlikely that they have any actual effect on the infection due to the barrier formed by the eardrum.

Dosage

To make mullein tea, add 1 to 2 teaspoons of dried leaves and flowers to 1 cup of boiling water and steep for 10 minutes. Make sure to strain the tea before drinking it because fuzzy bits of the herb can stick in your throat and cause an irritating tickle. You can also breathe the steam from a boiling pot of mullein tea.

Note: Mullein seeds contain the potentially toxic substance rotenone (see Safety Issues). For this reason, it is advisable to make sure there are no seeds in the mullein flowers that you use; or, alternatively, you can use only mullein leaf.

For ear infection pain, mullein oil products are brought to room temperature and dripped into the ear canal. However, it is advisable to make sure the eardrum isn't punctured before instilling mullein oil into the ear.

Safety Issues

Mullein leaves and flowers are on the FDA's GRAS (generally recognized as safe) list and there have been no credible reports of serious adverse effects. However, mullein seeds contain the insecticide and fish poison rotenone. While rotenone is relatively safe in humans, it does present some toxic risks. If mullein leaf products are contaminated with mullein seeds, long-term use might be harmful.

For this reason, as well as a complete lack of formal safety investigation of mullein, young children, pregnant or nursing women, or those with severe liver or kidney disease should not use mullein for a prolonged period of time.

N-Acetyl Cysteine

SUPPLEMENT FORMS/ALTERNATE NAMES: NAC

PRINCIPAL PROPOSED USES: *Angina Pectoris (in Combination with Conventional Treatment), Chronic Bronchitis, Female Infertility, Preventing Influenza*

OTHER PROPOSED USES: *Chemotherapy Support, Chronic Blepharitis, Colon Cancer Prevention, HIV Support, Liver Failure, Protection Against Kidney Damage Caused by Contrast Agents, Sjogren's Syndrome*

N-acetyl cysteine (NAC) is a specially modified form of the dietary amino acid cysteine. When taken orally, NAC is thought to help the body make the important **antioxidant** enzyme glutathione. It has shown promise for a number of conditions, especially chronic bronchitis.

Sources

There is no daily requirement for NAC and it is not found in food.

Therapeutic Dosages

Optimal levels of NAC have not been determined. The amount used in studies has varied from 250 to 1,500 mg daily.

It has been suggested that NAC may increase excretion of trace minerals; some evidence, however, suggests that this effect is too minimal to make a real difference. Prudence suggests that individuals taking NAC for an extended period of time should also consider taking a standard multivitamin/multimineral supplement.

Therapeutic Uses

Significant but not entirely consistent evidence suggests that regular use of NAC is helpful for individuals with **chronic bronchitis** (a condition commonly associated with smoking and emphysema) in reducing frequency of acute flare-ups of the condition.

Regular use of NAC may help prevent **influenza**, possibly by stimulating immunity.

One substantial study found that NAC can augment the effectiveness of clomiphene, a drug used for **female infertility**.

Mixed evidence suggests that NAC may enhance the effectiveness of the drug nitroglycerin, used for the treatment of **angina**. However, severe headaches may develop as a side effect.

NAC may be helpful in a life-threatening condition called *acute respiratory distress syndrome*. Very high dosages of NAC are used in hospitals as a conventional treatment for acetaminophen poisoning.

Note: Do not attempt to self-treat angina, acute respiratory distress syndrome, or acetaminophen poisoning! Medical supervision is absolutely essential because of the very real risk of death in these conditions.

In order to get more information from certain types of x-rays, radiologists often administer substances called *contrast agents*. Unfortunately, contrast agents can damage the kidney. Growing evidence indicates that NAC can help protect the kidney from such damage.

Some research has also suggested that NAC may be helpful for **Sjogren's syndrome** (a disease that causes dry eyes, among other symptoms), **chronic blepharitis** (ongoing infections of the eyelid), severe liver disease, and reducing the side effects of the **cancer chemotherapy** drug ifosfamide. Other evidence hints that NAC might help offset the carcinogenic effects of **smoking** and reduce colon **cancer** risk.

NAC has been proposed as supportive therapy for **HIV**, but despite some intriguing results, overall the evidence is inconsistent at best.

One double-blind trial failed to find NAC helpful for head and neck or lung cancer. Studies have also failed to find NAC helpful for treating **viral hepatitis**, **preeclampsia**, or **enhancing sports performance**.

What Is the Scientific Evidence for N-Acetyl Cysteine?

Chronic Bronchitis

Individuals who have smoked cigarettes for many years eventually develop deterioration in their lungs leading to various symptoms, including chronic production of thick mucus. This so-called chronic bronchitis (closely related to **chronic obstructive pulmonary disease**) tends to flare up periodically into severe acute attacks possibly requiring hospitalization.

Regular use of NAC may diminish the number of these attacks. A review and meta-analysis selected 8 double-blind, placebo-controlled trials of NAC for chronic bronchitis. The results of these studies, involving a total of about 1,400 individuals, suggest that NAC taken daily at a dose of 400 to 1,200 mg can reduce the number of acute attacks of severe bronchitis. However, the largest and best of these studies, a 3-year, double-blind, placebo-controlled trial of 523 people, failed to find that use of NAC at a dose of 600 mg daily reduced exacerbations or retarded the typical progressive worsening of lung function.

It is not clear how NAC works (if it does); the old concept that it acts by thinning mucus may not be correct.

Influenza

In a double-blind, placebo-controlled study of 262 seniors, regular use of NAC at a dose of 600 mg twice daily helped prevent the development of influenza-like illnesses. Over the 6-month study period, only 25% of participants taking NAC developed flu-like symptoms, as compared to 79% in the placebo group, a statistically significant difference.

Interestingly, blood tests suggested that NAC did not prevent influenza infection—about as many people showed antibodies indicating influenza infection in the NAC group as in the placebo group. Rather, the supplement seemed to reduce the rate at which influenza infection became severe enough to cause noticeable symptoms. Tests of immune function hinted that NAC functioned by increasing the strength of the immune response.

Angina Pectoris

Angina pectoris is a squeezing feeling in the chest caused by inadequate blood supply to the heart. It can be a precursor of heart attacks. People with angina often use the drug nitroglycerin to relieve symptoms. One 4-month, double-blind, placebo-controlled study of 200 people with **heart disease** found that the combination of nitroglycerin and NAC significantly reduced the incidence of heart attacks and other severe heart problems. NAC alone and nitroglycerin alone were not as effective. The only problem was that the combination of nitroglycerin and NAC caused severe headaches in many participants. This effect has been seen in other studies as well.

NAC may also help in cases of nitroglycerin tolerance, a condition in which the drug becomes less effective over time. In a small double-blind study of 32 people with angina, tolerance developed in 15 of 16 individuals who took nitroglycerin only, but in just 5 of 16 individuals who took nitroglycerin plus 2 g of NAC daily. However, other studies have found no benefit.

Female Infertility

In a double-blind, placebo-controlled study of 150 women suffering from infertility who had not responded to treatment with the fertility drug clomiphene, use of NAC at 1,200 mg daily significantly augmented the effectiveness of clomiphene. Treatment was begun on day 3 of the menstrual cycle and continued for 5 days. About 20% of women in the NAC plus clomiphene group became pregnant, as compared to 0% in the placebo plus clomiphene group.

Acute Respiratory Distress Syndrome

A double-blind, placebo-controlled clinical trial compared the effectiveness of NAC, Procysteine (a synthetic cysteine building-block drug), and placebo in 46 people with acute respiratory distress syndrome. This catastrophic lung condition can occur when an unconscious person inhales a small amount of his or her own vomit. Both NAC and Procysteine reduced the severity of the condition in some people (as compared with placebo). However, overall it did not reduce the number of deaths.

Colon Cancer Prevention

A preliminary double-blind, placebo-controlled study of NAC enrolled 62 individuals, each of whom had had a polyp removed from the colon. The abnormal growth of polyps is closely associated with the development of colon cancer. In this study, the potential anticancer benefits of NAC treatment were evaluated by taking a biopsy of the rectum. Individuals taking NAC at 800 mg daily for 12 weeks showed more normal cells in the biopsied tissue as compared to those in the placebo group.

Safety Issues

NAC appears to be a very safe supplement when taken alone, although one study in rats suggests that 60 to 100 times the normal dose can cause liver injury.

As mentioned above, the combination of nitroglycerin and NAC can cause severe headaches. Safety in young children, women who are pregnant or nursing, and individuals with severe liver or kidney disease has not been established.

Interactions You Should Know About

If you are taking **nitroglycerin**: NAC may cause severe headaches.

Neem

Azadirachta indica

PRINCIPAL PROPOSED USES: *None*

OTHER PROPOSED USES: *Fevers, Respiratory Diseases, Skin Diseases*

The neem tree has been called *the village pharmacy* because its bark, leaves, sap, fruit, seeds, and twigs have so many diverse uses in the traditional medicine of India. This member of the mahogany family has been used medicinally for at least 4,000 years and is held in such esteem that Indian poets called it *Sarva Roga Nivarini*, "The One That Can Cure All Ailments." Mohandas Gandhi encouraged scientific investigation of the neem tree as part of his program to revitalize Indian traditions, eventually leading to more than 2,000 research papers and intense commercial interest.

At least 50 patents have been filed on neem and neem-based products are licensed in the United States for control of insects in food and ornamental crops. However, the Indian government and many nongovernmental organizations have united to overthrow some patents of this type, which they regard as "folk-wisdom piracy." One fear is that if neem is patented, indigenous people who already use it will lose the right to continue to do so. Another point is the fundamental question: Who owns the genetic diversity of plants? The nations where the plants come from or the transnational corpo-

rations that pay for the research into those plants? Although this area of international law is rapidly evolving, a patent on the spice turmeric has already been overturned and neem may follow soon.

At least 100 bioactive substances have been found in neem, including nimbidin, azadiracthins, and other triterpenoids and limonoids. Although the scientific evidence for all of neem's uses in health care remains preliminary, the intense interest in the plant will eventually lead to proper double-blind, placebo-controlled trials.

What Is Neem Used for Today?

The uses of neem are remarkably diverse. In India, the sap is used for treating fevers, general debilitation, digestive disturbances, and skin diseases; the bark gum for respiratory diseases and other infections; the leaves for digestive problems, intestinal parasites, and viral infections; the fruit for debilitation, malaria, skin diseases, and intestinal parasites; and the seed and kernel oil for diabetes, fevers, fungal infections, bacterial infections, inflammatory diseases, fertility prevention, and as an insecticide. However, there is no reliable research evidence to support any of these uses.

As with many plant products, test-tube studies indicate that, on direct contact, neem can kill or inhibit the growth of bacteria, fungi and viruses. This does not mean, however, that neem acts as a systemic antibiotic if it is taken by mouth. Neem mouthwash or chewing gum might be helpful for preventing cavities because it can directly come in contact with cavity-causing bacteria, but this has not been proven.

On the basis of extremely preliminary evidence, neem has also been advocated as a treatment for **diabetes**.

Dosage

Because of the numerous parts of the neem tree used and the many different ways these can be prepared, the only advice we can give at this time is to follow the directions on the label of the neem product you purchase.

Safety Issues

Based on its extensive traditional use, neem seems to be quite safe. However, formal safety testing has only involved neem oil, the insecticide product made from the plant. While neem has been found adequately safe for use as an insecticide, animal studies suggest that long-term oral use of neem oil might produce toxic effects.

In addition, other animal studies suggest that whole neem extract (which includes more substances than neem oil) may damage chromosomes, at least when taken in high doses or for an extended period of time.

For all these reasons, as well as the lack of comprehensive safety investigation of neem products other than neem oil, we recommend that young children, pregnant or nursing women, or individuals with severe liver or kidney disease avoid use of neem.

Nettle

Urtica dioica

PRINCIPAL PROPOSED USES: *Allergies (Nettle Leaf), Benign Prostatic Hyperplasia (Nettle Root)*

Anyone who lives in a locale where nettle grows wild will eventually discover the powers of this dark green plant. Depending on the species, the fine hairs on its leaves and stem cause burning pain that lasts from hours to weeks. But this well-protected herb has also been used as medicine. Nettle juice was used in Hippocrates' time to treat bites and stings and European herbalists recommended nettle tea for lung disorders. Nettle tea was used by Native Americans as an aid in pregnancy, childbirth, and nursing.

What Is Nettle Used for Today?

Currently, nettle *root* is more commonly used medicinally than the above-ground portion of the herb. In Europe, nettle root is widely used for the treatment of **benign prostatic hyperplasia (BPH)**, or prostate enlargement. Like saw palmetto, pygeum, and beta-sitosterol, nettle appears to reduce obstruction to urinary flow and decrease the need for nighttime urination. However, the evidence is not as strong for nettle as it is for these other treatments.

Note: Before self-treating prostate symptoms with nettle root, be sure to get a proper medical evaluation to rule out prostate cancer.

Nettle leaf has become a popular treatment for **allergies** (hay fever) based on one preliminary double-blind study.

Nettle leaf is highly nutritious and in cooked form may be used as a general dietary supplement.

What Is the Scientific Evidence for Nettle?

The evidence is much better for nettle root and prostatic enlargement than for nettle leaf and allergies.

Nettle Root
Nettle root as a treatment for benign prostatic hyperplasia has not been as well studied as **saw palmetto**, but the evidence is still substantial.

In a double-blind, placebo-controlled study performed in Iran, 558 people were given either placebo or nettle root for 6 months. The results indicated that nettle root is significantly more effective than placebo on all major measures of BPH severity. Benefits were seen in three other double-blind studies as well, enrolling a total of more than 150 men.

There are theoretical reasons to believe that nettle root's effectiveness might be enhanced when it is combined with another herb used for prostate problems: **pygeum**. Nettle has also been studied in combination with saw palmetto, with mixed results.

Nettle root contains numerous biologically active chemicals that may influence the prostate indirectly by interacting with sex hormones or directly by altering the properties of prostate cells.

Nettle Leaf

One preliminary double-blind, placebo-controlled study following 69 people suggests that freeze-dried nettle leaf may at least slightly improve allergy symptoms.

One small double-blind study suggests that direct application of stinging nettle leaf to a painful joint may improve symptoms.

Dosage

Dosages of nettle root extract vary according to preparation and we recommend following label instructions. Some nettle root products are standardized to their content of the substance scopoletin, but since this substance is not established as an active ingredient, the significance of this standardization remains unclear.

For allergies, the studied dosage is 300 mg twice a day of freeze-dried nettle leaf.

Safety Issues

Because nettle leaf has a long history of food use, it is believed to be safe.

Nettle root does not have as extensive a history to go by. Although detailed safety studies have not been reported, no significant adverse effects have been noted in Germany where nettle root is widely used. In practice, it is nearly side-effect free. In one study of 4,087 people who took 600 to 1,200 mg of nettle root daily for 6 months, fewer than 1% reported mild gastrointestinal distress and only 0.19% experienced allergic reactions (skin rash).

For theoretical reasons, there are some concerns that nettle may interact with diabetes, blood pressure, anti-inflammatory, and sedative medications, although there are no reports of any problems occurring.

The safety of nettle root or leaf for pregnant or nursing mothers has not been established and there are concerns based on animal studies and its traditional use for inducing abortions. However, nettle leaf tea is a traditional drink for pregnant and nursing women.

Interactions You Should Know About

If you are taking **anti-inflammatory, antihypertensive, sedative**, or **blood sugar–lowering medications**: Nettle might conceivably interact with them, although this is unlikely.

Nicotinamide Adenine Dinucleotide

SUPPLEMENT FORMS/ALTERNATE NAMES: *NADH*

PRINCIPAL PROPOSED USES: *Jet Lag*

OTHER PROPOSED USES: *Alzheimer's Disease, Chronic Fatigue Syndrome, Depression, Parkinson's Disease, Sports Performance Enhancement*

NADH, short for *nicotinamide adenine dinucleotide*, is an important cofactor, or "assistant," that helps enzymes in the work they do throughout the body. NADH particularly plays a role in the production of en-

ergy. It also participates in the production of L-dopa, which the body turns into the important neurotransmitter dopamine.

Based on these basic biochemical facts, NADH has

been evaluated as a treatment for jet lag, Alzheimer's disease, Parkinson's disease, chronic fatigue syndrome, and depression and as a sports supplement. However, only the first of these uses has any meaningful scientific evidence behind it, and even that is highly preliminary.

Sources

Healthy bodies make all the NADH they need, using **vitamin B₃** (also known as niacin, or nicotinamide) as a starting point. The highest concentration of NADH in animals is found in muscle tissues, which means that meat might be a good source—were it not that most of the NADH in meat is destroyed during processing, cooking, and digestion. In reality, we don't get much NADH from our food.

Therapeutic Dosages

The typical dosage for supplemental NADH ranges from 5 to 50 mg daily, often taken sublingually (under the tongue). Products said to be "stabilized" are available.

Therapeutic Uses

Two small double-blind, placebo-controlled trials suggest that NADH may be useful for enhancing mental function under conditions of inadequate sleep, such as **jet lag**.

Supplemental NADH has also been proposed as a treatment for **Alzheimer's disease**, **chronic fatigue syndrome**, **depression**, and **Parkinson's disease**. Additionally, it has additionally been tried as a sports performance enhancer. However, although a few studies have been performed to evaluate these potential uses, none were designed in such a way as to produce scientifically meaningful results.

What Is the Scientific Evidence for Nicotinamide Adenine Dinucleotide?

In a double-blind, placebo-controlled trial, 35 individuals taking an overnight flight across four time zones were given either 20 mg of NADH or placebo sublingually (under the tongue) on the morning of arrival. Participants were twice given tests of wakefulness and mental function: first at 90 minutes and then at 5 hours after landing. Individuals given NADH scored significantly better on these tests than those given placebo.

The only other supporting evidence comes from an unpublished double-blind, placebo-controlled, crossover study funded by the makers of an NADH product. In this study, 25 people were kept awake all night and their cognitive function was tested the following day. People given NADH performed significantly better on various measures of mental function than those given placebo. NADH did not, however, reduce daytime sleepiness or enhance mood.

These small but promising studies suggest a need for further research.

Safety Issues

NADH appears to be quite safe when taken at a dosage of 5 mg daily or less. However, formal safety studies have not been completed, and safety in young children, pregnant or nursing women, or those with severe liver or kidney disease has not been established.

Noni

Morinda citrifolia

PRINCIPAL PROPOSED USES: *None*

OTHER PROPOSED USES: *Too Numerous to List*

Morinda citrifolia, also known as noni or Indian mulberry, is a small evergreen shrub or tree of the plant family Rubiaceae. Native to the Pacific islands, Polynesia, Asia, and Australia, it grows up to 10 feet high. The leaves are 8 or more inches long, dark green, oval shaped, and shiny, with deep veins. The flower heads are about an inch long and bear many small white flowers. These heads grow to become the mature fruit, 3 to 4 inches in diameter with a warty, pitted surface. Noni fruit starts out green, turns yellow with ripening, and has a foul odor, especially as it ripens to whiteness and falls to the ground.

Some cultures may eat noni fruit in times of scarcity (the unripened fruit is less noxious). Traditional Polynesian healers have apparently used the fruit for many purposes, including bowel disorders (constipation and diarrhea), skin inflammation, infection, mouth sores, fever, contusions, and sprains—but it is said that only sick and desperate people will take it due to its unpleasant odor and bitter taste. However, the primary indigenous use of this plant appears to be of the leaves, as a topical treatment for wound healing.

In Chinese medicine, the root of *M. officinalis* is also a standard medication (known as *bai ji tian* or *pa chi tien*) used for the digestive system, kidneys, heart, and liver.

Other traditional uses for the plant include making a red dye from the bark and a yellow dye from the root.

What Is Noni Used for Today?

Noni has been heavily promoted for an enormous range of uses, including abrasions, arthritis, atherosclerosis, bladder infections, boils, bowel disorders, burns, cancer, chronic fatigue syndrome, circulatory weakness, colds, cold sores, congestion, constipation, diabetes, drug addiction, eye inflammations, fever, fractures, gastric ulcers, gingivitis, headaches, heart disease, hypertension, improved digestion, immune weakness, indigestion, intestinal parasites, kidney disease, malaria, menstrual cramps, menstrual irregularities, mouth sores, respiratory disorders, ringworm, sinusitis, skin inflammation, sprains, stroke, thrush, and wounds. However, there is no real evidence that it is effective for any of these conditions.

Several animal studies have evaluated the effects of extracts derived from noni. The results suggest noni may have anti-cancer, immune-enhancing, and pain-relieving properties. However, most of these studies used unrealistically high doses that would be difficult to get from taking the juice itself. There have been no meaningful human trials of noni.

Dosage

Commercial products that contain noni juice or a juice concentrate are widely available and heavily promoted. These preparations have either eliminated the odor or altered the taste to make it more palatable. Tablets and capsules of the fruit and of the whole plant are also available.

The usual recommendation is the equivalent of 4 ounces of noni juice 30 minutes before breakfast. The typical recommendation is 2 tablespoons daily for liquid concentrates or 500 to 1,000 mg daily for powdered extracts.

According to noni promoters, it should be taken on an empty stomach and not together with coffee, tobacco, or alcohol. However, there is no scientific evidence for this recommendation.

Safety Issues

Although use of noni is not commonly associated with side effects, comprehensive safety studies have not been performed. A small number of case reports indicate that in rare cases use of noni might cause severe liver damage, potentially leading to a need for liver transplant. For this reason, people with liver disease, or who take medications that can harm the liver, or who consume alcohol to excess should not use noni. Due to the lack of evidence, use of noni by pregnant or nursing women is not recommended.

Nopal
Opuntia spp

ALTERNATE NAMES/RELATED TERMS: *Prickly Pear Cactus*
PRINCIPAL PROPOSED USES: *Diabetes, Hangover from Use of Alcohol*
OTHER PROPOSED USES: *High Cholesterol, Prostate Enlargement*

The nopal, or prickly-pear cactus, is one of the major national symbols of Mexico and appears on the Mexican flag.

This cactus has a long history of use as food and medicine. Its fleshy, leaf-like stems (*cladodes*), especially when young, are eaten as vegetables. The fruit is eaten raw, fermented into a beer, or turned into a cheese-like food. Medicinally, nopal fruit, stems, and flowers have been used to treat diabetes, stomach problems, fatigue, shortness of breath, easy bruising, prostate enlargement, and liver disease. Nopal is also a significant source of protein, vitamins, and minerals.

What Is Nopal Used for Today?

Although the results of animal studies and highly preliminary trials in humans are somewhat contradictory, taken together they suggest that nopal fruit and stems might have some benefit for **diabetes**. However, only properly designed and sufficiently large double-blind, placebo-controlled trials can tell us for sure whether nopal is effective, and none have been reported for this use of nopal.

The only properly designed study of nopal involved use of the cactus for treating hangover symptoms. In this double-blind, placebo-controlled study of 64 people, use of an extract made from the skin of nopal fruit significantly reduced hangover symptoms as compared to placebo. The greatest improvements were seen in symptoms of nausea, loss of appetite, and dry mouth. Overall, the rate of severe hangover symptoms was 50% lower in the treatment group as compared to the placebo group. The researchers involved in this study hypothesized that hangovers are caused by inflammation and that the herb reduced inflammation.

There is weak evidence that nopal fruit and stems might be helpful for reducing cholesterol levels. Other studies suggest that nopal stems and fruit might have anti-inflammatory, pain-relieving, and stomach-protective effects. Finally, test-tube studies suggest that the flower of the nopal cactus might be helpful for prostate enlargement (BPH).

Dosage

Neither the optimum dosage nor the most active species of nopal cactus has been established. The one double-blind study noted above used a special extract made from the skin of the fruit of *Opuntia ficus indica*.

Safety Issues

As a widely eaten food, nopal is presumed safe. However, safety in young children, pregnant or nursing women, or individuals with severe liver or kidney disease has not been established.

Nutritional Support (General)

SUPPLEMENT FORMS/ALTERNATE NAMES: *Vitamins and Minerals (General)*

PRINCIPAL PROPOSED USES: *Correct Nutrient Deficiencies*

OTHER PROPOSED USES: *Enhancing Mental Function, Female Infertility, Immune Support, Morning Sickness, Premenstrual Syndrome (PMS), Stress*

There are two main ways to use vitamins and mineral supplements: "megadose" and nutritional therapy.

The megadose approach involves taking supplements at doses far above nutritional needs in hopes of producing a specific medical benefit. This technique essentially uses nutrients as natural drugs. The individual supplement articles in this encyclopedia explain what is known about the potential risks and benefits of megadose therapy.

This article addresses the second approach: taking nutrients at the level of nutritional needs. We discuss general issues regarding such "nutritional insurance" and indicate which nutrients you should consider taking on a daily basis.

Requirements/Sources

There is no doubt that it's important to get enough of all necessary nutrients. However, the process of determining proper daily intake levels for vitamins and minerals is far from an exact science and the recommendations issued by experts in various countries often disagree to a certain extent.

In general, while it is fairly easy to determine the minimum nutrient intakes that are necessary to avoid frank malnutrition, there's no straightforward way to determine optimum intake levels. Furthermore, individual needs undoubtedly vary based on numerous factors, including age, genetics, lifestyle, other foods in the diet and many additional environmental influences; no schedule of official recommendations could possibly take all these factors into account, even if all the necessary data existed (which it doesn't).

Thus, all recommendations for daily nutrient intake must be regarded as approximate. The individual supplement articles in this encyclopedia summarize the current U.S. recommendations.

Common Nutritional Deficiencies

Severe deficiencies of vitamins or minerals are rare in the developed world. However, evidence suggests that slight deficiencies in certain nutrients may be relatively common. These include **calcium**, **chromium**, **folate**, **magnesium**, **vitamin B$_6$**, **vitamin C**, **vitamin B$_{12}$** (primarily in the elderly), **vitamin D**, **vitamin E**, and **zinc**.

While few people are so deficient in these nutrients to show symptoms of outright malnutrition, subtle deficiencies may increase the risk of a number of diseases. For example, insufficient intake of calcium and vitamin D may increase your chances of developing osteoporosis and inadequate folate and vitamin B$_6$ may speed the development of heart disease.

Thus, taking supplements to supply these important vitamins and minerals as a form of insurance may be a good idea. For standard dosage recommendations as well as safety issues, follow the links above to the full articles.

Besides vitamins and minerals, intake of essential fatty acids may be commonly inadequate. For more information, see the articles on **omega-6** and **omega-3 fatty acids**.

Women may develop **iron** deficiency, but men hardly ever do. Even in women, iron supplements are not beneficial in the absence of true deficiency. We recommend avoiding iron supplements unless tests show that you really need them.

Multivitamin/Mineral Supplements

The simplest way to support your nutrition is to take a general **multivitamin and mineral supplement** providing a broad range of nutrients at standard nutritional levels. However, there are a few caveats to keep in mind.

➤ **Some supplements include very high doses of certain nutrients, such as antioxidants. As described above, when you take nutrients in this fashion, you** are using them as drugs rather than nutrients; you are no longer in the world of nutritional supplementation and have passed into the riskier world of megadose treatment.

> We recommend that you use an iron-free multivitamin and mineral supplement unless you have been tested and found to be deficient in iron.

> The minerals calcium and magnesium are very bulky and few multivitamin/mineral supplements provide the daily requirement. These minerals generally must be taken in the form of additional pills. Note: It isn't possible for your body to absorb a day's worth of calcium in a single dose. At least two doses are necessary.

> Finally, note that food may contain many nonessential substances such as carotenoids and bioflavonoids that nonetheless enhance health. For this reason, no nutrient supplement should be regarded as a substitute for a healthy and varied diet.

Taking Individual Supplements

One problem with multivitamin/mineral supplements is that some nutrients may interfere with the absorption of others. For this reason, there may be advantages to taking supplements separately. (The hassle factor is a strong disadvantage!) In addition, this method allows one to avoid taking vitamins and minerals one doesn't need.

If you do use this approach, keep in mind the following:

> Minerals come in many different chemical forms, technically called *salts*. For example, you can purchase calcium as calcium carbonate, calcium citrate, calcium orotate, and in half a dozen or more other forms. In some cases, certain salts of minerals are known to be better absorbed than others. This is particularly the case with calcium, as described in the full article.

> When you take zinc, you should balance it with copper.

> There may be advantages to taking certain nutrients at levels a bit higher than the standard recommendations, but each nutrient presents its own issues. More is not necessarily better. See each individual nutrient article for details.

Natural versus Synthetic Vitamins

Many people wonder whether "natural" vitamins are better than "synthetic" ones. This question, however, is a bit of a red herring. Ultimately, no vitamin or mineral

supplement is "natural." Purified vitamins and minerals are refined, processed products analogous to white sugar or artificial fertilizer. It doesn't much matter whether they are extracted from foods or manufactured in a laboratory: the result is the same. For example, vitamin C made from rose hips is chemically identical to vitamin C synthesized from scratch. Both are ascorbic acid.

Rose hips themselves, however, supply many nutrients along with vitamin C. If you truly wish to get your vitamins naturally, you might consider taking them as freeze-dried or condensed whole food supplements rather than as purified vitamins. This might offer a specific advantage over purified vitamins: as we noted above, fruits and vegetables may provide substances that are not actually essential but that promote better health.

Therapeutic Uses

Under certain conditions, the need for many nutrients may increase. These include illnesses such as **diabetes**, **Crohn's disease**, **HIV**, and **ulcerative colitis**. Furthermore, individuals who **smoke cigarettes** or overuse **alcohol** may need additional nutrients.

Medications may increase the need for certain nutrients; if you look up your own medications in the **Drug Interaction** section of this book, you will find what is known about these so-called nutrient depletions.

Other potential uses of multivitamins generally lack strong support.

Some but not all studies suggest that multivitamin/multimineral supplements can **enhance mental function**. However, serious allegations of fraud have been raised regarding the work of one of the scientists involved in research on this and other uses of multivitamin/multimineral supplements.

Evidence is mixed on whether use of multivitamin/multimineral supplements may help prevent infections in seniors. Other studies have found evidence that supplementation with selenium, zinc, and copper may help prevent respiratory infections among people with diabetes and people suffering from severe burns.

Two studies found that multivitamin/multimineral tablets strengthen immune response to vaccines. Another study found a related effect: enhancement of immune response to skin testing. However, one well-designed study failed to find benefit and, in another, use of multivitamins *without* minerals actually impaired the immune response to vaccination.

Incomplete, and in some cases contradictory, evidence suggests that use of multivitamin and/or multimineral supplements may reduce antisocial behavior in children and young adults (especially those who are malnourished), prevent bedsores, lower **blood pressure**, improve **fertility in women**, improve **general well-being**, enhance growth in children, speed healing of **minor wounds**, reduce the pain of **osteoarthritis**, reduce **pregnancy-related nausea** ("morning sickness"), decrease symptoms of **premenstrual stress syndrome** (PMS) and ordinary **stress**, and reduce risk of prostate **cancer**.

Safety Issues

Standard multivitamin/multimineral tablets contain nutrients at levels believed to be safe for the majority of healthy people, as indicated by amounts at or below the recommended daily allowance. However, even these supplements could be harmful for people with certain diseases, such as kidney or liver disease, or for people taking certain medications, such as **warfarin** (Coumadin).

There are other multivitamin/multimineral tablets that contain high levels of certain nutrients far above nutritional needs. These could conceivably present risks for healthy people, particularly if they are taken in combination with additional specific supplements. Almost any mineral can be toxic if taken to excess, and there are also risks with excessive intake of vitamins A, B_6, and D.

One study found that use of multivitamin/mineral supplements may actually *increase* the infectivity of women with HIV. The reasons for this are unclear.

Nutrition Supplements: Vitamins, Minerals, and Non-Nutrient Supplements

SUPPLEMENT FORMS/ALTERNATE NAMES: *Supplements*

One of the great medical discoveries of the last century involved the identification of the nutritional substances necessary for life. Along with the *macronutrients* (fat, carbohydrate, and protein), these *micronutrients* make up the essential ingredients of a healthful diet.

Vitamins and minerals have been available as supplements since at least the 1930s. In the 1960s, however, a new way of using them came into vogue: so-called megadose therapy. The megadose approach involves taking supplements at doses far above nutrition needs in the hopes of producing a specific medical benefit—essentially, using nutrients as natural drugs. Each individual supplement article in the Collins Alternative Health Guide explains what is known about the potential risks and benefits of megadose therapy.

The original (and still important) method of using nutrients involves taking them at around the level of nutrition needs. This method may be considered nutrition insurance for the majority of us who don't get all the nutrients we need from foods. For information on which nutrients may be worth taking on a daily basis, see the **Nutritional Support (General)** article.

Finally, there are a number of substances sold as supplements that are not, in fact, nutritional in nature. While they might offer health benefits, you don't need them to stay alive. Examples include the following:

➤ **Isoflavones—Chemicals found in soy that may reduce the risk of cancer and some forms of heart disease**
➤ **Glucosamine—A substance found in gristle that's useful for osteoarthritis**
➤ **Melatonin—A hormone not found to any great extent in foods, but that is helpful for sleep**

These substances are also described in the individual supplement articles in the Collins Alternative Health Guide.

Specific Supplements

The Collins Alternative Health Guide has articles on all major supplements. For detailed information, see the herb and supplement index page.

Oak Bark

Quercus spp.

PRINCIPAL PROPOSED USES: *Diarrhea*

OTHER PROPOSED USES: *Canker Sores, Eczema, Hemorrhoids, Sore Throat*

The oak tree, respected for millennia as a source of strong, dense wood, also has a considerable tradition of medicinal use. The astringent, tannin-rich bark of the oak tree has been recommended for such diverse conditions as internal hemorrhage, diarrhea, dysentery, cancer, and pneumonia.

What Is Oak Bark Used for Today?

Currently, Germany's Commission E recommends oak bark internally for treatment of **diarrhea** and topically for **sore throat**, **mouth sores**, **hemorrhoids**, and **eczema**. However, there is no meaningful scientific evidence that oak bark offers any therapeutic benefit in these or any other conditions. Only double-blind, placebo-controlled studies can prove a treatment effective and none have been performed on oak bark. (For more information on why such studies are essential, see **Why Does This Book Rely on Double-blind Studies?**)

Oak bark contains numerous substances in the tannin family, especially ellagitannin, along with potentially active substances in the saponin family. Tannins are thought to have an astringent effect, meaning that they reduce tissue swelling and stop bleeding, and they are traditionally thought to be useful for diarrhea. However, oak bark has never been studied as a treatment for diarrhea. Saponins are often said to act as expectorants, enhancing the ability to cough up phlegm.

Again, however, there is no direct evidence that oak bark is useful for coughs or related conditions.

Very weak evidence (too weak to be relied upon at all) hints that oak bark may have value for **kidney stones**, possibly reducing pain and slowing stone growth. In addition, test-tube studies indicate that oak bark solutions applied topically might have activity against various microorganisms, including staphylococcus, and might also exert **cancer-preventive effects**. However, it is a long way from such studies to actual evidence of clinical benefit.

Dosage

A typical oral dose of oak bark is 1 g 3 times daily. For application as a treatment for eczema, an oak bark tea is made by boiling 1 to 2 tablespoons of the bark for 20 minutes in 2 cups of water and this is applied to the rash 3 to 5 times daily. Oak tinctures and extracts should be used according to label instructions.

Safety Issues

Although comprehensive safety testing has not been performed, use of oak bark is not generally associated with any side effects other than the occasional digestive upset or allergic reaction. Safety in young children, pregnant or nursing women, or people with severe liver or kidney disease has not been established.

Oat Straw

Avena sativa

ALTERNATE NAMES/RELATED TERMS: *Green Oats, Oat Straw, Wild Oat Extract*

PRINCIPAL PROPOSED USES: *None*

OTHER PROPOSED USES:

    Oat Straw Alone: *Enhancing Male Sexual Function, Stop-smoking Aid*

    In Combination with Saw Palmetto: *Benign Prostatic Hypertrophy (Prostate Enlargement), Enhancing Female Sexual Function*

When the oat plant matures, it produces a fruit that becomes the grain *oats*, a heart-healthy, high-fiber food. This article does not address this form of oat. Rather, it describes products made from the green, unripe oat straw, sold under the names *Avena sativa*, green oats, and wild oat extract.

Traditionally, oat straw was considered a mild *nervine*, an herb thought to calm and heal nervous symptoms. On this basis, it was used to treat insomnia, stress, anxiety, and nervousness. In addition, oat straw tea was used for arthritis, and an alcohol extract of oat straw for the treatment of narcotic and cigarette addiction. However, there is no evidence that it is effective when used for any of these purposes.

What Is Oat Straw Used for Today?

Oat straw is widely marketed for enhancing **male sexual function**, and a combination of oat straw and **saw palmetto** is said to help **sexual dysfunction in women**. The same combination is supposedly helpful for **enlargement of the prostate**. However, the only evidence for these claims comes from unpublished studies conducted by the manufacturer of oat straw products. Because these studies are not available in full, it is not possible to judge their validity.

For example, one double-blind, placebo-controlled trial of 75 men and women reportedly found that use of an oat straw product enhanced sexual experience for men but not for women. Unfortunately, it is not clear whether the results were statistically significant or exactly how the researchers arrived at their conclusions.

Another study discussed on the same web page supposedly found that oat straw combined with saw palmetto produced similar benefits for women, but it is not clear whether this trial was double-blind.

It has been claimed that oat straw works by increasing the amount of free testosterone in the blood. Many oat straw websites state that, with advancing age, testosterone in the body tends to become bound up and inactivated, that this leads to numerous problems including failing sexual function, and that oat straw reverses this process. However, none of the parts of this argument are fully substantiated: the argument is speculation piled on speculation.

Oat straw has also been advocated as a stop-smoking treatment. However, despite promising results in one rather informal study, reported in a letter to the journal *Nature* in 1971, the balance of the evidence suggests that alcohol tincture of wild oats is *not* helpful for **quitting smoking**.

Dosage

Oat straw extract should be taken according to the manufacturer's directions. Alcohol tincture of oat straw is typically used at a dose of 1/2 to 1 teaspoon 3 times per day.

Safety Issues

There are no known or suspected health risks with oat straw. However, comprehensive safety studies have not been reported.

Oligomeric Proanthocyanidins

SUPPLEMENT FORMS/ALTERNATE NAMES: *Grape Seed Extract, OPCs, Pine Bark Extract, Procyanidolic Oligomers (PCOs), Pycnogenol*

PRINCIPAL PROPOSED USES: *Easy Bruising, Edema (Swelling) Following Injury or Surgery, Traveler's Thrombosis (Blood Clots after Long Plane Travel), Varicose Veins, Weight Loss*

OTHER PROPOSED USES: *Aging Skin, Allergies, Asthma, Atherosclerosis Prevention, Cancer Prevention, Diabetes (Blood Sugar Control), Diabetic Neuropathy and Retinopathy, Hemorrhoids, Hypertension, Impaired Night Vision, Impotence, Liver Cirrhosis, Lupus, Periodontal Disease, Premenstrual Syndrome (PMS)*

One of the bestselling herbal products of the early 1990s was an extract of the bark of French maritime pine. This substance consists of a family of chemicals known scientifically as oligomeric proanthocyanidin complexes (OPCs) or procyanidolic oligomers (PCOs). Similar (but not identical) substances are also found in grape seed. The research record is complicated by the fact that certain identically named proprietary products have consisted at different times of various proportions of these related substances.

OPCs are marketed for a wide variety of uses. As yet, however, there is no solid evidence that they are effective for any medical condition.

Sources

OPCs aren't a single chemical, but a group of closely related compounds. Several food sources contain similar chemicals: red wine, cranberries, blueberries, bilberries, tea (green and black), black currant, onions, legumes, parsley, and the herb **hawthorn**. However, most OPC supplements are made from either grape seed or the bark of the maritime pine. These two OPC sources lead to products that are not necessarily identical in function, although there do seem to be many similarities. In the discussion of scientific studies below, we indicate the source of the OPCs used when it is possible to do so. In some cases, however, identifying the exact product is difficult, as both grape seed and pinebark OPCs, or their combination, have at various times been sold under the same name.

Therapeutic Dosages

For the treatment of specific medical conditions, studies have used doses of 150 to 300 mg daily. For use as a gen-

eral antioxidant, 50 mg of OPCs daily are often recommended; however, there is no evidence that this dose provides any health benefits.

Therapeutic Uses

The best-documented use of OPCs is to treat **chronic venous insufficiency**, a condition closely related to varicose veins. In both of these conditions, blood pools in the legs, causing aching, pain, heaviness, swelling, fatigue, and unsightly visible veins. Fairly good preliminary evidence suggests that OPCs from pine bark or grape seed can relieve the leg pain and swelling of chronic venous insufficiency. However, no studies have evaluated whether regular use of OPCs can make visible varicose veins disappear or prevent new ones from developing.

Other small double-blind trials suggest that OPCs may help reduce swelling caused by **injuries** or **surgery**.

Evidence from one small double-blind trial suggests that OPCs from bilberry and grape seed may reduce the general fluid retention and swelling that can occur in **premenstrual syndrome** (PMS).

One large study found some evidence that use of OPCs from pine bark might help prevent the leg blood clots that can develop on a long airplane flight.

Two preliminary studies found evidence that OPCs from pine bark, alone or with **arginine**, may be helpful for **male sexual dysfunction** (impotence).

Two small double-blind pilot studies suggest that OPCs from pine bark might help reduce **asthma** symptoms. OPCs are also often recommended for **allergies**, but an 8-week, double-blind trial of 49 individuals found no benefit with grape seed extract.

OPCs might marginally improve blood sugar control

in people with diabetes, according to a double-blind study of 77 people with type 2 diabetes.

Some evidence suggests that OPCs protect and strengthen collagen and elastin. Theoretically, this could mean that OPCs are helpful for **aging skin** and they are widely sold for this purpose, but there is as yet no direct evidence that they work.

On the basis of their use in the treatment of varicose veins, OPCs are often recommended as a treatment for **hemorrhoids** as well, but there is no direct evidence to support this use. (Hemorrhoids are varicose veins in and around the anus.)

One study suggests that while OPCs alone may not reduce levels of **cholesterol**, when taken in combination with chromium some benefits may occur.

OPCs are strong **antioxidants**. **Vitamin E** defends against fat-soluble oxidants and **vitamin C** neutralizes water-soluble ones, but OPCs are active against both types. Based on the (unproven) belief that antioxidants offer many health benefits, regular use of OPCs has been proposed as a measure to prevent **cancer**, **diabetic neuropathy and diabetic retinopathy**, and **heart disease**.

OPCs have been tried as a treatment for **impaired night vision**, **lupus** (systemic lupus erythematosus), **easy bruising**, **high blood pressure**, and **liver cirrhosis**. However, more research needs to be performed to discover whether it actually provides any benefits in these conditions.

One study failed to find OPCs significantly helpful for **weight loss**. Another failed to find OPCs helpful for reducing the side effects of **radiation therapy** for breast cancer.

What Is the Scientific Evidence for Oligomeric Proanthocyanidins?

Venous Insufficiency (Varicose Veins)

There is fairly good preliminary evidence for the use of OPCs to treat people with symptoms of venous insufficiency.

A double-blind, placebo-controlled study of 71 subjects found that grape seed OPCs, taken at a dose of 100 mg 3 times daily, significantly improved major symptoms, including heaviness, swelling, and leg discomfort. Over a period of 1 month, 75% of the participants treated with OPCs improved substantially. This result doesn't seem quite so impressive when you note that significant improvement was also seen in 41% of the placebo group; nonetheless, OPCs still did significantly better than placebo.

A 2-month, double-blind, placebo-controlled trial of 40 people with chronic venous insufficiency found that 100 mg of pine bark OPCs three times daily significantly reduced edema, pain, and the sensation of leg heaviness. A similar study of 20 individuals also found OPCs from pine bark effective.

A placebo-controlled study (blinding not stated) that enrolled 364 people with varicose veins found that treatment with grape seed OPCs produced statistically significant improvements as compared to baseline. There was a lesser response in the placebo group, but whether this difference was statistically significant was not stated.

OPCs have also been compared against other natural treatments for venous insufficiency. A double-blind study of 50 people with varicose veins of the legs found that doses of 150 mg per day of grape seed OPCs were more effective in reducing symptoms and signs than the bioflavonoid **diosmin**. Similarly, a double-blind study of 39 people found pine bark OPCs more effective than the herb **horse chestnut**.

Edema after Surgery or Injury

Breast cancer surgery often leads to swelling of the arm. A double-blind, placebo-controlled study of 63 postoperative breast cancer patients found that 600 mg of grape seed OPCs daily for 6 months reduced edema, pain, and peculiar sensations known as paresthesias. Also, in a double-blind, placebo-controlled study of 32 people who had received facial surgery, edema disappeared much faster in the group treated with grape seed OPCs.

Another 10-day, double-blind, placebo-controlled study enrolling 50 participants found that grape seed OPCs improved the rate at which edema disappeared following sports injuries.

Blood Clots after Plane Flights

It is commonly thought, though not proven, that the immobility endured during a long plane flight can lead to the development of potentially dangerous blood clots in the legs. Travelers at high risk are often recommended to take aspirin to "thin" their blood prior to flying.

One crossover study of 22 smokers found that 100 mg of OPCs had an equivalent blood thinning effect as 500 mg of aspirin. On the basis of this, a large double-blind study was performed to evaluate whether OPCs from pine bark could help reduce risk of blood clots on long airplane flights. The study followed 198 people thought to be at high risk for blood clots. Some participants were given 200 mg of OPCs 2 to 3 hours prior to the flight, 200 mg 6 hours later, and 100 mg the next day, while others received a placebo at the same schedule. The average flight length was about 8 hours. The results indicated that use of OPCs on this schedule can significantly reduce risk of blood clots.

Periodontal Disease

Inflammation of the gums (gingivitis) and plaque formation lead to periodontal disease, one of the most common causes of tooth loss. A 14-day, double-blind, placebo-controlled trial of 40 people evaluated the potential benefits of a chewing gum product containing 5 mg of OPCs from pine bark. Use of the OPC gum resulted in significant improvements in gum health and reductions in plaque formation; no similar benefits were seen in the placebo group.

Atherosclerosis

Although there are no reliable human studies, animal evidence suggests that OPCs can slow or reverse atherosclerosis. This suggests (but definitely does not prove) that OPCs might be helpful for preventing heart disease.

Safety Issues

OPCs have been extensively tested for safety and are generally considered to be essentially nontoxic. Side effects are rare, but when they do occur they are limited to occasional allergic reactions and mild digestive distress.

However, one study unexpectedly found that a combination of OPCs and vitamin C might slightly increase blood pressure in people with high blood pressure. Neither treatment alone had this effect. These results may have been a statistical fluke, but nonetheless people with hypertension should use the combination of vitamin C and OPCs only with caution.

Maximum safe dosages for young children, pregnant or nursing women, or those with severe liver or kidney disease have not been established.

OPCs may have some anticoagulant properties when taken in high doses, and therefore should be used only under medical supervision by individuals on blood-thinner drugs, such as Coumadin (warfarin), heparin, Plavix (clopidogrel), Ticlid (ticlopidine), Trental (pentoxifylline), or aspirin.

Interactions You Should Know About

If you are taking **warfarin** (Coumadin), **heparin**, **clopidogrel** (Plavix), **ticlopidine** (Ticlid), **pentoxifylline** (Trental), or **aspirin**: High doses of OPCs might cause a risk of excessive bleeding.

Olive Leaf

Olea europaea

PRINCIPAL PROPOSED USES: *None*

OTHER PROPOSED USES: *Antibiotic, Diabetes, Gout, High Blood Pressure*

What Is Olive Leaf Extract Used for Today?

Olive leaf contains a substance called *oleuropein* which breaks down in the body to another substance called *enolinate*. On websites that promote olive leaf extracts, it is stated that enolinate kills harmful bacteria, viruses, and fungi in the body, but at the same time nurtures microbes that are good for health. This remarkable claim, however, has no meaningful scientific justification.

It is true that oleuropein, enolinate, and other olive leaf constituents or their breakdown products can kill microbes in test-tube studies.

However, it is a long way from test-tube studies to evidence of efficacy in humans. Only double-blind, placebo-controlled studies can prove a treatment effective and the only study of this type reported for olive leaf was too flawed to prove anything. This small, poorly designed trial supposedly found that olive leaf extract reduces **blood pressure**. However, the study was too small and too poorly designed to produce meaningful results. The only other support for the widespread claim that olive leaf reduces blood pressure comes from test-tube and animal studies that are too preliminary to rely upon at all.

Other animal studies weakly suggest that olive leaf might help control blood sugar levels in **diabetes** and reduce symptoms of **gout**.

Dosage

Because olive leaf extracts vary widely, we recommend following label instructions.

Safety Issues

Olive leaf has not undergone comprehensive safety testing. However, based on the limited evidence available, it does not appear to commonly cause much more in the way of immediate side effects than occasional digestive distress. Safety in young children, pregnant or nursing women, or people with severe liver or kidney disease has not been established.

Oregano Oil
Origanum vulgare

PRINCIPAL PROPOSED USES: *Yeast Hypersensitivity Syndrome*
OTHER PROPOSED USES: *Colds and Flus, HIV, Intestinal Parasites*

The common food spice oregano grows wild in the mountains of Mediterranean countries. In ancient Greece, oregano or its **essential oil** was used for the treatment of wounds, snakebites, spider bites, and respiratory problems. Respiratory uses dominated the medicinal history of oregano in medieval Europe, but in the nineteenth century, physicians in the Eclectic school (a medical movement that emphasized herbal treatment) used oregano for promoting menstruation.

What Is Oregano Oil Used for Today?

In the 1990s, the concept of the **yeast hypersensitivity syndrome** (often called *systemic candidiasis*, or merely *candida*) became popular in alternative medicine circles. This theory states, in brief, that many people develop excessive levels of the yeast *Candida albicans* and subsequently experience allergic symptoms to the yeast in their body. The symptoms of this purported syndrome include common conditions, such as fatigue and headache, and a succession of anti-candidal treatments have been offered as treatment. Oregano oil is one of the more recent of these products.

It is true that oregano oil is toxic to many different types of microorganisms, including fungi and parasites.

However, the same is the case with hundreds of essential oils of herbs, not to mention vinegar, alcohol, and bleach. It is a long way from killing microorganisms in a test tube or on the surface of a block of cheese to medicinal effects in the body. Only double-blind, placebo-controlled studies in humans can prove a treatment effective and none have been performed on oregano oil.

Nonetheless, oregano oil is widely marketed as a treatment for candida. There is a related theory that many people suffer from undiagnosed intestinal parasites; oregano oil is marketed for treatment of this purported problem as well. Oregano oil is also advocated for dozens of other illnesses, ranging from **asthma** and **HIV infection** to **rheumatoid arthritis**, though without any reliable justification.

Websites selling oregano oil additionally point out that it has **antioxidant** properties. While true, this does not by itself indicate any health benefits; most major studies of antioxidants have failed to identify the specific benefits that were once seen as likely to result from supplementation with these substances.

Dosage

A typical dose of oregano oil is 100 mg 3 times daily of a product standardized to contain 55 to 65% of the presumed active ingredient carvacrol.

Safety Issues

There are no specific safety risks known to be associated with use of oregano oil products. However, in general, essential oils of herbs can be toxic when taken even in relatively small quantities. Allergic reactions are also possible.

Safety in young children, pregnant or nursing women, or people with severe liver or kidney disease has not been established.

Oregon Grape

Mahonia aquifolium, Berberis aquifolium

PRINCIPAL PROPOSED USES: *Psoriasis*

OTHER PROPOSED USES: *Acne, Athlete's Foot and Other Fungal Infections, Eczema*

The roots and bark of the shrub *Mahonia aquifolium* (also called *Oregon grape*) have traditionally been used both orally and topically to treat skin problems. They were also used for other conditions, such as gastritis, fever, hemorrhage, jaundice, gall bladder disease, and cancer. In addition, *Mahonia* was used as a bitter tonic to improve appetite.

According to some experts, *M. aquifolium* is identical to the plant named *Berberis aquifolium*, but others point to small distinctions. *Berberis vulgaris*, commonly called *barberry*, is a close relative of these herbs, but is not identical.

What Is Oregon Grape Used for Today?

Oregon grape is primarily used today as a topical treatment for **psoriasis**. Growing evidence suggests that it may help reduce symptoms, although it does not seem to be as effective for this purpose as standard medications.

Oregon grape has been proposed as a treatment for other skin diseases, such as fungal infections (for example, **athlete's foot**), **eczema**, and **acne**. However, the evidence is extremely preliminary and human trials must be conducted before we will know whether the herb is really effective for any of these conditions.

Many studies have been performed on purified berberine, a major chemical constituent of Oregon grape and other herbs such as **goldenseal**, but it is not clear whether their results apply to the whole herb. In addition, impossibly high dosages of herb would be required to duplicate the amount of berberine used in many of these studies.

What Is the Scientific Evidence for Oregon Grape?

Evidence from two double-blind, placebo-controlled studies and one comparative trial suggest that cream made from the herb Oregon grape may help reduce symptoms of psoriasis, although it does not seem to be as effective as standard medications.

In a double-blind study published in 2006, two hundred people were given either a cream containing 10% Oregon grape extract or placebo twice a day for 3 months. The results indicate that the people using Oregon grape experienced greater benefits than those in the placebo group, and the difference was statistically significant. The treatment was well tolerated, though in a few people it caused rash or burning sensation.

Benefits were also seen in a double-blind, placebo-controlled study of 82 people with psoriasis. However, the study design had a significant flaw: the treatment salve was darker in color than the placebo, possibly allowing participants to guess which was which.

Another study found that dithranol, a conventional drug used to treat psoriasis symptoms, was more effective than Oregon grape. Regrettably, the authors fail to state whether this study was double-blind. Forty-nine participants applied one treatment to their left side and the other to their right for 4 weeks. Skin biopsies were then analyzed and compared with samples taken at the beginning of the study. The physicians evaluating changes in skin tissue were unaware which treatments had been used on the samples. Greater improvements were seen in the dithranol group.

A large open study in which 443 participants with psoriasis used Oregon grape topically for 12 weeks found the herb to be helpful for 73.7% of the group. Without a placebo group, it's not possible to know whether Oregon grape was truly responsible for the improvement seen, but the trial does help to establish the herb's safety and tolerability (see Safety Issues below).

Laboratory research suggests Oregon grape has some effects at the cellular level that might be helpful in psoriasis, such as slowing the rate of abnormal cell growth and reducing inflammation.

Dosage

Topical ointments or creams containing 10% Oregon grape extract are generally applied 3 times daily to the affected areas.

Safety Issues

Oregon grape appears to be safe when used as directed. In the large open study described above, only 5 of the 443 participants reported side effects of burning, redness, and itching.

However, because Oregon grape contains berberine, which has been reported to cause uterine contractions and to increase levels of bilirubin, oral consumption of Oregon grape should be avoided by pregnant women. Safety in young children, nursing women, or people with severe liver or kidney disease has not been established.

There is an additional concern regarding the berberine content of Oregon grape. One study found that berberine impairs metabolism of the drug cyclosporine, thereby raising its levels. This could potentially cause toxicity.

Ornithine Alpha-Ketoglutarate

PRINCIPAL PROPOSED USES: *Recovery from Severe Injury*

OTHER PROPOSED USES: *Liver Cirrhosis, Sports Supplement*

Ornithine alpha-ketoglutarate (OKG) is manufactured from two amino acids, ornithine and glutamine. These amino acids are called *conditionally essential*. This means that ordinarily one does not need to consume them in food because the body can manufacture them from other nutrients. However, during periods of severe stress, such as recovery from major trauma or severe illness, the body may not be able to manufacture them in sufficient quantities and may require an external source.

Ornithine and glutamine are thought to have anabolic effects, meaning that they stimulate the body to build muscle and other tissues. These amino acids also appear to have anti-catabolic effects. This is a closely related but slightly different property; ornithine and glutamine appear to block the effect of hormones that break down muscle and other tissues (catabolic hormones).

Evidence suggests that use of OKG (and related amino acids) may offer benefits for hospitalized patients recovering from serious illness or injury.

Based on these findings (and a leap of logic), OKG has been extensively marketed as a sports supplement

for helping to build muscle. However, the fact that OKG helps seriously ill people build muscle does not mean that it will have the same effect in athletes and there is no direct evidence to indicate that it does.

Sources

The amino acids that make up OKG are found in high-protein foods such as meat, fish, and dairy products. Supplements are available in tablet or pill form.

Therapeutic Dosages

A typical dose of OKG is 5 to 25 g daily. It may be necessary to increase dosage slowly to avoid digestive upset.

Therapeutic Uses

OKG may play a role in the treatment of individuals recovering from severe physical trauma.

When the body experiences severe trauma—such

as injury, major surgery, or burns—it goes into what is called a *catabolic state*. In this temporary condition, the body tends to tear itself down rather than build itself up. The catabolic hormone cortisone plays a major role in inducing catabolism. In the catabolic state, the body fails to utilize protein found in the diet and high levels of protein breakdown products appear in the urine. Calcium levels in urine also rise, as bones begin to weaken.

The opposite of a catabolic state is an *anabolic state*, in which the body tends to build itself up. Studies of hospitalized patients recovering from severe illnesses or injuries suggest that OKG blocks the catabolic effects of cortisone and also directly stimulates anabolic activity. It is not clear how OKG accomplishes this. It may directly affect the enzymes involved in hormone metabolism. Another possibility is that OKG may increase levels of growth hormone (an anabolic hormone), at least when it is taken in high enough doses (12 mg a day or more). It has also been suggested that OKG increases insulin release, which would have anabolic effects; however, this has been disputed.

Based on these findings, OKG has become popular as a bodybuilding supplement. However, there are no reported double-blind studies of OKG alone as a sports supplement. One study evaluated a combined arginine and ornithine supplement and found some evidence of benefit.

OKG has shown some promise for hepatic encephalopathy, a life-threatening complication of **liver cirrhosis**.

Safety Issues

Because it is simply ornithine and glutamine, OKG is presumably safe. However, high doses (more than 5 to 10 g) can cause diarrhea and stomach cramps. The maximum safe dosages for young children, women who are pregnant or nursing, or those with serious liver or kidney disease have not been established.

Osha

Ligusticum porteri

PRINCIPAL PROPOSED USES: *Cough, Indigestion, Respiratory Infections*

Native to high altitudes in the Southwest and Rocky Mountain states, the root of the osha plant is a traditional Native American remedy for respiratory infections and digestive problems. A related plant, *Ligusticum wallichii*, has a long history of use in Chinese medicine, and most of the scientific studies on osha were actually performed on this species.

What Is Osha Used for Today?

Osha is frequently recommended for use at the first sign of a respiratory infection. Like a sauna, it will typically induce sweating and according to folk wisdom this may help avert the development of a full-blown **cold**. Osha is also taken during respiratory infections as a **cough** suppressant and expectorant, hence the common name "Colorado cough root." However, there have not been any double-blind, placebo-controlled studies to verify these proposed uses.

Chinese research suggests that *Ligusticum wallichii* can relax smooth muscle tissue (perhaps thereby moderating the cough reflex) and inhibit the growth of various bacteria. Whether these findings apply to osha as well is unknown.

Like other bitter herbs, osha is said to improve symptoms of indigestion and increase appetite.

Dosage

Osha products vary in their concentration and should be taken according to directions on the label.

Safety Issues

Osha is believed to be safe, although the scientific record is far from complete. Traditionally, it is not recommended for use in pregnancy. Safety in young children, nursing women, or those with severe liver or kidney disease has also not been established.

One potential risk with osha is contamination with hemlock parsley, a deadly plant with a similar appearance.

Oxerutins

SUPPLEMENT FORMS/ALTERNATE NAMES: *Hydroxyethylrutosides (HERs), Troxerutin*
PRINCIPAL PROPOSED USES: *Hemorrhoids, Venous Insufficiency*
OTHER PROPOSED USES: *Lower-leg Edema in People with Diabetes, Lymphedema, Postsurgical Edema, Vertigo*

Oxerutins are a group of chemicals derived from a naturally occurring bioflavonoid called *rutin*.

This supplement has been widely used in Europe since the mid-1960s, as a treatment for conditions in which blood or lymph vessels leak fluid. Considerable evidence suggests that oxerutins are effective, but, unfortunately, it is difficult to find this supplement in North America.

Requirements/Sources

Although they are closely related to a natural flavonoid, oxerutins are not found in food. The only way to take them is in a supplement.

Therapeutic Dosages

For varicose veins/venous insufficiency, oxerutins are usually taken in dosages ranging from 900 to 1,200 mg daily. A typical schedule is 1,000 mg daily, taken in two separate doses of 500 mg.

For treating lymphedema and postsurgical edema, a typical dosage is a good deal higher: 3,000 mg daily.

One particular oxerutin called *troxerutin* may be taken alone as a treatment for varicose veins, in similar dosages. There is no evidence as yet that rutin itself is effective.

Therapeutic Uses

Varicose means enlarged or distended. A varicose vein is abnormally enlarged, allowing blood to pool and stagnate instead of moving it efficiently toward the heart. Surface veins of the leg are those most vulnerable to becoming varicose. **Venous insufficiency** is a closely related condition affecting larger veins deep within the leg. In either case, blood pools within the vein and exerts pressure against the vein walls and capillaries, resulting in pain, aching, swelling, and feelings of heaviness and fatigue. In addition, varicose veins present a cosmetic problem: bulging, often ropy, blue or purple lines visible on the skin of the lower legs.

Strong evidence shows that oxerutins can be helpful for venous insufficiency/varicose veins, improving aching, swelling, and fatigue in the legs.

Mixed evidence suggests that oxerutins might also be helpful for the leg ulcers that can develop in venous insufficiency. There is no evidence as yet that oxerutins can improve the cosmetic appearance of varicose veins.

Oxerutins have also been found effective for treating varicose veins when they occur during **pregnancy**.

Hemorrhoids are a special type of varicose vein and oxerutins may be helpful for treating them as well, although there have been some negative studies.

Some evidence suggests that oxerutins may be helpful for lymphedema (chronic arm swelling caused by damage to the lymph drainage system) following **surgery** for breast cancer, as well as for **edema** in the immediate postsurgical period.

Preliminary evidence, including small double-blind trials, suggests that oxerutins might also be helpful for reducing lower extremity swelling in people with diabetes. In these trials, oxerutin therapy did not affect blood sugar control.

One small double-blind study suggests oxerutins may be helpful for reducing **vertigo** and other symptoms of Meniere's disease. This use is based on a theory that Meniere's disease is caused by excessive fluid leaking from capillaries in the inner ear.

Oxerutins

What Is the Scientific Evidence for Oxerutins?

Varicose Veins/Venous Insufficiency

About 20 double-blind, placebo-controlled studies, enrolling a total of more than 2,000 participants, have examined oxerutins' effectiveness for treating varicose veins and venous insufficiency. Virtually all found oxerutins significantly more effective than placebo, giving substantial relief from swelling, aching, leg pains, and other uncomfortable symptoms, while causing no significant side effects.

For example, one large double-blind, placebo-controlled study published in 1983 enrolled 660 people with symptoms of venous insufficiency. Three out of four participants were randomly assigned to receive oxerutins (1,000 mg daily) while one out of four was given placebo. After 4 weeks of treatment, those who took oxerutins reported less heaviness, aching, cramps, and "restless leg" or "pins and needles" symptoms than those who took placebo. According to the researchers' calculations, oxerutins had produced significantly better results than placebo. This report has been criticized, however, for omitting key information (such as whether or not any participants also wore support stockings) and for failing to present data in a usable form.

A more recent, better-designed study supported these positive findings. This 12-week, double-blind, placebo-controlled study enrolled 133 women with moderate chronic venous insufficiency. Half received 1,000 mg oxerutins daily and the rest took a matching placebo. All participants were also fitted with standard compression stockings and wore them for the duration of the study. The researchers measured subjective symptoms such as aches and pains, as well as objective measures of edema in the leg.

Those who took oxerutins had significantly less lower-leg edema than the placebo group. Furthermore, these results lasted through a 6-week follow-up period, even though participants were no longer taking oxerutins. Compression stockings, on the other hand, produced no lasting benefit after participants stopped wearing them. They gave symptomatic relief while they were worn, but they didn't improve capillary circulation in a lasting way, as oxerutins apparently did.

Regarding aching, sensations of heaviness, and other uncomfortable symptoms, however, there was little difference between the two groups. The authors theorized that the compression stockings gave both groups so much symptomatic relief that it was difficult to demonstrate a separate subjective benefit of oxerutin therapy.

Many other double-blind, placebo-controlled studies have also found benefits with oxerutins for varicose veins and venous insufficiency.

As mentioned above, there is some evidence that troxerutin—one of the compounds in the standardized mixture sold as oxerutins—may be effective when taken alone. One study found it more effective than placebo, but another (very small) study found it less effective than the standard oxerutin mixture.

Pregnant women are at especially high risk for varicose veins and venous insufficiency. A 1975 study examined 69 pregnant women with varicose leg veins and found that oxerutins (900 mg daily) were significantly more effective than placebo against pain as well as swelling. A more recent study also found positive results, but because it was neither placebo-controlled nor double-blind its results mean little (other than to suggest that oxerutins are safe in pregnancy).

Skin ulcers sometimes form on the legs of people with varicose veins or venous insufficiency, when capillary circulation has become too impaired to keep the skin healthy. A French study published in 1987 found that oxerutins combined with compression stockings were significantly more helpful for leg ulcers than the stockings alone. Other positive results have been reported as well.

However, some experiments found oxerutins to have no benefit in treating or preventing leg ulcers. Until more research is done, the most we can say is that oxerutins *might* be helpful for leg ulcers—especially if combined with compression stockings.

Hemorrhoids

Some evidence suggests that oxerutins might be helpful for hemorrhoids as well. A double-blind study enrolling 97 pregnant women found oxerutins (1,000 mg daily) significantly better than placebo in reducing the pain, bleeding, and inflammation of hemorrhoids.

Lymphedema

Women who have undergone surgery for breast cancer may experience a lasting and troublesome side effect: swelling in the arm caused by damage to the lymph system. Along with the veins, the lymph system is responsible for returning fluid to the heart, but when the system is damaged, fluid can accumulate. Three double-blind, placebo-controlled studies enrolling more than 100 people total have examined the effectiveness of oxerutins in this condition.

In one trial, oxerutins worked significantly better than placebo at reducing swelling, discomfort, immobility, and other measures of lymphedema over a 6-month treatment period, with better results appearing each month—suggesting that, for women with this condition, the full effect of oxerutins might take months to realize.

Two smaller studies also found oxerutins to be more effective than placebo, but the researchers were not sure that the improvement was large enough to make a real difference.

In all of these studies, the dosage used was 3 g daily—about 3 times the typical dosage for venous insufficiency.

Post-surgical Edema

Swelling often occurs in the recovery period following surgery. In one double-blind trial, researchers gave oxerutins or placebo for 5 days to 40 people recovering from minor surgery or other minor injuries and found oxerutins significantly helpful in reducing swelling and discomfort.

Safety Issues

Oxerutins appear to be safe and well tolerated. In most studies, oxerutins have produced no more side effects than placebo. For example, in a study of 104 elderly people with venous insufficiency, 26 participants taking oxerutins reported adverse events, compared with 25 in the placebo group. The most commonly observed side effects were gastrointestinal symptoms, headaches, and dizziness.

Oxerutins have been given to pregnant women in some studies, with no apparent harmful effects. However, their safety for pregnant or nursing women cannot be regarded as absolutely proven. In addition, the safety of oxerutins has not been established for people with severe liver or kidney disease.

Pantothenic Acid and Pantethine

PRINCIPAL PROPOSED USES: *High Cholesterol, High Triglycerides*

OTHER PROPOSED USES: *Performance Enhancement, Rheumatoid Arthritis, Stress*

The body uses pantothenic acid (better known as vitamin B_5) to make proteins as well as other important chemicals needed to metabolize fats and carbohydrates. Pantothenic acid is also used in the manufacture of hormones, red blood cells, and *acetylcholine*, an important neurotransmitter (signal carrier between nerve cells).

As a supplement, pantothenic acid has been proposed as a treatment for **rheumatoid arthritis, enhancing sports performance**, and fighting **stress** in general.

In the body, pantothenic acid is converted to a related chemical known as pantethine. For reasons that are not clear, pantethine supplements (but not pantothenic acid supplements) appear to reduce blood levels of triglycerides, and possibly also improve the **cholesterol** profile.

Requirements/Sources

The word *pantothenic* comes from the Greek word meaning "everywhere," and pantothenic acid is indeed found in a wide range of foods. For this reason, pantothenic acid deficiency is rare. The official U.S. and Canadian recommendations for daily intake of pantothenic acid are as follows:

> **Infants 0–6 months, 1.7 mg**
>   **7–12 months, 1.8 mg**
> **Children 1–3 years, 2 mg**
>   **4–8 years, 3 mg**
>   **9–13 years, 4 mg**
> **Males and females 14 years and older, 5 mg**
> **Pregnant women, 6 mg**
> **Nursing women, 7 mg**

Brewer's yeast, torula (nutritional) yeast, and calf liver are excellent sources of pantothenic acid. Peanuts, mushrooms, soybeans, split peas, pecans, oatmeal, buckwheat, sunflower seeds, lentils, rye flour, cashews, and other whole grains and nuts are good sources as well, as are red chili peppers and avocados. Pantethine is not found in foods in appreciable amounts.

Therapeutic Dosages

For lowering triglycerides, the typical recommended dosage of pantethine is 300 mg 3 times daily. Dosages of pantothenic acid as high as 660 mg 3 times daily are sometimes recommended for people with rheumatoid arthritis.

Therapeutic Uses

Inconsistent evidence from small double-blind trials suggest that pantethine might lower blood levels of triglycerides and, to a lesser extent, cholesterol. High triglycerides, like high cholesterol, increase risk of heart disease and strokes. Some people have only modestly elevated cholesterol but very high triglycerides, so pantethine may be especially useful for them.

Weak evidence hints that pantothenic acid might be helpful for rheumatoid arthritis.

Pantothenic acid is also recommended as an athletic performance enhancer, but there is no evidence at all that it works. It is also sometimes referred to as an anti-stress nutrient because it plays a role in the function of the adrenal glands, but whether it really helps the body withstand stress is not known.

What Is the Scientific Evidence for Pantothenic Acid and Pantethine?

Three small double-blind, placebo-controlled studies suggest that pantethine can reduce total blood triglycerides and perhaps improve cholesterol levels as well. For example, a double-blind placebo-controlled study followed 29 people with high cholesterol and triglycerides for 8 weeks. The dosage used was 300 mg 3 times daily, for a total daily dose of 900 mg. In this study, subjects taking pantethine experienced a 30% reduction in blood triglycerides, a 13.5% reduction in LDL ("bad") cholesterol, and a 10% rise in HDL ("good") cholesterol. However, other small studies have found no benefit. These contradictory results do not necessarily mean that pante-

thine is ineffective, as chance plays a considerable role in the outcome of small studies. Rather, they suggest that larger studies need to be performed to establish (or disprove) pantethine's potential efficacy.

Several open studies have specifically studied the use of pantethine to improve cholesterol and triglyceride levels in people with diabetes and found it effective without causing harmful effects.

These findings are supported by experiments in rabbits, which show that pantethine may prevent the buildup of plaque in major arteries. However, we don't know how pantethine acts in the body to reduce triglycerides.

Rheumatoid Arthritis

There is weak evidence for using pantothenic acid to treat rheumatoid arthritis. One observational study found 66 people with rheumatoid arthritis had less pantothenic acid in their blood than 29 healthy people. The more severe the arthritis, the lower the blood levels of pantothenic acid were. However, this result doesn't prove that pantothenic acid supplements can effectively reduce any of the symptoms of rheumatoid arthritis.

To follow up on this finding, researchers then conducted a small placebo-controlled trial involving 18 subjects to see whether pantothenic acid would help. This study found that 2 g daily of pantothenic acid (in the form of calcium pantothenate) reduced morning stiffness, pain, and disability significantly better than placebo. However, a study this small doesn't mean much on its own. More research is needed.

Safety Issues

No significant side effects have been reported for pantothenic acid or pantethine, used by themselves or with other medications. As noted above, pantethine has been used in people with diabetes, without apparent adverse effects. However, maximum safe dosages for young children, pregnant or nursing women, or people with serious liver or kidney disease have not been established.

Para-Aminobenzoic Acid

SUPPLEMENT FORMS/ALTERNATE NAMES: *PABA*

PRINCIPAL PROPOSED USES: *Peyronie's Disease*

OTHER PROPOSED USES: *Male Infertility, Scleroderma, Vitiligo*

Para-aminobenzoic acid (PABA) is best known as the active ingredient in sunblock. This use of PABA is not really medicinal: like a pair of sunglasses, PABA physically blocks ultraviolet rays when it is applied to the skin.

There are, however, some proposed medicinal uses of oral PABA supplements. PABA is sometimes suggested as a treatment for various diseases of the skin and connective tissue, as well as for male infertility. However, most of the clinical data on PABA comes from very old studies, some from the early 1940s.

Sources

PABA is not believed to be an essential nutrient. Nonetheless, it is found in foods, mainly in grains and meat. Small amounts of PABA are usually present in B vitamin supplements as well as in some multiple vitamins.

Therapeutic Dosages

A typical therapeutic dosage of PABA is 300 to 400 mg daily. Some studies have used much higher dosages. However, serious side effects have been found in dosages above 8 g daily (see Safety Issues below). You probably shouldn't take more than 400 mg daily except on medical advice.

Therapeutic Uses

PABA has been suggested as a treatment for **Peyronie's disease**, a condition in which the penis becomes bent owing to the accumulation of fibrous plaques. However, there has been only one reported double-blind, placebo-controlled study properly examining this use. (For information on why such studies are essential, see **Why Does This Book Rely on Double-blind Studies?**) This trial enrolled 103 men with Peyronie's disease and followed them for 1 year. The results showed that use of PABA at a dose of 3 g 4 times daily significantly slowed the progression of Peyronie's disease; it did not, however, reduce pre-existing plaque.

PABA has also been suggested as a treatment for **scleroderma**, a disease that creates fibrous tissue in the skin and internal organs. A 4-month double-blind, placebo-controlled study of 146 people with long-standing, stable scleroderma did not support this, failing to find any evidence of benefit. However, half the participants in this trial dropped out before the end, making the results unreliable.

Based on one small World War II–era study, PABA has been suggested for treating **male infertility** as well as **vitiligo**, a condition in which patches of skin lose their pigment, resulting in pale blotches. However, this study didn't have a control group, so its results aren't meaningful. Ironically, a recent study suggests that high dosages of PABA can *cause* vitiligo (see Safety Issues).

Safety Issues

PABA is probably safe when taken at a dosage up to 400 mg daily. Possible side effects at this dosage are minor, including skin rash and loss of appetite.

Higher doses are a different story, however. There has been one reported case of severe liver toxicity in a woman taking 12 g daily of PABA. Fortunately, her liver recovered completely after she discontinued her use of this supplement. Also, a recent study suggests that 8 g daily of PABA can cause vitiligo, the patchy skin disease described previously.

Clearly, there are questions that need to be answered about the safety of high-dose PABA therapy. You shouldn't take more than 400 mg daily except under medical supervision.

PABA may interfere with certain medications, including sulfa antibiotics.

Safety in young children, pregnant or nursing women, or those with serious liver or kidney disease has not been determined.

Interactions You Should Know About

If you are taking **sulfa antibiotics** such as Bactrim or Septra: Do not take PABA supplements except on medical advice.

Parsley

Petroselinum crispum, Petroselinum hartense, Petroselinum sativum

PRINCIPAL PROPOSED USES: *None*

OTHER PROPOSED USES: *Abortifacient, Amenorrhea, Colic, Flatulence, Indigestion, Kidney Stones*

Parsley is a culinary herb used in many types of cooking and as a nearly universal adornment to restaurant food. Originally a native plant of the Mediterranean region, parsley is grown today throughout the world. It is a nutritious food, providing dietary **calcium**, **iron**, carotenes, ascorbic acid, and **vitamin A**.

Parsley's traditional use for inducing menstruation may be explained by evidence that apiol and myristicin, two substances contained in parsley, stimulate contractions of the uterus. Indeed, extracted apiol has been tried for the purpose of causing abortions (see Safety Issues below).

A tea made from the "fruits" or seeds of parsley is also a traditional remedy for **colic**, **indigestion**, and **intestinal gas**.

What Is Parsley Used for Today?

Germany's Commission E suggests the use of parsley leaf or root to relieve irritation of the urinary tract (such as may occur in **bladder infections**) and to aid in passing **kidney stones**. Although there is no evidence that parsley is helpful for these conditions, parsley, due to its constituents apiol and myristicin, is believed to have a diuretic effect; because diuretics would increase the flow of urine, this might help the body to wash out bacteria as well as stones. However, no studies have as yet evaluated whether parsley is actually beneficial for either health problem.

A test-tube study evaluated parsley extract as a topical antibiotic, finding that the extract had a weak effect against *Staphylococcus* bacteria. However, it did not appear to be strong enough to be practically useful for this purpose.

Dosage

The usual dose of parsley leaf or root is 6 g of dried plant per day, consumed in 3 doses of 2 g, each steeped in 150 ml of water. Extract of parsley leaf and root are made at a ratio of 1 g of plant to 1 ml of liquid and used at a dose of 2 ml 3 times daily. Tea made from parsley seeds is used at a lower dosage of 2 to 3 g per day, using 1 g of seed per cup of tea.

Safety Issues

As a widely eaten food, parsley is generally regarded as safe. However, excessive quantities of parsley should be avoided during pregnancy, based on the evidence mentioned earlier that myristicin and apiol can stimulate the uterus. Myristicin may also cross the placenta and increase the heart rate of the fetus.

Parsley is known as a plant that can cause **photosensitivity**, which is an increased tendency to **sunburn**; this result, however, occurs from prolonged physical contact with the leaves, not from oral consumption of parsley.

Maximum safe intake of parsley in young children, pregnant or nursing women, or people with severe liver or kidney disease has not been established.

Interactions You Should Know About

If you are taking **lithium**: Use parsley only under doctor's supervision.

Passionflower

Passiflora incarnata

PRINCIPAL PROPOSED USES: *Anxiety, Drug Addiction*

OTHER PROPOSED USES: *Insomnia, Nervous Stomach*

The passionflower vine is a native of the Western hemisphere, named for symbolic connections drawn between its appearance and the crucifixion of Jesus. Native North Americans used passionflower primarily as a mild sedative. It quickly caught on as a folk remedy in Europe and was thereafter adopted by professional herbalists as a sedative and digestive aid.

What Is Passionflower Used for Today?

In 1985, Germany's Commission E officially approved passionflower as a treatment for "nervous unrest." The herb is considered to be a mildly effective treatment for **anxiety** and **insomnia**, less potent than **kava** and **valerian**, but nonetheless useful. Like **melissa** (lemon balm), **chamomile**, and valerian, passionflower is also used for nervous stomach.

However, there is only weak supporting scientific evidence that passionflower works for these purposes. Preliminary double-blind, comparative trials suggest that passionflower might be helpful for anxiety and **chemical dependency**. Animal studies suggest that passionflower extracts can reduce agitation and prolong sleep. However, there have not been any double-blind, placebo-controlled studies of passionflower reported.

The active ingredients in passionflower are not known.

What Is the Scientific Evidence for Passionflower?

Anxiety

A 4-week, double-blind study of 36 individuals with anxiety (specifically, generalized anxiety disorder) compared passionflower to the standard drug oxazepam. Oxazepam worked more quickly, but by the end of the 4-week trial, both treatments proved equally effective. Furthermore, passionflower showed a comparative advantage in terms of side-effects: use of oxazepam was associated with more job-related problems (such as, for example, daytime drowsiness). However, because this study lacked a placebo group, it would be premature to conclude from it that passionflower has been shown to be an effective treatment for anxiety.

Chemical Dependency

A 14-day, double-blind trial enrolled 65 men addicted to opiate drugs and compared the effectiveness of passionflower and the drug clonidine together against clonidine alone. Clonidine is a drug widely used to assist narcotic withdrawal. It effectively reduces physical symptoms, such as increased blood pressure. However, clonidine does not help emotional symptoms, such as drug craving, anxiety, irritability, agitation, and depression. These symptoms can be quite severe and often cause enrollees in drug treatment programs to end participation. In this 14-day study, the use of passionflower along with clonidine significantly eased the emotional aspects of withdrawal as compared to clonidine alone.

Dosage

The proper dosage of passionflower is 1 cup 3 times daily of a tea made by steeping 1 teaspoon of dried leaves for 10 to 15 minutes. Passionflower tinctures and powdered extracts should be taken according to the label instructions.

Safety Issues

Passionflower is on the FDA's GRAS (generally recognized as safe) list.

The alkaloids harman and harmaline found in passionflower have been found to act somewhat like the drugs known as MAO inhibitors and also to stimulate the uterus, but whether whole passionflower has these effects remains unknown. Passionflower might increase the action of sedative medications. Finally, there are five case reports from Norway of individuals becoming temporarily mentally impaired from a combination herbal product containing passionflower. It is not clear whether the other ingredients may have played a role.

Safety has not been established for pregnant or nursing mothers, very young children, or those with severe liver or kidney disease.

Interactions You Should Know About

If you are taking **sedative medications**: Passionflower might exaggerate their effect.

PC-SPES

Dendranthema morifolium Tzvel, Ganoderma lucidium Karst, Glycyrrhiza glabra L, Isatis indigotica Fort, Panax pseudo-ginseng Wall, Robdosia rubescens, Scutellaria baicalensis Georgi, and *Serenoa repens*

PRINCIPAL PROPOSED USES: *Prostate Cancer*

PC-SPES was, ostensibly, a formulation of eight natural products (seven herbs and one mushroom): *Isatis indigotica, Glycyrrhiza glabra* (**licorice**), *Panax pseudo-ginseng, Ganoderma lucidium* (**reishi mushroom**), *Scutellaria baicalensis, Dendranthema morifolium, Robdosia rubescens,* and *Serenoa repens* (**saw palmetto**).

The name PC-SPES was derived from the common abbreviation for prostate cancer (PC) and the Latin word *spes*, meaning "hope." After its commercial launch in 1996, PC-SPES received considerable interest from the general public and reputable medical researchers as a treatment for prostate cancer. Unfortunately, it turned out to be a fraud.

PC-SPES was not truly a purely herbal product; samples dating back to 1996 were found to contain a form of pharmaceutical estrogen, diethylstilbestrol (DES), as well as indomethacin (an anti-inflammatory medication in the ibuprofen family) and warfarin (a strong blood thinner). Samples subsequent to 1999 contained less DES; but they also showed less effectiveness in treating prostate cancer.

There is little doubt that DES is active against prostate cancer, but it presents a variety of risks, including blood clots in the legs. The other two pharmaceutical contaminants might actually reduce this risk (which may be why they were covertly added), but present various risks all on their own. For these reasons, we strongly recommend against using PC-SPES at all.

What Is PC-SPES Used for Today?

The only proposed use of PC-SPES was the treatment of **prostate cancer**. The formulation was tried at various stages of the disease, and preliminary research indicated that it had potential, particularly for treating prostate cancer that is no longer responsive to hormone therapies. Benefits were reported in the two main types of prostate cancer: hormone-sensitive and hormone-insensitive cancer. However, when the covert addition of pharmaceuticals was discovered, interest in this "herbal" combination ended.

What Is the Scientific Evidence for PC-SPES?

All the results reported in the following paragraphs are consistent with the known effects of hormones related to estrogen and may be due to the DES present in PC-SPES, rather than the herbal constituents.

Test-tube studies of cancer cells found that PC-SPES decreases cell growth, promotes tumor cell death, and reduces prostate-specific antigen (PSA) levels in both hormone-sensitive and hormone-insensitive prostate cancers, and exerts estrogenic effects.

In a rat study, PC-SPES treatment reduced the occurrence of prostate cancer tumors, inhibited their growth, and slowed the rate of cancer spread (metastasis) to the lungs.

In one uncontrolled human study, PC-SPES produced a significant decrease in PSA levels for most of the 33 volunteers tested. Similar results were seen in another study of 69 individuals by the same author and a study of 70 people conducted by another researcher. Benefits were seen in other uncontrolled trials, as well.

Dosage

The standard dosage of PC-SPES was 6 to 9 capsules (320 mg each) per day, taken on an empty stomach at least 2 hours before or after meals.

Safety Issues

Note: Due to the presence of unlisted pharmaceuticals, PC-SPES should not be used.

It's no surprise that side effects of PC-SPES closely resemble those of estrogen when taken by men for the treatment of prostate cancer; it may cause breast or nipple tenderness or swelling, loss of body hair, hot flashes, and loss of libido. Some individuals have also reported leg cramps, nausea and vomiting, and blood clots in the legs. Side effects of PC-SPES increase with dosage.

There is one case report of PC-SPES taken at twice the recommended dose causing internal bleeding, presumably due to the presence of **warfarin** (Coumadin), a strong blood thinner.

Pelargonium sidoides

ALTERNATE NAMES/RELATED TERMS: *Kalwerbossie, Rabassam, South African Geranium, Umckaloabo*
PRINCIPAL PROPOSED USES: *Acute Bronchitis, Sore Throat*
OTHER PROPOSED USES: *Colds and Flus, Sinusitis, Tonsillitis*

Pelargonium sidoides is a plant in the geranium family that grows in South Africa. It has heart-shaped leaves and narrow flowers of deep, saturated red. It has a long history of traditional use in southern Africa for treatment of respiratory problems. The root is the part used medicinally.

What Is *Pelargonium sidoides* Used for Today?

An alcohol extract made from *Pelargonium sidoides* has become popular in Germany as a treatment for various respiratory problems, including **acute bronchitis**, the **common cold**, sinusitis, **pharyngitis** (sore throat), and tonsillitis. Fairly large studies have been performed to substantiate some of these uses.

For example, in one double-blind, placebo-controlled study, 468 adults with recent onset of acute bronchitis were given either placebo or a standard alcohol extract of *Pelargonium sidoides* 3 times daily for a week. The results showed a significantly greater improvement in symptoms in the treatment group as com-

pared to the placebo group. On average, participants who received the real treatment were able to return to work 2 days earlier than those given placebo. A high dropout rate, however, somewhat diminishes the meaningfulness of these results.

Another double-blind, placebo-controlled study enrolled 143 children aged 6 to 10 years with a non-dangerous form of strep throat (technically, non–group A beta hemolytic strep tonsillopharyngitis). On average, the total duration of the illness was reduced by 2 days in the treatment group as compared to the placebo group.

Note: Only a medical test can distinguish between the relatively non-dangerous form of strep throat studied in this trial (non–group A strep) and strep throat of the potentially very dangerous A form (group A strep). For this reason, physician supervision is essential. See the **Strep Throat** article for more information.

It is not known how *Pelargonium sidoides* might work, but its action is hypothesized to involve both direct antibacterial effects and immune function modification.

Dosage

A typical adult dose of the tested standardized root extract is 30 drops 3 times daily. For children 6 to 11, this dose is typically reduced to 20 drops 3 times daily. However, other products besides the tested formulation may vary in strength. Therefore, we recommend that you follow the label instructions.

Safety Issues

In clinical trials enrolling a total of more than 2,500 adults and children, use of the tested standardized extract produced few side effects, other than the usual occasional allergic reactions or digestive upset. However, comprehensive safety testing has not been completed. There is no reliable evidence regarding safety in children under the age of 6, pregnant or nursing women, or people with severe liver or kidney disease.

Pennyroyal

Hedeoma pulegioides, Mentha pulegium

The name *pennyroyal* refers to two related plants: *Mentha pulegium* (European pennyroyal) and *Hedeoma pulegioides* (American pennyroyal). Pennroyal is a member of the mint family. Applied topically, pennyroyal has been used since the time of ancient Greece to repel fleas and other insects. Pennyroyal has been taken internally in Europe and North America for a variety of conditions, including colds and flus, coughs, kidney problems, headache, and upset stomach, as well as to induce abortion. Unfortunately, traditional herbalists do not appear to have noticed an essential fact about pennyroyal: it is toxic to the liver. In modern times, people have died as a consequence of using this herb according to traditional indications.

The essential oil of pennyroyal contains a substance called *pulegone*. In the body, pulegone is converted to the toxic chemical menthofuran. Low levels of menthofuran may not produce any untoward effects. At a certain point, however, depending on the individual, menthofuran poisons the nervous system, causing symptoms such as dizziness, vertigo, hallucinations, seizures, and possibly unconsciousness. Liver damage possibly leading to liver failure occurs subsequently.

Because of these safety risks and the fact that pennyroyal has not been proven effective for a single medical use, we recommend that you entirely avoid this herb. We do not even recommend using it topically as an insect repellant because it is possible that enough pulegone could be absorbed to cause harm.

Peppermint

Mentha piperita

PRINCIPAL PROPOSED USES:

Oral: *Dyspepsia, Irritable Bowel Syndrome, Other Forms of Spasms in the Digestive Tract*

OTHER PROPOSED USES:

Inhaled (Aromatherapy): *Nausea, Respiratory Congestion*

Topical: *Tension Headaches*

Oral: *Gallstones*

Peppermint is a relative of numerous wild mint plants, deliberately bred in the late 1600s in England to become the delightful tasting plant so well known today. It is widely used as a beverage tea and as a flavoring or scent in a wide variety of products.

Peppermint tea also has a long history of medicinal use, primarily as a digestive aid and for the symptomatic treatment of cough, colds, and fever. Peppermint oil is used for chest congestion (Vicks VapoRub), as a local anesthetic (Solarcaine, Ben-Gay), and most recently in the treatment of irritable bowel disease, also known as spastic colon.

What Is Peppermint Used for Today?

Some preliminary evidence suggests that peppermint oil may be helpful for **irritable bowel syndrome** and other conditions that involve spasms in the digestive tract.

The active ingredient of peppermint oil for this purpose is thought to be menthol. This substance relaxes the muscles of the small intestine in dilutions as low as 1:20,000 and has been found to counter the effect of drugs that cause intestinal spasm. Peppermint oil may also be helpful for **dyspepsia** (minor indigestion), as well as pain caused by medical examinations of the colon and stomach.

One study found that peppermint oil reduced pain after **surgery** (specifically, C-section), in part by reducing pain related to intestinal gas. (Intestinal gas is a common problem in the hours or days after major surgery.)

Oral peppermint oil has also shown some promise for helping to dissolve **gallstones**, but it is far from a proven treatment for this condition.

Peppermint oil is also used in another way: as **aromatherapy**. This means that it is inhaled, often by add-ing it to a humidifier. The Commission E has authorized inhaled peppermint oil for relief of mucus congestion of the lungs and sinuses; however, there is only weak supporting evidence for this use. Even weaker evidence hints that inhaled peppermint oil might relieve postsurgical **nausea**.

Similarly weak evidence hints that peppermint oil, applied to the forehead, might relieve **tension headaches**.

What Is the Scientific Evidence for Peppermint?

Irritable Bowel Syndrome

There have been a total of 12 double-blind, placebo-controlled studies of peppermint oil for irritable bowel syndrome. However, all of these studies were small and most were poorly designed and/or reported.

Of these, eight found benefit and four did not. In the largest of these studies, 110 people with irritable bowel syndrome were given either enteric-coated peppermint oil (187 mg) or placebo 3 to 4 times daily, 15 to 30 minutes before meals, for 4 weeks. The results in the 101 individuals who completed the trial showed significant improvements in abdominal pain and bloating, stool frequency, and flatulence.

Other Forms of Spasm in the Digestive Tract

A barium enema involves introducing a solution containing the metal barium into the lower intestines. It commonly causes intestinal pain and spasm. A double-blind study of 141 individuals found that adding peppermint oil to the barium reduced the severity of intestinal spasm that occurred. Benefits were also seen in a large study conducted by different researchers.

Another study found that peppermint oil reduced

Perilla frutescens

spasm in the stomach during a procedure called *upper endoscopy*.

Dyspepsia (Minor Indigestion)

Peppermint oil is often used in combination with other essential oils to treat minor indigestion.

A double-blind, placebo-controlled study including 39 individuals found that an enteric-coated peppermint-caraway oil combination taken 3 times daily for 4 weeks significantly reduced dyspepsia pain as compared to placebo. Of the treatment group, 63.2% were pain free after 4 weeks, compared to 25% of the placebo group.

Results from a double-blind, comparative study including 118 individuals suggest that the combination of peppermint and caraway oil is comparably effective to the no-longer-available drug cisapride. After 4 weeks, the herbal combination reduced dyspepsia pain by 69.7%, whereas the conventional treatment reduced pain by 70.2%.

A preparation of peppermint, caraway, fennel, and wormwood oils was compared to the drug metoclopramide in another double-blind study enrolling 60 individuals. After 7 days, 43.3% of the treatment group were pain free compared to 13.3% of the metoclopramide group.

Dosage

The proper dosage of peppermint oil when treating irritable bowel syndrome is 0.2 to 0.4 ml 3 times a day of an enteric-coated capsule. The capsule has to be enteric-coated to prevent stomach distress.

Safety Issues

At the normal dosage, enteric-coated peppermint oil is believed to be reasonably safe in healthy adults. However, case reports and one study in rats hint that peppermint might reduce **male fertility**. The species *Mentha spicata* may be more problematic in this regard than the more common *Mentha piperita*.

Excessive doses of peppermint oil can be toxic, causing kidney failure and even death. Very high intake of peppermint oil can also cause nausea, loss of appetite, heart problems, loss of balance, and other nervous system problems.

Safety in young children, pregnant or nursing women, or those with severe liver or kidney disease has not been established. In particular, peppermint can cause jaundice in newborn babies, so don't try to use it for colic.

Use of peppermint oil may increase levels of the drug cyclosporine in the body. If you are taking cyclosporine, and wish to take peppermint oil, notify your physician in advance, so that your blood levels of cyclosporine can be monitored and your dose adjusted if necessary. Conversely, if you are already taking both peppermint oil and cyclosporine, do not stop taking the peppermint without informing your physician. When you stop peppermint, your cyclosporine levels may fall.

Interactions You Should Know About

If you are taking **cyclosporine**: Do not use peppermint oil (or stop using it) except in consultation with your physician.

Perilla frutescens

ALTERNATE NAMES/RELATED TERMS: *Chinese Basil, Rosmarinic Acid*
PRINCIPAL PROPOSED USES: *Allergic Rhinitis (Hay Fever)*
OTHER PROPOSED USES: *Depression, Rheumatoid Arthritis*

A member of the mint family, perilla is used in a variety of Asian foods to add both flavor and color. It is also grown ornamentally in gardens.

The stem of the plant is used in Chinese medicine for treatment of morning sickness. The leaves are said to be helpful for asthma, colds and flus, and other lung problems.

What Is Perilla Used for Today?

Recently, extracts of perilla have undergone study as a treatment for **allergic rhinitis** (hay fever). Perilla contains high levels of the substance rosmarinic acid (also found in the herb rosemary and many other plants). Rosmarinic acid appears to have anti-inflammatory and anti-allergic actions. In a 3-week, double-blind, placebo-controlled study of 29 people with seasonal allergic rhinitis, participants were given one of three treatments: placebo, *Perilla frutescens* extract enriched to contain 50 mg of rosmarinic acid, or an extract enhanced to contain 200 mg of rosmarinic acid. The results showed that both perilla products reduced symptoms to a greater extent than placebo.

Animal studies hint that perilla might also be useful for a different type of allergy: the severe, rapid reaction known as *anaphylaxis*, commonly associated with shellfish, peanut, and bee-sting allergies.

Very weak evidence suggests that rosmarinic acid and/or perilla may have **anti-cancer effects** and might also have benefits for **rheumatoid arthritis** and other autoimmune diseases as well as **depression**.

Dosage

A typical dosage of perilla should supply 50 to 200 mg of rosmarinic acid daily. Perilla also contains luteolin, a substance that may also have anti-allergic actions. For this reason, perilla products are often enriched with luteolin as well, typically providing 5 to 10 mg daily.

Safety Issues

In the small clinical trials and animal studies conducted thus far, use of perilla and/or rosmarinic acid has not been associated with significant adverse effects. Due to the wide use of perilla in Asian cooking, as well as the prevalence of rosmarinic acid in many spices, these substances are assumed to have a relatively high level of safety. However, comprehensive safety testing has not been reported. Safety in young children, pregnant or nursing women, or people with severe liver or kidney disease has not been established.

Phaseolus vulgaris

ALTERNATE NAMES/RELATED TERMS: *Carbohydrate Blocker, Starch Blocker*
PRINCIPAL PROPOSED USES: *Weight Loss*

Supplements made from white kidney beans (*Phaseolus vulgaris*) are sold as starch blockers, supplements said to interfere with the digestion of carbohydrates and thereby promote weight loss.

Therapeutic Uses

Technically, starch blockers are *amylase inhibitors*. Amylase is one of the main enzymes the body uses to digest starch. In theory, when amylase is blocked, ingested starch can pass through the body undigested, contributing no calories.

However, theory is one thing, reality another. Studies of amylase inhibitors have generally failed to find them effective.

Several possible reasons for this discrepancy have been proposed, such as that the amylase inhibitor may be broken down in the stomach, the product may supply enough of its own amylase to counteract any benefit, and that another enzyme, glucoamylase, may be able to take over when amylase can't do the job. Whatever the cause, the net results in these studies were poor. Use of amylase inhibitors did not in fact block the digestion of starch.

However, according to the manufacturer of a current product, more concentrated extracts of *Phaseolus vulgaris*, taken in higher doses, do work. Unfortunately, the evidence for this claim rests entirely on unpublished studies that we are unable to verify.

In one of these studies, participants reportedly lost 3.9% of their total body weight and 10.45% of body fat mass in 30 days, without a reduction in lean tissue mass, as compared to those in the placebo group. Until these studies are published in a journal, and subject to proper review, it will be difficult to know how reliable they may be.

Dosage

The recommended dose of amylase inhibitors varies among products. Follow label instructions.

Safety Issues

On the basis of their widespread presence in commonly consumed foods (beans), amylase inhibitors are believed to be quite safe. One side effect, however, is to be expected: flatulence. It is the amylase inhibitors in beans that are responsible for their notorious gassiness.

Maximum safe doses in pregnant or nursing women, young children, or individuals with severe hepatic or renal disease have not been established.

Phenylalanine

SUPPLEMENT FORMS/ALTERNATE NAMES: *D-Phenylalanine, DL-Phenylalanine, L-Phenylalanine*
PRINCIPAL PROPOSED USES: *Depression*
OTHER PROPOSED USES: *Attention Deficit Disorder, Multiple Sclerosis, Pain (In General), Parkinson's Disease, Rheumatoid Arthritis, Vitiligo*

Phenylalanine occurs in two chemical forms: *L-phenylalanine*, a natural amino acid found in proteins; and its mirror image, *D-phenylalanine*, a form synthesized in a laboratory. Some research has involved the L-form, others the D-form, and still others a combination of the two known as DL-phenylalanine.

In the body, phenylalanine is converted into another amino acid called *tyrosine*. Tyrosine in turn is converted into L-dopa, norepinephrine, and epinephrine, three key *neurotransmitters* (chemicals that transmit signals between nerve cells). Because some antidepressants work by raising levels of norepinephrine, various forms of phenylalanine have been tried as a possible treatment for depression.

D-phenylalanine (but not L-phenylalanine) has been proposed to treat chronic pain. It blocks *enkephalinase*, an enzyme that may act to increase pain levels in the body.

Requirements/Sources

L-phenylalanine is an essential amino acid, meaning that we need it for life and our bodies can't manufacture it from other chemicals. It is found in protein-rich foods such as meat, fish, poultry, eggs, dairy products, and beans. Provided you eat enough protein, you are likely to get enough L-phenylalanine for your nutritional needs. There is no nutritional need for D-phenylalanine.

Therapeutic Dosages

D- and DL-phenylalanine are typically taken at a dose of 100 to 200 mg daily for the treatment of depression. For the treatment of chronic pain, studies have used D-phenylalanine in doses as high as 2,500 mg daily.

It is best not to take your phenylalanine supplement at the same time as a high-protein meal, as it may not be absorbed well.

Therapeutic Uses

Small double-blind comparative studies suggest (but do not prove) that both the D- and DL- forms of phenylalanine might be helpful for **depression**.

Weak and contradictory evidence has been used to advocate the use of D-phenylalanine as a general analgesic (pain relieving treatment).

Preliminary uncontrolled and double-blind studies found that L-phenylalanine may enhance the effectiveness of ultraviolet for **vitiligo**.

Highly preliminary evidence suggests that D-phenylalanine may be helpful for **multiple sclerosis** when combined with transcutaneous electrical nerve stimulation (TENS). D-phenylalanine has also been proposed as a treatment for **Parkinson's disease** (but see Safety Issues below).

Although D- and DL- phenylalanine are marketed as treatments for **attention deficit disorder**, they do not appear to be helpful. Some proponents claim that phenylalanine works better when combined with tyrosine, **glutamine**, and gamma-aminobutyric acid (GABA), but this has not been proven.

What Is the Scientific Evidence for Phenylalanine?

Depression

A pair of double-blind comparative studies found that D- or DL-phenylalanine may be as effective as the antidepressant drug imipramine and possibly work more quickly. The larger of the two studies compared the effectiveness of D-phenylalanine at 100 mg daily against the same daily dose of imipramine. Sixty people with depression were randomly assigned to take either imipramine or D-phenylalanine for 30 days. The results in both groups were statistically equivalent, meaning that phenylalanine was about as effective as imipramine. D-phenylalanine worked more rapidly, however, producing significant improvement in only 15 days. Like most antidepressant drugs, imipramine required several weeks to take effect.

The other double-blind study followed 27 people, half of whom received DL-phenylalanine (150 to 200 mg daily) and the other half imipramine (100 to 150 mg daily). When they were reevaluated after 30 days, both groups had improved by a statistically equal amount.

L-phenylalanine has also been tried as a treatment for depression, but not in studies that could provide a scientifically meaningful result.

Unfortunately, there have not been any double-blind, *placebo-controlled* studies of phenylalanine for depression. This is too bad, since without such evidence we can't be sure that the supplement is actually effective.

Chronic Pain

The enzyme enkephalinase breaks down enkephalins, naturally occurring substances that reduce pain. D-phenylalanine (but not L-phenylalanine) is thought to block enkephalinase; this could lead to increased enkephalin levels, which in turn would tend to reduce pain. On this basis, D-phenylalanine has been proposed as a pain-killing drug.

However, as yet there is no meaningful evidence that it really works in this way. A small double-blind, placebo-controlled study reported evidence for the effectiveness of D-phenylalanine in chronic pain, but a careful reexamination of the math involved showed that it actually proved little. Another small double-blind, placebo-controlled study failed to find any benefits at all. Another study commonly described as showing D-phenylalanine effective suffered from many flaws (including the fact that it lacked a control group) and therefore can't be trusted.

Safety Issues

The long-term safety of phenylalanine in any of its forms is not known. Both L- and D-phenylalanine must be avoided by those with the rare metabolic disease phenylketonuria (PKU).

The maximum safe dosages of phenylalanine have not been established for young children, pregnant or nursing women, or those with severe liver or kidney disease.

There are some indications that the combined use of phenylalanine with antipsychotic drugs might increase the risk of developing the long-term side effect known as tardive dyskinesia or worsen symptoms in those who already have it.

Like other amino acids, phenylalanine may interfere with the absorption or action of the drug levodopa which is used for Parkinson's disease.

Interactions You Should Know About

If you are taking:

- **Antipsychotic medications: Do not use phenylalanine.**
- **Levodopa: Like other amino acids, phenylalanine might interfere with its action.**

Phosphatidylserine

Phosphatidylserine

PRINCIPAL PROPOSED USES: *Age-related Memory Loss, Alzheimer's Disease*

OTHER PROPOSED USES: *Depression, Enhancing Mental Function in Young People, Performance Enhancement, Stress*

Phosphatidylserine, or PS for short, is a member of a class of chemical compounds known as *phospholipids*. PS is an essential component in all our cells; specifically, it is a major component of the cell membrane. The cell membrane is a kind of "skin" that surrounds living cells. Besides keeping cells intact, this membrane performs vital functions such as moving nutrients into cells and pumping waste products out of them. PS plays an important role in many of these functions.

Good evidence suggests that PS can help declining mental function and depression in the elderly and it is widely used for this purpose in Italy, Scandinavia, and other parts of Europe. PS has also been marketed as a "brain booster" for people of all ages, said to sharpen memory and increase thinking ability. However, the evidence to support this use is incomplete and inconsistent.

More recently, PS has been marketed as a sports supplement, said to help bodybuilders and power athletes develop larger and stronger muscles, a use that has no meaningful supporting evidence whatever.

Sources

Your body makes all the PS it needs. However, the only way to get a therapeutic dosage of PS is to take a supplement.

PS was originally manufactured from the brains of cows and all the studies described here used this form. However, because animal brain cells can harbor viruses, that form is no longer available. Most PS today is made from soybeans or other plant sources.

There are reasons to expect that plant-source PS should function very similarly to PS made from cows' brains, and some animal studies suggest that it is indeed effective. However, in preliminary trials, soy-based PS and cabbage-based PS failed to prove beneficial.

Therapeutic Dosages

For the purpose of improving mental function, PS is usually taken in dosages of 100 mg 2 to 3 times daily.

After maximum effect is achieved, the dosage can reportedly be reduced to 100 mg daily without losing benefit. PS can be taken with or without meals.

When taking PS for sports purposes, athletes sometimes take as much as 800 mg daily.

Therapeutic Uses

Meaningful evidence from numerous double-blind studies suggests that animal-source PS is an effective treatment for **Alzheimer's disease** and other forms of age-related mental decline. Vegetable-derived PS has little supporting evidence.

PS is widely marketed as a treatment for ordinary **age-related memory loss** as well. While there is little direct evidence that it works, in studies of severe mental decline, PS appears to have been equally effective whether the cause was Alzheimer's disease or something entirely unrelated, multiple small strokes. This certainly suggests that PS may have a positive impact on the brain that is not specific to any one condition. From this observation, it is not a great leap to suspect that it might be useful for much less severe problems with memory and mental function, such as those that seem to occur in nearly all of us who are older than 40. Indeed, one double-blind study did find that animal-source phosphatidylserine could improve mental function in individuals with relatively mild age-related memory loss; there is no supporting evidence for plant-based forms of PS at this time. However, two studies failed to find plant-source PS effective for this condition. PS has also been proposed for **enhancing mental function** in young people, but there is no direct evidence at all that any form is effective.

Animal-source PS has also shown a slight bit of promise for **depression**.

Recently, PS has become popular among athletes who hope it can help them **build muscle** more efficiently. This use is based on weak evidence that PS slows the release of cortisol following heavy exercise. Cortisol is a hormone that causes muscle tissue to break down. For reasons that are unclear, the body produces increased levels of cortisol after heavy exercise. Strength athletes believe that this natural cortisol release works against their efforts to rapidly build muscle mass and hope that PS will help them advance more quickly. However, only two double-blind, placebo-controlled studies of PS as a sports supplement have been reported, and neither one found effects on cortisol levels. Of these small trials, one found a possible ergogenic benefit and the other did not.

One study found preliminary evidence that a combination of soy-based PS and **lecithin** may moderate the body's reaction to mental **stress**.

What Is the Scientific Evidence for Phosphatidylserine?

Alzheimer's Disease and Other Forms of Dementia

Overall, the evidence for animal-source PS in dementia is fairly strong. Double-blind studies involving a total of more than 1,000 people suggest that phosphatidylserine is an effective treatment for Alzheimer's disease and other forms of dementia.

The largest of these studies followed 494 elderly subjects in northeastern Italy over a course of 6 months. All suffered from moderate to severe mental decline, as measured by standard tests. Treatment consisted of either 300 mg daily of PS or placebo. The group that took PS did significantly better in both behavior and mental function than the placebo group. Symptoms of depression also improved.

These results agree with those of numerous other smaller double-blind studies involving a total of more than 500 people with Alzheimer's and other types of age-related dementia. However, all these studies involved cow-brain PS; studies of plant-source PS for dementia have not been reported.

Ordinary Age-related Memory Loss

There is some evidence that PS can also help people with ordinary age-related memory loss. In one double-blind study that enrolled 149 people with memory loss but not dementia, phosphatidylserine provided significant benefits as compared with placebo. People with the most severe memory loss showed the most improvement.

However, another double-blind trial of 120 older people with memory complaints but not dementia failed to find benefits. This discrepancy may have to do with the type of phosphatidylserine used—the second trial used the more modern soy-derived form of the supplement (see Therapeutic Dosages above). A cabbage-based source of PS has also failed to prove effective for relatively mild memory loss.

Athletic Performance

Weak evidence suggests that PS might decrease the release of the hormone cortisol after intense exercise. Among its many effects, cortisol acts to break down muscle tissue—exactly the opposite of the effect desired by a strength athlete or bodybuilder. This double-blind, placebo-controlled study on 11 intensely trained athletes found that 800 mg of PS taken daily reduced the cortisol rise by 20% as compared with placebo. Another small study on 9 nonathletic males found that daily doses of 400 and 800 mg of PS reduced cortisol levels after exercise by 16% and 30%, respectively. Another study found that phosphatidylserine could relieve some overtraining symptoms, including muscle soreness, possibly due to effects on cortisol.

On the basis of these preliminary trials, PS has been proposed as a sports supplement. However, there is as yet no direct evidence to support the claims that PS actually helps athletes build muscles more quickly and with less training effort. Furthermore, the most recent and best-designed study, using vegetable-source PS, failed to find *any* effect on cortisol release, muscle soreness, or markers of muscle damage.

Safety Issues

Phosphatidylserine is generally regarded as safe when used at recommended dosages. Side effects are rare and when they do occur they usually consist of nothing much worse than mild gastrointestinal distress. One study found that use of phosphatidylserine did not alter results on standard medical screening tests. However, the maximum safe dosages for young children, pregnant or nursing women, or those with severe liver or kidney disease have not been established.

PS is sometimes taken with ginkgo because they both appear to enhance mental function. However, some caution might be in order: ginkgo is a "blood thinner," and PS might be one as well. PS is known to enhance the effect of heparin, a very strong prescription blood thinner. It is possible that combined use of PS and any drug or supplement that thins the blood could interfere with normal blood clotting enough to

Phyllanthus

cause problems. Some medications and supplements to consider include warfarin (Coumadin), aspirin, pentoxifylline (Trental), clopidogrel (Plavix), ticlopidine (Ticlid), garlic, ginkgo, and vitamin E.

Keep in mind, too, that Alzheimer's disease and other types of severe age-related mental impairment are too serious to treat on your own with PS or any other supplement. In some cases, the symptoms of these diseases could be confused with symptoms of other serious conditions. If you suspect that you or a loved one may have a severe age-related mental impairment, see your doctor for diagnosis and treatment.

Interactions You Should Know About

If you are taking:

- ➤ **Prescription blood thinners, such as warfarin (Coumadin), heparin, aspirin, pentoxifylline (Trental), clopidogrel (Plavix), or ticlopidine (Ticlid): Do not use phosphatidylserine except on a physician's advice.**
- ➤ **Ginkgo, garlic, or vitamin E: Taking phosphatidylserine at the same time might conceivably "thin" the blood too much.**

Phyllanthus

Phyllanthus amarus, Phyllanthus niruri, Phyllanthus urinaria

PRINCIPAL PROPOSED USES: *Chronic Hepatitis B*
OTHER PROPOSED USES: *Acute Hepatitis B*

Tropical plants in the genus *Phyllanthus* have a long history of use in **Ayurvedic** medicine (the traditional medicine of India) for the treatment of hepatitis, kidney and bladder problems, intestinal parasites, and diabetes. The most studied species is *Phyllanthus amarus*.

What Is Phyllanthus Used for Today?

Hepatitis B is a two-stage illness. It has an acute phase which causes jaundice, severe fatigue, and other symptoms. These symptoms usually resolve in a month or so; however, the infection may then become chronic. Long-term infection with hepatitis B can spread the disease to other people and can also lead to liver injury or liver cancer.

P. amarus has undergone considerable evaluation as a treatment for chronic hepatitis B and a bit of study for acute hepatitis. However, the results have not been promising. The current consensus is that the herb is not helpful for hepatitis. *P. urinaria* also appears to be ineffective.

What Is the Scientific Evidence for Phyllanthus?

Despite numerous test tube and animal studies showing efficacy against the hepatitis B virus, *P. amarus* has generally not done well in human trials.

Only one study clearly found benefits and it was seriously flawed. In this 30-day, double-blind, placebo-controlled trial of 60 people with chronic hepatitis B, treatment with phyllanthus (200 mg 3 times daily) dramatically increased the odds of full recovery. In the treated group, almost 60% were hepatitis B–negative at follow-up, as compared to only 4% in the placebo group.

However, the high drop-out rate in the placebo group significantly reduces the reliability of the results. Furthermore, multiple follow-up studies attempting to reproduce these findings have not found any benefits.

Another double-blind, placebo-controlled trial enrolled 57 people with acute hepatitis B to see whether treatment with *P. amarus* (300 mg 3 times daily for 1 week) could improve speed of recovery. The results showed no benefit. However, because acute hepatitis B usually lasts a month or more, the duration of treatment in this study was oddly short.

One highly preliminary study suggested that *P. urinaria*, a related species, might be more effective against hepatitis than other species of phyllanthus. However, a subsequent double-blind, placebo-controlled study designed to test this hypothesis failed to find benefit.

Dosage

The usual dose of *P. amarus* used in studies is 600 to 900 mg daily.

Safety Issues

There are no indications that *P. amarus* is toxic when used at recommended doses, but comprehensive safety studies have not been performed. In double-blind studies, significant side effects have not been reported. Safety in pregnant or nursing women, or individuals with severe liver or kidney disease, has not been established.

Plantain

Plantago lanceolata, Plantago major

PRINCIPAL PROPOSED USES: *None*

OTHER PROPOSED USES: *Anti-inflammatory, Chronic Bronchitis, Skin Conditions (Topical Use)*

Plantain (not to be confused with the relative of the banana known by the same name) is a small weed often found in cultivated fields and at the edge of lawns. Traditionally, the crushed leaves were applied to the skin to treat wounds and bites, a leaf tincture was used for coughs, and the dried leaf was taken internally for the treatment of bronchitis, ulcers, epilepsy, and liver problems.

What Is Plantain Used for Today?

Very weak evidence, too weak to rely upon at all, has been used to indicate that topical plantain is helpful for skin conditions, including poison ivy and **eczema**.

Similarly weak evidence from two studies performed in Bulgaria hint that oral plantain may be helpful for **chronic bronchitis**.

Plantain extracts do appear to have anti-inflammatory effects, at least in the test tube. However, unlike most pharmaceutical anti-inflammatory drugs, which work on the cyclooxygenase-1 (COX-1) and cyclooxygenase-2 (COX-2) systems, one study suggests that plantain may work in a different fashion, by decreasing levels of nitric oxide. Whether this indicates any real potential benefit in people remains unknown.

Other possible actions of plantain constituents based on test-tube studies include **anti-cancer** effects and antiviral actions.

Contrary to some reports, one study found that plantain does not have diuretic (kidney-stimulating) effects.

Dosage

A typical dose of plantain for oral use is 1 to 3 g 3 times daily. Syrups and tinctures are used for coughs.

Plantain contains active substances in the iridoid glycoside family, especially aucubin, catalpol, and acteoside. The highest levels are found when the plant is collected in mid-fall. Other potentially active ingredients fall in the phenolic category, such as caffeic acid. Some plantain products are standardized to levels of one or more of these ingredients, but it is not clear whether this produces a "better" product.

Safety Issues

Plantain appears to be relatively safe, but comprehensive safety studies have not been performed.

Plantain grown in soil contaminated with heavy metals, such as thallium or antimony, may develop relatively high concentrations of these potential toxins.

In 1997, the FDA reported that some "plantain" available for sale on the herb market was contaminated with similar-appearing foxglove (digitalis), an herb with potent and potentially toxic effects on the heart.

Safety in pregnant or nursing women, young children, or individuals with liver or kidney disease has not been established.

Pokeroot

Phytolacca americana

RELATED TERM: *Pokeweed*

PRINCIPAL PROPOSED USES: *We recommend against using pokeroot at all.*

The herb pokeroot grows wild in many parts of North America. The name comes from a Native American word, *pocan*, a term that indicates any plant used to provide a red-colored dye. Pokeroot is a source of a blood-red pigment. Medicinally, it was used as an *alterative*, a substance that supposedly removes toxins from the body and restores overall health. Like other alteratives, pokeroot was used for the treatment of cancer, skin conditions, and many other diseases attributed to toxins. Pokeroot causes vomiting and diarrhea, and these effects were also traditionally considered salutary. However, in modern times, it has become clear that pokeroot causes vomiting and diarrhea because it is toxic; it should not be used at all.

What Is Pokeroot Used for Today?

Pokeroot itself is not sold in the United States. However, substances found in pokeroot have shown promise for drug development. One of these, *pokeroot antiviral protein*, has shown potential as a treatment for **HIV** and other viral infections.

Note, however, that these findings on one ingredient of pokeroot do not indicate that the whole herb is useful for HIV infection.

Another substance in pokeroot, *pokeweed mitogen*, forces cells to divide, a property that has led to a great deal of scientific investigation.

These mitogenic effects are potentially quite dangerous and are more an argument against the use of pokeroot than for it.

Other pokeroot constituents have shown potential anti-inflammatory, diuretic, and blood pressure–lowering effects.

Dosage

We recommend against using pokeroot in any dosage.

Safety Issues

Pokeroot is a toxic herb. Ingestion can lead to symptoms such as nausea, vomiting (sometimes with blood), diarrhea, rapid heart rate, a dangerous fall in blood pressure, difficult breathing, confusion, and death. Symptoms may develop with one-time use or insidiously over time. Fresh root is more toxic than dried root. The juice of pokeweed berries is more toxic still and can cause severe damage to blood cells even when it is only applied to the skin. Pokeroot should definitely not be used by pregnant or nursing women or young children.

Policosanol

SUPPLEMENT FORMS/ALTERNATE NAMES: *1-Octacosanol, N-Octacosanol, Octacosanol, Octacosyl Alcohol, Wheat Germ Oil*

PRINCIPAL PROPOSED USES: *High Cholesterol*

OTHER PROPOSED USES: *Intermittent Claudication, Parkinson's Disease, Sports Performance Enhancement*

Policosanol is a mixture of waxy substances generally manufactured from sugarcane. It contains about 60% octacosanol, along with many related chemicals. In some

cases, the terms *octacosanol* and *policosanol* are used interchangeably.

Numerous studies have reported that sugarcane

policosanol can substantially improve cholesterol profile, with an efficacy approximately equal to that of the most effective drugs used for this purpose. On this basis, policosanol has been approved as a treatment for high cholesterol in about two dozen countries, most of them in Latin America. However, virtually all studies of policosanol were performed and reported by the single research group owning the patent on the substance, while the only reliable independent trial failed to find any benefit. Because of this, all evidence regarding policosanol is under a cloud of possible conflict of interest.

Policosanol is also marketed as a performance-enhancing dietary supplement. It is said to increase muscle strength and endurance and improve reaction time and stamina, but there is no reliable scientific evidence as yet to support these claims.

Requirements/Sources

The tested Cuban policosanol product is manufactured from sugarcane. Octacosanol and related substances are also found in wheat germ oil, vegetable oils, **alfalfa**, and various animal products.

Due to political and patent issues, sugarcane policosanol has not been widely available in the U.S. Products sold in the U.S. market as "policosanol" generally contain "policosanol" manufactured from beeswax or wheat germ. These products have a significantly different mixture of constituents and could have substantially different effects.

Therapeutic Dosages

Typical dosages of policosanol in Cuban studies have ranged from 5 to 10 mg twice daily. Results required up to 2 months to develop.

Therapeutic Uses

The Cuban research group that owns the patent on policosanol has published perhaps 80 double-blind studies on their product, involving a total of thousands of people and ranging in length from 6 weeks to 12 months. The cumulative results of these trials appear to indicate that policosanol can reduce LDL ("bad") cholesterol by 21 to 29% and total cholesterol by a slightly lower amount; in addition, policosanol appears to raise HDL ("good") cholesterol by 8 to 15%. However, in 2006 a set of independent researchers set out to replicate the Cubans' re-

sults and failed to find that policosanol, even at high doses, had *any* significant effect on lipid profile. A single study cannot invalidate an entire body of research and yet this finding has raised the specter of unreliable research.

A separate study failed to find benefit with wheat-germ policosanol.

The Bottom Line: Until there are positive studies originating from a reliable independent source, all therapeutic claims about policosanol must be regarded with skepticism.

According to the same patent-holding Cuban research group, policosanol is helpful for **intermittent claudication**.

The only evidence for policosanol as a **performance enhancer** comes from one small double-blind trial with marginal results.

Marginal benefits were also seen in a very small double-blind trial of individuals with **Parkinson's disease**. However, policosanol might interfere with the drug levodopa, used for Parkinson's disease.

In a small double-blind trial, policosanol failed to produce any benefits in **amyotrophic lateral sclerosis**.

Safety Issues

Note: Virtually all statements made in this section derive from the Cuban research group described above and are, therefore, open to doubt.

Policosanol appears to be safe at the maximum recommended dose. In the double-blind trials described above, only mild short-term side effects were reported, such as nervousness, headache, diarrhea, and insomnia. In a study that followed 27,879 participants for 2 to 4 years, policosanol reportedly produced adverse effects in only 0.31%, primarily weight loss, excessive urination, and insomnia.

No toxic signs were observed in animals given very high doses of policosanol (as much as 620 times the maximum recommended dose). In addition, the evidence of one human trial suggests that policosanol does not adversely affect the liver.

Policosanol has been found not to interact with three types of medications used for high blood pressure: calcium-channel antagonists, diuretics, and beta-blockers. However, policosanol appears to be a "blood thinner," and it reportedly enhances the blood-thinning effects of aspirin. This suggests that policosanol should not be combined with aspirin or other blood-thinning drugs, such as warfarin (Coumadin), heparin, clopidogrel

Policosanol

(Plavix), ticlopidine (Ticlid), or pentoxifylline (Trental). There is also at least a remote chance that it might cause excessive bleeding if combined with natural supplements that thin the blood, such as garlic, ginkgo, and high-dose vitamin E. Similarly, individuals with clotting problems should avoid policosanol and policosanol should not be used during the period immediately prior to or following surgery or labor and delivery.

One report suggests that policosanol might increase the action of levodopa, a medication used for Parkinson's disease, leading to increased side effects called *dyskinesias*.

The maximum safe dosages for young children, pregnant or nursing women, or individuals with severe liver or kidney disease have not been established.

Interactions You Should Know About

If you are taking:

> Blood-thinning medications such as aspirin, warfarin (Coumadin), heparin, clopidogrel (Plavix), ticlopidine (Ticlid), or pentoxifylline (Trental), or natural supplements that thin the blood, such as garlic, ginkgo, or high-dose vitamin E: Do not use policosanol except on medical advice.
> Levodopa: Keep in mind that policosanol may increase both the effects and side effects of the drug.

Potassium

SUPPLEMENT FORMS/ALTERNATE NAMES: , *Chelated Potassium (Potassium Aspartate, Potassium Citrate), Potassium Bicarbonate, Potassium Chloride*

PRINCIPAL PROPOSED USES: *Hypertension*

Potassium is a mineral found in many foods and supplements. But you will never see pure potassium in a health food store or pharmacy—it's a highly reactive metal that bursts into flame when exposed to water! The potassium you eat, or take as a supplement, is composed of potassium atoms bound to other nonmetallic substances—less exciting, perhaps, but chemically stable.

Potassium is one of the major electrolytes in your body, along with sodium and chloride. Potassium and sodium work together like a molecular seesaw: when the level of one goes up, the other goes down. All together, these three dissolved minerals play an intimate chemical role in every function of your body.

The most common use of potassium supplements is to make up for potassium depletion caused by diuretic drugs. These medications are often used to help regulate blood pressure, but by depleting the body of potassium they may inadvertently make blood pressure harder to control.

Requirements/Sources

Potassium is an essential mineral that we get from many common foods. True potassium deficiencies are rare except in cases of prolonged vomiting or diarrhea or with the use of diuretic drugs.

However, in one sense potassium deficiency is common, at least when compared to the amount of sodium we receive in our diets. It is probably healthy to take in at least five times as much potassium as sodium (and perhaps 50 to 100 times as much). But the standard American diet contains twice as much sodium as potassium. Therefore, taking extra potassium may be a good idea in order to balance the sodium we consume to such excess.

Bananas, orange juice, potatoes, avocados, lima beans, cantaloupes, peaches, tomatoes, flounder, salmon, and cod all contain more than 300 mg of potassium per serving. Other good sources include chicken, meat, and various other fruits, vegetables, and fish.

Over-the-counter potassium supplements typically contain 99 mg of potassium per tablet. There is some evidence that, of the different forms of potassium supplements, potassium citrate may be most helpful for those with high blood pressure.

Research indicates that it is important to get enough **magnesium**, too, when you are taking potassium. It might be wise to take extra **vitamin B$_{12}$** as well.

Therapeutic Dosages

When used by physicians, potassium is usually measured according to meq (milliequivalents) rather than the more common mg (milligrams). A typical therapeutic dosage of potassium is between 10 and 20 meq, taken 3 to 4 times daily.

Therapeutic Uses

Potassium may be mildly helpful for **hypertension**.

What Is the Scientific Evidence for Potassium?

According to a review of 33 double-blind studies, potassium supplements can produce a slight but definite drop in blood pressure. However, two large studies found *no* benefit. The explanation is probably that potassium is only slightly helpful. When a treatment has only a small effect, it's not unusual for some studies to show no effect while others find a modest benefit. It's possible that potassium may only help people who are at least a bit deficient in this mineral.

Evidence suggests that potassium supplements may be most effective for people who eat too much salt.

Safety Issues

As an essential nutrient, potassium is safe when taken at appropriate dosages. If you take a bit too much, your body will simply excrete it in the urine. However, people who have severe kidney disease cannot excrete potassium normally and should consult a physician before taking a potassium supplement. Similarly, individuals taking potassium-sparing diuretics (such as spironolactone), ACE inhibitors (such as captopril), or trimethoprim/sulfamethoxazole should also not take potassium supplements except under doctor supervision.

Potassium pills can cause injury to the esophagus if they get stuck on the way down, so make sure to take them with plenty of water.

Interactions You Should Know About

If you are taking:

- **Loop diuretics or thiazide diuretics: You may need more potassium.**
- **ACE inhibitors (such as captopril, lisinopril, enalapril), potassium-sparing diuretics (such as triamterene or spironolactone), or trimethoprim/sulfamethoxazole: You should not take potassium except on the advice of a physician.**
- **Potassium: You may need extra magnesium and vitamin B$_{12}$.**

Prickly Ash

Zanthoxylum clava-herculis, Zanthoxylum americanum

PRINCIPAL PROPOSED USES: *None*

OTHER PROPOSED USES: *Dry Mouth, Intermittent Claudication, Osteoarthritis, Raynaud's Syndrome, Toothache (Topical)*

The prickly ash tree has a long history of use in Native American medicine. The bark was used to treat intestinal cramps, dry mouth, muscle and joint pain, toothache, nervous disorders, arthritis, and leg ulcers. The berries were used for circulatory problems such as **intermittent claudication** and **Raynaud's syndrome**.

What Is Prickly Ash Used for Today?

There are no documented medical uses of prickly ash bark.

In test-tube studies, substances called *furanocoumarins* in prickly ash have shown anti-fungal properties. Another prickly ash constituent, *chelerythrine*, has shown activity against antibiotic-resistant staph bacteria. However, it is a long way from studies like these to actual evidence of efficacy. Only double-blind, placebo-controlled studies can actually show that a treatment works, and none have been performed on prickly ash. (For information on why such studies are essential, see **Why Does This Book Rely on Double-blind Studies?**.)

Dosage

Prickly ash is often taken in the form of tea, made by boiling 5 to 10 g of the bark in a cup of water for 10 to 15 minutes. For toothache, the pieces of the bark may be chewed. Tinctures are also available.

Safety Issues

Prickly ash has not undergone any modern scientific safety evaluation. It contains potentially toxic alkaloids; whether or not these lead to any harmful effects remains unknown. Safety in young children, pregnant or nursing women, or people with severe liver or kidney disease has not been established.

Progesterone

SUPPLEMENT FORMS/ALTERNATE NAMES: *Micronized Progesterone, Natural Progesterone, Progesterone Cream*

PRINCIPAL PROPOSED USES:

   Oral Uses: *Replacement for Standard Progestins*

OTHER PROPOSED USES:

   Topical Uses: *Menopausal Symptoms*

PROBABLY NOT EFFECTIVE USES:

   Topical Uses: *"Opposing" Estrogen, Preventing or Treating Osteoporosis*

Progesterone is one of the two primary female hormones. As the name implies, progesterone prepares ("pro") the womb for pregnancy (gestation). Progesterone works in tandem with **estrogen**; indeed, if estrogen is taken as a medication without being balanced by progesterone (so-called unopposed estrogen), there is an increased risk of uterine cancer.

However, progesterone is not well absorbed orally. For this reason, pharmaceutical manufacturers developed *progestins*, substances similar to progesterone which are more easily absorbed. Most of the time, a woman prescribed "progesterone" is really being given a progestin. Two of the most commonly used progestins are medroxyprogesterone and norethindrone. However, it has been suggested that actual progesterone may offer benefits over progestins, such as fewer side effects.

Progesterone can be absorbed through the skin to some extent and some alternative practitioners have, for years, promoted the use of progesterone creams. Such progesterone creams are typically, but misleadingly, said to contain "natural" progesterone. This is an oddly chosen term, as the progesterone in these creams is actually produced in a laboratory, just like other synthetic hormones. To avoid confusion in this article, we will call progesterone *true progesterone*, or just *progesterone*.

Besides creams, a special form of true progesterone that can be absorbed orally, micronized progesterone, has recently become available as a prescription drug.

Inconsistent evidence suggests that progesterone cream might help reduce menopausal symptoms. However, it does not appear to be strong enough to balance the effects of estrogen, thus reducing the risk of uterine cancer. (Oral micronized progesterone *is* strong enough for this purpose.) Contrary to numerous books and magazine articles, there is no more than weak, inconsistent evidence that progesterone cream offers any benefits for osteoporosis.

Requirements/Sources

Progesterone is synthesized in the body and is not found in appreciable quantities in food. For use as a drug or "dietary supplement," progesterone is synthesized from chemicals found in **soy** or **Mexican yam**.

Note: Another aspect of the widespread misinformation involving progesterone cream is the concept that Mexican yam itself contains progesterone or substances that the body can convert into progesterone. This is incorrect. Industrial chemists can convert a constituent of Mexican yam (diosgenin) into progesterone, but only by using chemical pathways not found in the body.

Therapeutic Dosages

The usual dose of progesterone in cream form is 20 mg daily. Although this dose might decrease **menopausal hot flashes**, most studies found that even doses as high as 64 mg daily do not provide enough progesterone to protect the uterus from the effects of estrogen. However, one study found that use of micronized progesterone *cream* at 80 mg daily produced similar progesterone levels in the body as an *oral* dose of 200 mg daily; oral micronized progesterone taken at a dose of 200 to 400 mg daily is approximately as effective as the standard dosage of the more commonly used progestins.

Therapeutic Uses

Progesterone cream was widely promoted in the 1990s as a treatment for **osteoporosis**, on the basis of meaningless "studies" whose designs were too poor to establish anything at all. When properly designed studies were performed, the results were at best inconsistent.

Studies conflict on whether progesterone cream can help hot flashes. One double-blind, placebo-controlled study failed to find any improvements in mood or **general well-being** in menopausal women using progesterone cream.

Like progestins, oral progesterone protects the uterus from the stimulating effects of unopposed estrogen. However, standard doses of progesterone cream probably provide too little progesterone to serve for this purpose (see next section).

What Is the Scientific Evidence for Progesterone?

Osteoporosis

Despite widespread reporting that true progesterone is effective for treating or preventing osteoporosis, the evidence for such an effect is at best inconsistent.

This notion began with test tube and other preliminary studies suggesting that progesterone or progestins can stimulate the activity of cells that build bone. Subsequently, a poorly designed and uncontrolled study (really, a series of case histories from one physician's practice) purportedly demonstrated that progesterone cream can slow or even reverse osteoporosis.

However, a 1-year, double-blind trial of 102 women given either progesterone cream (providing 20 mg progesterone daily) or placebo cream, along with calcium and multivitamins, found no evidence of any improvements in bone density attributable to progesterone. A smaller, short-term trial found that progesterone cream has no effect on bone metabolism.

In contrast to these negative results, benefits *were* seen in a small 2-year, double-blind, placebo-controlled study in which 22 women were given progesterone cream. (Interestingly, in this study, use of progesterone cream plus soy isoflavones produced inferior benefits to those of progesterone cream alone.) It is therefore at least possible that progesterone cream is helpful for osteoporosis if taken for a long enough period; however, more research is needed.

Menopausal Symptoms

In the 1-year, double-blind trial of 102 women described above, use of progesterone cream was found to significantly reduce hot flashes and related symptoms. However, a slightly smaller 12-week, double-blind trial failed to find progesterone cream helpful for reducing menopausal symptoms. The authors of this second study point out that the first study was statistically flawed.

Opposing Estrogen

Unless you have had a hysterectomy, if you take estrogen, you need to take progesterone too or you run the risk of uterine cancer. Two 12-week, double-blind studies enrolling a total of about 100 women found that progesterone cream (at doses up to 64 mg) did not have the required protective effect on the cells of the uterus.

One study, however, did find benefit at dosages of either 15 or 40 mg daily. The explanation for these disparate results may lie in the results of two other studies, which suggest that progesterone cream is erratically absorbed.

Safety Issues

Even though progesterone is sold as a dietary supplement, it is a hormone, not a food. We recommend that it *not* be used except under physician supervision.

Like progestins, true progesterone causes side effects. In one study, oral micronized progesterone at a dose of 400 mg per day was associated with dizziness, abdominal cramping, headache, breast pain, muscle pain, irritability, nausea, fatigue, diarrhea, and viral infections.

Proteolytic Enzymes

SUPPLEMENT FORMS/ALTERNATE NAMES: *Bromelain, Chymotrypsin, Digestive Enzymes, Pancreatin, Papain, Trypsin*

PRINCIPAL PROPOSED USES:

Pain Conditions: *Neck Pain and Other Forms of Chronic Musculoskeletal Pain, Osteoarthritis, Shingles (Herpes Zoster), Sports Injuries, Surgery Support*

Digestive Uses: *Dyspepsia, Pancreatic Insufficiency*

OTHER PROPOSED USES: *Breast Engorgement, Enhancing Sports Performance, Food Allergies, Reducing Side Effects of Radiation Therapy for Cancer, Rheumatoid Arthritis*

Proteolytic enzymes help you digest the proteins in food. Although your body produces these enzymes in the pancreas, certain foods also contain proteolytic enzymes.

Papaya and pineapple are two of the richest plant sources, as attested by their traditional use as natural "tenderizers" for meat. Papain and **bromelain** are the respective names for the proteolytic enzymes found in these fruits. The enzymes made in your body are called *trypsin* and *chymotrypsin*.

The primary use of proteolytic enzymes is as a digestive aid for people who have trouble digesting proteins. However, proteolytic enzymes may also be absorbed internally to some extent and may reduce pain and inflammation.

Sources

You don't need to get proteolytic enzymes from food because the body manufactures them (primarily trypsin and chymotrypsin). However, deficiencies in proteolytic enzymes do occur, usually resulting from diseases of the pancreas (pancreatic insufficiency). Symptoms include abdominal discomfort, gas, indigestion, poor absorption of nutrients, and passing undigested food in the stool.

For use as a supplement, trypsin and chymotrypsin are extracted from the pancreas of various animals. You can also purchase bromelain extracted from pineapple stems and papain made from papayas.

Therapeutic Dosages

When you purchase an enzyme, the amount is expressed not only in grams or milligrams but also in *activity units* or *international units*. These terms refer to the enzyme's potency (specifically, its digestive power).

Recommended dosages of proteolytic enzymes vary with the form used. Because of the wide variation, we suggest following label instructions.

Proteolytic enzymes can be broken down by stomach acid. To prevent this from happening, supplemental enzymes are often coated with a substance that doesn't dissolve until it reaches the intestine. Such a preparation is called *enteric coated*.

Therapeutic Uses

The most obvious use of proteolytic enzymes is to assist digestion. However, a small, double-blind, placebo-controlled trial found no benefit from proteolytic enzymes as a treatment for **dyspepsia** (indigestion).

Proteolytic enzymes can also be absorbed into the body whole and may help reduce inflammation and pain; however, the evidence is inconsistent. Several studies found that proteolytic enzymes might be helpful for **neck pain, osteoarthritis**, and **post-herpetic neuralgia** (an aftereffect of shingles). However, all of these studies suffer from significant limitations (such as the absence of a placebo group) and none provide substantially reliable information.

Studies performed decades ago suggest that proteolytic enzymes may help reduce the pain and discomfort that follows injuries (especially sports injuries). However, a more recent, better-designed, and far larger study failed to find benefit.

Proteolytic enzymes have also been evaluated as an aid to recovery from the pain and inflammation caused by **surgery**, but most studies are decades old and in any case the results were mixed.

One early double-blind, placebo-controlled trial found that use of proteolytic enzymes helped reduce the discomfort of breast engorgement in **lactating women**.

One recent study tested combination therapy with bromelain and ibuprofen for **enhancing recovery from heavy exercise** by decreasing delayed-onset muscle soreness, but found no benefits.

Another recent study failed to find proteolytic enzymes helpful for reducing side effects of **radiation therapy** for cancer.

Some alternative medicine practitioners believe that proteolytic enzymes may help reduce symptoms of **food allergies**, presumably by digesting the food so well that there is less to be allergic to; however, there is no scientific evidence for this proposed use.

Another theory popular in certain alternative medicine circles suggests that proteolytic enzymes can aid **rheumatoid arthritis, multiple sclerosis, lupus**, and other autoimmune diseases. Supposedly, these diseases are made worse when whole proteins from foods leak into the blood and cause immune reactions. Digestive enzymes are said to help foil this so-called leaky gut problem. Again, however, there is no meaningful evidence to substantiate this theory. Furthermore, one fairly large (301-participant) study failed to find proteolytic enzymes helpful for multiple sclerosis.

What Is the Scientific Evidence for Proteolytic Enzymes?

Most of the studies described in this section used combination products containing various proteolytic enzymes plus other substances, such as the **bioflavonoid** rutin.

Osteoarthritis and Other Forms of Chronic Musculoskeletal Pain

Several studies provide preliminary evidence that proteolytic enzymes might be helpful for various forms of chronic pain, including neck pain and osteoarthritis.

➣ *Neck Pain*

A double-blind, placebo-controlled trial of 30 people with chronic neck pain found that use of a proteolytic enzyme mixture modestly reduced pain symptoms as compared to placebo.

➣ *Osteoarthritis*

Studies enrolling a total of more than 400 people compared proteolytic enzymes to the standard anti-inflammatory drug diclofenac for the treatment of osteoarthritis-related conditions of the shoulder, back, or knee. The results generally showed equivalent benefits with the supplement as with the medication. However, all of these studies suffered from various flaws that limit their reliability; the most important was the absence of a placebo group.

Shingles *(Herpes Zoster)*

Herpes zoster (**shingles**) is an acute, painful infection caused by the varicella-zoster virus, the organism that causes chicken pox. Proteolytic enzymes have been suggested as treatment. However, there is little evidence to support their use.

A double-blind study of 190 people with shingles compared proteolytic enzymes to the standard antiviral drug acyclovir. Participants were treated for 14 days and their pain was assessed at intervals. Although both groups had similar pain relief, the enzyme-treated group experienced fewer side effects. However, since acyclovir offer minimal benefit at most, these results don't mean very much.

Similar results were seen in another double-blind study in which 90 people were given either an injection of acyclovir or enzymes, followed by a course of oral medication for 7 days.

Sports Injuries

Several small studies have found proteolytic enzyme combinations helpful for the treatment of sports injuries. However, the best and largest trial by far failed to find benefit.

A double-blind, placebo-controlled study of 44 people with sports-related ankle injuries found that treatment with proteolytic enzymes resulted in faster healing and reduced the time away from training by about 50%. Based on these results, a very large (721-participant) double-blind, placebo-controlled trial of people with sprained ankles was undertaken. Unfortunately, this study failed to find benefit with rutin, bromelain, or trypsin, separately or in combination.

Three other small double-blind studies, involving a total of about 80 athletes, found that treatment with proteolytic enzymes significantly speeded healing of bruises and other mild athletic injuries as compared to placebo. In another double-blind trial, 100 people were given an injection of their own blood under the skin to simulate bruising following an injury. Researchers found that treatment with a proteolytic enzyme combination significantly speeded up recovery. In addition, a double-blind, placebo-controlled trial of 71 people with finger fractures found that treatment with proteolytic enzymes significantly improved recovery. However, these studies were performed decades ago and are not quite up to modern standards.

Surgery

Numerous studies have evaluated various proteolytic enzymes as an aid to recovery from surgery, but the results have been mixed. Again, most of these studies are not up to modern standards.

A double-blind, placebo-controlled trial of 80 people undergoing knee surgery found that treatment with mixed proteolytic enzymes after surgery significantly improved rate of recovery, as measured by mobility and swelling.

Another double-blind, placebo-controlled trial evaluated the effects of a similar mixed proteolytic enzyme product in 80 individuals undergoing oral surgery. The results showed reduced pain, inflammation, and swelling in the treated group as compared to the placebo group. Benefits were also seen in another trial of mixed proteolytic enzymes for dental surgery, as well as in one study involving only bromelain.

A double-blind, placebo-controlled study of 204 women receiving episiotomies during **childbirth** found evidence that a mixed proteolytic enzyme product can reduce inflammation. Bromelain was also found helpful for reducing inflammation following episiotomy in one double-blind, placebo-controlled trial of 160 women, but a very similar study found no benefit.

Other double-blind, placebo-controlled studies have found that bromelain reduces inflammation and pain following nasal surgery, cataract removal, and foot surgery. However, a study of 154 individuals undergoing facial plastic surgery found no benefit.

Safety Issues

In studies, proteolytic enzymes are believed to have proven to be quite safe, although they can occasionally cause digestive upset and allergic reactions.

One proteolytic enzyme, pancreatin, may interfere with **folate** absorption. In addition, the proteolytic enzyme papain might increase the blood-thinning effects of warfarin and possibly other anticoagulants.

The proteolytic enzyme bromelain might also cause problems if combined with drugs that thin the blood. In addition, there are concerns that bromelain should not be mixed with sedative drugs. Finally, bromelain may increase blood concentrations of certain antibiotics.

Interactions You Should Know About

If you are taking:

- ➤ **The proteolytic enzyme pancreatin: You may need extra folate.**
- ➤ **Warfarin (Coumadin), aspirin, or other drugs that "thin" the blood: You should not take the proteolytic enzymes papain or bromelain except under a doctor's supervision.**
- ➤ **Sedative drugs: Do not take bromelain, except under a physician's supervision.**

Pumpkin Seed

Cucurbita pepo, Cucurbita maxima

PRINCIPAL PROPOSED USES: *Benign Prostatic Hyperplasia (BPH)*
OTHER PROPOSED USES: *Kidney Stones, Parasites*

The familiar Halloween pumpkin is a member of the squash family, native to North and Central America. The seeds of the pumpkin were used medicinally in Native American medicine, primarily for the treatment of kidney, bladder, and digestive problems. From 1863 to 1936, the United States Pharmacopoeia listed pumpkin seeds as a treatment for intestinal parasites.

What Is Pumpkin Seed Used for Today?

Pumpkin seed oil has become popular today as a treatment for **prostate enlargement** (benign prostatic hyperplasia, or BPH) and it was approved for this use in 1985 by Germany's Commission E. However, there is no meaningful evidence that pumpkin seed is helpful for this condition. Only double-blind, placebo-controlled studies can prove a treatment effective, and none have been reported for pumpkin seed oil alone. (For information on why this type of study is essential, see **Why Does This Book Rely on Double-blind Studies?**.) However, two such studies evaluated a combination product containing pumpkin seed oil and the herb **saw palmetto**.

These studies did suggest benefit with the combination product, but since saw palmetto is thought to be effective for BPH, it is not clear whether pumpkin seed oil made any additional contribution.

The only reported study on pumpkin seed oil alone lacked a placebo group and, for this reason, its results prove little. (BPH is a condition that responds greatly to the power of suggestion, so it could have been assumed even before conducting this trial that people given pumpkin seed oil would show improvement.)

In highly preliminary research, pumpkin seed or its constituent curcurbitin has shown some activity against intestinal parasites.

These studies, however, can only be regarded as highly preliminary investigations of a traditional use; they were not designed in such a way that they could prove effectiveness.

Two studies performed in Thailand hint that pumpkin seed snacks might help prevent **kidney stones** among children at high risk for developing them. However, this research only looked at chemical changes in the urine suggestive of a possible preventive effect, not actual reduction of stones. Furthermore, the design of the studies did not reach modern standards.

Dosage

In studies, the dose of pumpkin seed oil used for the treatment of BPH was 160 mg 3 times daily. For the prevention of kidney stones, the dose of pumpkin seed snack tried was 5 to 10 g per day.

Safety Issues

As a widely eaten food, pumpkin seeds are presumed to be safe (though there have been cases in which incompletely chewed up seeds have gotten stuck in the esophagus!). There are as yet no known or suspected safety risks with pumpkin seed oil.

Pygeum

Pygeum africanus

PRINCIPAL PROPOSED USES: *Benign Prostatic Hyperplasia (Prostate Enlargement)*

OTHER PROPOSED USES: *Impotence, Male Infertility, Prostatitis*

The pygeum tree (pronounced *pie-jee-um*) is a tall evergreen native to central and southern Africa. Its bark has been used since ancient times to treat problems with urination.

What Is Pygeum Used for Today?

Today, pygeum is primarily used as a treatment for benign prostatic hyperplasia (BPH), or prostate enlargement. This use is supported by scientific evidence about as strong as that for the more famous natural BPH remedy, **saw palmetto**. However, saw palmetto is probably the better treatment to use. The pygeum tree has been so devastated by collection for use in medicine that some regard it as a threatened species. Saw palmetto is cultivated rather than collected in the wild.

Besides BPH, pygeum is also sometimes proposed for **prostatitis**, as well as **impotence** and **male infertility**; however, there is little real evidence that it works for these conditions.

What Is the Scientific Evidence for Pygeum?

At least 17 double-blind trials of pygeum for BPH have been performed, involving a total of nearly 1,000 individuals and ranging in length from 45 to 90 days. Many of these studies were poorly reported and/or designed. Nonetheless, the results overall make a meaningful case that pygeum can reduce symptoms such as nighttime urination, urinary frequency, and residual urine volume.

The best of these studies was conducted at 8 sites in Europe and included 263 men between 50 and 85 years of age. Participants received 50 mg of a pygeum extract or placebo twice daily. The results showed significant improvements in residual urine volume, voided volume, urinary flow rate, nighttime urination, and daytime frequency.

We don't really know how pygeum works. Unlike the standard drug finasteride, it does not appear to work by affecting the conversion of testosterone to dihydrotestosterone. Rather it is thought to reduce inflammation in the prostate, and also to inhibit prostate growth factors, substances implicated in inappropriate prostate enlargement.

Dosage

The usual dosage of pygeum is 50 mg twice per day (occasionally 100 mg twice daily) of an extract standardized to contain 14% triterpenes and 0.5% n-docosanol. A dose of 100 mg once daily appears to be as effective as the most common dosage of 50 mg twice daily.

There is some reason to believe that pygeum's effectiveness might be enhanced when it is combined with **nettle root**, another natural treatment for BPH.

Safety Issues

Pygeum appears to be essentially nontoxic, both in the short and long term. The most common side effect is mild gastrointestinal distress. However, safety in young children, pregnant or nursing women, or those with severe liver or kidney disease has not been established.

Pyruvate

SUPPLEMENT FORMS/ALTERNATE NAMES: *Calcium Pyruvate, Dihydroxyacetone Pyruvate (DHAP), Magnesium Pyruvate, Potassium Pyruvate, Sodium Pyruvate*

PRINCIPAL PROPOSED USES: *Weight Loss*

OTHER PROPOSED USES: *Sports Performance Enhancement*

Pyruvate supplies the body with pyruvic acid, a natural compound that plays important roles in the manufacture and use of energy. Pyruvate supplements have become popular with bodybuilders and other athletes, based on claims that pyruvate can reduce body fat and enhance the ability to use energy efficiently. However, at the present time, there is only preliminary evidence that it really works.

Sources

Pyruvate is not an essential nutrient, since your body makes all it needs. But it can be found in food, with an average diet supplying anywhere from 100 mg to 2 g daily. Apples are the best source: a single apple contains about 450 mg of pyruvate. Beer and red wine contain about 75 mg per serving.

Therapeutic dosages are usually much higher than what you can get from food: you'd have to eat almost 70 apples a day to get the proper amount! To use pyruvate for therapeutic purposes, you must take a supplement.

Although most products on the market contain only (or almost only) pyruvate, some also contain a related compound, dihydroxyacetone, which the body converts to pyruvate. The combination of the two products is known as DHAP.

Therapeutic Dosages

A typical therapeutic dosage of pyruvate is 30 g daily, although 6 to 44 g daily have been used in studies. Dihydroxyacetone dosages in studies of DHAP (pyruvate plus dihydroxyacetone) have ranged from 12 to 75 g daily.

Therapeutic Uses

Evidence from several small placebo-controlled studies suggests that pyruvate may enhance **weight loss**.

Pyruvate is also marketed as a **sports performance supplement**, but the supporting evidence for this use is weak and contradictory at best.

What Is the Scientific Evidence for Pyruvate?

Several small studies enrolling a total of about 150 individuals have found evidence that pyruvate or DHAP can aid weight loss and/or improve body composition (the proportion of fat to muscle tissue).

For example, in a 6-week, double-blind, placebo-controlled trial, 51 individuals were given either pyruvate (6 g daily), placebo, or no treatment. All participated in an exercise program. In the treated group, significant decreases in fat mass (2.1 kg) and percentage body fat (2.6%) were seen, along with a significant increase in muscle mass (1.5 kg). No significant changes were seen in the placebo or non-treatment groups.

Another placebo-controlled study (blinding not stated) used a much higher dose of pyruvate, 22 to 44 g daily depending on total calorie intake. In this trial, 34 slightly overweight individuals were put on a mildly weight-reducing diet for 4 weeks. Subsequently, half were given a liquid dietary supplement containing pyruvate. Over the course of 6 weeks, individuals in the pyruvate group lost a small amount of weight (about 1.5 pounds) while those in the placebo group did not lose weight. Most of the weight loss came from fat.

A third placebo-controlled study evaluated the effects of combined dihydroxyacetone and pyruvate (DHAP) when individuals who had previously lost weight increased their calorie intake. Seventeen severely overweight women were put on a restricted diet as inpatients for 3 weeks, during which time they lost an average of approximately 17 pounds. They were then given a high-calorie diet. Approximately half of the women also received 15 g of pyruvate and 75 g of dihydroxyacetone daily. The results showed that after 3 weeks of this weight-gaining diet, individuals receiving the supplements gained only about 4 pounds, as compared to about 6 pounds in the placebo group. Close evaluation showed that pyruvate specifically blocked regain of fat weight.

While all these studies are intriguing, we really need large studies (100 participants or more) to establish the potential benefits of pyruvate for weight loss.

Safety Issues

Both pyruvate and dihydroxyacetone appear to be quite safe, aside from mild side effects, such as occasional stomach upset and diarrhea. Very weak evidence (too weak to get very concerned about) hints that pyruvate supplements might adversely affect **cholesterol** profile by negating the positive effects of exercise on HDL ("good" cholesterol).

Maximum safe dosages for children, women who are pregnant or nursing, or those with liver or kidney disease have not been established.

Keep in mind that if a contaminant were present even in very small percentages there could be harmful results due to the enormous doses of pyruvate used. For this reason, you should make sure to use a high-quality product.

Quercetin

SUPPLEMENT FORMS/ALTERNATE NAMES: *Quercetin Chalcone*

PRINCIPAL PROPOSED USES: *None*

OTHER PROPOSED USES: *Allergies (Hay Fever), Antiviral, Asthma, Cancer Prevention, Eczema, Heart Disease Prevention, Hives, Interstitial Cystitis, Prostatitis (Chronic Pelvic Pain Syndrome), Stroke Prevention*

You may have heard of the "French paradox." The French diet is very high in saturated fat and cholesterol (just think of *pate de fois gras* and croissants), yet France has one of the world's lowest rates of heart disease. One theory for this apparent discrepancy is that another major player in the French diet—red wine—protects the arteries of the heart.

Quercetin is a natural **antioxidant** found in red wine. Antioxidants protect cells in the body from damage by *free radicals*, naturally occurring but harmful substances that are thought to play a role in cardiovascular disease. On this basis, it has been suggested that quercetin might help protect against heart attacks as well as strokes.

Quercetin belongs to a class of water-soluble plant coloring substances called *bioflavonoids*. Although they don't seem to be essential to life, it's possible that we need bioflavonoids for optimal health.

Another intriguing finding is that quercetin may help prevent immune cells from releasing *histamine*, the chemical that initiates the itching, sneezing, and swelling of an allergic reaction. Based on this very preliminary research, quercetin is often recommended as a treatment for allergies and asthma.

Sources

Quercetin is not an essential nutrient. It is found in red wine, grapefruit, onions, apples, black tea, and, in lesser amounts, in leafy green vegetables and beans. However, to get a therapeutic dosage, you'll have to take a supplement.

Quercetin supplements are available in pill and tablet form.

Therapeutic Dosages

A typical dosage is 200 to 400 mg 3 times daily. A special type of quercetin, quercetin chalcone, is claimed to be absorbed better, but there is little reliable evidence to prove this.

Therapeutic Uses

Quercetin is widely marketed as a treatment for allergic conditions such as **asthma**, **hay fever**, **eczema**, and **hives**. These proposed uses are based on test-tube research showing that quercetin prevents certain immune cells from releasing histamine, the chemical that triggers an allergic reaction. Quercetin may also block other substances involved with allergies. However, this evidence is extremely preliminary, far too preliminary to rely upon at all. There is as yet no direct evidence as that taking quercetin supplements will reduce your allergy symptoms.

A different proposed use of quercetin does have some meaningful supporting evidence: **prostatitis**. This condition is an inflammation or infection of the prostate gland. The condition causes chronic pain and difficulty with urination and is sometimes called *chronic pelvic pain syndrome*. Conventional treatment for this condition is often unsatisfactory. One small double-blind, placebo-controlled study has found preliminary evidence that quercetin might help (see next section).

Another small double-blind, placebo-controlled trial found that a supplement containing quercetin reduced symptoms of **interstitial cystitis**.

As noted above, it has been suggested that quercetin's antioxidant properties might make it helpful for preventing **heart disease** and **strokes**. However, the evidence that it works is *highly* incomplete. Keep in mind that other powerful antioxidants such as **vitamin E** and **beta-carotene** have been ineffective for preventing these conditions.

Test-tube studies and animal research additionally suggest that quercetin might have **cancer preventive** properties.

An animal study found that quercetin might protect rodents with **diabetes** from forming **cataracts**. Another intriguing finding from test-tube research is that quercetin seems to prevent a wide range of viruses from infecting cells and reproducing once they are inside cells. One study found that quercetin produced this effect against *Herpes simplex*, polio virus, and various respiratory viruses, including **influenza**. However, such studies are too indirect to tell us whether humans taking quercetin supplements can hope for benefits against diseases caused by those viruses.

What Is the Scientific Evidence for Quercetin?

Prostatitis

A 1-month, double-blind, placebo-controlled trial of 30 men with chronic pelvic pain (prostatitis) tested the potential effectiveness of quercetin. Participants received either placebo or 500 mg of the supplement twice daily. The results showed that people who received quercetin experienced a statistically significant improvement in symptoms (such as pain), but those given placebo did not improve.

While these are promising results, the study was small and cannot be regarded as definitive. Furthermore, researchers failed to provide the usual statistical evaluation required for such studies (a statistical analysis that directly compares the results in the treatment group against those in the placebo group). Thus, further study will be necessary to discover whether quercetin is actually effective for prostatitis.

Interstitial Cystitis

People with interstitial cystitis experience pain and discomfort in the bladder that is reminiscent of a bladder infection, but without the actual presence of such an infection. In a 6-week, double-blind, placebo-controlled study, 20 people received either placebo or a supplement containing quercetin and other bioflavonoids. The results appeared to indicate better results in the quercetin group. However, this study has only been presented as an abstract and it is not clear from the write-up whether the results were statistically meaningful.

Safety Issues

Quercetin appears to be quite safe. However, concerns have been raised that, under some circumstances, it might raise cancer risk. Quercetin "fails" a standard laboratory test called the *Ames test*, which is designed to identify chemicals that might be carcinogenic. Nonetheless, a bad showing on the Ames test does not definitely mean a chemical causes cancer. Most other evidence suggests that quercetin does *not* cause cancer and may, in fact, help prevent cancer. Still, one highly preliminary study suggests that quercetin combined with other bioflavonoids in the diet of pregnant women might increase the risk of infant leukemia. On this basis, pregnant women should probably avoid quercetin supplements. Maximum safe dosages for young children, nursing women, or people with serious liver or kidney disease have not been established.

Evidence suggests that use of quercetin supplements can elevate urine and blood levels of the substance homovanillic acid. While this itself should be harmless, lab tests for homovanillic acid are used to diagnose a rare, dangerous condition called *neuroblastoma* and, for this reason, use of quercetin supplements could potentially cause a false positive diagnosis of this condition.

Red Clover

Trifolium pratense

PRINCIPAL PROPOSED USES: *Menopausal Symptoms*

OTHER PROPOSED USES: *Acne, Cyclic Mastalgia, Eczema, Enhancing Mental Function, High Blood Pressure, High Cholesterol, Osteoporosis, Psoriasis*

Red clover has been cultivated since ancient times, primarily to provide a favorite grazing food for animals. But, like many other herbs, red clover was also a valued medicine. Although it has been used for many purposes worldwide, the one condition most consistently associated with red clover is cancer. Chinese physicians and Russian folk healers also used it to treat respiratory problems.

In the nineteenth century, red clover became popular among herbalists as an "alternative" or "blood purifier." This medical term, long since defunct, refers to an ancient belief that toxins in the blood are the root cause of many illnesses. Cancer, eczema, and the eruptions of venereal disease were all seen as manifestations of toxic buildup.

Red clover was considered one of the best herbs to "purify" the blood. For this reason, it is included in many of the famous treatments for cancer, including Jason Winter's cancer-cure tea.

Recently, special red clover extracts high in substances called *isoflavones* have arrived on the market. These isoflavones produce effects in the body somewhat similar to those of estrogen and, for this reason, they are called *phytoestrogens* (*phyto* indicates a plant source). The major isoflavones in red clover include genistein and daidzen, also found in soy, as well as formononetin and biochanin.

What Is Red Clover Used for Today?

Evidence is inconsistent on whether red clover isoflavones are helpful for **menopausal hot flashes**, with the largest trial failing to find benefits.

A small and poorly reported double-blind, placebo-controlled study provides weak evidence that red clover isoflavones might be helpful for **cyclic mastalgia**.

Although soy and, possibly, soy isoflavones have been found to reduce cholesterol levels, two trials enrolling a total of more than 100 women failed to find red clover isoflavones helpful for this purpose. However, in a double-blind, placebo-controlled comparative study of 80 people (both men and women), a red clover extract modified to be rich in biochanin did reduce LDL ("bad") cholesterol, while one enriched in formononetin did not.

One very small double-blind study found hints that red clover isoflavones might slightly improve **blood pressure** in post-menopausal women with diabetes.

Preliminary evidence suggests that red clover isoflavones may help prevent or treat **osteoporosis**.

In a 6-month, double-blind study, use of red clover isoflavones failed to enhance or harm **mental function**.

There is no evidence that red clover can help **treat cancer**. However, its usage in many parts of the world as a traditional cancer remedy has prompted scientists to take a close look at the herb. It turns out that the isoflavones in red clover may possess antitumor activity in the test tube. However, such preliminary research does not prove that red clover can treat cancer.

Red clover is sometimes recommended for the treatment of **acne**, **eczema**, **psoriasis**, and other skin diseases.

What Is the Scientific Evidence for Red Clover?

In a 12-week, double-blind, placebo-controlled trial of 30 post-menopausal women, use of red clover isoflavones at a dose of 80 mg daily significantly reduced hot flash symptoms as compared to placebo. Benefits were also seen in a 90-day study of 60 postmenopausal women given placebo or 80 mg of red clover isoflavones. However, a much larger study (252 participants) failed to find benefit with 82 or 57 mg of red clover isoflavones daily.

Two other studies also failed to find benefit. One, a 28-week, double-blind, placebo-controlled crossover study of 51 post-menopausal women, found no reduction in hot flashes among those given 40 mg of red clover isoflavones daily. No benefits were seen in another double-blind, placebo-controlled trial, which involved 37 women given isoflavones from red clover at a dose of either 40 or 160 mg daily.

Dosage

A typical dosage of red clover extract provides 40 to 160 mg of isoflavones daily. In the positive study described above, 80 mg daily were sufficient to reduce menopausal hot flashes.

Safety Issues

Red clover is on the FDA's GRAS (generally recognized as safe) list and is included in many beverage teas. However, detailed safety studies have not been performed.

Because of its blood-thinning and estrogen-like constituents, red clover should not be used by pregnant or nursing women, or women who have had breast or uterine cancer. Safety in young children or those with severe liver or kidney disease has also not been established.

Based on their constituents, red clover extracts may conceivably interfere with hormone treatments and anticoagulant drugs (see the next section for specific drugs).

One double-blind study of post-menopausal women found the use of red clover isoflavones at a dose of 80 mg daily for 90 days resulted in increased levels of testosterone. The potential significance of this is unclear. The same study found that red clover isoflavones reduced the thickness of the uterine lining, a finding that suggests low possibility for endometrial cancer.

For other potential risks due to the isoflavones in red clover (especially in concentrated isoflavone-rich extracts of red clover), see the full article on **isoflavones**.

Interactions You Should Know About

If you are taking hormones or **blood-thinning drugs**, such as **warfarin** (Coumadin), **heparin**, **clopidogrel** (Plavix), **ticlopidine** (Ticlid), **pentoxifylline** (Trental), or even **aspirin**: Red clover should be used only under a physician's supervision.

Red Raspberry

Rubus idaeus

PRINCIPAL PROPOSED USES: *None*

OTHER PROPOSED USES: *Prevent Complications of Pregnancy*

Herbalists have long believed that raspberry leaf tea taken regularly during pregnancy can prevent complications and make delivery easier. Raspberry has also been used to reduce excessive menstruation and relieve symptoms of diarrhea. However, there is no evidence that it is safe or effective for these uses.

What Is Red Raspberry Used for Today?

Red raspberry tea is still commonly recommended for pregnant women. However, while there is weak preliminary evidence from animal studies that raspberry might have an effect on the uterus, the only real clinical study trial reported to date found no benefit. This double-blind, placebo-controlled study evaluated the effects of red raspberry in 192 pregnant women. Treatment (pla-

cebo or 2.4 g of raspberry leaf daily) began at the thirty-second week of pregnancy and was continued until the onset of labor. The results failed to show any statistically meaningful differences between the group. Red raspberry did not significantly shorten labor, reduce pain, or prevent complications. Thus, at present, it appears that red raspberry does *not* work in the manner ascribed to it by tradition.

Dosage

To make raspberry leaf tea, pour 1 cup of boiling water over 1 or 2 teaspoons of dried leaf, steep for 10 minutes, and then sweeten to taste. Unlike many medicinal herbs, raspberry leaf actually has a pleasant taste! During pregnancy, drink 2 to 3 cups daily.

Safety Issues

Raspberry is believed to be a safe herb. The double-blind placebo-controlled trial noted above found no evidence of harm in the 96 pregnant women given red raspberry. However, this does not exclude the possibility of rare side effects or toxicity with excessive dosages. Safety in young children or those with severe liver or kidney disease has also not been established.

Red Yeast Rice
Monascus purpureus

Hong Qu; Monacolin K
PRINCIPAL PROPOSED USES: *High Cholesterol*

Red yeast rice is a traditional Chinese substance made by fermenting a type of yeast called *Monascus purpureus* over rice. This product (called *Hong Qu*) has been used in China since at least 800 A.D. as a food and also as a medicinal substance. The ancient Chinese preparation contains naturally occurring substances similar (and, in some cases, identical) to cholesterol-lowering prescription drugs in the "statin" family.

What Is Red Yeast Rice Used for Today?

Because of its statin drug–like content, red yeast rice is most likely effective at **lowering cholesterol**. For example, an 8-week, double-blind, placebo-controlled trial of 83 people with high cholesterol evaluated red yeast rice. At the end of the 8-week treatment period, levels of total cholesterol decreased significantly in the red yeast rice group as compared to the placebo group. Benefits were also seen in LDL ("bad" cholesterol) and triglycerides as well. No significant differences were noted in HDL ("good" cholesterol) levels from baseline or between groups.

Similar benefits were also seen in an 8-week study of 79 people.

However, because red yeast rice is essentially a drug supplied by a natural product, and this drug has many potential side effects, we suggest that it should be used only under physician supervision.

Dosage

The dosage of red yeast rice used in most studies is 1.2 to 2.4g of red yeast rice powder daily. However, due to patent-infringement suits by the manufacturer of a statin drug that is naturally present in red yeast rice, the most studied red yeast rice product has been taken off the market and it is not clear whether the remaining products have greater or lesser potency.

Safety Issues

In clinical trials, use of red yeast rice has not been associated with any significant side effects. However, red yeast rice contains naturally occurring statin drugs and use of statin drugs can cause side effects ranging from minor to life-threatening. Some of the most common include muscle pain, joint pain, liver inflammation, and peripheral nerve damage; severe breakdown of muscle tissue (rhabdomyolysis) leading to kidney failure has also occurred. It is almost certain that red yeast rice can cause the same problems if it is used by enough people, and there are at least two case reports in the literature of muscle injury caused by red yeast rice; in one case, rhabdomyolosis developed. Due to the relative lack of regulation of supplement manufacture, the statin content of red yeast rice products is unpredictable and this could increase potential risk. In addition, red yeast rice may at times contain the toxic substance citrinin.

Based on the known effects of statins, pregnant or nursing women, women likely to become pregnant, young children, and people with liver or kidney disease should not use red yeast rice. Furthermore, red yeast rice should not be combined with fibrate drugs, cyclosporine, erythromycin-family drugs, antifungal drugs, or high-dose niacin. Finally, it would not make sense to combine red yeast rice with standard statin drugs.

Statin drugs are known to interfere with the body's ability to produce the natural substance **coenzymeQ$_{10}$**, and one animal study found the same effect with red yeast rice.

Interactions You Should Know About

If you are taking **fibrate drugs**, **cyclosporine**, erythromycin-family drugs, antifungal drugs, or high-dose **niacin**: Do not use red yeast rice.

Reishi

Ganoderma lucidum

PRINCIPAL PROPOSED USES: *Adaptogen (Improve Resistance to Stress)*
OTHER PROPOSED USES: *Altitude Sickness, Autoimmune Diseases, Cancer Prevention, Cancer Treatment, Diabetes, Enhancing Mental Function, High Blood Pressure, Immune Support, Insomnia, Multiple Sclerosis, Ulcers, Viral Infections*

The tree fungus known as reishi has a long history of use in China and Japan as a semi-magical healing herb. More revered than ginseng and, up until recently, more rare, many stories tell of people with severe illnesses journeying immense distances to find it. Presently, reishi is artificially cultivated and widely available in stores that sell herb products.

What Is Reishi Used for Today?

Reishi is marketed as a kind of cure-all, said to **strengthen immunity**, help **prevent cancer**, and also possibly **treat cancer** as well. It is also said to be useful for autoimmune diseases (such as myasthenia gravis and **multiple sclerosis**), viral infections, **high blood pressure**, **diabetes**, **enhancing mental function**, **altitude sickness**, **ulcers**, and **insomnia**. However, while there has been a great deal of basic scientific research into the chemical constituents of reishi, reliable, double-blind studies are lacking. (For information on why such studies are essential to show that a treatment works, see **Why Does This Book Rely on Double-blind Studies?**)

For example, test-tube studies indicate that reishi has *immunomodulatory* effects. This means that reishi may *affect* the immune system, but not necessarily that it *strengthens* it. (Alternative medicine proponents often blur the difference between these two ideas.) Other weak evidence hints that reishi may have chemopreven-

tive properties, suggesting that it may help prevent cancer. However, a great many substances fight cancer in the test tube, while few actually help people with the disease.

Other highly preliminary forms of evidence suggest that reishi may have antiviral effects and possibly antibacterial effects as well. However, it is a long way from studies of this type to meaningful clinical uses.

Contemporary herbalists regard reishi as an adaptogen, a substance believed to be capable of helping the body resist stress of all kinds. (For more information on adaptogens, see the article on **ginseng**.) However, there is no meaningful evidence to support this claim.

One questionable double-blind study performed in China reportedly found reishi helpful for neurasthenia. The term *neurasthenia* is seldom used in modern medicine; it generally indicates fatigue due to psychological causes.

Dosage

The usual dosage of reishi is 2 to 6 g per day of raw fungus, or an equivalent dosage of concentrated extract, taken with meals. In traditional Chinese medicine, reishi is often combined with related fungi, such as shiitake, hoelen, or polyporus. It is often taken continually for its presumed overall health benefits.

Resveratrol *(sidebar)*

Safety Issues

Because it is used as food in Asia, reishi is generally regarded as safe. However, one study suggests that reishi impairs blood clotting. For this reason, prudence suggests that individuals with bleeding problems should avoid reishi; the herb should also be avoided in the period just before and after surgery or labor and delivery. Furthermore, individuals taking medications that impair blood clotting, such as aspirin, warfarin (Coumadin), heparin, clopidogrel (Plavix), pentoxifyl-line (Trental), or ticlopidine (Ticlid), should only use reishi under a doctor's supervision.

Safety in young children, pregnant or nursing women, or those with severe liver or kidney disease has not been established.

Interactions You Should Know About

If you are taking blood-thinning medications, such as **aspirin**, **warfarin** (Coumadin), **heparin**, **clopidogrel** (Plavix), **pentoxifylline** (Trental), or **ticlopidine** (Ticlid): Use reishi only under a doctor's supervision.

Resveratrol

SUPPLEMENT FORMS/ALTERNATE NAMES: *Grape Skin*

PRINCIPAL PROPOSED USES: *None*

OTHER PROPOSED USES: *Cancer Prevention, Heart Disease*

You may have heard of the "French paradox." The French diet is very high in saturated fat and cholesterol (just think of *pate de fois gras* and croissants), yet France has one of the world's lowest rates of heart disease. One theory for this apparent discrepancy is that another major player in the French diet—red wine—protects the arteries of the heart. (Another possibility, perhaps even more likely, is that cutting down on saturated fat is less helpful than previously thought. See the **high cholesterol** article for more information.)

Resveratrol is a natural **antioxidant** found in red wine. Antioxidants protect cells in the body from damage by free radicals, naturally occurring but harmful substances that are thought to play a role in **cardiovascular disease**. Resveratrol is also a phytoestrogen, a substance that mimics some of the effects of estrogen, while blocking others. **Soy**, another phytoestrogen, is thought to help prevent heart disease as well as cancer, and resveratrol might have similar effects. However, as yet none of these potential benefits of resveratrol have been documented in any meaningful way and there is some evidence that resveratrol taken by mouth is broken down before it enters the bloodstream.

Sources

Resveratrol is not an essential nutrient. It is found in red wine as well as in red grape skins and seeds and purple grape juice. Peanuts also contain a small amount of resveratrol. Resveratrol supplements are available as well.

Therapeutic Dosages

Because there haven't been any clinical studies, the optimal therapeutic dosage hasn't been established for resveratrol. Based on animal studies, a reasonable therapeutic dosage of resveratrol might be about 500 mg daily.

Therapeutic Uses

Very preliminary evidence such as the results of test-tube studies suggests that resveratrol may help prevent **heart disease** and **cancer**. However, not all studies have been favorable. Furthermore, there is some evidence that resveratrol is immediately broken down by the human liver and thereby does not, in fact, enter the blood stream at any significant level. In any case, only double-blind studies can prove a treatment effective, and none have been reported with resveratrol. (For information on why such studies are essential, see **Why Does This Book Rely on Double-blind Studies?**.)

Safety Issues

Resveratrol has a chemical structure similar to that of the synthetic estrogenic hormone diethylstilbestrol and it has estrogenic effects. According to one study, it might stimulate the growth of breast cancer cells. For this reason, resveratrol should be avoided by women who have had breast cancer or are at high risk of developing it. Maximum safe dosages for children, pregnant or nursing women, or those with severe liver or kidney disease have not been determined.

Rhodiola rosea

PRINCIPAL PROPOSED USES: *Adaptogen, Enhancing Mental Function, Fatigue, Improving Sports Performance*

OTHER PROPOSED USES: *Altitude Sickness, Female Sexual Function, Liver Protection, Male Sexual Function*

The herb *Rhodiola rosea* has been used traditionally in Iceland, Norway, Sweden, Russia, and other European countries as a "tonic herb," said to fight fatigue, aid convalescence from illness, prevent infections, and enhance sexual function. In the twentieth century, Soviet physicians classified rhodiola as an **adaptogen**. This invented term refers to a hypothetical treatment described as follows: An adaptogen helps the body adapt to stresses of various kinds, whether heat, cold, exertion, trauma, sleep deprivation, toxic exposure, radiation, infection, or psychological stress. Furthermore, an adaptogen supposedly causes no side effects, treats a wide variety of illnesses, and helps return an organism toward balance no matter what may have gone wrong.

Perhaps the only indisputable example of an adaptogen is a healthful lifestyle. By eating right, exercising regularly, and generally living a life of balance and moderation, you will increase your physical fitness and ability to resist illnesses of all types. Multivitamin/multimineral supplements could offer similarly general benefits, at least in people whose diet is deficient in basic nutrients. Whether there are any herbs that offer adaptogenic benefits, however, remains unproven (and somewhat unlikely). Nonetheless, advocates of the adaptogen concept believe that rhodiola (as well as ginseng, ashwagandha, reishi, suma, and several other herbs) have this property.

What Is Rhodiola Used for Today?

Rhodiola is currently marketed as the "new ginseng," said to fight **fatigue**, **enhance mental function**, increase **general wellness**, improve sports performance, and **enhance sex drive in both men** and **women**. A few double-blind studies support the first two of these uses, finding that the use of rhodiola by people in stressful, fatiguing circumstances may help maintain normal mental function.

For example, a double-blind, placebo-controlled study of 56 physicians on night duty evaluated the potential benefits of rhodiola for maintaining mental acuity. Participants received either placebo or rhodiola extract (170 mg daily) for a period of 2 weeks. The results showed that participants taking rhodiola retained a higher level of mental function as measured by tests such as mental arithmetic.

Another double-blind, placebo-controlled study evaluated one-time use of rhodiola extract (at a dose of 370 mg or 555 mg) in 161 male military cadets undergoing sleep deprivation and stress. The results showed that rhodiola was more effective than placebo at fighting the effects of fatigue.

Finally, a third double-blind, placebo-controlled study examined the effects of a low dose of rhodiola extract (100 mg daily for 20 days) in 40 foreign students undergoing examinations (presumably a highly stressful situation). The results showed modest benefits on some measurements of fatigue and mental function and no significant benefit on others. The study authors considered the outcome relatively unimpressive and blamed this on the dose chosen.

Note, however, that while these results sound impressive, they were all performed in former Soviet republics and studies from these sources must be viewed with caution. For reasons that are not clear, double-blind studies performed in the former USSR (or China) almost always find the tested treatment effective. This consistent pattern of excessively positive results has made outside observers highly skeptical. For this reason, only if confirmation is obtained in a more reliable setting can rhodiola be considered to have real supporting evidence behind it.

One small double-blind trial performed in Belgium did find evidence that use of rhodiola extract at a dose of 200 mg 1 hour before endurance exercise may improve performance. However, another study failed to find benefit with a combination of **cordyceps** and rhodiola.

Very weak evidence hints that rhodiola might be helpful for preventing **altitude sickness**, and might aid **cancer chemotherapy** (by **protecting the liver**).

Dosage

Rhodiola extracts are standardized to their content of salidroside (also called *rhodioloside*). A typical dosage of 170 to 185 mg daily supplies 4.5 mg of salidroside. When rhodiola is used as a one-time treatment, 2 to 3 times this dose is often used.

Safety Issues

There are no known or suspected safety risks with rhodiola. However, comprehensive safety studies have not been performed. Safety in young children, pregnant or nursing women, or people with severe liver or kidney disease has not been established.

Ribose

PRINCIPAL PROPOSED USES: *None*

OTHER PROPOSED USES: AMPD *(Congenital Myoadenylate Deaminase Deficiency), Angina, Congestive Heart Failure*

PROBABLY NOT EFFECTIVE USES: *Duchenne Muscular Dystrophy, McArdle's Disease, Sports Performance Enhancement (High Intensity Exercise)*

Ribose is a carbohydrate vital for the body's manufacture of ATP (adenosine triphosphate), which is the major source of energy used by our cells.

Quite a few studies have been done on ribose, mostly relating to its potential usefulness for individuals with heart disease. When the heart is starved for oxygen, as can occur with a **heart attack** or **angina**, it loses much of its ATP and its ATP levels remain low for several days, even after blood flow is resumed. Scientists have found that supplying extra ribose in the blood helps restore the heart's normal ATP levels more quickly. This finding has raised hopes that ribose supplements might improve heart functioning and increase exercise capacity.

Ribose is better known as a **sports supplement**. However, current evidence indicates that it is *not* effective for this purpose.

Requirements/Sources

Ribose is not an essential nutrient. Although it is a common sugar present in the bodies of animals and plants, food sources don't supply recommended dosages.

Therapeutic Dosages

Typical doses recommended by sports supplement manufacturers are 1 to 10 g per day. Participants in a study of heart disease took 60 g of ribose in water (15 mg 4 times a day) by mouth for 3 days.

Typically provided as a powder to be dissolved in water or in liquid form, ribose is also available commercially in capsules. The dissolved powder has a sweetish taste that some people find unpleasant.

Therapeutic Uses

Ribose may be of benefit in improving exercise tolerance in people with angina by helping the heart regenerate its ATP, but the evidence that it works remains highly preliminary. One small study found evidence that ribose supplements might improve heart function in people with **congestive heart failure**.

Sports enthusiasts are more interested in ATP's effects on regular muscles than on the heart muscle. At least one animal study seems to show that skeletal muscle, like heart muscle, replenishes ATP more quickly when ribose is added to the blood. In theory, this could lead to enhanced performance in high intensity anaerobic exercise, such as sprinting. However, five small double-blind, placebo-controlled trials in humans failed to find any benefit. In one of these studies, dextrose (a form of ordinary sugar) proved effective while ribose did not.

In a few case reports, ribose apparently has produced an increase in exercise ability in people with a rare condition involving deficiency of the enzyme myoadenylate deaminase (AMPD). However, no double-blind studies of ribose in AMPD deficiency have been conducted. Small double-blind studies have failed to find ribose effective for another rare enzyme deficiency called *McArdle's disease* or for Duchenne's muscular dystrophy.

What Is the Scientific Evidence for Ribose?

Individuals with sufficiently severe coronary artery disease suffer reduced blood flow to the heart (ischemia) with exercise and experience angina pain. One small study examined whether giving ribose can improve exercise tolerance for people with angina. In the study, 20 men with severe coronary artery disease walked on a treadmill while researchers noted how long it took for signs of ischemia to develop. For the next 3 days, the men took either oral ribose (60 mg per day) or placebo, after which they repeated the treadmill test. Results of the final test showed that those taking ribose increased the time they were able to walk before developing EKG signs of ischemia, while those taking placebo had no such improvement. This preliminary study was too small to prove anything definitively, but it certainly suggests that further investigation would be worthwhile.

Another small placebo-controlled study enrolled people with coronary artery disease and congestive heart failure and found that use of ribose supplements improved objective measures of heart function and also enhanced subjective "quality of life."

Safety Issues

There are no reports of lasting or damaging side effects from ribose, but formal safety studies have not yet been conducted. Reported minor side effects include diarrhea, gastrointestinal discomfort, nausea, and headache.

Rose Hips

Rosa species

PRINCIPAL PROPOSED USES: *Natural Source of Vitamin C and Bioflavonoids*

OTHER PROPOSED USES: *Cancer Prevention, Kidney Stones (Prevention), Osteoarthritis*

A rose hip is the seed pod of a wild rose plant. Various wild rose species can be utilized as the source of rose hips. Traditionally, rose hips have been used to treat arthritis, colds and flus, indigestion, bladder stones, and gonorrhea.

What Are Rose Hips Used for Today?

Rose hips are primarily used today as a natural source of **vitamin C**. There is no evidence that the vitamin C in rose hips is any better than synthetic vitamin C (the most common form of the vitamin), but those who prefer to use truly natural products can do so by using the herb instead of the chemical. Like other plant sources of vitamin C, rose hips also contain substances in the **bioflavonoid** family. Information on the potential benefits of these two rose hips constituents can be found in the respective articles.

Weak evidence hints that rose hips might have value for **osteoarthritis**. Even weaker evidence hints that whole rose hips might be useful for prevention of **cancer**, and, possibly, treatment or prevention of **kidney stones**.

Dosage

Dosage of rose hips products is generally adjusted to supply the desired amount of vitamin C and bioflavonoids.

Safety Issues

As yet, there are no known or suspected safety issues with rose hips.

Rosemary

Rosmarinus officinalis

PRINCIPAL PROPOSED USES: *Dyspepsia*

OTHER PROPOSED USES: *Chemical Dependency, Muscle Aches (Topical)*

The herb rosemary has been used as a food spice and as a medicine since ancient times. Traditional medicinal uses of rosemary leaf preparations taken internally include digestive distress, headaches, and anxiety. The fragrance of rosemary leaf has been said to enhance memory. Rosemary oil was applied to the skin to treat muscle and joint pain and taken internally to promote abortions.

What Is Rosemary Used for Today?

Germany's Commission E has approved rosemary leaf for treatment of **dyspepsia** (non-specific digestive distress) and rosemary oil (used externally) for joint pain and poor circulation. However, there is no meaningful scientific evidence that rosemary is effective for any of these uses. Only double-blind, placebo-controlled studies can prove that a treatment really works, and no studies of this type have found rosemary effective. (For information on why such studies are essential, see **Why Does This Book Rely on Double-blind Studies?**)

Rosemary essential oil, like many essential oils, has antimicrobial properties when it comes in direct contact with bacteria and other microorganisms. Note, however, that this does not mean that rosemary oil is an antibiotic. Antibiotics are substances that can be taken internally to kill microorganisms throughout the body. Rosemary oil, rather, has shown potential antiseptic properties.

One animal study found evidence that rosemary might help **withdrawal from narcotics**.

Even weaker evidence hints that rosemary or its constituents may have antithrombotic (blood thinning), **anti-cancer**, diuretic, **liver-protective**, and **ulcer-protective** effects.

Rosmarinic acid from rosemary has shown potential anti-inflammatory and anti-allergic actions, but most published studies (including double-blind trials) have used a different plant source of the substance (the herb *Perilla frutescens*).

One controlled study failed to find rosemary cream protective against skin irritation caused by sodium laurylsulfate (a common ingredient of cosmetic products).

Rosemary essential oil has been used in **aromatherapy** (treating conditions through scent). One controlled study evaluated rosemary aromatherapy for enhancing memory, but found results that were mixed at best. Another study failed to find that rosemary aromatherapy reduced tension during an anxiety-provoking task; in fact, it appeared that use of rosemary actually increased anxiety.

Dosage

A typical dosage of rosemary leaf is 4 to 6 g daily. Rosemary essential oil should not be used internally.

Safety Issues

Although rosemary's use as a food spice suggests a relatively low level of toxicity, rosemary has not undergone comprehensive safety testing. Rosemary essential oil can be toxic if taken even in fairly low doses and the maximum safe dose is not known.

Based on its traditional use for abortion, as well as preliminary evidence showing embryotoxic effects, rosemary should not be used by pregnant women or women who wish to become pregnant.

One study suggests that rosemary may have diuretic effects. If it does, the herb could theoretically present risks in people taking the medication lithium.

Other weak evidence hints that rosemary may enhance the liver's rate of deactivating estrogen in the body. This suggests that rosemary might present risks for females, as well as anyone who uses medications containing estrogen.

Additionally, one study hints that rosemary might worsen blood sugar control in people with **diabetes**.

Interactions You Should Know About

If you are taking:

➤ **Lithium: Use rosemary only with caution.**
➤ **Medications containing estrogen: Rosemary may decrease their effect.**

S-Adenosylmethionine

SUPPLEMENT FORMS/ALTERNATE NAMES: *Ademetionine, SAM, SAMe*

PRINCIPAL PROPOSED USES: *Depression, Osteoarthritis*

OTHER PROPOSED USES: *Chronic Viral Hepatitis, Cirrhosis, Fibromyalgia, Other Forms of Liver Disease, Parkinson's Disease*

S-adenosylmethionine is quite a mouthful; the abbreviation SAMe (pronounced *samm-ee*) is easier to say. Its chemical structure and name are derived from two materials you may have heard about already: methionine, a sulfur-containing amino acid, and adenosine triphosphate (ATP), the body's main energy molecule.

SAMe was discovered in Italy in 1952. It was first investigated as a treatment for depression, but along the way it was accidentally noted to improve arthritis symptoms—a kind of positive side effect.

Unfortunately, SAMe is an extraordinarily expensive supplement at present. Full dosages can easily cost more than $200 per month.

Sources

The body makes all the SAMe it needs, so there is no dietary requirement. However, deficiencies in **methionine**, **folate**, or **vitamin B$_{12}$** can reduce SAMe levels.

SAMe is not found in appreciable quantities in foods, so it must be taken as a supplement.

It's been suggested that the supplement **TMG** might indirectly increase SAMe levels and provide similar benefits, but this effect has not been proven.

Therapeutic Dosages

A typical full dosage of SAMe is 400 mg taken 3 to 4 times per day. If this dosage works for you, take it for a few weeks and then try reducing the dosage. As little as 200 mg twice daily may suffice to keep you feeling better once the full dosage has "broken through" the symptoms.

However, some people develop mild stomach distress if they start full dosages of SAMe at once. To get around this, you may need to start low and work up to the full dosage gradually.

Recently, SAMe has come on the U.S. market at a recommended dosage of 200 mg twice daily. This dosage

S-Adenosylmethionine

labeling makes SAMe appear more affordable (if you're only taking 400 mg per day, you'll spend only about a third or a fourth of what you'd pay for the proper dosage), but it is unlikely that SAMe will actually work when taken at such a low dosage.

Therapeutic Uses

A substantial amount of evidence suggests that SAMe can be an effective treatment for **osteoarthritis**, the "wear and tear" type of arthritis that many people develop as they get older.

A moderate amount of evidence suggests that SAMe might be helpful for **depression**.

Weak and inconsistent evidence hints that SAMe might be helpful for a variety of **liver conditions**, such as **cirrhosis**, **chronic viral hepatitis**, **pregnancy-related jaundice**, and Gilbert's syndrome.

SAMe may help the painful muscle condition known as **fibromyalgia**.

SAMe has undergone some investigation as a possible supportive treatment for **Parkinson's disease**. One study suggests that it may reduce the depression so commonly associated with the disease. In addition, the drug levodopa, used for Parkinson's disease, depletes the body of SAMe. This suggests that taking extra SAMe might be helpful. However, it is also possible that SAMe could interfere with the effect of levodopa, requiring an increase in dosage.

Highly preliminary evidence suggests that SAMe can protect the stomach against damage caused by alcohol.

What Is the Scientific Evidence for S-Adenosylmethionine?

Osteoarthritis

A substantial body of scientific evidence supports the use of SAMe to treat osteoarthritis. Double-blind studies involving a total of more than 1,000 participants suggest that SAMe is about as effective as standard anti-inflammatory drugs. In addition, animal evidence suggests that SAMe may help protect cartilage from damage.

For example, a double-blind, placebo-controlled Italian study tracked 732 people taking SAMe, naproxen (a standard anti-inflammatory drug), or placebo. After 4 weeks, participants taking SAMe or naproxen showed about the same level of benefit as compared to each other and a superior level of benefit as compared to those in the placebo group.

A more recent double-blind study compared SAMe to celecoxib (Celebrex), a member of the newest class of non-steroidal anti-inflammatory drugs. Celecoxib produced more rapid effects than SAMe, but over time SAMe appeared to catch up. However, the lack of a placebo group makes these results less than fully reliable.

Another double-blind study compared SAMe with the anti-inflammatory drug piroxicam. A total of 45 individuals were followed for 84 days. The two treatments proved equally effective. However, the SAMe-treated individuals maintained their improvement long after the treatment was stopped, whereas those on piroxicam quickly started to hurt again.

Similarly long-lasting results have been seen with glucosamine and chondroitin. This pattern of response suggests that these treatments are somehow making a deeper impact on osteoarthritis than simply relieving symptoms. However, while we have some direct evidence that glucosamine and chondroitin can slow the progression of osteoarthritis, the evidence regarding SAMe is more hypothetical.

In other double-blind studies, oral SAMe has shown equivalent benefits to various doses of indomethacin, ibuprofen, and naproxen.

Depression

The evidence for SAMe for the treatment of depression is provocative but far from definitive.

Several double-blind, placebo-controlled studies have found SAMe effective in relieving depression, but most were small and poorly reported, and many used an injected form of the supplement. Furthermore, the most recent trial, a double-blind, placebo-controlled study of 133 depressed patients, failed to find intravenous SAMe more effective than placebo. Researchers resorted to questionable statistical manipulation of the data to show benefit.

Other trials compared SAMe to standard antidepressants rather than to placebo. The best of these was a 6-week, double-blind trial of 281 people with mild depression that compared oral SAMe to imipramine. The results indicated that the two treatments were about equally effective. However, the absence of a placebo group makes this study less than fully definitive.

Other studies have also compared the benefits of oral or intravenous SAMe to those of tricyclic antidepressants and have also found generally equivalent results; however, again, poor reporting and inadequacies of study design (such as too limited a treatment interval) mar the meaningfulness of the reported outcomes.

Fibromyalgia

Four double-blind trials have studied the use of SAMe for fibromyalgia, three of them finding it to be helpful. Unfortunately, most of these studies used SAMe given either intravenously or as an injection into the muscles, sometimes in combination with oral doses. When you inject a medication, the effects can be quite different than when you take it orally. For that reason, these studies are of questionable relevance.

Nonetheless, the one double-blind study that used only oral SAMe did find positive results. In this trial, 44 people with fibromyalgia took 800 mg of SAMe or placebo for 6 weeks. Compared to the group taking placebo, those taking SAMe had improvements in disease activity, pain at rest, fatigue, and morning stiffness, and in one measurement of mood. In other respects, such as the amount of tenderness in their tender points, the group taking SAMe did no better than those taking the placebo.

It isn't clear whether SAMe is helping fibromyalgia through its antidepressant effects, or by some other mechanism.

Parkinson's Disease

Evidence suggests that levodopa (the drug used to treat Parkinson's disease) can reduce brain levels of SAMe. This depletion may contribute to the side effects of levodopa treatment, as well as the depression sometimes seen with Parkinson's disease. One study found that SAMe taken orally improved depression without changing the effectiveness of levodopa. However, it is also possible that over time taking extra SAMe could interfere with levodopa's effectiveness (see Safety Issues).

Safety Issues

SAMe appears to be quite safe, according to both human and animal studies. The most common side effect is mild digestive distress. However, SAMe does not actually damage the stomach.

Like other substances with antidepressant activity, SAMe might trigger a manic episode in those with **bipolar disease** (manic-depressive illness).

Safety in young children, pregnant or nursing women, or those with severe liver or kidney disease has not been established.

SAMe might interfere with the action of the Parkinson's drug levodopa. In addition, there may also be risks involved in combining SAMe with standard antidepressants. For this reason, you shouldn't try either combination except under physician supervision.

Interactions You Should Know About

If you are taking:

> **Standard antidepressants, including MAO inhibitors, SSRIs, and tricyclics: Do not take SAMe except on a physician's advice.**
> **Levodopa for Parkinson's disease: SAMe might help relieve the side effects of this drug. However, it might also reduce its effectiveness over time.**

Saffron

Crocus sativus

PRINCIPAL PROPOSED USES: *Depression*

OTHER PROPOSED USES: *Cancer Prevention, Enhancing Mental Function, High Cholesterol*

The Mediterranean herb saffron, long used in cooking, is made from the dried stigma (top of the female portion) of the *Crocus sativa* flower. Each flower has only three small stigmas and it requires about 75,000 flowers to produce one pound of saffron. As a cooking herb, saffron is valued for its intense orange-yellow color and its subtle flavor. Medicinally, it has been used since ancient times for strengthening digestion, relieving coughs, smoothing menstruation, relaxing muscle spasms, improving mood, and calming anxiety. Saffron contains **vitamin B₂** along with a yellow flavonoid called *crocin*, a bitter glycoside called *picrocrocin*, and the volatile, aromatic substance *safranal*.

What Is Saffron Used for Today?

The best evidence for medicinal effects of saffron involve treatment of **depression**. According to three preliminary double-blind studies, use of saffron at 30 mg daily is more effective than placebo and equally effective as standard treatment for major depression. However, all these studies were small and were performed by a single research group (in Iran). Larger studies and independent confirmation will be necessary to determine whether saffron truly is effective for depression.

Other proposed uses of saffron have even weaker supporting evidence. Test-tube and animal studies hint that saffron and its constituents may help prevent or treat **cancer**, reduce **cholesterol levels**, protect against side effects of the drug **cisplatin**, and **enhance mental function**.

What Is the Scientific Evidence for Saffron?

Three small double-blind trials hint that saffron may be helpful for depression. However, all these studies were performed by a single research group, and only one of them used a placebo control. Because of these limitations, the evidence for saffron as an antidepressant remains highly preliminary.

In a 6-week, double-blind, placebo-controlled study of 40 people with major depression of mild to moderate severity, use of saffron at a dose of 30 mg daily proved more effective than placebo, according to standard methods of rating depression severity. Use of saffron was not associated with any significant side effects.

In a 6-week, double-blind study of 30 people with major depression of mild-to-moderate severity, use of saffron at a dose of 30 mg daily proved equally effective as the standard drug **imipramine** taken at a dose of 100 mg daily. This study, however, had no placebo group and therefore its meaningfulness is limited.

Finally, in a 6-week, double-blind, placebo-controlled study of 40 people with major depression of mild to moderate severity, use of saffron at 30 mg per day proved equally effective as **fluoxetine** (Prozac) at the standard dose of 20 mg daily. Once again, this study lacked a placebo group.

Dosage

In the studies of depression described above, saffron was used at a dose of 30 mg daily of an alcohol-based extract.

Safety Issues

Saffron appears to have a very low order of toxicity. It is often said that very high doses of saffron can cause abortion and possible toxic symptoms, but there is no scientific documentation of these supposed effects. However, the so-called meadow saffron, *Colchicum autumnale*, is highly toxic and sometimes people mistake one for the other.

Safety in young children, pregnant or nursing women, or people with severe liver or kidney disease has not been established.

Sage

Salvia lavandulaefolia, Salvia officinalis

PRINCIPAL PROPOSED USES: *Dyspepsia, Hyperhidrosis (Excessive Perspiration), Sore Throat*
OTHER PROPOSED USES: *Alzheimer's Disease, Anxiety, Breast-feeding Support (Reducing Breast Engorgement During Weaning), Enhancing Mental Function, Herpes*

The herb sage has a long history of use in food and medicine. In Mediterranean cultures it was used internally to treat excessive menstrual bleeding, increase fertility, aid memory, reduce symptoms of arthritis, and reduce breast engorgement during weaning. It was used topically for treatment of wounds, sprains, and muscle injuries, and as a gargle for sore throat, hoarseness, and cough.

What Is Sage Used for Today?

Sage has been approved by Germany's Commission E for internal use in the treatment of **dyspepsia** (non-specific digestive distress) and hyperhidrosis (excessive sweating), and for topical use in the treatment of inflammation of the mucous membranes of the throat and nose. However, only double-blind, placebo-controlled studies can prove that a treatment really works and no studies of this type have been performed using sage for any of these purposes other than sore throat. (For information on why such studies are essential, see **Why Does This Book Rely on Double-blind Studies?**.)

A double-blind study of 286 people found that a throat spray made using sage at a 15% concentration significantly reduced **sore throat** pain as compared to placebo.

Additionally, in a double-blind trial performed in Iran, 42 people with mild-to-moderate **Alzheimer's disease** were given either a sage extract or placebo for 4 months. The results appeared to suggest a modest improvement in mental function in the sage group as compared to the placebo group.

In another double-blind, placebo-controlled study, either placebo or sage **essential oil** was given to 24 healthy people using a crossover design. The results showed possible improvement in some aspects of **mental function**, but the design of the study was such that the results are difficult to trust. (The researchers tested too many aspects of memory, leading to a statistical likelihood that benefits would be seen on some of them by random chance.) A similar sized study (with similar flaws) found weak hints that sage leaf might improve mood and reduce **anxiety** level.

Much weaker evidence, too weak to rely upon at all, hints that sage might have **liver protective**, **anti-cancer**, immunomodulatory (alters immune function), antimicrobial, anti-anxiety, and anti-inflammatory activity.

One study failed to find that sage cream provided more than at most exceedingly modest benefits for treatment of **herpes**.

Dosage

For use as tea or gargle, 1 to 3 g of dried sage is steeped in a cup of water and taken 3 times daily. The equivalent dose of tincture or extract may also be used.

Safety Issues

As a widely used food spice, sage is thought to have a relatively high level of safety. However, comprehensive safety studies have not been performed. Sage essential oil contains the neurotoxic substance thujone. Maximum safe doses in young children, pregnant or nursing women, or people with severe liver or kidney disease have not been established.

Salt Bush

Atriplex halimus

PRINCIPAL PROPOSED USES: *Diabetes*

Salt bush is a shrub that grows throughout the Mediterranean region, in the Middle East, northern Africa, and southern Europe. As its name suggests, it is especially common in areas where the soil is saline. Salt bush is a nutritious plant, high in protein, **vitamins C, A,** and **D,** and minerals, such as **chromium**. It is also fairly tasty—shepherds as well as their flocks enjoy eating salt bush.

What Is Salt Bush Used for Today?

Salt bush may prove useful in the treatment of type 2 (non–insulin-dependent or adult onset) **diabetes**. This idea came to the attention of medical researchers in 1964, when they discovered that a rodent called the *sand rat* (*Psammomys obesus*) is highly susceptible to developing diabetes. Yet wild sand rats, which regularly consume salt bush, never show any signs of diabetes—they tend to develop it in response to being fed regular laboratory food! As a result, scientists have explored the possibility that salt bush has an antidiabetic effect.

The results of animal studies and preliminary human trials suggest that salt bush does indeed have antidiabetic effects. However, while these studies are certainly intriguing, only double-blind, placebo-controlled studies can prove a treatment effective and none have yet been reported. For this reason, the use of salt bush for diabetes remains highly speculative.

Some animal researchers speculate that the effect of salt bush (if, indeed, it has one) may be partly due to the chromium it contains. Considerable evidence indicates that **chromium** supplementation can improve blood sugar control, especially in type 2 diabetes. However, there could be other active ingredients in salt bush as well.

Dosage

No standard dosage of salt bush has been established.

Warning: Diabetes is a serious disease that should be treated only under medical supervision. Salt bush cannot be used as a substitute for insulin. Blood sugar levels should also be closely monitored. For more information, see Safety Issues.

Safety Issues

As a plant food commonly consumed by animals and humans, salt bush appears to be relatively safe. However, no comprehensive safety testing of salt bush has been performed. For this reason, it should not be used by young children, pregnant or nursing women, or people with severe liver or kidney disease.

Keep in mind that if salt bush is effective, the result might be excessive lowering of blood sugar levels. For this reason, people with diabetes who take salt bush should do so only under a physician's supervision.

Sandalwood

Santalum album

PRINCIPAL PROPOSED USES: *Bladder Infection*

OTHER PROPOSED USES: *Acne, Bronchitis, Cough, Dry Skin, Herpes, Rashes, Sore Throat*

Native to India, the sandalwood tree is used for many purposes—the wood for decorative carvings, the oil for fragrance in incense, perfumes, and soaps. Both its wood and oil have also been employed medicinally for a wide variety of conditions.

Unfortunately, harvesting of these trees is beginning to endanger the species. The Indian government has limited the amount of sandalwood that may be harvested each year, but has not restricted its export. Illegal harvesting of sandalwood has become very lucrative, as limits on legal harvesting have caused a price increase for sandalwood products.

In traditional Indian (**Ayurvedic**) medicine, sandalwood was used to treat gonorrhea and to decrease sex drive. Traditional Chinese medicine also lists sandalwood as a treatment for gonorrhea, as well as for stomachache and vomiting. In Europe, sandalwood was used to treat fever and pain, as we use aspirin today. However, no clinical evidence exists to support any of these applications.

What Is Sandalwood Used for Today?

Germany's Commission E has approved sandalwood for the treatment of bladder infections, not to be used alone, but along with other therapies. Sandalwood is said to act as an antiseptic in the urinary system; if this is correct, it might help to rid the body of the bacteria that cause these infections, but there is no reliable evidence as yet to verify this belief.

In test-tube studies, sandalwood was found to slow the growth of **herpes** virus. An intriguing animal study found that components isolated from sandalwood caused responses similar to those seen with medications used to treat **schizophrenia**. However, this evidence is far too weak to indicate that sandalwood is a useful treatment for either of these conditions.

Sandalwood is also advertised for other therapeutic uses, including **bronchitis**, sore throat, and persistent **cough**. External application of a sandalwood paste is sometimes suggested for **acne**, skin rashes, or dry skin. None of these proposed uses, however, have been scientifically studied.

Dosage

For urinary tract infections, the Commission E suggests 1 to 1.5 g of essential oil or 10 to 20 g of ground sandalwood daily, not to be taken for more than 6 weeks except on the advice of a physician. If the essential oil of sandalwood is used, an enteric-coated capsule is recommended (such capsules delay the release of a substance until it has passed through the stomach into the intestine, helping to avoid an upset stomach).

Safety Issues

The safety of sandalwood has not been formally evaluated. For this reason, it should not be used by pregnant or nursing women, young children, or individuals with severe kidney or liver disease.

Reported side effects include nausea and itching.

Sandalwood paste applied externally has been reported to cause skin irritation on rare occasions. There is also one case report of a man developing a skin rash after burning large quantities of sandalwood incense.

Sassafras

Santalum album

PRINCIPAL PROPOSED USES: *We strongly recommend against the use of sassafras in any form.*

The sassafras tree, a native of North America, has a long history of use both as flavoring and medicine. The oil extracted from its root was one of the original constituents of herbal root beer. As medicine, it was used to treat influenza and other fever-producing infections, as well as arthritis, urinary tract infections, and digestive disorders. It was also commonly used as a "spring tonic" or "blood purifier."

However, in the 1960s, it was discovered that sassafras oil contains high levels of a liver toxin named *safrole*. When given to animals, safrole causes liver cancer and even a single cup of sassafras tea contains dangerous levels of the substance.

Because of this, sassafras has been banned for human consumption. Only safrole-free products can be sold; however, there may be other carcinogens in sassafras besides safrole.

Sassafras oil is also immediately toxic; a few drops can kill an infant and a teaspoon can cause death in an adult.

For all these reasons, we strongly recommend against the use of sassafras for any purpose.

Saw Palmetto

Serenoa repens or Sabal serrulata

PRINCIPAL PROPOSED USES: *Benign Prostatic Hyperplasia (Prostate Enlargement)*

OTHER PROPOSED USES: *Hair Loss, Prostatitis (Prostate Infection)*

Saw palmetto is a native plant of North America and it is still primarily grown in the United States.

The saw palmetto tree grows only about 2 to 4 feet high, with fan-shaped serrated leaves and abundant berries. Native Americans used these berries for the treatment of various urinary problems in men, as well as for women with breast disorders. European and American physicians took up saw palmetto as a treatment for benign prostatic hyperplasia (BPH). In the 1960s, French researchers discovered that by concentrating the oils of saw palmetto berry they could maximize the herb's effectiveness.

Saw palmetto contains many biologically active chemicals. Unfortunately, we don't know which ones are the most important. We also don't really know how saw palmetto works; it appears to interact with various sex hormones, but it also has many other complex actions that could affect the prostate.

What Is Saw Palmetto Used for Today?

Saw palmetto oil is an accepted medical treatment for **benign prostatic hyperplasia** (BPH) in New Zealand and in France, Germany, Austria, Italy, Spain, and other European countries.

Typical symptoms of BPH include difficulty starting urination, weak urinary stream, frequent urination, dribbling after urination, and waking up several times at night to urinate. Most, though not all, research suggests that saw palmetto can markedly improve all these symptoms. Benefits require approximately 4 to 6 weeks of treatment to develop. It appears that about two-thirds of men respond reasonably well.

Furthermore, while the prostate tends to continue to grow when left untreated, saw palmetto causes a small but definite shrinkage. In other words, it isn't just relieving symptoms, but may actually be retarding prostate enlargement. The drug Proscar does this too (and to a greater extent than saw palmetto) but other standard medications for BPH have no effect on prostate size.

Research tells us that saw palmetto is equally effective for reducing BPH symptoms as Proscar and it has one meaningful advantage: it leaves PSA (prostate-specific antigen) levels unchanged. Cancer raises PSA levels, and lab tests that measure PSA are used to screen for prostate cancer. Proscar lowers PSA measurements and, therefore, its use may have the unintended effect of masking prostate cancer. Saw palmetto won't do this. On the other hand, Proscar has been shown to reduce the need for surgery, unlike saw palmetto or any of the other drugs used for BPH.

Saw palmetto also appears to be equally effective as another class of standard drugs known as alpha blockers, but may cause fewer side effects.

Note: Before self-treating with saw palmetto, be sure to get a proper medical evaluation to rule out prostate cancer.

Saw palmetto is also widely used to treat chronic prostatitis. An open trial that compared saw palmetto to the drug Proscar for the treatment of chronic nonbacterial prostatitis found that while the drug was effective, the herb was not. However, these results do *not* mean that saw palmetto is ineffective for prostatis. Because this was an open study, researchers and participants knew who was getting saw palmetto and who was getting the drug. If there was any expectation that the drug would be more powerful than the herb, this in itself would be sufficient to skew the results toward that outcome.

Saw palmetto is sometimes recommended as a treatment for hair loss, but there is no evidence at all that it is effective for this purpose.

What Is the Scientific Evidence for Saw Palmetto?

The science for the effectiveness of saw palmetto in treating prostate enlargement is reasonably strong.

At least 10 double-blind studies involving a total of about 900 people have compared the benefits of saw palmetto against placebo over periods of 1 to 12 months.

In all but three of these studies, the herb improved urinary flow rate and most other measures of prostate disease to a greater extent than placebo. However, in the most recent and perhaps best-designed of these studies, a 1-year trial of 225 men, a saw palmetto product failed to prove more effective than placebo.

A double-blind study followed 1,098 men who received either saw palmetto or the drug Proscar over a period of 6 months (unfortunately, there was no placebo group). The treatments were equally effective, but while Proscar lowered PSA levels and caused a slight worsening of sexual function on average, saw palmetto caused no significant side effects. Both treatments caused the prostate to shrink, but Proscar had a greater effect.

A 52-week, double-blind study of 811 men compared saw palmetto to a standard drug in another class: the alpha-blocker tamsulosin. Once again, both treatments proved equally effective. However, saw palmetto caused fewer side effects than the drug. In addition, the herb caused some prostate shrinkage, while the drug caused a slight prostate enlargement.

A study involving 435 men found that the benefits of saw palmetto endure for at least 3 years. However, there was no control group in this study, making the results unreliable.

A 48-week, double-blind trial of 543 men with early BPH compared combined saw palmetto and **nettle root** against Proscar and found equal benefits. Benefits were also seen with a combination of saw palmetto and nettle root in a 24-week, placebo-controlled study of 257 men.

Finally, a 6-month, double-blind, placebo-controlled trial of 44 men given a saw palmetto herbal blend (containing, in addition, nettle root and pumpkin seed oil) found shrinkage in prostate tissue. No significant improvement in symptoms was seen, but the authors pointed out that the study size was too small to statistically detect such improvements if they did occur.

Dosage

The standard dosage of saw palmetto for the treatment of BPH is 160 mg twice a day of an extract standardized to contain 85 to 95% fatty acids and sterols. A single daily dose of 320 mg may be just as effective for this condition. However, taking more than this amount does not, on average, seem to produce better results. As with many other herbs, the quality of commercial saw palmetto products may vary widely. For this reason, it is best to purchase a saw palmetto product that has been evaluated by an independent lab, such as Consumer Labs.

Safety Issues

Saw palmetto is generally thought to be essentially nontoxic. It is also nearly side-effect free. In a 3-year study, only 34 of the 435 participants complained of side effects—primarily the usual mild gastrointestinal distress.

However, there is one unexpected case report of saw palmetto apparently causing excessive bleeding during surgery. The significance of this isolated event isn't clear, but it definitely raises concerns. It is probably prudent to avoid saw palmetto prior to and just after surgery, and during the period surrounding labor and delivery. Individuals with bleeding problems (such as hemophilia) should also avoid saw palmetto, as should those taking any drug that "thins" the blood, such as **warfarin** (Coumadin), **heparin**, **aspirin**, **clopidogrel** (Plavix), **ticlopidine** (Ticlid), and **pentoxifylline** (Trental).

Saw palmetto has no known drug interactions. Safety for pregnant or nursing women, or those with severe kidney or liver disease, has not been established.

Schisandra

Schisandra chinensis

ALTERNATE NAMES/RELATED TERMS: *Fructus Schizandrae, Gomishi, Magnolia Vine, Wu-Wei-Zi*
PRINCIPAL PROPOSED USES: *None*
OTHER PROPOSED USES: *Cancer Prevention, Enhancing Mental Function, Hepatitis, Liver Protection, Sports Performance Enhancer*

Schisandra is a woody vine native to eastern Asia. It winds around the trunks of trees, covering the branches. The white flowers produce small red berries that may grow in clusters. Traditionally, the berries are harvested in the fall, dried, and then ground to make the powdered medicinal herb. The seeds of the fruit contain **lignans**, which are believed to be active constituents.

Schisandra has long been used in the traditional medicines of Russia and China for a wide variety of conditions, including asthma, coughs, and other respiratory ailments, diarrhea, insomnia, impotence, and kidney problems. Hunters and athletes have used schisandra in the belief that it will increase endurance and combat fatigue under physical stress.

More recently, schisandra has been studied for potential liver-protective effects.

What Is Schisandra Used for Today?

Schisandra has not been proven effective for any condition. Research on the herb is limited to studies in animals, as well as human trials that are not up to modern scientific standards.

Animal studies suggest schisandra may protect the liver from toxic damage, improve liver function, and stimulate liver cell regrowth. These findings led to its use in human trials for treating hepatitis. In a poorly designed and reported Chinese study of 189 people with hepatitis B, those given schisandra reportedly improved more rapidly than those given vitamins and liver extracts.

Other animal studies of schisandra have found possible anticancer properties.

Finally, weak evidence hints that schisandra or its extracts might enhance sports performance and improve mental function.

Dosage

Schisandra comes in capsules, tinctures, powder, tablets, and extracts. Common dosages are 1.5 to 6 g daily.

Safety Issues

Studies in mice, rats, and pigs have found schisandra to be relatively nontoxic. Noticeable side effects are apparently rare, though upset stomach and allergic reactions have been reported.

Safety in pregnant or nursing women, children, or people with severe liver or kidney disease has not been established.

Selenium

SUPPLEMENT FORMS/ALTERNATE NAMES: *Selenite, Selenium Dioxide, Selenized Yeast, Selenomethionine*

PRINCIPAL PROPOSED USES: *Cancer Prevention*

OTHER PROPOSED USES: *Acne, Anxiety, Asthma, Cataracts, Cervical Dysplasia, Diabetic Neuropathy, Fibromyalgia, General Well-being, Gout, Heart Disease Prevention, HIV Support, Male Infertility, Multiple Sclerosis, Osteoarthritis, Psoriasis, Rheumatoid Arthritis, Ulcers*

Selenium is a trace mineral that our bodies use to produce *glutathione peroxidase*. Glutathione peroxidase is part of the body's **antioxidant** defense system (see); it works with vitamin E to protect cell membranes from damage caused by dangerous, naturally occurring substances known as *free radicals*.

China has very low rates of colon cancer, presumably because of the nation's low-fat diet. However, in some parts of China where the soil is depleted of selenium, the incidence of various types of cancer is much higher than in the rest of the country. This fact has given rise to a theory that selenium deficiency is a common cause of cancer and that selenium supplements can reduce this risk.

As we will see, there is some preliminary evidence that selenium supplements might provide some protection against some types of cancer among people living in the U.S., but this evidence is far from definitive.

Requirements/Sources

The official U.S. and Canadian recommendations for daily intake of selenium are as follows:

- Infants 0–6 months, 15 mcg
  7–12 months, 20 mcg
- Children 1–3 years, 20 mcg
  4–8 years, 30 mcg
  9–13 years, 40 mcg
- Males and females 14 years and older, 55 mcg
- Pregnant women, 60 mcg
- Nursing women, 70 mcg

Selenium content of food varies depending on the selenium content of the soil in which it was grown. Studies suggest that many people in certain developed countries, including New Zealand, Belgium, and Scandinavia, do not get enough selenium in their diets. However,

most individuals in the U.S. and Canada are believed to consume more than enough selenium.

Foods containing significant and reliable amounts of selenium include animal products like meat, seafood, and dairy foods, as well as whole grains and vegetables grown in selenium-rich soils. These include wheat germ, nuts (particularly Brazil nuts), oats, whole-wheat bread, bran, red Swiss chard, brown rice, turnips, garlic, barley, and orange juice.

Certain digestive conditions, such as **Crohn's disease**, short-bowel syndrome, and **ulcerative colitis** may impair selenium absorption. In addition, medications that reduce stomach acid, such as proton pump inhibitors or H_2 blockers, may reduce absorption of selenium.

Therapeutic Dosages

In controlled trials of selenium, typical dosages were 100 to 200 mcg daily.

The two general types of selenium supplements available to consumers are organic and inorganic forms. These terms have a very specific chemical meaning and have nothing to do with "organic" foods. In chemistry, organic means that a substance's chemical structure includes carbon. Inorganic chemicals have no carbon atoms.

The inorganic form of selenium, selenite, is essentially selenium atoms bound to oxygen. Some research suggests that selenite is harder for the body to absorb than organic forms of selenium, such as selenomethionine (selenium bound to methionine, an essential amino acid) or high-selenium yeast (which contains selenomethionine). However, other research on both animals and humans suggests that selenite supplements are about as good as organic forms of selenium. These contradictory results suggest that any differences in absorption, if they exist at all, are relatively minor.

Therapeutic Uses

Preliminary evidence indicates that supplemental selenium may help prevent **cancer**.

Selenium is required for a well-functioning immune system. Based on this, selenium has been suggested as a treatment for people with **HIV**. However, the studies done so far have had mixed results at best. One study even hints that selenium deficiency may *increase* the infectiousness of women with HIV. On the positive side, another study found that selenium supplements decreased symptoms of psychological anxiety in patients undergoing HAART (highly active antiretroviral therapy), for reasons that are not clear.

One study of healthy people in the UK (where marginally low selenium intake is common) found that use of selenium supplements improved general immune function, as measured by response to poliovirus immunization.

A preliminary double-blind trial suggests that selenium supplements may improve **fertility in males** who are selenium deficient. Weak evidence suggests that selenium might be helpful for **diabetic neuropathy**.

Selenium has also been recommended for many other conditions, including **acne, anxiety, asthma, cataracts, cervical dysplasia, fibromyalgia, gout, multiple sclerosis, osteoarthritis, psoriasis**, and **ulcers**, but there is no real evidence as yet that it is actually helpful.

Current evidence regarding use of selenium for **preventing heart disease** is more negative than positive.

A large (about 500 participants) double-blind, placebo-controlled study failed to find that use of selenium supplements at 100, 200 or 300 mcg daily improved mood or **general well-being**.

Low selenium levels have been associated with increased likelihood of developing certain kinds of **rheumatoid arthritis**. However, selenium supplements *don't* appear to help rheumatoid arthritis once it has developed.

What Is the Scientific Evidence for Selenium?

Promising, but as yet preliminary, evidence hints that selenium supplements may help prevent cancer.

Evidence from observational studies indicates that low intake of selenium is tied to decreased risk of cancer. However, such studies are notoriously unreliable as guidelines to therapy. Only double-blind trials can truly determine whether selenium supplements can help prevent cancer. (For information on why this is

so, see **Why Does This Book Rely on Double-blind Studies?**)

The most important double-blind study on selenium and cancer was conducted by researchers at the University of Arizona Cancer Center. In this trial, which began in 1983, 1,312 people were divided into two groups. One group received 200 mcg of yeast-based selenium daily; the other received placebo. Participants were not deficient in selenium, although their selenium levels fell toward the bottom of the normal range. The researchers were trying to determine whether selenium could lower the incidence of skin cancers.

As it happened, no benefits for skin cancer were seen. (In fact, careful analysis of the data suggests that selenium supplements actually marginally *increased* risk of certain forms of skin cancer.) However, researchers saw dramatic declines in the incidence of several other cancers in the selenium group. For ethical reasons, researchers felt compelled to stop the study after several years and allow all participants to take selenium.

When all the results were tabulated, it became clear that the selenium-treated group developed almost 66% fewer prostate cancers, 50% fewer colorectal cancers, and about 40% fewer lung cancers as compared with the placebo group. (All these results were statistically significant.) Selenium-treated subjects also experienced a statistically significant (17%) decrease in overall mortality, a greater than 50% decrease in lung cancer deaths, and nearly a 50% decrease in total cancer deaths. A subsequent close look at the data showed that only study participants who were relatively low in selenium to begin with experienced protection from lung cancer or colon cancer; people with average or above average levels of selenium did not benefit significantly. It has not yet been reported whether this limitation of benefit to low-selenium participants was true of the other forms of cancer as well.

While this evidence is very promising, it has one major flaw. The laws of statistics tell us that when researchers start to deviate from the question their research was designed to answer, the results may not be trustworthy. Currently, other studies are underway in an attempt to validate the findings accidentally discovered in this trial.

Other evidence for the possible anticancer benefits of selenium comes from large-scale Chinese studies showing that giving selenium supplements to people who live in selenium-deficient areas reduces the incidence of cancer. In addition, animal trials have found anti-cancer benefits.

Safety Issues

The U.S. Institute of Medicine issues guidelines for the maximum total daily intake of various nutrients, based on estimations of what should be safe for virtually all healthy individuals. These tolerable upper intake levels (UL) are, thus, conservative guidelines. For selenium, they have been set as follows:

- Infants 0–6 months, 45 mcg
  7–12 months, 60 mcg
- Children 1–3 years, 90 mcg
  4–8 years, 150 mcg
  9–13 years, 280 mcg
- Males and females 14 years and older, 400 mcg
- Pregnant or nursing women, 400 mcg

Note that these dosages apply to combined dietary and supplemental intake of selenium; when deciding how much selenium it's safe to take, keep in mind that most adults already receive about 100 mcg of selenium in the daily diet.

Maximum safe doses of selenium for individuals with severe liver or kidney disease have not been established. Excessive selenium intake, beginning at about 900 mcg daily, can cause selenium toxicity. Signs include depression, nervousness, emotional instability, nausea, vomiting, and in some cases loss of hair and fingernails.

Interactions You Should Know About

If you are taking medications that reduce stomach acid, such as H_2 blockers or proton pump inhibitors: You may need extra selenium.

Senna

Cassia acutifolia, Cassia angustifolia, Cassia senna

PRINCIPAL PROPOSED USES: *Constipation*

Senna extract is an FDA-approved over-the-counter treatment for occasional constipation. Because there is no controversy regarding senna's effectiveness for this purpose, we do not present the supporting evidence here. Rather, we address the concerns that have been raised regarding senna's safety.

Senna contains chemicals in the anthranoid family, such as anthraquinones, anthrones, and dianthrones. Related substances are found in a variety of plants used for laxative purposes, such as cascara sagrada and turkey rhubarb. The mechanism of action of anthranoids, however, is somewhat worrisome: they seem to work primarily by damaging the cells lining the colon. In general, cell damage can be a precursor to cancer and, on this basis, concerns have been raised that senna might increase colon cancer risk.

Evaluating this possibility is more difficult than it sounds. The most obvious method is to survey a large population over time and see whether people who use senna have a higher incidence of colon cancer. However, studies of this type (observational studies) are inherently unreliable, because they don't show cause and effect. People with colon cancer or other precancerous conditions may become constipated and take senna and this would cause a statistical association between use of senna and colon cancer, even if senna did not cause cancer. In any case, the results of such studies have been mixed, and overall the association, if any, does not appear to be strong.

Studies in animals have generally been reassuring, but a few such trials, as well as test-tube studies, have found some evidence of possible increased risk with long-term use.

Senna does have one potential safety advantage over other herbal anthranoid laxatives: its particular anthranoids are not very absorbable. This reduces the potential risk of harm deeper in the body.

The bottom line: At present, it appears reasonable to conclude that short-term use of senna is quite safe, while long-term use might or might not be safe. However, senna is not recommended for long-term use. Chronic senna consumption can cause dependency, meaning that it becomes impossible to have a bowel movement without it. In addition, there have been sporadic reports of unusual reactions to chronic use of senna, such as hepatitis. Thus, if used appropriately, senna should be safe.

As is the case with all laxatives, people with significant colonic disease, such as **ulcerative colitis**, should not use senna.

If senna is taken to the point of diarrhea, the body may become depleted of the mineral **potassium**. This is particularly dangerous for people using drugs in the digoxin family, which can cause dangerous cardiac arrythmias if potassium levels in the blood are inadequate. People who use medications that themselves deplete the body of potassium, such as thiazide or loop diuretics, are at special risk of this complication of senna overuse.

The safety of senna during pregnancy has not been established, and pregnant women are advised to avoid senna during the first trimester. Nursing women should also avoid using senna.

Interactions You Should Know About

If you are taking **digoxin**, **thiazide diuretics**, or **loop diuretics**, it is especially important not to overuse senna.

Silicon

PRINCIPAL PROPOSED USES: *Aging Skin, Brittle Hair, Brittle Nails*

OTHER PROPOSED USES:

  Prevention: *Alzheimer's Disease, Atherosclerosis, Osteoporosis*

Silicon is one of the most prevalent elements on earth; it makes up more than a quarter of the earth's crust, mostly as silicon dioxide. Silicon is hypothesized to play an essential role in the body, but this is uncertain. Silicon supplements are currently marketed for improving the health of bone, skin, hair, and nails. The substance silicone, once used in breast implants, also contains silicon, but in an unusual synthetic form.

Requirements/Sources

Scientists have found it difficult to determine whether silicon is an essential nutrient in humans and, if it is, to identify the necessary daily intake. Silicon is found in whole grains, some root vegetables, and beer. Silicon-containing chemicals are also added to prevent caking in products such as salt and baking soda. The average intake of silicon is approximately 10 to 40 mg daily.

Therapeutic Dosages

When used as a supplement, common recommended dosage levels range from 10 to 30 mg per day.

Therapeutic Uses

Silicon is a constituent of the enzyme prolylhydrolase, which helps the body produce collagen and **glycosaminoglycans**. In addition, silicon is directly found in protein complexes that include glycosaminoglycans. These substances are essential for healthy bone, nails, hair, and skin.

Animal studies hint that silicon deprivation causes bone weakness as well as slowed wound healing. Artificial bone grafts containing silicon have been used successfully in surgical repair of damaged bones. Furthermore, in a major observational study, higher intake of silicon was associated with stronger bones. Based on these findings, silicon has been proposed as a bone-strengthening substance for preventing or treating **osteoporosis**. However, only double-blind, placebo-controlled studies can prove a treatment effective. (For information on why such studies are essential, see **Why Does This Book Rely on Double-blind Studies?**.) Only one such study has been performed on silicon as a treatment for osteoporosis and it found equivocal results at best.

One double-blind, placebo-controlled study did find potential benefits with silicon supplements for **aging skin, brittle nails**, and brittle hair. Fifty women with sun-damaged skin were give either 10 mg silicon daily (as orthosilicic acid) or placebo for 20 weeks. Measurements of skin roughness and elasticity showed improvement in the silicon group as compared to the placebo group. Brittleness of hair and nails also improved. However, this study, performed by the manufacturer of a silicon product, leaves much to be desired in design and reporting.

Silicon has also been claimed to help prevent **atherosclerosis**, but there is no meaningful evidence to support this claim.

Another potential use of silicon relates to the aluminum hypothesis of **Alzheimer's disease**, the theory that aluminum toxicity is a prominent contributor to the development of this condition. On some websites promoting silicon supplements, it is said that increased dietary silicon decreases aluminum absorption. However, whether or not silicon actually has this effect remains unclear. Furthermore, the hypothesis that aluminum is a major risk factor for Alzheimer's disease has lost ground in recent years.

Safety Issues

Silicon is thought to be a safe supplement when used at doses similar to the average daily intake. Based on conservative evaluation of data from animal studies, it has been estimated that even a much higher dose of 13 mg per kilogram of body weight should present little to no risk. (For an adult of average weight, this works out to 760 mg daily.) However, maximum safe doses in young children, pregnant or nursing women, or people with severe liver or kidney disease have not been established.

Silver

SUPPLEMENT FORMS/ALTERNATE NAMES: *Colloidal Silver*

PRINCIPAL PROPOSED USES: *We recommend against the use of oral silver products.*

The mineral silver has a long history of use in **Ayurveda**, the traditional medicine of India. Silver is toxic to many microbes and, on this basis, a suspension of finely ground silver granules called *colloidal silver* was once popular among U.S. physicians as an antiseptic. Currently, silver is used medically in the form of silver sulfadiazine, a cream used to prevent infection in burn victims. In addition, silver is used in some water purifiers to stop the growth of bacteria.

Oral colloidal silver is widely promoted on the Internet and elsewhere as a treatment for hundreds of conditions. Unfortunately, there is no evidence that this form of silver provides any medical benefits and it can lead to an unsightly and permanent discoloration of the skin called *argyria*.

Requirements/Sources

Silver is not an essential nutrient.

Therapeutic Dosages

A typical recommended dose of colloidal silver is 1 to 4 teaspoons a day, providing 25 to 100 mcg of silver.

Note: We strongly recommend against the use of oral silver products.

Therapeutic Uses

Colloidal silver kills microbes on contact and, for this reason, it can be properly described as an antiseptic. Despite widespread claims, however, it is not an antibiotic. The term *antibiotic*, as most commonly used, indicates a substance that is absorbed after administration and kills germs throughout the body. Colloidal silver does not have this property. When taken by mouth, it may destroy bacteria, fungi, and other organisms in the mouth and digestive tract, but it is not absorbed in sufficient concentrations to kill germs anywhere else. Colloidal silver is, thus, more analogous to bleach than to penicillin. Although both bleach and silver kill the germs that cause sinus infections, you can't treat a sinus infection by drinking either bleach or silver.

Confusion about the difference between an antibiotic and an antiseptic has led to an enormous number of false claims regarding silver's benefits. In fact, there is no reliable evidence that use of colloidal silver benefits any health condition.

Safety Issues

While oral use of silver is not believed to be toxic, it can cause a serious cosmetic problem known as *argyria*:

gray-black silver deposits that stain the skin and mucous membranes. The effect is unattractive and, to make matters worse, permanent: once it occurs, the discoloration never goes away. A growing number of cases of argyria have been reported in the United States due to the widespread marketing of colloidal silver products.

Safety in young children, pregnant or nursing women, or people with severe liver or kidney disease has not been established.

Skullcap, American/European

Scutellaria lateriflora

PRINCIPAL PROPOSED USES: *None*

OTHER PROPOSED USES: *Anxiety, Insomnia*

Native Americans as well as traditional European herbalists used skullcap to induce sleep, relieve nervousness, and moderate the symptoms of epilepsy, rabies, and other diseases related to the nervous system. In other words, skullcap was believed to function as an herbal sedative.

A relative of skullcap, *Scutellaria baicalensis*, is a common Chinese herb. However, the root instead of the above-the-ground portion of the plant is used and overall effects appear to be far different. The discussion below addresses American/European skullcap (*Scutellaria lateriflora*) only.

What Is Skullcap Used for Today?

Skullcap is still popular as a sedative. Unfortunately, there has been virtually no scientific investigation of how well the herb really works. The only meaningful reported study was a small double-blind, placebo-controlled trial that found indications that the herb might reduce anxiety levels in healthy volunteers.

Dosage

When taken by itself, the usual dosage of skullcap is approximately 1 to 2 g 3 times a day. However, skullcap is more often taken in combination with other sedative herbs such as **valerian**, **passionflower**, **hops**, and **melissa**, also called *lemon balm*. When using an herbal combination, follow the label instructions for dosage. Skullcap is usually not taken long term.

Safety Issues

Not much is known about the safety of skullcap. However, if you take too much, it can cause confusion and stupor. There have been reports of liver damage following consumption of products labeled skullcap; however, since skullcap has been known to be adulterated with germander, an herb toxic to the liver, it may not have been the skullcap that was at fault. Safety in young children, pregnant or nursing women, or those with severe liver or kidney disease has not been established.

Slippery Elm
Ulmus rubra, Ulmus fulva

PRINCIPAL PROPOSED USES: *None*

OTHER PROPOSED USES: *Cough, Dyspepsia, Esophageal Reflux, Gastritis, Hemorrhoids, Inflammatory Bowel Disease, Irritable Bowel Syndrome*

The dried inner bark of the slippery-elm tree was a favorite of many Native American tribes and was subsequently adopted by European colonists. Like **marshmallow** and **mullein**, slippery elm was used as a treatment for sore throat, coughs, dryness of the lungs, inflammations of the skin, wounds, and irritation of the digestive tract. It was also made into a kind of porridge to be taken by weaned infants and during convalescence from illness: various heroes of the Civil War are said to have credited slippery elm with their recovery from war wounds.

What Is Slippery Elm Used for Today?

Slippery elm has not been scientifically studied to any significant extent. It's primarily used today as a cough lozenge, widely available in pharmacies. Based on its soothing properties, slippery elm is also sometimes recommended for treating **irritable bowel syndrome**, inflammatory bowel disease (such as **Crohn's disease** and **ulcerative colitis**), **gastritis**, esophageal reflux (heartburn), and **hemorrhoids**. However, there is no meaningful evidence that it is helpful for any of these conditions.

Dosage

Suck cough lozenges as needed. For internal use, a typical dose is 500 to 1,000 mg 3 times daily.

Safety Issues

Other than occasional allergic reactions, slippery elm has not been associated with any toxicity. However, its safety has never been formally studied. Safety in young children, pregnant or nursing women, or those with severe liver or kidney disease has not been established.

Soy

SUPPLEMENT FORMS/ALTERNATE NAMES: *Hydrolyzed Soy Protein, Soy Protein, Soy Protein Extract*

PRINCIPAL PROPOSED USES: *High Cholesterol*

OTHER PROPOSED USES: *Allergic Rhinitis (Shoyu Polysaccharides), Cancer Prevention, Cyclic Mastitis, High Blood Pressure, Menopausal Symptoms, Menstrual Migraines, Osteoarthritis, Osteoporosis*

The soybean has been prized for centuries in Asia as a nutritious, high-protein food with a myriad of uses, and today it's popular in the United States, not only in Asian food, but also as a cholesterol-free meat and dairy substitute in traditional American foods. Soy burgers, soy yogurt, tofu hot dogs, and tofu cheese can be found in a growing number of grocery stores alongside the traditional white blocks of tofu, and soy is increasingly used as a protein filler in many prepared foods, including fast-food "hamburger."

Soy appears to reduce blood cholesterol levels, and the U.S. Food and Drug Administration has authorized allowing foods containing soy to carry a "heart-healthy" label.

Soy

Soybeans contain isoflavones, chemicals that are similar to estrogen. These are widely thought to be the active ingredients in soy, although, as discussed below, there is substantial evidence that other constituents may be equally or more important. Much of the information in this article overlaps with that in the **Isoflavone** article.

Sources

If you like Japanese, Chinese, Thai, or Vietnamese food, it's easy to get a healthy dose of soy. Tofu is one of the world's most versatile foods. It can be stir-fried, steamed, or added to soup. You can also mash a cake of tofu and use it in place of ricotta cheese in your lasagna. If you don't like tofu, there are many other soy products to try: plain soybeans, soy cheese, soy burgers, soy milk, or tempeh. Or, you can use a soy supplement instead.

Therapeutic Dosages

The FDA allows soy foods containing 6.5grams of soy to carry a heart-healthy label. Evidence suggests that a daily intake of 25 g of soy protein is adequate to noticeably reduce cholesterol. This amount is typically found in about 2.5 cups of soy milk or 0.5 pound of tofu.

Note: Soy is increasingly added to foods in the U.S. as a protein filler and there are concerns that some people here may be greatly exceeding the amount of soy eaten anywhere else in the world. Even the 25 g amount recommended for reducing cholesterol levels is relatively high. For comparison, in Asia, the average intake of soy is only about 10 g daily.

Therapeutic Uses

According to the combined evidence of numerous controlled studies, soy can reduce blood **cholesterol** levels and improve the ratio of LDL ("bad") versus HDL ("good") cholesterol. At an average dosage of 47 g daily, total cholesterol falls by about 9%, LDL cholesterol by 13%, and triglycerides by 10%. Soy's effects on HDL cholesterol itself are less impressive. Soy might also reduce **blood pressure**.

Soy may reduce the common **menopausal symptom** known as "hot flashes," but study results conflict. Soy has not been found helpful for improving the hot flashes that often occur in breast cancer survivors.

Unlike estrogen, soy appears to reduce the risk of uterine cancer. Its effect on breast cancer is not as well established, but there are reasons to believe that soy can help reduce breast **cancer** risk as well, possibly by reducing estrogen levels and lengthening the menstrual cycle. (For more information, see the **Isoflavone** article.) Soy has shown inconsistent promise for helping to prevent prostate and colon cancers.

One preliminary double-blind trial found evidence that soy protein can reduce symptoms of **osteoarthritis**. In addition, soy might help prevent **osteoporosis**.

In preliminary double-blind studies, a special extract of soy sauce called *Shoyu polysaccharides* has shown promise as a treatment for **allergic rhinitis** (hay fever).

The substance pinitol, found in soy, may improve blood sugar control in people with diabetes.

A product containing soy isoflavones and other herbs has shown some promise for **migraine headaches** associated with the menstrual cycle (menstrual migraines).

Weak evidence suggests that soy protein may be helpful for **cyclic breast pain**.

What Is the Scientific Evidence for Soy?

High Cholesterol

Numerous controlled studies indicate that soy can reduce LDL ("bad") cholesterol by about 10% and perhaps slightly raise HDL ("good") cholesterol as well.

Although there is some evidence that isoflavones are the active ingredients in soy responsible for improving cholesterol profile, in most studies purified isoflavones alone have failed to work. It is possible that non-isoflavone constituents of soy, such as proteins, fiber, and phospholipids, may be equally or perhaps even more important than the isoflavones in soy. For example, the substance pinitol appears to have cholesterol-lowering properties.

However, there are other possibilities as well. One study suggests that the isoflavone daidzein may be only effective for reducing cholesterol when it is converted by intestinal bacteria into a substance called *equol*. It appears that only about one-third of people have the right intestinal bacteria to make equol.

Another study found that soy products may at times have an unusual isoflavone profile—containing high levels of the isoflavone glycitein rather than the more usual **genistein** and daidzein. Glycitein could be inactive regarding cholesterol reduction; in other words, variations in the proportions of specific isoflavone constituents might have made some studied soy isoflavone products inactive.

Menopausal Symptoms ("Hot Flashes")

Although study results are not entirely consistent, soy may be helpful for symptoms of menopause, especially "hot flashes." For example, a double-blind, placebo-controlled study involving 104 women found that isoflavone-rich soy protein provided significant relief of hot flashes compared to placebo (milk protein). Improvements in hot flashes, as well as other symptoms, such as vaginal dryness, were seen in several other studies of soy or soy isoflavones as well. However, about as many studies have failed to find benefit with soy or concentrated isoflavones. Furthermore, in three double-blind, placebo-controlled trials, isoflavone-rich soy failed to reduce hot flashes among survivors of breast cancer.

To make matters even more complicated, a double-blind study of 241 women experiencing hot flashes found equivalent benefits whether isoflavone-free or isoflavone-rich soy products were used.

The high rate of the placebo effect seen in many studies of menopausal symptoms may account for these discrepancies. In addition, it is possible that certain formulations of soy contain as yet unidentified ingredients beyond isoflavones that play an important role.

Osteoporosis

In one study that evaluated the benefits of soy in osteoporosis, a total of 66 postmenopausal women took either placebo (soy protein with isoflavones removed) or soy protein with 56 or 90 mg of isoflavones daily for 6 months. The group that took the higher dosage of isoflavones showed significant gains in spinal bone density. There was little change in the placebo or low-dose isoflavone groups. This study suggests that the soy isoflavones in soy protein may be effective for osteoporosis.

Very nearly the same results were also seen in a similar study. This 24-week, double-blind study of 69 postmenopausal women found that soy can significantly reduce bone loss from the spine.

Similar benefits with soy or soy isoflavones have been seen in other human and animal trials, but other studies have failed to find benefit. On balance it is probably fair to say that isoflavones (either as soy, purified isoflavones, or tofu extract) are likely to have a modestly beneficial effect on bone density.

Interestingly, one small but long-term study suggests that **progesterone cream** (another treatment proposed for use in preventing or treating osteoporosis) may decrease the bone-sparing effect of soy isoflavones.

Estrogen and most other medications for osteoporosis work by fighting bone breakdown. It has been hypothesized that soy may also work in other ways, by helping to increase new bone formation.

Safety Issues

Studies in animals have found soy essentially nontoxic. However, soy or its isoflavones could conceivably have some potentially harmful effects in certain specific situations.

Soy appears to have numerous potential effects involving the thyroid gland. When given to individuals with **impaired thyroid function**, soy products have been observed to reduce absorption of thyroid medication. In addition, some evidence hints that soy isoflavones may directly inhibit the function of the thyroid gland, although this inhibition may only be significant in individuals who are deficient in iodine. However, to make matters even more confusing, studies of healthy humans and animals given soy isoflavones or other soy products have generally found that soy either had no effect on thyroid hormone levels or actually increased levels. The bottom line: In view of soy's complex effects regarding the thyroid, individuals with impaired thyroid function should not take large amounts of soy products except under the supervision of a physician.

One study found that soy products may decrease testosterone levels in men. This could conceivably cause problems for men with **infertility** or **erectile dysfunction**.

Soy may reduce the absorption of the nutrients zinc, iron, and calcium. To avoid absorption problems, you should probably take these minerals at least 2 hours apart from eating soy.

Other concerns relate to the estrogenic properties of soy isoflavones. For example, while soy is thought to reduce the risk of developing breast cancer, it is possible that soy might not be safe for women who have already had breast cancer. In addition, there are concerns that intensive use of soy products by pregnant women could exert a hormonal effect that impacts unborn fetuses. Finally, fears have been expressed by some experts that soy might interfere with the action of **oral contraceptives**.

Spirulina

However, one study of 36 women found reassuring results. For more information on these and other safety issues regarding the isoflavones in soy, see the full **Isoflavones** article.

One observational study raised concerns that soy might impair mental function. However, observational studies are highly unreliable by nature, and experts do not consider this a serious issue.

Interactions You Should Know About

If you are taking:

> ➤ Zinc, iron, or calcium supplements: It may be best to eat soy at a different time of day to avoid absorption problems.
> ➤ Thyroid hormone: You should consult your physician before increasing your intake of soy products.

Spirulina

SUPPLEMENT FORMS/ALTERNATE NAMES: *Blue-green Algae*
PRINCIPAL PROPOSED USES: *Nutritional Support*
OTHER PROPOSED USES: *Cancer Prevention, Fibromyalgia, Hay Fever, Herpes Infection, High Cholesterol, HIV Infection, Hives, Immune Support, Liver Protection, Weight Loss*

The supplement called *spirulina* consists of one or more members of a family of blue-green algae. The name was inspired by the spiral shapes in which these plants array themselves as they grow. Other blue-green algae products are also available on the market and they are discussed in this article as well.

Spirulina grows in the wild in salty lakes in Mexico and on the African continent. It reproduces quickly and, because the individual plants tend to stick together, it is easy to harvest. Records of the Spanish conquistadores suggest that the Aztecs used spirulina as a food source; we also know that the Kanembu people of Central Africa harvested it from what is now called Lake Chad.

This plant contains high levels of various B vitamins, **beta-carotene**, other carotenoids, and minerals, including **calcium, iron, magnesium, manganese, potassium,** and **zinc**. It is also a source of **gamma-linolenic acid** (GLA). Spirulina is a rich source of protein—dried spirulina contains up to 70% protein by weight—but you'd have to eat an awful lot of spirulina capsules to obtain a significant amount of protein this way. Spirulina also contains **vitamin B$_{12}$**, a nutrient otherwise found almost exclusively in animal foods. However, there's a catch: the vitamin B$_{12}$ in spirulina is not absorbable.

Spirulina has not been proven effective for any medical condition and there are significant safety concerns involving all forms of blue-green algae (see Safety Issues below).

Requirements/Sources

Unless you live within 35 degrees of the equator, and on the shores of an alkaline lake, you will have difficulty finding spirulina anywhere but in a health food store. Most carry a number of brands of spirulina that has been dried and processed into powder or tablets.

Therapeutic Dosages

Researchers studying spirulina's effects on health have used a variety of doses, ranging from 1 to 8.4 g daily.

Therapeutic Uses

There is no question that spirulina is a nutritious food, but it isn't cheap. Protein can be obtained much more easily and inexpensively from legumes, nuts, grains, and animal foods, iron from dark greens, prunes, and meat, and carotenes and vitamins from standard fruits and vegetables.

Spirulina might have other specific therapeutic uses beyond general nutritional support, but the evidence supporting these recommendations is highly preliminary at best.

Manufacturers of spirulina supplements sometimes claim that the plant can reduce appetite, thereby helping overweight individuals control their food intake. However, one small double-blind study of spirulina for **weight loss** failed to find a significant difference between spirulina and placebo treatment.

One small double-blind trial did find evidence that a blue-green algae called *Chlorella pyrenoidosa* might be useful for **fibromyalgia**.

It is commonly stated that spirulina and related products can **enhance immunity**. However, most of the evidence supporting this statement is too weak to mean much; the one meaningful trial, a double-blind study of 124 healthy adults, failed to find that chlorella supplements enhanced the immune response to influenza vaccine.

Evidence from animal studies, preliminary human trials and one small double-blind, placebo-controlled study suggests that spirulina or other forms of algae might improve cholesterol profile.

Very preliminary evidence hints that spirulina may help prevent **cancer**.

Test tube and animal studies suggest that spirulina might have some activity against the **HIV**, but much more research needs to be done before we could say that spirulina is helpful against HIV infection.

Highly preliminary evidence suggests that spirulina or other blue-green algae products may activate the counter allergic reactions, such as **hay fever** and **hives**, help **protect the liver** from toxic chemicals, reduce **blood pressure**, and control symptoms of **ulcerative colitis**.

Despite widespread publicity, there is no evidence that spirulina is useful for **attention deficit disorder**.

What Is the Scientific Evidence for Spirulina?

There are no well-documented uses of spirulina.

Fibromyalgia

Fibromyalgia is a common chronic condition whose main symptoms are specific tender points on various parts of the body, widespread musculoskeletal discomfort, morning stiffness, fatigue, and disturbed sleep. The cause of fibromyalgia is not known and current treatments are far from completely satisfactory.

A recent study suggests that the nutritious algae *Chlorella pyrenoidosa* might be helpful. In this double-blind, placebo-controlled trial 37 people with fibromyalgia

were given either placebo or chlorella supplements at a dose of 10 g daily. At the end of 3 months, individuals were switched to the opposite group, and then treated for an additional 3 months. The results showed significant improvements in symptoms when participants used chlorella as compared to placebo.

Weight Loss

A double-blind, placebo-controlled trial investigated the possible weight loss effects of spirulina. However, while individuals taking 8.4 g of spirulina daily lost weight, the difference between the spirulina group and the placebo group was not statistically significant. Larger and longer studies are needed to establish whether spirulina is indeed an effective treatment for obesity.

Safety Issues

Spirulina itself appears to be nontoxic. Studies in rats showed that high spirulina intake caused no weight reduction or toxicity symptoms in rats, nor did spirulina affect the rats' ability to reproduce normally.

Nevertheless, there are areas of serious concern for consumers.

Various forms of blue-green algae can be naturally contaminated with highly toxic substances called *microcystins*. Some states, such as Oregon, require producers to strictly limit the concentration of microcystins in blue-green algae products, but the same protections cannot be assumed to have been applied to all products on the market. Furthermore, the maximum safe intake of microcystins is not clear, and it is possible that when blue-green algae is used for a long time, toxic effects might build up. Long-term use by children raises particular concerns, especially in light of the widely popularized but unsubstantiated belief that blue-green algae is useful for attention deficit disorder.

Blue-green algae can also contain a different kind of highly toxic substance, called *anatoxin*.

In addition, when spirulina is grown with the use of fermented animal waste fertilizers, contamination with dangerous bacteria could occur. There are also concerns that spirulina might concentrate radioactive ions found in its environment. Probably of most concern is spirulina's ability to absorb and concentrate heavy metals, such as lead and mercury, if they are present in its environment. One study of spirulina samples grown in a number of locations found them to contain an unacceptably high content of these toxic metals. However, a second study on this topic claims that the first used an

Spleen Extract

unreliable method of analyzing heavy metal content and concludes that a person would have to eat more than 77 g daily of the most heavily contaminated spirulina to reach unsafe mercury and lead consumption levels.

These researchers, however, go on to suggest that it is not prudent to eat more than 50 g of spirulina daily. The reason they give is that the plant contains a high concentration of nucleic acids, substances related to DNA. When these are metabolized, they create uric acid, which could cause **gout** or **kidney stones**. This is of special concern to those who have already had uric acid stones or attacks of gout.

The safety of spirulina in pregnant and nursing women, young children, and individuals with kidney or liver disease has not been determined.

Spleen Extract

PRINCIPAL PROPOSED USES: *Immune Support*

The spleen is an organ located under the left side of the rib cage. Its functions in the body include removing "worn out" red blood cells and supplying certain types of white blood cells (immune cells). For use as a supplement, spleen extracts are made from the spleens of cows, pigs, or other animals.

According to a theory prevalent in some parts of alternative medicine, the consumption of spleen extracts can strengthen the function of an underperforming spleen. On this basis, spleen extracts are sometimes suggested for supporting the immune system. However, there is no meaningful scientific rationale or scientific evidence to indicate that this approach actually works.

Some manufacturers of glandular products claim that the animal version of an organ provides nutrients that support the corresponding organ in humans. However, there is no evidence that the human spleen requires any nutrients that are uniquely available in animal spleens.

It has been suggested by one manufacturer that consuming extracts of an organ might offer benefit in an indirect manner. According to this theory, some people may possess antibodies to certain of their own organs and, by consuming a similar organ, these antibodies will be diverted from their target. However, this explanation does not make a great deal of sense. Antibodies are primarily produced against proteins and, even if cow spleens had the same proteins as human spleens, which is unlikely, proteins are digested in the intestines and not absorbed whole into the bloodstream.

It may be that, on an unconscious level, those who recommend glandular extracts are being influenced by the ancient notion of *sympathetic magic*, the idea that eating a lion's heart, for example, will create courage. However, this is a prescientific form of reasoning that is difficult to take seriously in the modern era.

In any case, there is no meaningful scientific evidence to indicate that use of spleen extracts offers any benefits. Only double-blind, placebo-controlled studies can show a treatment effective and at present none have been reported for spleen extracts. (For information on why this type of study is essential, see **Why Does This Book Rely on Double-blind Studies?**) The only published studies on oral use of spleen glandular extracts date back to the 1930s and do not remotely reach current scientific standards. More recent studies have evaluated injected extracts of spleen, but these findings are not likely to apply to the oral product.

Sports Supplements, General

SUPPLEMENT FORMS/ALTERNATE NAMES: *Athletic Performance, Ergogenic Aids, Exercise, Fitness, Performance Enhancers*

In the competitive world of sports, the smallest advantage can make an enormous difference in the outcome of a contest. A substance that improves an athlete's strength, speed, or endurance is called an *ergogenic aid*. These are discussed in the Collins Alternative Health Guide article titled **Sports and Fitness Support: Enhancing Performance**.

Supplements could conceivably play another helpful role for athletes as well: aiding recovery from the "side effects" of intense exercise. While exercise of moderate intensity is almost undoubtedly a purely positive activity, high intensity endurance exercise can lead to respiratory infections. In addition, all forms of high intensity exercise can cause muscle soreness, which may get in the way of training. Herbs and supplements advocated for these problems are the subject of the article titled **Sports and Fitness Support: Enhancing Recovery**.

For information on natural treatments intended to aid recovery from injuries caused by sports, see the **Minor Injuries** article.

St. John's Wort

Hypericum perforatum

PRINCIPAL PROPOSED USES: *Mild to Moderate Depression*

OTHER PROPOSED USES: *Anxiety, Diabetic Neuropathy and Other Forms of Neuropathy, Eczema (Topical Cream), Insomnia, Menopause, Obsessive Compulsive Disorder, Premenstrual Syndrome (PMS), Seasonal Affective Disorder (SAD)*

PROBABLY INEFFECTIVE USES: *Viral Infections*

St. John's wort is a common perennial herb of many branches and bright yellow flowers that grows wild in much of the world. Its name derives from the herb's tendency to flower around the feast of St. John. (A *wort* simply means "plant" in Old English.) The species name *perforatum* derives from the watermarking of translucent dots that can be seen when the leaf is held up to the sun.

St. John's wort has a long history of use in treating emotional disorders. During the Middle Ages, St. John's wort was popular for "casting out demons." In the 1800s, the herb was classified as a *nervine*, or a treatment for "nervous disorders." When pharmaceutical antidepressants were invented, German researchers began to look for similar properties in St. John's wort.

What Is St. John's Wort Used for Today?

Today, St. John's wort is a widely used treatment for depression in Germany, other parts of Europe, and the United States. The evidence-base for its use approaches that of many modern prescription drugs at the time of their first approval.

Most studies of St. John's wort have evaluated individuals with major **depression** of mild to moderate intensity. This contradictory-sounding language indicates that the level of depression is more severe than simply feeling "blue." However, it is not as severe as the most severe forms of depression. Typical symptoms include depressed mood, lack of energy, sleep problems, anxiety, appetite disturbance, difficulty concentrating, and poor stress tolerance. Irritability can also be a sign of depression.

Taken as a whole, research suggests that St. John's wort is more effective than placebo and approximately as effective as standard drugs. Furthermore, St. John's wort appears to cause fewer side effects than many antidepressants. However, the herb does present one significant safety risk: it interacts harmfully with a great many standard medications (see Safety Issues below for details).

Warning: St. John's wort should never be relied on for the treatment of severe depression. If you or a loved one feels suicidal, unable to cope with daily life, paralyzed by anxiety, incapable of getting out of bed, unable to sleep, or uninterested in eating, see a physician at once. Professional care may be lifesaving.

Besides depression, St. John's wort has also been tried for many other conditions in which prescription antidepressants are thought useful, such as **attention deficit disorder**, **anxiety**, **insomnia**, **menopausal symptoms**, **premenstrual syndrome** (PMS), **seasonal affective disorder** (SAD), and social phobia. However, there is as yet no direct evidence that it offers any benefit for these conditions. One substantial double-blind study did find St. John's wort potentially helpful for somatoform disorders (commonly called *psychosomatic illnesses*).

Standard antidepressants are also often used for **diabetic neuropathy** and other forms of neuropathy (nerve pain). However, a small double-blind, placebo-controlled trial failed to find St. John's wort effective for this purpose. Another study failed to find St. John's wort helpful for obsessive-compulsive disorder.

St. John's wort contains, among other ingredients, the substances hypericin and hyperforin. Early reports suggested that St. John's wort or synthetic hypericin might be useful against viruses such as **HIV**, but these haven't panned out. However, there is some evidence hyperforin may be able to fight certain bacteria, including some that are resistant to antibiotics. **Note:** This evidence is far too preliminary to count St. John's wort as an effective antibiotic.

Based on weak evidence that hypericin might have anti-inflammatory properties, St. John's wort cream has been tried as a treatment for **eczema**, with some promising results.

One interesting double-blind study evaluated a combination therapy containing St. John's wort and **black cohosh** in 301 women with general **menopausal symptoms**, as well as depression. The results showed that use of the combination treatment was significantly more effective than placebo for both problems.

What Is the Scientific Evidence for St. John's Wort?

Depression

The results of numerous studies suggest St. John's wort is effective for mild to moderate depression.

There have been two main kinds of studies: those that compared St. John's wort to placebo and others that compared it to prescription antidepressants.

➢ St. John's Wort versus Placebo

Studies of St. John's wort (and other antidepressants) use a set of questions called the *Hamilton Depression Index* (HAM-D). This scale rates the extent of depression, with higher numbers indicating more serious symptoms.

Double-blind, placebo-controlled trials involving a total of more than 1,000 participants with major depression of mild to moderate severity have generally found that use of St. John's wort can significantly reduce HAM-D scores as compared to placebo.

For example, in a 6-week trial, 375 individuals with average 17-item HAM-D scores of about 22 (indicating major depression of moderate severity) were given either St. John's wort or placebo. Individuals taking St. John's wort showed significantly greater improvement than those taking placebo.

Three double-blind, placebo-controlled trials evaluating individuals with a similar level of depression have failed to find St. John's wort more effective than placebo. However, three studies cannot overturn a body of positive research. Keep in mind that 35% of double-blind studies involving pharmaceutical antidepressants have also failed to find the active agent significantly more effective than placebo. As if to illustrate this, in two of the three studies in which St. John's wort failed to prove effective, a conventional drug (Zoloft in one case, Prozac in the other) also failed to prove effective. The reason for these negative outcomes is not that Zoloft or Prozac does not work. Rather, statistical effects can easily hide the benefits of a drug, especially in a condition like depression where there is a high placebo effect and no really precise method of measuring symptoms. Thus, unless a whole series of studies find St. John's wort ineffective, especially trials in which a comparison drug treatment does prove effective, St. John's wort should still be regarded as probably effective for major depression of mild to moderate severity.

➣ *St. John's Wort versus Medications*

At least eight double-blind trials enrolling a total of more than 1,200 people have compared St. John's wort to fluoxetine (Prozac), citalopram (Celexa), paroxetine (Paxil), or sertraline (Zoloft). In all of these studies, the herb proved as effective as the drug, and generally caused fewer side effects.

In the largest of these trials, a 6-week study of 388 people with major depression of mild-to-moderate severity, St. John's wort proved equally effective as the drug citalopram (Celexa) and more effective than placebo. Additionally, Celexa caused a significantly higher rate of side effects than St. John's wort. There were also significantly more side effects in the placebo group than in the St. John's wort group—presumably because treatment of depression reduces physical symptoms of psychological origin.

St. John's wort has also been compared to older antidepressants, with generally favorable results.

➣ *How Does St. John's Wort Work for Depression?*

Like pharmaceutical antidepressants, St. John's wort is thought to raise levels of neurotransmitters in the brain, such as serotonin, norepinephrine, and dopamine.

The active ingredient of St. John's wort is not known. Extracts of St. John's wort are most often standardized to the substance hypericin, which has led to the widespread misconception that hypericin is the active ingredient. However, there is no evidence that hypericin itself is an antidepressant. Another ingredient of St. John's wort named hyperforin has shown considerable promise as the most important ingredient. Hyperforin was first identified as a constituent of *Hypericum perforatum* in 1971 by Russian researchers, but it was incorrectly believed to be too unstable to play a major role in the herb's action. However, subsequent evidence corrected this view. It now appears that standard St. John's wort extract contains about 1 to 6% hyperforin. Evidence from animal and human studies suggests that it is the hyperforin in St. John's wort that raises the levels of neurotransmitters. Nonetheless, there may be other active ingredients in St. John's wort also at work. In fact, two double-blind trials using a form of St. John's wort with low hyperforin content found it effective. The bottom line remains that more research is necessary to discover just how St. John's wort acts against depression.

Polyneuropathy

A double-blind, placebo-controlled trial of 54 people with diabetic neuropathy or other forms of neuropathy (pain, numbness and/or tingling caused by injury to nerves) did not find St. John's wort effective for this purpose.

Dosage

The typical dosage of St. John's wort is 300 mg 3 times a day of an extract standardized to contain 0.3% hypericin. Some products are standardized to hyperforin content (usually 2 to 3%) instead of hypericin. These are usually taken at the same dosage. Two studies found benefits with a single daily dose of 900 mg.

Yet another form of St. John's wort has also shown effectiveness in double-blind studies. This form contains little hyperforin and is taken at a dose of 250 mg twice daily. There is some evidence that this form of St. John's wort may be less likely to interact with medications. (See Drug Interactions below.)

If the herb bothers your stomach, take it with food.

Remember that the full effect takes 4 weeks to develop. Don't give up too soon!

Safety Issues

St. John's wort taken alone usually does not cause immediate side effects. In a study designed to look for side effects, 3,250 people took St. John's wort for 4 weeks. Overall, about 2.4% reported problems. The most common complaints were mild stomach discomfort (0.6%), allergic reactions—primarily rash—(0.5%), tiredness (0.4%), and restlessness (0.3%). Another study followed 313 individuals treated with St. John's wort for 1 year. The results showed a similarly low incidence of adverse effects.

In the extensive German experience with St. John's wort as a treatment for depression, there have been no published reports of serious adverse consequences from taking the herb alone. Animal studies involving enormous doses of St. John's wort extracts for 26 weeks have not shown any serious effects.

However, there are a number of potential safety risks with St. John's wort that should be considered. These are outlined in the following sections.

Photosensitivity

Cows and sheep grazing on St. John's wort have sometimes developed severe and even fatal sensitivity to the sun. In one study, highly sun-sensitive people were given twice the normal dose of the herb. The results showed a mild but measurable increase in reaction to ultraviolet radiation. Another trial found that a one-time dose of St. John's wort containing 2 or 6 times the normal daily dose did not cause an increased tendency to burn; nor did 7 days of treatment at the normal dose. However, there is a case report of severe and unexpected burning in an individual who used St. John's wort and then received ultraviolet therapy for psoriasis. In addition, two individuals using topical St. John's wort experienced severe reactions to sun exposure.

The morals of the story are as follows: if you are especially sensitive to the sun, don't exceed the recommended dose of St. John's wort, and continue to take your usual precautions against burning; if you are receiving UV treatment, do not use St. John's wort at all; and if you apply St. John's wort to your skin, keep that part of your body away from the sun.

In addition, you might get into problems if you combine St. John's wort with other medications that cause increased sun sensitivity, such as sulfa drugs and the anti-inflammatory medication Feldene (piroxicam). The medications Prilosec (omeprazole) and Prevacid (lansoprazole) may also increase the tendency of St. John's wort to cause photosensitivity.

Finally, a report suggests that regular use of St. John's wort might also increase the risk of sun-induced cataracts. While this is preliminary information, it may make sense to wear sunglasses when outdoors if you are taking this herb on a long-term basis.

Drug Interactions

Herbal experts have warned for some time that combining St. John's wort with drugs in the Prozac family (SSRIs) might raise serotonin too much and cause a number of serious problems. Recently, case reports of such events have begun to trickle in. This is a potentially serious risk. Do not combine St. John's wort with prescription antidepressants except on the specific advice of a physician. Since some antidepressants, such as Prozac, linger in the blood for quite some time, you also need to exercise caution when switching from a drug to St. John's wort.

Antimigraine drugs in the triptan family (such as sumatriptan, or Imitrex) and the pain-killing drug tramadol also raise serotonin levels and might interact similarly with St. John's wort.

However, perhaps the biggest concern with St. John's wort is that it appears to decrease the effectiveness of numerous medications, including protease inhibitors and reverse transcriptase inhibitors (for HIV infection), cyclosporine and tacrolimus (for organ transplants), digoxin (for heart disease), statin drugs (used for high cholesterol) warfarin (Coumadin) (a blood thinner), chemotherapy drugs, oral contraceptives, tricyclic antidepressants, protein pump inhibitors (like Prilosec), anesthetics, and olanzapine or clozapine (for schizophrenia).

There are theoretical reasons to believe that this herb might interact with about 50% of all medications.

These interactions could lead to catastrophic consequences. Indeed, St. John's wort appears to have caused several cases of heart, kidney, and liver transplant rejection by interfering with the action of cyclosporine. Also, many people with HIV take St. John's wort in the false belief that the herb will fight AIDS. The unintended result may be to reduce the potency of standard anti-HIV drugs. Furthermore, if you are taking St. John's wort and one of these medications at the same time and then stop taking the herb, blood levels of the drug may rise to dangerous levels.

The herb also appears to decrease the effectiveness of oral contraceptives and by doing so is thought to have caused unwanted pregnancies.

There is some evidence that low-hyperforin St. John's wort may have less potential for drug interactions than other forms of St. John's wort. Nonetheless, we recommend that people taking any oral or injected medication that is critical to their health or well-being should entirely avoid using any form of St. John's wort until more is known; if you are already taking the herb, you should not stop taking it until you can simultaneously have your drug levels monitored. On general principles, we also advise avoiding use of the herb prior to undergoing general anesthesia.

Safety in Special Circumstances

One animal study found no ill effects on the offspring of pregnant mice. However, these findings alone are not sufficient to establish St. John's wort as safe for use during pregnancy. Furthermore, the St. John's wort constituent hypericin can accumulate in the nucleus of cells and directly bind to DNA. For this reason, pregnant or nursing women should avoid St. John's wort. Furthermore, safety for use by young children or people with severe liver or kidney disease has not been established.

Like other antidepressants, case reports suggest that St. John's wort can cause episodes of mania in individuals with **bipolar disorder** (manic-depressive disease).

There is also one report of St. John's wort causing temporary psychosis in a person with **Alzheimer's disease**.

Other Concerns

Certain foods contain a substance named tyramine. These foods include aged cheeses, aged or cured meat, sauerkraut, soy sauce, other soy condiments, beer (especially beer on tap), and wine. Drugs in the MAO inhibitor family interact adversely with tyramine, causing severe side effects, such as high blood pressure, rapid heart rate, and delirium. One case report suggests that St. John's wort might present this risk as well. However, other studies suggest that normal doses of St. John's wort should not cause MAO-like effects. Until this issue is sorted out, we recommend that individuals taking St. John's wort avoid tyramine-containing foods. Since MAO inhibitors react adversely with stimulant drugs, such as Ritalin, ephedrine (found in the herb **ephedra**), and caffeine, we also recommend that you avoid combining St. John's wort with them.

One small study suggests that high doses of St. John's wort might slightly impair mental function.

One case report associates use of St. John's wort with hair loss. The authors note that standard antidepressants may also cause hair loss at times.

One study raised questions about possible antifertility effects of St. John's wort. When high concentrations of St. John's wort were placed in a test tube with hamster sperm and ova, the sperm were damaged and less able to penetrate the ova. However, since it is unlikely that this much St. John's wort can actually come in contact with sperm and ova when they are in the body rather than in a test tube, these results may not be meaningful in real life.

Transitioning from Medications to St. John's Wort

If you are taking a prescription drug for mild to moderate depression, switching to St. John's wort may be a reasonable idea if you would prefer taking an herb. To avoid overlapping treatments, the safest approach is to stop taking the drug and allow it to wash out of your system before starting St. John's wort. Consult with your doctor on how much time is necessary.

However, if you are taking medication for severe depression, switching over to St. John's wort is *not* a good idea. The herb probably won't work well enough and you may sink into a dangerous depression.

Interactions You Should Know About

If you are taking:

- Antidepressant drugs, including MAO inhibitors, SSRIs, and tricyclics, or possibly the drugs tramadol or sumatriptan (Imitrex): Do not take St. John's wort at the same time. Actually, you need to let the medication flush out of your system for a while (perhaps weeks, depending on the drug) before you start the herb.
- Digoxin, cyclosporine and tacrolimus, protease inhibitors or reverse transcriptase inhibitors, oral contraceptives, tricyclic antidepressants, warfarin (Coumadin), statin drugs, theophylline, chemotherapy drugs, newer antipsychotic medications (such as olanzapine and clozapine), anesthetics, or, indeed, any critical medication: St. John's wort might cause the drug to be less effective. Furthermore, if you are already taking St. John's wort and your physician adjusts your medication dosage to achieve proper blood levels, suddenly stopping St. John's wort could cause the level of the drug in your body to rebound to dangerously high levels.
- Medications that cause sun sensitivity, such as sulfa drugs and the anti-inflammatory medication piroxicam (Feldene), as well as omeprazole (Prilosec) or lansoprazole (Prevacid): Keep in mind that St. John's wort might have an additive effect.
- Stimulant drugs or herbs, such as Ritalin, caffeine, or ephedrine (ephedra): It is possible that St. John's wort might interact adversely with them.

Stanols/Sterols

SUPPLEMENT FORMS/ALTERNATE NAMES: *Campestanol, 5-Alpha-Stanols, Phytostanols, Phytosterols, Sitostanol, Stanol esters, Sterol esters, Sterols, Stigmastanol*

PRINCIPAL PROPOSED USES: *Lowering Cholesterol*

Stanols are substances that occur naturally in various plants. Their cholesterol-lowering effects were first observed in animals in the 1950s. Since then, a substantial amount of research suggests that plant stanols (usually modified into stanol esters) can help to lower cholesterol in individuals with normal or mildly to moderately elevated levels. Stanols are available in margarine spreads, salad dressings, and dietary supplement tablets.

Related substances called *sterols* or *phytosterols* (such as beta-sitosterol) and sterol esters appear to lower cholesterol in much the same manner as stanols. In this article, sterols and stanols and their ester forms are discussed together.

(**Note:** Use of beta-sitosterol for conditions other than high cholesterol is discussed in the **beta-sitosterol** article.)

Requirements/Sources

Sterols are found in most plant foods. Stanols occur naturally in wood pulp, tall oil (a byproduct of paper manufacturing), and soybean oil, and can also be manufactured from the sterols found in many foods. Stanol and sterol esters are manufactured by processing stanols or sterols with fatty acids from vegetable oils. Stanols and sterols and their esters are added to margarine spreads and salad dressings, and are also available as dietary supplement tablets.

Therapeutic Dosages

Typical dosages of stanol esters to lower cholesterol levels range from 3.4 , 5.1 g per day. One manufacturer of a commercially prepared margarine spread recommends taking 3 teaspoons (1.5 g of sitostanol ester per teaspoon) per day. The suggested use varies depending on the product and the quantity of sitostanol ester per serving. One study suggests that using stanol products once a day may be as effective as dividing up your intake throughout the day. It may take up to 3 months to show a substantial decrease in total cholesterol values.

The dosages of sterols and sterol esters have not been as well established, but are probably similar.

Therapeutic Uses

Strong evidence tells us that stanol esters and related substances taken on their own or in food products can significantly improve **cholesterol** levels. They are thought to work by attaching to cholesterol in the digestive tract and carrying it out of the body. This not only interferes with the absorption of cholesterol in food, it has the additional (and probably more important) effect of removing cholesterol from substances made in the liver that are recycled through the digestive tract.

What Is the Scientific Evidence for Stanols?

Plant stanol esters reduce serum cholesterol levels by inhibiting cholesterol absorption. Because they are structurally similar to cholesterol, stanols (and sterols) can displace cholesterol from the "packages" that deliver cholesterol for absorption from the intestines to the bloodstream. The displaced cholesterol is not absorbed and is excreted from the body.

Numerous double-blind, placebo-controlled studies, ranging in length from 30 days to 12 months and involving a total of more than 1,000 people, have found stanol esters and their chemical relatives effective for improving cholesterol levels. For long-term treatment, stanols may be more effective than sterols.

The combined results suggest that these substances can reduce total cholesterol and LDL ("bad") cholesterol by about 10 to 15%. Stanol esters did not have any significant effect on HDL ("good") cholesterol or triglycerides in most of these studies. However, when combined with a standard cholesterol-lowering diet, use of a spread enhanced with sterols improved total cholesterol, LDL cholesterol, HDL cholesterol, and triglycerides as compared to a normal reduced-fat spread.

For example, in a double-blind, placebo-controlled study, 153 people with mildly elevated cholesterol were given sitostanol esters in margarine (at 1.8 or 2.6 g of sitostanol per day), or margarine without sitostanol ester, for a total of 1 year. The results in the treated group receiving 2.6 g per day showed improvements in total cholesterol by 10.2% and LDL cholesterol by 14.1%—significantly better than the results in the control group. Neither triglycerides nor HDL cholesterol levels were affected.

Other studies have found evidence that people taking statin drugs may benefit from using stanols/sterols as well. According to one study, if you are on statins and start taking sterol ester margarine as well, your cholesterol will improve to the same effect as if you doubled the statin dose.

Three studies found stanols or sterols to be helpful for lowering cholesterol levels in people with type 2 (adult-onset) **diabetes**.

Safety Issues

Sterols are presumed safe because they are found in many foods. Stanols are also considered safe, but for a different reason: they are not absorbed. No adverse effects have been reported in any of the studies on lowering cholesterol, with the exception of one study that reported mild gastrointestinal complaints in a few preschool children. In addition, no toxic signs were observed in rats given stanol esters for 13 weeks at levels comparable to or exceeding those recommended for lowering cholesterol.

Although concerns have been expressed that stanol esters might impair absorption of the fat-soluble **vitamins A, D, and E**, this does not seem to occur at the dosages required to lower cholesterol. Stanol esters might, however, interfere with absorption of alpha- and **beta-carotene**, although some studies have found no such effect. Some evidence suggests that sterol supplements, especially sterol esters, *do* significantly decrease vitamin E and beta-carotene absorption. Until more is learned, it may be reasonable for people using stanol or sterol products to take a **multivitamin/multimineral tablet**.

Stevia

Stevia rebaudiana

PRINCIPAL PROPOSED USES: *Sweetener*

OTHER PROPOSED USES: *Diabetes, Hypertension*

This member of the Aster family has a long history of native use in Paraguay as a sweetener for teas and foods. It contains a substance known as *stevioside* that is 100 to 300 times sweeter than sugar, but provides no calories.

In the early 1970s, a consortium of Japanese food manufacturers developed stevia extracts for use as a zero-calorie sugar substitute. Subsequently, stevia extracts became a common ingredient in Asian soft drinks, desserts, chewing gum, and many other food products. Extensive Japanese research has found stevia to be extremely safe. However, there have not been enough U.S. studies for the FDA to approve stevia as a sugar substitute. Without identifying it as such, stevia is nonetheless widely used by savvy manufacturers to sweeten commercial beverage teas and other products.

Although stevia is best known as a sweetener, when stevia extracts are taken in very high doses they may reduce blood pressure, according to two large Chinese studies.

What Is Stevia Used for Today?

Stevia is primarily useful as a sweetening agent. In addition, two double-blind studies suggest that it may also offer potential benefits for **hypertension**.

Very weak evidence hints at potential benefits in diabetes.

What Is the Scientific Evidence for Stevia?

A 1-year, double-blind, placebo-controlled study of 106 individuals with high blood pressure evaluated the potential benefits of stevia for reducing blood pressure. In the treated group, the average blood pressure at the beginning of the study was about 166/102. Participants were given either placebo or stevioside (stevia extract) at a dose of 250 mg 3 times daily. By the end of the study, the average blood pressure had fallen to 153/90, a substantial if not quite adequate improvement. In contrast, no significant reductions were seen in the placebo group. (Note that this is a high dose of steviosides, the sweetness equivalent of more than one-third of a pound of sugar daily!)

A follow-up study tested a dose of 500 mg of steviosides 3 times daily over a 2-year period. This double-blind trial enrolled 174 people with more moderately high blood pressure (in the range of 150/95). The results showed that use of stevioside reduced blood pressure significantly, resulting in an average reading of 140/89.

Dosage

Stevia is sold as a powder to be added to foods as needed for appropriate sweetening effects. It tastes slightly bitter if placed directly in the mouth, but in liquids this is generally not noticeable and most people find the taste delightfully unique.

In the hypertension studies mentioned above, stevia was given as a standardized extract supplying 250 to 500 mg of stevioside 3 times daily (a dose considerably higher than any reasonable use of stevia as a sweetener).

Safety Issues

Animal tests and the extensive Japanese experience with stevia suggest that this is a safe herb. Based primarily on the apparently incorrect belief that stevia has been used traditionally to prevent pregnancy, some researchers have expressed concern that stevia might have an anti-fertility effect in men or women. However, evidence from most (though not all) animal studies suggests that this is not a concern at normal doses.

The two studies described above in which use of a stevia extract led to reductions in blood pressure raise at least theoretical concerns about stevia's safety. In theory, the herb could excessively reduce blood pressure in some people; furthermore, if stevia can reduce blood pressure, that means that it is, in some fashion, acting on the cardiovascular system. Since sugar substitutes are meant to be consumed in essentially unlimited quantities by a very wide variety of people, the highest levels of safety standards are appropriate and unknown effects on the heart and blood circulation are potentially worrisome. This concern is somewhat mitigated by the fact that the daily dose of stevioside used in those studies was considerably higher than is likely to be consumed if whole stevia is used for sweetening purposes.

Safety in young children, pregnant or nursing women, or those with severe liver or kidney disease has not been conclusively established; because of the concerns raised in the previous paragraph, individuals with cardiovascular disease should use high doses of stevia extracts only under physician supervision.

Strontium

PRINCIPAL PROPOSED USES: *Osteoporosis*

OTHER PROPOSED USES: *Cavities (Caries)*

Strontium is a trace element widely found in nature. It became famous in the 1960s when a radioactive form of strontium produced by atomic bomb testing, strontium-90, became prevalent in the environment. Nonradioactive strontium has recently undergone study as a treatment for osteoporosis, with some promising results.

Requirements/Sources

There is no known daily requirement for strontium.

Therapeutic Uses

Strontium has fundamental chemical similarities to calcium. When dietary intake of strontium is raised, strontium begins to take the place of calcium in developing bone. This replacement appears to be beneficial (at least with low doses of strontium—see Safety Issues below), leading to an increase in bone formation, a decrease in bone breakdown, and an overall rise in bone density.

The net result is a reduced incidence of of fractures due to **osteoporosis**, according to two very large studies.

In addition, highly preliminary evidence hints that strontium might also help prevent **cavities** by strengthening dental enamel.

What Is the Scientific Evidence for Strontium?

The major human studies of strontium for osteoporosis involved a special form of the mineral called *strontium ranelate*.

In a 3-year, double-blind, placebo-controlled study of 5,091 women with osteoporosis, use of strontium at a dose of 2 g daily significantly improved bone density and reduced incidence of all fractures as compared to placebo. Additionally, in a 3-year, double-blind, placebo-controlled study of 1,649 postmenopausal women with osteoporosis and a history of at least one vertebral fracture, use of strontium ranelate at a dose of 2 g daily reduced the incidence of new vertebral fractures by 49% in the first year and 41% in the full 3-year period (as compared to placebo). Use of strontium also significantly increased measured bone density. No significant side effects were seen.

Benefits were also seen in an earlier, smaller study.

A fourth study tested strontium ranelate for preventing osteoporosis in postmenopausal women who have not yet developed it. In this 2-year, double-blind, placebo-controlled study, 160 women received either placebo or strontium ranelate at a dose of 125 mg, 500 mg, or 1 g daily. The results showed greater gains in bone density the more strontium taken.

Other forms of strontium besides strontium ranelate, such as strontium chloride, have shown potential benefits in animal studies, but have not undergone significant testing in people.

Therapeutic Dosages

Based on current evidence strontium ranelate can be taken at a dose of 500 mg to 1 g daily to prevent osteoporosis and at a higher dose of 2 g daily to treat existing osteoporosis.

Note: It is not yet clear whether combining strontium with standard treatments for osteoporosis will enhance or diminish the ultimate benefits.

Safety Issues

When taken in recommended doses, strontium supplements appear to be safe and generally free of side effects. However, excessive intake of strontium can actually weaken bone by replacing too much of the bone's calcium with strontium.

Maximum safe doses of strontium in young children, pregnant or nursing women, or people with severe liver or kidney disease have not been established.

Interactions You Should Know About

If you are taking standard treatment for osteoporosis, it is not clear whether the addition of strontium will enhance or diminish the benefits.

Sulforaphane

PRINCIPAL PROPOSED USES: *Cancer Prevention*

Sulforaphane is a chemical found in broccoli sprouts, as well as other cabbage-family vegetables such as broccoli, Brussels sprouts, cabbage, cauliflower, and kale. Some evidence hints that sulforaphane might help **prevent cancer.**

Requirements/Sources

Sulforaphane is not an essential nutrient. It is found in especially high levels in broccoli sprouts.

Therapeutic Uses

Numerous observational studies have found that a high consumption of vegetables in the cabbage family is associated with a reduced risk of cancer, especially breast, prostate, lung, stomach, colon, and rectal cancer. On this basis, scientists have looked for anticancer substances in these foods. Sulforaphane is one such candidate substance (**indole-3-carbinol**, I3C, is another.) In test-tube and animal studies, sulforaphane exhibits properties that suggest it could indeed help prevent many forms of cancer.

However, it is a long way from such studies to reliable evidence of benefit. Observational studies are notoriously poor guides to treatment, sometimes leading to conclusions that are the reverse of what is ultimately found to be correct. The problem is that they can't show cause-and-effect—they only show association. It is possible, for example, that people who consume more cabbage-family vegetables share other traits that are responsible for reduced cancer rates. Consider the history of hormone replacement therapy. In the 1990s, scientists had concluded that estrogen prevents heart disease, based largely on observational studies that showed menopausal women who use hormone replacement have lower heart disease rates. When double-blind, placebo-controlled studies were performed, however, they showed that hormone replacement therapy actually *increases* heart disease risk. For all we know, we could be making a similar mistake with cabbage-family vegetables.

Certainly, it is too great a leap to jump to one constituent of such vegetables and advocate that substance for preventing cancer. Thousands of substances show anticancer properties in the test tube and fail to pan out in real life. The **beta-carotene** story is another instructive example. Not only did observational studies show that people who consume foods high in beta-carotene have less lung cancer, test-tube studies found that beta-carotene has anti-cancer properties. However, subsequent large double-blind studies found that beta-carotene supplements do not help prevent lung cancer and might even *increase* risk.

The bottom line: At present, we cannot recommend sulforaphane for preventing cancer.

Therapeutic Dosages

The proper daily intake (if there is any) of sulforaphane is not known. Typical recommendations range from 200 to 400 mcg daily.

Safety Issues

No major adverse effects have been reported with sulforaphane supplements, but comprehensive studies have not been performed. Maximum safe doses in young children, pregnant or nursing women, or people with severe liver or kidney disease are not known.

Note: Sulforaphane has shown the potential for interacting with numerous medications. For this reason, we recommend that people taking any oral or injected medication that is critical to their health or well-being avoid using sulforaphane supplements until more is known.

Interactions You Should Know About

If you are taking any medication that is critical to your health, do not take sulforaphane supplements except under physician supervision.

Suma

Pfaffia paniculata

PRINCIPAL PROPOSED USES: *None*

OTHER PROPOSED USES: *Adaptogen (Improve Resistance to Stress), Anxiety, Chronic Fatigue Syndrome, Immune Support, Menopausal Symptoms, Menstrual Problems, Sexual Dysfunction in Men, Sexual Dysfunction in Women, Sickle-Cell Disease, Sports Performance Enhancement, Ulcers*

Suma is a large ground vine native to Central and South America. Native peoples have long used suma, sometimes called *Brazilian ginseng*, to promote robust health as well as to treat practically all illnesses. They called it *Para Toda*, which means "for all things."

What Is Suma Used for Today?

Suma's ancient reputation has generated worldwide interest. However, there has been little formal scientific investigation of the herb at this time.

According to most contemporary herbalists, suma is best understood as an adaptogen, a substance that supposedly helps one adapt to **stress** and fight infection (see the article on **ginseng** for a more in-depth discussion about adaptogens). Russian Olympic athletes have reportedly used suma (as well as other adaptogens) in the belief that it will enhance sports performance. In the United States, suma is often recommended as a general strengthener of the body, as well as for the treatment of **chronic fatigue syndrome, menopausal symptoms, ul-** cers, **anxiety, menstrual problems, impotence,** and **immune support**. The herb also enjoys a considerable reputation as an aphrodisiac. However, there is no reliable scientific evidence that suma offers any benefits for these conditions. Finally, one test-tube study suggests that suma might be helpful for sickle-cell disease, but it is a long way from such preliminary investigations to evidence of efficacy.

Dosage

A typical dosage of suma is 500 mg twice daily. It is usually taken for an extended period of time.

Safety Issues

Suma has not been associated with any serious adverse reactions. However, comprehensive safety studies have not been undertaken. Safety in young children, pregnant or nursing women, or those with severe liver or kidney disease has not been established.

Superoxide Dismutase

SUPPLEMENT FORMS/ALTERNATE NAMES: SOD

PRINCIPAL PROPOSED USES: *None*

OTHER PROPOSED USES: *Anti-Aging, Radiation Therapy Support (Injected Form), Wound Healing (Topical Form)*

In the body, dangerous naturally occurring substances called *free radicals* pose a risk of harm to many tissues. The body deploys an "antioxidant defense system" to hold them in check. Superoxide dismutase (SOD) is one of the most important elements of this system. It controls levels of a chemical named *superoxide*. The body manufactures superoxide to kill bacteria, among other uses, but excess levels of superoxide can injure healthy cells. SOD converts superoxide to hydrogen peroxide. Then another enzyme, catalase, neutralizes hydrogen peroxide.

Nutrients such as **vitamin C** and **vitamin E** also help neutralize free radicals. In the 1990s, such **antioxidant** supplements were widely promoted for preventing a variety of diseases, including cancer and heart disease. During this period, oral SOD became popular as a supplemental antioxidant supplement. Unfortunately, the results of several large studies tended to dash these hopes. Compared to ordinary antioxidants, SOD suffers from the additional disadvantages of being expensive and poorly absorbed when taken by mouth.

Requirements/Sources

SOD is not an essential nutrient and it is not obtained through food.

Therapeutic Dosages

When taken orally, little to no SOD is absorbed. Some manufacturers advertise a sublingual (under the tongue) form of SOD to get around this problem. However, there does not appear to be any meaningful evidence that SOD can be absorbed any better this way.

Weak evidence hints that a form of SOD in which the substance is encapsulated in structures called *liposomes* may be absorbable. The optimum dose, if any, is not known.

Therapeutic Uses

Various websites promote SOD for a wide variety of health problems, from preventing aging to enhancing sports performance. However, as noted above, oral SOD supplements may be ineffective due to poor absorption.

A bit of evidence hints that SOD injections may reduce scarring caused by **radiation** therapy and also decrease symptoms of **osteoarthritis**.

SOD applied directly to wounds may enhance wound healing, according to experiments in animals.

In test-tube and animal studies, genetic manipulation has been used to increase SOD levels, in hopes of finding anti-aging effects, but the results have been mixed.

Inhaled SOD appears to be useful for premature infants, helping to prevent a condition called *respiratory distress syndrome*.

However, the only evidence for benefits with any oral form of SOD is a study in animals involving the special liposome form of the supplement mentioned above. It found possible anti-inflammatory effects.

Safety Issues

Oral SOD is presumably quite safe, since it is apparently not absorbable. The safety of other forms of SOD (including the possibly absorbable encapsulated form) has not been established.

Sweet Clover

Melilotus species

ALTERNATE NAMES/RELATED TERMS: *Melilot*
PRINCIPAL PROPOSED USES: *None*
OTHER PROPOSED USES: *Dyspepsia, Hemorrhoids, Injuries, Minor, Phlebitis, Varicose Veins*

Sweet clover, long popular as food for grazing animals, is used medicinally as well. It contains various substances in the coumarin family. These chemicals are thought to help strengthen the walls of blood and lymph vessels. However, there is no more than preliminary evidence that sweet clover is effective for any medical condition. In addition, use of sweet clover presents some safety concerns. (See Safety Issues below for more information.)

The name *Melilotus* originates from the Greek word

for honey, *meli*, and a term for clover-like plants, *lotos*. There are four common species in this genus of Eurasian origins: *Melilotus alba, M. indica, M. officinalis,* and *M. altissimus*.

The fresh or dried leaves and flowering stems of sweet clover were traditionally used as a diuretic.

What Is Sweet Clover Used for Today?

Germany's Commission E has authorized use of sweet clover extract for symptoms of **venous insufficiency** (a condition closely related to varicose veins), as well as for the treatment of **phlebitis** and **hemorrhoids**. When used for this purpose, however, sweet clover is generally combined with bioflavonoids, such as **oxerutin**. However, there is no meaningful evidence as yet that sweet clover taken *alone* is effective for these conditions.

Sweet clover contains coumarins, substances related to the prescription blood-thinner warfarin (Coumadin). Most scientific study relevant to sweet clover involves prescription drugs that combine coumarins and bioflavonoids. These medications have also been used to treat venous insufficiency, as well as numerous other conditions, including elephantiasis, hemorrhoids, mild digestive disturbances, and various forms of **edema**. However, it isn't clear whether sweet clover extracts containing coumarins would work in the same way as the coumarin portion of these pharmaceutical products.

Topical treatments made from sweet clover are sometimes recommended for the treatment of **hemorrhoids** and minor injuries, but as yet there is no real scientific evidence to support these proposed uses.

Dosage

Sweet clover products are standardized to their coumarin content. For treating symptoms of venous insufficiency/varicose veins, a daily dosage of a sweet clover preparation or extract providing 3 to 30 mg of coumarin is taken internally. (See Safety Issues below.)

Safety Issues

The safety of any medicinal use of sweet clover has not been established in humans. Sweet clover contains various substances in the coumarin family. Many (but not all) of these substances thin the blood and might cause excessive bleeding in some individuals. In particular, sweet clover should not be combined with blood-thinning drugs such as warfarin (Coumadin), heparin, or drugs in the aspirin family.

Safety in pregnant or nursing women, young children, or individuals with severe liver or kidney disease has not been established.

Interactions You Should Know About

If you are taking blood-thinning drugs such as **warfarin** (Coumadin), **heparin**, **clopidogrel** (Plavix), **pentoxifylline** (Trental), or drugs in the **aspirin** family: You should not use sweet clover.

Taurine

SUPPLEMENT FORMS/ALTERNATE NAMES: *L-Taurine*

PRINCIPAL PROPOSED USES: *Congestive Heart Failure, Viral Hepatitis*

OTHER PROPOSED USES: *Alcoholism, Cataracts, Diabetes, Epilepsy, Gallbladder Disease, Hypertension, Multiple Sclerosis, Psoriasis, Stroke*

Taurine is an amino acid, one of the building blocks of proteins. Found in the nervous system and muscles, taurine is one of the most abundant amino acids in the body. It is thought to help regulate heartbeat, maintain cell membranes, and affect the release of *neurotransmitters* (chemicals that carry signals between nerve cells) in the brain.

Sources

There is no dietary requirement for taurine, since the body can make it out of **vitamin B$_6$** and the amino acids **methionine** and cysteine. Deficiencies occasionally occur in vegetarians, whose diets may not provide the building blocks for making taurine.

People with diabetes have lower-than-average blood levels of taurine, but whether this means they should take extra taurine is unclear.

Meat, poultry, eggs, dairy products, and fish are good sources of taurine. Legumes and nuts don't contain taurine, but they do contain methionine and cysteine.

Therapeutic Dosages

A typical therapeutic dosage of taurine is 2 g 3 times daily.

Therapeutic Uses

Preliminary evidence suggests that taurine might be helpful in **congestive heart failure** (CHF), a condition in which the heart has trouble pumping blood, which leads to fluid accumulating in the legs and lungs. **Warning**: Keep in mind that CHF is too serious for self-treatment. If you're interested in trying taurine or any other supplement for CHF, you should first consult your doctor.

There is also some evidence that taurine may be helpful for acute **viral hepatitis**.

Taurine has additionally been proposed as a treatment for numerous other conditions, including **alcoholism**, **cataracts**, **diabetes**, **epilepsy**, gallbladder disease, **hypertension**, **multiple sclerosis**, **psoriasis**, and **stroke**, but the evidence for these uses is weak and, in some cases, contradictory. Taurine is also sometimes combined in an "amino acid cocktail" with other amino acids for treatment of **attention deficit disorder**, but there is no evidence as yet that it works for this purpose.

What Is the Scientific Evidence for Taurine?

Congestive Heart Failure

Several studies (primarily by one research group) suggest that taurine may be useful for congestive heart failure. For example, in one double-blind, placebo-controlled trial, 58 people with CHF took either placebo or 2 g of taurine 3 times daily for 4 weeks. Then the groups were switched. During taurine treatment, the study participants showed highly significant improvement in breathlessness, heart palpitations, fluid buildup, and heart x-ray, as well as standard scales of heart failure severity. Animal research as well as small blinded or open studies in humans have also found positive effects. Interestingly, one very small study compared taurine with another supplement commonly used for congestive heart failure, **coenzyme Q$_{10}$**. The results suggest that taurine is more effective.

Viral Hepatitis

There are several viruses that can cause acute viral hepatitis, a disabling and sometimes dangerous infection of the liver. The most common are hepatitis A and B, although there are others (with such imaginative names as C and D).

One double-blind study suggests that taurine supplements might be useful for acute viral hepatitis. In this double-blind, placebo-controlled study, 63 people with hepatitis were given either 12 g of taurine daily or placebo. (The report does not state what type of viral hepatitis they had.) According to blood tests, the taurine group experienced significant improvements in liver function as compared to the placebo group.

Acute hepatitis can also develop into a long-lasting or permanent condition known as *chronic hepatitis*. One small double-blind study suggests that taurine does not help chronic hepatitis. For this purpose, the herb **milk thistle** may be better.

Safety Issues

As an amino acid found in food, taurine is thought to be quite safe. However, maximum safe dosages of taurine supplements for children, pregnant or nursing women, or those with severe liver or kidney disease have not been determined.

As with any supplement taken in multigram doses, it is important to purchase a reputable product, because a contaminant present even in small percentages could add up to a real problem.

Tea Tree

Melaleuca alternifolia

PRINCIPAL PROPOSED USES: *Dandruff, Tinea Pedis (Athlete's Foot)*

OTHER PROPOSED USES: *Acne, Dandruff, Oral Herpes, Periodontal Disease, Thrush, Vaginal Infections*

Captain Cook named this tree after finding that its aromatic, resinous leaves made a satisfying substitute for proper tea. One hundred and fifty years later, an Australian government chemist named A. R. Penfold studied tea tree leaves and discovered their antiseptic properties. Tea tree oil subsequently became a standard treatment in Australia for the prevention and treatment of wound infections. During World War II, the Australian government classified tea tree oil as an essential commodity and exempted producers from military service.

However, tea tree oil fell out of favor when antibiotics became widely available.

What Is Tea Tree Used for Today?

Tea tree oil can kill many bacteria, viruses, and fungi on contact. This makes it an antiseptic, like betadine, hydrogen peroxide, and many other **essential oils**. It is not an antibiotic in the common sense because an antibiotic is absorbed throughout the body.

Preliminary double-blind studies suggest that tea tree oil might be useful for **athlete's foot** and other fungal infections of the skin and nails.

A single-blind study found evidence that tea tree oil may be helpful for **dandruff**.

Tea tree oil has also been proposed as a treatment for **acne**. However, it has not yet been proven effective for this purpose; the one published double-blind study on the topic merely found that tea tree oil is *less* effective than the standard treatment, benzoyl peroxide. (See What Is the Scientific Evidence for Tea Tree, below.)

One double-blind study found that tea tree oil gel may reduce gum inflammation in people with **periodontal disease**.

Tea tree oil may be as effective as standard antiseptics for removing resistant strains of staph bacteria from the skin of hospitalized patients. **Note:** This does not mean tea tree oil is effective as an *antibiotic* for staph. It is an *antiseptic*. Antiseptics work on the surface of the body, while antibiotics work from within.

Additionally, tea tree oil has been proposed as a treatment for **vaginal infections**, thrush, and **oral herpes** (cold sores). However, there is no reliable evidence to indicate that it is effective for these purposes.

What Is the Scientific Evidence for Tea Tree?

Athlete's Foot

In a double-blind, placebo-controlled trial, 158 people with athlete's foot were treated with placebo, 25% tea tree oil solution, or 50% tea tree oil solution, applied twice daily for 4 weeks. The results showed that the two tea tree oil solutions were more effective than placebo at eradicating infection. In the 50% tea tree oil group, 64% were cured; in the 25% tea tree oil group, 55% were cured; in the placebo group, 31% were cured. These differences were statistically significant. A few people developed dermatitis in response to the tea tree oil and had to drop out of the study, but most people did not experience any significant side effects.

Another double-blind, placebo-controlled trial followed 104 people with athlete's foot who were given either a 10% tea tree oil cream, the standard drug tolnaftate, or placebo. The results showed that tea tree oil reduced the symptoms of athlete's foot more effectively than placebo but less effectively than tolnaftate. Neither treatment cured the infection in 100% of the cases, but each treatment cured many cases.

A third double-blind study followed 112 people with fungal infections of the toenails, comparing 100% tea tree oil to a standard topical antifungal treatment, clotrimazole. The results showed equivalent benefits; however, because topical clotrimazole is not regarded as a particularly effective treatment for this condition, the results mean little.

Dandruff

In a 4-week, placebo-controlled study of 126 people with mild to moderate dandruff, use of 5% tea tree oil shampoo significantly reduced dandruff symptoms. Unfortunately, this study was not double-blind: The researchers knew which participants were receiving tea tree oil and which were receiving placebo. For this reason, its results can't be taken as completely reliable. (For more information on why double-blinding matters, see **Why Does This Book Rely on Double-blind Studies?**.)

Acne

A single-blind study of 124 people with acne compared a 5% tea tree oil against the standard acne treatment, benzoyl peroxide. Tea tree oil proved less effective than benzoyl peroxide.

People taking tea tree oil *did* improve to some extent. This does not, however, show that tea tree oil is effective for acne, as the researchers and some manufacturers claim. To show that tea tree oil is effective, this study would have needed a placebo group, which it did not have.

Dosage

Tea tree preparations contain various percentages of tea tree oil. For treating acne, the typical strength is 5 to 15%; for fungal infections, 70 to 100% is usually used; and for use as a vaginal douche (with medical supervision), 1 to 40% concentrations have been used. It is usually applied 2 to 3 times daily until symptoms resolve. However, tea tree oil can be irritating to the skin, so start with low concentrations until you know your tolerance.

The best tea tree products contain oil from the *alternifolia* species of *Melaleuca* only, standardized to contain not more than 10% cineole (an irritant) and at least 30% terpinen-4-ol. Oil from a specially bred variant of tea tree may have increased activity against microorganisms, while irritating the skin less.

Safety Issues

When used topically, tea tree oil is fairly safe. However, it can cause allergic inflammation of the skin.

Like other essential oils, tea tree oil can be toxic if taken orally in excessive doses.

Safety in young children, pregnant or nursing women, or those with severe liver or kidney disease has not been established.

Thymus Extract

SUPPLEMENT FORMS/ALTERNATE NAMES: *Calf Thymus Extract, Thymic Extract, Thymomodulin, Thymus Gland*

PRINCIPAL PROPOSED USES: *None*

OTHER PROPOSED USES: *Asthma, Eczema, Food Allergies, General Immune Support, Hay Fever*

The thymus gland is found behind the sternum in the middle of the chest. It plays a significant role in the immune system, especially in unborn and very young children. The theory behind the use of thymus extracts is that they might stimulate or normalize immunity. However, there is no reliable real evidence as yet that any thymus extracts are effective for any health condition. Furthermore, there are significant safety concerns with thymus products.

Requirements/Sources

Thymus extract is produced primarily from the thymus gland of cows. This has led to concerns regarding "mad cow" disease. (See Safety Issues below.) All the studies described below used a pharmaceutical-grade form of thymus called *Thymomodulin*. It is not known whether the thymus supplements available as a dietary supplement would have the same effect.

Therapeutic Dosages

The dosage of thymus extract used in studies has varied widely, depending on the particular thymus product used.

Therapeutic Uses

Two small double-blind, placebo-controlled trials enrolling children with frequent respiratory infections such as **colds** found that treatment with thymus extract reduced the rate of infection. In theory, this might indicate an immune boosting effect. However, small studies cannot provide reliable proof that a treatment is effective.

Weak evidence from a rather convoluted trial hints that thymus extract may also be helpful for preventing respiratory infections in adults.

Intensive athletic training can suppress immune function and lead to colds as well. However, a double-blind, placebo-controlled trial of 60 athletes failed to find any significant evidence of benefit with thymus extract.

Preliminary evidence hints that thymus extracts may be helpful for food allergies, asthma, hay fever, and **eczema**. If thymus extract really does help these conditions, it may do so not by boosting the immune system, but rather by calming it down and causing it to behave more normally.

Small double-blind trials of thymus extract for hepatitis B and C found marginal benefits at most.

Injectable forms of whole thymus extract or chemicals contained in it have been studied as a treatment for numerous other conditions, including **cancer**, cold sores, dermatomyositis, **eczema**, genital warts, **hepatitis**, HIV infection, leukopenia (low white cell count), **multiple sclerosis**, **psoriasis**, respiratory infections, **rheumatoid arthritis**, **scleroderma**, and **shingles** (*Herpes zoster*).

The results of these studies have been mixed. In any case, the results of trials involving injected thymus cannot be considered applicable to oral thymus products.

Safety Issues

Thymus extracts have not been definitely associated with any side effects. However, there are real concerns that any glandular extract might contain the virus causing "mad cow disease." Keep in mind that there is relatively little governmental regulation of thymus products sold as dietary supplements in the United States. Even when a ban is placed on importation of cow glands from a country where mad cow disease has been found, the ban does not apply to dietary supplements! For this reason, we recommend that you do not use thymus products sold as dietary supplements unless they are certified as free from risk of infection.

Tinospora cordifolia

ALTERNATE NAMES/RELATED TERMS: *Amrita, Guduchii*

PRINCIPAL PROPOSED USES: *Allergic Rhinitis*

OTHER PROPOSED USES: *Adaptogen, Cancer Prevention, Cancer Treatment Support, Diabetes, High Cholesterol, Liver Protection*

The herb *Tinospora cordifolia* has a long history of use in **Ayurvedic medicine** (the traditional medicine of India). It has been used to treat convalescence from severe illness, liver disease, arthritis, urinary problems, eye diseases, cancer, anemia, diabetes, and diarrhea. It is said to help remove toxins from the body and, on this basis, is often added to herbal formulas claimed to improve general health. Both the stem and the root are used medicinally.

What Is *Tinospora cordifolia* Used for Today?

According to some herbalists, tinospora has *adaptogenic effects*, a term that indicates it helps the body adapt to stress. However, there is no meaningful evidence to support this claim. Only double-blind, placebo-controlled studies can prove a treatment effective and the only such study performed on tinospora tested other effects.

In this study, 75 people with **allergic rhinitis** (hayfever) were given either tinospora or placebo for 8 weeks. According to the investigators, use of tinospora significantly decreased every measured symptom of allergic rhinitis in the majority of participants; in comparison, use of placebo provided almost no benefit at all. These results may sound promising, but they are, in fact, so excessively dramatic as to raise doubts about the study's overall validity. It is unusual for so few benefits to be seen in the placebo group of a study on a treatment for allergic rhinitis and it is nearly as unusual for almost universal benefits to be reported in the treatment group. Independent confirmation will be required to overcome the skepticism raised by these apparently "too good to be true" findings.

Besides anti-allergy effects, much very weak evidence hints that tinospora may have **anti-cancer**, **immune stimulating**, nerve cell protecting, **anti-diabetic**, **cholesterol-lowering**, and **liver-protective** actions. Tinospora has also shown some promise for decreasing the tissue damage caused by radiation and the side effects of some forms of **chemotherapy**. However, all these findings are far too preliminary to be relied upon.

Safety Issues

Use of tinospora has not been associated with significant side effects. However, comprehensive safety testing has not been conducted. One animal study found evidence that use of tinospora might decrease male fertility. Safety for pregnant or nursing women, young children, or individuals with severe liver or kidney disease has not been established.

Tocotrienols

PRINCIPAL PROPOSED USES: *None*

OTHER PROPOSED USES: *Cancer Prevention, Heart Disease Prevention, High Cholesterol*

Tocotrienols are fat-soluble substances closely related to **vitamin E**. Like vitamin E, they have **antioxidant** properties and help protect fatty substances in the body from being damaged by free radicals. In the 1990s, antioxidant supplements were thought to offer great potential for preventing a variety of diseases, including cancer and heart disease and, on this basis, tocotrienols were offered on the market as healthful supplements. Tocotrienols have also been proposed for reducing cholesterol. However, subsequent studies have tended to pour cold water on all these hopes. At present, there is no reliable evidence that tocotrienols offer any meaningful health benefits.

Requirements/Sources

Tocotrienols are not essential nutrients. They occur naturally in the oil extract of barley, palm fruit, rice bran, and wheat germ. Most commercially available supplements are made from rice bran oil or palm oil.

Therapeutic Dosages

A typical recommended dose of tocotrienols is 200 mg daily.

Therapeutic Uses

Test-tube and animal studies have found promising hints that tocotrienols may help prevent cancer.

However, only double-blind, placebo-controlled studies can prove a treatment effective and none have yet been performed on this potential use of tocotrienols. (For information on why such studies are essential, see **Why Does This Book Rely on Double-blind Studies?**.) In addition, there is a bad track record with antioxidants in this regard: the antioxidant **beta-carotene** also showed promise as an anti-cancer nutrient in preliminary studies, but proved useless (or even harmful) when it was properly evaluated.

Similarly, while test-tube studies, animal studies, and open human trials seemed to suggest that tocotrienols can correct **high cholesterol**, properly designed studies failed to find benefit.

The hypothesis that tocotrienols can prevent heart disease simply by virtue of their antioxidant actions has lost favor, since the same hypothesis proved incorrect with vitamin E and beta-carotene.

The bottom line: As experience has shown with related supplements, preliminary evidence can be misleading. The health benefits of tocotrienols, if there are any, remain to be established.

Safety Issues

Tocotrienols are thought to be safe substances. However, maximum safe doses have not been determined.

Tribulus terrestris

PRINCIPAL PROPOSED USES: *Sports Performance Enhancement*

OTHER PROPOSED USES: *Infertility (in Men and Women), Menopausal Symptoms, Sexual Dysfunction (in Men and Women); many others*

*T*ribulus terrestris (commonly known as puncture vine—the bane of bicycles in areas where it grows) has a long history of traditional medical use in China, India, and Greece. It was recommended as a treatment for female infertility, impotence and low libido in both men and women, and to aid rejuvenation after long illness. The herb became widely known in the West when medal-winning Bulgaria Olympic athletes claimed that use of tribulus had contributed to their success.

What Is *Tribulus terrestris* Used for Today?

Studies performed in Bulgaria are the primary source of most current health claims regarding tribulus. According to this research, tribulus increases levels of various hormones in the steroid family, including testosterone, DHEA, and estrogen, and for this reason improves **sports performance**, **fertility in men** and **women**, **sexual function** (again in men and women), and symptoms of **menopause** (such as hot flashes). Unfortunately, the design of these studies appears to fall far short of modern scientific standards and there has not been any trustworthy scientific confirmation of these supposed benefits. One well-designed study failed to find that tribulus affects male sex hormone levels in young men.

Other studies that are far too preliminary to prove anything at all are quoted as proving that tribulus is helpful for the treatment of **angina**, **high cholesterol**, **diabetes**, and muscle spasms, and for the prevention of **kidney stones**.

The best-designed and most recent human study compared the effects of tribulus (3.21 mg per kilogram of body weight—for example, 292 mg daily for a 200-lb man) against placebo (fake treatment) on body composition and endurance among 15 men engaged in resistance training. At the end of the 8-week study, the only significant difference between the treatment and placebo groups was that the *placebo* group showed greater gains in endurance.

Dosage

Tribulus terrestris is usually taken at a dose ranging from about 85 to 250 mg 3 times daily with meals. Some tribulus products are standardized to provide 40% furostanol saponins and taken at a dose providing 115 mg of saponins 2 to 3 times daily.

Safety Issues

No significant adverse effects have been noted in any of the clinical trials or human research studies of tribulus. Animal studies performed in Bulgaria are said to have found tribulus safe both in the short and long terms. However, it is not clear whether these studies were performed in such a way that their conclusions can be trusted.

Tribulus is known to have a toxic effect on sheep.

Note: Women who are pregnant or nursing should not use any tribulus product because if it works as described it might alter hormones in unsafe ways.

Trimethylglycine

SUPPLEMENT FORMS/ALTERNATE NAMES: *TMG*

RELATED TERMS: *Betaine*

PRINCIPAL PROPOSED USES: *High Homocysteine Levels*

OTHER PROPOSED USES: *Alcoholic Liver Disease, Enhancing Sports Performance, Non-alcoholic Steatosis, Substitute for SAMe*

TMG (trimethylglycine), also called *betaine*, is a substance manufactured by the body. It helps break down another naturally occurring substance called *homocysteine*.

In certain rare genetic conditions, the body cannot dispose of homocysteine, resulting in its accumulation to extremely high levels. This in turn leads to accelerated cardiovascular disease and other problems. Oral TMG is an FDA-approved treatment for this condition. It *methylates* homocysteine, removing it from circulation.

Meaningful, but not altogether consistent, evidence suggests that the relatively slight **elevation of homocysteine** that can occur in healthy people is also harmful. On this basis, it has been suggested that TMG might reduce heart disease risk in healthy people as well. However, this has not been proven and TMG has shown the potential for having adverse effects on cholesterol profile, which could counter any possible benefit via homocysteine.

Note: TMG is similar chemically to betaine hydrochloride, but it has entirely different actions.

Sources

TMG is not required in the diet because the body can manufacture it from other nutrients. Grains, nuts, seeds, and meats contain small amounts of TMG. However, most TMG in food is destroyed during cooking or processing, so food isn't a reliable way to get a therapeutic dosage.

After TMG has done its work on homocysteine, it is turned into another substance, dimethylglycine (DMG). Some manufacturers will tell you that DMG is identical to TMG, but this isn't true. DMG is not a methylating agent, so it can't have any effect on homocysteine (see also Therapeutic Uses below).

Therapeutic Dosages

Optimal therapeutic dosages of TMG are not known. Common recommendations range from 375 to 3,000 mg daily.

Therapeutic Uses

There is no doubt that TMG greatly reduces homocysteine levels and improves health among people with the rare disease cystathionine beta-synthase deficiency (as well as related conditions). TMG also appears to reduce relatively mild homocysteine elevations in people without genetic defects. However, as noted above, TMG also seems to worsen **cholesterol profile** and this may counteract any possible benefits. For this reason, if you have elevated levels of homocysteine, it may make more sense to reduce it by taking supplemental **folate**, **vitamin B$_6$**, and **vitamin B$_{12}$** ; these supplements are known to reduce homocysteine levels and, unlike TMG, they provide nutritional benefit as well.

TMG may help protect the liver against the effects of alcohol, perhaps by stimulating the formation of **SAMe**. In addition, it may be helpful for non-alcoholic forms of fatty liver (non-alcoholic steatosis) as well.

TMG has also been suggested as a less expensive substitute for SAMe in other conditions for which SAMe is used (such as **osteoarthritis** and **depression**). However, there is no evidence to show that it is effective.

A substance labeled *pangamic acid* or vitamin B$_{15}$ has been extensively used as a performance enhancer by Russian athletes and has also become popular among American athletes. However, it is not clear there really is any such substance; or, to state it another way, various substances have at various times been given that name. Most recently, the term has been associated with a mixture of calcium gluconate and DMG; one small study failed to find this form of pangamic acid effective for **enhancing sports performance**.

Safety Issues

The only known safety issue with TMG is regarding cholesterol profile, as already mentioned. People with high or borderline-high cholesterol should use TMG only with caution.

Maximum safe dosages for young children, pregnant or nursing mothers, or those with severe liver or kidney disease have not been established.

Tripterygium wilfordii

ALTERNATE NAMES/RELATED TERMS: *Lei Gong Teng, Thundergod Vine*
PRINCIPAL PROPOSED USES: *Rheumatoid Arthritis*
OTHER PROPOSED USES: *Lupus, Male Contraceptive*

Tripterygium is a climbing vine with a long history of use in **traditional Chinese herbal medicine**. It is used in mixtures intended for the treatment of arthritis, muscle injury, skin diseases, and other problems. The roots, leaves, and flowers are the parts used medicinally.

Tripterygium is thought to be toxic or even fatal if taken to excess. Extracts made with ethyl acetate or chorloroform-methanol came into use in China in the 1970s and were said to be less toxic. However, the safety of these extracts has not been conclusively established and we recommend against using tripterygium except in the context of a scientific trial.

What Is *Tripterygium wilfordii* Used for Today?

In animal, test-tube, and preliminary human trials, trypterygium has shown immunosuppressive and anti-inflammatory effects. Because drugs with these properties are useful for conditions in which the immune system is overactive, such as **rheumatoid arthritis** and **lupus**, trypterygium has been proposed for similar use. However, as yet there is only minimal evidence that it is effective.

One double-blind, placebo-controlled study performed in China in 1997 evaluated the topical use of a tripterygium extract in 61 people with rheumatoid arthritis. The extract was applied 5 to 6 times daily to the affected joints. The results appeared to indicate that use of the herbal tincture over 6 weeks significantly reduced rheumatoid arthritis symptoms as compared to placebo. However, due to problems in the study, researchers were compelled to use statistical methods that were somewhat questionable (technically, post-hoc analysis). For this reason, the results are only somewhat meaningful.

Another study compared placebo to oral trypterygium extract, taken in a low or high dose for 20 weeks. The results appeared to show benefit, but so many participants dropped out before the end of the study that the results are difficult to interpret.

At most, therefore, current evidence regarding tripterygium for rheumatoid arthritis remains preliminary. The U.S. National Institutes of Health (NIH) are currently conducting a much larger study on this herb that should provide more definitive information.

No other potential uses of tripterygium have undergone meaningful controlled clinical trials. Weak evidence hints that it might offer promise as a contraceptive for men.

Dosage

At present, we recommend that trypterygium should only be used in the context of a scientific trial.

Safety Issues

Trypterygium is a toxic herb: various components of trypterygium can cause liver injury, genetic damage, and birth defects. It is thought, but not proven, that certain chemical extracts of trypterygium are safe if used within proper dosage limits. All forms of the herb should be avoided by pregnant or nursing women, young children, and those with kidney or liver disease.

Turmeric

Curcuma longa

PRINCIPAL PROPOSED USES: *Dyspepsia (Indigestion)*

OTHER PROPOSED USES: *Alzheimer's Disease, Cancer Prevention, Cataract Prevention, Chronic Anterior Uveitis, High Cholesterol, Liver Protection, Menstrual Pain, Multiple Sclerosis, Osteoarthritis, Rheumatoid Arthritis*

Turmeric is a widely used tropical herb in the ginger family. Its stalk is used both in food and medicine, yielding the familiar yellow ingredient that colors and adds flavor to curry. In the traditional Indian system of herbal medicine known as **Ayurveda**, turmeric is believed to strengthen the overall energy of the body, relieve gas, dispel worms, improve digestion, regulate menstruation, dissolve gallstones, and relieve arthritis, among other uses.

Modern interest in turmeric began in 1971 when Indian researchers found evidence suggesting that turmeric may possess anti-inflammatory properties. Much of this observed activity appeared to be due to the presence of a constituent called *curcumin*. Curcumin is also an **antioxidant**. Many of the studies mentioned in this article used curcumin rather than turmeric.

What Is Turmeric Used for Today?

Turmeric's antioxidant abilities make it a good food preservative, provided that the food is already yellow in color, and it is widely used for this purpose.

Turmeric has been proposed as a treatment for dyspepsia. Dyspepsia is a catchall term that includes a variety of digestive problems, such as stomach discomfort, gas, bloating, belching, appetite loss, and nausea. Although many serious medical conditions can cause digestive distress, the term *dyspepsia* is most often used when no identifiable medical cause can be detected.

In Europe, dyspepsia is commonly attributed to inadequate bile flow from the gallbladder. While this has not been proven, turmeric does appear to stimulate the gallbladder. More importantly, one double-blind, placebo-controlled study suggests that turmeric does reduce dyspepsia symptoms.

Other proposed uses of turmeric or curcumin have little supporting evidence. Based on test tube and animal studies and on human trials too preliminary to provide any meaningful evidence, curcumin and turmeric are frequently described as anti-inflammatory drugs and recommended for the treatment of such conditions as **osteoarthritis** and menstrual pain. Some advocates go so far as to state that curcumin is superior to standard medications in the ibuprofen family because, at standard doses, it does not appear to harm the stomach. However, until turmeric is actually proven to meaningfully reduce pain and inflammation, such a comparison is rather premature. Not only that, high doses of curcumin might in fact increase the risk of **ulcers**. Contrary to some reports, turmeric does not appear to be effective for *treating* ulcers.

Animal and test-tube studies suggest (but definitely do not prove) that turmeric might help prevent cancer.

Some researchers have reported evidence that curcumin or turmeric might help protect the liver from damage. However, other researchers have failed to find any liver protective effects and there are even some indications that turmeric extracts can damage the liver when taken in high doses or for an extended period.

On the basis of even weaker evidence, curcumin or turmeric have also been recommended for preventing **cataracts** and for treating **high cholesterol**, **multiple sclerosis**, fungal infections, **Alzheimer's disease**, and chronic anterior uveitis (an inflammation of the iris of the eye).

What Is the Scientific Evidence for Turmeric?

A double-blind, placebo-controlled study performed in Thailand compared the effects of 500 mg curcumin 4 times daily against placebo, as well as against a locally popular over-the-counter treatment. A total of 116 people were enrolled in the study. After 7 days, 87% of the curcumin group experienced full or partial symptom relief from dyspepsia as compared to 53% of the placebo group and this difference was statistically significant.

Dosage

For medicinal purposes, turmeric is frequently taken in a form standardized to curcumin content at a dose that provides 400 to 600 mg of curcumin 3 times daily.

Safety Issues

Turmeric is on the FDA's GRAS (generally recognized as safe) list, and curcumin, too, is believed to be fairly nontoxic. Reported side effects are uncommon and are generally limited to mild stomach distress.

However, there is some evidence to suggest that turmeric extracts can be toxic to the liver when taken in high doses or for a prolonged period of time. For this reason, turmeric products should probably be avoided by individuals with liver disease and those who take medications that are hard on the liver.

In addition, due to curcumin's stimulating effects on the gallbladder, individuals with gallbladder disease should use curcumin only on the advice of a physician. However, safety in young children, pregnant or nursing women, and those with severe kidney disease have also not been established.

Tylophora

Tylophora asthmatica, Tylophora indica

PRINCIPAL PROPOSED USES: *Asthma*

OTHER PROPOSED USES: *Allergies (Hay Fever), Bronchitis, Colds*

T ylophora indica is a climbing perennial plant indigenous to India, where it grows wild in the southern and eastern regions and has a long-standing reputation as a remedy for asthma (hence the synonymous name, *T. asthmatica*).

The leaves and roots of tylophora have been included in the *Bengal Pharmacopoeia* since 1884. It is said to have laxative, expectorant, diaphoretic (sweating), and purgative (vomiting) properties. It has been used for the treatment of various respiratory problems besides asthma, including allergies, bronchitis, and colds, as well as dysentery and osteoarthritis pain.

What Is Tylophora Used for Today?

Tylophora has become an increasingly popular treatment for **asthma**, based on its traditional use for this purpose and several studies performed in the 1970s. However, the studies that found it effective were poorly designed and a better-designed study found no benefits.

Tylophora is also still recommended for some of its other traditional uses, including hay fever, **bronchitis**, and the **common cold**.

What Is the Scientific Evidence for Tylophora?

Weak preliminary evidence hints that tylophora might have anti-inflammatory, antiallergic, and antispasmodic actions. All these effects could make it useful for the treatment of asthma. However, only double-blind, placebo-controlled studies can actually show a treatment effective. For tylophora and asthma, the evidence from this type of study is mixed at best.

In 1972, researchers reported the results of a double-blind, placebo-controlled crossover trial of 195 individuals with asthma who were given either placebo or 40 mg of a tylophora alcohol extract daily for 6 days. The results showed that people taking tylophora had fewer asthma symptoms and the benefits endured for months after use

Tyrosine

of the herb was stopped. Similarly long-lasting results were seen in two double-blind, placebo-controlled studies involving more than 200 individuals with asthma.

Even the researchers involved in these trials expressed surprise that short-term use of tylophora could produce long-lasting benefits; to outside observers, such findings make the results difficult to believe at all. Furthermore, most of these studies suffered from poor design and reporting. In 1979, researchers published the results of a double-blind study designed to remedy these problems. A total of 135 people with asthma were given either tylophora or placebo. No benefits were seen and tylophora has not undergone much study since then.

The bottom line: Better studies that show benefit will be necessary before tylophora can be considered a promising herb for asthma.

Dosage

The typical dosage of tylophora leaf in dried or capsule form is 200 mg twice daily or 400 mg total in 2 doses.

Safety Issues

In the second study mentioned above, tylophora caused nausea, vomiting, mouth soreness, and alterations in taste sensation in more than half of the participants. The other two studies found similar side effects, but far less frequently. The difference may have been because the second study had people chew the whole leaves from the plant, whereas other studies have used dried leaves or powdered extract in capsule form.

Preliminary studies on animals have found tylophora extracts to be toxic only in extremely high doses; these extracts were apparently safe in the far smaller doses needed to produce a therapeutic effect.

Due to the lack of comprehensive safety studies on tylophora, the herb should not be used by children, pregnant or nursing women, or individuals with severe kidney or liver disease. Whether tylophora interacts with any drugs is unknown.

Tyrosine

SUPPLEMENT FORMS/ALTERNATE NAMES: *L-Tyrosine*

PRINCIPAL PROPOSED USES: *None*

OTHER PROPOSED USES: *Attention Deficit Disorder, Depression, Enhancing Mental Function, Enhancing Sports Performance, Fatigue, Jet Lag*

Tyrosine is an amino acid found in meat proteins. Your body uses it as a starting material to make several *neurotransmitters* (chemicals that help the brain and nervous system function). Based on this fact, tyrosine has been proposed as a treatment for various conditions in which mental function is impaired or slowed down, such as fatigue and depression. It has also been tried for attention deficit disorder (ADD).

Sources

Your body makes tyrosine from another common amino acid, **phenylalanine**, so deficiencies are rare; however, they can occur in certain forms of severe kidney disease as well as in phenylketonuria (PKU), a metabolic disorder that requires complete avoidance of phenylalanine.

Good sources of tyrosine include dairy products, meats, fish, and beans.

Therapeutic Dosages

The typical therapeutic dosage of tyrosine used in studies ranges from 7 to 30 g daily.

Therapeutic Uses

According to very preliminary evidence, tyrosine supplements may help fight **fatigue** and improve **memory and mental function** in people who are deprived of sleep or exposed to other forms of **stress**. Based on these findings, it can be inferred that tyrosine might enhance alertness in people suffering from **jet lag**, but this has not been studied directly.

Tyrosine may also provide some temporary benefit for **attention deficit disorder**, but the benefits appear to wear off in a couple of weeks. Tyrosine is said to work better for this purpose when it is combined in an "amino acid cocktail" along with gamma-aminobutyric acid (GABA), **phenylalanine**, and **glutamine**; however, there is no scientific evidence to support this use.

Although one extremely tiny study found tyrosine helpful for **depression**, a larger study found no evidence of benefit.

Tyrosine has also been suggested for **enhancing sports performance**. However, in a double-blind study of 20 men, one-time use of tyrosine at a dose of 150 mg per kilogram body weight failed to improve any measurement of muscular performance.

What Is the Scientific Evidence for Tyrosine?

Sleep Deprivation

A double-blind, placebo-controlled study that enrolled 20 U.S. Marines suggests that tyrosine can improve mental alertness during periods of sleep deprivation. In this study, the participants were deprived of sleep for a night and then tested frequently for their alertness throughout the day as they worked. Compared to placebo, 10 to 15 g of tyrosine given twice daily seemed to provide a "pick-up" for about 2 hours.

Similar benefits were seen with 2 g of tyrosine daily in a double-blind, placebo-controlled trial of 21 military cadets exposed to physical and psychological stress.

Depression

A pilot study that enrolled 9 individuals is widely quoted as proving that tyrosine can help depression. However, this study was too small to provide reliable results. A subsequent double-blind, placebo-controlled study of 65 people with depression failed to find any benefit.

Safety Issues

Tyrosine seems to be generally safe, though at high dosages some people have reported nausea, diarrhea, vomiting, or nervousness. As with any other supplement taken in multigram doses, it is important to use a high-quality product; even a very small percentage of contaminant in the product might add up to a dangerous amount.

Maximum safe dosages for young children, women who are pregnant or nursing, or those with severe liver or kidney disease have not been established.

Uva Ursi

Arctostaphylos uva-ursi

ALTERNATE NAMES/RELATED TERMS: *Bearberry*
PRINCIPAL PROPOSED USES: *Bladder Infection (Treatment, Not Prevention)*

The uva ursi plant is a low-lying evergreen bush whose berries are a favorite of bears, hence the name *bearberry*. However, it is the leaves that are used medicinally.

Uva ursi has a long history of use for treating urinary conditions in both America and Europe. Up until the development of sulfa antibiotics, its principal active component, arbutin, was frequently prescribed as a urinary antiseptic.

What Is Uva Ursi Used for Today?

Uva ursi is widely marketed today for the treatment of bladder infections. However, it has not been proven effective for this condition and there are significant safety concerns with its use.

What Is the Scientific Evidence for Uva Ursi?

Despite uva ursi's popularity for treating bladder infections, there is no meaningful evidence that it works. Two studies evaluated the antibacterial power of the urine of people who were taking uva ursi and found activity against most major bacteria that infect the urinary tract. However, while such findings are interesting, what is really needed is a double-blind, placebo-controlled trial to discover whether use of uva ursi actually helps people with established urinary tract infections. Unfortunately, not a single study of this type has been reported.

Rather strangely, one study evaluated continuous use of uva ursi for *prevention* of bladder infections. This double-blind, placebo-controlled trial followed 57 women for 1 year. Half were given a standardized dose of uva ursi (in combination with **dandelion** leaf, intended to promote urine flow), while the others received placebo. Over the course of the study, none of the women on uva ursi developed a bladder infection, whereas 5 of the untreated women did. However, this study is little more than a curiosity, because most experts do not believe that continuous treatment with uva ursi is safe! (See Safety Issues below.)

Dosage

European recommendations indicate that the dosage of uva ursi should be adjusted to provide 400 to 800 mg of arbutin daily. Due to fears of toxicity (see Safety Issues below) this dosage should not be exceeded; furthermore, the herb should not be used for more than 2 weeks and no more than 5 times a year.

Uva ursi should be taken with meals to minimize gastrointestinal upset. Uva ursi (based on its arbutin content) is thought to be most effective in alkaline urine and, for this reason, it should not be combined with **vitamin C** or **cranberry** juice. Some herbal experts recommend taking it along with calcium citrate to alkalinize the urine.

Uva ursi is also frequently sold in combination with other herbs traditionally thought to be helpful for bladder infections, including dandelion, cleavers, **juniper berry**, buchu, and parsley.

Safety Issues

There are significant safety concerns with uva ursi. The arbutin contained in uva ursi leaves is broken down in the intestine to another chemical, hydroquinone. This is altered a bit by the liver and then sent to the kidneys for excretion. Hydroquinone then acts as an antiseptic in the bladder. Unfortunately, hydroquinone is also a liver toxin, carcinogen, and irritant. For this reason, uva ursi is not recommended for long-term use. In addition, it should not be taken by young children, pregnant or nursing women, or those with severe liver or kidney disease.

Valerian
Valeriana officinalis

PRINCIPAL PROPOSED USES: *Insomnia*

OTHER PROPOSED USES: *Anxiety, Nervous Stomach*

More than 200 plant species belong to the genus *Valeriana*, but the one most commonly used as an herb is *Valeriana officinalis*. The root is used for medicinal purposes.

Galen recommended valerian for insomnia in the second century A.D. From the sixteenth century onward, this herb became popular as a sedative in Europe (and later, the United States). Scientific studies on valerian in humans began in the 1970s, leading to its approval as a sleep aid by Germany's Commission E in 1985. However, the scientific evidence showing that valerian really works remains incomplete.

As with most herbs, we are not exactly sure which ingredients in valerian are most important. Early research focused on a group of chemicals known as valepotriates, but they are no longer considered candidates.

A constituent called *valerenic acid* has also undergone study, but its role is far from clear. Another substance in valerian, linarin, has also attracted research interest.

Our understanding of how valerian might function remains similarly incomplete. Several studies suggest that valerian affects GABA, a naturally occurring amino acid that appears to be related to the experience of anxiety. Conventional tranquilizers in the Valium family are known to bind to GABA receptors in the brain and valerian may work similarly. However, there are some significant flaws in these hypotheses, and the reality is that we don't really know how valerian works (or if, indeed, it really does).

What Is Valerian Used for Today?

Valerian is commonly recommended as a mild treatment for occasional **insomnia**. However, evidence from the largest study on valerian suggests that it is most useful when taken over an extended period of time for chronic sleep disorders.

Like other treatments used for insomnia, valerian has also been proposed as a treatment for **anxiety**, but there is no reliable evidence as yet that it is effective.

Finally, valerian is sometimes suggested as a treatment for a nervous stomach; however, as of yet, there is no supporting scientific evidence for this use.

What Is the Scientific Evidence for Valerian?

Insomnia
The best study to date of valerian's effectiveness in treating insomnia involved 121 people followed for 28 days. Half of the participants took 600 mg of an alcohol-based valerian extract 1 hour before bedtime; the other half took placebo. At first, placebo and valerian were running neck and neck. But by the end of the study, the participants treated with valerian were definitely sleeping better than those on placebo.

Although positive, these results are a bit confusing because in another large study valerian was *immediately* more effective than placebo. This trial followed 128 subjects who had no sleeping problems. On nine nonconsecutive nights, each participant took one of three treatments: valerian, a valerian–hops combination, or placebo. The results showed that on the nights they took valerian alone, participants fell asleep faster than when they were taking placebo or the combination. (However, valerian–hops has been found effective in another trial, described below.) To make matters even more complex, other studies have failed

to find any immediate sedative effects with valerian, as one would expect with a substance that induces sleep. The explanation for these contradictory results remains elusive.

Additional evidence for valerian's effectiveness comes from a double-blind, placebo-controlled study of 78 elderly patients. In this case, sleep improved by the end of the study, at 14 days. A more recent study found that valerian improved sleep in children with developmental disabilities (specifically, intellectual impairment).

Furthermore, a 6-week, double-blind study of 202 people with insomnia compared valerian extract (600 mg at bedtime) with the standard drug oxazepam (10 mg at bedtime) and found equal efficacy. Equivalent benefits were also seen in a similar study of 75 people. However, the absence of a placebo group in these two studies decreases the reliability of the results.

In contrast, other studies have failed to find valerian more helpful than placebo for chronic insomnia.

A double-blind comparative study that enrolled 46 patients compared the effects of the standard drug bromazepam to a mixture of valerian and hops with either treatment taken one-half hour before bed. The results suggest that the two treatments were equally effective. One study found that this valerian–hops combination can antagonize the arousal produced by caffeine.

A combination of valerian and **lemon balm** has also been tried for insomnia. A rather poorly designed 30-day, double-blind, placebo-controlled study of 98 individuals without insomnia found marginal evidence that a valerian–lemon balm combination improved sleep quality as compared to placebo. However, a double-blind crossover study of 20 people with insomnia compared the benefits of the sleeping drug Halcion (0.125 mg) against placebo and a combination of valerian and lemon balm, and failed to find the herb effective. The drug, however, did prove effective.

Valerian has shown some promise for helping people sleep better after discontinuing conventional sleeping pills in the benzodiazepine family.

The most likely explanation for these contradictory results is that valerian offers mild benefits at most.

Anxiety
In a double-blind, placebo-controlled study, 36 people with generalized anxiety disorder were given either valerian extract, Valium, or placebo for a period of 4 weeks. The study failed to find statistically significant differences between the groups, presumably due to its small size.

In addition, a preliminary double-blind study found

that valerian may produce calming effects in stressful situations. Again, this study was too small to provide statistically meaningful results.

Dosage

For insomnia, the standard adult dosage of valerian is 2 to 3 g of dried herb, 270 to 450 mg of an aqueous valerian extract, or 600 mg of an ethanol extract, taken 30 to 60 minutes before bedtime. The same amount, or a reduced dose, can be taken twice daily for anxiety.

Because of valerian's unpleasant odor, European manufacturers have created odorless valerian products. However, these are not yet widely available in the United States.

Valerian is not recommended for children under 3 years old.

Safety Issues

Valerian is on the FDA's GRAS (generally recognized as safe) list and is approved for use as a food. In animals, it takes enormous doses of valerian to produce any serious adverse effects.

In a suicide attempt, one young woman took approximately 20 g of valerian (20 to 40 times the recommended dose). Only mild symptoms developed, including stomach cramps, fatigue, chest tightness, tremors, and lightheadedness. All of these resolved within 24 hours, after two treatments with activated charcoal. Her lab tests—including tests of her liver function—remained normal. Keep in mind that this does not mean that you can safely exceed the recommended dose.

One report did find toxic results from herbal remedies containing valerian mixed with several other herbal ingredients, including **skullcap**. Four individuals who took these remedies later developed liver problems. However, skullcap products are sometimes contaminated with the liver-toxic herb germander and this could have been the explanation.

There have also been about 50 reported cases of overdose with a combination preparation called *Sleep-Qik*, which contains valerian as well as conventional medications. Researchers specifically looked for liver injury, but found no evidence that it occurred.

There are some safety concerns about valepotriates, constituents of valerian, because in test-tube studies they have been found to affect DNA and cause other toxic effects. However, valepotriates are not present to a significant extent in any commercial preparations.

Although no animal studies or controlled human trials have found evidence that valerian causes withdrawal symptoms when stopped, one case report is sometimes cited in support of the possibility that this might occur. It concerns a 58-year-old man who developed delirium and rapid heartbeat after surgery. According to the patient's family, he had been taking high doses of valerian root extract (about 2.5 to 10 g per day) for many years. His physicians decided that he was suffering from valerian withdrawal. However, considering the many other factors involved (such as multiple medications and general anesthesia), it isn't really possible to conclude that valerian caused his symptoms.

In clinical trials use of valerian has not been associated with any significant side effects. A few people experience mild gastrointestinal distress and there have been rare reports of people developing a paradoxical mild stimulant effect from valerian.

Valerian does not appear to impair driving ability or produce morning drowsiness when taken at night. As noted above, most studies have failed to find any immediate sedative effect with valerian. However, one study reported finding mild impairment of attention for a couple of hours after taking valerian. For this reason, it isn't a good idea to drive immediately after taking it.

There have been no reported drug interactions with valerian and one study found reasons to believe that valerian should not raise or lower the blood levels of too many medications. Nonetheless, there are theoretical concerns that valerian might amplify the effects of sedative drugs. A 1995 study was somewhat reassuring on this score because it found no interaction between alcohol and valerian. However, animal studies have found that valerian extracts may prolong the effects of some sedatives and there have been some worrisome case reports suggesting that the combination of valerian and alcohol can lead to excessive sedation in some people. For this reason, we recommend that you do not combine valerian with central nervous system depressants except under doctor's supervision.

Safety in young children, pregnant or nursing women, or those with severe liver or kidney disease has not been established.

Interactions You Should Know About

If you are taking sedative drugs, such as **benzodiazepines**: Don't take valerian in addition to them, except under physician supervision.

Vanadium

SUPPLEMENT FORMS/ALTERNATE NAMES: *Vanadate, Vanadyl Sulfate*

PRINCIPAL PROPOSED USES: *None*

OTHER PROPOSED USES: *Bodybuilding, Diabetes, Osteoporosis*

Note: *There are serious safety concerns regarding vanadium use.*

Vanadium, a mineral, is named after the Scandinavian goddess of beauty, youth, and luster. Taking vanadium will not make you beautiful, youthful, and lustrous, but evidence from animal studies suggests it may be an essential micronutrient. That is, your body may need it, but in *very* low doses.

Based on promising animal studies, high doses of vanadium have been tested as an aid to controlling blood sugar levels in people with diabetes. Like **chromium**, another trace mineral used in diabetes, vanadium has also been recommended as an aid in bodybuilding. However, animal studies suggest that taking high doses of vanadium can be harmful.

Requirements/Sources

We don't know exactly how much vanadium people require, but estimates range from 10 to 30 mcg daily. (To realize how tiny this amount is, consider that it's about *one millionth* of the amount of calcium you need.) Human deficiencies have not been reported, but goats fed a low-vanadium diet have developed birth defects.

Vanadium is found in very small amounts in a wide variety of foods, including breakfast cereals, canned fruit juices, wine, beer, buckwheat, parsley, soy, oats, olive oil, sunflower seeds, corn, green beans, peanut oil, carrots, cabbage, and garlic. The average daily American diet provides between 10 and 60 mcg of vanadium.

Therapeutic Dosages

In various studies, vanadium has been used at doses thousands of times higher than is present in the diet, as high as 125 mg per day. However, there are serious safety concerns about taking vanadium at such high doses. We do not recommend exceeding the dose given in Safety Issues below.

Therapeutic Uses

Vanadium has been proposed as a treatment for **diabetes**, based on promising studies in animals and a few small human trials.

Vanadium is also sometimes used as a **sports supplement** by bodybuilders, but there is no evidence that it is effective.

Because studies in mice have found that vanadium is deposited in bone, some practitioners of nutritional medicine have suggested that it may be helpful for **osteoporosis**. However, since many toxic metals also accumulate in the bones without strengthening them, this doesn't prove that vanadium is good for bones.

What Is the Scientific Evidence for Vanadium?

Diabetes

Studies in rats with and without diabetes suggest that vanadium may have an insulin-like effect, reducing blood sugar levels. Based on these findings, preliminary studies involving humans have been conducted, with mostly promising results. However, no meaningful double-blind, placebo-controlled studies on vanadium as a treatment for diabetes have yet been reported. At present, it is not possible to say whether vanadium is helpful (or, for that matter, safe) for people with diabetes.

Bodybuilding

Vanadium has been promoted as a body-building sports supplement. However, a double-blind, placebo-controlled study involving 31 weight-trained athletes failed to find any benefit at a dosage more than 1,000 times the nutritional dose.

Safety Issues

Studies in humans and animals suggest that vanadium can cause toxic effects and might accumulate in the body if taken to excess. The safe upper intake level for adults has been set at 1.8 mg. Maximum safe doses for children have not yet been determined.

Another potential risk with vanadium involves its purported benefits. If vanadium does in fact improve blood sugar control in people with diabetes, the net re- sult could be a potentially dangerous fall in blood sugar levels (hypoglycemia). For this reason, medical supervi- sion is recommended before adding vanadium to a regi- men of standard diabetes medications.

Interactions You Should Know About

If you are taking **insulin** or **oral diabetes medications**: Seek medical supervision before taking vanadium be- cause you may need to reduce your dose of diabetes med- ication.

Vervain

Verbena officinalis

PRINCIPAL PROPOSED USES: *Stimulating Flow of Breast Milk*

OTHER PROPOSED USES: *Insomnia, Menstrual Pain*

The herb vervain is a common perennial wildflower in England, found growing at the edge of roads and in meadows. It has a long history of use in Celtic reli- gious tradition and has been used as medicine by many cultures. The leaf and flower are the parts used me- dicinally.

Like other bitter plants, vervain has been used to stimulate appetite and digestion. Other traditional uses include treating abdominal spasms, fevers, depression (especially following illness or childbirth), and inade- quate flow of breast milk.

What Is Vervain Used for Today?

Vervain is commonly recommended today to **increase flow of breast milk**, as well as to treat **insomnia** and **menstrual pain**. However, there is no meaningful evi- dence to support any of these uses.

One study in rats found possible sedative effects with a vervain extract. A test-tube study found hints of poten- tial **anti-cancer** effects. However, evidence like this is far, far too preliminary to show efficacy. Only double-blind, placebo-controlled studies can prove that a treatment re- ally works and no studies of this type have been performed on vervain. (For information on why such studies are es- sential, see **Why Does This Book Rely on Double-blind Studies?**.)

Dosage

A typical dosage of vervain is 2 to 3 g 3 times daily, taken as dry herb or made into tea. Equivalent dosages are also available in tincture form and may be more palatable.

Safety Issues

Although vervain is thought to be a relatively safe herb, it has not undergone any meaningful safety testing at a modern scientific level. There is some reason to believe it may not be safe for use in pregnancy. Despite its repu- tation for enhancing flow of breast milk, safety in nurs- ing women has also not been established. Additionally, safety in young children or people with severe liver or kidney disease remains unknown.

Vinpocetine

SUPPLEMENT FORMS/ALTERNATE NAMES: *Periwinkle*
PRINCIPAL PROPOSED USES: *Alzheimer's Disease and Other Forms of Dementia*
OTHER PROPOSED USES: *Enhancing Mental Function (In Healthy People), Strokes*

Vinpocetine is a chemical derived from vincamine, a constituent found in the leaves of common periwinkle (*Vinca minor* L.) as well as the seeds of various African plants. It is used as a treatment for memory loss and mental impairment.

Developed in Hungary over 20 years ago, vinpocetine is sold in Europe as a drug under the name Cavinton. In the United States it is available as a "dietary supplement," although the substance probably doesn't fit that category by any rational definition. Vinpocetine doesn't exist to any significant extent in nature. Producing it requires significant chemical work performed in the laboratory.

What Is Vinpocetine Used for Today?

Some evidence supports the idea that vinpocetine can **enhance memory** and mental function, especially in those with **Alzheimer's disease** and related conditions. It is also widely marketed for enhancing memory in healthy people, but there is no real evidence that it is helpful for this purpose.

It has been hypothesized that vinpocetine helps people with Alzheimer's disease by enhancing blood flow in the brain, safeguarding brain cells against damage, and inhibiting a substance known as phosphodiesterase.

Based on these proposed actions, vinpocetine has also been tried as a treatment for reducing brain damage following **strokes**.

What Is the Scientific Evidence for Vinpocetine?

Alzheimer's Disease and Related Conditions (Dementia)

A 16-week, double-blind, placebo-controlled trial of 203 individuals with mild to moderate dementia found significant benefit in the treated group. Benefits have been seen in other studies as well. However, a major review found that overall the evidence that it works remains too weak to rely upon, due to limitations in study quality.

Strokes

In a single-blind, placebo-controlled trial, 30 individuals who had just experienced a stroke received either placebo or vinpocetine along with conventional treatment for 30 days. The results showed that participants in the vinpocetine group experienced a significantly reduced level of residual disability as measured at 3 months.

A few other studies, some of poor design, also provide suggestive evidence that vinpocetine may be helpful for strokes. However, at present, the evidence is too preliminary to rely on.

Note: People who have had strokes are sometimes advised to take blood thinning drugs. There are concerns that vinpocetine may interact adversely with some medications of this type. See Safety Issues below.

Dosage

The usual dose of vinpocetine is 10-mg capsules 3 times per day, although dosages ranging from half to twice that amount have been used in studies. Vinpocetine reportedly is better absorbed when taken with a meal.

Safety Issues

No serious side effects have been reported in any of the clinical trials. However, there is one case report of vinpocetine apparently causing *agranulocytosis* (loss of certain white blood cells).

Vinpocetine inhibits blood platelets from forming clots and, for this reason, it could cause problems if it is taken by individuals with bleeding problems, during the period immediately before or after surgery or labor and delivery, or in combination with medications or natural substances that also affect platelet activity, such as aspirin, clopidogrel (Plavix), ticlopidine (Ticlid), pentoxifylline (Trental), garlic, ginkgo, policosanol, or high-dosage vitamin E.

The drug warfarin (Coumadin) affects blood clotting, but not through actions on platelets. One study found only a minimal interaction between warfarin and vinpocetine and, interestingly, it was in the direction of decreased clotting. Nonetheless, combination therapy with vinpocetine and warfarin should not be attempted except under the supervision of a physician.

Safety in pregnant or nursing women, young children, or those with severe liver or kidney disease has not been established.

Interactions You Should Know About

If you are taking:

➤ **Blood-thinning drugs, such as aspirin, clopidogrel (Plavix), ticlopidine (Ticlid), or pentoxifylline (Trental):** Simultaneous use of vinpocetine might cause bleeding problems.
➤ **Natural substances with blood-thinning properties, such as garlic, ginkgo, policosanol, or high-dose vitamin E:** Simultaneous use of vinpocetine might in theory cause bleeding problems.
➤ **Warfarin (Coumadin):** Vinpocetine might *impair* the blood-thinning actions.

Vitamin A

SUPPLEMENT FORMS/ALTERNATE NAMES: *Retinol*

PRINCIPAL PROPOSED USES: *Viral Infections in Children in Developing Countries*

OTHER PROPOSED USES: *Acne, Crohn's Disease, Diabetes, Eczema, HIV Support, Menorrhagia (Heavy Menstruation), Psoriasis, Rosacea, Seborrhea*

Vitamin A is a fat-soluble antioxidant that protects your cells against damaging free radicals and plays other vital roles in the body. However, it is potentially more dangerous than most other vitamins because it can build up to toxic levels. For this reason, it should be used with caution.

It has long been assumed that beta-carotene supplements taken at nutritional doses are a safer way to get the vitamin A you need. However, while this may be true in general, beta-carotene also appears to present some risks. See the full **Beta-Carotene** article for more information.

Requirements/Sources

Vitamin A is an essential nutrient—meaning you must get it in the diet. The official U.S. recommendations for daily intake of vitamin A are expressed in international units (IU) or retinol activity equivalents (RAE), which are measured in micrograms, as follows:

➤ **Infants 0–6 months, 400 mcg RAE or 1,330 IU 7–12 months, 500 mcg RAE or 1,665 IU**

➤ **Children 1–3 years, 300 mcg RAE or 1,000 IU 4–8 years, 400 mcg RAE or 1,330 IU**
➤ **Males 9–13 years, 600 mcg RAE or 2,000 IU 14 years and older, 900 mcg RAE or 3,000 IU**
➤ **Females 9–13 years, 600 mcg RAE or 2,000 IU 14 years and older, 700 mcg RAE or 2,330 IU**
➤ **Pregnant women, 770 mcg RAE or 2,560 IU (750 mcg RAE or 2,500 IUs if 18 years old or younger)**
➤ **Nursing women, 1,300 mcg RAE or 4,300 IU (1,200 mcg RAE or 4,000 IUs if 18 years old or younger)**

Warning: Pregnant women should not take vitamin A supplements. Instead they should take beta-carotene.

We get vitamin A from many foods, in the form of either vitamin A or beta-carotene. Liver and dairy products are excellent sources of vitamin A. Carrots, apricots, collard greens, kale, sweet potatoes, parsley, and spinach are good sources as well.

Deficiency in vitamin A is common in developing countries. In the developed world, deficiency is relatively

Vitamin A

rare. However, certain diseases can cause vitamin A deficiency by impairing the ability of the digestive tract to absorb nutrients. These include Crohn's disease, ulcerative colitis, and cystic fibrosis.

Therapeutic Dosages

Although some studies have used high doses of vitamin A, intake above the safe upper limit level is not recommended except on physician advice (see Safety Issues below).

Therapeutic Uses

There is some evidence that vitamin A supplements reduce deaths from measles and other infectious illnesses among children in developing countries, presumably because they correct a deficiency in the children's diets. This doesn't mean that vitamin A supplements above and beyond the basic nutritional requirement are a useful treatment for measles or any other childhood disease.

Vitamin A might improve blood sugar control in people with **diabetes**. Unfortunately, people with diabetes may also be especially vulnerable to liver damage from excessive amounts of vitamin A (see Safety Issues below). Therefore, if you have diabetes, you should take vitamin A only on the advice of a physician.

Vitamin A has shown some potential for preventing one type of skin cancer (squamous cell cancer). However, in these studies, doses above the standard safe upper limits have been used. With proper monitoring, this may be safe, but we do not recommend trying it without physician supervision. High-dose vitamin A has been tried for a variety of other skin diseases, including **acne**, **psoriasis**, **rosacea**, **seborrhea**, and **eczema**, as well as menorrhagia (heavy menstruation). However, the benefits seen have been modest at best and, again, the recommended dosages of vitamin A are so high as to raise concerns about toxic risk.

Incomplete and inconsistent evidence suggests that vitamin A or beta-carotene might be of benefit for people with **HIV** infection. On the basis of even weaker evidence, vitamin A has also been proposed as a treatment for a wide variety of other conditions, including Down's syndrome, **ear infections**, **eating disorders**, **glaucoma**, **gout**, impaired **night vision**, **kidney stones**, **lupus**, **multiple sclerosis**, **ulcerative colitis**, and **ulcers**.

One study suggests that vitamin A is *not* effective for **Crohn's disease**.

What Is the Scientific Evidence for Vitamin A?

Diabetes

According to many but not all studies, people with diabetes tend to be deficient in vitamin A.

An observational study suggests that vitamin A supplements may improve blood sugar control in people with diabetes. However, due to safety concerns, they should not supplement with vitamin A except under medical supervision (see Safety Issues below).

Menorrhagia (Heavy Menstruation)

One study suggests that women with heavy menstrual bleeding can benefit from taking 25,000 IU daily of vitamin A. But vitamin A cannot be recommended as an ongoing treatment for menorrhagia, since women who menstruate can become pregnant and even fairly low doses of supplemental vitamin A may cause birth defects.

HIV Support

One small double-blind study suggested that taking beta-carotene might raise white blood cell count in people with HIV. However, two subsequent larger controlled trials found no significant differences between those taking beta-carotene or placebo in white blood cell count, CD4+ count, or other measures of immune function.

Two observational studies lasting 6 to 8 years suggest that higher intakes of vitamin A or beta-carotene may be helpful, but they also found that caution is in order with regard to dosage. This group of researchers generally linked higher intake of vitamin A or beta-carotene to lower risk of AIDS and lower death rates, with an important exception: people with the highest intake of either nutrient (more than 11,179 IU per day of beta-carotene, more than 20,268 IU per day of vitamin A) did worse than those who took somewhat less.

Despite hopes that vitamin A given to pregnant, HIV-positive women might decrease the infection rate of their babies, two double-blind studies have found no significant differences between babies whose mothers took vitamin A compared to those whose mothers took placebo. In any case, vitamin A is not considered safe in pregnancy; beta-carotene is preferred.

Crohn's Disease

According to a double-blind study of 86 people with Crohn's disease, vitamin A does *not* help prevent flare-ups.

Safety Issues

The safe upper intake levels (ULs) of vitamin A have been set as follows:

➢ Infants 0–12 months, 600 mcg RAE or 2,000 IU
➢ Children 1–3 years, 600 mcg RAE or 2,000 IU
   4–8 years, 900 mcg RAE or 3,000 IU
➢ Males and females 9–13 years, 1,700 mcg RAE or 5,660 IU
   14–18 years, 2,800 mcg RAE or 9,320 IU
   19 years and older, 3,000 mcg RAE or 10,000 IU
➢ Pregnant women, 3,000 mcg RAE or 10,000 IU (2,800 mcg RAE or 9,320 IU if 18 years old or younger)
➢ Nursing women, 3,000 mcg RAE or 10,000 IU (2,800 mcg RAE or 9,320 IU if 18 years old or younger)

It is thought that dosages of vitamin A above 50,000 IU per day taken for several years can cause liver injury, bone problems, fatigue, hair loss, headaches, and dry skin. However, one recent study found no harm with dosages as high as 75,000 IU taken for 1 year. Nonetheless, we do not recommend using vitamin A at doses above the ULs, except under close physician supervision. Some people may be more likely to develop toxic symptoms than others.

If you already have liver disease, check with your doctor before taking vitamin A supplements, because even small doses may be harmful.

It is thought that people with diabetes may have trouble releasing vitamin A stored in the liver. This may mean that they are at greater risk for vitamin A toxicity.

Excessive intake of vitamin A (or beta-carotene) appears to accelerate liver injury in people with **alcoholism**. In addition, relatively high intake of vitamin A (but *not* beta-carotene) has been associated with increased risk of **osteoporosis**.

Women should avoid supplementing with vitamin A during pregnancy because at toxic levels it might increase the risk of birth defects. Pregnant women taking valproic acid medications (Depakote, Depacon, or Depakene) may be even more at risk of vitamin A toxicity.

Vitamin A may increase the anticoagulant effects of warfarin (Coumadin). In addition, because vitamin A chemically resembles the drug isotretinoin (Accutane), it may amplify its toxic effects.

Interactions You Should Know About

If you are taking:

➢ Isotretinoin (Accutane): Don't take vitamin A as the two might enhance each other's toxicity.
➢ Valproic acid (Depakote, Depacon, or Depakene) and you are pregnant: Do not take vitamin A supplements unless advised to do so by a physician.
➢ Warfarin (Coumadin): Do not take vitamin A supplements unless advised to do so by a physician.

Vitamin B₁

SUPPLEMENT FORMS/ALTERNATE NAMES: *Thiamin*

PRINCIPAL PROPOSED USES: *Congestive Heart Failure*

OTHER PROPOSED USES: *Alzheimer's Disease, Canker Sores, Enhancing Mental Function, Epilepsy, Fibromyalgia, HIV Support*

Vitamin B₁, also called *thiamin*, was the first B vitamin discovered. Every cell in your body needs thiamin to make adenosine triphosphate, or ATP, the body's main energy-carrying molecule. The heart, in particular, has considerable need for thiamin in order to keep up its constant work. Severe deficiency of thiamin results in beriberi, a disease common in the nineteenth century but rare today. Many of the principal symptoms of beriberi involve impaired heart function.

Vitamin B₁

Requirements/Sources

Your need for vitamin B_1 varies with age. The official U.S. and Canadian recommendations for daily intake are as follows:

- Infants 0–6 months, 0.2 mg
  7–12 months, 0.3 mg
- Children 1–3 years, 0.5 mg
  4–8 years, 0.6 mg
  9–13 years, 0.9 mg
- Males 14 years and older, 1.2 mg
- Females 14–18 years, 1.0 mg
  19 years and older, 1.1 mg
- Pregnant or nursing women, 1.4 mg

Although vitamin B_1 deficiency is rare in the developed world, it may occur in certain medical conditions, such as **alcoholism, Crohn's disease, anorexia,** and **folate** deficiency. People undergoing kidney dialysis or taking loop diuretics may also become deficient in vitamin B_1. Certain foods may impair your body's absorption of B_1 as well, including fish, shrimp, clams, mussels, and the herb **horsetail**.

Brewer's and nutritional yeast are the richest sources of B_1. Peas, beans, nuts, seeds, and whole grains also provide fairly good amounts.

Therapeutic Dosages

A typical dose of vitamin B_1 for therapeutic purposes is 200 mg daily, although much higher dosages have also been tried.

Some nutritional experts recommend taking B_1 with other B vitamins in the form of a **B-complex** supplement. However, there is no meaningful evidence that this offers any advantage.

Therapeutic Uses

Congestive heart failure (CHF) is a condition in which the pumping ability of the heart declines and fluid begins to accumulate in the lungs and legs. Standard treatment for CHF includes strong "water pills" called *loop diuretics*. These drugs, however, deplete the body of B_1. Since the heart depends on vitamin B_1 for its proper function, this is potentially quite worrisome. Preliminary evidence, including a small double-blind placebo-controlled trial, hints that supplementation with B_1 can improve symptoms.

One double-blind study suggests that thiamin taken at a dose of 50 mg daily might **enhance mental function**.

Other potential uses of thiamin have even less scientific support. Observational studies of people with **HIV** infection suggest (but definitely do not prove) that increased intake of vitamin B_1 might slow progression to AIDS and enhance overall survival rate. Weak and contradictory evidence hints that vitamin B_1 may be helpful for **Alzheimer's disease**. Vitamin B_1 has also been proposed as a treatment for **epilepsy, canker sores,** and **fibromyalgia**, but the evidence for these uses is too preliminary to cite.

Safety Issues

Vitamin B_1 appears to be quite safe even when taken in very high doses.

Interactions You Should Know About

If you are taking **loop diuretics**—for example, **furosemide** (Lasix): You may need extra vitamin B_1.

Vitamin B$_2$

SUPPLEMENT FORMS/ALTERNATE NAMES: *Riboflavin, Riboflavin-5-Phosphate*

PRINCIPAL PROPOSED USES: *Migraine Headaches*

OTHER PROPOSED USES: *Cataracts, HIV Support, Sickle-Cell Anemia, Sports Performance Enhancement*

Riboflavin, also known as vitamin B$_2$, is an essential nutrient required for life. This vitamin works with two enzymes critical to the body's production of adenosine triphosphate (ATP), its main energy source. Vitamin B$_2$ is also used to process amino acids and fats and to activate vitamin B$_6$ and folate.

Preliminary evidence suggests that riboflavin supplements may offer benefits for two illnesses: migraine headaches and cataracts.

Requirements/Sources

The official U.S. and Canadian recommendations for daily intake of riboflavin are as follows:

- Infants 0–6 months, 0.3 mg
  7–12 months, 0.4 mg
- Children 1–3 years, 0.5 mg
  4–8 years, 0.6 mg
  9–13 years, 0.9 mg
- Males 14 years and older, 1.3 mg
- Females, 14–18 years, 1.0 mg
  19 years and older, 1.1 mg
- Pregnant women, 1.4 mg
- Nursing women, 1.6 mg

Riboflavin is found in organ meats (such as liver, kidney, and heart) and in many vegetables, nuts, legumes, and leafy greens. The richest sources are torula (nutritional) yeast, brewer's yeast, and calf liver. Almonds, wheat germ, wild rice, and mushrooms are good sources as well.

Although serious riboflavin deficiencies are rare, slightly low levels can occur in children, the elderly, and those in poverty. Oral contraceptives used in the 1970s and 80s appeared to reduce levels of riboflavin, but it is not clear whether today's versions of those medications, which contain much lower levels of estrogen, would have the same effect.

Therapeutic Dosages

For migraine headaches, the typical recommended dosage of riboflavin is much higher than nutritional needs: 400 mg daily. For cataract prevention, riboflavin may be taken at the nutritional dosages described. Since the B vitamins tend to work together, many nutritional experts recommend taking B$_2$ with other B vitamins, perhaps in the form of a B-complex supplement.

Therapeutic Uses

Preliminary evidence suggests that riboflavin supplements taken at high dosages may reduce the frequency of **migraine headaches**.

One very large study suggests that riboflavin at nutritional doses may be helpful for **cataracts**, but in this study it was combined with another B vitamin, niacin or **vitamin B$_3$**, so it's hard to say which vitamin was responsible for the effect.

Riboflavin has also been proposed as a treatment for **sickle-cell anemia**, **HIV infection**, and as a performance enhancer for athletes, but there is no real evidence that it is effective for these uses.

What Is the Scientific Evidence for Vitamin B2?

Migraine Headaches

According to a 3-month, double-blind, placebo-controlled study of 55 people with migraines, riboflavin can significantly reduce the frequency and duration of migraine attacks. This study found that, when given at least 2 months to work, a daily dose of riboflavin (400 mg) can produce dramatic migraine relief. The majority of the participants experienced a greater than 50% decrease in the number of migraine attacks as well as the total days with headache pain. However, a larger and longer study is needed to follow up on these results.

Cataracts

Riboflavin supplements may help prevent cataracts, but the evidence isn't yet clear. In a large, double-blind, placebo-controlled study, 3,249 people were given either placebo or one of four nutrient combinations (**vitamin A –zinc**, riboflavin–niacin, **vitamin C**–molybdenum, or **selenium–beta-carotene–vitamin E**) for a period of 6 years. Those receiving the riboflavin–niacin supplement showed a significant (44%) reduction in the incidence of cataracts. However, it is unclear whether the benefits seen in this group were due to niacin, riboflavin, or the combination of the two. Strangely, there was a small but statistically significantly *higher* incidence of a special type of cataract (called a *subcapsular cataract*) in the riboflavin-niacin group.

Safety Issues

Riboflavin seems to be an extremely safe supplement.

Vitamin B₃

SUPPLEMENT FORMS/ALTERNATE NAMES: *Niacin, Niacinamide, Nicotinamide, Inositol Hexaniacinate*

PRINCIPAL PROPOSED USES:

Niacin: *High Cholesterol/Triglycerides*

Niacinamide: *Diabetes (Prevention and Treatment), Osteoarthritis, Photosensitivity*

Inositol Hexaniacinate: *Intermittent Claudication, Raynaud's Phenomenon*

OTHER PROPOSED USES: *Aging Skin, Cataracts, HIV Support, Pregnancy Support, Rosacea, Schizophrenia, Tardive Dyskinesia*

Vitamin B₃ is required for the proper function of more than 50 enzymes. Without it, your body would not be able to release energy or make fats from carbohydrates. Vitamin B₃ is also used to make sex hormones and other important chemical signal molecules.

Vitamin B₃ comes in two principal forms: niacin (nicotinic acid) and niacinamide (nicotinamide). When taken in low doses for nutritional purposes, these two forms of the vitamin are essentially identical. However, each has its own particular effects when taken in high doses. Additionally, a special form of niacin called *inositol hexaniacinate* has shown some promise as a treatment with special properties of its own.

Requirements/Sources

The official U.S. and Canadian recommendations for daily intake of niacin are as follows:

- Infants 0–6 months, 2 mg
  7–12 months, 4 mg
- Children 1–3 years, 6 mg
  4–8 years, 8 mg
  9–13 years, 12 mg
- Males 14 years and older, 16 mg
- Females 14 years and older, 14 mg
- Pregnant women, 18 mg
- Nursing women, 17 mg

Because the body can make niacin from the common amino acid tryptophan, niacin deficiencies are rare in developed countries. However, the antituberculosis drug isoniazid (INH) impairs the body's ability to produce niacin from tryptophan and may create symptoms of niacin deficiency.

Good food sources of niacin are seeds, yeast, bran, peanuts (especially with skins), wild rice, brown rice, whole wheat, barley, almonds, and peas. Tryptophan is found in protein foods (meat, poultry, dairy products, fish). Turkey and milk are particularly excellent sources of tryptophan.

Therapeutic Dosages

When used as therapy for a specific disease, niacin, niacinamide, and inositol hexaniacinate are taken in dosages much higher than nutritional needs, about 1 to 4 g daily. Because of the risk of liver inflammation at these doses, medical supervision is essential.

For prevention of diabetes in children, the usual dosage of niacinamide is 25 mg per kilogram body weight per day. There are 2.2 pounds in a kilogram, so a 40-pound child would get about 450 mg daily.

Warning: Medical supervision is essential before giving your child long-term niacinamide treatment.

Many people experience an unpleasant flushing sensation and headache when they take niacin. These symptoms can usually be reduced by gradually increasing the dosage over several weeks or by using slow-release niacin. However, slow-release niacin appears to be more likely to cause liver inflammation than other forms. Inositol hexaniacinate may also cause less flushing than plain niacin, and if you take an aspirin along with niacin, the flushing reaction will usually decrease.

Therapeutic Uses

There is no question that niacin (but not niacinamide) can significantly improve **cholesterol** profile, reducing levels of total and LDL ("bad") cholesterol and raising HDL ("good") cholesterol. However, unpleasant flushing reactions as well as a risk of liver inflammation and dangerous interactions with other cholesterol-lowering drugs have kept niacin from being widely used (see Safety Issues below).

Intriguing evidence suggests that regular use of niacinamide (but not niacin) may help prevent **diabetes** in children at special risk of developing it. Risk can be determined by measuring the ratio of antibodies to islet cells (ICA antibody test).

Niacinamide may improve blood sugar control in both children and adults who already have diabetes.

Furthermore, preliminary evidence suggests that niacinamide may be able to decrease symptoms of **osteoarthritis** and help control polymorphous light eruption, a type of **photosensitivity**.

Somewhat surprisingly, *topical* niacinamide has shown some promise for skin conditions. In a double-blind study of 50 women with signs of **aging skin**, use of a niacinamide cream significantly improved skin appearance and elasticity as compared to placebo cream. Niacinamide cream has also shown promise for **rosacea**.

The inositol hexaniacinate form of niacin (taken orally) may be helpful for **intermittent claudication** and **Raynaud's phenomenon**.

In addition, weak and in some cases contradictory evidence suggests one of the several forms of niacin might be helpful for people with **bursitis**, **cataracts**,

HIV infection, **pregnancy**, **schizophrenia**, and **tardive dyskinesia**.

What Is the Scientific Evidence for Vitamin B₃?

Niacin is one of the best researched of all the vitamins, and the evidence for using it to treat at least one condition—high cholesterol—is strong enough that it has become an accepted mainstream treatment.

High Cholesterol/Triglycerides

Niacin has been used since the 1950s to improve cholesterol profile. Several well-designed double-blind, placebo-controlled studies have found that niacin can reduce LDL ("bad") cholesterol by approximately 10% and triglycerides by 25% while raising HDL ("good") cholesterol by 20 to 30%. Niacin also lowers levels of lipoprotein(a)—another risk factor for atherosclerosis—by about 35%. Long-term studies have shown that use of niacin can significantly reduce death rates from cardiovascular disease.

Niacin appears to be a safe and effective treatment for high cholesterol in people with diabetes as well, and (contrary to previous reports) does not seem to raise blood sugar levels.

Preventing Diabetes

A large study conducted in New Zealand suggests that niacinamide can help prevent high-risk children from developing diabetes. In this study, more than 20,000 children were screened for diabetes risk by measuring ICA antibodies. It turned out that 185 of these children had detectable levels. About 170 were then given niacinamide for 7 years (not all parents agreed to give their children niacinamide or stay in the study for that long). About 10,000 other children were not screened, but they were followed to see whether they developed diabetes.

The results were positive. In the group in which children were screened and given niacinamide if they were positive for ICA antibodies, the incidence of diabetes was reduced by almost 60%.

These findings suggest that niacinamide is an effective treatment for preventing diabetes. (The results also indicate that tests for ICA antibodies can accurately identify children at risk for diabetes.)

At present, a very large, long-term trial called the European Nicotinamide Diabetes Intervention Trial is being conducted to definitively determine whether regular use of niacinamide can prevent diabetes. Results from the German portion of the study have been released and they are not positive. However, until the entire study is complete, it is not possible to draw conclusions.

Treating Diabetes

When a child develops diabetes, there is an interval called the *honeymoon period* in which the pancreas can still make some insulin and there is little to no need for injected insulin. Weak evidence suggests that niacinamide might slightly delay the onset of more severe symptoms. A cocktail of niacinamide plus **antioxidant** vitamins and minerals has also been tried, but the results were disappointing in one study. However, in another study, use of intensive insulin therapy along with niacinamide and vitamin E was more effective than insulin plus niacinamide alone in prolonging the honeymoon period.

A recent study suggests that niacinamide may also improve blood sugar control in type 2 (adult-onset) diabetes, but it did not use a double-blind design. (For information on why this is important, see **Why Does This Book Rely on Double-blind Studies?**.)

Intermittent Claudication

Double-blind studies involving a total of about 400 individuals have found that inositol hexaniacinate can improve walking distance for people with intermittent claudication. For example, in one study, 100 individuals were given either placebo or 4 g of inositol hexaniacinate daily. Over a period of 3 months, participants improved significantly in the number of steps they could take on a special device before experiencing excessive pain.

Osteoarthritis

There is some evidence that niacinamide may provide some benefits for those with osteoarthritis. In a double-blind study, 72 people with arthritis were given either 3,000 mg daily of niacinamide (in 6 equal doses) or placebo for 12 weeks. The results showed that treated participants experienced a 29% improvement in symptoms, whereas those given placebo worsened by 10%. However, at this dose, liver inflammation is a concern that must be taken seriously.

Raynaud's Phenomenon

According to one small double-blind study, the inositol hexaniacinate form of niacin may be helpful for Raynaud's phenomenon. The dosage used was 4 g daily—once again a dosage high enough for liver inflammation to be a real possibility.

Safety Issues

When taken at a dosage of more than 100 mg daily, niacin frequently causes annoying skin flushing, especially in the face, as well as stomach distress, itching, and headache. In studies, as many as 43% of individuals taking niacin quit because of unpleasant side effects.

A more dangerous effect of niacin is liver inflammation. Although some reports suggest that it occurs most commonly with slow-release niacin, it can occur with any type of niacin when taken at a daily dose of more than 500 mg (usually 3 g or more). Regular blood tests to evaluate liver function are therefore mandatory when using high-dose niacin (or niacinamide or inositol hexaniacinate). This reaction almost always goes away when niacin is stopped. **Note:** Contrary to claims on some manufacturers' websites, there is no reliable evidence that inositol hexaniacinate is safer than ordinary niacin.

If you have liver disease, ulcers (presently or in the past), or gout, or drink too much alcohol, do not take high-dose niacin except on medical advice.

Contrary to previous reports, niacin does not appear to raise blood-sugar levels in people with diabetes.

Combining high-dose niacin with statin drugs (the most effective medications for high cholesterol) further improves cholesterol profile by raising HDL ("good") cholesterol. Unfortunately, there are real concerns that this combination therapy could cause a potentially fatal condition called *rhabdomyolysis*.

A growing body of evidence, however, suggests that the risk is relatively slight in individuals with healthy kidneys. Furthermore, even much lower doses of niacin than the usual dose given to improve cholesterol levels (100 mg versus 1,000 mg or more) may provide a similar benefit. At this dose, the risk of rhabdomyolysis should be decreased.

Nonetheless, it is not safe to try this combination except under close physician supervision. Rhabdomyolysis can be fatal.

Another potential drug interaction involves the anticonvulsant drugs carbamazepine and primidone. Niacinamide might increase blood levels of these drugs, possibly requiring reduction in drug dosage. Do not use this combination except under physician supervision.

The maximum safe dosage of niacin for pregnant or nursing women has been set at 35 mg daily (30 mg if 18 years old or younger).

Interactions You Should Know About

If you are taking:

➤ Cholesterol-lowering drugs in the statin family, niacin might offer potential benefits; however, there are real dangers to this combination. Do not try it except under physician supervision.

➤ The antituberculosis drug isoniazid (INH): You may need extra niacin.

➤ Anticonvulsant drugs such as carbamazepine or primidone: Do not take niacinamide except under physician supervision.

If you drink alcohol excessively:

➤ Do not take niacin except under physician supervision.

Vitamin B$_6$

SUPPLEMENT FORMS/ALTERNATE NAMES: *Pyridoxal-5-Phosphate, Pyridoxine, Pyridoxine Hydrochloride*

PRINCIPAL PROPOSED USES: *Nausea of Pregnancy (Morning Sickness)*

OTHER PROPOSED USES: *Asthma, Depression, Heart Disease Prevention, HIV Support, Kidney Stones, MSG Sensitivity, Photosensitivity, Reducing Homocysteine Levels, Rheumatoid Arthritis, Schizophrenia, Seborrheic Dermatitis, Tardive Dyskinesia, Vertigo*

PROBABLY NOT EFFECTIVE USES: *Autism (B$_6$ Combined with Magnesium), Carpal Tunnel Syndrome, Diabetic Neuropathy, Eczema, Premenstrual Syndrome (PMS), Side Effects of Oral Contraceptives*

Vitamin B$_6$ plays a major role in making proteins, hormones, and *neurotransmitters* (chemicals that carry signals between nerve cells). Because mild deficiency of vitamin B$_6$ is common, this is one vitamin that is probably worth taking as insurance.

However, there is little evidence that taking vitamin B$_6$ above nutritional needs offers benefits in the treatment of any particular illnesses, except, possibly, nausea of pregnancy (morning sickness).

Requirements/Sources

Vitamin B$_6$ requirements increase with age. The official U.S. and Canadian recommendations for daily intake are as follows:

➤ Infants 0–6 months, 0.1 mg
    7–12 months, 0.3 mg
➤ Children 1–3 years, 0.5 mg
    4–8 years, 0.6 mg
    9–13 years, 1.0 mg

➤ Males 14–50 years, 1.3 mg
    51 years and older, 1.7 mg
➤ Females 14–18 years, 1.2 mg
    19–50 years, 1.3 mg
    51 years and older, 1.5 mg
➤ Pregnant women, 1.9 mg
➤ Nursing women, 2.0 mg

Severe deficiencies of vitamin B$_6$ are rare, but mild deficiencies are extremely common. In a survey of 11,658 adults, 71% of men and 90% of women were found to have diets deficient in B$_6$. Vitamin B$_6$ is the most commonly deficient water-soluble vitamin in the elderly, and children, too, often don't get enough. In addition, evidence has been presented that current recommended daily intakes should be increased.

Vitamin B$_6$ deficiency might be worsened by use of hydralazine (for high blood pressure), penicillamine (used for rheumatoid arthritis and certain rare diseases), theophylline (an older drug for asthma), MAO inhibitors, and the antituberculosis drug isoniazid (INH), all of which are thought to interfere with B$_6$ to some degree. Good sources of B$_6$ include nutritional (torula) yeast, brewer's yeast, sunflower seeds, wheat germ, soybeans, walnuts, lentils, lima beans, buckwheat flour, bananas, and avocados.

Therapeutic Dosages

One study found that 30 mg of vitamin B$_6$ daily was effective for symptoms of morning sickness. While far above nutritional needs, this dosage should be safe. However, for the treatment of other conditions, B$_6$ has been recommended at doses as high as 300 mg daily. There are potential risks at this level of vitamin B$_6$ intake (see the Safety Issues section below for more information).

Therapeutic Uses

The results of a large double-blind, placebo-controlled study suggest that vitamin B$_6$ at a dose of 30 mg daily may be helpful for treating **nausea in pregnancy** (morning sickness).

Vitamin B$_6$ has been proposed for numerous other uses as well, but without much (if any) scientific substantiation. For example, the two most famous uses of vitamin B$_6$, **carpal tunnel syndrome** and **premenstrual syndrome** (PMS), have no reliable supporting evidence at all, and the best-designed studies found it *ineffective* for either of these purposes.

Higher intake of vitamin B$_6$ reduces the level of **homocysteine** in the blood, a substance that might accelerate **cardiovascular disease** (heart disease, strokes, and related conditions). However, there is as yet no meaningful evidence that reducing homocysteine is beneficial and considerable evidence that it is not.

For the following other conditions, current evidence for benefit with vitamin B$_6$ remains incomplete and/or contradictory: allergy to monosodium glutamate (MSG), **asthma, depression, diabetes of pregnancy, HIV** infection, **photosensitivity,** preventing **kidney stones, schizophrenia, seborrheic dermatitis, tardive dyskinesia** and other side effects of anti-psychotic drugs, and **vertigo.**

Despite some claims in the media, vitamin B$_6$ has not shown benefit for **enhancing mental function.** One study failed to find B$_6$ at a dose of 50 mg daily helpful for rheumatoid arthritis (despite a general B$_6$ deficiency seen in people with this condition).

Vitamin B$_6$, alone or in combination with **magnesium,** showed some early promise for the treatment of **autism,** but the best-designed studies failed to find it effective.

Additionally, current evidence suggests that vitamin B$_6$ is *not* effective for treating **diabetic neuropathy** or **eczema** or for helping control the side effects of **oral contraceptives.**

What Is the Scientific Evidence for Vitamin B$_6$?

Morning Sickness (Nausea and Vomiting in Pregnancy)

Vitamin B$_6$ supplements have been used for years by conventional physicians as a treatment for morning sickness. In 1995, a large double-blind study validated this use. A total of 342 pregnant women were given placebo or 30 mg of vitamin B$_6$ daily. Subjects then graded their symptoms by noting the severity of their nausea and recording the number of vomiting episodes. The women in the B$_6$ group experienced significantly less nausea than those in the placebo group, suggesting that regular use of B$_6$ can be helpful for morning sickness. However, vomiting episodes were not significantly reduced.

Another study found vitamin B$_6$ and **ginger** equally effective for morning sickness. However, as ginger is not a proven treatment for this condition, this study by itself does not provide any additional evidence in favor of B$_6$.

Premenstrual Syndrome (PMS)

A recent, properly designed, double-blind study of 120 women found no benefit of vitamin B$_6$ for PMS. In this study, three prescription drugs were compared against vitamin B$_6$ (pyridoxine, at 300 mg daily) and placebo. All study participants received 3 months of treatment and 3 months of placebo. Vitamin B$_6$ proved to be no better than placebo.

Approximately a dozen other double-blind studies have investigated the effectiveness of vitamin B$_6$ for PMS, but none were well designed and overall the evidence for any benefit is weak at best. Some books on natural medicine report that the negative results in some of these studies were due to insufficient B$_6$ dosage, but in reality there was no clear link between dosage and effectiveness.

However, preliminary evidence suggests that the combination of B$_6$ and magnesium might be more effective than either treatment alone.

Autism

One double-blind, placebo-controlled crossover study found indications that very high doses of vitamin B$_6$ may produce beneficial effects in the treatment of autism. However, this study was small and poorly designed; furthermore, it used a dose of vitamin B$_6$ so high that it could cause toxicity.

It has been suggested that combining magnesium with vitamin B$_6$ could offer additional benefits, such as reducing side effects or allowing a reduced dose of the vitamin. However, the two reasonably well-designed studies using combined vitamin B$_6$ and magnesium have failed to find benefits. Therefore, it isn't possible at present to recommend vitamin B$_6$ with or without magnesium as a treatment for autism.

Asthma

A double-blind study of 76 children with asthma found significant benefit from vitamin B$_6$ after the second month of usage. Children in the vitamin B$_6$ group were able to reduce their doses of asthma medication (bronchodilators and steroids). However, a recent double-blind study of 31 adults who used either inhaled or oral steroids did *not* show any benefit. The dosages of B$_6$ used in these studies were quite high, in the range of 200 to 300 mg daily. Because of the risk of nerve injury, it is not advisable to take this much B$_6$ without medical supervision (see Safety Issues).

Safety Issues

The safe upper levels for daily intake of vitamin B$_6$ are as follows:

➤ Children 1–3 years, 30 mg
   4–8 years, 40 mg

➤ Males and females 9–13 years, 60 mg
   14–18 years, 80 mg
   19 years and older, 100 mg
➤ Pregnant or nursing women, 100 mg (80 mg if 18 years old or younger)

At higher dosages (especially above 2 g daily) there is a very real risk of nerve damage. Nerve-related symptoms have even been reported at doses as low as 200 mg. (This is a bit ironic, given that B$_6$ deficiency *also* causes nerve problems.) In some cases, very high doses of vitamin B$_6$ can cause or worsen **acne** symptoms.

In addition, doses of vitamin B$_6$ over 5 mg may interfere with the effects of the drug levodopa when it is taken alone. However, vitamin B$_6$ does not impair the effectiveness of drugs containing levodopa and carbidopa.

Maximum safe dosages for individuals with severe liver or kidney disease have not been established.

Interactions You Should Know About

If you are taking:

➤ Isoniazid (INH), penicillamine, hydralazine, theophylline, or MAO inhibitors : You may need extra vitamin B6, but take only nutritional doses. Higher doses of B6 might interfere with the action of the drug.
➤ Levodopa without carbidopa (for Parkinson's disease): Do not take more than 5mg of vitamin B6 daily, except on medical advice.
➤ Antipsychotic medications: B6 might reduce side effects.

Vitamin B$_{12}$

SUPPLEMENT FORMS/ALTERNATE NAMES: *Cobalamin, Cyanocobalamin, Hydrocobalamin, Methylcobalamin*

PRINCIPAL PROPOSED USES: *Correcting Deficiency*

OTHER PROPOSED USES: *Alzheimer's Disease, Amyotrophic Lateral Sclerosis (Lou Gehrig's Disease), Asthma, Bell's Palsy, Depression, Diabetic Neuropathy, Eczema, HIV Support, Male Infertility, Multiple Sclerosis, Osteoporosis, Periodontal Disease, Recurrent Miscarriage, Restless Legs Syndrome, Tinnitus, Vitiligo*

Vitamin B$_{12}$, an essential nutrient, is also known as cobalamin. The *cobal* in the name refers to the metal cobalt contained in B$_{12}$. Vitamin B$_{12}$ is required for the normal activity of nerve cells and works with folate and vitamin B$_6$ to lower blood levels of homocysteine, a chemical in the blood that might contribute to heart disease. B$_{12}$ also plays a role in the body's manufacture of **S-adenosylmethionine** (SAMe).

Anemia is usually (but not always) the first sign of B$_{12}$ deficiency. Earlier in this century, doctors coined the name "pernicious anemia" for a stubborn form of anemia that didn't improve even when the patient was given iron supplements. Today we know that pernicious anemia comes about when the stomach fails to excrete a special substance called *intrinsic factor*. The body needs the intrinsic factor for efficient absorption of vitamin B$_{12}$. In 1948, vitamin B$_{12}$ was identified as the cure for pernicious anemia. B$_{12}$ deficiency also causes nerve damage and this may, in some cases, occur without anemia first developing.

Vitamin B$_{12}$ has also been proposed as a treatment for numerous other conditions, but as yet there is no definitive evidence that it is effective for any purpose other than correcting deficiency.

Requirements/Sources

Extraordinarily small amounts of vitamin B$_{12}$ suffice for daily nutritional needs. The official U.S. and Canadian recommendations for daily intake are as follows:

> Infants 0–6 months, 0.4 mcg
> 7–12 months, 0.5 mcg
> Children 1–3 years, 0.9 mcg
> 4–8 years, 1.2 mcg
> 9–13 years, 1.8 mcg
> Males and females 14 years and older, 2.4 mcg
> Pregnant women, 2.6 mcg
> Nursing women, 2.8 mcg

Vitamin B$_{12}$ deficiency is rare in the young, but it's not unusual in older people: probably 10 to 20% of the elderly are deficient in B$_{12}$. This may be because older people have lower levels of stomach acid. The vitamin B$_{12}$ in our food comes attached to proteins and must be released by acid in the stomach in order to be absorbed. When stomach acid levels are low, we don't absorb as much vitamin B$_{12}$ from our food. Fortunately, vitamin B$_{12}$ supplements don't need acid for absorption and should therefore get around this problem. However, for reasons that are unclear, one study found that vitamin B$_{12}$–deficient seniors need very high dosages of B$_{12}$ supplements to normalize their levels, as high as 600 to 1,000 mcg daily.

Similarly, people who take medications that greatly reduce stomach acid, such as omeprazole (Prilosec) or ranitidine (Zantac), also may have trouble absorbing vitamin B$_{12}$ from food, and could benefit from B$_{12}$ supplements.

Stomach surgery and other conditions affecting the digestive tract can also lead to B$_{12}$ deficiency. Vitamin B$_{12}$ absorption or levels in the blood may also be impaired by colchicine (for gout), metformin and phenformin (for diabetes), and AZT (for AIDS). Exposure to nitrous oxide (such as may be experienced by dentists and dental hygienists) might cause B$_{12}$ deficiency, but studies disagree. Slow-release potassium supplements might impair B$_{12}$ absorption as well.

Vitamin B$_{12}$ is found in most animal foods; it is also found *only* in animal food. Beef, liver, clams, and lamb provide a whopping 80 to 100 mcg of B$_{12}$ per 3.5-ounce serving, at least 40 times the dietary requirement.

Sardines, chicken liver, beef kidney, and calf liver are also good sources, providing between 25 and 60 mcg per serving. Trout, salmon, tuna, eggs, whey, and many cheeses provide at least the recommended daily intake.

Note: Total vegetarians (vegans) must take vitamin B_{12} supplements or consume B_{12}-fortified foods, or they will eventually become deficient. Contrary to some reports, seaweed and tempeh do not provide B_{12}. (Some forms of blue-green algae, such as spirulina, contain B_{12}, but it is not in an absorbable state.)

Vitamin B_{12} is available in three forms: cyanocobalamin, hydrocobalamin, and methylcobalamin. The first is the most widely available and least expensive, but some experts think that the other two forms are preferable.

Severe B_{12} deficiency can cause anemia and, potentially, nerve damage. The latter may become permanent if the deficiency is not corrected in time. Anemia most often develops first, leading to treatment before permanent nerve damage develops. However, folate supplements can get in the way of this "early warning system." This is why people are cautioned against taking high doses of folate without medical supervision. When taken at a dosage higher than 400 mcg daily, folate can prevent anemia caused by B_{12} deficiency, thereby allowing permanent nerve damage to develop without any warning. More mild deficiencies of vitamin B_{12} may cause elevated levels of homocysteine in the blood, potentially increasing risk of heart disease. (See the **homocysteine** article for more information.) Mild B_{12} deficiency (too slight to cause anemia) may also impair brain function.

Therapeutic Dosages

For correcting absorption problems caused by medications, taking vitamin B_{12} at the level of dietary requirements should suffice.

For other purposes, enormously higher daily doses—ranging from 100 to 2,000 mcg—are sometimes recommended.

Therapeutic Uses

It appears that individuals who take medications that dramatically lower stomach acid, such as H_2 blockers or proton pump inhibitors, would benefit by taking B_{12} supplements. Other individuals likely to be deficient in B_{12}, such as the elderly, or those taking the medications listed in Requirements/Sources, might well benefit from a daily B_{12} supplement to prevent B_{12} deficiency.

For pernicious anemia, B_{12} injections are traditionally used but research has shown that oral B_{12} works just as well, provided you take enough of it (between 300 and 1,000 mcg daily).

Weak evidence suggests that B_{12} supplements may improve sperm activity and sperm count; on this basis, they could be useful for **male infertility**. Some cases of **recurrent miscarriage** might be due to vitamin B_{12} deficiency.

One double-blind, placebo-controlled study, enrolling 49 people with eczema, found benefit with a cream containing vitamin B_{12} at a concentration of 0.07%. Topical B_{12} is hypothesized to work for eczema by reducing local levels of the substance nitric oxide (not related to nitrous oxide).

On the basis of weak and sometimes contradictory evidence, vitamin B_{12} has been suggested for **HIV, amyotrophic lateral sclerosis, carpal tunnel syndrome, diabetic neuropathy, multiple sclerosis** (MS), **restless legs syndrome,** and **tinnitus.**

Some evidence suggests that people with **vitiligo** (splotchy loss of skin pigmentation) might be deficient in vitamin B_{12} and supplementation along with folate may be helpful. However, the evidence is very weak and not all studies agree.

Some alternative practitioners recommend the use of injected vitamin B_{12} for **Bell's palsy.** However, the only scientific support for this approach comes from one study that was not double-blind. (For information on the importance of a double-blind design, see **Why Does This Book Rely on Double-blind Studies?.**)

Vitamin B_{12} is also sometimes recommended for numerous other problems, including **asthma, depression, osteoporosis,** and **periodontal disease,** but there is essentially no evidence as yet that it really works.

A double-blind trial of vitamin B_{12} for seasonal affective disorder (SAD—a type of depression related to lack of light during the winter) failed to find evidence of benefit.

One double-blind, placebo-controlled study of 140 people with mildly low B_{12} levels failed to find B_{12} helpful for improving mental function and mood.

Another study failed to find evidence that vitamin B_{12} improved general sense of **well-being** among seniors with signs of mild B_{12} deficiency.

Although vitamin B_{12} has been proposed as a treatment for **Alzheimer's disease,** this recommendation is based solely on the results of one small, poorly designed study. More recent and better-designed studies found little to no benefit.

What Is the Scientific Evidence for Vitamin B$_{12}$?

Vitamin B$_{12}$ deficiencies in men can lead to reduced sperm counts and lowered sperm mobility. For this reason, B$_{12}$ supplements have been tried for improving fertility in men with abnormal sperm production. In one double-blind study of 375 infertile men, supplementation with vitamin B$_{12}$ produced no benefits on average in the group as a whole. However, in a particular subgroup of men with sufficiently low sperm count and sperm motility, B$_{12}$ appeared to be helpful. Such "dredging" of the data is suspect from a scientific point of view, however, and this study cannot be taken as proof of effectiveness.

Safety Issues

Vitamin B$_{12}$ appears to be extremely safe. However, in some cases, very high doses of vitamin B$_{12}$ can cause or worsen acne symptoms.

Interactions You Should Know About

If you are taking **colchicine**, **AZT**, medications that reduce stomach acid (such as the **H$_2$ blocker** ranitidine [Zantac] or the **proton pump inhibitor** omeprazole [Prilosec]), **oral hypoglycemics** (such as metformin or phenformin), or slow-release **potassium** supplements, or if you are exposed to nitrous oxide anesthesia: You may need extra B$_{12}$. Another option is to take extra **calcium**, which may, in turn, improve B$_{12}$ absorption.

Vitamin C

SUPPLEMENT FORMS/ALTERNATE NAMES: *Ascorbate, Ascorbic Acid*

PRINCIPAL PROPOSED USES: *None*

OTHER PROPOSED USES: *Acute Anterior Uveitis, Aging Skin, Allergies, Asthma, Autism, Bedsores, Cancer (Prevention), Cancer (Treatment), Cataracts, Colds (Treatment, Not Prevention), Easy Bruising, Gallbladder Disease Prevention, Glaucoma, Heart Disease Prevention, HIV Support, Hypertension, Insomnia, Low Sperm Count, Macular Degeneration, Maintaining Effectiveness of Nitrate Drugs, Menopausal Symptoms, Minor Injuries, Muscle Soreness after Exercise, Osteoarthritis, Photosensitivity, Preeclampsia (Prevention), Reflex Sympathetic Dystrophy (RSD) (Prevention), Sunburn (Prevention); Vascular Dementia (Prevention)*

PROBABLY NOT EFFECTIVE USES: *Cervical Dysplasia, Common Cold (Prevention)*

Although most animals can make vitamin C from scratch, humans have lost the ability over the course of evolution. We must get it from food, chiefly fresh fruits and vegetables. One of this vitamin's main functions is helping the body manufacture collagen, a key protein in our connective tissues, cartilage, and tendons.

From ancient times through the early nineteenth century, sailors and others deprived of fresh fruits and vegetables developed a disease called *scurvy*. Scurvy involves so-called scorbutic symptoms, which include nonhealing wounds, bleeding gums, bruising, and overall weakness. Now we know that scurvy is nothing more than vitamin C deficiency.

Scurvy was successfully treated with citrus fruit during the mid-1700s. In 1928, when Albert Szent-Gyorgyi isolated the active ingredient, he called it the *antiscorbutic principle*, or ascorbic acid. This, of course, is vitamin C.

Vitamin C is a powerful antioxidant that protects against damaging natural substances called *free radicals*. It works in water, both inside and outside of cells. Vitamin C complements another antioxidant vitamin, **vitamin E**, which works in lipid (fatty) parts of the body.

Vitamin C is the single most popular vitamin supplement in the United States and perhaps the most

Vitamin C

controversial as well. In the 1960s, two-time Nobel Prize winner Dr. Linus Pauling claimed that vitamin C could effectively treat both cancer and the common cold. Subsequent research has mostly discounted these claims, but hasn't dampened enthusiasm for this essential nutrient. The vitamin C movement has led to hundreds of clinical studies testing the vitamin on dozens of illnesses; at present, however, no dramatic benefits have been discerned.

Requirements/Sources

Vitamin C is an essential nutrient that must be obtained from food or supplements; the body cannot manufacture it. The official U.S. and Canadian recommendations for daily intake are as follows:

- ➤ Infants 0–6 months, 40 mg
  7–12 months, 50 mg
- ➤ Children 1–3 years, 15 mg
  4–8 years, 25 mg
  9–13 years, 45 mg
- ➤ Males 14–18 years, 75 mg
  19 years and older, 90 mg
- ➤ Females 14–18 years, 65 mg
  19 years and older, 75 mg
- ➤ Pregnant women 85 mg (80 mg if 18 years old or younger)
- ➤ Nursing women 120 mg (115 mg if 18 years old or younger)

Note: Smoking cigarettes significantly reduces levels of vitamin C in the body. The recommended daily intake for smokers is 35 mg higher across all age groups.

Scurvy, the classic vitamin C deficiency disease, is now a rarity in the developed world, although a more subtle deficiency of vitamin C is fairly common. According to one study, 40% of Americans do not get enough vitamin C. In fact, vitamin C deficiency sufficient to cause bleeding problems during surgery turns out to be more common than previously thought.

Aspirin and other anti-inflammatory drugs might lower body levels of vitamin C, as might oral contraceptives. Supplementation may be helpful if you are taking any of these medications.

Most of us think of orange juice as the quintessential source of vitamin C, but many vegetables are actually even richer sources. Red chili peppers, sweet peppers, kale, parsley, collard, and turnip greens are full of vitamin C, as are broccoli, Brussels sprouts, watercress,

cauliflower, cabbage, and strawberries. (Oranges and other citrus fruits are good sources, too.)

One great advantage of getting vitamin C from foods rather than from supplements is that you will get many other healthy nutrients at the same time, such as bioflavonoids and carotenes. However, vitamin C in food is partially destroyed by cooking and exposure to air, so for maximum nutritional benefit you might want to try freshly made salads rather than dishes that require a lot of cooking.

Vitamin C supplements are available in two forms: ascorbic acid and ascorbate. The latter is less intensely sour.

Therapeutic Dosages

Ever since Linus Pauling, proponents have recommended taking vitamin C in enormous doses, as high as 20,000 to 30,000 mg daily. However, some evidence suggests that there might not be any reason to take more than 200 mg of vitamin C daily (10 to 100 times less than the amount recommended by vitamin C proponents). The reason is that if you consume more than 200 mg daily (researchers have tested up to 2,500 mg) your kidneys begin to excrete the excess at a steadily increasing rate, matching the increased dose. Your digestive tract also stops absorbing it well. The net effect is that no matter how much you take, your blood levels of vitamin C don't increase very much.

However, there are some flaws in this research. It is possible that vitamin C levels might rise in other tissues even if they remain constant in the blood. Furthermore, this study did not evaluate the possible effects of taking vitamin C several times daily rather than once daily.

Many nutritional experts recommend a total of 500 mg of vitamin C daily. This dose is almost undoubtedly safe. Others recommend that you take as much vitamin C as you can, up to 30,000 mg daily, cutting back only when you start to develop stomach cramps and diarrhea. This recommendation seems based more on a semireligious enthusiasm for the vitamin C than on any evidence that such huge doses of the vitamin are good for you.

Intravenous vitamin C can easily raise vitamin C levels to a level 140 times higher than the maximum achievable with oral vitamin C. However, there is no meaningful evidence that intravenous vitamin C provides any medical benefits.

Therapeutic Uses

According to numerous double-blind, placebo-controlled studies, regular use of vitamin C supplements can slightly reduce symptoms of **colds** and modestly shorten the length of the illness. However, taking vitamin C at the onset of a cold probably will not work.

Regular use of vitamin C does not seem to help *prevent* colds. One exception is the *post-marathon sniffle*—colds that develop after heavy exercise. Vitamin C may be helpful for preventing this condition, although not all studies agree.

Two double-blind studies suggest that the use of vitamin C combined with **vitamin E** might slightly reduce the risk of developing **preeclampsia**, a complication of pregnancy. However, a much larger follow-up study failed to find benefits.

A small double-blind study suggests that vitamin C at a dose of 500 mg daily may help prevent **reflex sympathetic dystrophy (RSD)**, a poorly understood condition that can follow injuries such as fractures.

Over time, the body develops tolerance to drugs in the nitrate family (such as nitroglycerin). Some evidence suggests that use of vitamin C can help maintain the effectiveness of these medications.

Other small double-blind trials suggest that vitamin C might be helpful for **anterior uveitis** (when taken in combination with vitamin E), **autism**, **easy bruising**, **minor injuries**, reducing the **muscle soreness** that typically develops after exercise, protecting the liver in **non-alcoholic steatohepatitis**, speeding recovery from **bedsores**, treating **female infertility** (specifically, a condition called *luteal phase defect*), and for preventing early rupture of the chorioamniotic membranes ("the water breaking") in **pregnancy**.

Preliminary evidence suggests that cream containing vitamin C may improve the appearance of **aging or sun-damaged skin**. Inconsistent evidence suggests that oral or topical vitamin C, taken by itself or in combination with vitamin E, may also help *protect* the skin against sun damage.

Double-blind studies of vitamin C for the following conditions have yielded mixed results: **asthma**, **male infertility**, and **hypertension**. **Note**: Unexpectedly, one study found that a combination of vitamin C (500 mg daily) and grape seed **OPCs** (1,000 mg daily) slightly *increased* blood pressure. Whether this was a fluke of statistics or a real combined effect remains unclear.

Very weak and in some cases contradictory evidence suggests possible benefit in the prevention or treatment of liver-damage caused by general anesthetics, **gout**, **gallbladder disease** (in women), **vascular dementia**, **glaucoma**, and **allergies**. Intravaginal use of vitamin C tablets might be helpful for **non-specific vaginitis**.

Observational studies indicate that people with a higher intake of vitamin C have a lower incidence of **cataracts**, **macular degeneration**, **heart disease**, **cancer**, and **osteoarthritis**. However, these findings do not indicate that vitamin C *supplements* will help prevent or treat these conditions. Observational studies are notoriously unreliable for showing the efficacy of treatments; only double-blind studies can do that and none have been performed that directly examine vitamin C's potential benefits for preventing these conditions. (For more information on why double-blind studies are so important, see **Why Does This Book Rely on Double-blind Studies?**)

Vitamin C has been proposed as a *treatment* for cancer, but this claim is very controversial, and there is as yet no scientifically meaningful evidence that it works.

Massive doses of vitamin C have at times been popular among people with **HIV** infection based on highly preliminary evidence. An observational study linked high doses of vitamin C with slower progression to AIDS. However, a double-blind study of 49 people with HIV who took combined vitamins C and E or placebo for 3 months did not show any significant effects on the amount of HIV detected or the number of opportunistic infections. Furthermore, one study found that vitamin C at a dose of 1 g daily substantially reduced blood levels of the drug indinavir, a protease inhibitor used for the treatment of HIV infection. This could potentially cause the drug to fail.

One substantial study failed to find vitamin C useful for improving **high cholesterol**.

According to a double-blind, placebo-controlled study of 141 women with **cervical dysplasia** (early cervical cancer), vitamin C, taken at a dosage of 500 mg daily, does *not* help to reverse the dysplasia.

Vitamin C also does not appear to be helpful for treating **Raynaud's phenomenon** caused by **scleroderma**.

What Is the Scientific Evidence for Vitamin C?

Colds

As the most famous of all natural treatments for the common cold, vitamin C has been subjected to irresponsible hype from both proponents and opponents. Enthusiasts claim that if you take vitamin C daily, you will never get sick, while critics of the treatment insist that vitamin C has no benefit at all.

However, a cool-headed evaluation of the research indicates something in between. Numerous studies have found that vitamin C supplements taken at a dose of 1,000 mg daily or more throughout the cold season *can* modestly reduce symptoms of colds and help you get over a cold faster, but they do *not* generally help prevent colds.

Reducing Cold Symptoms

Most studies on vitamin C have evaluated the potential benefits to be gained by taking vitamin C throughout the cold season. The combined results of these trials suggest that use of vitamin C in this way can slightly reduce symptoms and marginally decrease the duration of colds.

Many people use vitamin C for colds in a different way: they only begin taking it when cold symptoms start. The limited body of evidence available suggests that vitamin C is probably not effective when used in this way. One double-blind trial enrolled 400 individuals with new-onset cold symptoms, and divided them into four different daily vitamin C dosage groups: 30 mg daily (a dose lower than the minimum daily requirement and used by the researchers as a placebo), 1,000 mg, 3,000 mg, or 3,000 mg with bioflavonoids. Participants were instructed to take the vitamin at the onset of symptoms and for the following 2 days.

The results showed no difference in the duration or severity of cold symptoms among the groups. High-dose vitamin C taken at the onset of a cold, in other words, didn't help. The bottom line: If you want to use vitamin C to take the edge off your colds, take the supplement throughout the winter. (There are numerous other natural treatments for the common cold as well, some of which may be more helpful than vitamin C. For more information, see the full **Colds and Flu** article.)

Preventing Colds

Although two relatively recent studies suggest that regular use of vitamin C throughout the cold season can help prevent colds, they suffer from a variety of flaws, and most other studies have found little to no benefit along these lines.

However, people who are truly vitamin C–deficient, such as elderly people in nursing homes, may show increased resistance to infection if they take vitamin C (or other nutrients).

In addition, vitamin C might be helpful for preventing the respiratory infections that can follow heavy endurance exercise. Marathon running and similar forms of exertion can temporarily weaken the immune system, leading to infections. Vitamin C may be helpful. According to a double-blind, placebo-controlled study involving 92 runners, taking 600 mg of vitamin C for 21 days prior to a race made a significant difference in the incidence of sickness afterward. Within 2 weeks of the race, 68% of the runners taking placebo developed cold symptoms versus only 33% of those taking the vitamin C supplement. As part of the same study, non-runners of similar age and gender to those running were also given vitamin C or placebo. Interestingly, the supplement had no apparent effect on the incidence of upper respiratory infections in this group. Vitamin C seemed to be effective in this capacity only for those who exercised intensively!

Two other studies found that vitamin C could reduce the number of colds experienced by groups of people involved in rigorous exercise in extremely cold environments. One study involved 139 children attending a skiing camp in the Swiss Alps, while the other enrolled 56 military men engaged in a training exercise in northern Canada during the winter months. In both cases, the participants took either 1 g of vitamin C or placebo daily at the time their training program began. Cold symptoms were monitored for 1 to 2 weeks following training and significant differences in favor of vitamin C were found.

However, one very large study of 674 U.S. Marine recruits in basic training found no such benefit. The results showed no difference in the number of colds between the treatment and placebo groups.

What's the explanation for this discrepancy? There are many possibilities. Perhaps basic training in the Marines is significantly different from the other forms of exercise studied. Another point to consider is that the Marines didn't start taking vitamin C right at the beginning of training, but waited 3 weeks. The study also lasted a bit longer than the positive studies mentioned above, continuing for 2 months; maybe vitamin C is more effective at preventing colds in the short term. Of course, another possibility is that it doesn't really work. More research is needed to know for sure.

Preeclampsia Prevention

Preeclampsia is a dangerous complication of pregnancy that involves high blood pressure, swelling of the whole body, and improper kidney function. A double-blind, placebo-controlled study of 283 women at increased risk for preeclampsia found that supplementation with vitamin C (1,000 mg daily) and vitamin E (400 IU daily) significantly reduced the chances of developing this disease.

While this research is promising, larger studies are necessary to confirm whether vitamins C and E will actually work. The authors of this study point out that similarly sized studies found benefits with other treatments, such as aspirin, that later proved to be ineffective when large-scale studies were performed. Furthermore, keep in mind that we don't know whether such high dosages of these vitamins are absolutely safe for pregnant women.

Cancer Treatment

Cancer treatment is one of the more controversial proposed uses of vitamin C. An early study tested vitamin C in 1,100 terminally ill cancer patients. One hundred patients received 10,000 mg daily of vitamin C, while 1,000 other patients (the control group) received no treatment. Those taking the vitamin survived more than four times longer on average (210 days) than those in the control group (50 days). A large (1,826 subjects) follow-up study by the same researchers found a nearly doubled survival rate (343 days versus 180 days) in vitamin C–treated patients whose cancers were deemed "incurable," as compared to untreated controls. However, these studies were poorly designed and other generally better-constructed studies have found no benefit of vitamin C in cancer. At the present time, vitamin C cannot be regarded as a proven treatment for cancer.

Reflex Sympathetic Dystrophy (RSD)

RSD is a set of symptoms that occasionally develops in the legs or arms after fractures and other injuries. The condition involves persistent pain, changes in skin temperature, redness, swelling, and difficulty in movement. Its cause is unknown and it is very difficult, if not impossible, to treat, creating significant suffering and disability.

A double-blind study set out to find whether vitamin C could prevent RSD from developing in individuals who had sustained wrist fractures. A total of 123 adults with wrist fractures were enrolled and followed for 1 year. All were given 500 mg of vitamin C or placebo daily for 50 days. The results showed significantly fewer cases of RSD in the treated group.

If these results hold up in larger studies, vitamin C treatment could become part of the standard treatment of fractures.

Easy Bruising

A 2-month, double-blind study of 94 elderly people with marginal vitamin C deficiency found that vitamin C supplements decreased their tendency to bruise.

Hypertension (High Blood Pressure)

According to a 30-day, double-blind study of 39 individuals taking medications for hypertension, treatment with 500 mg of vitamin C daily can reduce blood pressure by about 10%. Smaller benefits were seen in studies of individuals with normal blood pressure or borderline hypertension. However, other studies have failed to find any significant blood pressure–lowering effect. This mixed evidence suggests, on balance, that if vitamin C does have any blood pressure–lowering effect, it is at most quite small.

Maintaining the Effectiveness of Nitrate Drugs

Nitroglycerin and related nitrate medications are used for the treatment of angina. However, the effectiveness of these medications tends to diminish over time. According to a double-blind study of 48 individuals, use of vitamin C at a dose of 2,000 mg 3 times daily helped maintain the effectiveness of nitroglycerin. These findings are supported by other studies as well.

Note: Angina is too serious a disease for self-treatment. If you have angina, do not take vitamin C (or any other supplement) except on a physician's advice.

Safety Issues

The U.S. government has issued recommendations regarding tolerable upper intake levels (ULs) for vitamin C. The UL can be thought of as the highest daily intake over a prolonged time known to pose no risks to most members of a healthy population. The ULs for vitamin C are as follows:

- **Children 1–3 years, 400 mg**
  4–8 years, 650 mg
  9–13 years, 1,200 mg
- **Males and females 14–18 years, 1,800 mg**
  19 years and older, 2,000 mg
- **Pregnant women 2,000 mg (1,800 mg if 18 years old or younger)**
- **Nursing women 2,000 mg (1,800 mg if 18 years old or younger)**

Vitamin C

However, even within the safe intake range for vitamin C, some individuals may develop diarrhea. This side effect will likely go away with continued use of vitamin C, but you might have to cut down your dosage for a while and then gradually build up again.

Concerns have been raised that long-term vitamin C treatment can cause **kidney stones**. However, in large-scale observational studies, individuals who consume large amounts of vitamin C have shown either no change or a decreased risk of kidney stone formation. Still, there may be certain individuals who are particularly at risk for vitamin C–induced kidney stones. People with a history of kidney stones and those with kidney failure who have a defect in vitamin C or oxalate metabolism should probably restrict vitamin C intake to approximately 100 mg daily. You should also avoid high-dose vitamin C if you have glucose-6-phosphate dehydrogenase deficiency, iron overload, or a history of intestinal surgery.

Vitamin C supplements increase absorption of iron. Since it isn't good to get more iron than you need, individuals using iron supplements shouldn't take vitamin C at the same time except under a physician's supervision.

One study from the 1970s suggests that very high doses of vitamin C (3 g daily) might increase the levels of acetaminophen (such as Tylenol) in the body. This could potentially put you at higher risk for acetaminophen toxicity. This interaction is probably relatively unimportant when acetaminophen is taken in single doses for pain and fever or for a few days during a cold. However, if you use acetaminophen daily or have kidney or liver problems, simultaneous use of high-dose vitamin C is probably not advisable.

Weak evidence suggests that vitamin C, when taken in high doses, might reduce the blood-thinning effects of warfarin (Coumadin) and heparin.

As noted above, one study found that vitamin C at a dose of 1 g daily substantially reduced blood levels of the drug indinavir, a protease inhibitor used for the treatment of HIV infection.

Heated disagreement exists regarding whether it is safe or appropriate to combine antioxidants such as vitamin C with standard chemotherapy drugs. The reasoning behind the concern is that some chemotherapy drugs may work in part by creating free radicals that destroy cancer cells, and antioxidants might interfere with this beneficial effect. However, there is no good evidence that antioxidants actually interfere with chemotherapy drugs, but there is growing evidence that they do not.

The maximum safe dosages of vitamin C for people with severe liver or kidney disease have not been determined.

Interactions You Should Know About

If you are taking:

➤ Aspirin other anti-inflammatory drugs, or oral contraceptives: You may need more vitamin C.
➤ Acetaminophen (Tylenol): The risk of liver damage from high doses of acetaminophen may be increased if you also take large doses of vitamin C.
➤ Warfarin (Coumadin) or heparin: High-dose vitamin C might reduce their effectiveness.
➤ Iron supplements: High-dose vitamin C can cause you to absorb too much iron. This is especially a problem for people with diseases that cause them to store too much iron.
➤ Medications in the nitrate family: Vitamin C may help maintain their effectiveness. Note: Angina is too serious a disease for self-treatment. If you have angina, do not take vitamin C (or any other supplement) except on a physician's advice.
➤ Protease inhibitors for HIV: High-dose vitamin C may reduce their effectiveness.
➤ Cancer chemotherapy: Do not use vitamin C except on a physician's advice.

Vitamin D

SUPPLEMENT FORMS/ALTERNATE NAMES: *Cholecalciferol (Vitamin D₃), Ergocalciferol (Vitamin D₂)*
PRINCIPAL PROPOSED USES: *Osteoporosis (Prevention and Treatment)*
OTHER PROPOSED USES: *Cancer (Prevention), Diabetes (Prevention), Hypertension (Prevention), Polycystic Ovary Syndrome, Psoriasis, Seasonal Affective Disorder*

Vitamin D is both a vitamin and a hormone. It's a vitamin because your body cannot absorb calcium without it; it's a hormone because your body manufactures it in response to your skin's exposure to sunlight.

There are two major forms of vitamin D and both have the word *calciferol* in their names. In Latin, *calciferol* means "calcium carrier." Vitamin D₃ (cholecalciferol) is made by the body and is found in some foods. Vitamin D₂ (ergocalciferol) is the form most often added to milk and other foods and the form you're most likely to use as a supplement.

Strong evidence tells us that the combination of vitamin D and calcium supplements can be quite helpful for preventing and treating osteoporosis. Other potential uses of vitamin D have little supporting evidence.

Requirements/Sources

As with **vitamin A**, dosages of vitamin D are often expressed in terms of international units (IU) rather than milligrams. The official U.S. and Canadian recommendations for daily intake of vitamin D are as follows:

- Infants 0–12 months, 200 IU (5 mcg)
- Males and females 1–50 years, 200 IU (5 mcg)
  51–70 years, 400 IU (10 mcg)
  71 years and older, 600 IU (15 mcg)
- Pregnant women, 200 IU (5 mcg)
- Nursing women, 200 IU (5 mcg)

However, growing evidence suggests that these recommendations may be too low. In a study of military personnel in submarines, use of 400 IU of vitamin D daily was inadequate to maintain bone health, while 6 days of sun exposure proved capable of supplying enough vitamin D for 49 sunless days. In addition, a study of veiled Islamic women living in Denmark found that 600 IU of vitamin D daily was insufficient to raise vitamin D levels in the blood to normal levels. The authors of this study recommend that sun-deprived individuals should receive 1,000 IU of vitamin D daily.

There is very little vitamin D found naturally in the foods we eat (the best sources are coldwater fish). In many countries, vitamin D is added to milk and other foods, like breakfast cereals and margarine, contributing to our daily intake.

As indicated by the study of submarine personnel noted above, by far the best source of vitamin D is sunlight. However, current recommendations which stress sun avoidance and the use of sunblock may have the unintended effect of increasing the prevalence of vitamin D deficiency. Severe vitamin D deficiency was common in England in the 1800s due to coal smoke obscuring the sun. During that time, cod liver oil, which is high in vitamin D, became popular as a supplement for children to help prevent rickets. (Rickets is a disease caused by vitamin D deficiency in which developing bones soften and curve because they aren't receiving enough calcium.)

Vitamin D deficiency is known to occur today in the elderly (who often receive less sun exposure) as well as in people who live in northern latitudes and don't drink vitamin D–enriched milk. The consequences of this deficiency may be increased risk of hypertension, osteoporosis, and several forms of cancer.

Additionally, phenytoin (Dilantin), primidone (Mysoline), and phenobarbital for seizures; corticosteroids; cimetidine (Tagamet) for ulcers; the blood-thinning drug heparin; and the antituberculosis drugs isoniazid (INH) and rifampin may interfere with vitamin D absorption or activity.

Therapeutic Dosages

For therapeutic purposes, vitamin D is taken at the nutritional doses described in Requirements/Sources (and sometimes in even higher amounts). If you wish to exceed nutritional levels of vitamin D intake, physician supervision is recommended (see Safety Issues below).

Therapeutic Uses

Without question, if you are concerned about **osteoporosis**, you should take calcium and vitamin D. The combination appears to help prevent bone loss. This is true even if you are taking other treatments for osteoporosis; after all, you can't build bone without calcium and you can't properly absorb and utilize calcium without adequate intake of vitamin D. Interestingly, vitamin D may also help prevent the falls that lead to osteoporotic fractures.

Other uses of vitamin D are less well documented.

Some evidence suggests that getting adequate vitamin D may help prevent **cancer** of the breast, colon, pancreas, prostate, and skin, but the research on this question has yielded mixed results. One study suggests that combined use of calcium plus vitamin D, but not either supplement separately, can help reduce risk of colon cancer.

Adequate vitamin D might reduce the risk of **hypertension** and **diabetes**.

One preliminary study suggests that supplementation with vitamin D and calcium may be helpful for women with polycystic ovary syndrome.

Vitamin D is sometimes mentioned as a treatment for **psoriasis**. However, this recommendation is based on Danish studies using calcipotriol, a variation of vitamin D_3 that is used externally (applied to the skin). Calcipotriol does not affect your body's absorption of calcium, so it is a very different substance from the vitamin D you can purchase at a store.

It has been suggested that since vitamin D levels in the body drop in the wintertime, vitamin D supplements might be helpful for **seasonal affective disorder** ("winter blues"). A small double-blind, placebo-controlled trial conducted during winter on 44 people found that vitamin D supplements produced improvements in various measures of mood. However, a double-blind, placebo-controlled study of 2,217 women over 70 years old failed to find benefit. It has been hypothesized that light therapy (used successfully for SAD) works by raising vitamin D levels, but there is some evidence that this is not the case.

Vitamin D supplements also do *not* appear to help enhance growth in healthy children.

What Is the Scientific Evidence for Vitamin D?

Individuals with severe osteoporosis often have low levels of vitamin D. Supplementing with vitamin D alone may or may not be helpful, but the combination of calcium and vitamin D is probably more effective. (See the **calcium** article for more information.)

Interestingly, vitamin D may offer another benefit for osteoporosis in seniors: most (though not all) studies have found that vitamin D supplementation improves balance in seniors (especially female seniors) and reduces risk of falling. Since the most common adverse consequence of osteoporosis is a fracture due to a fall, this could be a meaningful benefit. Why vitamin D offers this benefit, however, remains a mystery.

Supplementation with vitamin D plus calcium may aid healing *after* a fracture has occurred.

Safety Issues

When taken at recommended dosages, vitamin D appears to be safe. However, when used at considerable excess, vitamin D can build up in the body and cause toxic symptoms. The precise dosage at which intake becomes toxic is a matter of dispute. Official safe upper limits for vitamin D daily intake have been set as follows:

- **Infants 0–12 months, 1,000 IU (25 mcg)**
- **Males and females 1 year and older, 2,000 IU (50 mcg)**
- **Pregnant and nursing women, 2,000 IU (50 mcg)**

People with sarcoidosis or hyperparathyroidism should never take vitamin D without first consulting a physician.

Taking vitamin D and calcium supplements might interfere with some of the effects of drugs in the calcium-channel blocker family. It is very important that you consult your physician before trying this combination.

The combination of calcium, vitamin D, and thiazide diuretics can lead to excessive calcium levels in the body. If you are taking thiazide diuretics, you should consult with a physician about the right doses of vitamin D and calcium for you.

Interactions You Should Know About

If you are taking:

- **Antiseizure drugs—such as phenobarbital, primidone (Mysoline), valproic acid (Depakene) or**

phenytoin (Dilantin)—corticosteroids, cimetidine (Tagamet), heparin, isoniazid (INH), or rifampin: You may need extra vitamin D.
➤ Calcium-channel blockers: Do not take high-dose

vitamin D (with calcium) except under physician supervision.
➤ Thiazide diuretics: Do not take calcium and vitamin D supplements unless under a doctor's supervision.

Vitamin E

SUPPLEMENT FORMS/ALTERNATE NAMES: *Alpha Tocopherol, D-Alpha-Tocopherol, D-Beta-Tocopherol, D-Delta-Tocopherol, D-Gamma-Tocopherol, DL-Alpha-Tocopherol, DL-Tocopherol, D-Tocopherol, Mixed Tocopherols, Tocopheryl Acetate, Tocopheryl Succinate*

PRINCIPAL PROPOSED USES: *Prostate Cancer (Prevention)*

OTHER PROPOSED USES: *Acute Anterior Uveitis (in Combination with Vitamin C), Alzheimer's Disease, Cataracts, Diabetic Neuropathy and Other Complications of Diabetes, Epilepsy, Immune Support, Macular Degeneration, Male Infertility, Menopausal Symptoms, Menstrual Pain, Preeclampsia (Prevention), Premenstrual Syndrome (PMS), Restless Legs Syndrome, Rheumatoid Arthritis, Sports Performance, Tardive Dyskinesia, Vascular Dementia*

PROBABLY NOT EFFECTIVE USES: *Amyotrophic Lateral Sclerosis, Cancer Prevention (Other than Prostate Cancer), Congestive Heart Failure, Fibrocystic Breast Disease, Heart Disease (Prevention), HIV Support, Kidney Damage in Diabetes, Macular Degeneration, Osteoarthritis, Parkinson's Disease*

Vitamin E is an **antioxidant** that fights damaging natural substances known as *free radicals*. It works in *lipids* (fats and oils), which makes it complementary to vitamin C, which fights free radicals dissolved in water. As an antioxidant, vitamin E has been widely advocated for preventing heart disease and cancer. However, the results of large, well-designed trials have generally not been encouraging. Many other proposed benefits of vitamin E have also failed to stand up in studies. There are no medicinal uses for vitamin E with solid scientific support.

Requirements/Sources

Vitamin E dosage recommendations are a bit complex, because the vitamin exists in many forms.

New vitamin E recommendations are in milligrams of alpha-tocopherol. Alpha-tocopherol can come from either natural vitamin E (called, somewhat incorrectly, *d-alpha-tocopherol*) or synthetic vitamin E (called, also somewhat incorrectly, *dl-alpha-tocopherol*). However, much of the alpha-tocopherol in synthetic vitamin E is inactive. For this reason, you have to take about twice as much of it to get the same effect.

There are other forms of vitamin E as well, such as beta-, delta-, and gamma-tocopherols, all of which occur in food. These other forms may be important; for example, preliminary evidence hints that gamma-tocopherol may be the most important form of vitamin E for preventing prostate cancer. On this basis, it has been suggested that the best vitamin E supplement would be a mixture of all these.

To make matters even more confusing, vitamin E dosages are commonly listed on labels as international units (IU). Here's how you make the conversion. One IU natural vitamin E equals 0.67 mg alpha-tocopherol; one IU synthetic vitamin E equals 0.45 mg alpha-tocopherol. Therefore, to meet the new dietary recommendations for vitamin E (15 mg per day), you need to get either 22 IU natural vitamin E (22 IU x 0.67 =15 mg) or 33 IU synthetic vitamin E (33 IU x 0.45 =15 mg). The official U.S. and Canadian recommendations for daily intake of vitamin E are as follows:

➤ **Infants 0–6 months, 4 mg**
   7–12 months, 5 mg
➤ **Children 1–3 years, 6 mg**

Vitamin E

4–8 years, 7 mg

9–13 years, 11 mg

➤ Males and females 14 years and older, 15 mg

➤ Pregnant women, 15 mg

➤ Nursing women, 19 mg

In developed countries, mild dietary deficiency of vitamin E is relatively common.

The best food sources of vitamin E are polyunsaturated vegetable oils, seeds, nuts, and whole grains. To get a therapeutic dosage, though, you need to take a supplement.

Therapeutic Dosages

The optimal therapeutic dosage of vitamin E has not been established. Most studies have used between 50 and 800 IU daily and some have used even higher doses. This would correspond to about 50 to 800 mg of synthetic vitamin E (dl-alpha-tocopherol) or 25 to 400 mg of natural vitamin E (d-alpha-tocopherol mixed tocopherols).

If you wish to purchase natural vitamin E, look for a label that says "mixed tocopherols." However, some manufacturers use this term to mean the synthetic dl-alpha-tocopherol, so you need to read the contents closely. Natural tocopherols come as d-alpha-, d-gamma-, d-delta-, and d-beta-tocopherol.

Therapeutic Uses

Observational studies raised hopes that vitamin E supplements could help prevent various forms of **cancer** as well as **heart disease**. However, observational studies are notoriously unreliable for determining the effectiveness of treatments. Only double-blind trials can do that (for information why, see **Why Does This Book Rely on Double-blind Studies?**), and such studies have, on balance, found vitamin E ineffective for preventing heart disease or any common form of cancer other than, possibly, prostate cancer.

Other potential uses of vitamin E have limited supporting evidence.

Intriguing but far from definitive studies suggest that vitamin E might help slow the progression of **cataracts**, improve **immune response** to vaccinations, decrease symptoms of **menstrual pain**, reduce symptoms of **premenstrual syndrome** (PMS), control symptoms of **restless legs syndrome**, reduce discomfort in **rheumatoid arthritis** (and possibly help prevent it), and help prevent **vascular dementia**.

Evidence regarding whether vitamin E can slow the progression of **Alzheimer's disease** is inconsistent.

Studies of vitamin E in combination with vitamin C for prevention of **preeclampsia** have yielded inconsistent results.

Vitamin E has also shown equivocal promise in **diabetes**. One double-blind trial found benefits for cardiac autonomic neuropathy, a complication of diabetes. Weaker evidence hints at possible benefits for diabetic peripheral neuropathy. However, the best-designed study of all, a long-term trial involving 3,654 people with diabetes, found that use of vitamin E did not protect against diabetes-induced kidney or heart damage. Similarly, while a few studies performed by one research group suggested that vitamin E might be helpful for improving glucose control in people with diabetes, subsequent evidence found that the benefits, if they exist at all, are short-term.

Similarly, studies on whether vitamin E is helpful for **allergic rhinitis** (hay fever) have produced conflicting results.

Vitamin E might help reduce the lung-related side effects caused by the drug amiodarone (used to prevent abnormal heart rhythms).

Studies have yielded mixed results on whether vitamin E is helpful for controlling seizures in people with **epilepsy**, reducing symptoms of **tardive dyskinesia**, aiding **recovery during heavy exercise**, and treating **male infertility**.

When combined with **vitamin C**, vitamin E may protect against sunburn to a small extent. The same combination has also shown promise for **acute anterior uveitis**. A separate study failed to find vitamin E alone (at the high dose of 1,600 mg daily) helpful for macular edema (swelling of the center of the retina) associated with uveitis.

Vitamin E has been tried for **amyotrophic lateral sclerosis** (Lou Gehrig's disease), but the results in the first reported double-blind study showed questionable benefits, if any. Some vitamin E proponents felt that the dose of vitamin E used in this study might have been too low. Accordingly, they conducted another study using *10 times* the dose, this one lasting 18 months and enrolling 160 people. Once again, vitamin E failed to prove significantly more effective than placebo.

In one observational study, high intake of vitamin E was linked to decreased risk of progression to AIDS in people with **HIV** infection. However, a double-blind study of 49 people with HIV who took combined vitamins C and E or placebo for 3 months did not show any significant effects on the amount of HIV virus detected or the number of opportunistic infections. It has been suggested that vitamin E may enhance the antiviral effects of AZT, but evidence for this is minimal.

Vitamin E is sometimes recommended for **osteoarthritis**. However, a 2-year, double-blind, placebo-controlled study of 136 people with osteoarthritis of the knee failed to find any benefit in terms of symptom control or slowing disease progression. A previous 6-month, double-blind, placebo-controlled trial of 77 individuals with osteoarthritis also failed to find benefit.

A 4-year, double-blind, placebo-controlled trial of 1,193 people with **macular degeneration** failed to find vitamin E alone helpful for preventing or treating macular degeneration. Vitamin E has also so far failed to prove helpful for preventing or treating **alcoholic hepatitis, asthma, congestive heart failure, fibrocystic breast disease**, or **Parkinson's disease**.

Although vitamin E is often recommended for **menopausal** hot flashes, there is no real evidence that it is effective. One 9-week, double-blind, placebo-controlled trial followed 104 women with hot flashes associated with breast cancer treatment, but it found marginal benefits at best.

What Is the Scientific Evidence for Vitamin E?

Cancer Prevention

The results of observational trials have been mixed, but on balance, they suggest that high intake of vitamin E and other antioxidants is associated with reduced risk of lung cancer and many other forms of cancer, including bladder, stomach, mouth, throat, laryngeal, liver, and prostate. Based on these and other results, researchers developed the hypothesis that antioxidants can help prevent cancer and set in motion very large, long-term, double-blind, placebo-controlled studies to verify it.

Unfortunately, these studies generally failed to find vitamin E helpful for the prevention of cancer in people at high risk for it.

The one positive note came in a double-blind trial of 29,133 smokers. In this study, 50 mg of synthetic vitamin E (dl-alpha-tocopherol) daily for 5 to 8 years caused a 32% reduction in the incidence of prostate cancer and a 41% drop in prostate cancer deaths.

Surprisingly, results were seen soon after the beginning of supplementation. This was unexpected because prostate cancer grows very slowly. A cancer that shows up today actually started to develop many years ago. The fact that vitamin E almost immediately lowered the incidence of prostate cancer suggests that it somehow blocks the step at which a hidden prostate cancer makes the leap to being detectable.

Nonetheless, the negative results regarding most other types of cancer have made scientists hesitant to place too much hope in these findings. It has been suggested that alpha-tocopherol alone is less effective than the multiple forms of tocopherol that occur in nature; in particular, it has been suggested that gamma-tocopherol rather than alpha-tocopherol might be the most relevant form of vitamin E for cancer prevention. However, this has not yet been tested. Interestingly, use of alpha-tocopherol supplements may deplete both gamma- and delta-tocopherol levels, potentially producing a negative effect.

Cardiovascular Disease

Most but not all observational studies have found associations between high intake of vitamin E and reduced risk of cardiovascular disease (heart disease and **strokes**). However, as we've explained, observational studies by themselves cannot be relied upon to identify useful treatments. Double-blind studies, which provide much more convincing evidence of effectiveness, have generally failed to find vitamin E supplements effective.

The Heart Outcomes Prevention Evaluation (HOPE) trial found that natural vitamin E (d-alpha-tocopherol) at a dose of 400 IU daily did not reduce the number of heart attacks, strokes, or deaths from heart disease any more than placebo. The trial followed more than 9,000 men and women who had existing heart disease or were at high risk for it.

Negative results were seen in numerous other large trials, as well.

When the results of these studies began to come in, some antioxidant proponents suggested that the people enrolled in these trials already had disease too advanced for vitamin E to help. However, a subsequent large trial found vitamin E ineffective for slowing the progression of heart disease in healthy people as well.

As with preventing cancer, critics have suggested that the form of vitamin E used in these studies (alpha-tocopherol) was not the best choice and that gamma-tocopherol might be more helpful. Gamma-tocopherol is present in the diet much more abundantly than alpha-tocopherol and it could be that the studies showing benefits with dietary vitamin E actually tracked the influence of gamma-tocopherol. However, an observational study specifically looking to see if gamma-tocopherol levels were associated with risk of heart attack found no relationship between the two. Nonetheless, intervention trials of gamma-tocopherol are currently underway.

Preeclampsia Prevention

Preeclampsia is a dangerous complication of pregnancy that involves high blood pressure, swelling of the whole body, and improper kidney function. A double-blind, placebo-controlled study of 283 women at increased risk for preeclampsia found that supplementation with vitamin E (400 IU daily of natural vitamin E) and vitamin C (1,000 mg daily) significantly reduced the chances of developing this disease.

While this research is promising, larger studies are necessary to confirm whether vitamins E and C will actually work. The authors of this study point out that studies of similar size found benefits with other treatments, such as aspirin, that later proved to be ineffective when large-scale studies were performed. Furthermore, keep in mind that we don't know whether such high dosages of these vitamins are absolutely safe for pregnant women.

Tardive Dyskinesia

Between 1987 and 1998, at least five double-blind studies were published that indicated vitamin E was beneficial in treating tardive dyskinesia (TD). Although most of these studies were small and lasted only 4 to 12 weeks, one 36-week study enrolled 40 individuals. Three small double-blind studies reported that vitamin E was not helpful. Nonetheless, a statistical analysis of the double-blind studies done before 1999 found good evidence that vitamin E was more effective than placebo. Most studies found that vitamin E worked best for TD of more recent onset.

However, in 1999, the picture on vitamin E changed with the publication of one more study—the largest and longest to date. This double-blind study included 107 participants from nine different research sites who took 1,600 IU of vitamin E or placebo daily for at least 1 year. In contrast to most of the previous studies, this trial did not find vitamin E effective in decreasing TD symptoms.

Why the discrepancy between this study and the earlier ones? The researchers, some of whom had worked on the earlier, positive studies of vitamin E, were at pains to develop an answer. They proposed a number of possible explanations. One was that the earlier studies were too small or too short to be accurate and that vita-

min E really didn't help at all. Another was the most complicated: that vitamin E might help only a subgroup of people who have TD—those with milder TD symptoms of more recent onset—and that fewer of these people had participated in the latest study. They also pointed to changes in schizophrenia treatment since the last study was done, including the growing use of antipsychotic medications that do not cause TD.

The bottom line: The effectiveness of vitamin E for a given individual is simply not known. Given the lack of other good treatments for TD and the general safety of the vitamin, it may be worth discussing with your physician.

Immune Support

Seniors often do not respond adequately to vaccinations. One double-blind study suggests that vitamin E may be able to strengthen the immune response to vaccines. In this trial, 88 people over the age of 65 were given either placebo or vitamin E at 60 IU, 200 IU, or 800 IU dl-alpha-tocopherol daily. The researchers then gave all participants immunizations against hepatitis B, tetanus, diphtheria, and pneumonia, and looked at subjects' immune response to these vaccinations. The researchers also used a skin test that evaluates the overall strength of the immune response.

The results were promising. Vitamin E at 200 mg per day and, to a lesser extent, at 800 mg per day significantly increased the strength of the immune response.

However, it is not clear whether vitamin E has a general immune support effect. One study in seniors found that use of vitamin E did not help prevent colds and other respiratory infections and, in fact, seemed to slightly increase the severity of infections that did occur. In a similar-sized double-blind study of long-term care residents, use of vitamin E at 200 IU daily failed to reduce incidence or number of days of respiratory infection or antibiotic use. The researchers managed to find some evidence of benefit by breaking down the respiratory infections by type, but such after-the-fact analysis is questionable from a statistical perspective. Subsequently, the same researchers repeated the study with a larger group, and did find a reduction in frequency of colds.

Alzheimer's Disease

Evidence is conflicting regarding whether high-dose vitamin E can slow the progression of Alzheimer's disease.

In a double-blind, placebo-controlled study, 341 people with Alzheimer's disease received either 2,000 IU daily of vitamin E (dl-alpha-tocopherol), the antioxidant drug selegiline, or placebo. Those given vitamin E took nearly 200 days longer to reach a severe state of the disease than the placebo group. (Selegiline was even more effective.)

However, negative results were seen in a study of 769 people at high risk of developing Alzheimer's disease based on early symptoms. Participants were given either 2,000 IU of vitamin E, the drug donepezil, or placebo for 3 years. Neither treatment reduced the percentage of people who went on to develop Alzheimer's disease.

Warning: Such high dosages of vitamin E should not be taken except under a doctor's supervision (see Safety Issues below).

Dysmenorrhea (Menstrual Pain)

In a double-blind, placebo-controlled trial, 100 young women complaining of significant menstrual pain were given either 500 IU of vitamin E or placebo for 5 days. Treatment began 2 days before and continued for 3 days after the expected onset of menstruation. While both groups showed significant improvement in pain over the 2 months of the study (presumably due to the power of placebo), pain reduction was greater in the treatment group as compared to the placebo group.

Benefits were also seen in an Iranian 4-month, double-blind, placebo-controlled study of 278 adolescent girls. The dose used in this study was 200 IU twice daily.

Low Sperm Count/Infertility

In a double-blind, placebo-controlled study of 110 men whose sperm showed subnormal activity, treatment with 100 IU of vitamin E daily resulted in improved sperm activity and higher actual fertility (measured in pregnancies). However, a smaller double-blind trial found no benefit.

Cardiac Autonomic Neuropathy

People with diabetes sometimes develop irregularities of their heartbeat called *cardiac autonomic neuropathy*. A 4-month, double-blind, placebo-controlled trial found that vitamin E at a dose of 600 mg daily might improve these symptoms.

Safety Issues

The adult safe upper intake level (UL) for vitamin E is set at 1,000 mg daily. The equivalent amounts are 1,500 IU of natural vitamin E and 1,100 IU of synthetic vitamin E. (For technical reasons, the conversion factor is a bit different than in the daily intake recommendations above.) For pregnant women under 19 years of age, the upper limit is 800 mg.

Vitamin E has a blood-thinning effect that could lead to problems in certain situations. In one study of 28,519 men, vitamin E supplementation at the low dose of about 50 IU synthetic vitamin E per day caused an increase in fatal hemorrhagic strokes, the kind of stroke caused by bleeding. (However, it reduced the risk of a more common type of stroke and the two effects essentially canceled out.) Based on its blood-thinning effects, there are concerns that vitamin E could cause problems if it is combined with medications that also thin the blood, such as warfarin (Coumadin), heparin, clopidogrel (Plavix), ticlopidine (Ticlid), pentoxifylline (Trental), and aspirin. Theoretically, the net result could be to thin the blood *too* much, causing bleeding problems. A study that evaluated vitamin E plus aspirin did in fact find an additive effect. In contrast, the results of a study on vitamin E and Coumadin found no evidence of interaction, but it would still not be advisable to combine these treatments except under a physician's supervision.

There is also at least a remote possibility that vitamin E could also interact with supplements that possess a mild blood-thinning effect, such as **garlic**, **policosanol**, and **ginkgo**. Individuals with bleeding disorders, such as hemophilia, and those about to undergo surgery or labor and delivery, should also approach vitamin E with caution.

In addition, vitamin E might at least temporarily enhance the body's sensitivity to its own insulin in individuals with adult-onset diabetes. This could lead to a risk of blood sugar levels falling too low. In addition, one study found that use of vitamin E can raise blood pressure in people with diabetes. The bottom line: If you have diabetes do not take high-dose vitamin E without first consulting your physician.

One widely reported meta-analysis (statistical review of studies) that claimed to find a slightly increased death rate among patients taking vitamin E was too statistically weak to get alarmed about; however, it does provide additional evidence that vitamin E is not the cure-all it was once claimed to be.

Finally, considerable controversy exists regarding whether it is safe or appropriate to combine vitamin E with standard chemotherapy drugs. The reasoning

Vitamin K

behind this concern is that some chemotherapy drugs may work in part by creating free radicals that destroy cancer cells. Antioxidants like vitamin E might interfere with this beneficial effect. However, there is no good evidence that antioxidants actually interfere with chemotherapy drugs, growing evidence that they do not, and some evidence of potential benefit under certain circumstances. Nonetheless, in view of the high stakes involved, we strongly recommend that you do not take any supplements while undergoing cancer chemotherapy, except on the advice of a physician.

One study appeared to find evidence that use of vitamin E plus **beta-carotene** may impair the effectiveness of radiation therapy for head and neck cancers.

Interactions You Should Know About

If you are taking:

> Blood-thinning drugs, such as warfarin (Coumadin), heparin, clopidogrel (Plavix), ticlopidine (Ticlid), pentoxifylline (Trental), or aspirin: Seek medical advice before taking vitamin E.
> Amiodarone: Vitamin E may help protect you from lung-related side effects.
> Phenothiazine drugs: Vitamin E may help reduce side effects.
> Chemotherapy drugs: Seek medical advice before taking vitamin E.
> Oral hypoglycemic medications: High-dose vitamin E might cause your blood sugar levels to fall too low, requiring an adjustment in medication dosage.

Vitamin K

SUPPLEMENT FORMS/ALTERNATE NAMES: *Vitamin K_1 (Phylloquinone), Vitamin K_2 (Menaquinone), Vitamin K_3 (Menadione)*

PRINCIPAL PROPOSED USES: *Osteoporosis, Treating Medication-induced Vitamin K Deficiency*

OTHER PROPOSED USES: *Menorrhagia (Heavy Menstruation), Nausea*

There's a good chance you haven't even heard of vitamin K. However, this obscure member of the vitamin clan is very important for good health. Without it, your blood wouldn't clot properly. There are three forms of vitamin K: K_1 (phylloquinone), found in plants; K_2 (menaquinone), produced by bacteria in your intestines; and K_3 (menadione), a synthetic form.

Vitamin K is used medically to reverse the effects of blood-thinning drugs, such as warfarin (Coumadin). Growing evidence suggests that it may also be helpful for osteoporosis.

Requirements/Sources

Vitamin K is an essential nutrient, but you need only a tiny amount of it. The official U.S. recommendations for daily intake have been set as follows:

> Infants 0–6 months, 2 mcg
> 7–12 months, 2.5 mcg

> Children 1–3 years, 30 mcg
> 4–8 years, 55 mcg
> Males 9–13 years, 60 mcg
> 14–18 years, 75 mcg
> 19 years and older, 120 mcg
> Females 9–13 years, 60 mcg
> 14–18 years, 75 mcg
> 19 years and older, 90 mcg
> Pregnant women, 90 mcg, preferably the K_1 variety (phylloquinone) (75 mcg if 18 years old or younger)
> Nursing women, 90 mcg, preferably the K_1 variety (75 mcg if 18 years old or younger)

Vitamin K (in the form of K_1) is found in green leafy vegetables. Kale and turnip greens are the best food sources, providing about 10 times the daily adult requirement in a single serving. Spinach, broccoli, lettuce, and cabbage are very rich sources as well and you can get perfectly respectable amounts of vitamin

K in such common foods as oats, green peas, whole wheat, and green beans, as well as watercress and asparagus.

Vitamin K (in the form of K_2) is also manufactured by bacteria in the intestines and is a major source of vitamin K. Long-term use of antibiotics can cause a vitamin K deficiency by killing these bacteria. However, this effect seems to be significant only in people who are deficient in vitamin K to begin with. Pregnant and postmenopausal women are also sometimes deficient in this vitamin. In addition, children born to women taking anticonvulsants while pregnant may be significantly deficient in vitamin K, causing them to have bleeding problems and facial bone abnormalities. Vitamin K supplementation during **pregnancy** may be helpful for preventing this.

The blood-thinning drug warfarin (Coumadin) works by antagonizing the effects of vitamin K. Conversely, vitamin K supplements, or intake of foods containing high levels of vitamin K, block the action of this medication and can be used as an antidote.

Cephalosporins and possibly other antibiotics may also interfere with vitamin K–dependent blood clotting. However, this interaction seems to be significant only in people who have vitamin K–poor diets.

People with disorders of the digestive tract, such as chronic **diarrhea**, celiac sprue, **ulcerative colitis**, or **Crohn's disease**, may become deficient in vitamin K. **Alcoholism** can also lead to vitamin K deficiency.

Therapeutic Dosages

In the study of osteoporosis described below, vitamin K was taken at the high dose of 1 g daily, more than 10 times the necessary nutritional intake.

Therapeutic Uses

Growing evidence suggests that vitamin K should be added to the list of nutrients helpful for preventing osteoporosis.

Based on its ability to help blood clot normally, vitamin K has been proposed as a treatment for excessive menstrual bleeding. However, the last actual study testing this idea was carried out more than 55 years ago. Vitamin K has also been recommended for **nausea**, although there is as yet no meaningful evidence that it really works.

Preliminary evidence suggests that vitamin K supplementation may help **prevent liver cancer**.

What Is the Scientific Evidence for Vitamin K?

Vitamin K plays a known biochemical role in the formation of bone. This has led researchers to look for relationships between vitamin K intake and osteoporosis.

Observational studies have found the people with osteoporosis often have low levels of vitamin K and that people with higher intake of vitamin K have a lower incidence of osteoporosis.

Research also suggests that supplemental vitamin K can reduce the amount of **calcium** lost in the urine. This is indirect evidence of a beneficial effect on bone.

However, while these studies are interesting, only double-blind, placebo-controlled trials can actually prove a treatment effective. (For the reasons why, see **Why Does This Book Rely on Double-blind Studies?**.) Two such studies have been performed on vitamin K for osteoporosis, with positive results.

One of these was a 3-year, double-blind, placebo-controlled trial of 181 women; it found that vitamin K significantly enhanced the effectiveness of supplementation with calcium, **vitamin D**, and **magnesium**. Participants, postmenopausal women between the ages of 50 and 60, were divided into three groups, receiving either placebo, calcium plus vitamin D plus magnesium, or calcium plus vitamin D plus magnesium plus vitamin K_1 (at the high dose of 1 g daily). Researchers monitored bone loss by using a standard DEXA bone density scan. The results showed that the study participants using vitamin K along with the other nutrients lost less bone than those in the other two groups.

The other study was a 48-week trial of 66 Indonesian women with osteoporosis. The results showed that calcium plus vitamin K was more effective in improving bone density than calcium plus placebo.

While these two studies don't provide definitive proof, they do strongly suggest that women at risk for osteoporosis should consider taking vitamin K along with other nutrients.

Some evidence hints that vitamin K works by reducing bone breakdown, rather than by enhancing bone formation.

For more information, see the **osteoporosis** article.

Safety Issues

Vitamin K is quite safe at the recommended therapeutic dosages.

Note: Vitamin K directly counters the effects of the anticoagulant warfarin (Coumadin). If you are taking warfarin, you should not take vitamin K supplements or alter your dietary intake of vitamin K without doctor supervision.

Newborns are commonly given vitamin K_1 injections to prevent bleeding problems. Although some have suggested that this practice may increase the risk of cancer, enormous observational studies have found no such connection (one such trial involved more than one million participants).

Interactions You Should Know About

If you are taking:

- **Warfarin (Coumadin):** Do not take vitamin K supplements or eat foods high in vitamin K except under the supervision of a physician. (You will need to have your medication dosage adjusted.)
- **Cephalosporins or other antibiotics:** You may need more vitamin K if you are already deficient in this nutrient.
- **Anticonvulsants—such as phenytoin (Dilantin), carbamazepine, phenobarbital, and primidone (Mysoline)—and are pregnant:** You may need more vitamin K.

Whey Protein

PRINCIPAL PROPOSED USES: *Raising Glutathione Levels*

OTHER PROPOSED USES: *Cancer Treatment Support, Cataracts, Diabetes, Enhancing Mental Function, Enhancing Sports Performance, HIV Support, Viral Hepatitis*

Whey is one of the two major classes of protein in milk. (The other is casein, the "curds" of "curds and whey.") Proteins are made of amino acids and whey contains high levels of the amino acid cysteine. This is the basis for many of its proposed uses. It also contains **branched-chain amino acids** (BCAAs). However, while there is no question that whey is a highly digestible and rich protein source, there is no meaningful supporting evidence that it provides any specific health benefits.

Requirements/Sources

When milk is converted into cheese, whey is the liquid that is left behind. There is no specific dietary requirement for whey, as the amino acids it contains are present in a wide variety of other foods as well.

Therapeutic Doses

A typical dose of whey protein is 20 to 30 g per day.

Therapeutic Uses

There are no well-documented medicinal uses of whey protein.

There is some evidence that whey can raise levels of **glutathione**. Glutathione is an **antioxidant** that the body manufactures to defend itself against free radicals. In certain diseases, glutathione levels may fall to below-normal levels. These conditions include **cataracts**, **HIV**, liver disease, **diabetes**, and various types of **cancer**. This reduction of glutathione might in turn contribute to the symptoms or progression of the disease. To solve this problem, glutathione supplements have been recommended, but glutathione is essentially not absorbed at all when it is taken by mouth. Whey protein may be a better solution. The body uses cysteine to make glutathione and whey is rich in cysteine. Meaningful preliminary evidence suggests that whey can raise glutathione levels in people with cancer, **hepatitis**, or HIV.

However, while these are promising findings, one essential piece of evidence is lacking: there is no evidence as yet that this rise in glutathione produces any meaningful health benefits.

Whey protein has also been proposed as a **body-building aid**, based partly on its high content of BCAAs. However, there is no more than minimal evidence that whey protein helps accelerate muscle mass development. Furthermore, there is no evidence that whey protein is more effective for this purpose than any other protein. For example, one small double-blind study found evidence that both casein and whey protein were more effective than placebo at promoting muscle growth after exercise, but whey was no more effective than the far less expensive casein.

One study looked at whether whey protein could help women with HIV build muscle mass. Participants were divided into three groups: those who undertook a course of resistance exercise (weight lifting), those who took whey, and those who did both. Resistance exercise alone was just as effective as resistance exercise plus whey, while whey alone was not effective.

Whey contains alpha-lactalbumin, a protein that in turn contains high levels of the amino acid tryptophan. Tryptophan is the body's precursor to serotonin and is thought to affect mental function. In a small double-blind study, use of alpha-lactalbumin in the evening **improved morning alertness**, perhaps by enhancing sleep quality. Another small double-blind study found weak evidence that alpha-lactalbumin improved mental function in people sensitive to stress. A third study failed to find that alpha-lactalbumin significantly improved memory in women experiencing **premenstrual symptoms**.

Very weak evidence hints that whey might help prevent cancer or augment the effectiveness of **cancer treatment**.

Infant formula based on pre-digested (hydrolyzed) whey protein is somewhat less allergenic than standard infant formula; this might reduce symptoms of **colic** and possibly decrease the risk that the infant will later develop allergies.

Safety Issues

As a constituent of milk, whey protein is presumed to be a safe substance. People with allergies to milk, however, are likely to be allergic to whey as well (even partially hydrolyzed forms of whey).

White Willow

Salix alba

PRINCIPAL PROPOSED USES: *Back Pain, Bursitis, Dysmenorrhea, Migraine Headaches, Musculoskeletal Pain, Osteoarthritis, Rheumatoid Arthritis, Tendonitis, Tension Headaches*

Willow bark has been used as a treatment for pain and fever in China since 500 B.C. In Europe, it was primarily used for altogether different purposes, such as stopping vomiting, removing warts, and suppressing sexual desire. However, in 1828, European chemists made a discovery that would bring together some of these different uses. They extracted the substance salicin from white willow, which was soon purified to salicylic acid. Salicylic acid is an effective treatment for pain and fever, but it is also sufficiently irritating to do a good job of burning off warts.

Chemists later modified salicylic acid (this time from the herb meadowsweet) to create acetylsalicylic acid, or aspirin.

What Is White Willow Used for Today?

As interest in natural medicine has grown, many people have begun to turn back to white willow as an alternative to aspirin. One double-blind, placebo-controlled trial found it effective for **back pain** and another found it helpful for **osteoarthritis**. It is also used for such conditions as **bursitis**, **dysmenorrhea**, tension headaches, **migraine headaches**, **rheumatoid arthritis**, and **tendonitis**. However, two recent studies

White Willow

failed to find it effective for rheumatoid arthritis or osteoarthritis.

Aspirin and related anti-inflammatory drugs are notorious for irritating or damaging the stomach. However, when taken in typical doses, willow does not appear to produce this side effect to the same extent. This may be partly due to the fact that most of the salicylic acid provided by white willow comes from salicin and other chemicals that are only converted to salicylic acid after absorption into the body. Other evidence suggests that standard doses of willow bark are the equivalent of one baby aspirin daily rather than a full dose.

This latter finding raises an interesting question: If willow provides only a small amount of salicylic acid, how can it work? The most likely answer seems to be that other constituents besides salicin play a role. Another possibility may be that the studies finding benefit were flawed and that it actually does not work.

What Is the Scientific Evidence for Willow?

In a 4-week, double-blind, placebo-controlled study of 210 individuals with back pain, two doses of willow bark extract were compared against placebo. The higher-dose group received extract supplying 240 mg of salicin daily; in this group, 39% were pain free for at least 5 days of the last week of the study. In the lower-dose group (120 mg salicin daily), 21% became pain free. In contrast, only 6% of those given placebo became pain free. Stomach distress did not occur in this study. The only significant side effect seen was an allergic reaction in one participant given willow.

Benefits were also seen in a double-blind, placebo-controlled trial of 78 individuals with osteoarthritis of the knee or hip.

However, two subsequent double-blind, placebo-controlled studies performed by a single research group failed to find white willow more effective than placebo. One enrolled 127 people with osteoarthritis (OA) of the hip or knee, the other 26 outpatients with active rheumatoid arthritis (RA). In the OA trial, participants received either willow bark extract (240 mg of salicin per day), the standard drug diclofenac (100 mg per day), or

placebo. In the RA trial, participants received either willow bark extract at the same dose or placebo. While diclofenac proved significantly more effective than placebo in the OA trial, willow bark did not. It also failed to prove more effective than placebo in the RA study.

The most likely interpretation of these conflicting findings is that willow provides at best no more than a modest level of pain relief.

Dosage

Standardized willow bark extracts should provide 120 to 240 mg of salicin daily.

Safety Issues

Evidence suggests that willow, taken at standard doses, is the equivalent of 50 mg of aspirin, a very small dose. Willow doesn't impair blood coagulation to the same extent as aspirin, and also doesn't appear to significantly irritate the stomach. Nonetheless, it seems reasonable to suppose that if it is used over the long term or in high doses willow could still cause the side effects associated with aspirin. All the risks of aspirin therapy potentially apply. For this reason, white willow should not be given to children, due to the risk of Reye's syndrome. It should also not be used by people with aspirin allergies, bleeding disorders, or kidney disease, and it may interact adversely with "blood thinners," other anti-inflammatory drugs, methotrexate, metoclopramide, phenytoin, probenecid, spironolactone, and valproate.

Safety in pregnant or nursing women, or those with severe liver or kidney disease, has not been established.

Interactions You Should Know About

If you are taking blood-thinning medications, such as **warfarin** (Coumadin), **heparin**, **clopidogrel** (Plavix), **ticlopidine** (Ticlid), **pentoxifylline** (Trental), or **aspirin**; **methotrexate**; **metoclopramide**; **phenytoin** (Dilantin); **sulfonamide drugs**; **spironolactone** and other **potassium-sparing diuretics**; or the antiseizure drug **valproic acid**: It may be wise to avoid taking white willow.

Wild Cherry

Prunus serotina

PRINCIPAL PROPOSED USES: *Cough*

The bark of the wild cherry tree is a traditional Native American remedy for two seemingly unrelated conditions: respiratory infections and anxiety. European settlers quickly adopted the herb for similar purposes.

What Is Wild Cherry Used for Today?

Over time, wild cherry has come to be used primarily as a component of cough syrups. It is tempting to connect the two traditional uses of wild cherry by imagining that it functions like codeine to affect both the mind and the cough reflex. However, this is just speculation, as there has been very little scientific evaluation of this herb.

Dosage

Syrups containing wild cherry should be taken as directed.

Safety Issues

Wild cherry is generally regarded as safe when used at recommended dosages. However, since it contains small amounts of cyanide, it should not be taken to excess. It is not recommended for use by young children, pregnant or nursing women, or those with severe liver or kidney disease. Some evidence suggests that wild cherry might interact with various medications by affecting their metabolism in the liver, but the extent of this effect has not been fully determined.

Wild Indigo

Baptisia tinctoria

PRINCIPAL PROPOSED USES: *Colds and Flus (In Combination with Echinacea and White Cedar), Chronic Bronchitis (Acute Exacerbation, along with Antibiotic Therapy), Immune Support*

Like its botanical relative true indigo (*Indigofera tinctoria*), wild indigo has historically been used as a source of a deep blue dye. It was also used medicinally: the natives of North America used it as a topical treatment for non-healing wounds and infections of the mouth and throat. The root is the part used.

What Is Wild Indigo Used for Today?

Currently, wild indigo is primarily used as part of a standardized four-herb combination said to improve immune function. This combination contains, besides wild indigo, *Echinacea purpurea* root, *Echinacea pallida* root, and white cedar (*Thuja occidentalis*). This combination is hypothesized to have immune-stimulating properties.

In a well-designed double-blind study of 263 people with recent onset of the **common cold**, use of this combination significantly improved cold symptoms as compared to placebo. Recovery occurred approximately 3 days earlier among people taking the herbal mixture as compared to those taking the placebo.

Benefits for the common cold were also seen in other double-blind, placebo-controlled studies involving a total of about 250 people.

The same combination therapy has also shown promise for augmenting the effects of antibiotics in people with bacterial infections. For example, in one study, 53 people experiencing an acute exacerbation of **chronic bronchitis** were given either antibiotics plus placebo or the same antibiotics plus this herbal combination. The results showed that participants receiving the herbal mixture recovered significantly more quickly than those given placebo.

Proponents of this combination therapy claim that it works by "balancing" or "strengthening" the immune system. However, while there is evidence that this herbal mixture affects the immune function, the current state of scientific knowledge is generally inadequate to determine whether any such effects are good, bad, or indifferent. See the article on **immune support** for more information on this widely misunderstood topic.

Dosage

Combination therapies containing wild indigo, echinacea, and white cedar should be taken according to label instructions.

Safety Issues

Wild indigo has not undergone comprehensive safety testing. However, in clinical studies, use of the standardized combination therapy has not been associated with any serious harmful effects. Safety in young children, pregnant or nursing women, or people with severe liver or kidney disease has not been established.

Wild Yam

Dioscorea species

ALTERNATE NAMES/RELATED TERMS: *Mexican Yam*
PRINCIPAL PROPOSED USES: *None*
INCORRECT USES: *Source of Women's Hormones*

Various species of wild yam grow throughout North and Central America and Asia. Traditionally, this herb has been used as a treatment for indigestion, coughs, morning sickness, gallbladder pain, menstrual cramps, joint pain, and nerve pain. The main use of wild yam in the U.S. today, however, is based on a fundamental misconception: that it contains women's hormones such as **progesterone** and **DHEA**.

In reality, there is no progesterone, DHEA, or any other hormone in wild yam, nor does wild yam contain any substances that have progesterone-like or estrogen-like effects.

To explain this widespread misunderstanding, we have to go back a number of years. When progesterone was first discovered, it was very expensive to produce. The first methods involved direct extraction of progesterone from cow ovaries, a process that required 50,000 cows to yield 20 mg of purified hormone! Other hormones such as estrogen and DHEA were also difficult to manufacture. Although doctors wanted to experiment with prescribing these treatments as medicine until a simpler production method could be developed, it simply wasn't feasible.

The race to discover a more economical source of hormones was won by a scientist/businessman named Russell Marker. In the 1940s, he perfected a method of synthesizing progesterone from a constituent of wild yam called *diosgenin*. This process involves several chemical transformations carried out in the laboratory.

Marker focused his attention on two species of yam found in Mexico, *Dioscorea macrostachya* and *Dioscorea barabasco*, the latter of which is richer in diosgenin, while the former is much easier to harvest in the wild. He formed a manufacturing company in Mexico that produced progesterone and DHEA from these raw materials.

Unfortunately, corporate competition and difficult labor conditions eventually forced him to close his plant. But Marker's method of synthesizing progesterone continued to be used, bringing the price down drastically and helping to pave the way for the modern birth control pill. Progesterone continued to be manufactured from wild yam for decades, until a cheaper source of raw material was found in cultivated soybeans.

But neither soybeans nor wild yam contain progesterone. They only contain chemicals that chemists can use as a starting point to manufacture progesterone. However, just because chemists can make progesterone out of diosgenin doesn't mean that the body can do the same. Actually, it's very unlikely, because the steps used by chemists to carry out this conversion don't even remotely resemble natural processes. Thus, any product that claims to contain "natural progesterone from wild yam" is misleading.

Studies involving cells in a test tube have found that wild yam does not act like estrogen or progesterone. Furthermore, in a double-blind, placebo-controlled study of 23 women with symptoms of menopause, use of wild yam did not reduce hot flashes nor raise levels of progesterone or estrogen in the body.

Nonetheless, some wild yam products do contain progesterone. Are we contradicting ourselves? Not at all: manufacturers add *synthetic* progesterone to these creams. There may be a value to taking progesterone in cream form, but the wild yam part of the product is a red herring!

Witch Hazel

Hamamelis virginiana

PRINCIPAL PROPOSED USES:

Skin Conditions, Including: *Eczema (Topical), Hemorrhoids (Topical)*

Topical: *Canker Sores, Cold Sores, Gum Inflammation, Minor Wounds, Varicose Veins*

Internal: *Diarrhea, Varicose Veins*

The bark, leaves, and twigs of the witch hazel shrub were widely used as medicinal treatments by native peoples of North America. Witch hazel was applied topically as a treatment for such conditions as skin wounds, insect bites, hemorrhoids, muscle aches, and back stiffness, and it was taken internally for colds, coughs, and digestive problems. It came into use among European colonists in the 1840s, when a businessman named Theron Pond marketed an extract of witch hazel under the name "Golden Treasure."

The most common witch hazel product available in the U.S. is made from the whole twigs of the shrub. Extracts of the bark alone are used in Europe.

What is Witch Hazel Used for Today?

Witch hazel is widely marketed for direct application to the skin to relieve pain, stop bleeding, control itching, reduce symptoms of **eczema**, and treat muscle aches. Pads, ointments, and suppositories containing witch hazel are used for treatment of **hemorrhoids**. Extracts of the bark and leaf are used in Europe to treat **diarrhea**, inflammation of the gums, **canker sores**, and **varicose veins**. However, there is no meaningful evidence that witch hazel is actually effective for any of these conditions.

One small double-blind study is commonly cited as evidence that witch hazel is effective for treatment of eczema. This study compared topical witch hazel ointment to the drug bufexamac, and found them equally effective. However, bufexamac itself has not been shown effective for the treatment of eczema, so this study proves little. A subsequent study failed to find witch hazel more effective than a placebo treatment for eczema.

There are no other meaningful studies of witch hazel. Extremely preliminary evidence hints that it may have anti-inflammatory properties, and even weaker evidence suggests that witch hazel may increase the contractility of veins (potentially making it useful in varicose veins). However, this evidence is far too weak to support using witch hazel for any of these conditions.

Dosage

Witch hazel preparations should be used according to label instructions.

Safety Issues

Witch hazel appears to be a relatively safe substance, but comprehensive safety studies have not been performed. When applied to the skin, it may cause allergic reactions. Witch hazel contains tannins, which can upset the stomach. Safety in pregnant or nursing women, young children, or people with severe liver or kidney disease is not established.

Wormwood

Artemisia absinthium

ALTERNATE NAMES/RELATED TERMS: *Common Wormwood*
PRINCIPAL PROPOSED USES: *None*
OTHER PROPOSED USES: *Dyspepsia, Esophageal Reflux, Irritable Bowel Syndrome, Parasites*

Artemisia absinthium, or common wormwood, is most famous as an ingredient of the alcoholic beverage absinthe. Wormwood is also found in vermouth, but at lower levels. Besides its common function as a flavoring, wormwood also has a long history of medicinal use. A reputed ability to kill intestinal worms gave rise to the herb's name. Other traditional uses include treating liver problems, joint pain, digestive discomfort, loss of appetite, insomnia, epilepsy, and menstrual problems. The leaves and flowers, and the essential oil extracted from them are the parts used medicinally.

Common wormwood is a relative of sweet wormwood (*Artemisia annua*), a source of the malaria drug artemisinin (also called *artemesin*).

What is Wormwood Used for Today?

Wormwood is sometimes recommended today for the treatment of digestive conditions such as intestinal parasites, **dyspepsia**, **esophageal reflux**, and **irritable bowel syndrome**. However, there is no meaningful evidence to indicate that it is effective for any of these conditions. Only double-blind, placebo-controlled studies can show a treatment effective and none have been performed using wormwood. (For information on why such studies are essential, see **Why Does This Book Rely on Double-blind Studies?**.)

Weak evidence, far too weak to rely upon at all, hints that wormwood essential oil (like many other essential oils) might have antifungal, antibacterial, and antiparasitic actions. Note, however, that is does not mean that wormwood oil is an antibiotic. Antibiotics are substances that can be taken internally to kill microorganisms throughout the body. Wormwood oil, rather, has shown potential antiseptic properties. Unfortunately, it is also potentially quite toxic (see Safety Issues below).

Other weak evidence hints that an alcohol extract of wormwood might have **liver-protective** actions.

Dosage

A typical dose of wormwood is 3 cups daily of a tea made by steeping 2.5 to 5 g of wormwood in hot water. Wormwood essential oil should not be used. Long-term use of any form of wormwood (more than 4 weeks) is considered unsafe.

Safety Issues

There are many unsolved questions about the toxicity of wormwood. When absinthe was popular in the late nineteenth and early twentieth centuries, a mental disorder known as *absinthism*—involving hallucinations, tremors, vertigo, sleeplessness, and seizures—was associated with it. Wormwood contains thujone, a substance thought to be toxic to nerves when taken at high doses, and thujone has been proposed as a factor contributing to absinthism. However, the symptoms of absinthism are also consistent with mere chronic overuse of alcohol and absinthe does not appear to contain sufficient thujone to cause harm. Furthermore, animal studies have generally failed to find

significant toxicity with wormwood even at relatively high doses.

Despite the absence of firm evidence, wormwood is still considered a potentially toxic herb, especially if taken over the long term. Wormwood essential oil contains thujone at much higher levels than those found in absinthe, and should be avoided. Wormwood should not be used by young children, pregnant or nursing women, or people with severe liver or kidney disease.

Xylitol

PRINCIPAL PROPOSED USES: *Cavities (Prevention)*

OTHER PROPOSED USES: *Ear Infections (Prevention), Periodontal Disease (Prevention)*

A natural sugar found in plums, strawberries, and raspberries, xylitol is used as a sweetener in some "sugarless" gums and candies. Not only does xylitol replace sugars that can lead to tooth decay, it also appears to help prevent cavities by inhibiting the growth of bacteria that cause cavities, such as *Streptococcus mutans*. Xylitol also inhibits the growth of a related species, *Streptococcus pneumoniae*, which is a cause of ear infections.

Gums, toothpaste, and candy containing high levels of xylitol are beginning to become available in the U.S.

What Is Xylitol Used for Today?

Many studies, including several under the auspices of the World Health Organization, have evaluated xylitol gums, toothpastes, and candies for **preventing dental cavities**, with good results. In all of these studies, xylitol users developed fewer cavities than those receiving either placebo or no treatment.

Xylitol is thought to prevent cavities by inhibiting the growth of the *Streptococcus mutans* bacteria. Since a related bacteria, *Streptococcus pneumoniae*, can cause **ear infections**, xylitol has been investigated as a preventive treatment for middle-ear infections, with some success.

In addition, preliminary evidence suggests that use of xylitol may offer some protection against **periodontal disease** (gum disease).

What Is the Scientific Evidence for Xylitol?

Preventing Cavities

Double-blind, placebo-controlled studies enrolling a total of almost 4,000 people, mostly children, have found that xylitol gum, candy, or toothpaste can help prevent cavities.

A double-blind, placebo-controlled study of 1,677 children compared a standard fluoride toothpaste with a similar toothpaste that also contained 10% xylitol. Over the 3-year study period, children given the xylitol-enriched toothpaste developed significantly fewer cavities than those in the fluoride-only group.

In another trial, a 40-month, double-blind study of 1,277 children, researchers studied gum products containing various concentrations of xylitol and/or sorbitol. Participants were divided into nine groups: xylitol gum in four different concentrations, two forms of xylitol/sorbitol gum, sorbitol-only gum, sucrose (ordinary sugar) gum, or no gum.

The gum with the highest xylitol concentration proved most effective at reducing cavities. However, children in every one of the xylitol and/or sorbitol gum groups showed significant reductions in cavities as compared to the sugar gum or no-gum groups.

Another series of studies suggests that children acquire cavity-causing bacteria from their mothers; regular use of xylitol by a mother of a newborn child may provide some protection to the child, as well.

Ear Infections

One large double-blind, placebo-controlled trial of 857 children investigated how well xylitol (in chewing gum, syrup, and lozenges) could prevent ear infections. The gum was most effective, reducing the risk of developing ear infections by a full 40%. Xylitol syrup was also effective, but less so. The lozenges weren't effective; researchers speculated that children got tired of sucking on the large candies and didn't get the proper dose of xylitol. (In addition, the children were able to distinguish between the xylitol and placebo lozenges by taste, making that portion of the study single-blind.)

Similarly positive results had been seen in an earlier double-blind study by the same researchers, evaluating about 300 children.

However, these studies were of short duration and did not test the long-term effect of xylitol in young children and infants, who are most at risk of contracting ear infections.

Dosage

In the studies described above, dosages for cavity prevention ranged from 4.3 to 10 g per day. The doses were divided throughout the day, usually after meals. For ear infections, children given xylitol-sweetened gum received 8.4 g of xylitol daily, also in divided doses. Those who took syrup received 10 g daily.

Safety Issues

Xylitol is believed to be safe, but doses higher than 30 g per day can cause stomach discomfort and possibly diarrhea. In studies, children taking xylitol syrup tended to have more such side effects than those using other forms of xylitol, possibly because it reached the stomach in a more concentrated dose.

Yarrow

Achillea millefolium

PRINCIPAL PROPOSED USES: *None*

OTHER PROPOSED USES: *Colds and Flus (Internal Use), Stopping Bleeding from Nosebleeds or Minor Wounds (Topical Use)*

According to legend, the Greek general Achilles used yarrow to stop the bleeding of his soldiers' wounds during the Trojan War: hence the scientific name *Achillea* and the common names soldier's wound-wort, bloodwort, and *herbe militaire*.

Yarrow has also been used traditionally as treatment for respiratory infections, menstrual pain, and digestive upsets.

What Is Yarrow Used for Today?

Like osha, yarrow tea is commonly taken at the first sign of a cold or flu to bring on sweating and, according to tradition, ward off infection. Crushed yarrow leaves and flower tops are also applied directly as first aid to stop **nosebleeds** and bleeding from **minor wounds**. However, there has not been any formal scientific study of how well yarrow works.

Dosage

To make yarrow tea, steep 1 to 2 teaspoons of dried herb per cup of water. Combination products should be taken according to label instructions.

Safety Issues

No clear toxicity has been associated with yarrow. The FDA has expressed concern about a toxic constituent of yarrow known as *thujone* and permits only thujone-free yarrow extracts for use in beverages. Nonetheless, the common spice sage contains more thujone than yarrow and the FDA lists sage as generally recognized as safe.

Safety in young children, pregnant or nursing women, or those with severe liver or kidney disease has not been established.

Yellow Dock

PRINCIPAL PROPOSED USES: *None*

OTHER PROPOSED USES: *Constipation, Diarrhea, Hemorrhoids, Minor Skin Wounds*

Yellow dock (*Rumex crispus*) is a perennial flowering herb, native to Europe, which grows throughout the United States. Its yellow roots were traditionally thought to have medicinal properties and its sour-sweet leaves can be used (in moderation) as a salad green.

Historically, the plant has been used to treat a variety of problems, including constipation *and* diarrhea, as well as dermatitis and venereal diseases. Powdered yellow dock root has also been used as a mouthwash or dentifrice.

What Is Yellow Dock Used for Today?

Yellow dock root has no established medical uses. However, it contains chemicals called *anthroquinones* (also found in the more famous herbal laxative senna), which stimulate bowel movements. For this reason, yellow dock is occasionally included in herbal laxative mixtures.

Like many other plants, yellow dock contains a substantial amount of tannins. These have astringent properties that may offer some benefit for treating minor skin **wounds** and **hemorrhoids**. Yellow dock is also sometimes recommended for nasal and lung congestion.

Dosage

Typical doses of yellow dock root are 2 to 4 g of the dried root, 2 to 4 ml of the liquid extract, or 1 to 2 ml of the tincture.

Safety Issues

Comprehensive safety studies of yellow dock have not been performed and, for this reason, it should not be used by pregnant or nursing women, young children, or individuals with severe liver or kidney disease.

As with any stimulant laxative, yellow dock should not be used if there is an intestinal obstruction. Possible side effects of overuse include cramps, diarrhea, nausea, intestinal dependence on the laxative, and excessive loss of **potassium**.

In addition, yellow dock (like spinach) contains oxalic acid. Consuming excessive quantities of oxalic acid can cause severe toxic symptoms, including vomiting and abdominal pain and, in extreme cases, **kidney stones** or kidney failure. One case of fatal yellow dock poisoning has been documented. The victim, who had diabetes, ingested one kilogram of the raw herb in a salad and died of liver and kidney failure. The liver failure was not explained.

Yerba Santa

Eriodictyon californicum

PRINCIPAL PROPOSED USES:

    Oral Uses: *Respiratory Problems (Asthma, Bronchitis, Common Cold)*

    Topical Uses: *Rash (Poison Ivy)*

Yerba santa is a sticky-leafed evergreen that is native to the American Southwest. It was given its name ("holy weed") by Spanish priests impressed with its medicinal properties. The aromatic leaves were boiled to make a tea to treat coughs, colds, asthma, pleurisy, tuberculosis, and pneumonia, and a poultice of the leaves was applied to painful joints.

Unlike many medicinal herbs, yerba santa actually has a pleasant taste. It has been used as a general food flavoring and in cough syrups to disguise the bad taste of other ingredients.

What Is Yerba Santa Used for Today?

Yerba santa is often used for the treatment of the **common cold**, as well as chronic respiratory problems, such as **bronchitis** and **asthma**. Unfortunately, there is no meaningful scientific evidence to indicate that it is effective. About the most that can be said scientifically is that one of its constituents, eriodictyol, might have mild expectorant properties.

Topical yerba santa has been recommended as a treatment for poison ivy.

Dosage

Yerba santa tea may be made by adding 1 teaspoon of crushed leaves to a cup of boiling water and steeping for half an hour. However, many of its resinous constituents do not dissolve in water and for that reason alcoholic tinctures of yerba santa are commonly used.

Safety Issues

Yerba santa is on the FDA's GRAS (generally recognized as safe) list for use as a food flavoring. There have been no reports of significant side effects or adverse reactions, except for the inevitable occasional allergic reaction. Nonetheless, safety in young children, pregnant or nursing women, or those with severe liver or kidney disease has not been established.

Yohimbe

Pausinystalia yohimbe

PRINCIPAL PROPOSED USES: *Impotence (Not Recommended)*

OTHER PROPOSED USES: *Sexual Dysfunction in Women*

The bark of the West African yohimbe tree is a traditional aphrodisiac and the source of yohimbine, a prescription drug for impotence. It appears to be modestly effective, but it also presents numerous safety risks. Yohimbe should not be used except under physician supervision.

What Is Yohimbe Used for Today?

Like the drug yohimbine, the bark of the yohimbe tree is widely used to treat **impotence**. Many herbalists report that the herb is more effective than the purified drug,

Yohimbe

perhaps due to the presence of other unidentified active ingredients. However, there have been no studies to evaluate this claim. Furthermore, due to the lack of supervision of herbal products, there are real concerns that herbal yohimbe might contain either too much or too little yohimbine. (See also Safety Issues below.)

Yohimbine (the drug) is only modestly effective at best; better than placebo but only successful in about 30 to 45% of the men who use it. Yohimbine has also been evaluated in combination with the supplement **arginine**. A double-blind, placebo-controlled trial of 45 men found that one-time use of this combination therapy an hour or two prior to intercourse improved erectile function, especially in those with only moderate erectile dysfunction scores. Arginine and yohimbine were both taken at a dose of 6 grams.

One small, double-blind study of yohimbine combined with arginine found an increase in measured physical arousal among 23 women with female sexual arousal disorder. However, the women themselves did not report any noticeable subjective effects. In addition, only the combination of yohimbine and arginine produced results; neither substance was effective when taken on its own.

An open trial of yohimbine alone to treat sexual dysfunction induced by the antidepressant fluoxetine (Prozac) found improvement in eight out of nine people, two of whom were women. However, in the absence of a placebo group, these results can't be considered reliable; in addition, there are concerns about the safety of combining yohimbe with antidepressants.

Yohimbe is also sometimes recommended for **depression**. However, its effectiveness is unknown and there are much safer herbs for this purpose, such as **St. John's wort**.

Dosage

Yohimbe bark is best taken in a form standardized to yohimbine content so you can properly control your dose of the drug. Unfortunately, label claims for yohimbine content have been frequently found to be inaccurate. The usual dose of yohimbine is 15 to 30 mg daily.

However, higher doses are not necessarily better and it appears that some people respond optimally to 10 or even 5 mg daily. Furthermore, while some people appear to respond immediately to a single dose, for others it takes 2 to 3 weeks of treatment to provide significant benefits.

Safety Issues

The following discussion applies to the drug yohimbine, rather than the herb yohimbe. All risks of the drug apply to the herb and there are additional risks to consider as well. For example, as noted above, the amount of yohimbine in a given sample of the herb may not be accurately reflected on the label. Furthermore, additional constituents contained in the herb besides yohimbine might present unique (and unknown) risks of their own.

Yohimbine in any form should not be used by pregnant or nursing women, or those with kidney, liver, or ulcer disease or high blood pressure. Intake of more than 40 mg a day of yohimbine can cause a severe drop in blood pressure, abdominal pain, fatigue, hallucinations, and paralysis. (Interestingly, lower dosages can cause an increase in blood pressure.) Since 40 mg is not very far above the typical recommended dose, yohimbine has what is known as a *narrow therapeutic index*. This means that there is a relatively small dosing range, below which the herb doesn't work and above which it is toxic.

Even when taken in normal dosages, side effects of dizziness, anxiety, hyperstimulation, and nausea are not uncommon.

Finally, yohimbine may interact adversely with numerous medications, including tricyclic antidepressants, phenothiazines, clonidine, and other drugs for lowering blood pressure.

Interactions You Should Know About

If you are taking **tricyclic antidepressants, phenothiazines, clonidine**, other drugs for lowering blood pressure, or central nervous system stimulants: Do not use yohimbine.

Yucca

Yucca schidigera (Mojave Yucca) and other species

PRINCIPAL PROPOSED USES: *Rheumatoid Arthritis, Osteoarthritis*

Various species of yucca plant were used as food by Native Americans and early California settlers. Yucca contains high levels of soapy compounds known as *saponins* that also made it a useful natural shampoo and soap.

What Is Yucca Used for Today?

One double-blind, placebo-controlled trial reported in 1975 concluded that use of yucca reduces arthritis symptoms (both **osteoarthritis** and **rheumatoid arthritis**). However, this study was highly preliminary in nature and there has not been any subsequent confirming evidence.

Animal and test-tube studies suggest that various yucca extracts may have antiviral, antifungal, antiprotozoal (for example *Giardia lamblia*) and antibacterial effects, but no human trials have been reported for potential uses based on these actions.

Yucca extracts are also widely used to enhance the foaming effect of carbonated beverages.

Dosage

The standard dosage is 2 to 4 tablets of concentrated yucca saponins daily.

Safety Issues

Yucca is generally accepted as safe based on its long history of use as a food. However, it sometimes causes diarrhea if taken to excess. Safety in young children, pregnant or nursing women, or those with severe liver or kidney disease has not been established. Yucca may have slight estrogen-like actions and, for this reason, should not be taken by women who have had breast cancer.

Zinc

SUPPLEMENT FORMS/ALTERNATE NAMES: *Zinc Sulfate, Zinc Gluconate, Zinc Citrate, Zinc Picolinate, Chelated Zinc*

PRINCIPAL PROPOSED USES: *Acne, Colds, General Nutritional Supplementation, Macular Degeneration, Sickle-cell Anemia, Attention Deficit and Hyperactivity Disorder (ADHD)*

OTHER PROPOSED USES: *Anorexia Nervosa, Benign Prostatic Hyperplasia (BPH), Cold Sores, Depression, Diabetes, Eczema, HIV Support, Impotence, Prostatitis, Radiation Therapy Support, Rheumatoid Arthritis, Tinnitus, Ulcers*

Zinc is an important element that is found in every cell in the body. More than 300 enzymes in the body need zinc in order to function properly. Although the amount of zinc we need in our daily diet is tiny, it's very important that we get it. However, the evidence suggests that many of us do *not* get enough. Mild zinc deficiency seems to be fairly common and, for this reason, taking a zinc supplement at nutritional doses may be a good idea.

However, taking too much zinc isn't a good idea—it can cause toxicity. In this article, we discuss the possible uses of zinc at various doses.

Zinc

Requirements/Sources

The official U.S. recommendations for daily intake of zinc are as follows:

- Infants 0–6 months, 2 mg
  7–12 months, 3 mg
- Children 1–3 years, 3 mg
  4–8 years, 5 mg
- Males 9–13 years, 8 mg
  14 years and older 11 mg
- Females 9–13 years, 8 mg
  14–18 years, 9 mg
  19 years and older, 8 mg
- Pregnant women, 11 mg (13 mg if 18 years old or younger)
- Nursing women, 12 mg (14 mg if 18 years old or younger)

The average diet in the developed world may provide insufficient zinc, especially in women, adolescents, infants, and the elderly. Thus, it may be a wise idea to increase your intake of zinc on general principles.

Various drugs may tend to reduce levels zinc in the body by inhibiting its absorption or increasing its excretion. These include captopril and possibly other ACE inhibitors, oral contraceptives, thiazide diuretics, and drugs that reduce stomach acid (including H_2 blockers and proton pump inhibitors). Certain nutrients may also inhibit zinc absorption, including calcium, soy, manganese, copper, and iron. Contrary to previous reports, folate is not likely to have this effect.

Oysters have a very high zinc content—one oyster provides at least the full daily dose of zinc (about 8 to 15 mg). Besides oysters, other types of shellfish, along with poultry and meat (especially organ meats), are high in zinc, providing 1 to 8 mg of zinc per serving. Whole grains, nuts, and seeds provide smaller amounts of zinc, ranging from 0.2 to about 3 mg per serving, and the zinc from them is not as absorbable. Breakfast cereals and nutrition bars are often fortified with substantial amounts of zinc.

Zinc can also be taken as a nutritional supplement, in one of many forms. Zinc citrate, zinc acetate, or zinc picolinate may be the best absorbed, although zinc sulfate is less expensive. When you purchase a supplement, you should be aware of the difference between the milligrams of actual zinc that the product contains (so-called elemental zinc) and the total milligrams of the zinc product, which includes the weight of the sulfate, picolinate, and so forth. All dosages given in this article refer to elemental zinc (unless otherwise stated).

Therapeutic Dosages

For most purposes, zinc should simply be taken at the recommended daily requirements listed previously.

Some evidence suggests that 30 mg of zinc daily may be helpful for acne. This is a safe dose for most people. However, in most studies of zinc for acne, a much higher dose was used: 90 mg daily or more. Doses this high should only be used under physician supervision (see Safety Issues below). Potentially dangerous doses of zinc have also been recommended for sickle-cell anemia, macular degeneration, and rheumatoid arthritis.

For best absorption, zinc supplements should not be taken at the same time as high-fiber foods. However, many high-fiber foods provide zinc in themselves.

Zinc gluconate may be slightly better absorbed than zinc oxide.

When taking zinc long-term, it is advisable to take 1 to 3 mg of copper daily as well, because zinc supplements can cause copper deficiency. Zinc may also interfere with magnesium and iron absorption.

Zinc is used topically in lozenge or nasal gel form for the treatment of colds. When using zinc this way, the purpose is not to increase zinc levels in your body, but to interfere with the action of viruses in the back of your throat or in the nose. It appears that of the common forms of zinc, only zinc gluconate and zinc acetate have the required antiviral properties. Certain sweeteners and flavorings used in lozenges can block zinc's antiviral action. Dextrose, sucrose, mannitol, and sorbitol appear to be fine, but citric acid and tartaric acid are not. The information on glycine as a flavoring agent is a bit equivocal.

Note: When using zinc nasal gel products, do not deeply inhale, as this may cause severe pain. Rather, simply squeeze the gel into the nose, according to the directions.

Therapeutic Uses

Use of zinc nasal spray or zinc lozenges at the beginning of a **cold** may reduce the duration and severity of symptoms, but study results are somewhat inconsistent. These treatments are thought to work by directly interfering with viruses in the nose and throat, and involve relatively high doses of zinc used for a short time.

Zinc

Zinc can also be taken long-term at nutritional doses orally to **improve overall immunity**; however, this approach probably only works if you are deficient in zinc to begin with.

A significant body of evidence suggests that oral zinc can reduce symptoms of **acne**, but in most studies potentially toxic doses were used and, in any case, the benefits appear to be rather slight.

Growing evidence suggests that oral zinc, especially in combination with antioxidants, can help slow the progression of **macular degeneration**. Oral zinc has also shown a bit of promise for **sickle-cell anemia**, **ADHD**, **stomach ulcers**, and dysgeusia (impaired taste). Topical zinc may be helpful for **cold sores**.

Radiation therapy in the vicinity of the mouth may cause alterations in taste sensation. In a small double-blind, placebo-controlled trial, use of zinc supplements tended to protect taste sensation. However, another study failed to find zinc supplements helpful for improving taste sensation among people undergoing kidney dialysis.

Weak and/or contradictory results have been seen in studies of zinc for **anorexia nervosa**, **depression**, **rheumatoid arthritis**, enhancing **sexual function** in men on kidney dialysis, **tinnitus**, and **warts**.

Some, but not all, studies have found that **HIV-positive** people tend to be deficient in zinc, with levels dropping lower in more severe disease. Higher zinc levels have been linked to better immune function and higher CD4+ cell counts, whereas zinc deficiency has been linked to increased risk of dying from HIV. One preliminary study among people taking AZT found that 30 days of zinc supplementation led to decreased rates of opportunistic infection over the following 2 years. However, other research has linked higher zinc intake to more rapid development of AIDS. The bottom line: If you have HIV, consult your physician before supplementing with zinc.

Although the evidence that it works is not yet meaningful, zinc is sometimes recommended for the following conditions as well: **Alzheimer's disease**, **benign prostatic hyperplasia**, **bladder infection**, **cataracts**, **diabetes**, Down's syndrome, **infertility in men**, **inflammatory bowel disease** (**ulcerative colitis** and **Crohn's disease**), **osteoporosis**, **periodontal disease**, **prostatitis**, **psoriasis**, and **wound** and **burn** healing.

An 8-week, double-blind trial of zinc at 67 mg daily failed to find any benefit for **eczema** symptoms.

What Is the Scientific Evidence for Zinc?

Colds

Use of lozenges containing zinc gluconate or zinc acetate have shown somewhat inconsistent but generally positive results for reducing the severity and duration of the common cold. For example, in a double-blind trial, 100 people who were experiencing the early symptoms of a cold were given a lozenge that either contained 13.3 mg of zinc from zinc gluconate or was just a placebo. Participants took the lozenges several times daily until their cold symptoms subsided. The results were impressive. Coughing disappeared within 2.2 days in the treated group versus 4 days in the placebo group. Sore throat disappeared after 1 day versus 3 days in the placebo group, nasal drainage in 4 days (versus 7 days), and headache in 2 days (versus 3 days).

Positive results have also been seen in double-blind studies of zinc acetate. Not all studies have shown such positive results. However, the overall results appear to be favorable.

It has been suggested that the exact formulation of the zinc lozenge plays a significant role. Flavoring agents, such as citric acid and tartaric acid, appear to prevent zinc from inhibiting viruses, and chemical forms of zinc other than zinc gluconate or zinc acetate may not work; in particular, zinc sulfate may be ineffective. Sweeteners such as sorbitol, sucrose, dextrose, and mannitol are fine, but the information on glycine as a flavoring agent is equivocal.

Use of zinc in the nose is somewhat more controversial. In addition to showing inconsistent results in studies, use of zinc nasal gel can cause pain and possibly loss of sense of smell (see Safety Issues below).

For example, in a double-blind, placebo-controlled trial of a widely available zinc nasal gel product, 213 people with a newly starting cold used one squirt of zinc gluconate gel or placebo gel in each nostril every 4 hours while awake. The results were significant: treated participants stayed sick an average of 2.3 days, while those receiving placebo were sick for an average of 9 days, a 75% reduction in the duration of symptoms. Somewhat more modest, but still significant relative benefits were seen with zinc nasal gel in a double-blind, placebo-controlled study of 80 people with colds. However, another study, this one involving 77 people, failed to find benefit even with near-constant saturation of the nasal passages with zinc gluconate nasal spray. Furthermore, a study of 91 people using the standard commercially available nasal spray failed to find benefit. Yet another double-blind, placebo-controlled trial, this one enrolling 185 individuals, failed to find benefit with zinc nasal spray. However, this study used a much lower amount of zinc per squirt of spray than was used in the two studies just described: 50 times lower.

Besides using zinc to directly interfere with viruses, supplementation at nutritional dosages may also help reduce the frequency of colds by generally enhancing immunity.

In a 2-year study of nursing home residents, participants given zinc and selenium developed illnesses much less frequently than those given placebo. Of course, it isn't clear from this study which was more helpful, the zinc or the selenium. However, we do know that chronic zinc deficiency weakens the immune system, and studies performed in developing countries using zinc alone have found benefits. For example, a 6-month, double-blind, placebo-controlled study of 609 preschool children in India found that zinc supplements reduced the rate of respiratory infections by 45%. Nine other studies have also found zinc supplements helpful for preventing illness.

Cold Sores

Cold sores are infections caused by the herpes virus. One study suggests that topical zinc may be helpful. In this trial, 46 individuals with cold sores were treated with a zinc oxide cream or placebo every 2 hours until cold sores resolved. The results showed that individuals using the cream experienced a reduction in severity of symptoms and a shorter time to full recovery.

Zinc is thought to interfere with the ability of the herpes virus to reproduce itself. As with colds, the formulation of zinc must be properly designed to release active zinc ions. This study used a special zinc oxide and glycine formulation.

Some participants in this study experienced burning and inflammation caused by the zinc itself, but this seldom caused a serious problem.

Macular Degeneration

Macular degeneration is one of the most common causes of vision loss in the elderly.

A double-blind, placebo-controlled trial evaluated the effects of zinc with or without antioxidants on the progression of macular degeneration in 3,640 individuals in the early stage of the disease. Participants were randomly assigned to receive one of the following: **antioxidants** (**vitamin C** 500 mg, **vitamin E** 400 IU, and **beta-carotene** 15 mg), or **zinc** (80 mg) and **copper** (2 mg), or antioxidants plus zinc, or placebo. (Copper was administered along with zinc to prevent zinc-induced copper deficiency.)

The results suggest that zinc (alone or, even better, with antioxidants) significantly slowed the progression of the disease.

Previous studies of zinc for macular degeneration found mixed results, but they were much smaller.

There is also some evidence that making sure to get your dietary requirement of zinc on a daily basis over many years might reduce the risk of developing macular degeneration later in life.

Keep in mind that the dosages of zinc used in most of these studies are rather high and should be used only under a physician's supervision.

Attention Deficit/Hyperactivity Disorder

Zinc has shown some promise for treatment of ADHD. In a large (approximately 400-participant) double-blind, placebo-controlled study, use of zinc at a dose of 40 mg daily produced statistically significant benefits as compared to placebo among children not using any other treatment. This dose of zinc, while higher than nutritional needs, should be safe. However, the benefits seen were quite modest: about 28% of the participants given zinc showed improvement as compared to 20% in the placebo group.

Another, much smaller double-blind, placebo-controlled study evaluated whether zinc at 15 mg per day could enhance the effect of Ritalin. Again, modest benefits were seen.

Finally, extremely weak evidence hints that zinc might enhance the effectiveness of **evening primrose oil** for ADHD.

Acne

Studies suggest that people with acne have lower-than-normal levels of zinc in their bodies. This fact alone does not prove that taking zinc supplements will help acne, but several small double-blind studies involving a total of more than 300 people have found generally positive results.

In one of these studies, 54 people were given either placebo or 135 mg of zinc as zinc sulfate daily. Zinc produced slight but measurable benefits. Similar results have been seen in other studies using 90 to 135 mg of zinc daily. Some evidence suggests that a lower and safer dose, 30 mg daily, may offer some benefits. In some studies, however, no benefits were seen.

Two studies have compared zinc against a standard treatment for acne, the antibiotic tetracycline. One found that zinc was as effective as tetracycline taken at 250 mg daily, but another found the antibiotic far more effective when taken at 500 mg daily.

Keep in mind that the dosages of zinc used in most of these studies are rather high; case reports indicate that people have made themselves extremely ill by taking zinc in hopes of treating their acne symptoms. Doses of zinc higher than the recommended safe levels (see Safety Issues below) should be used only under a physician's supervision.

Sickle-cell Disease

Children with sickle-cell disease often do not grow normally. There is some evidence that people with sickle-cell disease are more likely than others to be deficient in zinc. Since zinc deficiency can also cause growth retardation, zinc supplementation at nutritional doses has been suggested for children with sickle-cell disease. In a placebo-controlled study, 42 children (ages 4 to 10) with sickle-cell disease were given either zinc supplements (10 mg of zinc daily) or placebo for a period of 1 year. Results showed that by the end of the study, the participants given zinc showed enhanced growth compared to those given placebo. Curiously, researchers did not find any solid connection between the severity of zinc deficiency and the extent of response to treatment.

Zinc is thought to have a stabilizing effect on the cell membrane of red blood cells in people with sickle-cell disease. For this reason, it has been tried as an aid for preventing sickle-cell crisis. In a double-blind, placebo-controlled study of 145 people with sickle-cell disease conducted in India, participants received either placebo or about 50 mg of zinc 3 times daily. During 18 months of treatment, the zinc-treated subjects had an average of 2.5 crises, compared to 5.3 for the placebo group. However, zinc didn't seem to reduce the severity of a crisis, as measured by the number of days spent in the hospital for each crisis.

Sickle-cell disease can also cause skin ulcers (non-healing sores). In a 12-week, placebo-controlled trial, use of zinc at 88 mg 3 times per day for 12 weeks enhanced the rate of ulcer healing. **Warning:** The high dosages of zinc used in the last two studies can cause dangerous toxicity and should be taken (if at all) only

under the supervision of a doctor. The nutritional dose described in the first study, however, is safe (see Safety Issues).

Safety Issues

Zinc taken orally seldom causes any immediate side effects other than occasional stomach upset, usually when it's taken on an empty stomach. Some forms do have an unpleasant metallic taste. Use of zinc nasal gel, however, has been associated with anosmia (loss of sense of smell). Furthermore, if the gel is inhaled too deeply, severe pain may occur.

Long-term use of oral zinc at dosages of 100 mg or more daily can cause a number of toxic effects, including severe copper deficiency, impaired immunity, heart problems, and anemia. The U.S. government has issued recommendations regarding tolerable upper intake levels (ULs) for zinc. The UL can be thought of as the highest daily intake over a prolonged time known to pose no risks to most members of a healthy population. The ULs for zinc are as follows:

- **Infants 0–6 months, 4 mg**
  7–12 months, 5 mg
- **Children 1 to 3 years, 7 mg**
  4 to 8 years, 12 mg
  9 to 13 years, 23 mg
- **Males and females 14 to 18 years, 34 mg**
  19 years and older, 40 mg
- **Pregnant or nursing women, 40 mg (34 mg if 18 years old or younger)**

Very weak evidence hints that use of zinc supplements might increase risk of prostate cancer in men.

There are also some interactions between zinc and certain medications to consider:

- **Use of zinc can interfere with the absorption of the drug penicillamine and also antibiotics in the tetracycline or fluoroquinolone (Cipro, Floxin) families.**
- **The potassium-sparing diuretic amiloride was found to significantly reduce zinc excretion from the body. This means that if you take zinc supplements at the same time as amiloride, zinc accumulation could occur. This could lead to toxic side effects. However, the potassium-sparing diuretic triamterene does not seem to cause this problem.**

Zinc

Interactions You Should Know About

If you are taking:

- ACE inhibitors, oral contraceptives, estrogen-replacement therapy, thiazide diuretics, or medications that reduce stomach acid (such as H2 blockers [Zantac] or proton pump inhibitors [Prilosec]): You may need to take extra zinc.
- Manganese, calcium, copper, iron, antacids, soy, or antibiotics in the fluoroquinolone (such as, Cipro, Floxin) or tetracycline families: It may be advisable to separate your doses of zinc and these substances by at least 2 hours.
- Zinc supplements: You should also take extra copper and perhaps magnesium as well because zinc interferes with their absorption. Zinc interferes with iron absorption, too, but you shouldn't take iron supplements unless you know you are deficient.
- Penicillamine: Zinc interferes with penicillamine's absorption so it may be advisable to take zinc and penicillamine at least 2 hours apart.
- Amiloride: It could reduce zinc excretion from the body, leading to zinc accumulation, which could cause toxic side effects. Do not take zinc supplements unless advised by a physician.

ALTERNATIVE
THERAPIES

Acupressure

A cupressure is a method closely related to **acupuncture** that involves pressure stimulation, instead of needle stimulation, applied to acupuncture points. Acupressure is also closely related to Shiatsu, a form of Asian massage.

Acupuncture

FEMALE INFERTILITY: *Acupressure, Electroacupuncture*

EVIDENCE-BASED USES: *Nausea and Vomiting, Tendonitis, Osteoarthritis*

OTHER STUDIED USES: *Alcoholism, Anxiety, Asthma, Back Pain, Bell's Palsy, Bladder Infections, Breast-feeding Support, Cancer Chemotherapy Support, Childbirth, Cigarette Addiction, Crohn's Disease, Dental Procedures, Depression, Dysmenorrhea, Epilepsy, Female Infertility, Fibromyalgia, Headache, Insomnia, Irritable Bowel Syndrome, Menopause, Migraine Headache, Narcotic Addiction, Neck Pain, Pain During Medical Procedures, Peripheral Neuropathy in HIV, Pregnancy Support, Psoriasis, Raynaud's Phenomenon, Rheumatoid Arthritis, Shingles (Post-herpetic Neuralgia), Sports Performance Enhancement, Stroke, Surgery Support, Tension Headache, Tinnitus, Temporomandibular Joint (TMJ) Pain, Weight Loss*

Overview

Acupuncture has been part of the medical mainstream in countries such as China and Japan for centuries. It is also one of the most widely utilized forms of alternative therapy in the United States. More than 10 million acupuncture treatments are administered annually in the U.S. alone. In addition, third-party insurance reimbursement and managed care coverage for acupuncture are increasing.

Due to its popularity, scientific investigation of acupuncture has grown dramatically in recent years, with many new studies reported every week. However, the results have been mixed at best.

What Is Acupuncture?

Simply defined, acupuncture is a treatment method aimed at eliciting a response (such as pain relief) through insertion of very fine needles in the body surface at sites called *acupuncture points*. A related technique called *acupuncture* (or *shiatsu*) uses pressure on these points; a related therapy known as *electroacupuncture* applies electricity to the points.

A wide variety of treatment methods, approaches, techniques, styles, and theoretical frameworks exist within the very broad scope of the term *acupuncture*. Differences in forms of acupuncture are often cultural; the system of acupuncture practiced in Japan, for example, is quite different from that found in China. Many acupuncturists practice a more or less traditional style called **Traditional Chinese Medicine** (TCM). Others have adopted modern styles that have little or no reliance on traditional principles.

Acupuncture needles are most often inserted at specific locations on the skin called *acupuncture points*. These points are located on specific lines outlined by tradition, referred to as *meridians* or *channels*. According to Chinese medical theory, there are 14 major meridians that form an invisible network connecting the body surface with the internal organs. Meridians are to conduct *Qi*, the energy or vital force of the body. Pain or illness is said to result from imbalances or blockages in the flow of *Qi* through the meridians. Acupuncture is traditionally thought to remove such blockages, restore the normal circulation of *Qi*, and improve overall health by promoting the balance of energy in the system. However, there is no scientific evidence for the existence of the meridians or Qi itself. (Meridians are not visible under a microscope and, contrary to popular belief, they do not match major nerve pathways.)

In addition to meridians and Qi, the concept of yin and yang is central to acupuncture theory, as it is to all of traditional Chinese philosophy. The terms *yin* and *yang* do not represent forces or substances; rather, they are a way to look at the world in terms of the interaction of polar opposites. According to this viewpoint, all movement, growth, and change in the world is a manifestation of the push and pull of these forces. Although seemingly in opposition, these forces are thought to complement and support each other. For example, without rest one cannot exert energy; without becoming tired by exerting energy, it is difficult to sleep. This is just one illustration of the harmony and interaction of yin and yang.

Yang is traditionally associated with heat, power, daylight, summer, and many other active or energetic aspects of life; yin is cold, quiet, and dark. Many illnesses are characterized in terms of an excess or deficiency of either yin or yang, or of both at the same time. For example, when the body is feverish, it is too yang as a whole. There is also a yin and yang balance in each individual organ and part of the body; these can become excessive or deficient too.

Thus, in TCM, illnesses are described as complex patterns of imbalances and blockages. Treatment is based not on medical diagnosis, but on identifying these problems in the body's energy and seeking to correct them. Does this traditional analysis contain truths about human health or is it just archaic thinking? The answer, as yet, remains unknown.

History of Acupuncture

Primitive acupuncture needles dating back to around 1000 B.C. have been discovered in archeological finds of the Shan dynasty in China. The theoretical framework underlying the practice of acupuncture was first set forth in the *Inner Classic of Medicine* or *Nei Jing*, first published in 206 B.C. during the Han dynasty.

As an active and growing tradition, the theory and practice of TCM evolved over the centuries, at times undergoing rapid changes. Acupuncture reached perhaps its golden age under the Ming dynasty in the late sixteenth and early seventeenth centuries. Subsequently, it took second place to an ascending practice of **herbal medicine**. By the time acupuncture came back in vogue in twentieth-century China, it had undergone a major transformation sometimes called the *herbalization of acupuncture*. Current acupuncture methods given the name Traditional Chinese Medicine are derived to a great extent from this relatively modern revision of the theory. Present-day Japanese acupuncture, however, dates back to earlier versions of acupuncture.

Another major change occurred after the Communist Revolution in 1949. The new leadership, while wanting to carry through a process of modernization, decided to support and preserve traditional medicine. During the Cultural Revolution, the famous "barefoot doctors" were trained in both modern and traditional medicine and sent out to the rural areas to provide medical care for the masses. Today, in the largest and most modern Chinese hospitals, Western medicine and TCM, including acupuncture and herbal treatments, are practiced side by side.

Acupuncture was virtually unheard of and unavailable in the U.S. until 1972, when President Nixon made his historic visit to China. Among the accompanying press was the well-known journalist James Reston, who was hospitalized while in China and received acupuncture anesthesia. Upon returning to the U.S., Reston published an article about his experience, stimulating new interest in acupuncture among the public and the medical community. Although it was later discovered that the drugs used along with acupuncture anesthesia probably played a major role, the perception of acupuncture as a powerful treatment caused it to gain respect in the U.S. Acupuncture schools began to open in the late 1970s and 1980s. With training available in the U.S., the number of acupuncturists in this country began to grow rapidly and today there are many thousands of certified and/or licensed acupuncturists.

How Does Acupuncture Work?

The exact mechanisms by which acupuncture might produce effects on the body remain unknown. Weak preliminary evidence from the 1970s hints that acupuncture encourages the release of endorphins (morphine-like compounds that function as the body's internal pain-regulating substances). Support for this theory comes from a study in which use of the drug naloxone, which opposes the effects of endorphins, was found to block pain relief from acupuncture. However, the body releases endorphins in response to any sort of pain and it may be that it is needle-insertion per se, and not acupuncture, that is responsible for the rise in endorphins. Furthermore, there is some evidence that the placebo effect itself works by means of endorphins—in one study, naloxone blocked the ability of a placebo treatment to reduce pain.

It has also been proposed that acupuncture may influence other chemicals in the body that control various physiologic activities. Preliminary studies have shown possible effects of acupuncture on norepinephrine, acetylcholine, and cyclic AMP, all of which are "chemical messengers" that regulate key systems in the body. However, none of this evidence is strong.

What Is the Scientific Evidence for Acupuncture?

Although there have been numerous controlled studies of acupuncture, there is no condition for which acupuncture's supporting evidence is strong. There are several reasons for this, but one is fundamental: even with the best of intentions, it is difficult to properly ascertain the effectiveness of a hands-on therapy such as acupuncture.

Only one form of study can truly prove that a treatment is effective: the double-blind, placebo-controlled trial. However, it isn't easy to fit acupuncture into a study design of this type. One problem is designing a form of placebo acupuncture and an even more challenging problem is to keep participants and practitioners in the dark regarding who is receiving real acupuncture and who is receiving fake. But without such blinding, the results of the study can be skewed by numerous factors. For a discussion of these factors, see **Why Does This Book Rely on Double-blind Studies?**.

In an attempt to approximate double-blind studies of acupuncture, researchers have resorted to a number of clever techniques. Perhaps the most common involves sham acupuncture. In such studies, a fake version of acupuncture is used to keep participants in the dark. However, because the acupuncturist knows that this is a fake treatment, he or she may subtly convey a lack of confidence in the outcome. Such studies are called *single-blind* and are not fully trustworthy. (The only exception are studies in which the patient is anesthetized prior to the acupuncture and is, therefore, presumably incapable of receiving this sort of "top spin.")

To get around this problem and produce a truly double-blind study, some studies may employ technicians trained only to insert needles, rather than real acupuncturists. Such technicians might be given a list of real acupuncture points or phony acupuncture points,

without being told which is which. However, it is not reasonable to suppose that an essentially untrained technician can give an acupuncture treatment as effective as that of a real acupuncturist. Furthermore, using a fixed set of points to treat a problem is not true to traditional acupuncture, which always individualizes treatment to the person.

Another approach is to use real acupuncturists to deliver treatment, but to have a separate person evaluate the effects of that treatment. Such studies may be described as partially double-blind (or *observer-blind*); they prevent researchers from biasing their own observations, but they still don't eliminate the problem that the acupuncturist might communicate confidence (or lack of it) to the participants. The placebo effect in acupuncture is very sensitive to expectation; in one study, patients who believed they were getting real acupuncture experienced benefits and those who believed they were getting fake acupuncture failed to experience benefits. Whether or not they were *actually* receiving real or fake acupuncture proved to be irrelevant; it was the belief that mattered. One naturally doubts whether acupuncturists are sufficiently adept at hiding their true feelings from their patients. Osteopathic physician Kerry Kamer suggested a whimsical approach to testing acupuncture: for the placebo group, use actors trained to convey confidence while performing fake acupuncture. However, such studies have not yet been reported.

Despite their limitations, most of the best studies available at present are the single-blind or partially double-blind designs described earlier. Although imperfect, they at least can give us some idea whether true acupuncture might be effective.

There is another problem to consider as well: acupuncture causes a very strong placebo effect, whether it's real or fake. This phenomenon tends to diminish the difference in results between the treatment group and the placebo group and can potentially hide a true benefit by making it too small to reach statistical significance. As an example, consider a study in which 67 people with hip arthritis received either random needle placement or actual acupuncture. The results showed improvement in both groups, but to the same extent. Does this mean that traditional acupuncture is actually no better than random acupuncture? Not necessarily. The study could simply have been too small to identify benefits that did occur. In studies that show a strong placebo effect, it may be necessary to enroll hundreds of participants to show benefit above statistical "background noise." Keep this in mind regarding all of the negative trials described below. A small study can fail to find benefit, but it cannot actually prove lack of benefit.

There is one additional problem in evaluating the evidence for acupuncture: many of the studies were performed in China, and there is evidence of systematic bias in the Chinese medical literature. Researchers evaluating the acupuncture studies from China discovered that every one found acupuncture effective! This led them to look further into other Chinese medical research. Upon review of controlled trials involving other therapies, such as standard drugs, it was noted that Chinese trials reported positive results 99% of the time. By comparison, trials published in England were positive only 85% of the time. Although some bias exists in all medical publications, this finding suggests a particularly high rate of bias in the Chinese research record.

Some studies have compared acupuncture to other therapies, such as physical therapy or **massage**. Trials of this kind are good for determining relative cost effectiveness, but they can't be taken as proof of efficacy for one simple reason: these other therapies have never been proven effective themselves.

Numerous acupuncture studies failed to use placebo treatment or had no control group at all. Such studies prove nothing and generally are not reported here.

The following sections begin with conditions in which acupuncture research has been most positive, continue with those for which the record is mixed, and conclude with those in which the tested form of acupuncture has not proved effective. Note that we also include studies of acupressure and electroacupuncture.

Evidence-based Uses
➣ *Nausea and Vomiting*
Numerous studies have evaluated treatment on a single acupuncture point—P6—traditionally thought to be effective for relief of various forms of nausea and vomiting. This point is located on the inside of the forearm, about 2 inches above the wrist crease. Most studies have investigated the effects of pressure on this point (acupressure) rather than needling. The most common methods involve a wristband with a pearl-sized bead in it situated over P6. The band exerts pressure on the bead while it is worn, and the user can press on the bead for extra stimulation.

Although the research record is mixed, on balance it appears that P6 stimulation offers at least modest benefits for nausea. This approach has been studied in

anesthesia-induced nausea, the nausea and vomiting of pregnancy, and other forms of nausea.

Anesthesia-induced Nausea General anesthetics and other medications used for **surgery** frequently cause nausea. At least nine controlled studies enrolling a total of more than 750 women undergoing gynecologic surgery found that P6 stimulation of various types reduced such postsurgical nausea as compared to placebo.

On the negative side, a double-blind, placebo-controlled study of 410 women undergoing gynecologic surgery failed to find P6 acupressure more effective than fake acupressure (both were more effective than no treatment). A small trial of acupuncture in gynecological surgery also failed to find benefit, as did three studies of acupressure for women undergoing C-section.

Studies of acupuncture or acupressure in other forms of surgery have produced about as many negative results as positive ones.

A 2004 review of the entire literature regarding P6 stimulation for postoperative nausea found a total of 26 studies. All of these studies suffered from significant flaws; however, on balance the reviewers found that they suggest stimulation of P6 does reduce postoperative nausea as compared to placebo.

One particularly interesting aspect of studies of acupressure for postsurgical nausea is that here a single-blind study is probably as good as a double-blind study. If the acupressure wrist band is not put on till after anesthesia has begun, no amount of confidence or lack of it by the practitioner is likely to alter the placebo effect experienced by the unconscious patient. Thus, studies of acupressure/acupuncture for this condition have a higher potential validity than studies for any of the other conditions listed below. The fact that benefits have been seen strongly suggests that stimulation of P6 does in fact affect nausea. That there is no clear physiological reason why this should be so makes this an intriguing finding, even if the benefit is too slight to make much real difference in postoperative care.

Nausea and Vomiting of Pregnancy Several controlled studies have evaluated the benefits of acupressure or acupuncture in the **nausea and vomiting of pregnancy**, commonly called *morning sickness*. The results for acupressure have generally been more positive than for acupuncture.

For example, a double-blind, placebo-controlled study of 97 women found evidence that wristband

Acupuncture

acupressure may work. Participants wore either a real wristband or a phony one that appeared identical. Both real and fake acupressure caused noticeable improvement in more than half of the participants. However, women using the real wristband showed better results in terms of the duration of nausea. Intensity of the nausea symptoms was not significantly different between groups.

These results are consistent with other studies of acupressure for morning sickness, though two studies failed to find benefit for severe morning sickness.

However, one large trial of *acupuncture* instead of acupressure failed to find benefit. This single-blind, placebo-controlled study of 593 pregnant women with morning sickness compared the effects of traditional acupuncture, acupuncture at P6 only, acupuncture at "wrong" points (sham acupuncture), and no treatment. As noted earlier, the placebo effect of acupuncture is very strong. Women in all three treatment groups (including the fake acupuncture group) showed significant improvements in nausea and dry retching compared to the no-treatment group. However, neither form of real acupuncture proved markedly more effective than fake acupuncture.

Other Forms of Nausea A single-blind, placebo-controlled study found acupressure helpful for **motion sickness**, though a similar study did not.

A single-blind, placebo-controlled trial of 104 people undergoing high-dose **chemotherapy** for breast cancer found that electrical stimulation on P6 significantly reduced episodes of vomiting. Similar improvements were found in a pilot study. In a small sham-controlled study, acupressure wristbands showed promise, although the benefit seen just missed the conventional cutoff for statistical significance. Equivocal or absent effectiveness were also seen in three other studies of wristbands and one study failed to find more benefit with real acupuncture than fake acupuncture.

⤞ Tendonitis
Several small controlled studies have found acupuncture helpful for **tendonitis**. For example, a single-blind, placebo-controlled trial of 52 people with rotator cuff (shoulder) tendonitis found evidence that acupuncture is more effective than placebo. Benefits were also seen in three other studies of people with shoulder or elbow tendonitis. However, one study failed to find benefit.

In a study of 82 people with elbow tendonitis, deep acupuncture was more effective than shallow acupuncture placebo in the short term, but by 3 months there was no difference between the groups.

A comparative trial of 20 people found weak evidence that electroacupuncture may be more effective than ordinary acupuncture for elbow tendonitis. Another trial failed to find laser acupuncture effective.

A 2004 systematic review found a total of five positive controlled studies on acupuncture for tennis elbow and concluded that "strong evidence" supports the use of acupuncture for this condition. However, this characterization of the evidence as strong would seem to be premature. For the reasons described in the beginning of this section, virtually all studies of acupuncture are single-blind and such studies (except when performed on anesthetized patients) cannot exclude the possible effect of confidence conveyed by practitioners performing valid treatment as compared to lack of confidence by those delivering sham treatment.

⤞ Osteoarthritis
Acupuncture has shown considerable promise for treatment of **osteoarthritis**. A review published in 2001 evaluated the results of studies of acupuncture for osteoarthritis of the knee. The reviewers found seven studies they rated as meaningful, involving a total of 393 participants. Although not all studies were positive, overall the reviewers concluded that "strong evidence" indicates that acupuncture is more effective for knee arthritis than sham acupuncture. Again, however, the characterization "strong" would seem to be premature for evidence involving single-blind studies.

A subsequent study of 294 people with osteoarthritis of the knee compared acupuncture, fake acupuncture, and no treatment. The results indicated that real acupuncture is more effective than fake acupuncture, but that the benefits fade with time after acupuncture is stopped. Another study, enrolling a total of about 100 people, found that acupuncture plus a standard anti-inflammatory drug was more effective than placebo acupuncture plus the drug. A study of 570 people also found benefit, but the dropout rate was so high as to make the results questionable.

Benefits have been seen in other forms of osteoarthritis as well. For example, a single-blind, controlled trial of 67 people with osteoarthritis of the hip found that acupuncture significantly improved symptoms, with relief lasting for months after the end of treatment. One small study found acupuncture more effective than advice and exercises for hip pain. However, yet another study found that insertion of needles at random spots in the general vicinity of the hip was just as effective as traditional acupuncture. Larger trials will be necessary to fully sort out acupuncture's effectiveness for hip pain.

Acupuncture for osteoarthritis in various joints has also been compared to anti-inflammatory drugs, steroid injections, and diazepam (Valium) with mixed results.

➣ Pregnancy Support

As noted above, acupuncture has shown some promise for reducing symptoms of morning sickness. Acupuncture has additionally shown promise for aiding **other aspects of pregnancy** as well.

A controlled study of 210 women giving birth found that real acupuncture was more effective than sham acupuncture at reducing labor pain. (Another study on this use of acupuncture was invalid because it lacked a placebo group—pain would be expected to respond well to acupuncture as a placebo treatment.)

A study of 45 pregnant women found that use of acupuncture on the expected birth due date significantly speeded up the actual date of delivery. However, this trial used a no-treatment control group instead of sham acupuncture.

Acupuncture has also been studied for converting breech presentation of the unborn infant to normal positioning. In a study of 240 women at 33 to 35 weeks gestation, acupuncture combined with **moxibustion** caused the breech presentation to convert in 54% of women, while only 37% of women in the no-treatment control converted. Again, placebo acupuncture would have been better than no treatment. A much smaller study also found benefits with acupressure.

➣ Headache

Acupuncture has shown some promise for various types of headaches, including **migraines** and **tension headaches**; however, the research record remains mixed and the more recent and better-designed studies have generally failed to find benefit. At present, it is unclear whether acupuncture offers any benefit for headaches beyond the placebo effect.

➣ Neck Pain

A 1999 literature review found one double-blind and eight single-blind, placebo-controlled trials of acupuncture for various forms of **neck pain**, enrolling a total of more than 250 participants. The results of these small trials are almost equally balanced: approximately as many found acupuncture superior to placebo as found it no better than placebo.

A subsequent study of 177 people with chronic neck pain compared acupuncture to placebo acupuncture, as well as massage. The results after five sessions showed no significant difference between real and fake acupuncture. Interestingly, even fake acupuncture produced better results than massage. Another study found acupuncture more effective than fake acupuncture, but only minimally.

Most studies of acupuncture have used the Chinese style called *TCM*. A single-blind, placebo-controlled trial of 45 people evaluated Japanese-style acupuncture in chronic neck pain and found benefit. Participants received twice-weekly treatments for 4 weeks, once-weekly treatments for 4 weeks, and then treatments every other week for 2 weeks. The results showed significant improvement in the group receiving actual treatment as compared to those in the control group.

In another study, use of laser acupuncture failed to provide benefit for whiplash injuries.

➣ Dental Procedures

The evidence regarding acupuncture treatment of dental pain is mixed. A literature review identified four meaningful studies on acupuncture for reducing pain during dental procedures. Three of the studies found positive results, but the largest (with 110 participants) found no benefit.

A more recent single-blind, controlled trial of 39 people, conducted by the author of two of the positive studies just mentioned, found acupuncture beneficial for pain control after oral surgery.

Although there are more studies with positive results than negative results, large trials are more meaningful than small ones. For this reason, it is difficult to draw any firm conclusions from this set of studies.

➣ Chemical Dependency

Although some animal studies suggest that ear acupuncture or electroacupuncture may have some benefits for **chemical dependency**, study results in humans have been mixed at best, with the largest studies reporting no benefits.

For example, a single-blind, placebo-controlled trial that evaluated 620 cocaine-dependent adults found acupuncture no more effective than sham acupuncture or relaxation training. Similarly, a single-blind, placebo-controlled study enrolling 236 residential clients found no benefit for cocaine addiction from ear acupuncture.

However, benefits were seen in a much smaller single-blind trial.

The situation is much the same for **alcohol addiction**. A single-blind, placebo-controlled study of 503 alcoholics failed to find evidence of benefit with 3 weeks of ear acupuncture. In addition, a 10-week, single-blind, placebo-controlled study of 72 alcoholics found no difference in drinking patterns or cravings between sham acupuncture and real acupuncture groups. Two other small trials also failed to find significant benefits. However, one single-blind trial of 54 people did find some evidence of improvement.

A single-blind, controlled trial of 100 people with heroin addiction evaluated the potential benefits of ear acupuncture. However, a high dropout rate makes the results difficult to interpret.

In a meta-analysis of 12 placebo-controlled trials, acupuncture was not found more effective than sham acupuncture for **smoking cessation**. A more recent observer-blind, sham-controlled study of 330 adolescent smokers also found no benefit. One study found that acupuncture may not be effective on its own, but may (in some unknown manner) increase the effectiveness of stop-smoking education. In this sham-controlled study of 141 adults, acupuncture plus education was twice as effective as sham acupuncture plus education and four times as effective as acupuncture alone. However, these benefits were only seen in the short term; at long-term follow-ups, the relative advantage of acupuncture disappeared.

➢ Back Pain

Thus far, research has not produced convincing evidence that acupuncture is effective for **back pain**. Many studies widely cited as providing such evidence were actually invalid due to lack of a proper control group. There is no doubt that people with back pain given acupuncture report benefits, but the problem is that people given fake acupuncture also experience benefits, often to a similar degree.

For example, in a single-blind, controlled trial of 113 people with back pain, 20 sessions of traditional acupuncture generally failed to produce significantly more benefit than sham acupuncture. Both sham and real acupuncture, however, were far more effective than no treatment, demonstrating once again the placebo power of acupuncture.

In a single-blind, controlled study (using sham acupuncture and no treatment) of 298 people with chronic back pain, use of real acupuncture failed to prove significantly more effective than sham acupuncture. Other studies enrolling a total of about 200 people have also failed to find benefit.

A trial compared the effects of acupuncture, massage, and education (such as videotapes on back care) in 262 people with chronic back pain over a 10-week period. The exact type of acupuncture and massage was left to practitioners, but only 10 visits were permitted. At the 10-week point, evaluations showed benefit with massage but not with acupuncture. One year later, massage and education were nearly equivalent and both were superior to acupuncture.

One small study found chiropractic spinal manipulation *more* effective than anti-inflammatory medication or acupuncture for low back pain.

In another trial, acupressure-style massage was found to be more effective for back pain than Swedish massage. However, Swedish massage has not been proven effective for back pain, so this does not prove that acupressure-style massage is effective.

Two single-blind, placebo-controlled trials, one with 30 participants and another with 60, also failed to find evidence of benefit.

Two studies did find possible slight benefits with electrical acupuncture for chronic low back pain. An additional study found acupressure more effective than physical therapy for low back pain and another found some potential benefit with electric acupuncture.

Several other studies have compared acupuncture to other treatments for back pain, such as TENS, physical therapy, and chiropractic care, and found them equally effective. However, because TENS, physical therapy, and chiropractic care have not been proven effective for back pain, studies of this type cannot be taken as evidence that acupuncture is effective. One study did find acupressure massage more effective than standard physical therapy; however, it was performed in a Chinese population that may have had more faith in this traditional approach than in physical therapy.

➢ Stroke

Acupuncture is widely used in China for treatment of acute **stroke**. A few controlled studies have been published over the last 10 years, but the best-designed and largest studies failed to find benefit.

For example, a single-blind, placebo-controlled trial of 104 people who had just experienced a stroke failed to find any benefit with 10 weeks of twice-weekly acupuncture.

Similarly, a single-blind, controlled study of 150 people recovering from stroke compared acupuncture (including electroacupuncture), high-intensity muscle stimulation, and sham treatment. All participants received 20 treatments over a 10-week period. Neither acupuncture nor muscle stimulation produced any benefits. A 10-week study of 106 people, which provided a total of 35 traditional acupuncture sessions, also failed to find benefit.

A few studies did find benefit, but they were very small and some did not use a placebo group.

Other Studied Uses

Acupressure and acupuncture have been tried for **insomnia**, with mixed results. A single-blind, placebo-controlled study involving 84 nursing home residents found that real acupressure was superior to sham acupressure for improving sleep quality. Treated participants fell asleep faster and slept more soundly. Another single-blind, controlled study reported benefits with acupuncture, but failed to include a proper statistical analysis of the results. For this reason, no conclusions can be drawn from the report. In a third study, 98 people with severe kidney disease were divided into three groups: no extra treatment, 12 sessions of fake acupressure (not using actual acupuncture points), and 12 sessions of real acupressure. Participants receiving real acupressure experienced significantly improved sleep as compared to those receiving no extra treatment. However, fake acupressure was just as effective as real acupressure. In one study, magnetic pearls used to stimulate acupuncture points in the ear seemed to show some benefit as compared to nonmagnetic stimulation of ear points.

One small double-blind, placebo-controlled study found real acupuncture more effective than sham acupuncture for **menstrual pain**. (This study used non-acupuncturists given real or fake acupuncture protocols to apply, unbeknownst to them.) In addition, a controlled study of 61 women evaluated the effects of a special garment designed to stimulate acupuncture points related to menstrual pain. Unfortunately, in this latter study, researchers chose to compare treatment to no treatment, rather than to sham treatment. For this reason, the results (which were positive) mean little.

Although anesthesia apparently performed entirely with acupuncture first raised Western interest in acupuncture, the original demonstrations of acupuncture anesthesia have been discredited. It now appears that if acupuncture has any anesthetic effect, it is extremely modest, at most capable of slightly decreasing the required dose of general anesthetic necessary to induce anesthesia (but even this has not been consistently seen in studies). One double-blind study failed to find electroacupuncture effective for reducing anesthesia requirements during surgery.

One study found possible marginal benefit with acupuncture and moxibustion for the treatment of **Crohn's disease**.

A 6-month, single-blind, controlled study of 67 women with frequent **bladder infections** found that acupuncture therapy reduced the frequency of infection. Another study found that acupuncture may be helpful for hyperactive bladder (frequent need to urinate without the presence of an infection).

A study of 52 people with **allergic rhinitis** (hay fever) found that acupuncture plus Traditional Chinese herbal treatment was slightly more effective than fake acupuncture plus fake Chinese herbal treatment. However, another study failed to find acupuncture alone beneficial for allergic rhinitis.

A Chinese study found that acupuncture plus moxibustion was more effective for **Bell's palsy** than drug treatment.

A review of acupuncture for **fibromyalgia** found three controlled studies, only one of which was of adequate quality. This trial enrolled 70 people and followed them for 3 weeks; some evidence of benefit was seen. A subsequent study (published only in abstract form) also found acupuncture more effective than placebo acupuncture in amplifying the effects of standard treatment (antidepressants), However, the largest and most rigorous studies have failed to find acupuncture more effective than fake acupuncture for fibromyalgia.

Two small controlled studies found preliminary evidence that acupuncture can improve **menopausal symptoms**. Another study failed to find benefits with electroacupuncture.

A sham-acupuncture controlled trial evaluated 43 people with **depression** and 13 with generalized **anxiety disorder**. The results suggest that 10 (but not 5) acupuncture sessions can significantly improve symptoms.

Another trial compared real and sham ear acupuncture in healthy people and found some evidence that real acupuncture can relieve normal daily **stress**.

A small study found acupuncture more effective than sham acupuncture for **impotence**.

Although open trials appeared to show benefit, a placebo-controlled study failed to find acupuncture helpful for improving the success rate of in vitro fertilization.

Acupuncture has been explored as a means of reducing pain after **surgery**, but the results so far have been equivocal. A double-blind, placebo-controlled study of 42 people undergoing arthroscopic knee surgery found that the use of acupuncture during surgery did not reduce pain levels during the subsequent 24 hours. Another double-blind, placebo-controlled trial of 50 women undergoing hysterectomy found no benefit with electroacupuncture, and a double-blind study of 71 people undergoing abdominal surgery failed to find acupressure helpful. However, some benefits of acupressure were reported in a single-blind trial of 40 patients undergoing arthroscopic knee surgery. In addition, a special form of needle insertion called *intradermal acupuncture* reduced postsurgical pain in 107 people undergoing abdominal surgery. Ear acupuncture has also shown promise.

Acupuncture may be as effective as standard treatments for **Temporomandibular joint (TMJ) pain**. For example, a study of 110 people with TMJ pain found acupuncture at least as effective as standard occlusal splint therapy.

Although acupuncture is widely used for **weight loss**, there is only weak, inconsistent evidence that it works.

A single-blind trial tested acupuncture on a group of 36 healthy young men and found some evidence of improvement in **sports performance**. However, a single-blind, controlled study of 48 people found that use of acupuncture did not reduce **muscle soreness caused by exercise**.

Although case reports suggest that acupuncture might be helpful for **psoriasis**, a controlled trial failed to find acupuncture more effective than fake acupuncture.

One study purportedly found that acupressure reduced fatigue in people with severe kidney disease. In fact, however, it found that both sham acupuncture and real acupuncture reduced fatigue as compared to no treatment but that real acupuncture was *not* more effective than fake acupuncture.

One study found minimal benefits for **Parkinson's disease**. Another study failed to find any benefits.

A Chinese study reported that acupuncture is helpful for vocal cord dysfunction.

After an acute attack of shingles, pain may linger for months or years, causing what is known as **post-herpetic neuralgia**. A single-blind, placebo-controlled study of 62 people with pain of this type failed to find any benefit with acupuncture.

A double-blind, placebo-controlled study tested the effect of single-point acupuncture versus placebo acupuncture in 56 people with **rheumatoid arthritis**. There

was no difference in results between the real treatment and placebo groups. However, using a single acupuncture point to treat a complex disease such as rheumatoid arthritis must be regarded as highly questionable; normally, acupuncture for such a complex condition would involve many needles.

There have been numerous reports about acupuncture treatment for **asthma**, but most published studies are of low quality and the results have been contradictory at best. One study failed to find acupuncture helpful for shortness of breath associated with advanced cancer.

Peripheral neuropathy (nerve pain in the extremities) is a common complaint in **HIV** infection. A placebo-controlled trial of 239 people with HIV found acupuncture no more effective than placebo in peripheral neuropathy. Interestingly, the study also tested drug therapy for peripheral neuropathy and found it ineffective as well.

A single-blind, controlled trial of individualized acupuncture for 34 people with severe **epilepsy** found no benefit. Another small study found no benefit with standardized acupuncture for **Raynaud's phenomenon**.

One controlled study failed to find electroacupuncture effective for reducing discomfort during colonoscopy.

A controlled study purportedly found acupuncture helpful for speeding recovery in people with spinal cord injuries, but it failed to use a sham-acupuncture control group.

Several controlled and open trials of acupuncture for **tinnitus** (ringing in the ear) found no benefit.

A well-designed, single-blind, placebo-controlled study of 60 people with **irritable bowel syndrome** compared traditional acupuncture to sham acupuncture. Over the 13-week study period, both groups improved to the same extent. Two other studies have also failed to find acupuncture more effective than placebo acupuncture.

In a placebo-controlled trial, 60 **nursing** women received needle acupuncture, 56 women received laser acupuncture, and 60 women received placebo acupuncture. The results showed no differences in milk production.

What to Expect During an Acupuncture Treatment

Acupuncture therapy has its own style and atmosphere, both like and unlike an ordinary medical encounter. Your first session will begin with a thorough analysis of your condition and health history. If the acupuncturist practices according to the principles of TCM, you will be asked a number of questions about your specific complaint and your general health, including how well you sleep, digest your food, eliminate, and breathe; your energy level; and so forth. All of these factors are considered relevant. The acupuncturist may ask questions that seem to have little bearing on your condition, such as, "Do you tend to feel cold or hot most of the time?" TCM looks for overall patterns in both physical and emotional well-being, which guide the acupuncturist in developing a treatment plan that is specific not only for your symptoms, but for your overall health pattern.

Depending on your specific complaint and your individual symptom pattern, the acupuncturist may use only a few needles or as many as 20 or more. Acupuncture needle sizes are typically 32 to 36 gauge, which means they are about ¼ mm in diameter, much smaller than a hypodermic needle. Unlike hollow hypodermic needles, acupuncture needles are solid, which allows them to penetrate the skin easily and relatively painlessly. Acupuncture needles may produce a mild pricking sensation when inserted, but sometimes you will feel nothing at all as the needle is inserted. The needles are generally inserted to a depth ranging from a few millimeters to ½ inch or so. Insertion depth is deeper at the more fleshy areas of the body, such as the thighs and buttocks.

Acupuncture needles are typically inserted through a plastic tube that guides the needle into the skin. This is a fairly modern needle insertion technique. Traditional freehand insertion is also used; most acupuncturists are trained in this method. Virtually all acupuncturists in the United States now use presterilized, one-time-use disposable needles, which eliminates any risk of cross-infection.

The acupuncturist may twirl the inserted needles and ask you to say when you feel a mild achy, heavy sensation; or the area may feel slightly numb or tingly. These sensations, described in TCM as the *arrival of Qi*, are regarded as a positive response that will enhance the effectiveness of the treatment.

Whatever you feel, the sensation should be mild, not overly unpleasant, and should subside within a few minutes. If any needles are genuinely painful, inform the practitioner so he or she can adjust the depth or remove the needle altogether. The needles are generally left in place for 20 to 30 minutes. During this time, you should feel comfortable and relaxed and you may fall asleep.

Acupuncturists may also employ a technique known as *electroacupuncture*, in which electrodes are attached to the needles and a mild current is applied. This is in-

tended to increase the stimulation of the needle and is generally used for more painful conditions. Electroacupuncture produces a tingly, pulsating sensation. The acupuncturist can control the intensity and adjust it to a level that is comfortable for you.

Traditionally trained acupuncturists often use heat as well as needles to stimulate acupuncture points with a procedure called *moxibustion*, which involves a mixture of herbs rolled into a cigarlike shape. The moxa roll is lit and the burning end is held over the skin, allowing the heat to penetrate the area around the acupressure point. The roll never touches the skin, so you will not be burned. The acupuncturist will ask you to let him/her know before it gets too hot. Moxibustion is generally quite pleasant. It is regarded as a "tonifying" treatment, which means it is intended to strengthen function.

How to Choose a Qualified Acupuncturist

Acupuncture is a licensed health profession in 39 states and the District of Columbia. Most states require at least 3 years of training at an accredited school of acupuncture and passage of a national board certification exam administered by the National Certification Commission for Acupuncture and Oriental Medicine (NCCAOM). Most states grant the title Licensed Acupuncturist, Certified Acupuncturist, Registered Acupuncturist, or simply Acupuncturist. A few states allow acupuncturists who have a doctorate from an approved or accredited college to use the title Doctor of Oriental Medicine (D.O.M.) or Oriental Medical Doctor (O.M.D.).

In most states, medical doctors can practice acupuncture with no training; in many states, chiropractors may practice acupuncture with 100 or fewer hours of training.

Approximately one-third of the states that license acupuncturists require their clients to have a referral from a Western medical practitioner (an M.D., osteopath, chiropractor, or dentist) prior to or in conjunction with acupuncture treatment. In the remaining states, acupuncturists may accept patients without prior referral.

Training programs have become fairly standardized in recent years, so an acupuncturist with qualifications in one state has essentially the same training as in other states. If you are in a state that does not license acupuncturists, ask to see evidence that the acupuncturist has completed at least 3 years of training at an accredited institution. Check with your state medical board for the exact licensure title and requirements in your state.

States that License Acupuncturists:

The following states license acupuncturists:

Alaska	Idaho	Montana	Rhode Island
Arizona	Illinois	Nevada	South Carolina
Arkansas	Indiana	New Hampshire	Tennessee
California	Iowa	New Jersey	Texas
Colorado	Lousiana	New Mexico	Utah
Connecticut	Maine	New York	Vermont
District of Columbia	Maryland	North Carolina	Virginia
Florida	Massachuetts	Ohio	Washington
Georgia	Minnesota	Oregon	West Virginia
Hawaii	Missouri	Pennsylvania	Wisconsin

For a list of licensed acupuncturists in your area, contact the National Acupuncture and Oriental Medicine Alliance at P.O. Box 738, Gig Harbor, Washington 98335; phone: (253) 238-8133.

This organization also has an informative Web site (www.aomalliance.org) with an acupuncturist referral list and other useful information about training and qualifications.

Safety Issues

Serious adverse effects associated with the use of acupuncture are rare. The most commonly reported problems include short-term pain from needle insertion, tiredness, and minor bleeding. There is one report of infection caused by acupuncture given to a person with diabetes.

Some acupuncture points lie over the lungs and insertion to excessive depth could conceivably cause a pneumothorax (punctured lung). Because acupuncturists are trained to avoid this complication, it is a rare occurrence.

A recent report from China contained an example of another complication caused by excessively deep needling. A 44-year-old man was needled on the back of the neck at a commonly used acupuncture point just below the bony protuberance at the base of the skull. However, the acupuncturist inserted the needle too deeply and punctured a blood vessel in the skull. The client developed a severe headache with nausea and vomiting; a CAT scan showed bleeding in the brain and a spinal tap found a small amount of blood in the cerebrospinal fluid. The severe headache, along with neck stiffness, continued for 28 days. The man was treated with standard pain medication and the condition resolved itself without any permanent effects.

Infection due to the use of unclean needles has been reported in the past, but the modern practice of using disposable sterile needles appears to have eliminated this risk.

Aromatherapy

ALTERNATE NAME: *Essential Oils*

PRINCIPAL PROPOSED USES:

Inhaled: *Reducing Anxiety, Decreasing Agitation in People with Alzheimer's Disease or Other Forms of Dementia*

Oral: *Acute Bronchitis, Acute Sinusitis, Chronic Bronchitis, Common Cold*

OTHER PROPOSED USES:

Inhaled: *Chronic Bronchitis, Common Cold, Enhancing Memory and Mental Function, Insomnia, Nausea, Pregnancy Support, Smoking Cessation*

Topical: *Alopecia, Athlete's Foot, Insect Bites, Pregnancy Support, Tension Headaches, Vaginal Infections*

Oral: *Dyspepsia, Irritable Bowel Syndrome*

Overview

Aromatherapy is actually a form of herbal medicine. However, instead of using the entire herb, it employs the fragrant "essential oil" that is released when a fresh herb is compressed or subjected to chemical extraction. Essential oils are also often used as fragrances in cosmetics and bath products.

When employed medicinally, essential oils are often evaporated into the air through the use of a humidifier. The famous Vicks VapoRub® is a gel form of the essential oils of peppermint, eucalyptus, and camphor. Essential oils may also be applied directly to the skin or clothes so they will release their odor near the patient.

Essential oils may be inhaled, taken by mouth, or applied to the skin.

What Is Aromatherapy Used For?

Inhaled aromatherapy has become a popular, gentle treatment to reduce mild anxiety. It has also been tried for a variety of respiratory conditions, post-surgical nausea, and tension headaches.

Topical treatment with essential oils has shown possible value for fungal infections and hair loss. Oral use of essential oils has shown promise for various digestive and respiratory problems.

What Is the Scientific Evidence for Aromatherapy?

There is a major difficulty in studying aromatherapy by inhalation: how to conduct a double-blind, placebo-controlled trial. For the results of a study to be truly reliable, both participants and researchers must be kept in the dark regarding participants who received real treatment and who received placebo. (For more information on why this is so crucial, see **Why Does This Book Depend on Double-blind Studies?**.) Although it may be possible to keep researchers in the dark regarding which group is which, participants will certainly be aware of whether they smell something or not! Researchers have used various clever compromises in an effort to partially solve this problem. For example, some studies used a control group that received an aromatic substance believed to be ineffective. Unfortunately, it's just as hard to prove that an aromatic substance is ineffective as it is to prove that it's effective! If the placebo in a study is just as effective as the tested treatment, the study will falsely indicate that the tested treatment is ineffective.

In other studies, researchers tricked participants in the control group and told them that they might be receiving an active but odorless treatment, when in fact they were simply given an inactive treatment without much in it. Compromises such as these are necessary. Unfortunately, most published studies on aromatherapy were also poorly designed in various unnecessary ways, making their results unreliable.

These problems do not arise to the same extent in studies of essential oils taken by mouth or applied directly to the skin.

Inhalation of Essential Oils
➤ *Calming Effects*

Preliminary controlled trials suggest that aromatherapy might be helpful for calming people with **Alzheimer's disease and other forms of dementia**. For example, in one interestingly designed, but very small study, a hospital ward was suffused with either lavender oil or water for two hours. An investigator who was unaware of the study's design and who wore a device to block inhalation of odors entered the ward and evaluated the behavior of the 15 residents, all of whom had dementia. The results indicated that use of lavender oil aromatherapy modestly decreased agitated behavior. Furthermore, in a double-blind study of 71 people with severe dementia, use of a lotion containing essential oil of **lemon balm** reduced agitation compared to placebo lotion. Another set of researchers, however, point out that the ability to detect odors greatly decreases in Alzheimer's disease and suggest that the benefits seen in the second study involved absorption of the herb through the skin rather than a true influence via aroma. This does not explain the results seen in the first study, however, and somewhat casts doubt on the results.

Several relatively poorly designed studies hint that aromatherapy combined with **massage** may help to relieve **anxiety** in people without Alzheimer's disease. Another study suggests that aromatherapy with geranium oil might modestly reduce anxiety levels (again in people without Alzheimer's). However, in a trial of 66 women waiting to undergo abortions, 10 minutes of inhaling the essential oils of vetivert, bergamot, and geranium failed to reduce anxiety significantly more than placebo treatment. In another study, **rosemary** oil failed to reduce tension during an anxiety-provoking task and might have actually *increased* anxiety.

➤ *Cigarette Addiction*

A controlled study suggests that inhalation of black pepper vapor may reduce the craving for cigarettes. In this trial, a total of 48 smokers used cigarette substitute devices that delivered black pepper vapor, menthol, or no fragrance. The results showed that use of the black pepper–based dummy cigarette reduced symptoms of craving for the first morning cigarette.

➤ *Tension Headaches*

Weak evidence hints that **peppermint** oil applied to the forehead might relieve **tension headaches**.

A topical ointment known as Tiger Balm has also shown promise for headaches. Tiger Balm contains camphor, menthol, cajaput, and clove oil. A double-blind study enrolling 57 people with acute tension headache compared the application of Tiger Balm to the forehead against placebo ointment as well as the drug acetaminophen (Tylenol). The placebo ointment contained mint essence to make it smell similar to Tiger Balm. Real Tiger Balm proved more effective than placebo and just as effective and more rapid-acting than acetaminophen.

➤ *Other Conditions*

Weak evidence suggests that inhaled peppermint oil might relieve **post-surgical nausea**.

Inhaled peppermint oil may also be helpful for relieving mucus congestion of the lungs and sinuses; however, there is only weak supporting evidence for this use.

Controlled studies have evaluated proprietary-inhaled aromatherapy preparations for treating the **common cold** and preventing flare-ups of **chronic bronchitis**, but the results were marginal at best.

A controlled study evaluated rosemary and also lavender aromatherapy for **enhancing memory and mental function**, but found results that were mixed at best.

In a large, controlled trial (more than 600 participants), lavender oil in bathwater failed to improve pain after **childbirth**. However, lavender oil has shown a bit of promise for **insomnia**.

Another large study failed to find aromatherapy more helpful than placebo for reducing psychological distress among people undergoing **radiation therapy for cancer**.

Oral Use of Essential Oils
➤ *Respiratory Problems*

Eucalyptus is a standard ingredient in cough drops and cough syrups, as well as in oils added to humidifiers. A standardized combination of eucalyptus oil plus two other essential oils has been studied for effectiveness in a variety of respiratory conditions. This combination therapy contains cineole from eucalyptus, d-limonene from citrus fruit, and alpha-pinene from pine. Because these oils are all in a chemical family called *monoterpenes*, the treatment is called **essential oil monoterpenes**.

Most, though not all, double-blind studies, some of which were quite large, indicate that oral use of essential oil monoterpenes can help colds, sinus infections, and acute bronchitis. For example, a 3-month, double-blind trial of 246 people with chronic bronchitis found that consumption of essential oil monoterpenes helped prevent the typical worsening of chronic bronchitis that occurs during the winter. Another study evaluated 676 male and female outpatients with *acute* bronchitis and found that essential oil monoterpenes were more effective than placebo. Essential oil monoterpenes are thought to work by thinning mucus, though they may have other effects.

Eucalyptus oil alone may be helpful for respiratory problems as well. In a double-blind trial, 32 people on steroids to control severe **asthma** (steroid-dependent asthma) were given either placebo or essential oil of eucalyptus for 12 weeks. The results showed that people using eucalyptus were able to gradually reduce their steroid dosage to a greater extent than those taking placebo. In another study, eucalyptus oil proved helpful for the treatment of "head cold" symptoms (technically, nonpurulent rhinosinusitis). In this double-blind, placebo-controlled study of 152 people, use of cineole at a dose of 200 mg 3 times daily markedly improved cold symptoms as compared to placebo.

➢ Digestive Problems

A double-blind, placebo-controlled study of 39 people found that an enteric-coated peppermint-**caraway** oil combination taken 3 times daily by mouth for 4 weeks significantly reduced **dyspepsia** pain as compared to placebo. Of the treatment group, 63.2% of participants were pain-free after 4 weeks, compared to 25% of the placebo group. Similarly, results from a double-blind comparative study of 118 people suggest that the combination of peppermint and caraway oil is comparably effective to the standard drug cisapride, which is no longer available. After 4 weeks, the herbal combination reduced dyspepsia pain by 69.7%, whereas the conventional treatment reduced pain by 70.2%.

A preparation of peppermint, caraway, fennel, and **wormwood** oil was compared to the drug metoclopramide in a double-blind study enrolling 60 people. After 7 days, 43.3% of the treatment group was pain-free, compared to 13.3% of the metoclopramide group.

Oral use of peppermint oil has shown considerable promise for **irritable bowel syndrome**. However, most studies were relatively poorly designed.

One study found preliminary evidence that a complicated mixture of essential oils (taken by gargle or mouth spray) might be helpful for reducing snoring symptoms.

Topical Use of Essential Oils

Tea tree oil, an essential oil from the plant *Melaleuca alternifolia*, possesses antibacterial and antifungal properties. It has been tried for various forms of **vaginal infection**, but the only supporting evidence for this use comes from an uncontrolled trial. There is slightly better evidence to support the use of tea tree oil for the treatment of **athlete's foot** and related fungal infections. One open study hints that oil of **bitter orange**, a flavoring agent from dried bitter orange peel, might have some effectiveness against athlete's foot when applied topically.

Topical essential oils might be helpful for **alopecia areata**, a form of hair loss that can occur in men and women. In a 7-month, double-blind, placebo-controlled trial, 84 people with alopecia areata massaged either essential oils or a non-treatment oil into their scalps each night for 7 months. The treatment oil contained essential oils of thyme, rosemary, lavender, and cedarwood. The results showed that 44% of the treatment group experienced new hair growth, compared to only 15% of the control group.

Cineol (from eucalyptus) has shown some effectiveness for repelling **mosquito bites**.

One study in rats indicates that under some circumstances essential oils instilled into the ear may be able to penetrate the eardrum. This supports the idea of treating **otitis media**, the typical ear infection of childhood, with herbal ear drops, it also raises concerns about possible harm to the middle ear.

Finally, for literally hundreds of essential oils, test-tube studies show antimicrobial effects (activity against fungi, bacteria, and/or viruses). Presumably, essential oils are part of the plants' own defenses against such organisms. However, contrary to widespread claims, such studies do *not* indicate that these essential oils can work as antibiotics; innumerable substances kill microorganisms in the test tube but not when taken orally by people. (Bleach would be one good example!)

How Might Aromatherapy Work?

It's not clear how inhaled aromatherapy works (assuming that it does). Possibly, enough is inhaled through the lungs to produce meaningful concentrations of herbal chemicals in the body. It is also possible that aromatherapy might work through the olfactory centers of the brain. In other words, a pleasant fragrance may be soothing, refreshing, calming, and stimulating—hardly a revolutionary concept!

How to Choose an Aromatherapy Practitioner

For all intents and purposes, licensure in aromatherapy does not exist. For this reason, the best way to find a qualified practitioner is to seek a referral from a health care professional.

Safety Issues

Essential oils can be toxic when taken internally, producing unpleasant and even fatal effects. Toxicity studies have not been performed for many essential oil products and maximum safe dosages remain unknown. Infants, children, seniors, and people with severe illnesses should not use essential oils internally except under the supervision of a physician; healthy adults should only use well-established products (such as peppermint oil) for which safe dosages have been determined.

Inhaled or topical use of essential oils is much safer than oral use. However, allergic reactions to inhaled or topical plant fragrances are not uncommon. Furthermore, when applied to the skin, some essential oils might also promote sunburning (photosensitization), raise the risk of skin cancer, or be absorbed sufficiently to cause toxic effects.

Ayurveda

RELATED TERMS: *Ayurvedic Herbs*

PRINCIPLE PROPOSED USES:

Acne: *Fixed combination containing oral and topical* Aloe barbadensis, Azardirachta indica, Curcuma longa, Hemidesmus indicus, Terminalia chebula, Terminalia arjuna, *and* Withania somnifera

Allergies: *Septilin—fixed combination containing* Commiphora mukul, Tinospora cordifolia, Rubia cordifolia, Emblica officinalis, Moringa pterygosperma, *and* Glycyrrhiza glabra

Angina: Terminalia arjuna, *Alba—fixed herbal combination containing* Terminalia arjuna *and approximately 40 other herbs*

Asthma: *Boswellia, Tylophora*

Bed-wetting: *Mentat—fixed herbal combination containing* Bacopa monniera *and approximately 30 other ingredients*

Colds and Flus: *Andrographis*

Diabetes: *Fenugreek, Gymnema, Diabecon—fixed herbal combination containing* Gymnema sylvestre, Eugenia jambolana, Tinospora cordifolia, Pterocarpus marsupium, Ficus glomerata, Momordica charantia, *and* Ocimum sanctum

Enhancing Immunity: *Septilin—fixed combination containing* Commiphora mukul, Tinospora cordifolia, Rubia cordifolia, Emblica officinalis, Moringa pterygosperma, *and* Glycyrrhiza glabra

Enhancing Memory: Bacopa monniera, *Mentat—fixed herbal combination containing* Bacopa monniera *and approximately 30 other ingredients*

Hemorrhoids: *Pilex—fixed combination oral and topical herbal treatment*

Hepatitis: *Phyllanthus, Picrorhiza kurroa, Kamalahar—fixed combination containing* Tecoma undulate, Phyllanthus urinaria, Embelia ribes, Taraxacum officinale, Nyctanthes arbortistis, *and* Terminalia arjuna

Nausea: *Ginger*

Osteoarthritis: *Articulin-F—fixed combination containing* Boswellia serrata, Withania somnifera, Curcuma longa, *and zinc*

Rheumatoid Arthritis: *Boswellia*

Rotator Cuff Injury: *Rumalaya—fixed oral and topical combination containing nearly 15 herbs*

Ayurveda (continued)

Stress and Fatigue: *Mentat—fixed herbal combination containing* Bacopa monniera *and approximately 30 other ingredients*

Varicose Veins: *Gotu Kola*

Weight Loss and Cholesterol Reduction: *Three fixed herbal combinations*

OTHER PROPOSED USES:

Aging: *Geriforte—fixed herbal combination containing approximately 40 herbs,*

Asthma: *Astha-15—fixed herb combination containing 15 herbal ingredients*

Atherosclerosis: *Garlic*

Attention Deficit Disorder: *Mentat—fixed herbal combination containing* Bacopa monniera *and nearly 30 other ingredients*

Depression: *Mentat—fixed herbal combination containing* Bacopa monniera *and nearly 30 other ingredients*

Dyspepsia: *Turmeric*

Epilepsy: *Mentat—fixed herbal combination containing* Bacopa monniera *and nearly 30 other ingredients*

Fluid Retention: *Dandelion*

Heart Disease: *Garlic*

Hypertension: *Alba—fixed herbal combination containing* Terminalia arjuna *and approximately 40 other herbs*

Febrile Seizures: *Mentat—fixed herbal combination containing* Bacopa monniera *and nearly 30 other ingredients*

Improving Immunity: *DefensePlus™—fixed combination containing* Tinospora cordifolia, Withania somnifera, Ocimum sanctum, *and* Emblica officinalis

Reducing Cholesterol: *Garlic, Guggul*

Rheumatoid Arthritis: *RA-1—fixed combination containing ashwagandha, boswellia, ginger, and turmeric*

Stroke: *Mentat—fixed herbal combination containing* Bacopa monniera *and nearly 30 other ingredients*

Overview

Ayurveda, the ancient healing system of India, is one of the great healing traditions of the world. Like traditional Chinese medicine, with which it has many historical connections, Ayurveda is a holistic medical system grounded in a comprehensive philosophical/spiritual view of life.

Ayurvedic treatment is highly individualized and incorporates a wide range of methods, including dietary changes, herbal therapy, exercise, massage, meditation, and numerous special procedures such as cleansing of the nasal passages. Although the scientific base for Ayurveda is not yet strong, some of its methods have undergone meaningful scientific evaluation, and worldwide interest continues to increase.

The History of Ayurveda

The roots of Ayurveda lie in the ancient Sankhya school of Indian philosophy, developed many thousands of years ago. The first major classic of Ayurveda, the *Caraka Samhita*, was written down between the second and fourth centuries B.C., but it is believed to be based on a much older oral tradition. This text sets out all the fundamental principles of Ayurveda but concentrates most of its attention on digestion (described as internal fire, or *agni*). Another early classic, the Susruta Samhita, focuses on surgical techniques. The *Astanga Hridayam*, written in about 500 A.D., sets out most of the detailed principles of Ayurveda, including the *dosha* and *subdosha*. (See The Principles of Ayurveda for more information.)

Ayurvedic thinking exerted a strong influence during the formation of traditional Chinese medicine, which in turn influenced Ayurveda's further development. The Ayurvedic technique of pulse-taking may have been derived from Chinese medical theory. Furthermore, translations of Ayurvedic texts influenced Islamic and European medicine.

In modern India, Ayurveda is one of three widely available forms of medicine, along with **homeopathy** and conventional medicine. It has become increasingly popular in the West as well, largely through the work of Deepak Chopra, Vasant Lad, and Maharishi Mahesh Yogi (the founder of transcendental meditation, or TM).

The Principles of Ayurveda

Even a basic introduction to the principles of Ayurveda exceeds the scope of this article. Consider the following information as nothing more than a taste of this vast medical system.

In Ayurvedic theory, the body is said to contain three primal forces (*tridosha*) that work in tandem: *vata*, *pitta*, and *kapha*. These *dosha*, in turn, are formed from combinations of five elements that control the universe: space, air, fire, water, and earth. The *dosha vata* includes space and air; it controls movement. *Pitta* is made of fire and water; it controls digestion and metabolism. *Kapha* is composed of earth and water; it forms the body's structures. Each person can be said to be dominated by one or two of these *dosha*, and may therefore be called a *vata*, *pitta*, *kapha*, *vata-pitta*, *vata-kapha*, or *pitta-kapha* type.

There are many other aspects of the body considered in Ayurveda as well. These include 20 attributes, 5 sub-*doshas*, 7 tissues, 4 states of *agni*, and 14 bodily systems. Health exists when all aspects of the body are in proper balance; disease occurs when that balance is disturbed. Excess *vata*, for example, might lead to arthritis, anxiety, and fatigue. Excess *kapha*, on the other hand, is said to cause obesity and diabetes.

The Practice of Ayurveda

The practice of Ayurveda is intrinsically holistic and preventive in intent. Perfect health in the Ayurvedic system involves not only physical wellness, but also emotional, mental, and spiritual perfection. Treatment aims to promote and maintain balance in order to prevent or, when necessary, cure disease.

One of the primary methods of healing in Ayurveda involves diet. Foods are thought specifically to strengthen or weaken various *doshas*; therefore, people are prescribed a diet according to their constitutions. This method is different from the dietary approaches used in conventional medicine or the natural medicine systems that arose in the West (such as naturopathy). We tend to see certain foods as healthy and others as unhealthy; in Ayurveda, what's good for one person is bad for another and vice versa. For example, a person tending toward an excess of *vata* might be advised to avoid raw vegetables but consume nuts and seeds in abundance; someone with an excess of *kapha* would be given the opposite recommendation. To make matters more complex, dietary recommendations may vary from season to season, and frequently include numerous details about the optimal ways to prepare and consume foods.

Herbs (both culinary and medicinal) are another mainstay of Ayurvedic treatment. For example, people with a *vata* constitution are thought to benefit from turmeric, cumin, coriander, ginger, **garlic**, and **fenugreek**. But again, some of these herbs might not be healthy for a person with a different constitution.

In addition to cooking spices, Ayurveda also uses purely medicinal herbs, which include **andrographis**, ashwagandha, *Bacopa monnieri* (Brahmi), *Boswellia serrata*, *Coleus forskohlii*, **dandelion**, **gotu kola**, gymnema, **guggul**, **neem**, phyllanthus, and **tylophora**. Minerals such as silver, mercury, and lead may be used as well (see Safety Issues below).

Ayurvedic therapy also has an exercise component known as hatha yoga. In general, the practice of yoga is believed to promote good health; in addition, certain postures are believed to offer assistance in specific medical conditions.

Like Chinese medicine with its acupuncture needles, Ayurveda has additional characteristic methods. One set of its therapies is collectively called *panchakarma*. This is a method of purification that may involve massage, *shirodhara* (extended pouring of warm oil on the "third eye" point in the center of the forehead), emetics, purgatives, enemas, cleansing of the nasal passages with various substances, and bloodletting. Additionally, the drinking of urine is recommended in certain situations.

What Is the Scientific Evidence for Ayurveda?

It is undoubtedly true that all people are different, and that the ideal form of medicine should take such differences into account. Ayurveda's strength in this regard is one of its sources of appeal. However, the mere fact that medicine ought to treat people individually doesn't imply that Ayurveda's individualized treatment techniques are actually grounded in reality. They could be wishful thinking rather than an insight into the truth.

It is very difficult to scientifically validate entire systems of health. In medicine, only double-blind, placebo-controlled trials produce scientifically reliable results. However, there is really no way to fit Ayurvedic medicine into such a format. Try to invent a method for keeping people in the dark regarding whether or not they are, for example, taking enemas, and you will see the difficulty.

Thus, it isn't possible to make a scientifically grounded statement regarding the effectiveness of Ayurveda as a whole. We do have some evidence for a subset of Ayurveda: its herbal therapies.

Many Ayurvedic herbs taken alone have undergone varying levels of study. Most of these are described elsewhere in this book, under the articles titled andrographis (for colds and flus), ashwagandha, boswellia (for rheumatoid arthritis, asthma), *Coleus forskohlii* (for asthma), dandelion (for diuretic, to help treat fluid retention), fenugreek (for diabetes), garlic (for high cholesterol, heart disease), gymnema (for diabetes), ginger (for nausea), gotu kola (for varicose veins), guggul (for high cholesterol), neem, phyllanthus (for hepatitis), turmeric (for dyspepsia), and *tylophora* (for asthma).

Other Ayurvedic herbs that have been studied in double-blind, placebo-controlled trials are discussed below. In addition, we discuss fixed combinations of multiple herbs that have undergone such trials.

Many other Ayurvedic herbal combinations have been studied in trials of lower quality, but because only double-blind, placebo-controlled studies can actually prove the effectiveness of a treatment, those studies are not reported here.

Even the double-blind, placebo-controlled studies we report below fall far short of modern scientific standards and independent confirmation of results is usually lacking. Nonetheless, the results described below are at least somewhat encouraging.

Single Herbs
➣ *Angina:* Terminalia arjuna
In a double-blind study, 58 men with chronic stable **angina** received either *Terminalia arjuna* (500 mg every 8 hours), the drug isosorbide mononitrate (40 mg daily), or a matching placebo for 1 week each. The results indicated that use of *T. arjuna* was more effective than placebo for angina and approximately as effective as the medication.

In another study, 105 men with coronary heart disease received either placebo, vitamin E, or *T. arjuna* (500 mg daily) for 30 days. The results indicated that the herb reduced cholesterol levels. However, the researchers inexplicably decided to make this an "open label" study, meaning that participants and researchers knew which treatment was which. Because of this, the results are essentially meaningless.

➣ *Hepatitis:* Picrorhiza kurroa
In a double-blind trial of 33 people with acute viral **hepatitis**, use of *Picrorhiza kurroa* at a dose of 375 mg 3 times daily significantly speeded recovery time as compared to placebo.

➣ *Memory and Mental Function:* Bacopa monniera (*brahmi*)
The Ayurvedic herb *Bacopa monniera* (brahmi) has a traditional reputation for **improving memory**. However, a 12-week, double-blind, placebo-controlled trial of 76 people that tested the potential memory-enhancing benefits of brahmi generally failed to find much evidence of benefit. The only significant improvement seen among the many measures used was in one that evaluated retention of new information. Although this may sound at least a little positive, in fact it means little. Here's why: When a study uses many different techniques to assess improvement, mere chance ensures that at least one of them will come up with results. Properly designed studies should focus on one test of benefit alone (the primary outcome measure) that is selected prior to running the trial. The use of multiple tests is sometimes called "fishing for results" and it is frowned upon.

However, if several independent studies use multiple tests of improvement and the pattern of response is reliably maintained, then the results begin to appear more significant. In a previous double-blind, placebo-controlled study

Ayurveda

enrolling 46 people, use of brahmi over a 2-week period produced quite a different pattern of benefits. In another double-blind, placebo-controlled study of 38 people, short-term use of brahmi failed to produce any measurable improvements in memory.

In yet another study, one-time combined treatment with *Ginkgo biloba* (120 mg) and brahmi (300 mg) failed to improve mental function.

Combination Therapies
➢ Allergies and Immunity: Septilin
Septilin is a fixed combination containing the following ingredients:

➢ *Commiphora mukul*
➢ *Tinospora cordifolia*
➢ *Rubia cordifolia*
➢ *Emblica officinalis*
➢ *Moringa pterygosperma*
➢ *Glycyrrhiza glabra*

This combination therapy has shown promise for the treatment of **allergic rhinitis**. In a double-blind study, 190 people were given either the herbal combination or a standard antihistamine (chlorpheniramine). The results over 7 days indicated that the two treatments were equally effective.

Another study found general evidence for an antihistamine-like effect. In this double-blind, placebo-controlled trial of 32 healthy people, use of Septilin for 4 weeks significantly reduced the allergic reaction caused by injection of histamine under the skin.

Septilin has also been tried as a treatment for improving immunity. In a double-blind, placebo-controlled study of 40 children with persistent low-grade infections (such as chronic sore throat or sinus infection), use of Septilin for 1 month led to significant improvement compared to placebo.

➢ Various Brain-related Disorders: Mentat—Fixed herbal combination containing Bacopa monniera *and almost* 30 *other ingredients*
The proprietary Ayurvedic mixture Mentat has been studied for numerous brain-related conditions. For example, in a 3-month, double-blind, placebo-controlled study of 50 adult students, use of Mentat appeared to improve memory and attention and **reduce stress**. Similarly, in a 3-month, double-blind, placebo-controlled trial of 42 people in high-stress jobs who complained of **fatigue**, use of Mentat decreased symptoms.

In several double-blind, placebo-controlled trials, Mentat has shown promise for normalizing the behavior of children with **attention deficit disorder**, developmental disabilities, or brain damage.

Other double-blind, placebo-controlled trials found evidence that this combination therapy might be helpful for **depression**, **epilepsy**, decreasing amnesia caused by ECT (electroconvulsive therapy), reducing frequency of febrile seizures (seizures caused by fever), enhancing recovery from aphasia (loss of speech caused by stroke), and improving memory in people with **anxiety**. Mentat has also shown promise for **bed-wetting**.

➢ Acute Hepatitis: Kamalahar
Kamalahar is a fixed combination containing the following ingredients:

➢ *Tecoma undulata*
➢ *Phyllanthus urinaria*
➢ *Embelia ribes*
➢ *Taraxacum officinale*
➢ *Nyctanthes arbortistis*
➢ *Terminalia arjuna*

In a double-blind, placebo-controlled study, 52 people with acute hepatitis were randomly assigned to receive placebo or this combination herbal therapy at a dose of 500 mg, 3 times daily for 15 days. The results indicate that the herbal combination improved liver function to a significantly greater extent than placebo.

➢ Other Liver-Related Conditions: Liv.52
Liv.52 is a fixed combination containing the following ingredients:

➢ *Capparis spinosa*
➢ *Cichorium intybus*
➢ *Solanum nigrum*
➢ *Terminalia arjuna*
➢ *Cassia occidentalis*
➢ *Achillea millefolium*
➢ *Tamarix gallica*

In a poorly reported, 5-week, double-blind, placebo-controlled study of 30 children with hepatitis A, use of this combination formula apparently improved the rate of recovery compared to placebo. Benefits were also seen in a 6-week study of 34 people with acute hepatitis A.

Another double-blind, placebo-controlled study evaluated the effectiveness of Liv.52 in a variety of liver conditions. A total of 104 people were enrolled in this trial and divided into three groups depending on the liver condition they had: **cirrhosis**, acute hepatitis, and chronic hepatitis (type not stated). Participants with cirrhosis were treated for 24 months, those with chronic active hepatitis were treated for 12 months, and participants with hepatitis A were treated for only 6 weeks. Use of Liv.52 was associated with substantially better outcomes than placebo. Apparent benefits were also seen in a 6-month, double-blind, placebo-controlled study of 36 people with cirrhosis. However, in a 6-month, double-blind study of 80 people with alcoholic liver disease (alcoholic hepatitis or cirrhosis), Liv.52 failed to provide any benefits.

➣ *Frozen Shoulder: Rumalaya—Fixed oral and topical combination containing almost 15 herbs*

In a placebo-controlled trial of 100 people with rotator-cuff injury ("frozen shoulder"), use of this tablet and cream combination significantly improved results, compared to little improvement in the placebo group.

➣ *Weight Loss and Cholesterol Reduction: Three different fixed combinations*

In a 3-month, double-blind, placebo-controlled study, 70 overweight people were divided into four groups: placebo; triphala guggul (a mixture of five Ayurvedic ingredients) plus Gokshuradi guggul (a mixture of eight Ayurvedic ingredients); triphala guggul plus Sinhanad guggul (a mixture of six Ayurvedic herbs); or triphala guggul plus Chandraprabha vati (a mixture of 36 Ayurvedic ingredients). Reportedly, all three Ayurvedic ingredients produced significant **weight loss** and **improvements in cholesterol** relative to placebo; furthermore, the improvements produced by each of the treatments were close to identical.

➣ *Osteoarthritis: Articulin-F*

Articulin-F is a fixed combination containing the following ingredients:

- ➣ *Boswellia serrata*
- ➣ *Withania somnifera*
- ➣ *Curcuma longa*
- ➣ *Zinc*

In a 3-month, double-blind, placebo-controlled trial of 42 people with **osteoarthritis**, use of this combination therapy significantly improved pain and disability compared to placebo.

➣ *Diabetes: Diabecon*

Diabecon is a fixed herbal combination containing the following ingredients:

- ➣ *Gymnema sylvestre*
- ➣ *Eugenia jambolana*
- ➣ *Tinospora cordifolia*
- ➣ *Pterocarpus marsupium*
- ➣ *Ficus glomerata*
- ➣ *Momordica charantia*
- ➣ *Ocimum sanctum*

In a 6-month, double-blind, placebo-controlled trial, 40 people with type 2 **diabetes** who had failed to respond fully to oral drugs received either this combination of Ayurvedic herbal therapy or placebo. The results indicated that the herbal therapy was modestly helpful.

➣ *Acne: Fixed topical and oral combination*

This fixed topical and oral combination contains the following ingredients:

- ➣ *Aloe barbadensis*
- ➣ *Azadirachta indica*
- ➣ *Curcuma longa*
- ➣ *Hemidesmus indicus*
- ➣ *Terminalia chebula*
- ➣ *Terminalia arjuna*
- ➣ *Withania somnifera*

In a 4-week, double-blind study, 53 people with **acne** received one of four therapies: real herb in oral tablets and as topical cream; real herb in oral tablets and as topical gel; real herb in oral tablets with placebo gel; or placebo tablet with placebo topical treatment. The results appear to indicate that while oral herb alone is not helpful, oral herb plus topical herb can improve acne symptoms.

➣ *Improving Immunity: DefensePlus™*

DefensePlus™ is a fixed combination containing the following ingredients:

- ➣ *Tinospora cordifolia*
- ➣ *Withania somnifera*
- ➣ *Ocimum sanctum*
- ➣ *Emblica officinalis*

Test tube and animal trials suggest that this combination product may strengthen the **immune response**. Promising results have also been seen in two unpublished human trials. One was a double-blind, placebo-controlled trial of children ages 5 to 18 who experienced recurring bouts of tonsillitis. The results showed that participants taking the herbal combination were less likely to require surgical treatment for the condition (tonsillectomy). The other double-blind, placebo-controlled study found that use of this herbal combination along with standard therapy improved recovery from eye conditions requiring antibiotics.

➢ *Rheumatoid Arthritis: RA-1*

RA-1 is a fixed combination containing extracts of **ashwagandha**, boswellia, **ginger**, and **turmeric**.

A 16-week, double-blind, placebo-controlled trial of 182 people with **rheumatoid arthritis** evaluated the potential effectiveness of this formula. Participants in both groups improved significantly; however, according to most measures of disease severity, the benefits of the herbal combination were no greater than those of placebo.

➢ *Hemorrhoids: PILEX—Fixed combination oral and topical herbal treatment*

This combination therapy was evaluated in a double-blind, placebo-controlled trial of 100 people with **hemorrhoids**. The results indicated that the benefits were seen in 50% of those using the herbal treatment as compared to only 20% in the placebo group.

➢ *Hypertension and Angina: Alba— Terminalia arjuna and approximately 40 other herbs*

In a double-blind study of 43 men and women with **hypertension**, use of the proprietary herbal combination Alba proved approximately as effective for controlling blood pressure as the drug methyldopa. Additionally, in a double-blind, placebo-controlled trial of 25 people with angina, use of this combination therapy reduced chest pain and improved heart function.

➢ *Aging: Geriforte—Fixed herb combination containing approximately 40 herbs*

A fixed combination of Ayurvedic herbs has been marketed as a general "tonic" for seniors. Several poorly designed and/or incompletely reported placebo-controlled trials suggest that this herbal combination might possibly improve cholesterol levels, general well-being, and mood in seniors.

➢ *Astha 15—Fixed herb combination containing 15 herbs*

One double-blind comparative study provides weak evidence that the herbal combination called Astha 15 might be helpful for mild **asthma**.

How to Choose a Practitioner of Ayurvedic Medicine

There is no widely accepted licensure for the practice of Ayurvedic medicine. However, there are several schools that offer extensive training. These schools generally require from 500 to 3,500 hours of training. Some of the better-known schools include the following:

The Ayurvedic Institute
11311 Menaul NE, Albuquerque, NM, 87112
Phone: (505) 291-9698
Web site: *http://www.ayurveda.com*
E-Mail: *info@ayurveda.com*

California College of Ayurveda
1117A East Main Street, Grass Valley, CA, 95945
Enrollment: (866) 541-6699
General Information: (530) 274-9100
Web site: *http://www.ayurvedacollege.com*
E-Mail: *info@ayurvedacollege.com*

American Institute of Vedic Studies
P.O. Box 8357, Santa Fe, NM, 87504-8357
Phone: (505) 983-9385
Web site: *http://www.vedanet.com*
E-Mail: *Vedicinst@aol.com*

Safety Issues

Ayurvedic therapy presents numerous potential safety concerns. One serious problem is that many Ayurvedic herbs have never undergone a formal safety evaluation, and those that have been evaluated have not necessarily been proven harmless. For more information on safety risks with individual Ayurvedic herbs, see the following articles: **androgrphis, ashwagandha, boswellia, *Coleus forskohlii*, dandelion, fenugreek, garlic, ginger, gotu kola, guggul, gymnema, neem, phyllanthus, turmeric,** and **tylophora.**

Most of the proprietary herbal formulas described in this article have undergone a certain amount of safety testing by the manufacturer and were found reassuringly non-toxic; however, verification of safety by independent laboratories that maintain modern standards remains limited.

There are other concerns as well. For example, oral silver, a traditional Ayurvedic remedy, can cause permanent gray-black staining of the skin and mucous membranes.

In addition, some traditional Ayurvedic formulas may contain toxic levels of heavy metals; in one case report, a brain-damaged child born to a mother using an Ayurvedic formula was found to have the highest bloods levels of lead ever recorded in a living newborn. Analysis of the formula revealed a very high lead content, along with toxic levels of mercury.

The dietary recommendations made within the context of Ayurvedic theory could conceivably lead to inadequate intake of essential nutrients, and hence malnutrition. However, most reputable Ayurvedic practitioners are well aware of modern nutrition knowledge and take care to make reasonable recommendations within that context.

Finally, various traditional Ayurvedic techniques, such as blood-letting and drinking urine, clearly suggest possible health risks. Fortunately, most modern Ayurvedic practitioners shun the most worrisome of these methods.

Bach Flower Remedies

In the early part of the twentieth century, a British physician named Edward Bach developed a system of healing based on flowers. Each of these "Bach flower remedies" was created by dipping a particular type of flower in water and then preserving the fragrant liquid with brandy. According to Dr. Bach, the appropriately chosen flower could be used to treat emotional problems, such as shyness, anxiety, and grief. Bach flower remedies are sometimes compared to **homeopathy**, but they differ because they do not use extreme dilutions.

Numerous additional remedies were added to the original repertory proposed by Bach and this form of treatment is widely used today. However, there is no scientific evidence that any Bach flower remedy produces a medicinal effect and there is some evidence that the method does not work.

In 2001, a double-blind, placebo-controlled study tested whether a particular combination of Bach flower remedies could relieve the **anxiety** that students experience while taking exams. The trial used a mixture containing 10 flower extracts: impatiens, mimulus, gentian,

chestnut bud, rock rose, larch, cherry plum, white chestnut, scleranthus, and elm. (An expert in the use of Bach flower remedies suggested this particular combination.) A total of 61 students were enrolled in the study; 55 completed it. Each participant received either the Bach flower remedy or placebo for a period of 2 weeks leading up to an exam. Participants answered a questionnaire to assess their anxiety levels before starting treatment and just prior to the test. Unfortunately, the use of Bach flower remedies did not measurably reduce anxiety levels compared to placebo.

A previous study also evaluated the use of a Bach flower remedy (Rescue Remedy) for treating test anxiety and found no benefit. However, more than 50% of the participants dropped out, making the results of that trial unreliable.

A double-blind study reported in 2005 failed to find Bach flower remedies more effective than placebo for treatment of **attention deficit disorder**.

At the very least, Bach flower remedies should be harmless because they are sufficiently diluted to minimize the presence of any active ingredients.

Biofeedback

PRINCIPAL PROPOSED USES: *High Blood Pressure*

OTHER PROPOSED USES: *Anxiety, Back Pain, Defecation Problems in Children and Adults, Female Stress Incontinence, Insomnia, Migraine Headaches, Pain in General (Many Types), Raynaud's Disease, Rehabilitation from Strokes, Stress*

Overview

Some functions in the body occur automatically, outside of conscious control (such as heart rate and blood pressure). Biofeedback is a method of making those "involuntary" processes something you can do at will.

The basic method is quite simple. In biofeedback, a machine gives you direct information regarding the bodily process in question (the "feedback" part of the term "biofeedback"). Given this information, you can find a way to control it, just like you can learn to wiggle your ears if you try hard enough.

For example, your blood pressure might be displayed on a screen. Blood pressure naturally goes up and down from time to time. When it goes down, you'll notice that and feel pleased; when it goes up, you'll feel displeased. Pleasure and displeasure act like the reward-and-punishment technique used for training animals. When a rat in a maze is rewarded with food for going the right way and given an electric shock for going the wrong way, it will soon learn to go the right way. Similarly, the unconscious parts of the nervous system figure out a way to get a "reward" instead of receive "punishment." In the case just described, this means reducing blood pressure.

The display screen provides the feedback because normally we can't detect our own blood pressure. Using a machine to provide that information allows the person to achieve conscious control. This process generally works, at least to a modest extent. After a number of sessions, most people reach a place where they can lower their blood pressure simply by thinking, "I want my blood pressure to fall." They don't know how they're doing it (any more than ear wigglers know how they've accomplished that); nonetheless, they can cause the desired effect.

In addition to measuring blood pressure and heart rate, there are biofeedback machines in fairly common use that measure muscle tension, skin temperature, skin resistance to electricity, and brain-wave activity.

What Is Biofeedback Used For?

Probably the most common use of biofeedback is to treat **stress** and stress-related conditions, including **anxiety**, **insomnia**, **high blood pressure**, **fibromyalgia**, muscle pain, **migraine headaches**, and **tension headaches**.

What Is the Scientific Evidence for Biofeedback?

Although many studies have evaluated biofeedback, most of them suffer from inadequate design. Only one form of study can truly prove that a treatment is effective: the double-blind, placebo-controlled trial. (For more information on why such studies are so crucial, see **Why Does This Book Rely on Double-blind Studies?**.)

However, it is somewhat tricky to fit biofeedback into a study design of this type. The main problem is finding a placebo for biofeedback treatment. In the best-designed studies of biofeedback, people in the placebo group practice biofeedback with a machine that produces carefully garbled information. Study participants in this group believe they are practicing biofeedback, but in fact they are not learning any conscious control over the body process in question.

Many biofeedback studies do not use placebo biofeedback; they compare biofeedback to no treatment. Studies of this type cannot provide reliable evidence about the efficacy of a treatment. If a benefit is seen, there is no way to determine whether biofeedback caused it or whether it was caused generically by attention. (Attention alone will almost always produce some reported benefit.)

Other trials used intentionally neutral therapies, such as the use of a home diary. These are better than studies with a no-treatment control group. However, when the placebo is so different in form than the treatment under study, any apparent differences in outcome could simply represent differences in the power of suggestion in each approach.

Still other studies simply involved giving people biofeedback and seeing whether they improved. Such trials are almost completely meaningless; numerous studies have shown that both participants and examining physicians will frequently think they observe improvement in people given a treatment, regardless of whether the treatment does anything on its own. For example, early studies of biofeedback for stroke rehabilitation that did not use blinding or a control group reported miraculous successes equivalent to the "throw down your crutches and walk" cliché. However, when controlled trials were performed, it turned out that biofeedback did not provide much more than marginal benefit, if any. For this reason, we do not even report uncontrolled studies below.

Given these caveats, the following is a summary of what science knows about the medical benefits of biofeedback.

Possible Effects of Biofeedback

Of all the medical conditions for which biofeedback has been advocated, the best studied is **hypertension**. One review of the literature found 23 controlled trials of acceptable quality. Taken as a whole, these studies suggest that biofeedback can reduce blood pressure by approximately 5%, a modest but useful improvement.

In one of the best of these studies, 30 people with mild hypertension received 8 sessions of real or placebo biofeedback in the laboratory, followed by 12 home sessions. After 4 weeks, the results showed that blood pressure measurements in the treated group decreased by an average of 11 mm systolic (the upper number in the blood pressure reading) compared to only 4 mm improvement in the placebo group, for a net improvement of 7 mm. This difference was statistically significant.

In another study, this ability was found to be fostered by true biofeedback but, not surprisingly, suppressed over time by false biofeedback.

The evidence is less positive for several other conditions. The balance of the evidence suggests that biofeedback is *not* effective for **asthma** or defecation problems in children and adults, and that it is no more than marginally effective for **Raynaud's disease**.

Biofeedback has been studied for numerous other medical conditions as well. At least one controlled study supports the use of biofeedback for each of the following: **Anxiety**, **chronic low back pain**, female stress incontinence, **insomnia**, headaches (including **migraine** and **tension** headaches), and, possibly, rehabilitation from **strokes**. Note that the evidence of benefit with biofeedback is not definitive for any of these conditions and, in many cases, there are also studies with negative outcomes.

What to Expect During a Biofeedback Session

As described above, biofeedback training involves the use of a machine that relays information about the aspect of the body that you wish to control. In early stages, the trick is finding the "muscles" necessary to produce the desired effect. Typically, a biofeedback practitioner will teach a series of visualizations and other mental exercises in the hope that it will facilitate the process. For example, if you have high blood pressure, you might be asked to imagine the blood vessels in your body opening up and dilating. (It is not precisely clear that such methods work, but at the very least they give you something to do consciously while your brain solves the problem.)

Ability in biofeedback comes in fits and starts and grows with practice. The initial sessions are done with a practitioner, but once your abilities start to develop you will be asked to continue to work with a biofeedback machine at home. Ordinarily, several sessions of training and weeks of daily home practice are required to achieve the desired effect.

How to Choose a Biofeedback Practitioner

As with all medical therapies, it is best to choose a licensed practitioner in states where a biofeedback license is available. Where licensure is not available, seek a referral from a qualified and knowledgeable health care provider.

Safety Issues

There are no known safety risks with biofeedback.

Chelation Therapy

ALTERNATE NAME: *EDTA Chelation*

Overview

When medical researchers first investigated the phenomenon known as *hardening of the arteries* (closely related to **atherosclerosis**), they discovered that the damaged, brittle vessels found in people with heart disease were lined with calcium deposits. Naturally, this finding inspired the notion that calcium deposits were the cause of the problem.

Some early researchers investigated the possible therapeutic effect of removing such deposits. However, subsequent research indicated that the calcium deposits of atherosclerosis were a symptom rather than a cause and mainstream interest turned elsewhere. Certain physicians nonetheless maintained an interest in removing calcium; thus chelation therapy was born.

Chelation therapy for heart disease consists of intravenous infusions of a chemical called *ethylenediaminetetraacetic acid* (EDTA). This synthetic substance is used in conventional medicine to remove heavy metals, such as lead, from the body, but it also has an effect on calcium, which is why it came into use in chelation therapy.

Proponents claim that EDTA chelation is an effective alternative to heart surgery and that it also offers many other health benefits. To support this, they cite numerous anecdotes of cures apparently brought about by its use. However, anecdotes cannot possibly prove a treatment effective. (For a detailed explanation of why this is the case, see **Why Does This Book Rely on Double-blind Studies?**) Only double-blind, placebo-controlled trials can do so and, thus far, such studies have failed to find chelation therapy effective.

In 2000, a highly respected researcher reviewed the literature on chelation therapy and concluded, "The most striking finding is the almost total lack of convincing evidence for efficacy. . . . Only two controlled clinical trials were located. They provide no evidence that chelation therapy is efficacious beyond a powerful placebo effect. . . . Given the potential of chelation therapy to cause severe adverse effects, this treatment should now be considered obsolete."

Subsequent to this review, a well-designed study compared chelation therapy to placebo in 84 people with coronary artery disease. People receiving EDTA chelation showed improvement; however, those receiving placebo also improved—to the same extent! This finding reminds us why double-blind, placebo-controlled studies are necessary to establish the effectiveness of a treatment. If researchers had performed this study without a placebo group, they might have concluded that EDTA chelation really works. Instead, the fact that the same level of benefits was seen in the fake-treatment group indicates that chelation therapy does not work.

Another double-blind study evaluated the potential benefits of chelation therapy when added to conventional therapy in the treatment of people with coronary artery disease. Researchers were looking for improvements in the ability of a blood vessel in the arm (the brachial artery) to dilate, but did not find any. However, this study had several limitations in its design, making its results less meaningful than they might have been.

Safety Issues

Not only does it appear to be ineffective, EDTA chelation therapy may present some safety risks. This treatment is generally given in a series of 10 to 30 sessions. If the practitioner fails to take proper precautions, severe adverse consequences, such as kidney damage, may result. While it appears to be the case that properly performed chelation therapy is unlikely to cause harm, we do not see any justification for using such an invasive method, in the absence of evidence that it will help.

Chiropractic

RELATED TERMS: *Spinal Manipulation; Manipulation, Spinal*

PRINCIPAL PROPOSED USES: *Back Pain, Migraine Headaches, Neck Pain, Tension Headaches*

OTHER PROPOSED USES: *Asthma, Bedwetting, Dysmenorrhea (Menstrual Pain), High Blood Pressure, Infantile Colic, Phobias, Premenstrual Syndrome (PMS)*

Overview

Chiropractic is one of the most widely used health services today. It has gained increasing acceptance as a treatment for back and neck pain and is covered by many health insurance plans. Millions of people would report that chiropractic spinal manipulation has brought them relief. Nonetheless, at present the research record for its effectiveness is inconclusive at best.

History of Chiropractic

Daniel David Palmer founded chiropractic in 1895, after an experience in which he apparently believed he cured a man's deafness by manipulating his back. He opened the Palmer School of Chiropractic and began teaching spinal manipulation. This college still exists today, with a fully accredited program.

One of Palmer's first students was his son, Bartlett Joshua (B.J.) Palmer. It was B.J. Palmer who truly popularized the technique. Later, Willard Carver, an Oklahoma City lawyer, opened a competing school. He believed that chiropractic physicians needed to offer other methods of treatment in addition to spinal manipulation. This opened a schism in the chiropractic world that still exists today. Followers of Palmer and his methods focus only on spinal adjustments, an approach called *straight* chiropractic. Those who, like Carver, use various approaches to healing are called *mixers*. Mixers may use vitamins, herbs, and any other treatment methods they find useful (and are allowed to practice by law).

Medical treatments in the nineteenth and early twentieth centuries were not based on scientific evidence of effectiveness and chiropractic treatment was no exception. It became a widespread technique long before there was any real evidence that it worked. Chiropractic schools utilized all of their profits and resources to further develop programs for training people in chiropractic techniques—not for verifying the theory and practice of chiropractic. However, in the 1970s proper scientific research into chiropractic began to draw interest. In 1977, the Foundation for Chiropractic Education and Research (FCER) established a program to train chiropractic researchers. Since then, efforts have been made to fund scientific trials testing the effectiveness of chiropractic techniques and to establish a scientific foundation for the practice.

Forms of Spinal Manipulation

There are many different chiropractic techniques in use today, some with proprietary names such as the Gonstead and Maitland techniques. In general, most involve rapid (high-velocity) short (low-amplitude) thrusts. Manipulation may be purely manual or mechanically assisted. For example, some chiropractors use an *activator*—a small metal tool that applies a force directly to one vertebra.

In addition, some chiropractors use a related therapy called *spinal mobilization*. This method involves gentle, extended movements (low-velocity, high-amplitude), rather than the "back-cracking" of classic chiropractic spinal manipulation.

How Does Chiropractic Spinal Manipulation Work?

Since its origin, chiropractic theory has based itself on *subluxations*, or vertebrae that have shifted position in the spine. These subluxations are said to impede nerve outflow and cause disease in various organs. A chiropractic treatment is supposed to "put back in" these "popped out" vertebrae; for this reason, it is called an *adjustment*.

However, no real evidence has ever been presented showing that a given chiropractic treatment alters the position of any vertebrae. In addition, there is as yet no real evidence that impairment of nerve outflow is a major contributor to common illnesses or that spinal manipulation changes nerve outflow in such a way as to affect organ function.

More recent theories suggest that chiropractic manipulation may relieve pain by "loosening" vertebrae that have become relatively immobile rather than by changing their position. In addition, the sudden movements of manipulation may alter the response patterns of nerves in the spine (technically, dorsal horn neurons), again relieving pain.

What Is Chiropractic Used For?

Chiropractic spinal manipulation is widely used for the treatment of back pain, neck pain, and headaches, whether acute or chronic. It is also frequently tried for pain in other areas, such as the shoulders, knees, and jaw, as well as for breech birth positioning of a baby, infantile colic, frequent colds, and many other conditions.

Some chiropractic physicians promote "comprehensive chiropractic care" as a means of staying healthy. This approach may include diet, exercise, and supplements, along with regular chiropractic manipulation.

What Is the Scientific Evidence for Chiropractic Spinal Manipulation?

Chiropractic spinal manipulation has been evaluated scientifically to determine its efficacy, as well as its costs comparative to other forms of health care. However, the evidence is not compelling in either case.

Efficacy

Although there is some evidence that chiropractic spinal manipulation may be helpful for various medical purposes, in general the evidence is not strong. There are several reasons for this, but one is fundamental: Even with the best of intentions, it is difficult to properly ascertain the effectiveness of a hands-on therapy like chiropractic.

Only one form of study can truly prove that a treatment is effective: the double-blind, placebo-controlled trial. (For more information on why such studies are so crucial, see **Why Does This Book Rely on Double-blind Studies?**.) However, it isn't easy to fit chiropractic into a study design of this type. Consider the obstacles: What could researchers use for placebo chiropractic treatment? And how could they make sure that both participants and practitioners would be kept in the dark

regarding who was receiving real chiropractic manipulation and who was receiving fake manipulation?

Because of these problems, all studies of chiropractic manipulation fall short of optimum design. Many have compared chiropractic treatment against no treatment. However, studies of this type cannot provide reliable evidence about the efficacy of a treatment. If a benefit is seen, there is no way to determine whether it was caused by chiropractic manipulation specifically or just attention generally. (Attention alone will almost always produce some reported benefit.)

More meaningful trials used some sort of unrelated fake treatment for the control group, such as phony laser acupuncture. However, it is less than ideal to use a placebo treatment that is so very different in form from the treatment under study.

Better studies compare real chiropractic manipulation against sham forms of manipulation, such as light touch. Studies of this type are a definite step forward. However, it is quite likely that the practitioners at least unconsciously conveyed more enthusiasm and optimism when performing the real therapy than the fake therapy; this, too, could affect the outcome.

It has been suggested that the only way to get around this problem would be to compare the effectiveness of trained practitioners to actors trained only enough to provide a simulation of treatment; however, such studies have not been reported.

Still other studies have simply involved treating people with chiropractic spinal manipulation and seeing whether they improve. These trials are particularly meaningless; it has been long since proven that both participants and examining physicians will at least think that they observe improvement in people given a treatment, regardless of whether the treatment does anything on its own.

Finally, other trials have compared chiropractic manipulation to competing therapies, such as **massage therapy** or conventional physical therapy. However, neither of these therapies has been proven effective. When you compare unproven therapies to each other, the results cannot possibly prove that any of the tested treatments are effective.

Given these caveats, we discuss below what science knows about the effects of chiropractic.

Costs

Besides effectiveness, another important consideration is cost of care. There are many aspects to the cost of treatment, including number of visits to the chosen provider,

Chiropractic

real evidence that impairment of nerve outflow is a major contributor to common illnesses or that spinal manipulation changes nerve outflow in such a way as to affect organ function.

More recent theories suggest that chiropractic manipulation may relieve pain by "loosening" vertebrae that have become relatively immobile rather than by changing their position. In addition, the sudden movements of manipulation may alter the response patterns of nerves in the spine (technically, dorsal horn neurons), again relieving pain.

What Is Chiropractic Used For?

Chiropractic spinal manipulation is widely used for the treatment of back pain, neck pain, and headaches, whether acute or chronic. It is also frequently tried for pain in other areas, such as the shoulders, knees, and jaw, as well as for breech birth positioning of a baby, infantile colic, frequent colds, and many other conditions.

Some chiropractic physicians promote "comprehensive chiropractic care" as a means of staying healthy. This approach may include diet, exercise, and supplements, along with regular chiropractic manipulation.

What Is the Scientific Evidence for Chiropractic Spinal Manipulation?

Chiropractic spinal manipulation has been evaluated scientifically to determine its efficacy, as well as its costs comparative to other forms of health care. However, the evidence is not compelling in either case.

Efficacy
Although there is some evidence that chiropractic spinal manipulation may be helpful for various medical purposes, in general the evidence is not strong. There are several reasons for this, but one is fundamental: Even with the best of intentions, it is difficult to properly ascertain the effectiveness of a hands-on therapy like chiropractic.

Only one form of study can truly prove that a treatment is effective: the double-blind, placebo-controlled trial. (For more information on why such studies are so crucial, see **Why Does This Book Rely on Double-blind Studies?**) However, it isn't easy to fit chiropractic into a study design of this type. Consider the obstacles: What could researchers use for placebo chiropractic treatment? And how could they make sure that both participants and practitioners would be kept in the dark

regarding who was receiving real chiropractic manipulation and who was receiving fake manipulation?

Because of these problems, all studies of chiropractic manipulation fall short of optimum design. Many have compared chiropractic treatment against no treatment. However, studies of this type cannot provide reliable evidence about the efficacy of a treatment. If a benefit is seen, there is no way to determine whether it was caused by chiropractic manipulation specifically or just attention generally. (Attention alone will almost always produce some reported benefit.)

More meaningful trials used some sort of unrelated fake treatment for the control group, such as phony laser acupuncture. However, it is less than ideal to use a placebo treatment that is so very different in form from the treatment under study.

Better studies compare real chiropractic manipulation against sham forms of manipulation, such as light touch. Studies of this type are a definite step forward. However, it is quite likely that the practitioners at least unconsciously conveyed more enthusiasm and optimism when performing the real therapy than the fake therapy; this, too, could affect the outcome.

It has been suggested that the only way to get around this problem would be to compare the effectiveness of trained practitioners to actors trained only enough to provide a simulation of treatment; however, such studies have not been reported.

Still other studies have simply involved treating people with chiropractic spinal manipulation and seeing whether they improve. These trials are particularly meaningless; it has been long since proven that both participants and examining physicians will at least think that they observe improvement in people given a treatment, regardless of whether the treatment does anything on its own.

Finally, other trials have compared chiropractic manipulation to competing therapies, such as **massage therapy** or conventional physical therapy. However, neither of these therapies has been proven effective. When you compare unproven therapies to each other, the results cannot possibly prove that any of the tested treatments are effective.

Given these caveats, we discuss below what science knows about the effects of chiropractic.

Costs
Besides effectiveness, another important consideration is cost of care. There are many aspects to the cost of treatment, including number of visits to the chosen provider,

Biofeedback

Still other studies simply involved giving people biofeedback and seeing whether they improved. Such trials are almost completely meaningless; numerous studies have shown that both participants and examining physicians will frequently think they observe improvement in people given a treatment, regardless of whether the treatment does anything on its own. For example, early studies of biofeedback for stroke rehabilitation that did not use blinding or a control group reported miraculous successes equivalent to the "throw down your crutches and walk" cliché. However, when controlled trials were performed, it turned out that biofeedback did not provide much more than marginal benefit, if any. For this reason, we do not even report uncontrolled studies below.

Given these caveats, the following is a summary of what science knows about the medical benefits of biofeedback.

Possible Effects of Biofeedback

Of all the medical conditions for which biofeedback has been advocated, the best studied is **hypertension**. One review of the literature found 23 controlled trials of acceptable quality. Taken as a whole, these studies suggest that biofeedback can reduce blood pressure by approximately 5%, a modest but useful improvement.

In one of the best of these studies, 30 people with mild hypertension received 8 sessions of real or placebo biofeedback in the laboratory, followed by 12 home sessions. After 4 weeks, the results showed that blood pressure measurements in the treated group decreased by an average of 11 mm systolic (the upper number in the blood pressure reading) compared to only 4 mm improvement in the placebo group, for a net improvement of 7 mm. This difference was statistically significant.

In another study, this ability was found to be fostered by true biofeedback but, not surprisingly, suppressed over time by false biofeedback.

The evidence is less positive for several other conditions. The balance of the evidence suggests that biofeedback is *not* effective for **asthma** or defecation problems in children and adults, and that it is no more than marginally effective for **Raynaud's disease**.

Biofeedback has been studied for numerous other

medical conditions as well. At least one controlled study supports the use of biofeedback for each of the following: **Anxiety**, **chronic low back pain**, female stress incontinence, **insomnia**, headaches (including **migraine** and **tension** headaches), and, possibly, rehabilitation from **strokes**. Note that the evidence of benefit with biofeedback is not definitive for any of these conditions and, in many cases, there are also studies with negative outcomes.

What to Expect During a Biofeedback Session

As described above, biofeedback training involves the use of a machine that relays information about the aspect of the body that you wish to control. In early stages, the trick is finding the "muscles" necessary to produce the desired effect. Typically, a biofeedback practitioner will teach a series of visualizations and other mental exercises in the hope that it will facilitate the process. For example, if you have high blood pressure, you might be asked to imagine the blood vessels in your body opening up and dilating. (It is not precisely clear that such methods work, but at the very least they give you something to do consciously while your brain solves the problem.)

Ability in biofeedback comes in fits and starts and grows with practice. The initial sessions are done with a practitioner, but once your abilities start to develop you will be asked to continue to work with a biofeedback machine at home. Ordinarily, several sessions of training and weeks of daily home practice are required to achieve the desired effect.

How to Choose a Biofeedback Practitioner

As with all medical therapies, it is best to choose a licensed practitioner in states where a biofeedback license is available. Where licensure is not available, seek a referral from a qualified and knowledgeable health care provider.

Safety Issues

There are no known safety risks with biofeedback.

Chelation Therapy

ALTERNATE NAME: *EDTA Chelation*

Overview

When medical researchers first investigated the phenomenon known as *hardening of the arteries* (closely related to **atherosclerosis**), they discovered that the damaged, brittle vessels found in people with heart disease were lined with calcium deposits. Naturally, this finding inspired the notion that calcium deposits were the cause of the problem.

Some early researchers investigated the possible therapeutic effect of removing such deposits. However, subsequent research indicated that the calcium deposits of atherosclerosis were a symptom rather than a cause and mainstream interest turned elsewhere. Certain physicians nonetheless maintained an interest in removing calcium; thus chelation therapy was born.

Chelation therapy for heart disease consists of intravenous infusions of a chemical called *ethylenediaminetetraacetic acid* (EDTA). This synthetic substance is used in conventional medicine to remove heavy metals, such as lead, from the body, but it also has an effect on calcium, which is why it came into use in chelation therapy.

Proponents claim that EDTA chelation is an effective alternative to heart surgery and that it also offers many other health benefits. To support this, they cite numerous anecdotes of cures apparently brought about by its use. However, anecdotes cannot possibly prove a treatment effective. (For a detailed explanation of why this is the case, see **Why Does This Book Rely on Double-blind Studies?**) Only double-blind, placebo-controlled trials can do so and, thus far, such studies have failed to find chelation therapy effective.

In 2000, a highly respected researcher reviewed the literature on chelation therapy and concluded, "The most striking finding is the almost total lack of convincing evidence for efficacy. . . . Only two controlled clinical trials were located. They provide no evidence that chelation therapy is efficacious beyond a powerful placebo effect. . . . Given the potential of chelation therapy to cause severe adverse effects, this treatment should now be considered obsolete."

Subsequent to this review, a well-designed study compared chelation therapy to placebo in 84 people with coronary artery disease. People receiving EDTA chelation showed improvement; however, those receiving placebo also improved—to the same extent! This finding reminds us why double-blind, placebo-controlled studies are necessary to establish the effectiveness of a treatment. If researchers had performed this study without a placebo group, they might have concluded that EDTA chelation really works. Instead, the fact that the same level of benefits was seen in the fake-treatment group indicates that chelation therapy does not work.

Another double-blind study evaluated the potential benefits of chelation therapy when added to conventional therapy in the treatment of people with coronary artery disease. Researchers were looking for improvements in the ability of a blood vessel in the arm (the brachial artery) to dilate, but did not find any. However, this study had several limitations in its design, making its results less meaningful than they might have been.

Safety Issues

Not only does it appear to be ineffective, EDTA chelation therapy may present some safety risks. This treatment is generally given in a series of 10 to 30 sessions. If the practitioner fails to take proper precautions, severe adverse consequences, such as kidney damage, may result. While it appears to be the case that properly performed chelation therapy is unlikely to cause harm, we do not see any justification for using such an invasive method, in the absence of evidence that it will help.

Chiropractic

RELATED TERMS: *Spinal Manipulation; Manipulation, Spinal*

PRINCIPAL PROPOSED USES: *Back Pain, Migraine Headaches, Neck Pain, Tension Headaches*

OTHER PROPOSED USES: *Asthma, Bedwetting, Dysmenorrhea (Menstrual Pain), High Blood Pressure, Infantile Colic, Phobias, Premenstrual Syndrome (PMS)*

Overview

Chiropractic is one of the most widely used health services today. It has gained increasing acceptance as a treatment for back and neck pain and is covered by many health insurance plans. Millions of people would report that chiropractic spinal manipulation has brought them relief. Nonetheless, at present the research record for its effectiveness is inconclusive at best.

History of Chiropractic

Daniel David Palmer founded chiropractic in 1895, after an experience in which he apparently believed he cured a man's deafness by manipulating his back. He opened the Palmer School of Chiropractic and began teaching spinal manipulation. This college still exists today, with a fully accredited program.

One of Palmer's first students was his son, Bartlett Joshua (B.J.) Palmer. It was B.J. Palmer who truly popularized the technique. Later, Willard Carver, an Oklahoma City lawyer, opened a competing school. He believed that chiropractic physicians needed to offer other methods of treatment in addition to spinal manipulation. This opened a schism in the chiropractic world that still exists today. Followers of Palmer and his methods focus only on spinal adjustments, an approach called *straight* chiropractic. Those who, like Carver, use various approaches to healing are called *mixers*. Mixers may use vitamins, herbs, and any other treatment methods they find useful (and are allowed to practice by law).

Medical treatments in the nineteenth and early twentieth centuries were not based on scientific evidence of effectiveness and chiropractic treatment was no exception. It became a widespread technique long before there was any real evidence that it worked. Chiropractic schools utilized all of their profits and resources to further develop programs for training people in chiropractic techniques—not for verifying the theory and practice of chiropractic. However, in the 1970s proper scientific research into chiropractic began to draw interest. In 1977, the Foundation for Chiropractic Education and Research (FCER) established a program to train chiropractic researchers. Since then, efforts have been made to fund scientific trials testing the effectiveness of chiropractic techniques and to establish a scientific foundation for the practice.

Forms of Spinal Manipulation

There are many different chiropractic techniques in use today, some with proprietary names such as the Gonstead and Maitland techniques. In general, most involve rapid (high-velocity) short (low-amplitude) thrusts. Manipulation may be purely manual or mechanically assisted. For example, some chiropractors use an *activator*—a small metal tool that applies a force directly to one vertebra.

In addition, some chiropractors use a related therapy called *spinal mobilization*. This method involves gentle, extended movements (low-velocity, high-amplitude), rather than the "back-cracking" of classic chiropractic spinal manipulation.

How Does Chiropractic Spinal Manipulation Work?

Since its origin, chiropractic theory has based itself on *subluxations*, or vertebrae that have shifted position in the spine. These subluxations are said to impede nerve outflow and cause disease in various organs. A chiropractic treatment is supposed to "put back in" these "popped out" vertebrae; for this reason, it is called an *adjustment*.

However, no real evidence has ever been presented showing that a given chiropractic treatment alters the position of any vertebrae. In addition, there is as yet no cost of evaluation procedures such as x-rays, insurance reimbursement versus patient out-of-pocket expense, and costs for missed work time.

However, it is difficult to develop accurate cost-comparison figures because there are many complicating factors in research on the subject. For example, one approach is to simply identify people with similar injuries who choose one treatment or another and add up the total cost. Unfortunately, the results of such a study can be misleading. People with more or less severe back pain might tend to choose different forms of treatment; if those with more severe pain usually chose surgical treatment, this would tend to inflate the comparative costs of conventional care and make chiropractic seem less expensive.

Another potentially complicating factor is that, to a great extent, insurance companies control utilization of treatment; if they are less inclined to authorize chiropractic visits, people who choose chiropractic care might find their care cut off more rapidly than others who choose, say, physical therapy. This too would lead to artificially low costs of chiropractic treatment compared to physical therapy, skewing the results of the study.

These problems could be solved by conducting a study in which researchers randomly assign participants to certain treatments, with the length of treatment determined entirely by the treating physician. Unfortunately, studies of this type have not yet been conducted.

Because of these and other limitations, any estimate of comparative costs must be regarded as an approximation. Nonetheless, because this is potentially such an important issue, in the following sections we discuss what is known about the comparative costs of chiropractic and other forms of care for various conditions.

Back Pain

Although chiropractic spinal manipulation is commonly used for the treatment of **back pain**, there is as yet little evidence that it is effective. Furthermore, despite widespread claims that spinal manipulation is a more cost-effective treatment for back pain than conventional methods, the studies cited to bolster these claims suffer from significant flaws that make the apparent results unreliable.

➢ *Efficacy*

Chiropractic spinal manipulation is one of the most popular treatments for acute and chronic back pain in the U.S., and it may in fact provide at least modest benefit;

however, as yet, research evidence has failed to find chiropractic manipulation convincingly more effective than standard medical care.

Chiropractic does seem to be more effective than placebo, if not by a great deal. For example, a single-blind controlled study of 84 people suffering from low back pain compared manipulation to treatment with a diathermy machine (a physical therapy machine that uses microwaves to create heat beneath the skin) that was not actually functioning. The researchers asked the participants to assess their own pain levels within 15 minutes of the first treatment, then 3 and 7 days after treatment. The only statistically significant difference between the two groups was within 15 minutes of the manipulation. (Chiropractic had better results at that point.)

In another single-blind, placebo-controlled study, researchers assigned 209 participants to one of three groups: a high-velocity, low-amplitude (HVLA) spinal manipulation; a sham manipulation; or a back-education program. Although this has been reported as a positive study, most of the differences seen between the groups were not statistically significant. In addition, because almost half the participants dropped out of the study before the end, the results can't be regarded as meaningful.

Unimpressive results were also seen in a well-designed study of 321 people with back pain comparing chiropractic manipulation, a special form of physical therapy (the Mackenzie method), and the provision of an educational booklet in treating low back pain. All groups improved to about the same extent.

Several studies evaluated the effectiveness of chiropractic manipulation combined with a different kind of treatment called *mobilization*, but they too found little to no benefit.

On a positive note, one study of 100 people with back pain and sciatica symptoms (pain down the leg due to disc protrusion) found that chiropractic manipulation was significantly more effective at relieving symptoms than sham chiropractic manipulation.

Several studies have found that chiropractic is at least as helpful as other commonly used therapies for low back pain, such as muscle relaxants, anti-inflammatory medication, soft-tissue massage, conventional medical care, and physical therapy. For example, a large, well-designed study found chiropractic manipulation more effective than general medical care and exercise therapy.

Note: The main conventional therapy for back pain, physical therapy, also lacks consistent supporting evidence.

For example, in one large study of people with back pain, a single session of advice proved equally effective as a full course of physical therapy for back pain.

≽ Costs

At present, there is no conclusive evidence regarding the relative costs of chiropractic and other forms of care for back pain. For the general obstacles to evaluating this, please see Costs on page 802.

In one recent study, the mean costs of care for low back pain were about the same for physical therapy and chiropractic over a 2-year period: $437 for physical therapy and $429 for chiropractic.

In some studies comparing chiropractic to other forms of care for low back pain, chiropractic care cost more than conventional care. The researchers theorize that the higher cost of chiropractic care was because of the large number of visits and the extensive use of x-rays.

In another cost comparison, however, chiropractic medical expenses were significantly lower than conventional care for certain categories of back injury. This study observed data from 3,062 claims (chosen from a total of 7,551 back injury claims) from the Workers Compensation Fund in Utah in 1986. Investigators compared data for six different conditions ranging from "nonspecific sprain" to "lumbosacral disc." Although visits to the chiropractic physician were often more frequent, the cost of each visit was much lower than one visit to a conventional physician and the net effect was a significant cost savings. Also, people seen by conventional physicians were paid for almost 10 times as many days of lost work as those in the chiropractic group.

However, two hidden factors were also at work. First, the Workers' Compensation System sets arbitrary limits on chiropractic costs; when these are reached, an injured person is referred to a conventional medical provider. Perhaps due in part to this fact, only two chiropractic claims in this study exceeded $5,000, whereas 100 conventional medical cases did. The second important point of consideration is that in a study of this kind it is impossible to determine whether the medical and chiropractic patient groups were comparable. Perhaps the conventional physicians saw more of the most severely injured people, or vice versa. As noted earlier, a study of this type simply can't yield definitive conclusions.

Neck Pain

As with back pain, despite the widespread use of chiropractic spinal manipulation for neck pain, there is as yet no reliable evidence that it works. Of the limited number of studies performed, most have failed to find manipulation (with or without mobilization or massage) convincingly more effective than placebo or no treatment. One large study (almost 200 participants) found that a special exercise program (MedX) was more effective than manipulation.

Tension Headaches and Cervicogenic Headaches

Many people experience headaches caused by muscle tension, neck problems, or a combination of the two. Because these so-called **tension headaches** and cervicogenic headaches (caused by neck problems) overlap, we discuss them together here. Chiropractic spinal manipulation has shown some promise for these conditions, but the evidence remains incomplete and somewhat contradictory. In a controlled trial of 150 people, investigators compared spinal manipulation to the drug amitriptyline for the treatment of chronic tension-type headaches. By the end of the 6-week treatment period, participants in both groups had improved similarly. However, 4 weeks after treatment was stopped, people who had received spinal manipulation showed greater reduction in headache intensity and frequency and over-the-counter medication usage than those who used the medication, and the difference in the amount of improvement between the groups was statistically significant.

In another positive trial, 53 people with cervicogenic headaches received chiropractic spinal manipulation or laser acupuncture plus massage. Chiropractic manipulation was more effective. However, a similar study of 75 people with recurrent tension headaches found no difference between the two groups. Other, smaller studies of spinal manipulation have been reported as well, with mixed results.

Finally, in a controlled trial, 200 people with cervicogenic headaches were randomly assigned to receive one of four therapies: manipulation, a special exercise technique, exercise plus manipulation, or no therapy. Each participant received at least 8 to 12 treatments over a period of 6 weeks. All three treatment approaches produced better results than no treatment and approximately the same effect as each other. However, these results prove little because, as noted earlier, any treatment whatsoever will generally produce better results than no treatment for a number of reasons having nothing to do with the treatment itself.

Migraine Headaches

There is some evidence that chiropractic manipulation may provide both long- and short-term benefits for **migraine headaches**.

In a double-blind, placebo-controlled study, 123 participants suffering from migraine headaches were treated for 2 months with chiropractic manipulations or fake electrical therapy (electrodes placed on the body without electrical current sent between them) as placebo. The study lasted a total of 6 months: 2 months pretreatment, 2 months of treatment, and 2 months posttreatment.

After 2 months of treatment, those receiving chiropractic manipulation showed statistically significant improvement in headache severity and frequency compared to the control group. Furthermore, these benefits persisted to a 2-month follow-up evaluation.

Chiropractic manipulation also produced relatively prolonged benefits in another trial as well. In this study, 218 people with migraine headaches were divided into three groups: manipulation, medication (amitriptyline), or manipulation plus medication. During the 4 weeks of treatment, all three groups experienced comparable benefits. During the follow-up 4-week period, however, people who had received manipulation alone experienced more benefit than those who had been in the other two groups.

However, a study of 85 people with migraines compared spinal manipulation against two other treatments: manipulation performed by a non-chiropractor and mobilization. The results showed no difference between groups.

Other Conditions

Chiropractic has been evaluated for many other conditions as well, but the results as yet provide little evidence of benefit.

➣ Infantile Colic

Infantile colic is a common and frustrating problem. Although chiropractic manipulation has been promoted as a treatment for this condition, there is as yet little evidence that it offers specific benefits.

In a single-blind, placebo-controlled trial, a total of 86 infants either received three chiropractic treatments or were held for 10 minutes by a nurse. While a high percentage of infants improved, there was no significant difference between the two groups.

Another trial compared spinal manipulation to the drug dimethicone. While chiropractic proved more effective than the medication, dimethicone itself has never been proven effective for infantile colic and the study did not use a placebo group. For this reason, the results of this study indicate little about the effectiveness of chiropractic treatment for infantile colic.

➣ Premenstrual Syndrome

A small crossover trial of chiropractic for **premenstrual syndrome** (PMS) symptoms found equivocal results.

➣ Phobias

A small trial compared real and sham activator-style chiropractic treatment in people with phobias and found some evidence of benefit.

➣ Asthma

In two controlled studies comparing spinal manipulation to sham manipulation for treatment of people with **asthma**, the results showed equal improvement for participants in the two groups. These results suggest that the benefits were most likely caused by the attention given by the chiropractor and not due to the spinal manipulation itself. However, one of these studies has been sharply criticized for using as a sham treatment a chiropractic method perfectly capable of producing a therapeutic effect. This could hide real benefits of the tested form of chiropractic. (If the "placebo" treatment used in a study is actually better than placebo and the tested treatment does no better than this "placebo," the results would appear to indicate that the tested treatment is no better than placebo, and, hence, ineffective.)

➣ Dysmenorrhea (Menstrual Pain)

A single-blind, placebo-controlled study of 138 women complaining of **menstrual pain** compared spinal manipulation to sham manipulation for four menstrual cycles and found no differences between the two groups.

➣ High Blood Pressure

In a study of 148 people with mild **high blood pressure**, use of chiropractic spinal manipulation plus dietary changes failed to prove more effective for reducing blood pressure than dietary changes alone.

➣ Bedwetting

A single-blind, placebo-controlled trial compared real and sham chiropractic (activator technique) in 46 children with **bedwetting** problems, but failed to find a statistically significant difference between the groups.

What to Expect with Chiropractic Treatment

Depending on the condition, chiropractic treatment is usually conducted on a two- or three-times-a-week basis, for a month or more. Chiropractic is also sometimes used on an as-needed basis, or in a once- or twice-a-month maintenance form. For many chiropractors, x-rays are essential at the first visit and at some follow-up visits.

Each session involves hands-on manipulation following the methods of whatever manipulation technique the practitioner chooses to use. Sometimes other modalities may be used as well, such as massage or hot or cold packs.

Chiropractic physicians may also provide general wellness counseling and prescribe herbs or supplements.

Safety Issues

Chiropractic manipulation appears to be generally safe—rarely causing serious side effects. However, a temporary increase of symptoms may occur relatively frequently. Other side effects include temporary headache, tiredness, and discomfort radiating from the site of the adjustment.

More serious complications may occur on rare occasions. These are primarily associated with manipulation of the neck. Articles have been published that document a total of almost 200 cases of more serious complications associated with neck manipulation, including stroke, vertebral fracture, disc herniation, severely increased sensation of nerve pinching, and rupture of the windpipe. More than half of these reports involve some form of stroke, often due to a tear in a major blood vessel at the base of the neck (the vertebral artery).

Although attempts have been made to determine in advance who will experience strokes following chiropractic, they have not been successful. Thus, stroke must be considered an unpredictable, though rare, side effect of chiropractic manipulation of the neck. To put this in perspective, however, the rate of complications from chiropractic is extremely low; according to one estimate, only one complication per million individual sessions occurs. Among people receiving a course of treatment involving manipulation of the neck, the rate of stroke is perhaps one per 100,000 people; the rate of death is one per 400,000. By comparison, serious medical complications involving common drugs in the ibuprofen family (non-steroidal anti-inflammatory drugs, or NSAIDs) are far more common. Among people using them for arthritis, NSAIDs result in hospitalizations at a rate of about four in 1,000 people, and death at a rate of four in 10,000. To put it another way, the rate of complications with these common over-the-counter drugs is perhaps 100 to 400 times greater than with chiropractic.

Certain health conditions preclude spinal manipulation, such as nerve impingement causing severe nerve damage, or significant disease of the spinal bones.

Detoxification

Overview

The concept of detoxification plays a major role in many schools of alternative medicine, including Ayurveda, naturopathy, and chiropractic. In this context, the term refers to a belief that toxins accumulated in the body are a major cause of disease and that health can be promoted by removing them through various means.

The toxins referred to in this theory are said to have several major sources:

➤ Chemicals added to processed foods, such as preservatives
➤ Chemicals that enter the food chain through the use of pesticides, artificial fertilizers, and drugs given to cows, chickens, and other food animals
➤ Toxins produced in the intestines due to improper digestion
➤ Toxins produced in the bloodstream due to stress
➤ Pharmaceutical medications, nearly all of which are regarded as essentially toxic by proponents of detoxification

➤ Toxins present in the general environment, such as automobile exhaust, cigarette smoke, the aluminum in antiperspirants, and the formaldehyde released by new carpet

➤ Toxins in water

➤ Toxins introduced through the use of mercury fillings and other medical procedures

These toxins are said to cause a wide variety of chronic illnesses, from **multiple sclerosis** and **migraine headaches** to **cancer** and **rheumatoid arthritis**, and alternative practitioners use various methods with the intention of removing the toxins. One such recommendation has made it into conventional wisdom: drinking at least a quart (or a half-gallon) of water per day. Other detoxification methods include fasting (on juice, water, fruit, or brown rice), using "cleansing" herbs and supplements (such as olive oil and lemon juice to flush the liver, dandelion root to purge the gallbladder, or psyllium seed to cleanse the colon), taking high colonics, receiving intravenous vitamin C, and/or removing mercury fillings.

Removing toxins is often said to cause a temporary flare-up of illness. This reaction is generally interpreted as a positive sign, but also as a call for careful medical management to avoid causing harm on the way to healing.

Is There Scientific Support for Detoxification Methods?

In general, there is little to no scientific support for detoxification methods. Aside from specific toxicities, such as lead or arsenic, medical researchers have observed no general phenomenon of toxification. For this reason, it is difficult to scientifically validate whether detoxification methods actually work.

Most detoxification approaches essentially remain unexamined, rather than proven or disproven, and rely on reasonable concepts but no hard evidence for their justification. Mercury-filling removal is a typical example. Many alternative practitioners believe that the mercury in silver fillings is a cause of numerous health problems and should be removed to prevent or treat disease. However, although it is a matter of indisputable fact that mercury can be toxic, scientific evaluation generally indicates that mercury levels in people with mercury fillings are far below those necessary to cause toxic

symptoms. Anti-mercury advocates respond that some people are sensitive to mercury in very low amounts and that those people will therefore benefit from filling removal even if they are not experiencing actual toxicity. This could certainly be true. However, despite numerous unreliable anecdotes, there is as yet no meaningful evidence that removing mercury fillings can treat or prevent any disease.

Much the same can be said about all of the other popular detoxification methods. However, in the case of one form of detoxification, colon cleansing, the theory behind the technique is definitely wrong. According to this nineteenth-century theory known as *colon health* or *colon hygiene*, years of bad diet cause the colon to become caked with layer upon layer of accumulated toxins. This accumulation is said to resemble sedimentary rock. High colonics, which are essentially enemas that reach far up into the large intestine, are said to release the accumulated buildup and thereby restore health. However, in recent decades, physicians have performed colon examinations to search for colon cancer in millions of patients, and their findings do not support the theory. Most of the patients given these examinations are at least middle-aged and not very many have devoted their lives to healthy diets and clean colons. According to the colonic hygiene theory, colon examinations on such patients should turn up concretelike deposits. However, all that shows up during a typical colonoscopy is fresh, pink flesh. Unfortunately, proponents of colonics do not seem to have assimilated this information; they continue to recount theories about the colon that were shown to be untrue decades ago.

Safety Issues

The safety of detoxification methods varies widely. While drinking a quart of water a day is undoubtedly benign and mercury-filling removal is unlikely to harm anything but one's pocketbook, other methods might be risky. High colonics have occasionally resulted in serious internal injury, and intravenous therapies, being highly invasive, must be handled with a certain degree of sophistication to avoid causing harm. Considering that detoxification has not been proven useful, we recommend sticking to the more moderate of its various methods if you wish to try it at all.

Functional Foods

Increasingly, foods sold in the supermarkets come with health claims on the label. To name just a few, oatmeal and soy are said to help prevent heart disease, milk and calcium-fortified orange juice to fight osteoporosis, and folate-enriched flour to prevent birth defects. These are all "functional foods"—foods marketed as offering specific health benefits.

There are two main categories of functional foods. The first (and largest) category consists of ordinary foods that contain health-promoting substances. This category essentially includes all fruits, vegetables, and whole grains, soy and other legumes, and numerous other foods such as herbal teas, yogurt, and cold-water fish. When these foods are presented as functional foods, their specific health benefits and healthy constituents are highlighted, such as fiber, vitamins, minerals, and non-nutrient chemicals with potential health benefits.

The second category of functional foods consists of foods that have been enriched with a potentially health-promoting ingredient. Examples include margarines containing **stanol esters**, orange juice enriched with **calcium** and other nutrients, and beverages to which **echinacea** and other herbs have been added.

Some of these functional food products are based on good, solid science. For others, however, the supporting evidence is weak or speculative. Furthermore, the requirement for good taste sometimes forces manufacturers to limit the amount of herbs and other additives to a level so low that they are unlikely to have any effect.

In the following table, we list some of the more promising functional foods, as well as natural products that are added to food products to create functional foods.

Cancer prevention	Diindolylemethane (found in broccoli-family vegetables)
	Fish oil (found in salmon and other cold-water fish)
	Flaxseed (contains lignans)
	Folate
	Garlic
	Green tea
	I3C (found in broccoli-family vegetables)
	IP6 (found in nuts, seeds, beans, whole grains, cantaloupe, and citrus fruits)
	Lycopene (found in tomatoes)
	Resveratrol (found in grape skin)
	Selenium
	Soy foods
	Turmeric (added to many foods as a preservative)
	Vitamin C
	Vitamin E
Cataracts	Lutein (found in dark-green vegetables)
Cavities	Xylitol (added to chewing gum and candy)
Colds and flus	Echinacea (herbal tea)
	Garlic
Diabetes	Chromium (whole grains, brewer's yeast, fortified nutritional yeast, liver)
	Evening primrose oil
Diarrhea	Probiotics ("friendly bacteria") (found in yogurt)

Digestive problems	Probiotics ("friendly bacteria") (found in yogurt)
Ear infections	Xylitol (added to chewing gum and candy)
Easy bruising	Bioflavonoids (found in citrus fruits, buckwheat, and most fruits and vegetables)
Eczema	Probiotics ("friendly bacteria") (found in yogurt)
General nutrition	Fortified grains and beverages
Heart disease prevention	Alpha-linolenic acid (found in flaxseed oil)
	Calcium (added to beverages; found in milk and other dairy products)
	Garlic
	Fish oil (found in salmon and other cold-water fish)
	Potassium (found in orange juice, bananas, and other foods)
	Soy products
	Stanols/Sterols (added to margarine and other spreads)
	Fiber (found in oats, glucomannan, as well all whole grains and fruits, legumes, and vegetables)
	Wine and other alcoholic beverages (in moderation)
High cholesterol	Fiber (found in whole grains and fruits, legumes, and vegetables)
	Garlic
	Krill oil
	Soy products
	Stanols (added to margarine and other spreads)
Menopausal symptoms	Soy products
Nausea	Ginger (beverages)
Osteoporosis	Calcium (added to beverages; found in milk and other dairy products)
	Vitamin D (added to butter, milk, and other beverages)
	Soy foods
Premenstrual syndrome (PMS)	Calcium (added to beverages; found in milk and other dairy products)
	Krill oil
Ulcerative colitis	Probiotics ("friendly bacteria") (found in yogurt)
Urinary tract infections	Cranberry juice
Vaginal infection	Probiotics ("friendly bacteria") (found in yogurt)

A Note About Labeling

The FDA allows labels on foods similar to those used on dietary supplements. These do not require very much scientific validation and they formally state that the claims made are not approved by the FDA.

In some cases, however, the FDA has specifically authorized higher level health claims such as "heart healthy." These claims may be taken as representing scientific consensus. Because this is such a rapidly growing field, an increasing number of these labels should be expected.

Hatha Yoga

ALTERNATE NAME: *Yoga*

PRINCIPAL PROPOSED USES: *Increasing Strength, Balance, and Flexibility; Reducing Tension and Stress*

OTHER PROPOSED USES: *Asthma, Carpal Tunnel Syndrome, Chemical Dependency, Depression, Epilepsy, High Blood Pressure, Osteoarthritis, Well-Being in General*

Overview

Hatha yoga, or, as it is commonly called in the U.S., simply *yoga*, is an exercise system derived from ancient traditions in India. There are many schools or varieties of hatha yoga, but all of them involve *asanas*, or postures. Many asanas function as gentle stretching exercises, increasing flexibility. Others encourage the development of strength and balance.

The practice of hatha yoga goes beyond exercise, however. Special breathing techniques are almost always part of the process. In addition, hatha yoga originated in traditional Hindu spiritual practice and therefore can involve meditation, chanting, and consideration of philosophical and religious points of view. (**Note**: Completely secular versions of hatha yoga are widely available.)

Hatha yoga is believed by its practitioners to provide benefits above and beyond simple exercise. For example, certain asanas are said to address specific health problems. However, there is only minimal scientific evidence that the practice of hatha yoga actually provides any well-defined medical benefits.

How Is Hatha Yoga Used Today?

There are numerous specific schools of hatha yoga, including Iyengar yoga, Ashtanga yoga, Kriya yoga, Vini yoga, and Bikram yoga, as well as "generic" hatha yoga. Yoga is ordinarily learned through inexpensive group lessons, but regular at-home practice is necessary to progress in skill (and to derive potential health benefits). Lessons are commonly available at hospital wellness centers, health clubs, city recreation departments, and private yoga studios. There are also a wealth of do-it-yourself yoga videotapes and books, but most serious yoga practitioners caution against learning the technique without an instructor present.

What Is the Scientific Evidence for Hatha Yoga?

Although there is some evidence that yoga may offer medical benefits, in general this evidence is not strong. There are several reasons for this (including funding obstacles), but one is fundamental: Even with the best of intentions, it is difficult to properly ascertain the effectiveness of an exercise therapy like yoga.

Only one form of study can truly prove that a treatment is effective: the double-blind, placebo-controlled trial. However, it isn't possible to fit yoga into a study design of this type. While it might be possible to design a placebo form of yoga, it would be quite difficult to keep participants and researchers in the dark regarding who is practicing real yoga and who is practicing fake yoga!

Some compromise with the highest research standards is, therefore, inevitable. Unfortunately, the compromise used in most studies is less than optimal. In these trials, yoga has been compared to no treatment. The problem with such studies is that a treatment—any treatment—frequently appears to better than no treatment, due to a host of factors. (See **Why Does This Book Rely on Double-blind Studies?**) It would be better to compare yoga to generic forms of exercise, such as daily walking, but thus far this method has not seen much use.

Given these caveats, the following is a summary of what science has found out about the possible medical benefits of yoga.

Possible Benefits of Hatha Yoga

Yoga, like **Tai Chi**, has been advocated as a means of increasing strength, balance, and physical function in seniors. However, there is as yet little scientific proof that yoga offers such benefits or that it is superior to generic exercises such as walking. Hatha yoga is also said to relieve **tension and stress**. While this has not been quantified scientifically, most people do feel relaxed after a yoga session. There is little doubt that yoga, like any form of stretching, will increase flexibility if it practiced consistently and over a long period of time.

Weak evidence hints that hatha yoga may offer modest benefits for people with **asthma**. For example, in one controlled study, 59 people with mild asthma were randomly assigned to practice yoga and attend a general class or simply to attend the general class. The results showed slight improvements in asthma in the treated group compared to the untreated group. However, even these modest benefits did not last; assessment 2 months later showed no difference between the groups. Furthermore, as noted above, studies in which the participants in the control group do not receive placebo treatment are inherently unreliable.

In another study, 42 people with **carpal tunnel syndrome** were randomly assigned to receive either yoga or a wrist splint for a period of 8 weeks. The results indicated that use of yoga was more effective than the wrist splint. However, participants in the control group were simply offered the wrist splint and given the choice of using it or not; it would have been preferable for them to have received an option with more "glamour," such as fake laser acupuncture or, even better, phony yoga postures.

Similarly weak evidence has been reported regarding the possible usefulness of yoga for **depression, low back pain, general well-being**, and **osteoarthritis**.

Hatha yoga has also been promoted as a treatment for **epilepsy** (seizure disorder), but a review of all published scientific trials concluded that there is as yet no meaningful evidence that it is effective.

Some evidence suggests that hatha yoga is *not* helpful for **chemical dependency** or **high blood pressure**.

What to Expect from a Hatha Yoga Class

Yoga classes typically last about 1 to 2 hours. Most of that time is spent practicing various asanas; however, other activities, such as breathing exercises, may take place as well. Hatha yoga is generally a gentle, nonaerobic form of exercise. However, some types of yoga, such as Iyengar yoga, are more physically vigorous.

By the end of a yoga class, many people report feeling relaxed and comfortable, and consider this a meaningful benefit in itself. However, without regular home practice, it is unlikely that performing yoga will provide any long-term benefit. For this reason, instructors generally encourage daily practice, ranging from a few minutes to an hour or more.

Safety Issues

Hatha yoga is generally at least as safe as any other stretching-based exercise program. However there are a few hatha yoga positions, such as the headstand, that can cause injury when they are performed by a person who isn't yet sufficiently advanced in yoga or who has certain health problems, such as a detached retina. A properly qualified instructor can help you avoid injury, taking your own individual health status into account.

Herbal Medicine

ALTERNATE NAMES: *Herbology, Western Herbal Medicine*

Overview

Along with massage therapy, herbal treatment is undoubtedly one of the most ancient forms of medicine. By the time written history began, herbal medicine was already in full swing and being used in all parts of the world.

There are several major surviving schools of herbal medicine. Two of the most complex systems are **Ayurveda** (the traditional herbal medicine of India) and **Traditional Chinese Herbal Medicine** (TCHM). Both

Herbal Medicine

Ayurveda and TCHM make use of combinations of herbs. However, the herbal tradition in the West focuses more on individual herbs, sometimes known as *simples*. That is the form of herbology discussed here.

History of Herbal Medicine

Originally, herbal medicine in Europe was primarily a women's art. The classic image of witches boiling herbs in a cauldron stems to a large extent from this period. Beginning in about the thirteenth century, however, graduates of male-only medical schools and members of barber-surgeon guilds began to displace the traditional female village herbalists. Ultimately, much of the original lore was lost. (So-called traditional herbal compendiums, such as *Culpeppers Herbal*, are actually of fairly recent vintage.)

Another major change took place in the nineteenth century, when chemistry had advanced far enough to allow extraction of active ingredients from herbs. The old French word for herb, *drogue*, became the name for chemical drugs. Subsequently, these chemical extracts displaced herbs as the standard of care. There were several forces leading to the predominance of chemicals over herbs, but one of the most important remains a major issue today: the problem of reproducibility.

Herbal Medicine's Greatest Problem: Reproducibility

When you purchase a drug, you generally know exactly what you are getting. Drugs are single chemicals that can be measured and quantified down to their molecular structure. Thus, a tablet of extra-strength Tylenol contains 500 mg of acetaminophen, no matter where or when you buy it. Although a vitamin, not a drug, the same is true of a vitamin C tablet, provided that it is correctly labeled.

Herbs, however, are living organisms comprised of thousands of ingredients and the proportions of all these ingredients may differ dramatically between two plants. Numerous influences can affect the nature of a given crop. Whether it was grown at the top or bottom of a hill, what the weather was like, what time of year it was picked, what other plants lived nearby, and what kind of soil predominated are only a few of the factors that can affect an herb's chemical makeup.

This presents a real problem for people who wish to use herbs medicinally (as opposed to, say, for taste or fragrance). Since so much variation is possible, it's difficult to know whether one batch of an herb is equivalent in effectiveness to another.

The desire to overcome this problem provided the main initial motivation for finding the active principles of herbs and purifying them into single-chemical drugs. However, by now most of the common herbs that possess an identifiable active ingredient have long since been turned into drugs. Today's popular herbs do not contain any known, single active ingredients. For this reason, there's no simple way to determine the effectiveness of a given herbal batch.

This difficulty can be partially overcome by a method called *herbal standardization*. In this process, manufacturers make an extract of the whole herb and boil off the liquid until the concentration of some ingredient reaches a certain percentage. Contrary to popular belief, this ingredient is not usually the active ingredient; it is merely a "tag" or "handle" used for standardization purposes.

The extract is then made into tablets or capsules or bottled as a liquid, with the concentration of the tag ingredient listed on the label. This method is far from perfect because two products with the same concentration of tag ingredients may still differ widely in other unlisted or even unidentified active constituents. Nonetheless, this form of partial standardization is better than nothing and it allows a certain amount of reproducibility. For this reason, we recommend that whenever possible, you should use standardized herbal extracts. Even better, use the actual products that were tested in double-blind studies.

Effectiveness of Herbs

There is no doubt that herbs can be effective treatments in principle, if for no other reason than that up through perhaps the 1970s, most drugs used in medicine came from herbs. Many of today's medicinal herbs have been studied in meaningful double-blind, placebo-controlled trials that provide a rational basis for believing them effective. Some of the best substantiated include **ginkgo** for **Alzheimer's disease**, **St. John's wort** for mild to moderate **depression**, and **saw palmetto** for **benign prostatic hypertrophy**.

However, even the best-documented herbs have less supporting evidence than the majority of drugs for one simple reason: You cannot patent an herb; therefore, no single company has the financial incentive to invest millions of dollars in research when another company can "steal" the product after it is proved to work. In addition, the problem of reproducibility always makes it difficult or impossible to know whether the batch of herbs you are buying is as effective as the one tested in published studies.

Each herb entry in the *Collins Alternative Health Guide* analyzes the body of scientific evidence for its effectiveness. We also note the traditional uses of each herb, but keep in mind that such uses are not reliable indicators of an herb's effectiveness. For many reasons, it simply isn't possible to accurately evaluate the effectiveness of a medical treatment without performing double-blind, placebo-controlled studies, and many herbs lack these.

Safety Issues

There is a common belief that herbs are by nature safer and gentler than drugs. However, there is no rational justification for this belief; an herb is simply a plant that contains one or more drugs, and it is just as prone to side effects as any medicine, especially when taken in doses high enough to cause significant benefits.

Nonetheless, the majority of the most popular medicinal herbs are at least fairly safe. The biggest concern in practice tends to involve interactions with medications. Many herbs are known to interact with drugs, and as research into this area expands, more such interactions will certainly be discovered. Each herb entry in the *Collins Alternative Health Guide* lists what is known about all safety risks. See also the article on which **herbs and supplements to avoid in pregnancy**.

Specific Herbs

The *Collins Alternative Health Guide* has articles on all major herbal therapies. For detailed information, see the **herbs and supplement index page**.

Homeopathy

What Is Homeopathy?

In the opinion of most U.S. medical professionals, homeopathy is nothing but quackery. While herbs and supplements have remained largely outside of mainstream medicine, physicians have no problem accepting in principle that these could have effects in the body. In contrast, homeopathy is an approach to healing that sounds quasi-magical: Homeopathic remedies are so phenomenally diluted that they contain no material substance in them except pure sugar (see below). Proponents of homeopathy claim that these so-called high-potency remedies possess some sort of healing energy field—a concept that does not sit well with medical professionals accustomed to seeing the world from a scientific perspective.

Nonetheless, homeopathy is used widely even today, especially in the United Kingdom, but also in the U.S. and other countries. Some studies seem to provide evidence that homeopathic remedies can be effective.

The term *homeopathy* is formed from the combination of two Greek words: *omio* meaning "same" and *pathos* meaning "suffering." This etymology reflects the homeopathic belief that a substance that causes certain symptoms in a healthy person can cure an ailing person of similar symptoms. Although this theory sounds superficially similar to the principle behind vaccines, homeopathy actually functions in a distinctly different manner. The homeopathic theory has some relationship to ancient healing traditions, but in many ways stands uniquely on its own ground, unrelated to other approaches.

The Origin of Homeopathy

Homeopathy is the invention of Samuel Christian Hahnemann, born in 1755 in Dresden, Germany, and educated as a physician.

The medical practices of the eighteenth century

were remarkably unhelpful and invasive. A good example is bloodletting. Doctors commonly bled their patients of a pint of blood or more per treatment, in the belief that it would accelerate healing. More likely, however, bloodletting impaired the patients' ability to recover, rather than strengthened it, and the practice is undoubtedly responsible for many deaths.

Physicians also used strong laxatives to "cleanse" the body. These purgatives included very toxic drugs containing mercury or arsenic and they, too, contributed to the great danger attendant on being visited by a doctor.

Samuel Hahnemann quickly became disillusioned by the standard medical procedures of his time; he gave up his medical practice and supported his family in part by translating old scientific and medical texts into German. In 1790, while translating William Cullen's *Materia Medica*, he was struck by the lack of experimental basis for Cullen's suggested uses for drugs. Hahnemann wondered how doctors could justify prescribing toxic substances without even knowing their effects on healthy people. He came to believe there was a correlation between the resulting symptoms of toxic doses of a given substance and the symptoms that the substance was being used to cure.

To explore his new theory, Hahnemann began collecting reports of accidental poisonings. Later, he tested various substances on himself and documented his reactions to them.

For example, he had read that *Cinchona officinalis*, or Peruvian bark, was used by South American Indians to treat malaria. Hahnemann took a high dose of *Cinchona officinalis* and his body reacted by breaking out in fever. Since malaria is characterized by fever, he perceived his own fever as evidence that a substance used to treat an ailment produced similar symptoms in a healthy individual.

Hahnemann then set out to experiment systematically with this hypothesis, ingesting other substances and carefully noting his reactions to them. He also gave substances to other healthy people. Hahnemann took detailed notes of the reactions. He recorded not only major physical symptoms, such as fever, but practically any sensation experienced by the person, including such details as a desire to lie down on one's left side and restlessness that is worse in the early evening.

These *provings*, as he called them, were recorded in homeopathic medical texts (such as the *Homeopathic Materia Medica*) and became the basis for homeopathic treatment.

Currently, provings are done in a different manner, using homeopathic dilutions of substances rather than the substances themselves. Currently, provings are more often done using high dilutions of substances; in other words, the homeopathic remedy is tested, not the underlying substance. This method is safer, even if not entirely consistent with the original theory.

The Three Laws

Based on his observations, Hahnemann postulated three major laws of homeopathy: the first two proposed early in his practice, the third after 20 years of practicing. (There are at least six other relatively minor laws as well.)

The first law is known as the Law of Similars, or "like cures like." This law states that "a substance that produces a certain set of symptoms in a healthy person has the power to cure a sick person manifesting those same symptoms." The second law, or Law of Infinitesimals, states that diluting a remedy makes it more powerful.

These two laws in combination define the method of creating homeopathic remedies. Following is an example: the substance ipecac (today, an over-the-counter household remedy for poisoning) causes vomiting. According to the first and second laws of homeopathy, diluted ipecac would potentially treat vomiting and the more it were diluted, the more effective it would be.

Hahnemann's third law, the Law of Chronic Disease, states that "when disease persists despite treatment, it is the result of one or more conditions that affect many people and have been driven deep inside the body by earlier allopathic therapy."

The word *allopathic*, today sometimes used to describe conventional medicine, was also a creation of Hahnemann and was used as the opposite of *homeopathic*. *Allopathic* means "other than the disease," while homeopathic means "same as the disease." In other words, homeopathy uses remedies that, when taken in high doses by healthy people (according to the first law), cause symptoms similar to those of the disease it is intended to treat. However, the allopathic remedies used by conventional physicians, such as prednisone for asthma, do not have the same relationship. They simply relieve the symptoms and, for that reason (according to homeopathic theory), don't get to the heart of the problem.

Hahnemann felt that allopathic treatments were actually harmful. A person with a skin rash provides an example. To Hahnemann, such a condition represents the body's attempt to "release" a deeper illness. Homeopathic treatment would seek to facilitate such a release. In contrast, allopathic remedies, like cortisone cream, "suppress" the rash and thereby drive the illness back into the body.

Note that herbal remedies are also allopathic, according to this principle. Taking St. John's wort for depression, according to homeopathy, is just as likely to worsen the underlying problem as using Prozac. Furthermore, herbs, like drugs, are said to interfere with the effectiveness of homeopathic remedies. Thus, contrary to popular opinion, homeopathy and herbal medicine are not compatible.

In further work developing the third law, Hahnemann elaborated on the various types of deeply buried diseases that could be the roots of many illnesses. He focused ultimately on psoriasis and syphilis as the primary underlying *miasms* beneath many health problems. However, this feature of his theory is less popular with today's practitioners of homeopathy.

Homeopathic Dilutions

As mentioned above, the second law of homeopathy requires that a homeopathic treatment be diluted for maximum effect. Hahnemann developed techniques to control the concentration, or dilution, of substances to create homeopathic remedies. First, he took the substance and preserved it in a solvent, usually alcohol. The substances he used were plants and minerals. After letting the substance stand for a month, he poured off the liquid, which became the *mother tincture*. Next, he took one drop of tincture and added it to 99 drops of pure alcohol. He then mixed the liquid by banging the container on a hard surface, a process called *succussion*. Homeopathic practitioners believe that succussion is essential to creating an effective remedy.

This first step creates a remedy with a dilution of one part in 10^2, or 100. This dilution would be noted by "c," for centesimal (indicating a dilution of two factors of 10), or by the terms 2x or D2 (x and D each indicate one factor of 10). The dilution is then continued, always adding one part of tincture to 99 parts alcohol, and succussing at each step. Such a process carried out six times leads to a 6c remedy (or 12x or D12), and so forth.

Sometimes homeopathic remedies are made with substances that are insoluble. In this case, they are ground up, mixed with lactose, and then made into remedies. At times, people make homeopathic remedies by diluting one part of tincture to nine drops of alcohol at each step, to make a 1x or D1 dilution.

The complete process of creating homeopathic remedies is called *potentization*, based on the theory that each successive dilution makes the remedy more potent. Today, you can buy homeopathic remedies that consist of small white milk sugar pills into which the potentized solution has been absorbed. Other remedies are in the form of liquids to ingest or creams to use externally.

Special Forms of Homeopathic Remedies

In addition to standard homeopathic remedies that use unrelated substances that happen to produce a similar symptom, there are two special forms of homeopathic remedies that use substances specifically related to the condition.

Isopathic remedies are made from the actual substance that causes the condition. For example, homeopathically prepared cat dander (containing zero molecules of cat dander) might be used to treat cat allergy.

Nosodes are made from infected animal tissues or bodily secretions. For example, tuberculosis-infected glands from a cow could be homeopathically diluted to create a remedy for human tuberculosis.

The Practice of Homeopathy: Constitutional Homeopathy vs. Disease-Oriented Homeopathy

Based on Hahnemann's theory of homeopathy, a practice developed that is now known as *constitutional* (or *classical*) homeopathy. This holistic art looks at the *symptom picture* of a person, including psychological, emotional, physical, and hereditary information, and tries to choose an appropriate remedy. Recently, however, a simplified form of homeopathy has developed, *disease-oriented* (or *symptomatic*) homeopathy, in which remedies are given based solely on specific diseases.

Both types of homeopathy have been studied scientifically, although disease-oriented homeopathy has received more attention for the simple reason that it is easier to study.

Homeopathy Today

Homeopathy is highly respected in Britain, where it is part of the national health care system. It is also

Homeopathy

widely used in India and, to a lesser extent, France, Germany, the Netherlands, Greece, South Africa, and South America. In the United States, homeopathy is becoming more widespread again after a period of decline.

In the U.S., over-the-counter homeopathic remedies are available in pharmacies and health food stores. Unlike herbs and supplements, manufacturers of homeopathic products are allowed to make strong healing claims on the labels, in part because one of the founders of the organization that became the Food and Drug Administration, Senator Royal Copeland, was a homeopathic physician. He made sure that homeopathic medicines were given a specially protected status.

Scientific Evaluation of Homeopathy

Despite its widespread acceptance in some countries, most modern scientific authorities do not take homeopathy seriously, putting it in the same category as perpetual motion machines, ghosts, and E.S.P. There are several reasons for this intense skepticism, but the most important focuses on a basic fact of chemistry. Simply put, there's absolutely nothing material in a "high-potency" homeopathic remedy; some force of nature unknown to modern science would have to be involved if homeopathy is effective.

Here's why: In the process of making a 30X homeopathic remedy, the original substance is diluted by a factor of one part in 10^{30}. This is such an enormous dilution that not even one single molecule is likely to remain. Such a remedy is merely pure sugar (if the form is a sugar pill) or pure water (if the form is a tincture). Even higher dilutions are in use, some so vast that you could use the entire earth as the starting material and still not end up with a single molecule of the original material in the resulting remedy.

Because of this chemical reality, the comparison of homeopathy to vaccinations, as advanced by many homeopathic practitioners, falls short. Vaccinations contain a great deal of substance, an amount that can be measured and weighed and which stimulates the immune system. High-potency homeopathic remedies, by contrast, contain nothing at all. (Low-potency remedies do contain a measurable amount of substance, but they are supposedly less effective than the high-potency forms, which are physically content-free.)

Some researchers have speculated that homeopathic remedies produce subtle alterations in the structure of the water in which they are dissolved. However, studies with highly sensitive equipment have failed to find any evidence of such structural changes, and chemistry as it has been understood, both before and after the development of quantum mechanics, makes it highly implausible that liquid water could retain any changes of the type hypothesized.

There are other problems with homeopathy as well. For one, it is hard to understand why a substance that produces certain symptoms when taken in overdose should cure a disease that just coincidentally happens to possess the same symptoms. This hypothesis appears too pat, too tidy and perfect, to reflect the messy world of human illness.

Furthermore, the detailed symptom pictures upon which constitutional homeopathy are based seem to be far too specific and personal to offer any likelihood of universal truth. For example, the homeopathic remedy *sulphur* is said to be useful for people who have red lips, stooped posture, and a tendency toward untidiness in personal affairs. A small selection of other supposed characteristics of this remedy include mid-morning hunger and a tendency for increased discomfort of whatever physical symptoms they may be experiencing between 10:00 and 11:00 a.m. and after exposure to cold air or motion.

As noted above, these symptoms were assembled through multiple experiences of overdose (homeopathic provings). However, from a scientific perspective, it is difficult to believe that the majority of people who overdose on sulphur experience symptoms largely similar to these (as well as to the several pages of other symptoms commonly associated with the remedy). In any case, modern knowledge of the difficulties involved in evaluating the effects of medical treatments indicates that provings must be conducted in a double-blind and placebo-controlled manner to be valid. Otherwise, participants are likely to experience symptoms simply because they expect to and observers will tend to observe the expected symptom picture as well. Unfortunately, few of the provings used to define the treatments chosen by homeopaths were performed in a scientifically reliable way. Large, rigorous studies have failed to find any difference in symptoms or biochemical measures between healthy people given homeopathic treatments or placebo.

Thus, on the face of it, homeopathy seems to be a method that shouldn't have a ghost of a chance of being true. However, some studies have found evidence that homeopathic remedies do, in fact, relieve symptoms of illness. Many of these were double-blind, placebo-controlled studies, the most meaningful kind of study. This presents a conundrum to impartial scientists.

How can this contradiction be resolved?

One possibility is that homeopathy operates via some mysterious new force that science has yet failed to discover. Another, less optimistic interpretation, is that the positive trials may be too flawed to mean anything—even though they were double-blind.

In 1997, scientists Klaus Linde, Nicola Clausius, and others published a groundbreaking review of all placebo-controlled trials of homeopathic remedies. This article appeared in a prestigious British journal, *The Lancet*. The authors wanted to determine whether there was enough evidence in total to say that homeopathy has benefits beyond the placebo effect. The results of this meta-analysis were positive, and have been widely quoted by advocates of homeopathy to conclude that the method has been proven effective.

However, not all double-blind, placebo-controlled trials are created equal. Fairly subtle design flaws can invalidate the results of a study that, on first glance, seems rigorous. In 1999 the authors reanalyzed the data and noticed a direct relationship between the quality of the study and the amount of benefit seen: the higher the quality, the less the benefit. Based on this, Linde et al. concluded that their original meta-analysis overestimated the extent to which homeopathy has been proven more effective than placebo. A 2005 evaluation of all the evidence regarding homeopathy also failed to find convincing evidence that homeopathy is more effective than placebo.

Since then, however, further positive studies have been reported, some of which appear to be quite well designed. So does homeopathy actually work?

Maybe. But when a method seems, on the face of it, scientifically impossible, it properly requires a high level of evidence before it can be accepted as true. Homeopathy has certainly not yet achieved this level of evidence and therefore must be regarded at present as unproven therapy.

What to Expect From a Session With a Homeopathic Physician

To understand how a visit to a homeopathic physician works, consider the following imaginary scenario: Sam has felt tense and nervous for months. His workload has increased dramatically since he started a new job last year. He has not been sleeping well and he's lost weight. His conventional physician recommends a stress-reduction program consisting of gentle exercise and regular relaxation, but he decides to try classical homeopathy instead.

His initial homeopathic consultation consists of a lengthy interview. The homeopath makes note of small nuances that would not be considered important by a conventional physician. Aside from his nervousness, Sam has been suffering from frequent nosebleeds, easy bruising, dry cough, hoarseness of voice at times, and occasional diarrhea and stomach aches.

The doctor asks whether cold drinks relieve his stomach pain and Sam nods. Next, the homeopath asks him several questions about his family history, personality, and psychological tendencies. Sam says that he is outgoing and friendly and likes company. "You wouldn't happen to be afraid of thunderstorms," she asks, and Sam answers that, in fact, he is. The interview continues for an hour.

Based on her analysis of Sam's *constitution* as revealed by close questioning, the homeopath carefully selects a homeopathic remedy that matches, based on the classic description in the *Homeopathic Materia Medica*. This text reports the symptoms to be expected when taking an overdose of various substances. These descriptions are complex and elaborate, covering physical and psychological symptoms that developed in the people who undertook the experiment; taken together, they represent the symptom picture of the remedy.

Sam's homeopath chooses the remedy *phosphorus*, because its symptom picture matches him closely. He is told to take the remedy for 3 months. During the period of treatment, he is advised to avoid the use of any pharmaceutical drugs, medicinal herbs (such as St. John's wort), or foods with druglike properties (such as coffee) because they have properties that might *antidote* (counteract) the effect of treatment. At the end of 3 months, he is advised to call for a follow-up visit, at which point he may be given a new remedy to treat "deeper" problems that may emerge.

Note: This description applies to practitioners using classical or constitutional homeopathy. Many alternative practitioners use homeopathic remedies to treat particular diseases and use herbs and supplements in conjunction with them.

A Note About Safety

Although serious objections remain regarding the possible efficacy of homeopathy, there is little doubt that in one respect, at least, Samuel Hahnemann achieved his aim when he invented the treatment: even if it doesn't work, it cannot possibly cause direct harm.

As described earlier, homeopathy came into being during a period in history when conventional medicine was very often more harmful than helpful. It was the age of "heroic medicine," during which treatments were chosen more for the drama of their effects than any evidence of efficacy. The most dramatic effects, however, were frequently the most dangerous. Bleeding sick patients or inducing vomiting or diarrhea were more likely to kill people than help them.

Today, conventional medicine is far safer (not to mention more effective). Nonetheless, most pharmaceutical medications present at least some risk. Not so with homeopathic treatments. On a chemical basis there is nothing in them (or, for low potency formulations, next to nothing); for this reason, it is as difficult to conceive of any manner in which homeopathic remedies could cause harm as it is to believe that they can cure. Homeopathic tablets are, by nature, completely nontoxic.

However, according to the principles of classical (or constitutional) homeopathy, versus disease-oriented (or symptomatic) homeopathy, these remedies can cause problems. On the way toward a cure, temporary exacerbation of symptoms are said to occur frequently. Such *homeopathic aggravations* are supposed to indicate a "release" of underlying problems and are therefore seen as ultimately helpful, if temporarily unpleasant. However, there is no meaningful scientific evidence that such aggravations take place at any higher rate than could be accounted for by chance (and patient's expectation).

Conclusion

Because the theories of homeopathy seem to contradict basic laws of physics, it appears reasonable to insist that homeopathy pass a higher standard of proof than other forms of alternative medicine and it has not yet done so. As we shall see in subsequent pages, some apparently rigorous studies do appear to have found homeopathic methods effective. However, many more studies have failed to find it effective and, overall, the body of supporting evidence is too weak to overcome the reasonable presumption that it does not work. Proponents of homeopathy have considerable work to do before their method can be given scientific credence.

Hypnotherapy

ALTERNATIVE NAMES: *Ericksonian hypnosis, Hypnosis, Neurolinguistic Programming, Self-hypnosis*

PRINCIPAL PROPOSED USES: *Cancer Treatment (Reducing Side Effects), Surgery Support, Warts*

OTHER PROPOSED USES: *Asthma, Burn Injury (Reducing Pain), Fibromyalgia, Hay Fever, Irritable Bowel Syndrome, Labor and Delivery, Nocturnal Enuresis (Bedwetting), Psoriasis, Smoking Cessation, Tension Headache and Other Forms of Headache, Weight Loss*

Overview

Hypnotherapy is a poorly understood technique that has multiple definitions, descriptions, and forms. It is generally agreed that the hypnotic state is different from both sleep and ordinary wakefulness, but just exactly what it consists of remains unclear. Hypnosis is sometimes described as a form of heightened attention combined with deep relaxation, uncritical openness, and voluntarily lowered resistance to suggestion. Thus, one might say that when you watch an engrossing movie and allow yourself to surrender to it as if it were reality, you are undergoing something indistinguishable from hypnosis.

In therapeutic hypnosis, the hypnotherapist uses one of several techniques to induce a hypnotic state. The most famous (and dated) technique is the swinging watch accompanied by the suggestion to fall asleep. Such *fixed gaze* hypnosis is no longer the mainstay.

More often, hypnotists use progressive relaxation methods, such as those described in the article on **relaxation therapies**. Other methods include *mental misdirection* (think of a suspense movie that leads you down the wrong path) and *deliberate mental confusion*. The net effect is the same: the person being hypnotized is in a state of heightened willingness to accept outside suggestions.

Once the client is in this state, the hypnotherapist can make a suggestion aimed at producing therapeutic benefit. At its most straightforward, this involves direct affirmation of the desired health benefit, such as "You are now relaxing the muscles of your neck and you will keep them relaxed." Indirect or paradoxical suggestions may be used as well, especially in schools of hypnotherapy such as Ericksonian hypnosis and Neurolinguistic Programming (NLP).

It is also possible to learn to give oneself suggestions by inducing a state of hypnosis; this is called *self-hypnosis*.

Uses of Hypnotherapy

Hypnotherapy is commonly used for the treatment of addictions, as well as for reducing fear and anxiety surrounding stressful situations, such as surgery or severe illness. Other relatively common uses for hypnotherapy include insomnia, childbirth, pain control in general, and nocturnal enuresis (bedwetting). However, the evidence that hypnotherapy is effective for these uses remains incomplete at best.

What Is the Scientific Evidence for Hypnotherapy?

It is more difficult to ascertain the effectiveness of a therapy like hypnosis than a drug or a pill for one simple reason: it is not easy to design a proper double-blind, placebo-controlled study of this therapy.

Researchers studying the herb St. John's wort, for example, can use placebo pills that are indistinguishable from the real thing. However, it's difficult to conceive of a form of placebo hypnosis that can't be detected as such by both practitioners and patients. For this reason, all studies of hypnosis have made various compromises to the double-blind design. Some randomly assigned participants to receive either hypnosis or no treatment. In the

best of these studies, results were rated by examiners who didn't know which participants were in which group (in other words, blinded observers). However, it isn't clear whether benefits reported in such studies are due to the hypnosis or less specific factors, such as mere attention.

Other studies have compared hypnosis to various psychological techniques, including relaxation therapy and cognitive psychotherapy. However, the same issues arise when trying to study these latter therapies as with hypnosis, and the results of a study that compares an unproven treatment to an unproven treatment are not very meaningful.

In some studies, participants were allowed to choose whether they received hypnosis or some other therapy. Such nonrandomized studies are highly unreliable; the people who chose hypnosis, for example, might have been different in another way.

Even less meaningful studies of hypnotism simply involved giving people hypnosis and monitoring them to see whether they improved. Studies of this type have been used to support the use of hypnotherapy for hundreds of medical conditions. However, for at least a dozen reasons, such open-label trials prove nothing at all, and we do not report them here. The reasons why are discussed in the article **Why Does This Book Rely on Double-blind Studies?** Note, however, that one criticism of open-label studies discussed in that article does not apply here: concerns regarding the placebo effect.

In studies of most medical therapies, researchers must take pains to eliminate the possibility of a placebo effect. This concern, however, loses its relevance when hypnotism is in question. It isn't a criticism of a study on hypnosis if an observed benefit turns out to be caused by the power of suggestion. After all, hypnosis consists precisely of the power of suggestion! (The placebo effect is only one of many problems with open-label studies, however. For more information, see the article referenced above.)

Given these caveats, the following is a summary of what science knows about the medical benefits of hypnotherapy.

The Possible Benefits of Hypnotherapy

At least 20 controlled studies, enrolling a total of more than 1,500 people, have evaluated the potential benefit of hypnosis for people undergoing **surgery**. Their combined results suggest that hypnosis may provide benefits both during and after surgery, including reducing anxiety, pain, and nausea; normalizing blood pressure and heart rate; minimizing blood loss; speeding recovery;

and shortening hospitalization. Unfortunately, many of these studies were of very poor quality.

Hypnosis has also shown some promise for reducing nausea, pain, and anxiety in adults and children undergoing **treatment for cancer**.

Numerous anecdotal reports suggest that **warts** can sometimes disappear in response to suggestion. In three controlled studies enrolling a total of 180 people with warts, use of hypnosis showed superior results compared to no treatment. In one of these, hypnosis was also superior to salicylic acid (a standard treatment for warts)! In that trial, hypnosis was also superior to fake salicylic acid, hinting that the power of suggestion with hypnosis is greater than with an ordinary placebo.

Other conditions for which hypnosis has shown promise in controlled trials include the following:

➤ **Asthma**
➤ **Burn injury (reducing pain)**
➤ **Fibromyalgia**
➤ **Hay fever**
➤ **Irritable bowel syndrome**
➤ **Labor and delivery**
➤ **Nocturnal enuresis**
➤ **Chest pain of unknown cause (unrelated to the heart)**
➤ **Peptic ulcers**
➤ **Psoriasis**
➤ **Smoking cessation**
➤ **Tension headache and other forms of headache**
➤ **Vertigo and headache caused by head injury**

However, the quality of many of the supporting studies is poor and their results are frequently inconsistent.

Hypnosis is particularly popular as an aid to **weight loss**. However, a careful analysis of published studies throws cold water on the belief that hypnosis has been shown to be highly effective for this condition; at best, the evidence only points toward a marginal benefit.

What to Expect in a Hypnotherapy Session

Hypnotherapy sessions usually last 30 to 60 minutes. They typically involve some questions and answers, followed by the hypnosis itself. Some hypnotists teach their clients self-hypnosis so they can reinforce the formal session.

How to Choose a Hypnotherapist

As with all medical therapies, it is best to choose a licensed practitioner in states where a hypnotherapy license is available. Where licensure is not available, seek a referral from a qualified and knowledgeable medical provider.

Safety Issues

In the hands of a competent practitioner, hypnotherapy should present no more risks than any other form of psychotherapy. These risks might include worsening of the original problem and temporary fluctuations in mood.

Contrary to various works of fiction, hypnosis does not give the hypnotist absolute power over his or her subject. However, as with all forms of psychotherapy, the hypnotherapist does gain some power over the client through the client's trust; an unethical therapist can abuse this.

Low Glycemic Index Diets

ALTERNATE NAMES: *Diet, Low-GI*; *Diet, Low Glycemic Index*; *GI Diet*; Glucose Revolution; Sugar Busters

Overview

Mainstream groups such as the American Heart Association and the American Dietetic Association endorse a unified set of guidelines for the optimum diet. According to these organizations, the majority of calories in the daily diet should come from carbohydrates (55 to 60%); fat should provide no more than 30% of total calories; and protein should be kept to 10 to 15%.

However, many popular diet books turn the standard diet on its head. As described in the entry on **low-carbohydrate diets**, the Atkins diet, the Zone diet, Protein Power, and other "alternative" dietary approaches turn thumbs down on carbohydrates and advocate increased consumption of fat and/or protein. According to theory, the low-carb approach aids in weight loss (and provides a variety of other health benefits) by reducing the body's production of insulin.

The low glycemic index (low-GI) diet splits the difference between the low-carb and low-fat approaches. It maintains the low-carb diet's focus on insulin, but it suggests choosing certain carbohydrates over others rather than restricting carbohydrate intake.

Evidence suggests that carbohydrates are not created equal. Some carbohydrates, such as pure glucose, are absorbed quickly and create a rapid, strong rise in both blood sugar and insulin. However, others (such as brown rice) are absorbed much more slowly and produce only a modest blood sugar and insulin response. According to proponents of the low-GI diet, eating foods in the latter category will enhance weight loss and improve health. However, as we shall see, despite some promising theory there is as yet no solid evidence that low-GI diets enhance weight loss.

Besides weight loss, preliminary evidence suggests that the low-GI approach (or, even better, a related method called *low glycemic load*) may help prevent heart disease. The low-GI approach has also shown promise for treating and possibly preventing diabetes.

What Is the Glycemic Index?

The precise measurement of the glucose-stimulating effect of a food is called its *glycemic index*. The lower a food's glycemic index, the less potent its effects on blood sugar (and therefore insulin).

The glycemic index of glucose is arbitrarily set at 100. The ratings of other foods are determined as follows. First, researchers calculate a portion size for the food to supply 50 g of carbohydrates. Next, they give that amount of the food to at least eight to ten people and measure the blood sugar response. (By using a group of people rather than one person, researchers can ensure that the idiosyncrasies of one individual don't skew the results.) On another occasion, researchers also give each participant an equivalent amount of glucose and perform the same measurements. The glycemic index of a food is then determined by comparing the two outcomes. For example, if a food causes half of the blood

sugar rise of glucose, it is assigned a GI of 50; if it causes one-quarter of the rise, it is assigned a GI of 25. The lower the glycemic index, the better.

When scientists first began to determine the glycemic index of foods, some of the results caused eyebrows to rise. It didn't surprise anyone when jellybeans turned out to have a high glycemic index of 80—after all, jellybeans are mostly sugar. Nor was it unexpected that kidney beans have a low glycemic index of 27 because they are notoriously hard to digest. But when baked potatoes came back with a reading of 93, researchers were taken aback. This rating is higher than that of almost all other foods, including ice cream (61), sweet potatoes (54), and white bread (70). Based on this finding, low-GI diets recommend that you stay largely away from potatoes. (However, the concern regarding potatoes is probably unnecessary. See the discussion of glycemic load below.)

There are other surprises hidden in the glycemic index tables. For example, fructose (the sweetener in honey) has an extraordinarily low glycemic index of 23—lower than brown rice and almost three times lower than white sugar. Candy bars also tend to have a relatively good (low) glycemic index, presumably because their fat content makes them digest slowly.

It's difficult to predict the glycemic index of a food without specifically testing it, but there are some general factors that can be recognized. Fiber content tends to reduce the glycemic index of a food, presumably by slowing down digestion. For this reason, whole grains usually have a lower GI score than refined, processed grains. Fat content also reduces GI score. Simple carbohydrates (such as sugar) often have a higher GI score than complex carbohydrates (such as brown rice).

However, there are numerous exceptions to these rules. Factors such as the acid content of food; the size of the food particles; and the precise mixture of fats, proteins, and carbohydrates can substantially change the GI measurement. For a measurement like the glycemic index to be meaningful, it has to be generally reproducible between people. In other words, if a potato has a glycemic index of 93 in one person, it should have pretty much the same glycemic index when given to another person. Science suggests that the GI passes this test. The glycemic index of individual foods is fairly constant between people and even mixed meals have a fairly predictable effect according to most (but not all) studies.

Thus, the GI of a food really does indicate its propensity to raise insulin levels. Whether a diet based on the index will aid in weight loss, however, is another story.

How to Follow a Low Glycemic Index Diet

Following a low glycemic index diet is fairly easy. Basically, you follow the typical diet endorsed by authorities such as the American Dietetic Association, but you choose carbohydrates that fall toward the lower end of the glycemic index scale. Books such as *The Glucose Revolution* give a great deal of information on how to make these choices.

Do Low Glycemic Index Diets Aid in Weight Loss? Problems with the Theory

There are two primary theoretical reasons given why low-GI diets should help reduce weight. The most prominent reason given in books on the low-GI approach involves insulin levels. Basically, these books show that low-GI diets reduce insulin release and then take almost for granted the idea that reduced insulin levels should aid in weight loss. However, there is little justification for the second part of this argument. Excess weight is known to lead to elevated insulin levels, but there is little meaningful evidence for the reverse: that reducing insulin levels will help remove excess weight. For more information on this very complicated subject, see the article on **low-carb diets**.

Books on the low-GI diet give another reason for using their approach as well: they state that low-GI foods fill you up more quickly than high-GI foods and also keep you feeling full for longer. Unfortunately, as we shall see, there is more evidence against this belief than for it.

The Satiety Index

A measurement called the *Satiety Index* assigns a numerical quantity to the filling quality of a food. These numbers are determined by feeding people fixed caloric amounts of those foods and then determining how soon they get hungry again and how much they eat at subsequent meals. The process is similar to the methods used to establish the GI index.

The results of these measurements do not corroborate the expectations of low-GI diet proponents. As it happens, foods with the worst (highest) GI index are often the most satiating—exactly the reverse of what low-GI theory proponents would say.

For example, the Satiety Index tells us that potatoes are among the most satiating of foods. However, as noted above, the GI analysis gave potatoes a bad rating. According to the low-GI theory, you should feel hunger pangs shortly after eating a big baked potato. In real life, that doesn't happen (even without the sour cream!).

There are numerous other contradictions between research findings and the low-GI/high-satiety theory. For example, one study found no difference in satiety between fructose (fruit sugar) and glucose when taken as part of a mixed meal, even though fructose has a GI more than four times lower than glucose.

A few studies do seem to suggest that certain low-GI foods are more filling than high-GI foods. However, in these studies the bulkiness and lack of palatability of the low-GI foods chosen may have played a more important role than the food's glycemic index.

Thus, the satiety argument for low-GI diets doesn't appear to hold up to scrutiny.

Is the Glycemic Index Even the Right Measurement?

There's another problem with the low-GI approach: It's probably the wrong way to assess the insulin-related effects of food.

The glycemic index measures blood sugar response per gram of carbohydrate contained in a food, not per gram of the food. This leads to some odd numbers. For example, a parsnip has a glycemic index of 98, almost as high as pure sugar. If taken at face value, this figure suggests that dieters should avoid parsnips like the plague; however, if you've ever eaten a parsnip, you know that it's not exactly candy. In fact, parsnips are mostly indigestible fiber and you would have to eat a few bushels to trigger a major glucose and insulin response.

The reason for the high number is that the glycemic index rates the effects per gram of carbohydrate rather than per gram of total parsnip, and the sugar present in minute amounts in a parsnip itself is highly absorbable. The high glycemic index rating of parsnips is thus extremely misleading. Books such as *The Glucose Revolution* take care of issues like this on a case-by-case basis by saying, for example, that you can consider most vegetables "free foods" regardless of their glycemic index. But in fact the same considerations apply to all foods and distort the meaningfulness of the scale as a whole.

A different measurement, the *glycemic load* (GL), takes this into account. The GL is derived by multiplying the glycemic index by the percent of carbohydrate content of a food. In other words, it measures the glucose/insulin response per gram of food rather than per gram of carbohydrate in that food. Using this system, the glycemic load of a parsnip is 10, while glucose has a relative load of 100. And remember the potato problem, that terrible bogey of GI diets? The glycemic load of a typical serving of potato is only 27—not such a bogeyman at all. Such numbers make a lot more sense.

What Is the Direct Evidence Regarding Whether Low-GI Diets Enhance Weight Loss?

Theory is one thing and practice is another. It is certainly possible that making sure to focus on low–glycemic index or low–glycemic load foods will help you lose weight, even if the theoretical justification for the idea is weak. However, there is only preliminary evidence to support this possibility. The studies commonly cited, although promising, are too preliminary to prove much.

In one of these studies, 107 overweight adolescents were divided into two groups: a low-GI group and a low-fat group. The low-GI group was counseled to follow a diet consisting of 45 to 50% carbohydrates (preferably low-GI carbohydrates), 20 to 25% protein, and 30 to 35% fat. Calorie restriction was not emphasized. The low-fat group received instructions for a standard low-fat, low-calorie diet divided up into 55 to 60% carbohydrates, 15 to 20% protein, and 25 to 30% fat. Over a period of about 4 months, participants on the low-GI diet lost about 4.5 pounds, while those on the standard diet lost just fewer than 3 pounds.

Unfortunately, this study does not say as much about the low-GI approach as it might seem. Perhaps the most obvious problem is that the low-GI diet used here was also a high-protein diet. It is possible that high-protein diets might help weight loss regardless of the glycemic index of the foods consumed. (In fact, that is precisely what proponents of high-protein diets claim.)

Another problem is that participants were not assigned to the two groups randomly. Rather, researchers consciously picked which group each participant should join. This is a major flaw because it introduces the possibility of intentional or unintentional bias. It is quite possible, for example, that researchers placed adolescents with greater self-motivation into the low-GI group, based on an unconscious desire to see results from the study. This is not an academic problem and modern medical studies always use randomization to circumvent it.

Finally, researchers made no effort to determine how well participants followed their diets. It might be that those in the low-fat diet group simply didn't stick to the rules as well as those in the low-GI diet group because the rules were more challenging.

Despite these many flaws, the study results are still promising. Losing weight without deliberately cutting calories is potentially a great thing.

In the other study, 30 overweight women with excessively high insulin levels were put on either a normal low-calorie diet or one that supplied the same amount of calories but used low-GI foods. The results over 12 weeks showed that women following the low-GI diet lost several pounds more than those following the normal diet.

In yet another small study, this one involving overweight adolescents, a conventional reduced calorie diet was compared against a low-glycemic load diet that did not have any calorie restrictions. The results showed that simply by sticking to low-GI foods, without regard for calories, the participants on the low-GI diet were able to lose as much or more weight as those on the low-calorie diet.

Does the Low-GI Diet Offer Any Health Benefits?

There is some evidence that a low–glycemic index diet (or, even better, a low–glycemic load diet) might help prevent cancer and heart disease. The low-GI approach has also shown promise for preventing or treating diabetes.

Heart Disease Prevention

One large observational study evaluated the diets of more than 75,000 women and found that those women whose diets provided a lower glycemic load had a lower incidence of **heart disease**. In this study, 75,521 women aged 38 to 63 years were followed for 10 years. Each filled out detailed questionnaires regarding her diet. Using this data, researchers calculated the average glycemic load of each participant. The results showed that women who consumed a diet with a high GL were more likely to experience heart disease than those who consumed a diet of low GL.

Other observational studies suggest that consumption of foods with lower GL may lead to reduced triglyceride levels and higher HDL ("good" cholesterol) levels. These effects in turn might lead to decreased risk of heart disease.

However, other observational studies have found little or no relationship between heart disease and GI or GL.

These contradictory results are not surprising, but even if the observational study results were entirely consistent, that wouldn't prove the case for a low-GI approach. Conclusions based on observational studies are notoriously unreliable due to the possible presence of unidentified confounding factors. For example, because there is an approximate correlation between fiber in the diet and glycemic load, it is possible that benefits, when seen, are really due to fiber intake instead. Factors such as this one may easily obscure the effects of the factor under study, leading to contradictory or misleading results.

Intervention trials (studies in which researchers actually intervene in participants' lives) are more reliable and some have been conducted to evaluate the low-GI diet. For example, a 3-month study followed 30 people with high lipid levels. During the second month, low-GI foods were substituted for higher-GI foods, while other nutrients were kept similar. Improvements were seen in total cholesterol, LDL cholesterol, and triglycerides, but not in HDL. Interestingly, a close analysis of the results showed that only patients who had high triglycerides at the beginning of the study showed benefit.

Another approach to the issue involves analysis of effects on insulin resistance. Evidence suggests that increased resistance of the body to its own insulin raises the risk of heart disease. One study found that use of a low-GI diet versus a high-GI diet improved the body's sensitivity to insulin in women at risk for heart disease. Similar results were seen in a group of people with severe heart disease and a group of healthy people.

While these results are preliminary, taken together they do suggest that consumption of low-GI foods might have a beneficial effect on heart disease risk.

Low-GI Diet and Diabetes

Two large observational studies, one involving men and the other involving women, found that diets with lower glycemic loads were associated with a lower rate of **diabetes**. For example, one trial followed 65,173 women for a period of 6 years. Women whose diets had a high glycemic load had a 47% increased risk of developing diabetes compared with those whose diets had the lowest glycemic load. Fiber content of diet also makes a difference. People who consumed a diet that was both low in fiber and high in glycemic load had a 250% increased incidence of diabetes.

However, as always, the results of these observational studies have to be taken with a grain of salt. It's quite possible that unrecognized factors are responsible for the results seen. For example, **magnesium** deficiency is widespread and may contribute to the development of diabetes; whole grains contain magnesium and are also low-GI foods. Therefore, it could be that the benefits seen in these studies are actually caused by increased magnesium intake in the low-GI group, rather than effects on blood sugar and insulin.

Furthermore, one observational study found no connection between the glycemic values of foods and the incidence of diabetes. Another observational study did find a correlation between carbohydrate intake (especially pastries) and the onset of diabetes, but no consistent relationship with glycemic index. Other studies have found no relationship between sugar consumption (a high-GI food) and diabetes onset.

Thus, reducing dietary glycemic load may help prevent diabetes, but we don't know this for sure.

Whether or not low-GI diets can prevent diabetes, for people who already have diabetes, going on a low GI diet might improve blood sugar control. However, the benefits seem to be small at most.

Other Uses of Low Glycemic Index Diet

Weak evidence hints that a low glycemic index diet might help prevent **macular degeneration**. Although there are theoretical reasons to believe that use of white sugar and other high glycemic index foods might promote colon cancer, a large observational study failed to find any association between colon cancer rates and diets high in sugar, carbohydrates, or glycemic load.

It has been proposed that low-GI foods may **enhance sports performance**. However, one study involving a simulated 64-km bicycle race found no performance differences between use of honey (low GI) or dextrose (high GI) as a carbohydrate source.

The Bottom Line

As you have seen, the evidence that a low-GI diet will help you lose weight is not yet very impressive. Its theoretical foundation is weak and it appears to be using the wrong method of ranking foods regarding their effects on insulin. Conversely, however, there's no reason to believe a low-GI diet causes harm. If you find that you lose weight with a low-GI diet, stick with it.

Note: While the most popular low-GI diet books (*The

Glucose Revolution, Sugar Busters) recommend a diet that is generally reasonable and should be safe, it is easy to design some fairly extreme low-GI diets. For example, a diet consisting of nothing but lard would be a very, very low-GI diet, since the glycemic index of lard is 0. While it no longer seems that saturated fat is as harmful as once thought, a pure lard diet is probably not a good idea. If you run across a diet book that recommends achieving a low–glycemic index by consuming an extreme diet, approach it with caution.

Low-Carbohydrate Diet

RELATED TERMS: *Atkins Diet; Diet, Atkins; Diet, High-Protein; Diet, Low-Carb; Diet, Zone; High-Protein Diet; Zone Diet*

Overview

Mainstream groups such as the American Heart Association and the American Dietetic Association endorse a unified set of dietary guidelines for people who wish to lose weight—eat a low-fat diet and cut calories.

However, many popular diet books take a very different approach. The Atkins diet, the Zone diet, *Protein Power*, and numerous other dietary approaches turn thumbs down on low-fat. Instead, these methods recommend cutting down on carbohydrates. According to proponents of these theories, when you reduce the carbohydrates in your diet (and, correspondingly, increase protein and/or fat), you will find it much easier to reduce your calorie intake and you may even lose weight without cutting calories.

The controversy over these contradictions has grown heated. Proponents of the low-fat diet claim that low-carbohydrate diets are ineffective and even dangerous, while low-carb proponents say much the same about the low-fat approach. However, an article published in the *Journal of the American Medical Association* suggests that neither side has a strong case. Researchers concluded, essentially, that a calorie is a calorie, regardless of whether it comes from a low-carbohydrate or a low-fat diet. They did not find any consistent evidence that the low-carb diet makes it easier to lose weight than the low-fat diet, but neither did they find any consistent evidence for the reverse. Furthermore, the authors of the *JAMA* review did not find any compelling reason to conclude that low-carb diets are unsafe, although they did point out that the long-term safety of such diets remains unknown.

Subsequent studies have tended to confirm these findings for a variety of low-carb diets. In general, it appears that weight loss leads to improvement in cholesterol profile, regardless of the diet used to achieve the weight loss. Low-carb, high-fat diets appear to be equally effective as low-carb, high-protein diets. Contrary to claims by some low-carb proponents, low-fat, high-carb diets do not seem to promote weight gain.

Proponents of low-carb diets claim that their approaches offer various health benefits beyond weight loss, such as preventing diabetes and enhancing energy. However, the justification for these claims rests almost entirely on theoretical arguments. There is a little evidence, however, that diets high in meat protein can reduce blood pressure in people with **high blood pressure**; however, any diet that causes weight loss is likely to lower blood pressure.

Therefore, based on the current state of information, it seems that the most sensible course is as follows: if you need to lose weight, experiment with different diets and see which one allows you to most easily cut calories (and keep them cut). If the low-carb diet approach works for you, stick with it. However, if it does not help you lose weight, you probably should not continue it indefinitely.

Note: Any form of extreme dieting can cause serious side effects or even death. We strongly recommend that all people who intend to adopt an unconventional diet should first seek medical advice. Furthermore, people with kidney failure should not use low-carb, high-protein diets, as high protein intake can easily overstress failing kidneys. (High-protein diets are probably not harmful for people with healthy kidneys.)

In addition, people who take the blood thinner **warfarin** (Coumadin) may need to have their blood coagulation tested after beginning a high-protein, low-carbohydrate diet. Two case reports suggest that such diets may decrease the effectiveness of warfarin, requiring a higher dose. Conversely, if you are already on warfarin and a high-protein, low-carbohydrate diet and go off the diet, you may need to reduce your warfarin dose.

Magnet Therapy

RELATED TERMS: *Electromagnetic Therapy, Magnetic Stimulation, PEMF, rTMS, Static Magnets, TMS, Transcranial Magnetic Stimulation*

PRINCIPAL PROPOSED USES:

Static Magnets: *Rheumatoid Arthritis, Post-polio Syndrome, Fibromyalgia, Diabetic Peripheral Neuropathy (and Other Forms of Peripheral Neuropathy), Low Back Pain and Other Forms of Chronic Musculoskeletal Pain, Wound Healing after Plastic Surgery*

Electromagnetic Therapy—PEMF: *Nonhealing Bone Fractures, Osteoarthritis, Stress Incontinence, Migraines*

Electromagnetic Therapy—RTMS: *Depression*

OTHER PROPOSED USES:

Static Magnets: *Carpal Tunnel Syndrome, Chronic Pelvic Pain in Women (Caused by Various Conditions, such as Endometriosis and Chronic Cystitis), Edema, Fatigue, Insomnia, Menstrual Pain, Osteoarthritis, Rheumatoid Arthritis, Scar Tissue, Sports and Fitness Support: Enhancing Recovery; Sports and Fitness Support: Enhancing Performance, Tinnitus*

Electromagnetic Therapy—PEMF: *Multiple Sclerosis, Erectile Dysfunction*

Electromagnetic Therapy—RTMS: *Epilepsy, Schizophrenia, Parkinson's Disease, Obsessive-compulsive Disorder, Myofascial Pain Syndrome, Post-traumatic Stress Disorder*

Overview

Long popular in Japan, magnet therapy has entered public awareness in the United States, stimulated by golfers and tennis players extolling the virtues of magnets in the treatment of sports-related injuries. Magnetic knee, shoulder, and ankle pads, as well as insoles and mattress pads, are widely available and are touted as providing myriad healing benefits.

Despite this enthusiasm, as yet there is little scientific evidence to support the use of magnets for any medical condition. However, some small studies completed in the last few years suggest that various forms of magnet therapy might have a therapeutic effect in certain conditions. More studies are underway.

History of Magnet Therapy

Magnet therapy has a long history in traditional folk medicine. Reliable documentation tells us that Chinese doctors believed in the therapeutic value of magnets at least 2,000 years ago and probably earlier than that. In sixteenth-century Europe, Paracelsus used magnets to treat a variety of ailments. Two centuries later, Mesmer became famous for treating various disorders with magnets.

In the middle decades of the twentieth century, scientists in various parts of the world began performing studies on the therapeutic use of magnets. From the 1940s on, magnets became increasingly popular in Japan. Yoshio Manaka, one of the influential Japanese acupuncturists of the twentieth century, used magnets in conjunction with **acupuncture**. Magnet therapy also became a commonly used technique of self-administered medicine in Japan. For example, a type of plaster containing a small magnet became popular for treating aches and pains, especially among the elderly. Magnetic mattress pads, bracelets, and necklaces also became popular—again, mainly among the elderly. During the 1970s, both magnets and electromagnetic machines became popular among athletes in many countries for treating sports-related injuries.

These developments led to a rapidly growing industry creating magnetic products for a variety of conditions. However, the development of this industry preceded any reliable scientific evidence that static magnets actually work for the purposes intended. In the United States, it was only in 1997 that properly designed clinical trials of magnets began to be reported. Subsequently, results of several preliminary studies (detailed in the Scientific Evidence section below) suggested that both static magnets and electromagnetic therapy may indeed offer therapeutic benefits for several disorders. These findings have escalated research interest in magnet therapy.

Types of Magnet Therapy and Their Uses

The term *magnet therapy* usually refers to the use of static magnets placed directly on the body, generally over regions of pain. Static magnets are either attached to the body by tape or encapsulated in specially designed products such as belts, wraps, or mattress pads. Static magnets are also sometimes known as *permanent magnets*.

Static magnets come in various strengths. The units of measuring magnet strength are *gauss* and *tesla*. One tesla equals 10,000 gauss. A refrigerator magnet, for example, is around 200 gauss. Therapeutic magnets measure anywhere from 200 to 10,000 gauss, but the most commonly used measure 400 to 800 gauss.

Therapeutic magnets come in two different types of polarity arrangements: *unipolar magnets* and *alternating-pole devices*. Magnets that have north on one side and south on the other are known, rather confusingly, as unipolar magnets. Bipolar or alternating-pole magnets are made from a sheet of magnetic material with north and south magnets arranged in an alternating pattern, so that both north and south face the skin. This type of magnet exerts a weaker magnetic field because the alternating magnets tend to oppose each other. Each type of magnet has its own recommended uses and enthusiasts. (There are many heated opinions—with no supporting evidence—on this matter.)

More complex magnetic devices have also been studied—not for home use, but for use in physicians' offices and hospitals. Electromagnetic therapy (usually as *pulsed electromagnetic field therapy*, or PEMF) has been used to treat nonhealing fractures since the 1970s and is now being investigated experimentally for **osteoarthritis**, stress incontinence, **migraines**, and other conditions.

A special form of electromagnetic therapy, repetitive transcranial magnetic stimulation (rTMS), is undergoing particularly close study. rTMS is designed specifically to treat the brain with low-frequency magnetic pulses. A large body of small studies suggest that rTMS might be beneficial for **depression**. It is also being studied for the treatment of **Parkinson's disease**, **epilepsy**, **schizophrenia**, and **obsessive-compulsive disorder**.

How Does Magnet Therapy Work?

Many commercial magnets have such a weak field that it is hard to believe they could affect the body at all. Some, however, are quite powerful and could conceivably cause effects at some depth. Nonetheless, biophysicists are skeptical that static magnets could significantly affect the body. (The moving magnetic fields of rTMS and PEMF act differently and there is little doubt that they can affect nerve tissue and possibly other parts of the body as well.)

A commonly held misconception is that magnets attract the iron in blood cells, thus moving the blood and stimulating circulation. However, the iron in the blood is not in a magnetic form. Static magnets *could* affect charged particles in the blood, nerves, and cell membranes or subtly alter biochemical reactions, although whether the effect is strong enough to make a difference remains to be shown. Some research results suggest that static magnets affect local blood circulation, but a rigorously designed double-blind trial found that commercially available static magnets have no effect on blood flow. Another well-designed trial also failed to find effects on blood circulation. However, there is some weak evidence that static magnets may affect muscle metabolism. Further research will be necessary to sort out these possibilities.

What Is the Scientific Evidence for Magnet Therapy?

Static Magnets

In double-blind, placebo-controlled trials, static magnets have shown promise for a number of conditions, but in no case is the evidence strong enough to be relied upon. **Note:** Some magnet proponents claim that it is impossible to carry out a truly double-blinded study on magnets because participants can simply use a metal pin or a similar object to discover whether they have a real magnet applied to or not. Some researchers have gotten around this by using a weak magnet as the placebo treatment. Other researchers have designed more complicated placebo devices that patients have been found unable to identify as fake treatments.

⇛ *Rheumatoid Arthritis*

A double-blind, controlled trial of 64 people with **rheumatoid arthritis** of the knee compared the effects of strong alternating polarity magnets (see Types of Magnet Therapy and Their Uses for definition) with the effects of a deliberately weak unipolar magnet. Researchers used the weakened magnet as a control group so that participants wouldn't find it easy to break the blind by testing the magnetism of their treatment.

After 1 week of therapy, 68% of the participants using the strong magnets (called the treatment group) reported relief, compared to 27% in the control group. This difference was statistically significant. Two out of four other subjective measurements of disease severity also showed statistically significant improvements. However, no significant improvements were seen in objective evaluations of the condition, such as blood tests for inflammation severity or physician's assessment of joint tenderness, swelling, or range of motion. This study suggests that magnet therapy may reduce the pain of rheumatoid arthritis without altering actual inflammation. However, the mixture of statistically significant and insignificant results indicates that a larger trial is necessary to factor out "statistical noise."

⇛ *Post-polio Syndrome*

A double-blind, placebo-controlled study of 50 people with post-polio syndrome found evidence that magnets are effective for relieving pain. The magnets or placebo magnets were placed on previously determined trigger points (one per person) for 45 minutes. (Trigger points are sore areas within muscle that, when pressed, cause relief in other areas of the muscle and conversely, when inflamed, cause pain in other parts of the muscle.) In the treatment group, 76% of the participants reported improvement, compared to 19% in the placebo group.

⇛ *Fibromyalgia*

A 6-month, double-blind, placebo-controlled trial of 119 people with **fibromyalgia** compared two commercially available magnetic mattress pads against sham treatment and no treatment. Group 1 used a mattress pad designed to create a uniform magnetic field of negative polarity. Group 2 used a mattress pad that varied in polarity. In both groups, manufacturer's instructions were followed. Groups 3 and 4 used sham treatments designed to match in appearance the magnets used in Groups 1 and 2. Group 5 received no treatment.

On average, participants in all groups showed improvement over the 6 months of the study. Participants in the treatment groups, especially Group 1, showed a trend toward greater improvement; however, the differences between real treatment and sham or no treatment failed to reach statistical significance in most measures. This outcome suggests that magnetic mattress pads might be helpful for fibromyalgia, but a larger study would be necessary to identify benefits.

A previous double-blind, placebo-controlled study of 30 women with fibromyalgia did find significant improvement with magnets compared to placebo. The women slept on magnetic mattress pads (or sham pads for the control group) every night for 4 months. Of the 25 women who completed the trial, participants sleeping on the experimental mattress pads experienced a significant decrease in pain and fatigue compared to the placebo group, along with significant improvement in sleep and physical functioning.

⇛ *Peripheral Neuropathy*

A 4-month, double-blind, placebo-controlled crossover study of 19 people with **peripheral neuropathy** found a significant reduction in symptoms compared to placebo. Participants wore magnetic foot insoles during the day throughout the trial period. Reduction in the symptoms of burning, numbness, and tingling were especially marked in those cases of neuropathy associated with diabetes.

Based on these results, a far larger randomized, placebo-controlled, follow-up study was performed by the same researchers. This trial enrolled 375 people with peripheral neuropathy caused by diabetes and tested the effectiveness of 4 months of treatment with magnetic insoles. The results indicated that the insoles produced benefits beyond that of the placebo effect, reducing such symptoms as burning pain, numbness, tingling, and exercise-induced pain.

⇛ *Wound Healing After Plastic Surgery*

A double-blind, placebo-controlled study looked at the effect of magnets on healing after plastic **surgery**. The study examined the use of magnets on 20 patients who had had suction lipectomy (commonly known as *liposuction*). Magnets contained in patches were placed over the operative region immediately after surgery and left in place for 14 days. The treatment group experienced statistically significant reduction of pain and swelling on postoperative days 1 through 4 and in discoloration on days 1 through 3 compared to the control group.

➢ Low Back Pain and Other Forms of Chronic Musculoskeletal Pain

A double-blind, placebo-controlled crossover trial of 54 people with knee or **back pain** compared a complex static magnet array against a sham magnet array. Participants used either the real or sham device for 24 hours; then, after a 7-day rest period, they used the opposite therapy for another 24 hours. Evaluations showed that use of the real magnet was associated with greater improvements than the sham treatment.

Benefits were also seen in a double-blind, placebo-controlled trial of 43 people with chronic knee pain who used fairly high-power but otherwise ordinary static magnets continuously for 2 weeks.

A double-blind, placebo-controlled crossover study of 20 people who had chronic low back pain for at least 6 months' duration failed to find any evidence of benefit. However, the alternating pole magnet used in this study produced a very weak magnetic field.

In a double-blind study of 101 people with chronic neck and shoulder pain, use of a magnetic necklace failed to prove more effective than placebo treatment.

Another study failed to find magnetic insoles helpful for heel pain.

➢ Osteoarthritis

A widely publicized 12-week study of 194 people reportedly found that use of magnetic bracelets reduced osteoarthritis pain in the hip and knee. However, the study actually found statistically similar benefits among participants given a placebo treatment. The researchers suggest that this failure to show superior effects may have been due, in part, to an unfortunate error: the study utilized weak magnets as the placebo treatments, but 34 patients in the placebo group accidentally received strong magnets instead. This would tend to decrease the difference in outcome seen between the treatment and the placebo group and could therefore hide a real treatment benefit. Nonetheless, as matters currently stand, this study does not provide evidence

that magnetic bracelets offer any benefit for osteoarthritis beyond that of the placebo effect.

A much smaller study also failed to find statistically significant benefit, but it was too small to be able to produce statistically meaningful results. Rather, it was designed to evaluate a special placebo magnet device. After the study, researchers polled the participants to see if they could correctly identify whether they'd been given the real treatment or the placebo: they could not.

➢ Pelvic Pain

A double-blind, placebo-controlled study of 14 women with chronic pelvic pain (due to **endometriosis** or other causes) found no significant benefit when magnets were applied to abdominal trigger points for 2 weeks. However, statistical analysis showed that it would have been necessary to enroll a larger number of participants to detect an effect. A larger study did find some evidence of benefit after 4 weeks of treatment, but a high dropout rate and other design problems compromise the meaningfulness of the results. Another small study found possible evidence of benefit in **menstrual pain**.

➢ Carpal Tunnel Syndrome

A double-blind, placebo-controlled study of 30 people with **carpal tunnel syndrome** found that a single treatment with a static magnet produced dramatic and longlasting benefits. However, identical dramatic benefits were seen in the placebo group! Thus, this study supports other trials that found placebo treatment quite effective for the treatment of pain, but provides no evidence for the effectiveness of magnets per se.

➢ Sports Performance

People who undergo intense exercise often experience muscle soreness afterward. (See **Sports and Fitness Support: Enhancing Recovery.**) One study tested magnet therapy for reducing this symptom. However, while use of magnets did reduce muscle soreness, so did placebo treatment, and there was no significant difference between the effectiveness of magnets and placebo. Another study, of more complex design, also failed to find benefit.

Magnetic insoles have also been advocated for increasing **sports performance**. However, a study of 14 college athletes failed to find that magnetic insoles improved vertical jump, bench squat, 40-yard dash, or a soccer-specific fitness test performance.

Electromagnetic Therapy: Pulsed Electromagnetic Field Therapy (PEMF)

Electromagnetic therapy is used in two main ways: pulsed electromagnetic field therapy (PEMF) or a special version of PEMF called repetitive transcranial magnetic stimulation (rTMS). In this section, we discuss PEMF.

Although bone has a remarkable capacity to heal from injury, in some cases the broken ends do not join: these are called non-union fractures. PEMF therapy has been used to stimulate bone repair in non-union and other fractures since the 1970s; this is a relatively accepted use and will not be discussed here. More controversially, PEMF has shown promise for osteoarthritis, stress incontinence, and possibly other conditions as well.

➢ *Osteoarthritis*

Three double-blind, placebo-controlled studies enrolling a total of more than 350 people suggest that pulsed electromagnetic field therapy can improve symptoms of osteoarthritis.

For example, a double-blind, placebo-controlled study tested PEMF in 86 people with osteoarthritis of the knee and 81 with osteoarthritis of the cervical spine. Participants received 18 half-hour sessions with either a PEMF machine or a sham device. The treated participants showed significantly greater improvements in disease severity than those given placebo. For both osteoarthritis conditions, benefits lasted for at least 1 month after treatment was stopped.

A more recent double-blind trial evaluated low-power, extremely low-frequency pulsed electromagnetic fields for the treatment of knee osteoarthritis. A total of 176 people received eight sessions of either sham or real treatment over a period of 2 weeks. The results showed significantly greater pain reduction in the treated group.

➢ *Stress Incontinence*

Many women experience stress incontinence, the leakage of urine following any action that puts pressure on the bladder. Laughter, physical exercise, and coughing can all trigger this unpleasant occurrence. A recent study suggests that PEMF treatment might be helpful. In this placebo-controlled study, researchers applied high-intensity pulsating magnetic fields to 62 women with stress incontinence. The intention was to stimulate the nerves that control the pelvic muscles.

The results showed that one session of magnetic stimulation significantly reduced episodes of urinary leakage over the following week, compared to placebo. In the treated group, 74% experienced significant improvement, compared to only 32% in the placebo group. Presumably, the high-intensity magnetic field used in this treatment created electrical currents in the pelvic muscles and nerves. This was confirmed by objective examination of 13 patients, which found that magnetic stimulation was, in fact, increasing the strength of closure at the exit from the bladder. However, there was one serious flaw in this study: it does not appear to have been double-blind. (For more information on why this is important, see **Why Does This Book Rely on Double-blind Studies?**.) Researchers apparently knew which participants were getting real treatment and which were not and, therefore, might have unconsciously biased their observations to conform to their expectations. Thus, the promise of electromagnetic therapy for stress incontinence still needs to be validated in properly designed trials.

➢ *Multiple Sclerosis*

A 2-month, double-blind, placebo-controlled study of 30 people with **multiple sclerosis** was conducted using a PEMF device. Participants were instructed to tape the device to one of three different acupuncture points on the shoulder, back, or hip. The study found statistically significant improvements in the treatment group, most notably in bladder control, hand function, and muscle spasticity. Benefits were seen in another small study too.

➢ *Erectile Dysfunction*

In a 3-week, double-blind, placebo-controlled trial, 20 men with **erectile dysfunction** received PEMF therapy or placebo. The magnetic therapy was administered by means of a small box worn near the genital area and kept in place as continuously as possible over the study period; neither participants nor observers knew whether the device was actually activated or not. The results showed that use of PEMF significantly improved sexual function compared to placebo.

➢ *Migraines*

In a double-blind trial, 42 people with migraine headaches were given treatment with real or placebo pulsed electromagnetic therapy to the inner thighs for 1 hour 5 times per week for 2 weeks. The results showed benefits in headache frequency and severity. However, the study design was rather convoluted and nonstandard and, therefore, the results are difficult to interpret.

Electromagnetic Therapy: Repetitive Transcranial Magnetic Stimulation

Repetitive transcranial magnetic stimulation (rTMS), a form of PEMF that specifically involves applying low-frequency magnetic pulses to the brain, has been investigated for treating emotional illnesses and other conditions that originate in the brain. The results of preliminary studies have been generally promising.

⇛ *Depression*

About 20 small studies have evaluated rTMS for the treatment of depression (including severe depression that does not respond to standard treatment, as well as the depressive phase of **bipolar illness**) and most found it effective.

In one of the best of these studies, 70 people with major depression were given rTMS or sham rTMS in a double-blind setting over a period of 2 weeks. The results showed that participants who had received actual treatment experienced significantly greater improvement than did those receiving sham treatment.

Another study evaluated the effects of rTMS in 20 people whose depression did not respond to standard drug therapy (treatment-resistant depression) and also found benefits. This suggests that rTMS might be an option for the 20% to 30% of depressed people for whom conventional drug therapy is not successful. ECT (electroconvulsive therapy, or shock treatment) is often used for people who fall in this category, but rTMS may be an equally effective and less traumatic alternative.

After all these small trials, it is time for a large one!

⇛ *Epilepsy*

In a double-blind, placebo-controlled trial, 24 people with epilepsy (technically, partial complex seizures or secondarily generalized seizures) not fully responsive to drug treatment were given treatment with rTMS or sham rTMS twice daily for a week. The results showed a mild reduction in seizures among the people given real rTMS. However, the benefits rapidly disappeared when treatment was stopped. Similarly short-lived effects were seen in an open trial.

⇛ *Schizophrenia*

A double-blind, placebo-controlled crossover trial looked at the use of low-frequency rTMS in 12 people diagnosed with schizophrenia and manifesting frequent and treatment-resistant auditory hallucinations (hearing voices). Participants received rTMS for 4 days, with length of treatment building from 4 minutes on the first day to 16 on the fourth day. Active stimulation significantly reduced the incidence of auditory hallucinations compared to sham stimulation. The extent of the benefit varied widely, lasting from 1 day in one participant to 2 months in another. Possible benefits were seen in other small studies as well.

⇛ *Parkinson's Disease*

A 2-month, double-blind, placebo-controlled trial of 18 people with Parkinson's disease compared rTMS against placebo. The results suggest that rTMS therapy can improve Parkinson's symptoms. Benefits were seen in two other small studies too.

⇛ *Myofascial Pain Syndrome*

Myofascial pain syndrome is a condition similar to fibromyalgia but more localized; while fibromyalgia involves tender trigger points all over the body, myofascial pain syndrome involves trigger points clustered in one portion of the body only. One controlled trial found indications that a form of rTMS applied to the painful area (rather than to the brain) may be effective for myofascial pain syndrome of the trapezius muscle.

⇛ *Tinnitus*

One preliminary study found indications that rTMS may be helpful for **tinnitus** (ringing in the ear).

⇛ *Post-traumatic Stress Disorder*

A small double-blind, placebo-controlled study found that use of rTMS may be able to reduce symptoms of post-traumatic stress disorder.

⇛ *Cigarette Addiction*

A very small double-blind, placebo-controlled study found evidence that rTMS may reduce craving for cigarettes in people attempting to **quit smoking**.

⇛ *Obsessive-compulsive Disorder*

A double-blind, placebo-controlled study of 18 people with obsessive-compulsive disorder found no evidence of benefit with rTMS.

How to Use Magnet Therapy

The following is a brief description of the use of magnet therapy. However, keep in mind that the current ways that magnets are used have yet to be fully evaluated by long-term clinical testing.

A full medical evaluation is advisable before using magnets. You don't want to be treating a painful back with magnets if the underlying cause of pain is a fracture or a tumor! Other concerns are discussed in the Safety Issues section below.

Types of Magnets

If you have decided you do wish to try magnet therapy, you will have to choose among many different types of magnets and magnetic devices on the market today. There are a number of theories on the size and type of magnets to use and where to apply them, based on the type of condition being treated and other factors. Because unipolar magnets have greater depth of magnetic field penetration, some researchers consider these more effective in treating deeper tissues. Conversely, it is considered that alternating-pole magnet devices might be more effective at stimulating surface tissue. Thus, it might be appropriate to use a unipolar high-gauss magnet for low back pain that originates deep in the tissue and an alternating-pole configuration for an injury closer to the surface, such as a wrist sprain. However, there is no meaningful scientific evidence to support these distinctions.

In addition, some practitioners hold that the north side of the magnet calms and the south side excites, and that using the correct side of the magnet is crucial. However, from a scientific perspective, it is difficult to see how there could be any difference between the two poles of the magnet in terms of the effect upon body tissue.

There is general consensus that the magnet should be placed as close to the affected part of the body as possible. This can be done by taping the magnet to the skin, slipping the magnet inside a bandage over the affected area, or using a wrap device that has magnets embedded in it.

Tape holding magnets to the body might irritate the skin; in addition, some research scientists and practitioners suspect that the body may accommodate to the magnetic field over time, thus reducing the therapeutic effect. In order to prevent both the irritation and the accommodation, practitioners usually recommend intermittent use, such as 5 days on, 2 days off; or 12 hours on, 12 hours off.

Magnetic Devices Available

Manufacturers make a wide range of magnetic devices. For treating large areas of the body, wraps and belts containing magnets are available. Wraps are specifically designed for the wrist, elbow, knee, ankle, neck, shoulder,

and back, and are often made out of thermal material to have the added effect of warming the area. These wraps are often recommended in cases of injury and arthritis where heat feels better. Proponents of magnet therapy often recommend the use of magnetic mattress pads and mattresses for people with problems affecting several areas of the body, such as fibromyalgia or arthritis; they also recommend magnetic mattress pads for insomnia and fatigue.

Proponents of magnet therapy recommend magnetic foot insoles for people with diabetic peripheral neuropathy, leg aches and pains, circulatory problems of the lower extremities, or foot injuries and problems, and for people who stand all day.

Magnetic necklaces are said to be useful for neck and shoulder pain as well as for generalized aches and pains, and magnetic bracelets are advocated for wrist pain and general problems.

Safety Issues

In general, magnets appear to be safe; the biggest risk appears to be irritation from tape holding them in place. MRI machines, for example, expose the body to gigantic magnetic fields and extensive investigation has found no evidence of harm. However, during the MRI, the patient is subjected to a high level of magnetism for a short period of time, whereas people who use static magnets daily or sleep on them every night are subjected to a low level of magnetism over a long period of time. So far, it is not known whether this type of exposure has any deleterious effects. Nonetheless, one study in which participants slept on a magnetic mattress pad every night for 4 months found no side effects. In addition, a safety study of rTMS found no evidence of harm.

It was previously thought that people with implantable cardioverter defibrillators (ICDs) and pacemakers should not use magnetic devices at all, but this recommendation has been adjusted. One study found that with the exception of magnetic mattresses and mattress pads, most magnets sold for therapeutic purposes do not interfere with the magnetically activated switches present in most pacemakers. Magnetic mattress pads can deactivate and alter the function of ICDs and pacemakers, but other therapeutic magnets are safe if kept 6 inches or further from these devices.

There are theoretical concerns that magnets might be risky for people with epilepsy. Similarly, until the physiological effects of magnet treatments are better understood, pregnant women should avoid them.

Massage Therapy

RELATED TERMS: *St. John's Neuromuscular, Rolfing®, Swedish Massage, Neuromuscular Massage, Deep-tissue Massage, Shiatsu, Acupressure, Structural Integration, Reflexology*

PRINCIPAL PROPOSED USES: *Low Back Pain, Other Forms of Muscular Pain, General Stress Reduction*

OTHER PROPOSED USES: *Attention Deficit Disorder (ADD), Anorexia, Anxiety, Asthma, Autism, Bulimia, Cystic Fibrosis, Depression, Diabetes, Eczema, Fibromyalgia, HIV Support, Iliotibial Band Pain, Juvenile Rheumatoid Arthritis, Migraine Headaches, Neck Pain, Premenstrual Syndrome (PMS), Pregnancy Support, Quitting Smoking, Recovery from Severe Burns, Spinal Cord Injury*

Overview

Along with **herbal treatment**, touch-based therapy is undoubtedly one of the most ancient forms of medical care. We instinctively stroke and rub areas of our body that hurt; massage therapy develops this instinct into a professional treatment. There is no doubt that massage relieves pain and induces relaxation at least temporarily; besides that, it feels good! Whether it offers any lasting benefits, however, remains unclear.

Forms of Massage

There are many schools of massage. In most cases, massage therapists combine several techniques, although there are also purists who stick to one method. The most common technique is Swedish massage, which combines long strokes and gentle kneading movements that primarily affect surface muscle tissues. Deep-tissue massage utilizes greater pressure to reach deeper levels of muscles. This may be called the "hurts-good-and-feels-great-after" approach. Shiatsu or acupressure massage also use deep pressure, but according to the principles of acupuncture theory. (Acupuncture is so similar to acupressure that we have elected to discuss studies of acupressure in the **acupuncture** article rather than here.) Neuromuscular massage (such as the St. John Method of Neuromuscular Therapy) applies strong pressure to tender spots, technically known as trigger points.

Several other techniques are best described as relatives of massage. Rolfing Structural Integration® aims to affect not muscles, but the connective tissue (fascia) surrounding muscles and everything else in the body. This highly organized technique aims to permanently improve the body's structure. Reflexology is a form of foot massage based on the theory that the whole body is reflected in the foot.

How Does Massage Work?

There are many theories about how massage might work, but none have been proved true. Little doubt exists that massage temporarily increases blood circulation in the massaged area, but it is not clear that this makes any lasting difference. Some massage therapists and massage therapy schools promote the notion that massage breaks up calcium deposits in the muscle, but there is no objective substantiation for this claim.

A completely different explanation is that massage promotes healing in a more general way, by reducing stress and inducing relaxation. Massage also satisfies the basic human need to be touched.

Some forms of massage, such as Rolfing Structural Integration, acupressure, and reflexology have elaborate theories behind them. However, there is little to no scientific evidence for these theories; moreover, there is some evidence that the theory behind reflexology is incorrect.

What Is Massage Therapy Used For?

Massage is most commonly used to relieve muscular tension and promote relaxation. It is also said to be helpful as an aid to the treatment of various conditions, including **attention deficit disorder** (ADD), **asthma**, **autism**, bedsores, **bulimia**, cystic fibrosis, **diabetes**, **eczema**, **fibromyalgia**, **HIV**, **iliotibial band pain**, juvenile rheumatoid arthritis, **low back pain**, **lymphedema**, **neck pain**, **premenstrual syndrome** (PMS), **pregnancy**, severe burns, and spinal cord injury.

What Is the Scientific Evidence for Massage Therapy?

Although there is some evidence that massage may be helpful for various medical purposes, in general the evidence is not strong. There are several reasons for this, but one is most fundamental: even with the best of intentions, it is difficult to properly ascertain the effectiveness of a hands-on therapy like massage.

Only one form of study can truly prove that a treatment is effective: the double-blind, placebo-controlled trial. (For more information on why such studies are so crucial, see **Why Does This Book Rely on Double-blind Studies?**) However, it isn't possible to fit massage into a study design of this type. What could researchers use for placebo massage? And how could they make sure that both participants and practitioners would be kept in the dark regarding who was receiving real massage and who was receiving fake massage? The fact is, they can't.

Because of these problems, all studies of massage fall short of optimum design. Many have compared massage to no treatment. However, studies of this type cannot provide reliable evidence about the efficacy of a treatment. If a benefit is seen, there is no way to determine whether it was caused by massage specifically, or just attention generally. (Attention alone will almost always produce some reported benefit.)

More meaningful trials used some sort of fake treatment for the control group, such as phony laser acupuncture. However, using a placebo treatment that is very different in form from the treatment under study is less than ideal. One study (discussed below) compared real reflexology against fake reflexology. However, it is quite likely that the reflexologists at least unconsciously conveyed more enthusiasm and optimism when performing the real therapy than the fake therapy; this, too, could affect the outcome. It has been suggested that the only way to get around this last problem would be to compare the effectiveness of trained practitioners against actors trained only enough to provide a simulation of treatment; however, such studies have not been reported.

Still other studies have simply involved giving people massages and seeing whether they improved. These trials are particularly meaningless; it has been long since proven that both participants and examining physicians will at least think that they observe improvement in people given a treatment, whether or not the treatment does anything on its own.

Finally, other trials have compared massage to competing therapies, such as acupuncture or **relaxation therapy**. Unfortunately, when you compare unproven therapies to each other, the results cannot possibly prove that any of the tested treatments are effective.

Given these caveats, the following is a summary of what science knows about the effects of massage.

Low Back Pain

Although the evidence is far from complete, it does appear that massage may offer benefits for low back pain. However, these benefits may last for only the short term.

One of the more recent studies compared massage to fake laser therapy in 107 people with low-back pain. The results indicate that massage is more effective than fake laser therapy for relieving low back pain and that massage therapy combined with exercise and posture training is even more effective.

Another study compared acupuncture, massage, and self-care education in 262 people with persistent back pain. By the end of the 10-week treatment period, massage had shown itself more effective than self-care (or acupuncture). However, at a 1-year follow-up, there was no difference in symptoms between the massage group and the self-care group.

In another study, acupressure-style massage was more effective than Swedish massage for the treatment of low back pain.

Other Conditions

Preliminary controlled trials of varying quality suggest that massage may provide benefit in a number of conditions, including the following:

➤ **ADD**
➤ **Anorexia nervosa**
➤ **Asthma in children**
➤ **Autism**
➤ **Bulimia**
➤ **Cystic fibrosis**
➤ **Depression and anxiety in children**
➤ **Diabetes**
➤ **Eczema**
➤ **Fibromyalgia**
➤ **Iliotibial band pain (a form of tendonitis that can cause knee or hip pain)**
➤ **Juvenile rheumatoid arthritis**
➤ **Migraine headaches**
➤ **Pregnancy and childbirth**

> Quitting smoking
> Burn recovery
> Spinal cord injury

One study commonly cited as evidence that ordinary massage therapy is helpful for premenstrual syndrome (PMS) was flawed by the absence of a control group. However, a better-designed trial compared reflexology against fake reflexology in 38 women with PMS symptoms and found evidence that real reflexology was more effective.

Study results are mixed on whether massage can improve measures of immune function in people with HIV.

One study found that massage is less effective than acupuncture for chronic neck pain. In fact, in this trial massage was no more effective than *fake* acupuncture.

A review of the literature published in 1997 suggests that massage is not helpful for preventing pressure sores (bedsores).

Several studies indicate that massage combined with **aromatherapy** may be helpful for relieving anxiety.

How to Choose a Massage Therapist

As with all medical therapies, it is best to choose a licensed practitioner. Where licensure is not available, your best bet is to seek a referral from a qualified and knowledgeable medical practitioner. However, most states license massage therapists.

Note that massage, like other hands-on therapies, involves personal talents that go beyond specific training, certification, or licensure: Some people are simply gifted with their hands. Furthermore, what works for one person may not work for another. For these reasons, some trial and error is often necessary to find the best massage therapist for you.

Safety Issues

Massage is generally safe. However, it can sometimes exacerbate pain temporarily, even when properly performed. In addition, if massage is performed too forcefully on fragile people, bone fractures and other internal injuries are possible. However, licensed massage therapists have been trained in ways to avoid causing these problems. Machines designed to perform elements of massage may be less safe.

Naturopathy

ALTERNATE NAMES: *Adrenal Support, Natural Medicine, Naturopathic Doctor, Naturopathic Medicine, N.D.*

PRINCIPAL PROPOSED USES: *None*

What Is Naturopathy?

Naturopathy, or "natural medicine," is one of the most important branches of alternative medicine, exerting an influence far beyond the actual numbers of its formal practitioners. Named by Benedict Lust at the turn of the century, its immediate roots go back to the spa treatments of nineteenth-century Germany, but its founding principles can be found in the writings of Hippocrates and other healers of the ancient world.

The defining principle of naturopathy is *vis medica-trix naturae*, or nature's healing power. From this perspective, disease is caused by departing from the natural way of living and health is established by returning to it.

Much of conventional medicine's current interest in diet and lifestyle came into being through the influence of naturopathic practitioners. There is little doubt that their general recommendations are health-promoting: eat a well-balanced diet rich in fruits and vegetables, exercise regularly, maintain a healthful weight, and avoid toxic habits, such as smoking. It is less clear, however, whether the more specific dietary suggestions sometimes made by naturopathic practitioners will actually enhance health. Some of these suggestions include drinking 64 ounces of water daily, eating organic fruits and vegetables, and avoiding certain food combinations (such as starches and protein).

Herbal Medicine

Naturopathic medicine is also largely responsible for the resurgence in interest in herbal medicine. Growing scientific evidence tells us that some herbs have real healing properties (although no magic cures have yet appeared). The considerable evidence for and against the use of herbs for various conditions is discussed in the **herb articles** in this book.

Vitamins, Minerals, and Supplements

Naturopathic practitioners are also famous for emphasizing the use of vitamins and supplements. Ironically, early practitioners of naturopathy were quite opposed to the use of vitamins and supplements, considering them refined processed foods (which they are). Matters changed in the 1960s when Linus Pauling promoted vitamin C as a cure for many illnesses, leading to the development of *orthomolecular medicine*. This approach, now incorporated into naturopathy, believes that the roots of many diseases may be found in a subtle form of malnutrition caused by a combination of the following factors: poor diet, inability to absorb nutrients, increased need for nutrients, and difficulties metabolizing or using nutrients. When nutrient levels in the body are increased, the theory goes, the body will have the means to heal itself.

On this principle, naturopathic practitioners often recommend that people take relatively high doses of certain nutrients in the form of supplements. In addition, they believe that many non-nutrient substances found in plants can contribute to health. For more information on the evidence regarding the health-promoting effects of various food supplements, see the **supplement articles** in this book.

Detoxification

Another traditional naturopathic emphasis revolves around the concept of **detoxification**. This term refers to the belief that modern life, with its chemical pollutants, poor lifestyle habits, and psychological stresses, causes toxins to accumulate in the body. These toxins are said to be a major cause of disease and removing them from the body is believed to promote health. Detoxification methods include adopting a healthful diet, drinking large quantities of water, using cleansing herbs and supplements, and undergoing special processes such as colon-cleansing, liver-flushing, and removal of mercury fillings. As yet there is little scientific evidence that any of these methods enhance general health.

Immune Support

Immune support is another characteristic naturopathic interest. Based on the indisputable fact that the body's susceptibility to illness is at least as important a factor as its accidental exposure to microorganisms, naturopathic practitioners utilize a number of treatments that they believe will enhance immunity. These include a wide variety of herbs and supplements, as well as elimination of certain foods from the diet, such as white sugar. However, it has proved difficult to establish scientifically that any treatment does indeed "boost" immunity.

Adrenal Support

Adrenal support is also commonly recommended by naturopathic practitioners. This method is based on classic studies performed in the early- to mid-twentieth century that found a relationship between stress, illness, and adrenal function. Naturopathic practitioners frequently recommend treatments they believe will help the adrenals, including removing sugar and stimulants from the diet while adding **adrenal supplements** and various other herbs and supplements said to strengthen adrenal function. Adrenal support is said to be helpful for a variety of conditions, including allergies, anxiety, fatigue, and stress. However, the theory of adrenal support has only a limited scientific foundation and it does not by itself justify the common therapies used in conjunction with the diagnosis. Furthermore, there is little in the way of specific scientific evidence to indicate that methods used to support the adrenals are beneficial for any disease.

Other Treatments Related to Naturopathic Medicine

Various other treatments have gathered under the umbrella of naturopathic medicine more for historical reasons than for a close connection to *vis medicatrix naturae*, including an emphasis on the following:

➤ Food allergies
➤ The belief that low (rather than high) stomach acid is a cause of many illnesses
➤ An interest in the yeast *Candida* and other intestinal parasites

➤ An interest in certain animal-based hormones, such as thyroid supplements
➤ An attitude of caution toward many interventions recommended by conventional medicine (such as vaccinations)

Diagnostic Techniques

Besides its unique treatment approaches, naturopathic medicine also makes use of a number of characteristic diagnostic techniques, such as hair and saliva analysis, and a more fine-grained analysis of standard blood tests than conventional medicine believes to be warranted.

How to Choose a Qualified Naturopathic Practitioner

Principles of naturopathic medicine are used by "holistic" medical doctors (M.D.'s) and doctors of osteopathy (D.O.'s), chiropractors, massage therapists, herbalists, and nutritionists. However, the premier practitioners of this form of medicine are naturopathic physicians (N.D.'s). Several states offer the N.D. licensure; they are listed in the table below. Most major Canadian provinces also license N.D.'s. In states where the N.D. li-

cense is not granted, N.D.'s may still practice, although in something of a legal gray zone.

U.S. States and Territories that Offer N.D. Licensure

Alaska	New Hampshire
Arizona	Oregon
Connecticut	Utah
Hawaii	Vermont
Kansas	Washington
Maine	Puerto Rico
Montana	U.S. Virgin Islands

There are a few accredited colleges in North America granting the N.D. degree. These include:

➤ Bastyr University in Washington state
➤ The Southwest College of Naturopathic Medicine in Arizona
➤ The College of Naturopathic Medicine in Oregon
➤ The Canadian College of Naturopathic Medicine in Ontario

Osteopathic Manipulation

ALTERNATE NAMES: *Cranial Osteopathy, Cranial-sacral Therapy, Doctor of Osteopathy (D.O.),*
Greenman Muscle-energy, Jones Counterstrain, Mobilization, Myofascial Release, Osteopathic
Medicine, Osteopathy, Strain-counterstrain
PRINCIPLE PROPOSED USES: *Back Pain, Enhancing Recovery from Surgery or Serious Illness,*
Fibromyalgia, General Health, Musculoskeletal Pain, Neck Pain
OTHER STUDIED USES: *Asthma, General Health, Sinus Infections*

Overview

Osteopathy originated as a nineteenth-century alternative medical approach focusing on physical manipulation. Today, osteopathic physicians study and practice the same types of medical and surgical techniques as conventional medical doctors. Some of osteopathy's original techniques still persist, however; these, taken together, are called *os-*

teopathic manipulation (OM). OM is less well known to the public than chiropractic spinal manipulation, but it has shown promise for many of the same conditions: for example, back pain and tension headaches.

History of Osteopathic Manipulation

Osteopathic medicine was founded in 1874 by Andrew Taylor Still, a U.S. physician. Physicians educated in this method were called *doctors of osteopathy*, or D.O.'s. Subsequently, however, schools of osteopathic medicine became integrated with conventional medical schools and today the license of D.O. is legally equivalent to that of M.D.

Forms of Osteopathic Manipulation

Osteopathic and chiropractic techniques overlap, but they are not identical. As a general rule, chiropractors focus most of their attention on the spine, while osteopathic practitioners devote more of the their efforts to the manipulation of soft tissues and joints outside the spine. Another general difference is that chiropractic spinal manipulation tends to make use of rapid short movements (spinal manipulation, which is a high-velocity, low-amplitude technique), while OM typically concentrates on gentle, larger movements (mobilization, which is a low-velocity, high-amplitude technique). But neither of these distinctions is absolute and many chiropractic and osteopathic methods do not fit neatly into these categories.

There are several specific osteopathic techniques in wide use, many of which are named after their founders. Some of the more popular are Greenman muscle-energy, Jones counterstrain (also known as strain-counterstrain), myofascial release, and cranial-sacral therapy (formally known as osteopathy in the cranial field).

Greenman Muscle-energy Technique

Greenman muscle-energy technique involves bending a joint just up to the point where muscular resistance to movement begins ("the barrier") and then holding it there while the patient gently resists. The pressure is maintained for a few seconds and then released. After a brief pause to allow the affected muscles to relax, the practitioner then moves the joint a little farther into the barrier, which will usually have shifted slightly toward improved mobility during the interval.

Strain-counterstrain Technique (Jones Counterstrain)

Strain-counterstrain technique (Jones counterstrain) involves finding tender points and then manipulating the joint connected to them in order to find a position where the tenderness decreases toward zero. Once this precise angle is found, it is held for 90 seconds and then released. Like muscle-energy work, strain-counterstrain progressively increases range of motion and, it is hoped, decreases muscle spasm and pain.

Myofascial Release

Myofascial release focuses on the fascial tissues that surround muscles. The practitioner first positions the painful area either at the edge of the barrier to movement or, alternatively, at the opposite extreme (the area of greatest comfort). Next, while the patient breathes slowly and easily, the practitioner palpates the fascial tissues, looking for a subtle sensation that indicates the tissues are ready to "unwind." After receiving this indication, the practitioner then helps the tissue to follow a pattern of spontaneous movement. This process is repeated over several sessions until a full release is achieved. Myofascial release is said to be especially useful in pain conditions that have persisted for months or years.

Cranial-sacral Therapy

Cranial-sacral therapy, more properly called *cranial osteopathy* (or just cranial for short), is a very specialized technique based on the scientifically unconfirmed belief that the tissues surrounding the brain and spinal cord undergo a rhythmic pulsation. This "cranial rhythm" is supposed to cause subtle movements of the bones of the skull. A practitioner of cranial-sacral therapy gently manipulates these bones in time with the rhythm (as determined by the practitioner's awareness), in order to repair "cranial lesions." This therapy is said to be helpful for numerous conditions ranging from headaches and sinus allergies to multiple sclerosis and asthma. However, many researchers have serious doubts that the cranial rhythm even exists.

What is Osteopathic Manipulation Used For?

Osteopathic manipulation is primarily used to treat **musculoskeletal pain** conditions, such as **back pain**, shoulder pain, and **tension headaches**. OM is often said to be specifically effective for conditions that have persisted for some time, as opposed to chiropractic spinal manipulation, which, according to this view, is most effective for treatment of injuries that have occurred recently. However, there is no meaningful scientific support for this belief.

Some advocates of OM believe that it has numerous additional benefits, including the enhancement of overall health and well-being.

What Is the Scientific Evidence for Osteopathic Manipulation?

There is little evidence as yet that osteopathic manipulation is helpful for the treatment of any medical condition. There are several possible reasons for this, but one is fundamental: even with the best of intentions, it is difficult to properly ascertain the effectiveness of a hands-on therapy like OM.

Only one form of study can truly prove that a treatment is effective: the double-blind, placebo-controlled trial. However, it isn't possible to fit OM into a study design of this type. What could researchers use as a placebo OM? And how could they make sure that both participants and practitioners would be kept in the dark regarding who is receiving real OM and who is receiving fake OM? The fact is, they can't.

Because of these problems, all studies of OM fall short of optimum design. Many have compared OM against no treatment. However, studies of that type cannot provide reliable evidence about the efficacy of a treatment: if a benefit is seen, there is no way to determine whether it was a result of OM specifically or just attention generally. (Attention alone will almost always produce some reported benefit.)

More meaningful trials used fake osteopathy for the control group. Such studies are single-blind, because the practitioner is aware of applying phony treatment. However, this design can introduce potential bias in the form of subtle unconscious communication between practitioner and patient.

Still other studies have simply involved giving people OM and seeing if they improve. These trials are particularly meaningless; it has long since been proven that both participants and examining physicians will think, at least, that they observe improvement in people given a treatment, whether or not the treatment does anything on its own; such studies are not reported here.

Given these caveats, the following is a summary of what science knows about the effects of OM.

Possible Effects of OM

Most studies of OM have involved its potential use for various pain conditions.

In a study of 183 people with neck pain, use of osteopathic methods provided greater benefits than standard physical therapy or general medical care. Participants receiving OM showed faster recovery and experienced fewer days off work. OM appeared to be less expensive overall than the other two approaches; however, researchers strictly limited the allowed OM sessions, making direct cost comparisons questionable. Another study evaluated a rather ambitious combined therapy for the treatment of chronic pain resulting from whiplash injury (craniosacral therapy along with Rosen Bodywork and Gestalt psychotherapy). The results failed to find this assembly of treatments more effective than no treatment.

In a 14-week, single-blind study of 29 elderly people with **shoulder pain**, real OM proved more effective than placebo OM. Although participants in both groups improved, those in the treated group showed relatively greater increase in range of motion in the shoulder.

In another study, 24 women with **fibromyalgia** were divided into five groups: standard care, standard care plus OM, standard care plus an educational approach, standard care plus moist heat, and standard care plus moist heat and OM. The results indicate that OM plus standard care is better than standard care alone, and that OM is more effective than less specific treatments, such as moist heat or general education. However, because this was not a blinded study (participants knew which group they were in), the results can't be taken as reliable.

A study of 28 people with tension headaches compared one session of OM against two forms of sham treatment and found evidence that real treatment provided a greater improvement in headache pain.

Although OM has shown some promise for the treatment of **back pain**, one of the best-designed trials failed to find it a superior alternative to conventional medical care. In this 12-week study of 178 people, OM proved no more effective than standard treatment for back pain. Another study, this one enrolling 199 people and following them for 6 months, also failed to find OM more effective than fake OM. This study also included a no-treatment group. Both real and fake OM were more effective than no treatment.

A much smaller study reportedly found that muscle-energy technique enhances recovery from back pain, but this study does not appear to have used a meaningful placebo treatment.

Some studies have evaluated the potential benefits of OM for speeding healing in people recovering from **surgery** or serious illness. The best of these studies compared OM against light touch in 58 elderly people hospitalized for pneumonia. The results indicate that use of osteopathy aided recovery.

In a much less meaningful study, OM was compared to no treatment in people recovering from knee or hip surgery. While the people receiving OM recovered more quickly, these results mean very little, since, as noted above, any form of attention should be expected to produce greater apparent benefits than no attention.

A similarly weak study suggests that OM might also be helpful for people hospitalized with pancreatitis.

A small study found some evidence that OM might be helpful for childhood **asthma**.

Finding a Qualified Practitioner of Osteopathic Manipulation

Although there are many licensed doctors of osteopathy (D.O.'s), most practice conventional medicine and do not specialize in OM. Some do, and many of those have been certified by the American Osteopathic Board of Neuromusculoskeletal Medicine.

In addition, many physical therapists and massage therapists use some osteopathic techniques, with variable amounts of training.

Safety of Osteopathic Manipulation

Most forms of OM, because of their gentle nature, are believed to be quite safe. However, mild short-term pain may occur immediately following treatment. In addition, some osteopathic practitioners use the high-velocity thrusts common to chiropractic and might, therefore, incur some slight safety risks. (See the **Chiropractic** article for more information.)

Prolotherapy

RELATED TERMS: *Sclerotherapy*

PRINCIPAL PROPOSED USES: *Back Pain, Osteoarthritis*

OTHER PROPOSED USES: *Fibromyalgia, Plantar Fasciitis, Sciatica, Sports Injuries, Temporomandibular Joint (TMJ) Disorder, Tendinitis, Tension Headaches*

What Is Prolotherapy?

Invented in the 1950s by George Hackett, prolotherapy is based on the theory that chronic pain is often caused by laxness of the ligaments that are responsible for keeping a joint stable. When ligaments and associated tendons are loose, the body is said to compensate by using muscles to stabilize the joint. The net result, according to prolotherapy theory, is muscle spasms and pain.

Prolotherapy treatment involves injections of chemical irritant solutions into the area around such ligaments. These solutions cause tissue to proliferate (grow), increasing the strength and thickness of ligaments. In turn, this tightens up the joint and presumably relieves the burden on associated muscles, stopping muscle spasms. In the case of arthritic joints, increased ligament strength may allow the joint to function more efficiently, thus reducing pain.

Prolotherapy has not yet been widely accepted in conventional medicine. However, highly respected institutions have studied it and standard textbooks of orthopedics and rehabilitation medicine mention it. The technique is used by prolotherapy practitioners to treat many conditions, including back pain, osteoarthritis, fibromyalgia, plantar fasciitis, sciatica, sports injuries, temporomandibular joint (TMJ) disorder, tendinitis, and tension headaches. The best evidence at present is for its use in back pain and osteoarthritis.

How Is Prolotherapy Performed?

Prolotherapy is generally administered at intervals of 4 to 6 weeks, although studies have used a more frequent schedule. The treatment involves injection of a mixture containing an irritant and a local anesthetic. A total of four to six treatments is typical.

When treating back pain, prolotherapy practitioners frequently use a form of manipulation somewhat similar

Prolotherapy

to chiropractic. However, it is applied after local anesthetic has been injected and is somewhat intense.

There are several irritant solutions used in prolotherapy. Concentrated dextrose or glucose has become increasingly popular because it is completely non-toxic. Phenol (a potentially toxic substance) and glycerin are also sometimes used. Other non-irritant substances may be added to the solution, such as vitamin B_{12}, corn extracts, cod liver oil extracts, zinc, and manganese; however, there is no evidence that these substances add any benefit.

What Is the Scientific Evidence for Prolotherapy?

Animal and human studies have found that prolotherapy injections increase strength and thickness of ligaments.

Six double-blind human trials of prolotherapy have been reported: four involving back pain (with mixed results) and the other two involving osteoarthritis (with positive results).

Back Pain

In a double-blind study, 81 people with **low back pain** of many years' duration were given either prolotherapy or placebo injections 6 times per week. The prolotherapy group received a mixture of dextrose, glycerin, and phenol, thought to irritate tissues and stimulate ligament growth. The placebo group received saline (salt-water) injections. Both groups also received spinal manipulation with local anesthetic on the first visit, although in the treatment group this was more extensive.

The results were positive for prolotherapy. Treated participants showed significantly less pain and disability within a month as compared to those in the placebo group and the relative benefit continued for the full 6 months of the study. One possible complicating factor in this study is that the more extensive manipulation applied to the treatment group might have contributed to the benefit.

A subsequent double-blind study of nearly identical size and design, performed by many of the same researchers, found similar benefits.

However, another study conducted by independent researchers failed to find prolotherapy with 20% glucose more effective than saline injections for low back pain. This study involved treatment for 6 months and a subsequent follow-up of 2 years.

A fourth study also failed to find benefit. At present, therefore, it is unclear whether prolotherapy provides any real benefit for back pain beyond that of the placebo effect.

Osteoarthritis

A double-blind, placebo-controlled study evaluated the effects of 3 prolotherapy injections (using a 10% dextrose solution) at 2-month intervals in 68 people with **osteoarthritis** of the knee. At the 6-month follow-up, participants who had received prolotherapy showed significant improvements in pain at rest and while walking, reduction in swelling, episodes of "buckling," and range of flexion, as compared to those who had received placebo treatment.

The same research group performed a similar double-blind trial of 27 people with osteoarthritis in the hands. The results at the 6-month follow-up showed that range of motion and pain with movement improved significantly in the treated group as compared to the placebo group.

Safety Issues

In studies, prolotherapy has not caused any serious injury. There is usually discomfort after each injection that lasts for a few minutes to several days, but this discomfort is seldom severe. Severe headaches have been reported in treatment of low back pain. Because phenol is a potentially toxic substance, treatment with a dextrose solution alone may be preferable.

Finding a Qualified Prolotherapy Practitioner

Prolotherapy is practiced by a medical doctor (M.D.) or doctor of osteopathy (D.O.). Generally, physicians specializing in orthopedics or physical medicine and rehabilitation are most likely to practice prolotherapy. To find a qualified practitioner, contact the following groups:

American College of Osteopathic Sclerotherapeutic Pain Management, Inc.
303 S. Ingram Court
Middletown, DE 19709
(800) 471-6114

American Association of Orthopaedic Medicine
600 Pembrook Drive
Woodland Park, CO 80863
(800) 992-2063

Reiki

PRINCIPAL PROPOSED USES: *None*

OTHER PROPOSED USES: *Increasing Wellness, Treating Diseases of All Types*

Overview

The Japanese word *Reiki* can be translated to "life-force energy." The term refers to a form of spiritual healing that involves holding the hands above the body. There are many people who have taken training in Reiki and the service is provided in a variety of settings. However, there has as yet been no meaningful scientific evaluation of this healing technique.

History of Reiki

There are two principle stories regarding the origin of Reiki. In both versions, the method was invented in Japan by Mikao Usui. Many American Reiki practitioners believe that Mikao Usui was a Christian monk who invented the technique in the mid-1800s. However, according to the more traditional Japanese schools of Reiki, Usui was a member of a Japanese spiritual organization called *Rei Jyutsu Ka* and he developed the technique around 1915. (The story that he was a Christian may have been invented to facilitate the acceptance of Reiki in the West.) Both versions of Reiki's history agree that Usui based his technique on methods and philosophies drawn from numerous traditional Asian healing methods.

After Usui's death, various forms of Reiki continued to be taught by his students. One of these students, Dr. Chujiro Hayashi, systematized Reiki into three levels and added a great many hand movements to the technique. In turn, one of Hayashi's students, Hawayo Takata, brought Reiki to the United States.

In the early 1980s, Takata's granddaughter, Phyllis Furumoto, took on the mantle of Hayashi and Takata's line of Reiki and popularized it widely in the West. However, many other forms of Reiki continue to exist as well, descending through different lineages of teachers. There are considerable differences between the various approaches and certain groups strongly challenge the validity of others.

What Is Reiki?

Most forms of Asian medicine make use of the concept of *Qi*, a form of vital energy that flows through the body. Free-flowing, abundant Qi is said to create health, while stagnant or deficient Qi is thought to lead to illness. Reiki practitioners believe that they can improve this energy by holding their hands in certain positions over parts of the patient's body; advanced practitioners believe they can produce this effect from a remote distance. The net result, according to the theory, is accelerated healing and increased wellness.

In many ways, Reiki resembles Therapeutic Touch, except that the instructions given to its practitioners are more specific. A certified practitioner of Reiki has spent time learning specified hand movements and positions and has also undergone an *attunement* to an already-certified Reiki practitioner. This chain of attunements goes back to Mikao Usui, the method's founder.

In its most popular Western form, Reiki is learned in three stages. The first stage involves an attunement that permits physical healing. The second stage grants the ability to carry out healing over a distance. The third degree of training allows the practitioner to perform healing on a spiritual level and to give attunements to students. Generally, each level is obtained by paying a fee and completing a weekend course.

What Is Reiki Used For?

Reiki is promoted as a treatment that can accelerate physical, emotional, or spiritual healing in every conceivable situation. It is used as a support for conventional medical care, rather than as a replacement for it.

What Is the Scientific Evidence for Reiki?

The only truly meaningful way to determine whether a medical therapy works is to perform a double-blind, placebo-controlled trial. (For the reasons why this is true, see **Why Does This Book Rely on Double-blind Trials?**.) For hands-on therapies such as Reiki, however, a truly double-blind study is not possible—the Reiki practitioner will inevitably know whether he or she is administering real Reiki rather than fake Reiki! The best that can be hoped for is a single-blind study in which participants do not know whether they received real or fake Reiki and in which their medical outcome is evaluated by an observer who is also kept in the dark (a blinded observer). However, only one such study has been reported.

A simpler study design compares Reiki to no treatment. However, studies of that type cannot provide reliable evidence about the efficacy of a treatment: If a benefit is seen, there is no way to determine whether it was caused by Reiki specifically or just attention generally. (Attention alone will almost always produce some reported benefit.)

Finally, there are many case reports in which people are given Reiki and then seem to improve. Such reports, unfortunately, do not mean anything at all; numerous people receiving placebo in placebo-controlled studies also seem to improve. Thus, such reports cannot say anything about whether Reiki itself offers any benefit, and we do not report them here.

In one study, which we have only been able to obtain in an incomplete abstract form, female nursing students received either real Reiki or a placebo form of the treatment called *mimic Reiki*. Before and after tests failed to find any improvement in general well-being attributable to Reiki treatment.

In another study, researchers evaluated the effectiveness of Reiki (in combination with a related technique called *LeShan*) in 21 people undergoing oral surgery for impacted wisdom teeth. Each participant received two surgeries, one with Reiki and the other without (in random order). People reported less pain when they received Reiki than when they received no treatment; however, due to the lack of a fake treatment group, the results mean little.

One series of studies commonly described as an attempt to determine whether Reiki treatments improved wound healing actually involved Therapeutic Touch.

How to Find a Qualified Reiki Practitioner

There are several competing organizations that issue certifications to Reiki practitioners. These include the following:

Usui Reiki, The Reiki Alliance
(208) 783-3535
http://www.reikialliance.org

The Reiki Foundation
East Coast office: (845) 278-3038
Southeast office: ReikiWend@aol.com
Midwest office: (248) 354-0178
Southwest office: (435) 586-6985
Northwest office: (206) 522-1643
http://www.asunam.com/reiki_foundation.htm

Safety Issues

There are no known or proposed safety risks with Reiki unless a person chooses to use Reiki *instead* of, rather than as a *support* to, standard medical care.

Relaxation Therapies

ALTERNATE NAMES: *Autogenic Training; Guided Imagery; Guided Visualizations; Imagery, Guided; Jacobsen's Relaxation Technique; Meditation; Progressive Muscular Relaxation (PMR); Relaxation Response; Transcendental Meditation (TM); Visualizations, Guided*

PRINCIPAL PROPOSED USES: *Cancer Chemotherapy Support, Chronic Pain of Various Kinds, General Stress, Insomnia, Surgery Support*

OTHER PROPOSED USES: *Angina, Asthma, Anxiety of Various Types, Bulimia Nervosa, Colds (Prevention), Fibromyalgia, Herpes (Prevention), Hypertension, Immune Support, Irritable Bowel Syndrome, Menopause, Premenstrual Syndrome (PMS), Pregnancy Support, Psoriasis, Rheumatoid Arthritis, Stroke Rehabilitation, Tension Headaches, Ulcerative Colitis*

Overview

Constant stress is one of the defining features of modern life and the source of many common health problems. Stress plays an obvious role in nervousness, anxiety, and insomnia, but it is also thought to contribute to a vast number of other illnesses.

In the past, most people engaged in many hours of physical exercise daily, an activity that reduces the effects of psychological stress. Life was also slower then and more in harmony with the natural cycles of day and season. Today, however, our bodies are relatively sedentary, while our minds are forced to respond to the rapid pace of a society that never stops. The result is high levels of stress and reduced ability to cope with it.

There are several ways to mitigate the damage caused by stress. Increased physical exercise can help, as can simple, common-sense steps like taking relaxation breaks and vacations. If these approaches do not have adequate results, there are more formal methods that may be helpful.

This article discusses a group of stress-reduction techniques often called *relaxation therapies*. In addition to these methods, **yoga**, **Tai Chi**, **hypnosis**, **massage**, and **biofeedback** can also help induce a relaxed state. For potentially helpful herb and supplement options, see the article on **stress**.

What Are Relaxation Therapies?

There are many types of relaxation therapies and they use a variety of techniques. However, most of them share certain related features.

In a great many relaxation techniques, one begins by either lying down or assuming a relaxed, seated posture in a quiet place and closing the eyes. The next step differs depending on the method. In autogenic training, Relaxation Response, and certain forms of meditation, one focuses one's mind on internal sensations, such as the breath. Guided-imagery techniques employ deliberate visualization of scenes or actions, such as walking on a quiet beach. Progressive relaxation techniques involve gradual relaxation of the muscles. Finally, some schools of meditation incorporate the repetition of a phrase or sound silently or aloud.

All of these techniques are best learned with the aid of a trained practitioner. The usual format is a group class supplemented by regular home practice. If you are diligent enough, experience suggests that you can develop the ability to call on a relaxed state at will, even in the middle of a very stressful situation.

What Are Relaxation Therapies Used For?

Relaxation therapies are most commonly tried in medical circumstances in which stress is believed to play a particularly large role. These include **insomnia**, **surgery**, chronic pain, and **cancer chemotherapy**.

A very specific form of guided visualization (described below) has also been used in an attempt to actually treat cancer.

What Is the Scientific Evidence for Relaxation Therapies?

Although many studies have been performed on relaxation therapies, most of them suffer from inadequate design. To be fair, there are considerable difficulties in the path of any researcher who wishes to scientifically assess the effectiveness of a relaxation therapy such as hypnosis. There are several factors involved, but the most important is fairly fundamental: it isn't easy to design a proper double-blind, placebo-controlled study of relaxation therapy. Researchers studying the herb St. John's wort, for example, can use placebo pills that are indistinguishable from the real thing. However, it's difficult to design a form of placebo relaxation therapy that can't be detected as such by both practitioners and patients.

One very clever method used by some researchers involves the use of intentionally neutral visualizations. Instead of imagining lying in bed and sleeping peacefully, patients in the placebo group might be told to visualize something like a green box. The problem here is that researchers teaching the visualization method to participants may inadvertently convey a sense of disbelief in the placebo treatment. This can be solved by using relatively untrained people who are themselves deceived by experimenters to teach the method, but the practical obstacles are significant.

For this reason, many studies of relaxation therapy have made major compromises to the double-blind, placebo-controlled model. Some randomly assigned participants to receive either relaxation therapy or no treatment. In the best of these studies, results were rated by examiners who didn't know which participants were in which group (in other words, "blinded observers"). However, it isn't clear whether benefits reported in such studies are due to the relaxation therapy or less specific factors, such as mere attention.

Other studies have compared relaxation therapies to different techniques, such as hypnosis or cognitive psychotherapy. However, the same difficulties arise when trying to study these latter therapies and the results of a study that compares an unproven treatment to one that is also imperfectly documented are not very meaningful.

Even less meaningful studies of relaxation therapies simply involved giving people the therapy and monitoring them to see whether they improved. For at least a dozen reasons, such open-label trials prove nothing at all, and we do not report them here. (The reasons are discussed in the article **Why Does This Book Rely on Double-blind Studies?**.)

Given these caveats, the following is a summary of what science knows about the medical benefits of relaxation therapy.

The Possible Benefits of Relaxation Therapy

Numerous controlled studies have evaluated relaxation therapies for the treatment of insomnia. These studies are difficult to summarize because many involved therapy combined with other methods, such as biofeedback, sleep restriction, and paradoxical intent (trying *not* to sleep). The type of relaxation therapy used in the majority of these trials was progressive muscle relaxation (PMR). Many of these trials used the clever form of placebo treatment described above; others simply compared relaxation therapy to no treatment.

Overall, the evidence indicates that relaxation therapies may be somewhat helpful for insomnia, although not dramatically so. For example, in a controlled study of 70 people with insomnia, participants using progressive relaxation showed no meaningful improvement in the time to fall asleep or the duration of sleep, but they reported feeling more rested in the morning. In another study, 20 minutes of relaxation practice was required to increase sleeping time by 30 minutes.

The supporting evidence for the effectiveness of relaxation therapies in other conditions remains quite limited. A review article published in 2002 found 15 published controlled trials that evaluated relaxation therapies for the treatment of **asthma**. Most of the studies were rated as very poor or poor quality. Overall the results failed to demonstrate improvement, although a muscular relaxation technique called *Jacobsen's relaxation* did show a hint of benefit.

Other conditions that have at least minimal supporting evidence for response to relaxation therapy include the following:

➤ **Angina**
➤ **Anxiety of various types**
➤ **Bulimia nervosa**
➤ **Cancer treatment support**
➤ **Chronic pain in general**
➤ **Fibromyalgia**
➤ **Hypertension and other heart disease risk factors**
➤ **Irritable bowel syndrome**
➤ **Menopause**
➤ **Premenstrual syndrome (PMS)**
➤ **Pregnancy support (reducing sense of stress)**
➤ **Psoriasis**
➤ **Rheumatoid arthritis**
➤ **Stress in general**

➤ Stroke rehabilitation
➤ Surgery support (primarily reducing pain and stress before or after surgery)
➤ Tension headaches
➤ Ulcerative colitis

In many cases the results are marginal at best, and contradictory outcomes between trials are common.

One study suggests that the use of visualizations prior to surgery can not only reduce the need for pain medications, it can also help prevent hematomas (collections of blood under the skin). However, more study would be needed to verify this somewhat difficult-to-believe result. A more easily accepted study found that either relaxation therapy or aerobic exercise can improve symptoms of fatigue after cancer surgery and that each approach is about as effective as the other.

Some studies have evaluated highly specific guided visualizations, rather than general relaxation. For example, it has been suggested that a systematic program of imagining microscopic soldiers shooting down one's cancer cells can improve the chances of **surviving cancer**. Unfortunately, despite much enthusiasm shown by some patients and practitioners, there is still no meaningful evidence to support this appealing idea at present. Nonetheless, there is some evidence from a set of small trials that specific immune-oriented visualizations can provide enhanced protection against **herpes** flare-ups and winter **colds**.

Contrary to common claims, published evidence does *not* demonstrate that transcendental meditation (TM) improves mental functioning.

How to Choose a Relaxation Therapist

There is no widely accepted license for practicing relaxation therapy. However, it is often practiced by therapists and psychologists.

Safety Issues

There are no known or proposed safety risks with relaxation therapies.

Tai Chi

RELATED TERMS: *Tai Chi Chuan, Taijiquan*
PRINCIPAL PROPOSED USES: *Improving Balance and Preventing Falls in Seniors*
OTHER PROPOSED USES: *Improving Overall Health, Enhancing Immunity*

Overview

Tai Chi (Tai Chi Chuan, Taijiquan) is a traditional form of martial art used more for promoting health than for fighting. Its gentle, dancelike moves are said to strengthen and balance the body's "energy." The net results, according to tradition, include increased physical stamina, enhanced sense of well-being and comfort, and improved resistance to illness.

Tai Chi is said to have been invented by the Taoist monk Chang San-Feng sometime in the Middle Ages. (The exact dates and even the existence of this monk are disputed.) Various schools of Tai Chi developed over subsequent centuries, each with their own particular movements and postures, but all conforming to the same underlying principles.

In the 1950s, the Chinese government began to develop a series of standardized Tai Chi forms. One of these has become the most popular form of Tai Chi in the West, a 37-posture form abbreviated from a traditional approach to Tai Chi called the *Yang Style*.

How Is Tai Chi Used Today?

Tai Chi is an extremely popular form of exercise among older Asians in China and other Asian countries. In the U.S., it is gaining widespread use as a method of improving balance and preventing falls among seniors. The slow movements of Tai Chi provide a gentle framework for enhancing physical control and improving balance.

Tai Chi is also advertised to improve overall health and enhance immunity, but this has not been evaluated scientifically to any significant extent.

What Is the Scientific Evidence for Tai Chi?

Although there is some evidence that Tai Chi may offer medical benefits, in general this evidence is not strong. There are several reasons for this (including funding obstacles), but one is fundamental: Even with the best of intentions, it is difficult to properly ascertain the effectiveness of an exercise therapy like Tai Chi.

Only one form of study can truly prove that a treatment is effective: the double-blind, placebo-controlled trial. However, it isn't possible to fit Tai Chi into a study design of this type. While it might be possible to design a placebo form of Tai Chi, it would be quite difficult to keep participants and researchers in the dark regarding who is practicing real Tai Chi and who is practicing fake Tai Chi! Therefore, some compromise with the highest research standards is inevitable. Unfortunately, the compromise used in most studies is less than optimal. In these trials, Tai Chi was compared to no treatment. The problem with such studies is that a treatment—*any* treatment—frequently appears to be better than no treatment, due to a host of factors. (See **Why Does This Book Rely on Double-blind Studies?** for more information.) It would be better to compare Tai Chi to generic forms of exercise, such as daily walking, but thus far this method has not seen much use.

Given these caveats, the following is a summary of what science has found out about Tai Chi.

Most controlled trials of Tai Chi published in English have evaluated its potential benefits for improving balance in seniors. Falling is one of the most common causes of injury in seniors, leading to fractures, head injuries, and even death. Recovery from fall-related injuries may involve extensive immobilization in bed, which in turn increases the risk of osteoporosis, pneumonia, and depression. According to most (but not all) studies, Tai Chi can improve balance and decrease risk of falling. For example, in a 10-week study, 24 seniors practiced Tai Chi (one class weekly, plus daily home practice), while a control group of 22 volunteers did not change their activity. The results showed that people practicing Tai Chi experienced substantially improved balance (measured by the ability to stand on one leg) compared to the control group. Some studies failed to find benefit; however, this is typical of treatments for which all studies have been small in size. For statistical reasons, small studies commonly fail to identify benefit even when there is one.

Besides balance, Tai Chi may mildly improve flexibility and cardiovascular health, presumably because it is a form of moderate exercise. However, one fairly large (207-participant) and long-term (1-year) study that compared Tai Chi to resistance exercise (weight lifting) found that while resistance exercises measurably improved one measure of cardiovascular risk (insulin sensitivity), Tai Chi did not affect *any* measures of cardiovascular risk.

What Should You Expect in a Tai Chi Class?

A Tai Chi class consists of progressive training in the movements of a Tai Chi form. Each subsequent class adds more moves to your repertoire, until you finally know how to perform the entire series. The Tai Chi instructor will gently correct your movements, helping you to make your stances and transitions between them more precise, graceful, and balanced.

Expect to feel pretty awkward at first. Even if you were a world-class ballet dancer, you wouldn't immediately be able to do Tai Chi as well as someone who has taught and practiced it for years. However, the intricate, often beautiful movements of Tai Chi have a strong intrinsic charm; they are pleasant to perform and, as with all things, they respond to practice. If you can give yourself 15 minutes a day to practice at home, you'll improve rapidly; soon you may wish to spend even more time at it.

Therapeutic Touch

PRINCIPLE PROPOSED USES: *None*

OTHER PROPOSED USES: *Anxiety, HIV Support, Osteoarthritis, Pregnancy Support, Promoting General Wellness, Sports Injuries, Stress, Surgery Support, Tension Headaches, Wound Healing*

Overview

Therapeutic Touch (TT) is a form of "energy healing" popular in the American nursing community. In the words of its official organization, "Therapeutic Touch is an intentionally directed process of energy exchange during which the practitioner uses the hands as a focus to facilitate the healing process." TT is used by nurses in a variety of settings, from the office to the Intensive Care Unit (ICU). However, there is as yet no meaningful evidence that it is effective.

What Is Therapeutic Touch?

Therapeutic Touch was developed in the early 1970s by two people: Dolores Krieger, Ph.D., R.N., and a self-professed healer named Dora Van Gelder Kunz. At first, TT involved setting the hands lightly on the body of the patient, but the method rapidly evolved into a non-contact, "energy healing" method. Today certified practitioners can be found in virtually all parts of the U.S. and in much of the world. TT is available in mainstream health care facilities, including hospices, hospital-based alternative health programs, and even ICUs.

Therapeutic Touch is sometimes described as a scientific version of "laying on of hands," a technique practiced by faith healers. However, there is more spirituality than science to this method; it makes use of beliefs and principles common in spiritual healing traditions but alien to current science culture.

According to TT, the body has an "energy field" and, without physical contact, the energy field of one person can substantially affect the energy field of another. The practitioner is said to heal, balance, replenish, and improve the flow of the patient's energy field, thereby leading to enhanced overall **wellness**. However, there is no meaningful scientific evidence for any of these beliefs.

What Is the Scientific Evidence Regarding Therapeutic Touch?

There has been considerable research interest in TT. However, as yet the evidence for benefit is no more than weakly positive at best. A 1999 review of all published studies concluded that many of the studies had serious design flaws that could bias the results; in addition, the manner in which they were reported did not meet adequate scientific standards.

To be fair, proper study of TT presents researchers with some serious obstacles. The only truly meaningful way to determine whether a medical therapy works is to perform a double-blind, placebo-controlled trial. (For the reasons why this is true, see **Why Does This Book Rely on Double-blind Studies?**) For hands-on therapies such as TT, however, a truly double-blind study is not possible—the TT practitioner will inevitably know whether he or she is administering real TT or fake TT!

The best type of study that can be performed on TT is a single-blind study with blinded observers. In such studies, participants do not know whether they received real or fake TT and an observer who is also kept in the dark evaluates their medical outcome. However, such a study still has potential bias in it; practitioners could very well communicate a kind of cynicism when they administer fake TT and this problem appears to be insurmountable.

Further problems are involved in the choice of fake treatment. In most of the studies described below, sham TT involved practitioners counting backward in their heads by subtracting seven serially from 100. The intent of this method was to avoid any possibility of projecting a healing concentration. It has been pointed out that this somewhat stressful effort would cause the practitioner to communicate tension rather than relaxation to study participants and this too could bias results. However, it is difficult to suggest what should have been used instead for placebo.

Some studies compared TT to no treatment. However, it has been well established that any therapy whatsoever will seem to produce benefit compared to no treatment for various non-specific reasons; because of this, such studies say little to nothing about the specific benefits of TT. Finally, numerous trials have simply involved enrolling people with a medical problem, applying TT, and seeing whether they improve. Trials of this type prove absolutely nothing at all; for at least a dozen reasons, it would be rather surprising if benefit were *not* seen.

Given these caveats, here is a summary of the research available thus far.

At the time of the 1999 review noted above, many published studies of TT were of unacceptably low quality and, in any case, the results were quite inconsistent.

For example, in one trial, 31 inpatients in a Veterans Affairs psychiatric facility received Therapeutic Touch, relaxation therapy, or sham TT. The study was designed to evaluate the effectiveness of TT for reducing **anxiety** and **stress**. The results appear to indicate that TT was more effective for this purpose than sham TT. However, there are some very serious design problems in this study that make the results hard to trust. The real TT was administered by a woman in street clothes and the placebo treatment by a woman in nursing garb; to make matters more complex, the relaxation therapy was administered by a man dressed as a clergyman. These large differences in appearance could only be expected to considerably influence the results in ways that cannot be predicted.

In a better study, 60 people with **tension headaches** were randomly assigned to receive either TT or placebo touch. TT proved to be significantly more effective than placebo touch.

However, in a reasonably well-designed study published in 1993, use of TT in 108 people undergoing **surgery** failed to reduce post-operative pain to a greater extent than sham TT.

A series of studies evaluated TT for aiding **wound healing**. Some found TT more effective than placebo, others found no significant effect, and still others found placebo more effective than real treatment. These results suggest that the effects seen were due to chance.

Subsequent to the 1999 review, several better-quality trials were published. One such study compared real TT and sham TT in 99 men and women recovering from severe burns. Researchers hypothesized that use of TT would decrease pain and anxiety during that arduous and traumatic process and, indeed, some evidence of benefit was seen.

In a smaller study (25 participants), real TT appeared to reduce the pain of knee **osteoarthritis** compared to sham TT. Furthermore, in a study of 20 HIV-infected children, use of TT improved anxiety while sham TT did not.

Taking all these studies together, it appears that real TT may be more effective than sham TT (using the serial subtraction technique described above). However, whether these apparent benefits are due to the energy-healing effects claimed by practitioners or more of an emotional communication of relaxation remains unclear.

Some studies provide preliminary evidence that TT does *not* work in the manner practitioners believe it does. For example, in one well-designed study, TT produced no effect when conducted without eye contact. The researcher, an influential person in the history of TT, had hypothesized that TT involved a kind of energy transfer that would not need eye contact. The fact that no effects were seen without the addition of eye contact suggests that it might be focused attention that makes the difference, not energy transmitted through the hands.

Furthermore, if TT actually involves contact with the "energy field" of a patient, it would seem that the practitioners would be able to sense the presence of such a field. However, in a widely publicized study, 21 practitioners who had practiced TT for 1 to 27 years proved unable to do this. In this trial, TT practitioners placed their hands face up through holes in a barrier. The experimenter (a 9-year-old student) held a hand above one of the practitioner's hands and the practitioner was asked to sense its presence. The practitioners' guesses proved to be no more accurate than chance would allow. This study has been strongly criticized by proponents of TT. Some have said that the experimenter was in the throes of puberty and, for that reason, her energy field was too disturbed to detect; others have complained about the disturbing presence of video cameras. While these criticisms are potentially valid, the burden is actually on proponents of TT to prove that there really is such a thing as a human "energy field."

Nonetheless, the studies already performed do indicate that, at the very least, concentrated, positive attention provided by one human being to another is consoling and calming. This is a wonderful fact, even if there is no special "energy field" involved.

What to Expect During a Therapeutic Touch Session

Therapeutic Touch is generally administered in a session that lasts about 20 minutes. You will be asked to lie still, relax, and remain quiet. The practitioner will place his or her hands a few inches above your body and move them slowly and rhythmically.

Some people experience a variety of subjective sensations while receiving TT, such as heat and moving energy. Most people find TT generally relaxing, but some undergo cathartic emotional experiences.

How to Find a Qualified Therapeutic Touch Practitioner

The original and most well-established Therapeutic Touch organization is Nurse Healers–Professional Associates International, Inc. (NH-PAI). This organization certifies training programs in TT. For more information, call them at (877) 32NHPAI ([877] 326-4724), contact them by e-mail at nhpai@therapeutic-touch.org, or visit their Web site at http://www.therapeutic-touch.org.

Safety Issues

There are no known or suspected safety risks with TT.

Traditional Chinese Herbal Medicine

ALTERNATE NAMES: *Aristolochia Clematis; Banxia Houpo Tang; Biminne; Bing Gan Tang; Bupleurum, Minor; Chinese Herbs; Chinese Patent Remedies; Coptis Formula; Daio-Kanzo-To; Fuzheng Jiedu Tang; Hange Koboku-To; Herbs, Chinese; Hochu-Ekki-To; Jianpi Wenshen Recipe; Kampo; Magnolia and Pinelliae Formula; Minor Bupleurum; PC-SPES; Saiboku-To; Saiko-Keishi-To; Shakuyaku-Kanzo-To; Shosaiko-To; Sho-Seiryu-To; Shuang Huang Lian; Toki-Shakuyaku-San; Yi Zhu Decoction; Zemaphyte*

PRINCIPAL PROPOSED USES: *Liver Conditions*

OTHER PROPOSED USES: *Allergies, Asthma, Chronic Fatigue Syndrome, Constipation, Dementia, Diabetes, Eczema, Epilepsy, HIV Support, Infertility in Women, Insomnia, Irregular Menstruation, Irritable Bowel Syndrome, Menopause, Menstrual Pain, Muscle Spasms, Osteoarthritis, Respiratory Infections, Sexual Dysfunction in Men, Stress, Stroke Rehabilitation, Tension Headache, Weight Loss*

Overview

The system of herbal medicine that developed in China differs in several significant ways from European herbal medicine. The most obvious difference is that the Western herbal tradition focuses on *simples*, or herbs taken by themselves. In contrast, traditional Chinese herbal medicine (TCHM) makes almost exclusive use of herbal combinations. More importantly, these formulas are not designed to treat symptoms of a specific illness; rather, they are tailored specifically to the individual according to the complex principles of traditional Chinese medicine. For this reason, TCHM is potentially a deeply holistic healing approach. On the other hand, it is both more difficult to use and to study than its Western counterpart.

TCHM is widely used in Asian countries, both in its traditional holistic form and in a simplified disease-oriented version. There have been a few properly designed scientific trials of TCHM, but the evidence base remains highly inadequate. In addition to questions regarding effectiveness, there remain serious safety concerns to be resolved.

History of Chinese Herbal Medicine

Chinese herbal medicine has a long historical tradition, although it is not quite as ancient as popularly believed. Ancient herbology in China focused on potions whose function was part medicinal and part magical and it lacked a substantial theoretical base. Sometime between the second century B.C.E. and the second century A.D., the theoretical foundations of traditional Chinese medicine were laid, but the focus was more on acupuncture than on herbs. Only by about the twelfth century A.D. were the deeper principles of Chinese medicine fully applied to herbal treatment, forming a method that can be called TCHM. This was further refined and elaborated during various periods of active theorizing in the fourteenth through the nineteenth centuries. Western disease concepts entered the picture in the twentieth century, leading to further changes.

In China today, TCHM is used alongside conventional pharmaceutical treatment. Considerable attempts have been made to subject TCHM to scientific evaluation; however, most of the published Chinese studies on the subject fall far short of current scientific standards. (For example, they generally lack a placebo group.)

In neighboring Japan, a variation of the TCHM system known as *Kampo* has become popular and the Japanese Health Ministry has approved many Kampo remedies for medical use. The scientific basis for these remedies remains incomplete, but several studies of moderately good quality have been reported.

Principles of Traditional Chinese Herbal Medicine

Even a basic introduction to the principles of TCHM exceeds the scope of this article. Consider the following nothing more than a taste of this vast medical system.

According to the principles of all Chinese medicine, health exists when the body is balanced and its energy is freely flowing. The term *energy* refers to Qi, the life energy that is said to animate the body. The term *balance* refers to the relative factors of yin and yang—the classic Taoist opposing forces of the universe. Yin and yang find their expression in various subsidiary antagonists such as cold versus heat, dampness versus dryness, descending versus ascending, at rest versus active, and full versus empty.

In an ideal state, yin and yang in all their forms are perfectly balanced in every part of the body. However, external or internal factors can upset this balance, leading to disease. Chinese medical diagnosis and treatment involves identifying the factors that are out of balance and attempting to bring them back into harmony. Diagnosis is carried out by means of *listening* to the pulse (in other words, taking the pulse with extraordinary care and sensitivity), observing and palpating various parts of the body, and asking a long series of questions.

It is important to realize that diagnosis according to TCHM differs greatly from Western diagnosis. To understand this, consider two hypothetical patients with the single Western diagnosis of migraine headaches. The first might be said to have "dryness in the liver and ascending Qi," while another might be diagnosed with "exogenous wind-cold." Based on these differing diagnoses, entirely different remedies might be applied. In other words, there is no such thing as a TCHM remedy for migraines per se; rather, treatment must be individualized to the imbalance determined by traditional theory.

The herbal formulas used in TCHM consist of four categories of herbs: *ministerial, deputy, assistant,* and *envoy.* The ministerial herb addresses the principal pattern of the disease. Deputy herbs assist the ministerial herb or address coexisting conditions. Assistant herbs are designed to reduce the side effects of the first two classes of herbs, and envoy herbs direct the therapy to a particular part of the body. For example, in the case of "dryness in the liver and ascending Qi" described above, an herbalist might employ a ministerial herb to reverse ascending Qi, a deputy herb to exert a moistening effect, an assistant herb to prevent the stagnation of Qi (Qi stagnation is said to be a side effect of moistening herbs), and an envoy to carry these effects to the liver.

TCHM remedies can also be designed to fit all common causes of migraines simultaneously, mostly by multiplying the number of ingredients. Practitioners of TCHM frown upon this "one-size-fits-all" approach, but it is often popular among consumers and it is easier to test scientifically.

Types of Chinese Herbal Remedies

To use Chinese herbal medicine in the most traditional fashion, you must visit an herbalist's shop. There, experienced herb preparers will chop, grind, fry, and slice dried herbs according to the prescription given by an experienced herbalist. You will walk home with a packet of dried herbs that need to be prepared according to the instructions, which typically involve adding water, boiling for several hours in a ceramic pot, pouring off the liquid, adding more water, and repeating the process twice more. Certain herbs are supposed to be added right at the end, while others require extra-long preparation.

If you don't wish to carry out such a complex process or if a classic herbal shop is not available, you may wish to move one step away from tradition and purchase an already-prepared Kampo formula. There are several hundred such formulas designed to match the most commonly seen forms of imbalance. Available in powder, capsule, or tablet form, they can be used much more conveniently than fully traditional herbs. Many Kampo combinations are licensed in Japan and are manufactured there on a large scale by reputable manufacturers.

The lowest level of TCHM, scarcely deserving the name at all, involves so-called Chinese Patent Remedies, which consist most commonly of tiny brown spheres in small brown bottles. They are marketed both for classical imbalances and western disease categories. Patent remedies are inexpensive and widely available. However, there have been so many scandals involving dangerous contaminants not listed on the label that we recommend avoiding this form of treatment entirely. (See Safety Issues below.)

In the West, herbal medicine is part of folk medicine. However, in China there is a distinct tradition of Chinese folk medicine that is separate from the orthodox, rather academic TCHM approach. In this Chinese folk medicine, herbs are used more simply, somewhat in the manner of Western herbal medicine. Herbs most commonly used in this manner include **astragalus**, **dong quai**, **ginger**, **kudzu** (*Pueraria lobata*), **licorice**, *Panax ginseng*, and **schisandra**. For more information on the use of these herbs, see the appropriate individual articles.

What Is Chinese Herbal Medicine Used for Today?

In the traditional system of Chinese herbal medicine, herbal formulas can be used to treat virtually any condition. Some of the most common uses in China include liver disease (**hepatitis** and **cirrhosis**), **sexual dysfunction in men**, **infertility in women**, **insomnia**, **colds and flus**, **menstrual pain**, irregular menstruation, and **menopause**. **Acupuncture** is often used along with herbs as a supplemental treatment; in addition, extraordinarily de-

tailed lifestyle suggestions are common. It is not unusual for a traditional practitioner to "prescribe" dinner, as well as counsel changes in living situation (for example, move from the basement to the first floor or face the bed south rather than north). Exercise systems, such as **Tai Chi** and Chi Gung, may also be recommended.

What Is the Scientific Evidence for Traditional Chinese Herbal Medicine?

To establish the effectiveness of a treatment, it must be put through a double-blind, placebo-controlled trial. For this reason, the *Collins Alternative Health Guide* is organized around such studies. However, there are a few issues that make it a bit difficult to study TCHM in this way.

The first problem involves diagnosis. As described above, there is no such thing as a TCHM remedy for migraine headaches, for example. Each person with migraines receives individualized treatment. This introduces an extra wrinkle for experimenters.

The best way to address this issue is as follows. People are chosen to participate in a study based on a Western diagnosis. Next, all participants are diagnosed by a classic herbal practitioner and prescribed a formula specific to their individual constitutions according to the principles of TCHM. Finally, another party steps in and provides participants with either the real formula or a placebo formula, under conditions whereby neither practitioners nor participants know which is which.

Other studies utilize a fixed remedy for all participants, in hopes that it will still prove effective on average. Such an approach doesn't really test the effectiveness of true TCHM; rather, it tests a much-simplified form of it. Still, trials of this type are valid as far as they go.

Numerous other studies simply involve enrolling people with a certain condition and giving each participant an herbal remedy. Researchers then record the extent of improvement. Such open-label trials, however, prove virtually nothing because even phony treatments will appear to cause benefits. (For more information, see **Why Does This Book Rely on Double-blind Trials?**) We do not report open-label trials here.

Chronic Hepatitis

Hepatitis is a serious problem in many Asian countries and conventional care leaves much to be desired. For this reason, herbal remedies are widely used.

The herbal combination Shosaiko-to (Minor Bupleurum) has been approved as a treatment for chronic hepatitis by the Japanese Health Ministry and it enjoys wide use in that country and elsewhere. However, a search of the literature uncovered only one large-scale, double-blind, placebo-controlled study supporting its effectiveness. In this 24-week trial, the efficacy of Shosaiko-to was tested in 222 people with chronic active hepatitis using a double-blind, placebo-controlled crossover design. Results showed that use of Shosaiko-to significantly improved liver function measurements compared to placebo. Although these results are promising, an absence of long-term evaluation limits their meaningfulness. (Researchers only followed participants for 3 months.)

Other Chinese herbal remedies have been tested as adjuncts to conventional interferon treatment with promising results. However, published trials are of generally poor quality.

Note: If you are on interferon therapy, you should not use Chinese herbal formulas (or any herbs or supplements) except under the supervision of a physician (see Safety Issues below).

Other combination Chinese herbal therapies have shown a bit of promise for the treatment of chronic hepatitis, including Bing Gan Tang, Yi Zhu decoction, Fuzheng Jiedu Tang, and Jianpi Wenshen recipe. However, the quality of most of these studies was again quite poor—the results are mixed and, overall, the evidence for these remedies remains far too weak to rely upon. One study failed to find Chinese herbal treatment helpful for hepatitis C.

Note: There have been numerous cases of hepatitis and other forms of liver injury caused by Chinese herbs. See Safety Issues below for more information.

Liver Cirrhosis

Shosaiko-to, mentioned in the previous section, has also shown some promise for preventing liver cancer and liver fibrosis in people with liver cirrhosis or chronic hepatitis. However, the evidence remains marginal. For example, in a double-blind, placebo-controlled study, 260 people with cirrhosis were randomly assigned to take Shosaiko-to or placebo, along with conventional treatment. Over 5 years of evaluation, people taking the herb appeared to be less likely to develop cancer or die, but the results just missed the ordinary cutoff for statistical significance. For the subgroup of participants without hepatitis B infection, the benefits *were* statistically significant at the usual cutoff point.

Irritable Bowel Syndrome

In a double-blind, placebo-controlled trial, 116 people with **irritable bowel syndrome** (IBS) were randomly as-

signed to receive individualized Chinese herbal formulations, a "one-size-fits-all" Chinese herbal formulation, or placebo. Treatment consisted of 5 capsules 3 times daily, taken for 16 weeks. The results showed that both forms of active treatment were superior to placebo, significantly reducing IBS symptoms. Interestingly, the individualized treatment was no more effective than the "generic" treatment.

Constipation

The Kampo formula known as Daio-kanzo-to is a mixture of rhubarb and licorice. In a 2-week, double-blind, placebo-controlled trial, 132 people complaining of constipation were randomly assigned to one of three groups: placebo, low-dose Daio-kanzo-to, or high-dose Daio-kanzo-to. The results indicate that the higher-dose group, but not the lower-dose group, experienced statistically significant improvements in constipation compared to placebo.

These finding are not surprising because rhubarb contains known laxative constituents (anthraquinones) similar to those found in approved over-the-counter laxative preparations. The licorice constituent of this formula is said to reduce side effects by protecting mucous membranes. However, there is no meaningful evidence for any such protective effect, nor indication that such a protective effect is needed. Furthermore, licorice presents significant safety risks (see Safety Issues below).

Allergies

In a double-blind, placebo-controlled trial, 220 people with **allergic rhinitis** were given either placebo or the Kampo remedy Sho-seiryu-to for a period of 2 weeks. The results showed that use of the herbal formula significantly relieved all major symptoms of allergic rhinitis compared to placebo. Based on this and other more preliminary studies, Sho-seiryu-to has been approved by the Japanese Health Ministry for the treatment of allergic rhinitis and allergic conjunctivitis.

Another combination herbal therapy has shown promise for allergic rhinitis as well. In a 12-week, double-blind, placebo-controlled trial, 58 people with allergic rhinitis were given either placebo or an 11-herb combination remedy called Biminne. This combination therapy contains the following herbs:

➤ *Rehmannia glutinosa*
➤ *Scutellaria baicalensis*
➤ *Polygonatum sibiricum*

➤ *Ginkgo biloba*
➤ *Epimedium sagittatum*
➤ *Psoralea corylifolia*
➤ *Schisandra chinensis*
➤ *Prunus mume*
➤ *Ledebouriella divaricata*
➤ *Angelica dahurica*
➤ *Astragalus membranaceus*

Use of Biminne produced significant improvements in some symptoms of allergic rhinitis, while other symptoms showed a trend toward improvement that was not statistically significant. A follow-up evaluation suggested that the results persisted for a year after treatment was stopped.

Benefits have been seen in small studies of other formulations as well. However, one study failed to find that use of herbal treatments augmented the effectiveness of acupuncture for allergic rhinitis.

Osteoarthritis

A double-blind, placebo-controlled study of 96 people with osteoarthritis of the knee tested the effectiveness of a mixture of three Chinese herbs (*Clematis mandshurica*, *Trichosanthes kirilowii*, and *Prunella vulgaris*). Participants were randomly assigned to placebo group or one of three other groups: 200 mg, 400 mg, or 600 mg of the herbal formula 3 times daily. After 4 weeks of treatment, significant improvement in arthritis symptoms was seen in all three treatment groups compared to placebo. No dose appeared conclusively superior to the others.

Muscle Spasms

The Kampo remedy Shakuyaku-kanzo-to is a combination of peony root and licorice, commonly used for the treatment of muscle spasms in general. In a double-blind, placebo-controlled study, 101 people with liver cirrhosis who also suffered from severe muscular spasms at least twice per week were given either Shakuyaku-kanzo-to or placebo 3 times daily for 2 weeks. (The herb combination is not specifically aimed at liver cirrhosis. However, people with liver cirrhosis often have muscle spasms, so it made sense to try an anti-muscle-spasm formula on them.) The results showed significant reduction in frequency and severity of spasms among the participants using the herb compared to those taking placebo. However, some participants using the herb developed edema (swelling caused by excess fluid) and weight gain. Researchers attributed this side effect to the licorice constituent. (See Safety Issues below for risks associated with the use of licorice.)

Menstrual Pain

In a double-blind trial of 40 women complaining of menstrual pain, the Kampo formula Toki-shakuyaku-san was compared to placebo with good results. The design of this study was interesting because researchers preselected women who, according to the principles of traditional Chinese medicine, would be expected to respond to this Kampo treatment. Over six menstrual cycles, women using the real herbal formula experienced significantly less menstrual pain compared to those in the placebo group. Benefits took three menstrual cycles to develop.

Diabetes

A double-blind study of more than 200 people evaluated the effectiveness of Coptis Formula (a traditional combination therapy) with or without the drug glibenclamide for the treatment of **diabetes**. Coptis Formula appeared to significantly enhance the effectiveness of the drug; however, the herbs produced marginal benefits at best when taken alone.

Asthma

The Kampo remedy Saiboku-to has been approved by the Japanese Health Ministry for the treatment of **asthma**. However, meaningful supporting evidence appears to be limited to one small trial. In this double-blind, placebo-controlled crossover study, 33 people with mild to moderate asthma received Saiboku-to or placebo 3 times daily for 4 weeks. Treatment with the herbal remedy improved symptoms of asthma to a greater extent than placebo. Additional measurements suggested that Saiboku-to works by reducing asthmatic inflammation (technically, eosinophilia)

A Chinese study using a proprietary formulation reported benefits as well.

Eczema

A Chinese herbal mixture sold under the name Zemaphyte has shown promise as a treatment for **eczema**. This formula, based on herbs traditionally used for skin conditions, contains the following:

➤ *Ledebouriella seseloides*
➤ *Potentilla chinensis*
➤ *Akebia clematidis*
➤ *Rehmannia glutinosa*
➤ *Paeonia lactiflora*

➤ *Lophatherum gracile*
➤ *Dictamnus dasycarpus*
➤ *Tribulus terrestris*
➤ *Glycyrrhiza uralensis*
➤ *Schizonepeta tenuifolia*

In paired double-blind, placebo-controlled trials carried out by one research group, Zemaphyte produced significantly better effects than placebo for both adults and children. Each study enrolled approximately 40 people and used a crossover design in which all participants received the real treatment and placebo for 8 weeks each. Use of the herb significantly reduced eczema symptoms compared to placebo.

However, a subsequent study of similar design performed by a different research group failed to find significant benefit with Zemaphyte. The reason for this discrepancy is not clear.

Tension Headache

A topical ointment known as Tiger Balm is a popular treatment for headaches and other conditions. Tiger Balm contains camphor, menthol, cajaput, and clove oil. A double-blind study enrolling 57 people with acute **tension headache** compared the application of Tiger Balm to the forehead against placebo ointment, as well as against the drug acetaminophen (Tylenol). The placebo ointment contained mint essence to make it smell similar to Tiger Balm. Real Tiger Balm proved more effective than placebo and just as effective and more rapid-acting than acetaminophen.

HIV

Chinese herbal therapies have been investigated for the treatment of **HIV**, but the results have not been very promising. In a 12-week, double-blind, placebo-controlled trial, 30 HIV-infected adults with CD4 counts of 200 to 500 were given a Chinese herbal formula containing 31 herbs. The results hint that use of the herbal combination might have improved various symptoms compared to placebo, but none of the differences were statistically significant. Interestingly, people who believed they were taking the real treatment showed significant benefit regardless of whether they were in the placebo group or the real treatment group.

In another double-blind, placebo-controlled trial, 68 HIV-infected adults were given either placebo or a preparation of 35 Chinese herbs for a period of 6 months. The results indicate that use of Chinese herbs did not improve symptoms or objective measurements of HIV

severity. In fact, people using the herbs reported *more* digestive problems than those given placebo!

Prostate Cancer

For several years, the Chinese herbal combination PC-SPES underwent significant investigation as a treatment for prostate cancer, with apparently impressive results. However, subsequent investigation revealed that PC-SPES contained undisclosed pharmaceutical ingredients (principally, a form of estrogen and the strong blood thinner warfarin [Coumadin]) and that these were probably responsible for its benefits. The treatment has since been withdrawn.

Other Uses for Traditional Chinese Herbal Medicine

In a small, double-blind, placebo-controlled trial, use of the herbal combination Banxia Houpo Tang (also called Hange Koboku-To or Magnolia and Pinelliae Formula) was tested for the treatment of impaired cough reflex in people who had suffered a **stroke**. The results indicated that the herbal combination was more effective than placebo treatment for improving the coughing response.

Various Chinese herbal formulas have been evaluated for the treatment of respiratory infections. The results of published studies appear to indicate that these formulas are more effective than standard antibiotics, but the poor design of most of these trials precludes placing much faith in their outcomes. One combination therapy called Shuang Huang Lian has better supporting evidence than most.

Numerous studies have evaluated traditional Chinese herbal medicine for treatment of liver cancer with generally positive results. However, study design and reporting were markedly substandard.

A double-blind, placebo-controlled study of 29 people with **chronic fatigue syndrome** found indications that use of the Kampo remedy Hochu-ekki-to significantly improved symptoms compared to placebo.

The Kampo remedies Saiko-keishi-to and Shosaiko-to have been suggested for the treatment of **epilepsy**, but the supporting evidence is too preliminary to be relied upon. Both of these combination treatments consist of bupleurum, peony root, pinellia root, cassia bark, ginger root, jujube fruit, Asian ginseng root, **Asian skullcap root**, and licorice root, but the proportions are different.

Other traditional herbal combinations with some

supporting evidence (often from studies of questionable quality) include Mai-Men-Dong-Tang for allergic **asthma**, Yi-Gan San for **dementia**, Bofu-tsusho-san for **weight loss** and diabetes-impaired glucose tolerance, Chang Ji Tai for irritable bowel syndrome, and Ondamtanggamibang (a Korean formulation) for reducing symptoms of **stress**.

In one study, the herbal formula Duhuo Jisheng Wan, widely used for osteoarthritis, proved to be as effective as the standard anti-inflammatory drug diclofenac. However, the herb caused as many side effects as the drug and was slower to act. (It was so slow, in fact, that its benefits could have been due solely to the placebo effect.) This study did not use a placebo control group.

One double-blind, placebo-controlled study tested the remedy Hochu-ekki-to for enhancing immune response to influenza vaccine, but failed to find benefit.

One study quoted as showing that a Chinese herbal formula can reduce **blood pressure** actually failed to find any effect on blood pressure.

How to Choose a Practitioner of Traditional Chinese Herbal Medicine

There is no general certification for the practice of TCHM. Many people who are certified in acupuncture, however, have significant training in herbal medicine as well. (In general, 500 hours of specific training is considered necessary.) Some states offer the license of O.M.D. (Doctor of Oriental Medicine); licensed O.M.D.'s are generally well versed in TCHM.

Safety Issues

There are several serious safety concerns with the use of TCHM.

One concern involves the use of multiple herbs typical in this approach. In general, conventional medicine makes a point of using as few medications as possible (in theory, at least) because the greater the number of medications, the greater the risk of harm. (Also, when medications are used together and harm does result, it's hard to know which drug was at fault.) From this perspective, formulas consisting of 5, 10, or 30 herbs are quite worrisome.

Interestingly, such combinations are actually designed for the purpose of *reducing* risks. According to TCHM theory, the various herbs in a formula balance and moderate each other. Unfortunately, this theory has never been put to the test and there are reasons not to trust it. Simply put, it is very difficult to get an accurate picture of the risks of a treatment if you don't keep systematic records of adverse effects and the ancient Chinese government had no such system in place. In any case, the individualized nature of treatment would make it almost impossible to track harm. Herbalists would be expected to notice immediate, dramatic reactions to herbal formulas and one can assume with some confidence that treatments used for thousands of years are at least unlikely to cause such problems in very many people who take them. However, certain types of harm could be expected to easily elude the detection of traditional herbalists. These include safety problems that are delayed, occur relatively rarely, or are difficult to detect without scientific instruments. How would a traditional herbalist ever know, for example, if a treatment caused liver failure in one out of 100,000 people who used it, especially if such failure took 2 or more years to develop? If such a death did occur in the herbalist's patient population, it would probably be attributed to hepatitis or some other common cause.

These factors may explain why Chinese herbal medicine traditionally uses treatments that are now recognized as potentially dangerous, such as mercury, arsenic, lead, licorice, coltsfoot, and *Aristolochia*.

Mercury, arsenic, and lead accumulate slowly in the body and for many years their harm can only be detected by lab tests. Licorice (used in many herb formulas to "harmonize" the ingredients) can raise blood pressure and disturb blood chemistry. These effects were presumably undetectable to traditional practitioners unless they became quite severe. The herb *Aristolochia* can cause severe kidney damage and kidney cancer, but only rarely. Modern medical surveillance has uncovered quite a few such cases, but traditional herbology considered the herb worth using. *Aristolochia* contains aristolochic acid, a substance shown in animal studies to damage the kidney when taken in high enough doses. Chinese herbal products generally list *Aristolochia* on the label when it is present, but in some cases *Aristolochia* was apparently added accidentally—it is similar in appearance to a much safer herb.

Coltsfoot (*Tussilago farfara*), used in Chinese cough syrups and other formulations, contains pyrrolizidine alkaloids, substances that can over time damage the liver. This also does not appear to have been noticed by traditional herbalists. Under modern conditions of medical surveillance, many incidents have been reported in which use of Chinese herbs appears to have various forms of liver injury, including acute hepatitis, chronic hepatitis, hepatic fibrosis, and acute liver failure. Ancient herbal practitioners might not have been able to distinguish these herb-induced illnesses from the effects of infectious hepatitis, a widely prevalent condition, and therefore failed to make the connection.

Other reported complications of Chinese herbal treatments include movement disorders and ovarian failure.

Another set of potential problems arises from the fact that Chinese herbal medicine does not restrict itself to plant products with subtle effects. Many traditional Chinese herbal remedies are, simply put, poisons. When taken in proper doses, they may be safe for use, but dosage miscalculation or use in a particularly susceptible person may lead to serious consequences, including death. For example, in Hong Kong poisoning caused by the herb aconite (used in numerous Chinese herbal formulas) was sufficiently widespread that public health authorities felt it necessary to launch an information campaign to combat the problem.

Besides toxicity caused by Chinese herbs, other problems have been caused by adulteration of herbal products with unlisted ingredients. For example, the Chinese herbal formula PC-SPES, used for prostate cancer, turned out to contain three pharmaceutical drugs—diethylstilbestrol (DES), warfarin (Coumadin), and indomethacin. This appears to have been an inten-

tional adulteration designed somewhat along the lines of a traditional Chinese formula, with one pharmaceutical adulterant that treated prostate cancer balanced by two others to offset the side effects of the first. Unfortunately, the combination is dangerous and has caused at least one case of severe bleeding.

In another episode, 8 out of 11 Chinese herbal creams sold in the United Kingdom for the treatment of eczema were found to contain strong pharmaceutical steroids. Other studies have also found steroids in eczema preparations. In addition, Chinese herbal weight-loss aids have also been found to contain an unlisted chemical related to the appetite suppressant drug fenfluramine (of fen-phen fame).

Herbal products approved by the Japanese government have undergone meaningful safety testing and are very unlikely to contain known toxins or unlisted drugs. However, this does not mean they are completely safe. For example, several case reports suggest that therapy for chronic hepatitis combining an approved herbal formula with the standard drug interferon can cause severe inflammation of the lungs.

The bottom line: TCHM is a potentially dangerous form of treatment that should only be used under the supervision of a physician.

Vega Test

RELATED TERMS: *Electrodermal Testing, EDT, Electroacupuncture According to Voll, EAV*

Overview

An unconventional device called the *Vega-test machine* is promoted by some alternative medicine practitioners for diagnosing illnesses and determining appropriate treatments. Other names for this approach include electrodermal testing (EDT) and electroacupuncture according to Voll (EAV). The method, which has many variations, generally involves measuring the body's electrical resistance at acupuncture points. Possible allergens or toxins, or prospective treatments, are placed within a device called a *honeycomb* that is said to test the effects of that substance on the body. More recent

devices use a computer that supposedly simulates the presence of test substances.

There is no obvious commonly accepted scientific basis for the use of this method. To the limited extent that it has been tested, it has not proven itself a valid diagnostic technique.

What Is the Scientific Evidence for the Vega Test?

Four Vega-test practitioners, each with at least 10 years experience, agreed to participate in a study conducted by a proponent of EDT testing. Thirty people volunteered to participate as patients. Half the volunteers had known allergies to house dust mites or cat dander (as determined by skin testing), while the others were not allergic to these allergens. Each participant was tested with six items in three separate sessions by each of three different operators of the Vega machine, resulting in a total of more than 1,500 separate allergy tests over the course of the study. The results showed that the Vega-test practitioners were unable to distinguish between allergic and non-allergic participants. In addition, no individual operator of the machine was more accurate than any other.

In another study, the Vega test failed to distinguish between people with respiratory allergies to a defined set of substances and those without them.

One smaller double-blind study did find the Vega test capable of distinguishing between allergens and non-allergens. However, one of the authors of this study felt that it suffered from significant flaws and went on to conduct the first trial discussed above.

On the basis of this information, the only fair assessment at present is that the Vega test has not been shown to be a meaningful method of identifying allergies to dust mites or cat dander. Proponents of the Vega device and other EDT techniques object that identifying respiratory allergens is not the device's primary use. However, at present there is no reliable evidence that the method has validity for *any* use.

DRUG INTERACTIONS

Acetaminophen

ALTERNATE NAMES: *APAP*

TRADE NAMES: *Apacet, Arthritis Foundation Aspirin Free, Arthritis Foundation Nighttime, Acephen, Aceta, Amaphen, Anoquan, Aspirin Free Anacin, Aspirin Free Excedrin, Bayer Select, Dapacin, Dynafed, Endolor, Esgic, Excedrin P.M., Fem-Etts, Femcet, Feverall, Fioricet, Fiorpap, Genapap, Genebs, Halenol, Isocet, Liquiprin, Mapap, Maranox, Meda, Medigesic, Midol, Multi-Symptom Pamprin, Neopap, Nighttime Pamprin, Oraphen-PD, Panadol, Phrenilin, Repan, Ridenol, Sedapap, Silapap, Sominex Pain Relief, Tapanol, Tempra, Tylenol, Uni-Ace, Unisom with Pain Relief*

Milk Thistle, Coenzyme Q$_{10}$, and Methionine—Possible Helpful Interactions

Vitamin C—Possible Increased Risk of Toxicity

Chaparral, Comfrey, and Coltsfoot—Possible Harmful Interaction

Citrate—Possible Harmful Interaction

Acetaminophen is widely used to reduce pain and fever.

Milk Thistle, Coenzyme Q$_{10}$ (CoQ$_{10}$), Methionine

Possible Helpful Interactions

The herb **milk thistle** and the supplements coenzyme Q$_{10}$ (CoQ$_{10}$) and methionine might help protect the liver against damage caused by excessive use of acetaminophen. However, it is extremely dangerous to take excessive amounts of acetaminophen, and we certainly wouldn't count on any of these supplements to protect you from harm if you do so!

Vitamin C

Possible Increased Risk of Toxicity

One study from the 1970s suggests that very high doses of **vitamin C** (3 g daily) might increase the levels of acetaminophen in the body. This could potentially put you at higher risk for acetaminophen toxicity. You probably don't need to be overly concerned if you take acetaminophen in recommended doses now and then for pain or fever. However, a problem might occur if you take higher-than-recommended doses or if you take high doses of acetaminophen on a regular basis, such as for osteoarthritis. The risk increases if you have liver or kidney impairment or if you drink alcoholic beverages regularly, which taxes the liver even more.

Chaparral, Comfrey, and Coltsfoot

Possible Harmful Interaction

The herbs chaparral (*Larrea tridentata* or *L. mexicana*), comfrey (*Symphytum officinale*), and coltsfoot (*Tussilago farfara*) contain liver-toxic substances. Combined use with acetaminophen could accentuate the liver toxicity of the medication.

Citrate

Possible Harmful Interaction

Potassium citrate, sodium citrate, and potassium-magnesium citrate are sometimes used to prevent kidney stones. These supplements reduce urinary acidity, and can therefore lead to decreased blood levels and effectiveness of acetaminophen.

Amiloride/Hydrochlorothiazide

TRADE NAMES: *Moduretic*

This medication is a combination of the following drugs:

➤ Potassium-Sparing Diuretics
➤ Thiazide Diuretics

Please see the separate articles on each one to find out about potential drug interactions. The interactions for each may be different, so read both articles carefully to find out the whole story.

Aminoglycosides

TRADE NAMES: *Amikacin, Gentamycin, Tobramycin*
Ginkgo—Possible Harmful Interaction
Minerals: Magnesium and Calcium—Possible Harmful Interaction
Vitamin B$_{12}$—Supplementation Possibly Helpful
N-acteylcysteine—May Decrease Activity of Drug

Aminoglycosides are antibiotics given intravenously to treat certain infections. These drugs can damage the kidneys as well as the nerve supplying the ear (the auditory nerve).

Ginkgo

Possible Harmful Interaction

The herb **ginkgo** is thought to increase circulation and protect nerve cells from damage. On this basis, it has been proposed as a possible treatment to help protect the auditory nerve from damage caused by aminoglycosides. However, the one animal study performed to evaluate this potential benefit found instead that the herb *increased* damage to the auditory nerve. Based on this finding, individuals using aminoglycoside drugs should avoid ginkgo.

Minerals: Magnesium and Calcium

Possible Harmful Interaction

Weak evidence from animal studies hints that use of gentamycin may reduce levels of **magnesium** and **calcium**. Supplementation may therefore be helpful on general principles if gentamicin treatment is used for a long time. One animal study suggests that calcium supplements in particular might help prevent gentamicin-induced kidney damage.

Vitamin B$_{12}$

Supplementation Possibly Helpful

One animal study weakly hints that **vitamin B$_{12}$** might help prevent hearing damage caused by gentamicin.

N-acteylcysteine

May Decrease Effectiveness of the Drug

One exceedingly preliminary animal study suggests that **N-acetylcysteine** might help protect the kidneys from damage caused by gentamicin.

Amiodarone

TRADE NAMES: *Cordarone, Pacerone*

Vitamin E—May Protect Against Side Effects

Chaparral, Comfrey, and Coltsfoot—Possible Harmful Interaction

St. John's Wort, Dong Quai—Possible Harmful Interaction

Amiodarone is used to restore normal heart rhythm.

Vitamin E

May Protect Against Side Effects

One of the problems with amiodarone is that it can cause injury to the lungs. One study suggests that vitamin E supplements might help prevent this side effect.

Chaparral, Comfrey, and Coltsfoot

Possible Harmful Interaction

The herbs chaparral (*Larrea tridentata* or *L. mexicana*), comfrey (*Symphytum officinale*), and coltsfoot (*Tussilago farfara*) contain liver-toxic substances. Because amiodarone also can be hard on the liver, combining these herbs with the medication is not advisable.

Dong Quai, St. John's Wort

Possible Harmful Interaction

Amiodarone has been reported to cause increased sensitivity to the sun, amplifying the risk of sunburn or skin rash. Because **St. John's wort** and **dong quai** may also cause this problem, taking these herbal supplements during amiodarone therapy might add to this risk.

It may be a good idea to wear a sunscreen or protective clothing during sun exposure if you take one of these herbs while using amiodarone.

Amlodipine/Benazepril

TRADE NAMES: *Lotrel*

This medication is a combination of the following drugs:

➤ Angiotensin-Converting Enzyme Inhibitors
➤ Calcium Channel Blockers

Please see the separate articles on each one to find out about potential drug interactions. The interactions for each may be different, so read both articles carefully to find out the whole story.

Amoxicillin

TRADE NAMES: *Amoxil, Trimox, Wymox*
Bromelain—Possible Helpful Interaction
Vitamin K—Possible Nutritional Depletion
See also *Antibiotics (General).*

Amoxicillin is a relative of the antibiotic penicillin, but has been modified to have a broader spectrum of effect.

Bromelain

Possible Helpful Interaction

According to two studies, the supplement **bromelain** (from pineapple stems) may increase the absorption of amoxicillin. This effect might help the antibiotic work better.

Vitamin K

Possible Nutritional Depletion

There are concerns that antibiotic treatment might reduce levels of **vitamin K** in the body. However, this effect seems to be slight, and only significant, if at all, in individuals who are already considerably deficient in vitamin K.

Angiotensin-Converting Enzyme Inhibitors

Arginine—Possible Harmful Interaction
Licorice—Possible Harmful Interaction
Potassium—Possible Harmful Interaction
St. John's Wort, Dong Quai—Possible Harmful Interaction
Iron—Possible Benefits and Risks
Zinc—Supplementation Possibly Helpful

Angiotensin-converting enzyme inhibitors (ACE inhibitors) block the conversion of a naturally occurring substance, angiotensin, to a more active form. These medications are widely used to treat hypertension as well as congestive heart failure and other conditions. Drugs in this category include

> benazepril hydrochloride (Lotensin, Lotrel),
> captopril (Capoten),
> enalapril maleate (Lexxel, Teczem, Vaseretic, Vasotec),
> fosinopril (Monopril),
> lisinopril (Prinivil, Prinzide, Zestril, Zestoretic),
> moexipril hydrochloride (Uniretic, Univasc),
> quinapril hydrochloride (Accupril),
> ramipril (Altace),
> trandolapril (Mavik, Tarka),
> and others.

Arginine

Possible Harmful Interaction

Arginine is an amino acid that has been used to improve immunity in hospitalized patients as well as for many other conditions.

Based on experience with intravenous arginine, it is possible that the use of high-dose oral arginine might alter potassium levels in the body, especially in people with severe liver disease. This is a potential concern for individuals who take ACE inhibitors.

Licorice

Possible Harmful Interaction

Licorice root, a member of the pea family, has been used since ancient times as both food and medicine.

Whole licorice (*Glycyrrhiza glabra* or *G. uralensis*) can cause sodium retention and increase blood pressure, thus counteracting the intended effects of ACE inhibitors. An often unrecognized source of licorice is chewing tobacco.

A special form of licorice known as DGL (deglycyrrhizinated licorice) is a deliberately altered form of the herb that should not cause these problems.

Potassium

Possible Harmful Interaction

ACE inhibitors cause the body to retain more **potassium** than usual. This could raise your blood levels of potassium too high, a condition called hyperkalemia, which can be dangerous. Depending on how high your potassium levels are, the symptoms you might experience include irregular heart rhythm, muscle weakness, nausea, vomiting, irritability, and diarrhea. If you are on one of these medications, do not take potassium supplements except on medical advice.

Because ingesting more potassium makes the problem worse, it is important to be aware of the various sources of extra potassium. Besides potassium supplements, sources include high-potassium diets, salt substitutes containing potassium, and potassium-sparing diuretics (diuretics that cause your body to retain potassium).

Your physician will want to keep an eye on the levels of potassium in your blood and let you know if you need to adjust your potassium intake.

Dong Quai, St. John's Wort

Possible Harmful Interaction

St. John's wort (*Hypericum perforatum*) is primarily used to treat mild to moderate depression.

The herb **dong quai** (*Angelica sinensis*) is often recommended for menstrual disorders such as dysmenorrhea, PMS, and irregular menstruation.

ACE inhibitors have been reported to cause increased sensitivity to the sun, amplifying the risk of sunburn or skin rash. Because St. John's wort and dong quai may also cause this problem, taking these herbal supplements during treatment with ACE inhibitors might add to this risk.

It may be a good idea to wear a sunscreen or protective clothing during sun exposure if you take one of these herbs while using an ACE inhibitor.

Iron

Possible Benefits and Risks

Individuals taking ACE inhibitors frequently develop a dry cough as a side effect. One study suggests that **iron** supplementation can alleviate this symptom. In this 4-week, double-blind, placebo-controlled trial of 19 individuals, use of iron as ferrous sulfate significantly reduced cough symptoms as compared to placebo.

Keep in mind that it is not healthy to get too much iron. For this reason, we recommend that you seek medical advice before starting iron supplements.

However, remember that iron supplements can interfere with the absorption of captopril and perhaps other ACE inhibitors. Iron appears to bind with captopril, resulting in a compound that the body cannot absorb. This, of course, also impairs iron absorption. To minimize any potential problems, take iron supplements and ACE inhibitors 2 to 3 hours apart.

Zinc

Supplementation Possibly Helpful

ACE inhibitors may cause **zinc** depletion. The ACE inhibitors captopril and enalapril attach to the trace mineral zinc. Because zinc in this bound form cannot replace the zinc that the body uses to meet its normal needs, a gradual loss of zinc from body tissues may result. Continued drug therapy could lead to zinc deficiency.

It has been suggested, though not proven, that zinc deficiency might account for some of the side effects seen with ACE inhibitors, such as taste disturbances, poor appetite, and skin numbness or tingling.

Whether zinc supplementation will prevent ACE inhibitor–induced zinc deficiency has not been examined, but it seems reasonable to think that taking extra zinc might help. Generally, zinc supplements should also contain copper to prevent zinc-induced copper deficiency.

Antacids

Folate—Supplementation Possibly Helpful

Minerals—Supplementation Possibly Helpful, but Take at a Different Time of Day

Calcium Citrate—May Increase Aluminum Absorption

The term *antacid* is used to describe certain compounds that directly neutralize stomach acid. Tums, Maalox, and Mylanta all fall into this category. The active ingredients in most antacids are various forms of calcium, magnesium, and aluminum. Antacids are useful mostly for symptomatic relief of uncomfortable "acid stomach" and also may be helpful for heartburn.

Many antacids are available today, including

➤ aluminum carbonate (Basaljel),

➤ aluminum hydroxide (ALternaGEL, Alu-Cap, Alu-Tab, Amphojel, Dialume, Nephrox),

➤ aluminum hydroxide/magnesium carbonate (Duracid),

➤ aluminum hydroxide/magnesium hydroxide (Alamag, Almacone, Aludrox, Gaviscon Liquid, Gelusil, Kudrox, Maalox, Magalox, Magnox, Mintox, Mylanta, Rulox),

➤ aluminum hydroxide/magnesium hydroxide/calcium carbonate (Tempo),

➤ aluminum hydroxide/magnesium trisilicate (Alenic Alka, Gaviscon, Genaton, Foamicon),

➤ calcium carbonate (Alkets, Amitone, Chooz, Equilet, Gas-Ban, Maalox Antacid Caplets, Mallamint, Mylanta Lozenges, Titralac, Tums),

➤ calcium carbonate/magnesium carbonate (Marblen, Mi-Acid Gelcaps, Mylanta Gelcaps, Mylagen Gelcaps),

➤ magnesium hydroxide (Milk of Magnesia, Phillips' Chewable),

➤ magaldrate or aluminum magnesium hydroxide sulfate (Iosopan, Riopan),

➤ magnesium oxide (Mag-Ox, Maox, Uro-Mag),

➤ sodium bicarbonate (Bell/ans, Bromo Seltzer), and sodium citrate (Citra pH).

Other drugs work by reducing the stomach's production of acid. These are discussed separately in the articles on **H₂ Blockers** (for example, Zantac [ranitidine], Axid [nizatidine], Tagamet [cimetidine], Pepcid [famotidine]) and **Proton Pump Inhibitors** (Prilosec [omeprazole], Prevacid [lansoprazole]). These drugs produce a more powerful effect than antacids and are used for ulcers as well as for the treatment of esophageal reflux, commonly known as heartburn.

Folate

Supplementation Possibly Helpful

Research suggests that antacids physically bind to **folate** and reduce its absorption by the body. However, the decrease in folate absorption is relatively small and this interaction may be clinically significant only in individuals who take antacids regularly and whose diets are low in folate content.

Minerals

Supplementation Possibly Helpful, but Take at a Different Time of Day

Different types of antacids can interfere with the absorption of various minerals. Supplements containing the U.S. Dietary Reference Intake (formerly known as the Recommended Dietary Allowance) of these minerals should be helpful, especially if you take them at a different time of day from when you take antacids, at least 2 hours before or after taking your antacid.

Any antacid can interfere with the absorption of **iron, zinc,** and possibly other minerals by neutralizing stomach acid.

Aluminum-containing antacids can bind with phosphorus and interfere with its absorption, and this can further lead to calcium depletion.

Antacids that contain calcium may also compete for absorption with iron. Although calcium antacids may alter the absorption of magnesium, the clinical importance of this effect appears to be minimal. Calcium-containing antacids, when taken with zinc supplements, might substantially decrease zinc absorption. However, the presence of a meal appears to mitigate this effect. Finally, calcium antacids might also impair the absorption of manganese and chromium.

Citrate

May Increase Aluminum Absorption

Concerns have been raised that the aluminum in some antacids may not be good for you. Since there is some evidence that calcium citrate supplements might increase the absorption of aluminum, it might not be a good idea to take calcium citrate at the same time of day as aluminum-containing antacids. Another option is to use other forms of calcium, or to avoid antacids containing aluminum.

Antibiotics (General)

See also *Amoxicillin, Cephalosporins, Ethambutol, Fluoroquinolones, Isoniazid, Nitrofurantoin, Rifampin, Tetracyclines,* and *Trimethoprim/Sulfamethoxazole.*

There are an enormous number of antibiotics in use today. Issues common to antibiotics in general are discussed below.

Some of the drugs that fall into this family include

➤ amoxicillin (Amoxil, Trimox, Wymox),
➤ amoxicillin/potassium clavulanate (Augmentin),
➤ ampicillin (Omnipen, Principen, Totacillin, Marcillin),
➤ azithromycin (Zithromax),
➤ bacampicillin (Spectrobid),
➤ carbenicillin indanyl sodium (Geocillin),
➤ chloramphenicol (Chloromycetin Kapseals),
➤ cinoxacin (Cinobac),
➤ clarithromycin (Biaxin),
➤ clindamycin (Cleocin),
➤ clofazimine (Lamprene),
➤ cloxacillin sodium (Cloxapen),
➤ colistin sulfate (Coly-Mycin S),
➤ dapsone,
➤ dicloxacillin sodium (Dycill, Dynapen, Pathocil),
➤ dirithromycin (Dynabac),
➤ erythromycin (E-Base, Ilosone, EryPed, E.E.S., Ery-Tab, E-Mycin, Eryc, Erythrocin, PCE),
➤ fosfomycin tromethamine (Monurol),
➤ kanamycin (Kantrex),
➤ lincomycin (Lincocin),
➤ metronidazole (Flagyl, Protostat),
➤ nafcillin sodium (Unipen),
➤ nalidixic acid (NegGram),
➤ neomycin (Neo-Tabs, Mycifradin, Neo-fradin),
➤ novobiocin (Albamycin),
➤ oxacillin sodium,
➤ paromomycin (Humatin),
➤ penicillin V (Pen Vee K Beepen-VK, Penicillin VK, Veetids),
➤ troleandomycin (Tao),
➤ vancomycin (Vancocin),
➤ and others.

Vitamin K

Possible Nutritional Depletion

Vitamin K plays a crucial role in blood clotting and also seems to be important for proper bone formation.

There are concerns that antibiotic treatment might reduce levels of vitamin K in the body. However, this effect seems to be slight, and only significant, if at all, in individuals who are already considerably deficient in vitamin K.

Acidophilus and Other Probiotics

Probable Helpful Interactions

One common side effect of antibiotic therapy is diarrhea (about 25 to 30% of people taking antibiotics report this problem). It is primarily caused by the antibiotic killing many of the bacteria that normally live in the intestines. Changes in bacteria can also cause yeast infections. However, if you take "friendly" microorganisms such as *Saccharomyces boulardii*, **L.acidophilus**, or *Bifidobacterium longum* at the same time you start antibiotics, and continue for some time afterward, you may be able to significantly reduce the risk of these complications.

Anticonvulsant Drugs

See *Carbamazepine (Tegretol), Phenobarbital, Phenytoin (Dilantin), Primidone (Mysoline), and Valproic Acid (Depakene).*

Anti-Inflammatory Drugs

See also *Corticosteroids and Nonsteroidal Anti-Inflammatory Drugs (NSAIDs).*

Antipsychotics

Drugs in this class are used primarily to treat schizophrenia and other forms of psychosis. Many of these medications fall in the class known as phenothiazines. This category includes

➤ chlorpromazine hydrochloride (Thorazine),
➤ fluphenazine (Permitil, Prolixin),
➤ mesoridazine besylate (Serentil),
➤ perphenazine (Trilafon),
➤ prochlorperazine (Compazine),
➤ promazine hydrochloride (Sparine),
➤ promethazine hydrochloride (Anergan [injectable], Phenergan),
➤ thioridazine hydrochloride (Mellaril),
➤ trifluoperazine hydrochloride (Stelazine),
➤ triflupromazine hydrochloride (Vesprin [injectable]),
➤ and others.

Newer medications, risperidone (Risperdal), quetiapine (Seroquel), ziprasidone (Geodon), aripiprazole (Abilify), olanzapine (Zyprexa) and clozapine (Clozaril), are called **atypical antipsychotics**.

See **Phenothiazines** or **Atypical Antipsychotics** for more information.

Aspirin/Acetaminophen

TRADE NAMES: *Buffets Vanquish, Extra Strength Excedrin, Gelpirin, Goody's, Maximum Pain Relief Pamprin, Menoplex, Supac.*

This medication is a combination of the following drugs:

➤ Acetaminophen
➤ Nonsteroidal Anti-Inflammatory Drugs

Please see the separate articles on each one to find out about potential drug interactions. The interactions for each may be different, so read both articles carefully to find out the whole story.

Atypical Antipsychotics

St. John's Wort—Possible Harmful Interaction
Glycine—Possible Benefits and Risks
Ginkgo—Possible Helpful Interaction

The medications olanzapine (Zyprexa), risperidone (Risperdal), clozapine (Clozaril) quetiapine (Seroquel), ziprasidone (Geodon), and aripiprazole (Abilify) are used to treat schizophrenia and other forms of psychosis. Most medications used for schizophrenia are in the **phenothiazine** family. The atypical antipsychotics are so called because they are chemically quite different.

St. John's Wort

Possible Harmful Interaction

The herb **St. John's wort** might reduce levels of these medications in the blood. This could lead to an increase in the severity of psychotic symptoms.

Perhaps even more dangerously, if medication levels are adjusted for an individual already taking St. John's wort, stopping the herb could cause these levels to rise, potentially causing dangerous toxic symptoms.

Glycine

Possible Benefits and Risks

Some evidence suggests that the amino acid **glycine** may augment the action of phenothiazine antipsychotic drugs. It may also augment the action of olanzapine and risperidone; whether it augments or decreases the effectiveness of clozapine remains unclear.

Ginkgo

Possible Helpful Interaction

Preliminary evidence suggests that **ginkgo** might reduce the side effects and increase the efficacy of various antipsychotic medications, including atypical antipsychotic drugs.

Bendroflumethiazide/Nadolol

TRADE NAMES: *Corzide*

This medication is a combination of the following drugs:

➤ Beta-Blockers
➤ Thiazide Diuretics

Please see the separate articles on each one to find out about potential drug interactions. The interactions for each may be different, so read both articles carefully to find out the whole story.

Benzodiazepines

Grapefruit Juice—Possible Harmful Interaction

Kava, Valerian, Passionflower, Hops—Possible Harmful Interaction

Melatonin—Supplementation Possibly Helpful

Pregnenolone—May Decrease Activity of Drug

Kava—Possibly Helpful

Medications in the benzodiazepine family exert calming and sedative effects and are used to treat anxiety and insomnia. Benzodiazepines are also used as muscle relaxants and anticonvulsants. They work by increasing the effects of the neurotransmitter (a chemical messenger) GABA. Benzodiazepine drugs include

➤ alprazolam (Xanax),
➤ chlordiazepoxide hydrochloride (Libritabs, Librium, Limbitrol, Lipoxide, Mitran, Reposans-10, Sereen),
➤ clonazepam (Klonopin),
➤ clorazepate dipotassium (Gen-XENE, Tranxene-T, Tranxene-SD),
➤ diazepam (Diastat, Valium, Valrelease, Vazepam),
➤ estazolam (ProSom),
➤ flurazepam hydrochloride (Dalmane, Durapam),
➤ halazepam (Paxipam),
➤ lorazepam (Ativan),
➤ oxazepam (Serax),
➤ quazepam (Doral),
➤ temazepam (Razepam, Restoril, Temaz),
➤ triazolam (Halcion),
➤ and others.

Grapefruit Juice

Possible Harmful Interaction

Grapefruit juice slows the body's normal breakdown of several drugs, including some benzodiazepines, allowing them to build up to potentially dangerous levels in the blood. A recent study indicates that this effect can last for 3 days or more following the last glass of juice.

Because of this risk, if you take benzodiazepines, the safest approach is to avoid grapefruit juice altogether.

Hops, Kava, Passionflower, Valerian

Possible Harmful Interaction

The herb **kava** (*Piper methysticum*) has a sedative effect and is used for anxiety and insomnia.

Combining kava with drugs in the benzodiazepine family, which possess similar effects, could result in "add-on" or excessive physical depression, sedation, and impairment. In one case report of a 54-year-old man hospitalized for lethargy and disorientation, these side effects were attributed to his having taken the combination of kava and alprazolam for 3 days.

Experimental studies suggest that kava, similarly to benzodiazepines, exerts its sedative effects at binding sites in the brain called GABA receptors.

Other herbs with a sedative effect that might cause problems when combined with benzodiazepines include **ashwagandha** (*Withania somnifera*), **calendula** (*Calendula officinalis*), **catnip** (*Nepeta cataria*), **hops** (*Humulus lupulus*), lady's slipper (*Cypripedium*), **lemon balm** (*Melissa officinalis*), **passionflower** (*Passiflora incarnata*), sassafras (*Sassifras officinale*), **skullcap** (*Scutellaria lateriflora*), **valerian** (*Valeriana officinalis*), and yerba mansa (*Anemopsis californica*).

Because of the potentially serious consequences, you should avoid combining these herbs with benzodiazepines or other drugs that also have sedative or depressant effects unless advised by your physician.

Melatonin

Supplementation Possibly Helpful

Melatonin is a natural hormone that regulates sleep.

Many people who take conventional sleeping pills (most of which are in the benzodiazepine family) find it difficult to quit. The reason is that when you try to stop the medication, you may experience severe insomnia or interrupted sleep. A double-blind, placebo-controlled study of 34 individuals who regularly used such medications found that melatonin at a dose of 2 mg nightly (in a controlled-release formulation) could help them discontinue the use of the drugs.

Warning: It can be dangerous to stop using benzodiazepines if you have taken them for a while. Consult your physician before trying melatonin to help handle benzodiazepine withdrawal or before trying to stop benzodiazepine medication under any conditions.

Pregnenolone

Supplementation May Decrease Effectiveness of the Drug

The hormone **pregnenolone** is widely sold as a kind of "fountain of youth." However, the only direct evidence that pregenolone supplements have any effect at all relates to a potential interaction between the hormone and benzodiazepine drugs. In a carefully designed clinical trial, regular use of pregnenolone was found to greatly decrease the sedative effects of diazepam (Valium). The reasons for this interaction are not known. However, people who rely upon benzodiazepine drugs may find them less effective if pregnenolone is added into the mix.

Kava

Possibly Helpful

Although they are highly effective for anxiety, benzodiazepine drugs can cause unpleasant and dangerous withdrawal symptoms when they are discontinued.

A 6-week, double-blind, placebo-controlled trial of 40 people who had been taking benzodiazepines found that use of **kava** significantly reduced withdrawal symptoms and helped maintain control of anxiety.

Note: This trial involved close medical supervision and very gradual tapering of benzodiazepine dosages. Do not discontinue antianxiety medications except on the advice of a physician, as withdrawal symptoms can be life threatening.

Beta-Blockers

Coenzyme Q$_{10}$ (CoQ$_{10}$)—Supplementation Possibly Helpful

Chromium—Possible Helpful Interaction

Coleus forskohlii—Theoretical Interaction

Beta-blockers are used for hypertension as well as for a variety of heart conditions.

Drugs that fall into this family include

➤ acebutolol hydrochloride (Sectral),
➤ atenolol (Tenormin),
➤ alprenolol,
➤ betaxolol hydrochloride (Kerlone),
➤ bisoprolol fumarate (Zebeta),
➤ carteolol (Cartrol),
➤ carvedilol (Coreg),
➤ esmolol hydrochloride (Brevibloc),
➤ labetalol hydrochloride (Normodyne, Trandate),
➤ metoprolol (Lopressor, Toprol XL),
➤ nadolol (Corgard),
➤ penbutolol (Levatol),
➤ pindolol (Visken),
➤ propranolol hydrochloride (Betachron E-R, Inderal, Inderal LA),
➤ sotalol (Betapace),
➤ timolol maleate (Blocadren),
➤ and others.

Coenzyme Q$_{10}$ (CoQ$_{10}$)

Supplementation Possibly Helpful

There is some evidence that beta-blockers (specifically propranolol, metoprolol, and alprenolol) might impair the body's ability to utilize the substance **coenzyme Q$_{10}$** (CoQ$_{10}$). This is particularly worrisome, because CoQ$_{10}$ appears to play a significant role in normal heart function. Depletion of CoQ$_{10}$ might be responsible for some of the side effects of beta-blockers. In one study, CoQ$_{10}$ supplements reduced side effects caused by the beta-blocker propranolol. The beta-blocker timolol may interfere with CoQ$_{10}$ production to a lesser extent than other beta-blockers.

Chromium

Possible Helpful Interaction

Beta-blockers have been known to reduce levels of HDL ("good") cholesterol. According to one study, **chromium** supplementation can offset this adverse effect.

Coleus forskohlii

Theoretical Interaction

The herb *Coleus forskohlii* relaxes blood vessels and might have unpredictable effects on blood pressure if combined with beta-blockers.

Bile Acid Sequestrant Drugs

Many Nutrients—Supplementation Likely Helpful

The **bile acid sequestrant drugs** are among the earliest class of medications used to lower cholesterol. They are seldom prescribed today because of their many side effects.

Medications in the bile acid sequestrant family include cholestyramine resin (Locholest, Prevalite, Questran, Questran Light) and colestipol hydrochloride (Colestid), among others.

Many Nutrients

Supplementation Likely Helpful

Bile acid sequestrants have been reported to impair the absorption of numerous nutrients, including **calcium**, **folate**, **iron**, **vitamin A**, **vitamin B₁₂**, and **vitamin E**. It appears, however, that only folate supplementation may be needed by individuals on long-term therapy with bile acid sequestrants. Although the bile acid sequestrant used in the studies interfered with the absorption of the other nutrients, their levels remained in the normal range. Just to be safe, though, making sure to get enough vitamin E and vitamin A (in the form of beta-carotene) would make sense.

Blood Pressure Drugs

See *ACE Inhibitors, Beta-Blockers, Calcium Channel–Blockers, Clonidine, Hydralazine, Loop Diuretics, Methyldopa, Potassium-Sparing Diuretics, Thiazide Diuretics.*

Bromocriptine

TRADE NAMES: *Parlodel*
Chasteberry—Theoretical Interference with Drug Action

Bromocriptine reduces the level of the hormone prolactin by affecting the pituitary gland. It is sometimes used to treat conditions in which there is too much prolactin, such as certain forms of PMS and infertility.

Chasteberry

Theoretical Interference with Drug Action

The herb **chasteberry** inhibits prolactin secretion and might have unpredictable effects if combined with bromocriptine.

Calcium Channel Blockers

Calcium and Vitamin D—Possible Decreased Action of Drug
Ginkgo Biloba—Possible Decreased Action of Drug

Calcium channel–blockers are used to treat hypertension, angina, heart arrhythmias, and other heart-related conditions.

Drugs in this family include

➤ amlodipine (Norvasc),
➤ bepridil hydrochloride (Vascor),
➤ diltiazem (Cardizem, Cardizem CD, Cardizem SR, Dilacor XR, Tiamate, Tiazac),
➤ felodipine (Plendil),
➤ isradipine (DynaCirc, DynaCirc CR),
➤ nicardipine hydrochloride (Cardene, Cardene SR),
➤ nifedipine (Procardia, Procardia XL, Adalat, Adalat CC),

➤ nimodipine (Nimotop),

➤ nisoldipine (Sular),

➤ verapamil (Calan, Calan SR, Covera-HS, Isoptin, Isoptin SR, Verelan),

➤ and others.

Calcium, Vitamin D

Possible Decreased Action of Drug

Taking **calcium** and **vitamin D** supplements might interfere with some of the effects of calcium channel–blockers.

Ginkgo Biloba

Possible Decreased Action of Drug

According to a study in rats, **ginkgo** extract may cause the body to metabolize nicardipine (a calcium channel-blocker) more rapidly, thereby decreasing its effects.

Carbamazepine

TRADE NAMES: *Atretol, Carbatrol, Epitol, Tegretol, Tegretol XR*

Ginkgo—Possible Harmful Interaction

Glutamine—Possible Harmful Interaction

Grapefruit Juice—Possible Harmful Interaction

Ipriflavone—Possible Harmful Interaction

Hops, Kava, Passionflower, Valerian—Possible Harmful Interaction

Nicotinamide—Possible Harmful Interaction

Dong Quai, St. John's Wort—Possible Harmful Interaction

Biotin—Supplementation Possibly Helpful, but Take at a Different Time of Day

Folate—Supplementation Possibly Helpful

Calcium—Supplementation Probably Helpful, but Take at a Different Time of Day

Carnitine—Supplementation Possibly Helpful

Vitamin D—Supplementation Possibly Helpful

Vitamin K—Supplementation Possibly Helpful for Pregnant Women

Carbamazepine is an anticonvulsant agent used primarily to prevent seizures in conditions such as epilepsy.

Other anticonvulsant agents include **phenobarbital**, **phenytoin**, **primidone**, and **valproic acid**. In some cases, combination therapy with two or more anticonvulsant drugs may be used.

Ginkgo

Possible Harmful Interaction

The herb **ginkgo** (*Ginkgo biloba*) has been used to treat Alzheimer's disease and ordinary age-related memory loss, among many other conditions.

This interaction involves potential contaminants in ginkgo, not ginkgo itself.

A recent study found that a natural nerve toxin present in the seeds of *Ginkgo biloba* made its way into standardized ginkgo extracts prepared from the leaves. This toxin has been associated with convulsions and death in laboratory animals.

Fortunately, the detected amounts of this toxic substance are considered harmless. However, given the lack of satisfactory standardization of herbal formulations in the United States, it is possible that some batches of product might contain higher contents of the toxin depending on the season of harvest.

In light of these findings, taking a ginkgo product that happened to contain significant levels of the nerve toxin might theoretically prevent an anticonvulsant from working as well as expected.

Glutamine

Possible Harmful Interaction

The amino acid **glutamine** is converted to glutamate in the body. Glutamate is thought to act as a neurotransmitter (chemical that enables nerve transmission). Because anticonvulsants work (at least in part) by blocking glutamate pathways in the brain, high dosages of the amino acid glutamine might theoretically diminish an anticonvulsant's effect and increase the risk of seizures.

Grapefruit Juice

Possible Harmful Interaction

Grapefruit juice slows the body's normal breakdown of several drugs, including the anticonvulsant carbamazepine, allowing it to build up to potentially dangerous levels in the blood. A recent study indicates this effect can last for 3 days or more following the last glass of juice.

Because of this risk, if you use carbamazepine, the safest approach is to avoid grapefruit juice altogether.

Ipriflavone

Possible Harmful Interaction

Ipriflavone, a synthetic isoflavone that slows bone breakdown, is used to treat osteoporosis.

Test-tube studies indicate that ipriflavone might increase blood levels of the anticonvulsants carbamazepine and phenytoin when they are taken therapeutically. Ipriflavone was found to inhibit a liver enzyme involved in the body's normal breakdown of these drugs, thus allowing them to build up in the blood. Higher drug levels increase the risk of adverse effects.

Because anticonvulsants are known to contribute to the development of osteoporosis, a concern is that the use of ipriflavone for this drug-induced osteoporosis could result in higher blood levels of the drugs with potentially serious consequences.

Individuals taking either of these drugs should use ipriflavone only under medical supervision.

Hops, Kava, Passionflower, Valerian

Possible Harmful Interaction

The herb **kava** (*Piper methysticum*) has a sedative effect and is used for anxiety and insomnia.

Combining kava with anticonvulsants, which possess similar depressant effects, could result in "add-on" or excessive physical depression, sedation, and impairment. In one case report, a 54-year-old man was hospitalized for lethargy and disorientation, side effects attributed to his having taken the combination of kava and the antianxiety agent alprazolam (Xanax) for 3 days.

Other herbs having a sedative effect that might cause problems when combined with anticonvulsants include **ashwagandha** (*Withania somnifera*), **calendula** (*Calendula officinalis*), **catnip** (*Nepeta cataria*), **hops** (*Humulus lupulus*), **lady's slipper** (*Cypripedium* species), **lemon balm** (*Melissa officinalis*), **passionflower** (*Passiflora incarnata*), sassafras (*Sassafras officinale*), **skullcap** (*Scutellaria lateriflora*), **valerian** (*Valeriana officinalis*), and yerba mansa (*Anemopsis californica*).

Because of the potentially serious consequences, you should avoid combining these herbs with anticonvulsants or other drugs that also have sedative or depressant effects unless advised by your physician.

Nicotinamide

Possible Harmful Interaction

Nicotinamide (also called niacinamide) is a compound produced by the body's breakdown of niacin (**vitamin B$_3$**). It is a supplemental form that does not possess the flushing side effect or the cholesterol-lowering ability of niacin.

Nicotinamide appears to increase blood levels of carbamazepine and primidone, possibly requiring a reduction in drug dosage to prevent toxic effects.

Carbamazepine blood levels increased in two children with epilepsy after they were given nicotinamide, but the fact that the children were on several anticonvulsant drugs clouds the issue somewhat. Similarly, nicotinamide given to three children on primidone therapy increased blood levels of primidone. It is thought that nicotinamide may interfere with the body's normal breakdown of these anticonvulsant agents, allowing them to build up in the blood.

Dong Quai, St. John's Wort

Possible Harmful Interaction

St. John's wort (*Hypericum perforatum*) is primarily used to treat mild to moderate depression.

The herb **dong quai** (*Angelica sinensis*) is often recommended for menstrual disorders such as dysmenorrhea, PMS, and irregular menstruation.

The anticonvulsant agents carbamazepine, phenobarbital, and valproic acid have been reported to cause increased sensitivity to the sun, amplifying the risk of sunburn or skin rash. Because St. John's wort and dong quai may also cause this problem, taking them during treatment with these drugs might add to this risk.

It may be a good idea to wear a sunscreen or protective clothing during sun exposure if you take one of these herbs while using these anticonvulsants.

Biotin

Supplementation Possibly Helpful, but Take at a Different Time of Day

Anticonvulsants may deplete **biotin**, an essential water-soluble B vitamin, possibly by competing with it for absorption in the intestine. It is not clear, however, whether this effect is great enough to be harmful.

Blood levels of biotin were found to be substantially lower in 404 people with epilepsy on long-term treatment with anticonvulsants compared to 112 untreated people with epilepsy. The effect occurred with phenytoin, carbamazepine, phenobarbital, and primidone. Valproic acid appears to affect biotin to a lesser extent than other anticonvulsants.

A test-tube study suggested that anticonvulsants might lower biotin levels by interfering with the way biotin is transported in the intestine.

Biotin supplementation may be beneficial if you are on long-term anticonvulsant therapy. To avoid a potential interaction, take the supplement 2 to 3 hours apart from the drug. It has been suggested that the action of anticonvulsant drugs may be at least partly related to their effect of reducing biotin levels. For this reason, it may be desirable to take enough biotin to prevent a deficiency, but not an excessive amount.

Folate

Supplementation Possibly Helpful

Folate (also known as folic acid) is a B vitamin that plays an important role in many vital aspects of health. Carbamazepine appears to lower blood levels of folate by speeding up its normal breakdown by the body and also by decreasing its absorption. Other antiseizure drugs can also reduce levels of folate in the body.

Low folate can lead to anemia and reduced white blood cell count, and folate supplements have been shown to help prevent these complications of carmabazepine treatment.

Adequate folate intake is also necessary to prevent neural tube birth defects such as spina bifida and anencephaly. Because anticonvulsant drugs deplete folate, babies born to women taking anticonvulsants are at increased risk for such birth defects. Anticonvulsants may also play a more direct role in the development of birth defects.

The low serum folate caused by anticonvulsants can raise **homocysteine** levels, a condition hypothesized to increase the risk of heart disease.

However, the case for taking extra folate during anticonvulsant therapy is not as simple as it might seem. It is possible that folate supplementation itself might impair the effectiveness of anticonvulsant drugs, and physician supervision is necessary.

Calcium

Supplementation Probably Helpful, but Take at a Different Time of Day

Anticonvulsant drugs may impair **calcium** absorption and in this way increase the risk of osteoporosis and other bone disorders.

Calcium absorption was compared in 12 people on anticonvulsant therapy (all taking phenytoin and some also taking carbamazepine, phenobarbital, and/or primidone) and 12 people who received no treatment. Calcium absorption was found to be 27% lower in the treated participants.

An observational study found low calcium blood levels in 48% of 109 people taking anticonvulsants. Other findings in this study suggested that anticonvulsants might also reduce calcium levels by directly interfering with parathyroid hormone, a substance that helps keep calcium levels in proper balance.

A low blood level of calcium can itself trigger seizures, and this might reduce the effectiveness of anticonvulsants.

Calcium supplementation may be beneficial for people taking anticonvulsant drugs. However, some studies indicate that antacids containing calcium carbonate may interfere with the absorption of phenytoin and perhaps other anticonvulsants. For this reason, take calcium supplements and anticonvulsant drugs several hours apart if possible.

Carnitine

Supplementation Possibly Helpful

Carnitine is an amino acid that has been used for heart conditions, Alzheimer's disease, and intermittent claudication (a possible complication of atherosclerosis in which impaired blood circulation causes severe pain in calf muscles during walking or exercising).

Long-term therapy with anticonvulsant agents, particularly valproic acid, is associated with low levels of carnitine. However, it isn't clear whether the anticonvulsants cause the carnitine deficiency or whether it occurs for other reasons. It has been hypothesized that low carnitine levels may contribute to valproic acid's damaging effects on the liver. The risk of this liver damage increases in children younger than 24 months, and carnitine supplementation may be protective. However, in one double-blind crossover study, carnitine supplementation produced no real improvement in "well-being" as assessed by parents of children receiving either valproic acid or carbamazepine.

L-carnitine supplementation may be advisable in certain cases, such as in infants and young children (especially those younger than 2 years) who have neurologic disorders and are receiving valproic acid and multiple anticonvulsants.

Vitamin D

Supplementation Possibly Helpful

Anticonvulsant drugs may interfere with the activity of **vitamin D**. As proper handling of calcium by the body depends on vitamin D, this may be another way that these drugs increase the risk of osteoporosis and related bone disorders (see the previous Calcium topic).

Anticonvulsants appear to speed up the body's normal breakdown of vitamin D, decreasing the amount of the vitamin in the blood. A survey of 48 people taking both phenytoin and phenobarbital found significantly lower levels of calcium and vitamin D in many of them as compared to 38 untreated individuals. Similar but lesser changes were seen in 13 people taking phenytoin or phenobarbital alone. This effect may be apparent only after several weeks of treatment.

Another study found decreased blood levels of one form of vitamin D but normal levels of another. Because there are multiple forms of vitamin D circulating in the blood, the body might be able to adjust in some cases to keep vitamin D in balance, at least for a time, despite the influence of anticonvulsants.

Adequate sunlight exposure may help overcome the effects of anticonvulsants on vitamin D by stimulating the skin to manufacture the vitamin. Of 450 people on anticonvulsants residing in a Florida facility, none were found to have low blood levels of vitamin D or evidence of bone disease. This suggests that environments providing regular sun exposure may be protective.

Individuals regularly taking anticonvulsants, especially those taking combination therapy and those with limited exposure to sunlight, may benefit from vitamin D supplementation.

Vitamin K

Supplementation Possibly Helpful for Pregnant Women

Phenytoin, carbamazepine, phenobarbital, and primidone speed up the normal breakdown of vitamin K into inactive byproducts, thus depriving the body of active **vitamin K**. This can lead to bone problems such as osteoporosis. Also, use of these anticonvulsants can lead to a vitamin K deficiency in babies born to mothers taking the drugs, resulting in bleeding disorders or facial bone abnormalities in the newborns.

Mothers who take these anticonvulsants may need vitamin K supplementation during pregnancy to prevent these conditions in their newborns.

Cephalosporins

Vitamin K—Supplementation Possibly Helpful
See also *Antibiotics (General).*

These antibiotics work somewhat similarly to penicillin, but have been chemically modified to have a broader spectrum of effect.

Drugs in this family include

- cefadroxil (Duricef),
- cephalexin (Cefanex, Keflex, Keftab, Biocef),
- cephradine (Velosef),
- cefaclor (Ceclor, Ceclor CD),
- cefprozil (Cefzil),
- cefuroxime (Ceftin),
- loracarbef (Lorabid),
- cefdinir (Omnicef),
- cefixime (Suprax),
- cefpodoxime proxetil (Vantin),
- ceftibuten (Cedax),
- and others.

Vitamin K

Supplementation Possibly Helpful

Like all other antibiotics, cephalosporins might interfere with **vitamin K** levels by killing vitamin K–producing bacteria in the intestines. In addition, antibiotics in the cephalosporin family may also interfere with the way vitamin K works. For this reason, taking extra vitamin K may be a good idea when using cephalosporins over the long term.

Chlorothiazide/Methyldopa

TRADE NAMES: *Aldoclor*

This medication is a combination of the following drugs:

- Methyldopa
- Thiazide Diuretics

Please see the separate articles on each one to find out about potential drug interactions. The interactions for each may be different, so read both articles carefully to find out the whole story.

Chlorthalidone/Atenolol

TRADE NAMES: *Tenoretic*

This medication is a combination of the following drugs:

- Beta-Blockers
- Thiazide Diuretics

Please see the separate articles on each one to find out about potential drug interactions. The interactions for each may be different, so read both articles carefully to find out the whole story.

Chlorthalidone/Clonidine

TRADE NAMES: *Combipres*

This medication is a combination of the following drugs:

➤ Clonidine
➤ Thiazide Diuretics

Please see the separate articles on each one to find out about potential drug interactions. The interactions for each may be different, so read both articles carefully to find out the whole story.

Cilostazol

TRADE NAMES: *Pletal*

Interactions—Possible Increased Risk of Bleeding

Cilostazol, a drug that makes the blood clot less easily, is used to reduce the risk of strokes, heart attacks, and other conditions caused by blood clots.

Interactions

Possible Increased Risk of Bleeding

For information on potentially harmful interactions with cilostazol, see the article on the related drug pentoxifylline.

Cisplatin

TRADE NAME: *Platinol*

Black Cohosh—Possible Harmful Interaction

Magnesium and Potassium—Possibly Helpful Interaction

Melatonin—Possibly Helpful Interaction

Antioxidants—Possibly Helpful Interaction

Milk Thistle—Possible Helpful Interaction

Acetyl-L-Carnitine—Possible Helpful Interaction

Ginger—No Benefit

Cisplatin is a chemotherapy drug used to treat cancer of the testicles, bladder, lung, stomach, esophagus, and ovaries, as well as other forms of cancer. Cisplatin can cause numerous side effects, including:

➤ Nausea and vomiting
➤ Kidney or liver damage
➤ Peripheral neuropathy (numbness or tingling of the extremities)

➤ **Hearing loss**
➤ **Ringing in the ear**
➤ **Loss of appetite**
➤ **Abnormal taste sensations**
➤ **Hair loss**

Some of the treatments mentioned below have been advocated for preventing or treating cisplatin side effects. For information on the use of natural treatments as a support to cancer chemotherapy in general, see the **Cancer Treatment** article.

Black Cohosh

Possible Harmful Interaction

The herb **black cohosh** is often used for menopausal symptoms. Because women receiving cancer chemotherapy may experience menopausal symptoms, black cohosh may appear to be a promising option. However, one test-tube study found that use of black cohosh may decrease the effectiveness of cisplatin.

Magnesium and Potassium

Possibly Helpful Interaction

There is some evidence that use of cisplatin may cause the body to develop potentially dangerous deficiencies of **potassium** and **magnesium**. Taking supplements of these nutrients may be advisable.

Melatonin

Possible Helpful Interaction

Weak preliminary evidence hints that use of **melatonin** may reduce side effects and increase efficacy of chemotherapy regimens that include cisplatin.

Antioxidants

Possible Helpful Interaction

It has been suggested that many of the undesired effects of cisplatin are due to creation of free radicals, dangerous, naturally occurring substances that can damage many cells. For this reason, treatment with antioxidants has been proposed for preventing toxic side effects. However, as yet there is no more than minimal evidence for benefit.

One animal study tested a combination of substances with strong antioxidant properties (**vitamin E**, *Crocus sativus*, and *Nigella sativa*) and found evidence that this mixture reduced the kidney toxicity of cisplatin.

A small human trial found evidence that use of vitamin E might help prevent nerve injury (peripheral neuropathy) caused by cisplatin, but because this was an open study, its results are not very reliable.

Another open study found possible benefits with **selenium**.

Unfortunately, in open studies, the placebo effect and other confounding factors can play a significant role. (For more information on why this is the case, see **Why Does This Book Rely on Double-blind Studies?**.)

In a better-designed, double-blind, placebo-controlled study of 48 people undergoing cancer treatment with cisplatin, participants were given either placebo or a combination of vitamin E, **vitamin C**, and selenium in hopes of reducing toxicity to the ears and kidneys. No significant benefits were seen.

Note that there are concerns that use of antioxidants could potential decrease the effectiveness of some forms of chemotherapy. For this reason, we strongly suggest that people on cancer chemotherapy do not use antioxidants, or any herbs or supplements, except in consultation with their physician.

Milk Thistle

Possible Helpful Interaction

Animal and test-tube studies hint that the herb **milk thistle** might decrease the kidney toxicity of cisplatin and also possibly increase cisplatin efficacy.

However, no studies in humans have been reported.

Acetyl-L-Carnitine

Possible Helpful Interaction

One study found evidence that the supplement **acetyl-L-carnitine** might reduce symptoms of peripheral neuropathy caused by cisplatin.

Ginger

No Benefit

The herb **ginger** is widely used for treatment of **nausea**. However, one study failed to find ginger helpful for nausea caused by cisplatin.

Clonidine

TRADE NAMES: *Catapres*

Coenzyme Q$_{10}$ (CoQ$_{10}$)—Supplementation Possibly Helpful

Yohimbe—Probable Dangerous Interaction

Coleus forskohlii—Theoretical Interaction

Clonidine is often used to reduce blood pressure as well as to counter symptoms that occur during withdrawal from alcohol and other addictive substances.

Coenzyme Q$_{10}$ (CoQ$_{10}$)

Supplementation Possibly Helpful

There is some evidence that clonidine might impair the body's ability to manufacture the substance **coenzyme Q$_{10}$ (CoQ$_{10}$)**. However, it has not yet been shown that CoQ$_{10}$ supplements offer any particular benefit to those taking this medication.

Yohimbe

Probable Dangerous Interaction

If you are taking clonidine, it is not safe to take **yohimbe**.

Coleus forskohlii

Theoretical Interaction

The herb *Coleus forskohlii* relaxes blood vessels and might have unpredictable effects if combined with clonidine.

Clopidogrel

TRADE NAMES: *Plavix*

Clopidogrel, a drug that makes the blood clot less easily, is used to reduce the risk of strokes, heart attacks, and other conditions caused by blood clots.

Numerous herbs and natural supplements might interfere with the ability of the blood to clot as well. If they are taken with clopidogrel, excess bleeding might occur. For a discussion of all these natural products, see the **Warfarin** article.

Colchicine

Vitamin B$_{12}$—Supplementation Possibly Helpful

Although primarily used on a short-term basis to treat attacks of gout, colchicine is increasingly being prescribed for longer periods as a gout preventive.

This practice may heighten the chance of developing the nutritional deficiency discussed here.

Vitamin B$_{12}$

Supplementation Possibly Helpful

Colchicine can impair intestinal absorption of **vitamin B$_{12}$**, so taking a B$_{12}$ supplement during extended colchicine therapy may be warranted.

Corticosteroids

ALTERNATE NAMES: *Glucocorticoids*

Calcium and Vitamin D—Helpful Interactions

Aloe and Licorice (Topical)—Possible Supportive Interactions with Topical Steroids

Creatine—Possible Helpful Interaction

DHEA (Dehydroepiandrosterone)—Possible Helpful Interaction

Chromium—Supplementation Possibly Helpful

Ipriflavone—Possible Harmful Interaction

Licorice (Internal)—Possible Harmful Interaction

Corticosteroid drugs (also known as glucocorticoids) act like the naturally occurring adrenal hormone cortisone in the body. They are strong anti-inflammatory and immune-suppressant medications used in many inflammatory and autoimmune conditions, such as **rheumatoid arthritis**, **asthma**, **inflammatory bowel disease**, and **systemic lupus erythematosus**. Corticosteroids are also prescribed to suppress transplant rejection.

Drugs in this family include

➤ betamethasone (Celestone),
➤ cortisone acetate (Cortone Acetate),
➤ dexamethasone (Decadron, Dexameth, Dexone, Hexadrol),
➤ hydrocortisone (Cortef, Hydrocortone),
➤ methylprednisolone (Medrol),
➤ prednisolone (Delta-Cortef, Pediapred, Prelone),
➤ prednisone (Deltasone, Liquid Pred, Meticorten, Orasone, Panasol-S, Prednicen-M, Sterapred DS),
➤ triamcinolone (Aristocort, Atolone, Kenacort),
➤ and others.

Calcium, Vitamin D

Helpful Interactions

One of the most serious side effects of long-term corticosteroid use is accelerated osteoporosis. Although we don't fully understand how this works, corticosteroid interference with calcium and vitamin D is known to play a major role.

Calcium and vitamin D supplements are definitely beneficial for fighting ordinary osteoporosis; in addition, there is good evidence that they also protect against osteoporosis brought on by corticosteroids. A review of five trials enrolling a total of 274 participants found that calcium and vitamin D supplementation significantly prevented bone loss at the lumbar spine and forearm in corticosteroid-treated individuals. For example, in a 2-year, double-blind, placebo-controlled study of 130 individuals, supplementation with 1,000 mg of calcium and 500 IU of vitamin D daily actually reversed steroid-induced bone loss, causing a net bone gain.

Aloe and Licorice (Topical)

Possible Supportive Interactions with Topical Corticosteroids

Aloe and **licorice** are two herbs sometimes used topically for skin problems. Preliminary evidence suggests that each one might help topical corticosteroids, such as hydrocortisone, work better.

DHEA (Dehydroepiandrosterone)

Possible Helpful Interaction

There are theoretical reasons (but little direct evidence) to believe that individuals taking corticosteroids (such as prednisone) might be protected from some side effects by taking **DHEA** at the same time.

Chromium

Supplementation Possibly Helpful

Long-term, high-dose corticosteroid treatment can cause diabetes. This may be at least partly caused by **chromium** deficiency. A very preliminary study found treatment with corticosteroids caused increased loss of chromium in the urine. Another preliminary study found that individuals with corticosteroid-induced diabetes could improve blood sugar control by taking chromium supplements.

Creatine

Possible Helpful Interaction

Long-term use of corticosteroids, whether orally, or, possibly, by inhalation, can slow a child's growth. One animal study suggests that use of the supplement **creatine** may help prevent this side effect.

Ipriflavone

Possible Harmful Interaction

The supplement **ipriflavone** is used to treat osteoporosis (see). A 3-year, double-blind trial of almost 500 women, as well as a small study, found worrisome evidence that ipriflavone can reduce white blood cell count in some people. For this reason, anyone taking medications that suppress the immune system should avoid using ipriflavone except under physician supervision.

Licorice (Internal)

Possible Harmful Interaction

When taken by mouth, the herb **licorice** appears to enhance some actions of oral corticosteroids, but interfere with others. Because of the unpredictable nature of this interaction, individuals using oral corticosteroids should avoid licorice.

Cyclosporine

TRADE NAMES: *Neoral; Sandimmune*

Grapefruit Juice—Possible Harmful Interaction

Citrus Aurantium—Possible Harmful Interaction

Berberine—Possible Harmful Interaction

St. John's Wort—Possible Harmful Interaction

Ipriflavone—Possible Harmful Interaction

Peppermint—Possible Harmful Interaction

Scutellaria baicalensis—Possible Harmful Interaction

Cyclosporine helps prevent rejection of a transplanted organ by suppressing the immune system.

Grapefruit Juice

Possible Harmful Interaction

Grapefruit juice slows the body's normal breakdown of several drugs, including cyclosporine, allowing it to build up to potentially excessive levels in the blood. A recent study indicates this effect can last for three days or more following the last glass of juice.

If you take cyclosporine, the safest approach is to avoid grapefruit juice altogether.

Citrus Aurantium

Possible Harmful Interaction

Like grapefruit juice, bitter orange (*citrus aurantium*) may raise levels of cyclosporine.

If you take cyclosporine, the safest approach is to avoid *citrus aurantium* altogether.

Berberine

Possible Harmful Interaction

The substance berberine, found in **goldenseal**, **oregon grape**, and **barberry**, may increase levels of cyclosporine.

St. John's Wort

Possible Harmful Interaction

The herb **St. John's wort** (*Hypericum perforatum*) is primarily used to treat mild to moderate depression.

St. John's wort has the potential to accelerate the body's normal breakdown of certain drugs including cyclosporine, resulting in lower blood levels of these drugs.

This interaction appears to have occurred in two heart transplant patients taking cyclosporine, leading to heart transplant rejection. These individuals had been doing well after transplantation while taking standard immunosuppressive therapy that included cyclosporine. After starting St. John's wort for depression, however, they began experiencing problems and their blood levels of cyclosporine were found to have dipped below the therapeutic range. After St. John's wort was discontinued, cyclosporine levels returned to normal and no further episodes of rejection occurred.

Numerous cases of transplant rejection episodes involving the heart, kidney, and liver have also been reported in people using the herb.

Based on this evidence, if you are taking cyclosporine, you should not take St. John's wort.

Ipriflavone

Possible Harmful Interaction

The supplement **ipriflavone** is used to treat osteoporosis. A 3-year, double-blind trial of almost 500 women, as well as a small study, found worrisome evidence that ipriflavone can reduce white blood cell count in some people. For this reason, anyone taking medications that suppress the immune system should avoid taking ipriflavone.

Peppermint

Possible Harmful Interaction

An animal study indicates that use of peppermint oil may increase cyclosporine levels in the body. If you are taking cyclosporine and wish to use peppermint oil as well, notify your physician in advance, so that your blood levels of cyclosporine can be monitored and your dose adjusted if necessary. If you are already taking both peppermint oil and cyclosporine and stop taking the peppermint, your cyclosporine levels may fall. Again, consult your physician to make the necessary dosage adjustment.

Scutellaria baicalensis

Possible Harmful Interaction

The herb *Scutellaria baicalensis* (Chinese skullcap) may impair absorption of cyclosporine, according to a study in animals.

Digoxin

ALTERNATE NAMES: *Digitoxin*

TRADE NAMES: *Crystodigin, Lanoxicaps, Lanoxin*

Magnesium—Supplementation Possibly Helpful, but Take at a Different Time of Day

Calcium—Supplementation Possibly Helpful

Hawthorn—Possible Increased Action of Drug

Licorice—Possible Dangerous Interaction

Eleutherococcus senticosus—Possible Interaction

Horsetail—Possible Dangerous Interaction

St. John's Wort—Possible Reduction of Effectiveness of Drug

Uzara—Possible Harmful Effect

Gingko biloba—No Interaction

The digitalis drugs digoxin and digitoxin are used for congestive heart failure and other heart conditions. The concerns described below apply equally to both medications.

Magnesium

Supplementation Possibly Helpful, but Take at a Different Time of Day

Magnesium deficiency can increase the risk of toxicity from digoxin. However, taking magnesium supplements at the same time as digoxin might impair the absorption of the drug. The solution? Do not take your magnesium supplement during the two hours before or after your digoxin dose.

Calcium

Supplementation Possibly Helpful

Although the evidence is quite weak, digoxin might cause a tendency toward **calcium** deficiency. Taking calcium supplements couldn't hurt.

Hawthorn

Possible Increased Action of Drug

Because **hawthorn** has effects on the heart somewhat similar to those of digoxin, you shouldn't combine the two treatments except under the supervision of a physician.

Licorice

Possible Dangerous Interaction

Licorice root can lower potassium levels in the body, which can be dangerous for an individual taking digoxin. The special form of licorice known as DGL (deglycyrrhizinated licorice) is a deliberately altered form of the herb that should not affect potassium levels.

Eleutherococcus senticosus

Possible Interaction

There has been one report of an apparent elevation in digoxin level caused by the herb *Eleutherococcus senticosus* (so-called "Siberian ginseng") (see). However, the details of the case suggest that the eleutherococcus product might actually have interfered with a *test* for digoxin, rather than the digoxin levels themselves.

Horsetail

Possible Dangerous Interaction

Because **horsetail** can deplete the body of potassium, it may not be safe to combine this herb with digitalis drugs.

St. John's Wort

Possible Reduction of Effectiveness of Drug

Evidence suggests that **St. John's wort** may interact with digoxin, possibly requiring an increased dosage to maintain the proper effect. Conversely, if you are taking St. John's wort already and your physician adjusts your dose of medication, suddenly stopping the herb could cause blood levels of the drug to rise dangerously high.

Uzara

Possible Harmful Effect

Uzara root (*Xysmalobium undulatum*) is used to treat diarrhea. It contains substances similar to digoxin and may cause false readings on tests designed to measure digoxin levels. These substances also might alter (either increase or decrease) the effectiveness of digoxin.

Gingko biloba

No Interaction

One study found that simultaneous use of the herb *Ginkgo biloba* (80 mg three times daily of the typical standardized extract) does *not* change digoxin levels.

Diltiazem/Enalapril

TRADE NAMES: *Teczem*

This medication is a combination of the following drugs:

➤ **Angiotensin-Converting Enzyme Inhibitors**
➤ **Calcium Channel Blockers**

Please see the separate articles on each one to find out about potential drug interactions. The interactions for each may be different, so read both articles carefully to find out the whole story.

Dipyridamole

TRADE NAMES: *Persantine*
Interactions—Possible Increased Risk of Bleeding

Dipyridamole, a drug that makes the blood clot less easily, is used to reduce the risk of strokes, heart attacks, and other conditions caused by blood clots.

Interactions

Possible Increased Risk of Bleeding

For information on potential interactions with dipyridamole, see the article on the related drug **pentoxifylline**.

Diuretics

See *Loop Diuretics, Potassium-Sparing Diuretics, and Thiazide Diuretics.*

Each of these three major types of diuretics has its own particular concerns regarding herb and drug interactions.

Enalapril/Felodipine

TRADE NAMES: *Lexxel*

This medication is a combination of the following drugs:

➤ ACE Inhibitors (Angiotensin-Converting Enzyme Inhibitors)
➤ Calcium Channel Blockers

Please see the separate articles on each one to find out about potential drug interactions. The interactions for each may be different, so read both articles carefully to find out the whole story.

Erythromycin/Sulfisoxazole

TRADE NAMES: *Eryzole, Pediazole*

This medication is a combination of the following drugs:

➤ Antibiotics (General)
➤ Trimethoprim/Sulfamethoxazole

Please see the separate articles on each one to find out about potential drug interactions. The interactions for each may be different, so read both articles carefully to find out the whole story.

Estrogen

Folate—Supplementation Possibly Helpful

Ipriflavone—Potential Benefits and Risks

Other Nutrients—Supplementation Possibly Helpful

Boron—Theoretical Harmful Interaction

Resveratrol—Possible Harmful Interaction

Rosemary—Possible Harmful Interaction

Indole-3-Carbinol—Theoretical Harmful Interaction

Chasteberry—Theoretical Harmful Interaction

Dong Quai—Interaction Unlikely or Probably Insignificant

Estrogen is used as a component of birth control pills as well as for preventing osteoporosis and heart disease in menopausal women.

Some estrogen products contain the hormone in different forms. For example, certain products such as Ortho Dienestrol Vaginal Cream contain estrogen as *dienestrol*. Medications containing a form of estrogen called *estradiol* include

- Alora,
- Climara,
- Combipatch,
- Delestrogen (injectable),
- depGynogen (injectable),
- Depo-Estradiol Cypionate (injectable),
- Depogen (injectable),
- Esclim,
- Estrace,
- Estraderm,
- Estra-L (injectable),
- Estring,
- Fempatch,
- Gynogen L.A. (injectable),
- Vagifem,
- Valergen (injectable),
- Vivelle,
- and others.

Premarin, Cenestin, Prempro, and Premphase contain another form of estrogen called *conjugated estrogens*. Other forms of estrogen and some of their brand names include *diethylstilbestrol diphosphate* (Stilphostrol), *estrone* (Kestrone-5), *esterified estrogens* (Estratab, Menest),

estropipate (Ogen, Ortho-Est), and *ethinyl estradiol* (Estinyl) among others.

Folate

Supplementation Possibly Helpful

Some evidence suggests that estrogen may interfere with the absorption of **folate**. Since folate deficiency is fairly common even among those not taking estrogen, taking a folate supplement on general principle is probably a good idea.

Ipriflavone

Potential Benefits and Risks

When the two are taken together, **ipriflavone** may increase estrogen's ability to protect bone (see). This may allow you to use a lower dose of estrogen and still receive its beneficial effects.

However, there may be risks involved. Although ipriflavone itself probably does not affect tissues other than bone, some evidence suggests that when it is combined with estrogen, estrogen's effects on the uterus are increased. This might mean that risk of uterine cancer would be elevated by the combination.

It should be possible to overcome this risk by taking **progesterone** along with estrogen, which is standard medical practice in any case. However, this finding does make one wonder whether ipriflavone–estrogen combinations raise the risk of breast cancer as well, an estrogen side effect that has no easy solution. At present, there is no available information on this important subject.

Estrogen

Other Nutrients

Supplementation Possibly Helpful

Estrogen use may decrease blood levels of **magnesium**, **vitamin C**, and **zinc**. This may mean that supplementation is advisable.

Boron

Theoretical Harmful Interaction

In some studies, **boron** has been found to elevate levels of the body's own estrogen. This might lead to an increased risk of estrogen side effects if boron is combined with estrogen therapy.

Resveratrol

Possible Harmful Interaction

The supplement **resveratrol** has a chemical structure similar to that of the synthetic estrogen diethylstilbestrol and produces estrogenic-like effects. For this reason, it should not be combined with prescription estrogen products.

Rosemary

Possible Harmful Interaction

Weak evidence hints that the herb **rosemary** may enhance the liver's rate of deactivating estrogen in the body. This could potentially interfere with the activity of medications that contain estrogen.

Indole-3-Carbinol

Theoretical Harmful Interaction

Indole-3-carbinol (I3C) is a substance found in broccoli that is thought to have cancer preventive effects. One of its mechanisms of action is thought to involve facilitating the inactivation of estrogen, as well as blocking its effects on cells. The net result could be decreased effectiveness of medications containing estrogen.

Chasteberry

Theoretical Harmful Interaction

Because of its effects on the pituitary gland, **chasteberry** might unpredictably alter the effects of estrogen-replacement therapy.

Dong Quai

Interaction Unlikely or Probably Insignificant

The herb **dong quai** (*Angelica sinensis*) is used for menstrual disorders.

Because dong quai contains beta-sitosterol, a phytoestrogen, there have been concerns that taking the herb with estrogen might add to estrogen-related side effects. However, a 24-week, placebo-controlled study of 74 postmenopausal women found no estrogen-like effects or reduction of menopausal symptoms associated with taking dong quai.

Therefore, dong quai seems unlikely to increase estrogen-related side effects.

Ethambutol

TRADE NAMES: *Myambutol*
Copper and Zinc—Take at a Different Time of Day
See also *Antibiotics (General).*

Ethambutol is often used along with isoniazid in the treatment of tuberculosis.

Copper, Zinc

Take at a Different Time of Day

Ethambutol may interfere with the absorption of copper and zinc by binding to them. In order to avoid deficiency, you may wish to take supplements of these essential minerals. Make sure to separate your ethambutol dose and your mineral supplements by at least 2 hours.

Fibrate Drugs

B Vitamins—Possible Helpful Interaction
Blood Thinning Supplements—Possible Harmful Interaction

Drugs in the fibrate family are used to improve levels of cholesterol and related lipids found in the blood. Fibrates are particularly helpful for individuals with high levels of triglycerides.

Medications in this category include:

➤ Clofibrate (Atromid-S)
➤ Gemfibrozil (Lopid)
➤ Fenofibrate (Tricor)

B Vitamins

Possible Helpful Interaction

Fibrate drugs are known to raise homocysteine levels in the blood. High levels of homocycsteine have been associated with increased risk of heart disease, although a direct connection has not been proven.

In a double-blind, placebo-controlled trial of 29 men taking fenofibrate, use of the B-vitamins **folate** (650 mcg), **vitamin B$_{12}$** (50 mcg), and **vitamin B$_6$** (50 mg) once daily for 6 weeks restored homocysteine levels to nearly normal values.

Blood Thinning Supplements

Possible Harmful Interaction

Fibrate drugs are known to increase the "blood thinning" effects of drugs in the **warfarin** (Coumadin) family. Certain herbs, such as garlic, danshen, devil's claw, dong quai, papaya, PC-SPES, and red clover, may thin the blood in a manner somewhat similar to warfarin. Although no such interactions have yet been reported, it is at least theoretically possible that combined use of these herbs and fibrate drugs could pose a risk of bleeding problems.

Fluoroquinolones

Minerals—Take at a Different Time of Day
Fennel—Possible Harmful Interaction
St. John's Wort, Dong Quai—Possible Harmful Interaction

Drugs in the fluoroquinolone family are used for treating urinary tract infections as well as other infectious diseases.

Fluoroquinolone drugs include

➤ ciprofloxacin (Cipro),
➤ enoxacin (Penetrex),
➤ lomefloxacin (Maxaquin),
➤ norfloxacin (Noroxin),
➤ ofloxacin (Floxin),
➤ sparfloxacin (Zagam),
➤ levofloxacin (Levaquin),
➤ grepafloxacin (Raxar),
➤ trovafloxacin/alatrofloxacin (Trovan),
➤ and others.

Minerals

Take at a Different Time of Day
The minerals **calcium**, **iron**, **magnesium**, and **zinc** can interfere with the absorption of fluoroquinolones (and vice versa). Therefore, if you take supplements of these minerals, you should take them at least 2 hours before or after your fluoroquinolone dose.

Fennel

Possible Harmful Interaction
The herb fennel appears to reduce blood levels of ciprofloxacin, possibly impairing its effectiveness. This finding comes from a placebo-controlled study in rats. Fennel might be expected to interfere similarly with other fluoroquinolone antibiotics.

Allowing 2 hours between taking ciprofloxacin and fennel should reduce the potential for an interaction, but may not eliminate it. For this reason, it may be advisable to avoid fennel supplementation during therapy with ciprofloxacin or other antibiotics in this family.

Dong Quai, St. John's Wort

Possible Harmful Interaction
Fluoroquinolone antibiotics have been reported to cause increased sensitivity to the sun, amplifying the risk of sunburn or skin rash. Because **St. John's wort** and **dong quai** may also cause this problem, taking these herbal supplements during treatment with fluoroquinolone drugs might add to the risk.

It may be a good idea to wear a sunscreen or protective clothing during sun exposure if you take one of these herbs with a fluoroquinolone antibiotic.

H₂ Blockers

Vitamin B₁₂—Probable Need for Supplementation
Folate—Supplementation Possibly Helpful
Minerals—Supplementation Possibly Helpful
Magnesium—Take at a Different Time of Day
Vitamin D—Possible Inhibition by Cimetidine

Medications in this family sharply decrease stomach acid production. They are widely used for the treatment of ulcers as well as for mild cases of esophageal reflux (heartburn).

Drugs that fall into this family include

➤ cimetidine (Tagamet, Tagamet HB),
➤ famotidine (Pepcid, Pepcid AC, Pepcid RPD),
➤ nizatidine (Axid, Axid AR),
➤ ranitidine hydrochloride (Zantac, Zantac EFFER-dose, Zantac GELdose, Zantac 75),
➤ and others.

Vitamin B₁₂

Probable Need for Supplementation

H₂-receptor blockers appear to impair the absorption of **vitamin B₁₂** from food. This is thought to occur because the vitamin B₁₂ in food is attached to proteins. Stomach acid separates them and allows the B₁₂ to be absorbed.

The solution? If you regularly use H₂ blockers, take B₁₂ supplements. They can be absorbed easily because they are not attached to proteins.

Folate

Supplementation Possibly Helpful

There is some evidence that H₂ blockers may slightly reduce the absorption of **folate**. Folate is an important nutrient and one that is commonly deficient in the diet; so if you are taking H₂ blockers, you should probably take folate supplements, too.

Minerals

Supplementation Possibly Helpful

By reducing stomach acid levels, H₂ blockers might interfere with the absorption of **iron, zinc**, and perhaps other minerals. Taking mineral supplements that provide the U.S. Dietary Reference Intake (formerly known as the Recommended Dietary Allowance) of these substances should help.

Magnesium

Take at a Different Time of Day

Magnesium supplements may interfere with the absorption of H₂ blockers. However, the interference may be too minor to cause a real problem. If you think your magnesium supplements are interfering with your medication, you can get around the problem by taking these minerals at least 2 hours before or after you take an H₂-blocking medication.

Vitamin D

Possible Inhibition by Cimetidine

Cimetidine may interfere with **vitamin D** metabolism. Other H₂ blockers may not interact. Whether taking more vitamin D is useful remains unknown.

Heparin

Chondroitin—Possible Harmful Interaction

Garlic—Possible Harmful Interaction

Ginkgo—Possible Harmful Interaction

PC-SPES—Possible Harmful Interaction

Phosphatidylserine—Possible Harmful Interaction

Policosanol—Possible Harmful Interaction

Vitamin C—Possible Harmful Interaction

White Willow—Possible Harmful Interaction

Other Herbs and Supplements—Possible Harmful Interaction

Vitamin D—Supplementation Possibly Helpful

Heparin is a very strong blood-thinning drug that is delivered by injection. If you receive heparin, make sure you check with your doctor before taking any type of supplement.

Chondroitin

Possible Harmful Interaction

Based on **chondroitin's** chemical similarity to the anticoagulant drug heparin, it has been suggested that chondroitin might have anticoagulant effects as well. There are no case reports of any problems relating to this and studies suggest that chondroitin has at most a mild anticoagulant effect. Nonetheless, prudence suggests that chondroitin should not be combined with heparin except under physician supervision.

Garlic

Possible Harmful Interaction

The herb **garlic** (*Allium sativum*) is taken to lower cholesterol, among many other proposed uses.

Because garlic has a blood-thinning effect itself, it might be dangerous to combine garlic with heparin.

Two cases have been reported in which the combination of garlic and the blood-thinner warfarin doubled the time it took for blood to clot. Though warfarin thins the blood in a different way than heparin, there are concerns that garlic might interact similarly with heparin.

Ginkgo

Possible Harmful Interaction

The herb **ginkgo** (*Ginkgo biloba*) has been used to treat Alzheimer's disease and ordinary age-related memory loss, among many other conditions.

Ginkgo thins the blood by reducing the ability of blood-clotting cells called platelets to stick together. Because case reports have implicated use of *Ginkgo biloba* in the development of serious bleeding abnormalities, combining ginkgo with heparin might be expected to intensify the danger.

PC-SPES

Possible Harmful Interaction

PC-SPES is an herbal combination that has shown promise for the treatment of prostate cancer. One case report suggests that PC-SPES might increase risk of bleeding complications if combined with blood-thinning medications.

Phosphatidylserine

Possible Harmful Interaction

The supplement **phosphatidylserine** is promoted to treat Alzheimer's disease and ordinary age-related memory loss.

A test-tube study suggests that phosphatidylserine might amplify heparin's blood-thinning effects. If this effect were to occur inside the body, it could increase the risk of abnormal bleeding. If you receive heparin, make sure you check with your doctor before taking phosphatidylserine.

Policosanol

Possible Harmful Interaction

Policosanol, derived from sugarcane, has been taken for hyperlipidemia and intermittent claudication.

Human trials suggest that policosanol makes blood platelets more slippery, an action that could potentiate the blood-thinning effects of heparin, possibly causing a risk of abnormal bleeding episodes. A 30-day, double-blind, placebo-controlled trial of 27 individuals with high cholesterol levels found that policosanol at 10mg daily markedly reduced the ability of blood platelets to clump together. Another double-blind, placebo-controlled study of 37 healthy volunteers found evidence that the blood-thinning effect of policosanol increased as the dose was increased—the larger the policosanol dose, the greater the effect. Yet another double-blind, placebo-controlled study of 43 healthy volunteers compared the effects of policosanol (20mg daily), the blood-thinner aspirin (100mg daily), and policosanol and aspirin combined at these same doses. The results again showed that policosanol substantially reduced the ability of blood platelets to stick together and that the combined therapy exhibited additive effects.

Based on these findings, you should not combine heparin and policosanol except under medical supervision.

Vitamin C

Possible Harmful Interaction

Test-tube studies suggest that high amounts of **vitamin C** may reduce the blood-thinning effect of heparin. However, it is not clear whether the interaction is significant enough to make a practical difference.

White Willow

Possible Harmful Interaction

The herb **white willow** (*Salix alba*), also known as willow bark, is used to treat pain and fever. White willow

contains a substance that is converted by the body into a salicylate similar to aspirin.

Since combining aspirin with heparin increases the risk of abnormal bleeding, it would be advisable not to combine white willow with heparin.

Other Herbs and Supplements

Possible Harmful Interaction

Based on their known effects or constituents, the following herbs and supplements might not be safe to combine with heparin, though this has not been proven: **bromelain** (in the fruit and stem of pineapple, *Ananas comosus*), papaya (*Carica papaya*), **chamomile** (*Matricaria recutita*), ***Coleus forskohlii***, danshen (*Salvia miltorrhiza*), **devil's claw** (*Harpogophytum procumbens*), **dong quai** (*Angelica sinensis*), **feverfew** (*Tanacetum parthenium*), **ginger** (*Zingiber officinale*), **horse chestnut** (*Aesculus hippocastanum*), **red clover** (*Trifolium pratense*), **reishi** (*Ganoderma lucidum*), **mesoglycan**, **fish oil**, **OPCs** (oligomeric proanthocyanidins), and **vitamin E**.

Vitamin D

Supplementation Possibly Helpful

High doses or long-term use of heparin may interfere with the proper handling of **vitamin D** by the body; because vitamin D is needed for calcium absorption and utilization, this may in turn lead to bone loss and osteoporosis. Additionally, heparin may directly interfere with bone formation.

This interaction is of special concern during pregnancy, when there is a greater calcium demand and diminished levels of a hormone that pushes calcium into bones. In fact, there have been several reports of fractured and collapsed vertebrae in pregnant women on heparin therapy.

Supplementary calcium and vitamin D may help prevent heparin-induced osteoporosis. It might also be advisable to have your bone density checked during long-term heparin therapy.

Hydralazine

TRADE NAMES: *Apresoline*

Vitamin B$_6$—Supplementation Likely Helpful

Coenzyme Q$_{10}$ (CoQ$_{10}$)—Supplementation Possibly Helpful

Coleus forskohlii—Theoretical Interaction

Hydralazine causes dilation of the walls of blood vessels and is sometimes used to treat hypertension.

Vitamin B$_6$

Supplementation Likely Helpful

Hydralazine is known to deplete the blood of **vitamin B$_6$**. Taking B$_6$ supplements may prevent or reverse side effects of the medication.

Coenzyme Q$_{10}$ (CoQ$_{10}$)

Supplementation Possibly Helpful

There is some evidence that hydralazine might impair the body's ability to manufacture the substance coenzyme Q$_{10}$ (CoQ$_{10}$). This suggests (but definitely does not prove) that taking CoQ$_{10}$ supplements may produce a beneficial effect.

Coleus forskohlii

Theoretical Interaction

The herb *Coleus forskohlii* relaxes blood vessels and might have unpredictable effects if combined with hydralazine.

Hydrochlorothiazide/Benazepril

TRADE NAMES: *Lotensin HCT*

This medication is a combination of the following drugs:

➤ ACE Inhibitors (Angiotensin-Converting Enzyme Inhibitors)
➤ Thiazide Diuretics

Please see the separate articles on each one to find out about potential drug interactions. The interactions for each may be different, so read both articles carefully to find out the whole story.

Hydrochlorothiazide/Bisoprolol

TRADE NAMES: *Ziac*

This medication is a combination of the following drugs:

➤ Beta-Blockers
➤ Thiazide Diuretics

Please see the separate articles on each one to find out about potential drug interactions. The interactions for each may be different, so read both articles carefully to find out the whole story.

Hydrochlorothiazide/Captopril

TRADE NAMES: *Capozide*

This medication is a combination of the following drugs:

➤ ACE Inhibitors (Angiotensin-Converting Enzyme Inhibitors)
➤ Thiazide Diuretics

Please see the separate articles on each one to find out about potential drug interactions. The interactions for each may be different, so read both articles carefully to find out the whole story.

Hydrochlorothiazide/Enalapril

TRADE NAMES: *Vaseretic*

This medication is a combination of the following drugs:

➤ Angiotensin-Converting Enzyme Inhibitors
➤ Thiazide Diuretics

Please see the separate articles on each one to find out about potential drug interactions. The interactions for each may be different, so read both articles carefully to find out the whole story.

Hydrochlorothiazide/Hydralazine

TRADE NAMES: *Apresazide*

This medication is a combination of the following drugs:

➤ Hydralazine
➤ Thiazide Diuretics

Please see the separate articles on each one to find out about potential drug interactions. The interactions for each may be different, so read both articles carefully to find out the whole story.

Hydrochlorothiazide/Lisinopril

TRADE NAMES: *Prinzide, Zestoretic*

This medication is a combination of the following drugs:

➤ ACE Inhibitors (Angiotensin-Converting Enzyme Inhibitors)
➤ Thiazide Diuretics

Please see the separate articles on each one to find out about potential drug interactions. The interactions for each may be different, so read both articles carefully to find out the whole story.

Hydrochlorothiazide/Methyldopa

TRADE NAMES: *Aldoril*

This medication is a combination of the following drugs:

➤ Methyldopa
➤ Thiazide Diuretics

Please see the separate articles on each one to find out about potential drug interactions. The interactions for each may be different, so read both articles carefully to find out the whole story.

Hydrochlorothiazide/Metoprolol

TRADE NAMES: *Lopressor HCT*

This medication is a combination of the following drugs:

➤ Beta-Blockers
➤ Thiazide Diuretics

Please see the separate articles on each one to find out about potential drug interactions. The interactions for each may be different, so read both articles carefully to find out the whole story.

Hydrochlorothiazide/Moexipril

TRADE NAMES: *Uniretic*

This medication is a combination of the following drugs:

➤ ACE Inhibitors (Angiotensin-Converting Enzyme Inhibitors)
➤ Thiazide Diuretics

Please see the separate articles on each one to find out about potential drug interactions. The interactions for each may be different, so read both articles carefully to find out the whole story.

Hydrochlorothiazide/Propranolol

TRADE NAMES: *Inderide*

This medication is a combination of the following drugs:

➤ Beta-Blockers
➤ Thiazide Diuretics

Please see the separate articles on each one to find out about potential drug interactions. The interactions for each may be different, so read both articles carefully to find out the whole story.

Hydrochlorothiazide/Timolol

TRADE NAMES: *Timolide*

This medication is a combination of the following drugs:

➤ Beta-Blockers
➤ Thiazide Diuretics

Please see the separate articles on each one to find out about potential drug interactions. The interactions for each may be different, so read both articles carefully to find out the whole story.

Influenza Vaccine

TRADE NAMES: *FluShield, Fluvirin, Fluzone*
Ginseng—May Increase Effectiveness of Vaccine

The influenza vaccine, while not perfect, significantly decreases the risk of catching the annual flu epidemic. It may also lead to less severe symptoms if influenza does develop.

Ginseng

May Increase Effectiveness of Vaccine

A double-blind study of 227 individuals found that **ginseng** might help the vaccine work more effectively, increasing antibody production and decreasing the frequency of colds and flus. The dose used in the study was 100 mg of Asian ginseng (*Panax ginseng*) taken twice daily for 1 month prior and 2 months after the vaccine was administered.

Insulin

TRADE NAMES: *Humalog, Humulin, Iletin, Novolin, Velosulin*
Herbs and Supplements—Might Require Reduced Insulin Dosage

Insulin injections are used to regulate blood sugar in people with childhood-onset diabetes as well as those with severe adult-onset diabetes.

Herbs and Supplements

Might Require Reduced Insulin Dosage

Meaningful preliminary evidence suggests that use of the following herbs and supplements could potentially improve blood sugar control and require you to reduce your insulin dosage: **aloe, chromium, fenugreek, ginseng, gymnema, coenzyme Q**$_{10}$, and **vanadium**.

Weaker evidence suggests that the following herbs and supplements could potentially have the same effect under certain circumstances: *Anemarrhena asphodeloides,* **arginine,** *Azadirachta indica* (**neem**), bilberry leaf, **biotin, bitter melon, carnitine,** *Catharanthus roseus, Coccinia indica,* **coenzyme Q**$_{10}$, **conjugated linoleic acid (CLA),** *Cucumis sativus,* *Cucurbita ficifolia, Cuminum cyminum* (cumin), *Euphorbia prostrata,* **garlic, glucomannan,** *Guaiacum coulteri, Guazuma ulmifolia,* **guggul,** holy basil, *Lepechinia caulescens,* **lipoic acid,** *Medicago sativa* (**alfalfa**), *Musa sapientum* L. (banana), niacinamide, nopal cactus, onion, *Phaseolus vulgaris, Psacalium peltatum,* pterocarpus, *Rhizophora mangle,* **salt bush,** *Spinacea oleracea, Tournefortia hirsutissima, Turnera diffusa,* and **vitamin E.**

Isoniazid

ALTERNATE NAMES: *INH*

TRADE NAMES: *Laniazid, Nydrazid*

Vitamin B$_6$—Supplementation Likely Helpful

Vitamin B$_3$—Supplementation Possibly Helpful

Vitamin D—Supplementation Possibly Helpful

See also *Antibiotics (General).*

Used for the treatment of tuberculosis, isoniazid can interfere with the absorption or metabolism of numerous nutrients. Since this antibiotic is commonly taken for a very long period of time, deficiencies can mount up over the course of treatment, impairing overall health.

Vitamin B$_6$

Supplementation Likely Helpful

Individuals who take isoniazid may develop nerve problems such as tingling or numbness in the arms, hands, legs, and feet. The cause is believed to be the drug's interference with the action of **vitamin B$_6$**. In fact, use of isoniazid is one cause of the few occasions in which vitamin B$_6$ deficiency is seen in the developed world.

To prevent these complications, it may make sense to take vitamin B$_6$ supplements at a dose of 15 to 30 mg per day when using isoniazid.

Vitamin B$_3$

Supplementation Possibly Helpful

According to animal studies, isoniazid can interfere with the body's ability to produce **vitamin B$_3$** (niacin) by blocking a key enzyme. This can produce either a subtle or an all-out niacin deficiency (known as *pellagra*). Taking niacin supplements at standard U.S. Dietary Reference Intake (formerly known as the Recommended Dietary Allowance) doses should help you get the niacin you need.

Vitamin D

Supplementation Possibly Helpful

Isoniazid may interfere with the body's ability to use **vitamin D**.

Although it is not clear whether this actually causes symptoms of vitamin D deficiency, it still might be a good idea to take vitamin D supplements at standard U.S. Adequate Intake (AI) dosages.

Isoniazid/Rifampin

TRADE NAMES: *Rifamate*

This medication is a combination of the following drugs:

➤ Isoniazid
➤ Rifampin

Please see the separate articles on each one to find out about potential drug interactions. The interactions for each may be different, so read both articles carefully to find out the whole story.

Isoniazid/Rifampin/Pyrazinamide

TRADE NAMES: *Rifater, Rimactane/INH Dual Pack*

This medication is a combination of the following drugs:

➤ Isoniazid
➤ Rifampin

Please see the separate articles on each one to find out about potential drug interactions. The interactions for each may be different, so read both articles carefully to find out the whole story.

Isotretinoin

TRADE NAMES: *Accutane*

Vitamin A—Probable Dangerous Interaction
St. John's Wort, Dong Quai—Possible Harmful Interaction

Chemically related to vitamin A, isotretinoin is used for the treatment of acne and other skin conditions.

Vitamin A

Probable Dangerous Interaction

Do not combine **vitamin A** and isotretinoin, as they might increase each other's toxicity.

Dong Quai, St. John's Wort

Possible Harmful Interaction

Isotretinoin has been reported to cause increased sensitivity to the sun, amplifying the risk of sunburn or skin rash.

Because **St. John's wort** and **dong quai** may also cause this problem, taking these herbal supplements during isotretinoin therapy might add to this risk.

It may be a good idea to wear a sunscreen or protective clothing during sun exposure if you take one of these herbs while using isotretinoin.

Levodopa/Carbidopa

TRADE NAMES: *Sinemet*

5-Hydroxytryptophan (5-HTP)—Possible Harmful Interaction

BCAAs—Possible Harmful Interaction

Iron—Take at a Different Time of Day

Kava—Possible Harmful Interaction

Vitamin B$_6$—Possible Reduced Action of Drug

Policosanol—Possible Benefits and Risks

S-Adenosylmethionine (SAMe)—Possible Benefits and Risks

Carbidopa in combination with levodopa is used in treating Parkinson's disease. This disease is associated with a deficit of dopamine, a neurotransmitter (a chemical messenger in the brain). By preventing the breakdown of levodopa in the general circulation, carbidopa enables more levodopa to enter the brain, where it is converted into dopamine.

5-Hydroxytryptophan (5-HTP)

Possible Harmful Interaction

The body uses the natural substance **5-hydroxytryptophan** (5-HTP) to manufacture serotonin, and supplemental forms of 5-HTP have been used for treating depression and migraine headaches. Since it is converted by the body to serotonin, 5-HTP might have antidepressant properties. For this reason, some people with Parkinson's-related depression have tried it.

However, the combination of 5-HTP and carbidopa might cause a scleroderma-like condition in which the skin becomes hard and tight. Because of the risk of this side effect, if you take levodopa/carbidopa for Parkinson's disease, avoid supplemental 5-HTP.

BCAAs

Possible Harmful Interaction

Branched-chain amino acids (BCAAs) in supplement form have been used to improve appetite in cancer patients and to slow the progression of amyotrophic lateral sclerosis (ALS, or Lou Gehrig's disease).

Dietary protein can decrease the effectiveness of levodopa in Parkinson's disease. Because it is the amino acids in proteins that affect levodopa, BCAAs might cause the same problem. Therefore, if you take levodopa/carbi-

dopa for Parkinson's, it may be advisable to avoid BCAAs and other amino acid supplements.

Iron

Take at a Different Time of Day

Iron appears to interfere with the absorption of both levodopa and carbidopa by binding to them. Studies have found that blood levels of levodopa and carbidopa are reduced 30 to 51% and 75%, respectively, by iron supplementation, resulting in a worsening of symptoms of Parkinson's disease. Based on this finding, you should separate the times you take iron and these drugs by as long as possible.

Kava

Possible Harmful Interaction

The herb **kava** (*Piper methysticum*) has a sedative effect and is used for anxiety and insomnia.

A few case reports suggest that kava might interfere with the action of dopamine in the body. This could at least partially neutralize the therapeutic effects of levodopa. In one individual, parkinsonism symptoms got worse following supplementation with kava extract (150 mg twice daily for 10 days).

Based on these reports, it may be advisable to avoid kava during levodopa/carbidopa therapy.

Vitamin B$_6$

Possible Reduced Action of Drug

If you are taking levodopa alone, you shouldn't take more than 5 mg per day of **vitamin B$_6$** or it might impair the effectiveness of the drug. But if you use levodopa/

carbidopa combinations that provide a total daily dose of at least 75 mg of carbidopa, this issue is not a concern.

Policosanol

Possible Benefits and Risks

Policosanol may increase both the effects and side effects of levodopa.

S-Adenosylmethionine (SAMe)

Possible Benefits and Risks

S-adenosylmethionine (SAMe) is a naturally occurring compound derived from the amino acid methionine and the energy molecule adenosine triphosphate (ATP).

SAMe is widely used as a supplement for treatment of osteoarthritis and depression.

Preliminary evidence suggests that levodopa might deplete levels of SAMe in the body. This suggests (but definitely does not prove) that individuals taking levodopa/carbidopa might benefit from SAMe supplements.

One short-term (30-day), double-blind study suggests that such combination treatment is safe and might help depression related to Parkinson's disease. However, there are also concerns that SAMe could cause levodopa to be less effective over time.

The bottom line: If you are taking levodopa/carbidopa, consult your physician about whether you should take SAMe as well.

Lithium

TRADE NAMES: *Eskalith, Eskalith CR, Lithane, Lithobid, Lithonate, Lithotabs*
Inositol—Possible Helpful Interaction
Herbal Diuretic—Possible Harmful Interaction
Citrate—Possible Harmful Interaction

Lithium is a medication used to treat bipolar disorder (manic-depressive illness). While it is quite effective, use of lithium creates some risks, especially related to dehydration.

Inositol

Possible Helpful Interaction

Lithium may cause or exacerbate symptoms of psoriasis. One very small, double-blind study found that use of supplemental inositol may help alleviate this problem. For more information, including dosage and safety issues, see the full **Inositol** article.

Herbal Diuretic

Possible Harmful Interaction

The use of lithium as a therapy requires careful attention to lithium levels in the blood. If there's too little lithium, the treatment won't work; if lithium levels get too high, toxicity may result.

One cause of excessively high lithium levels is dehydration. When the amount of water in the blood decreases, lithium levels proportionally rise, just as the Great Salt Lake becomes saltier as its water evaporates. For this reason, individuals taking lithium are warned that they must make sure to drink sufficient liquids when they are exposed to heat. Diuretic drugs ("water pills") can also cause problems, by causing the body to excrete water.

A recent case report suggests that herbal diuretics can also lead to increased lithium levels. Certain herbs are thought to act as diuretics, including **buchu**, celery seed, **cleavers**, corn silk, couchgrass, **dandelion**, **goldenrod**, gravel root, **horsetail**, **juniper**, **parsley**, **rosemary**, and wild carrot.

This report noted the case of a 26-year-old woman who had been taking a constant dose of lithium for 5 months without any problems. When she suddenly developed drowsiness, tremor, unsteadiness in walking, and rapid involuntary movements of the eyes, doctors conducted a laboratory examination and found that her lithium level had skyrocketed. It turned out that a few weeks before this episode she had started taking an herbal weight-loss formula that included numerous herbal diuretics.

Manufacturers frequently add herbal diuretics to weight-loss formulas in order to cause short-term loss of water weight. This has no value for long-term weight loss, but it does cause some immediate sense of success. However, in this case, the herbal diuretics also caused lithium levels to rise.

The bottom line: If you are taking lithium, avoid herbal diuretics.

Citrate

Possible Harmful Interaction

Potassium citrate, sodium citrate, and potassium-magnesium citrate are sometimes used to prevent kidney stones. These supplements reduce urinary acidity and can therefore lead to decreased blood levels and effectiveness of lithium.

Loop Diuretics

Potassium—Probable Need for Supplementation

Magnesium—Probable Need for Supplementation

Vitamin B$_1$—Probable Need for Supplementation

Licorice—Possible Dangerous Interaction

St. John's Wort, Dong Quai—Possible Harmful Interaction

These powerful diuretics are used to reduce fluid accumulation in the body. Drugs in this family include

➤ bumetanide (Bumex),
➤ ethacrynic acid (Edecrin),
➤ furosemide (Lasix),
➤ and torsemide (Demadex).

Potassium

Probable Need for Supplementation

Loop diuretics cause a constant and significant loss of potassium. The classic treatment for this is to eat bananas and drink orange juice. Potassium supplements are also frequently prescribed.

Magnesium

Probable Need for Supplementation

Long-term use (more than 6 months) of loop diuretics might lead to **magnesium** deficiency. In turn, magnesium depletion can increase loss of potassium.

Since magnesium deficiency is common anyway, taking a magnesium supplement at standard U.S. Di-

etary Reference Intake (formerly known as the Recommended Dietary Allowance) levels might make sense.

Vitamin B$_1$

Probable Need for Supplementation

Evidence suggests that loop diuretics interfere with the body's metabolism of **vitamin B$_1$** (thiamin).

This effect may cause adverse consequences in one group of individuals who commonly take loop diuretics: people with heart failure. The heart depends on B$_1$ for proper function; therefore, this finding suggests that taking a B$_1$ supplement may be advisable. In fact, preliminary evidence suggests that thiamin supplementation does indeed improve heart function in individuals with congestive heart failure (CHF).

Licorice

Possible Dangerous Interaction

Licorice, too, affects potassium, and the combination of licorice and loop diuretics might cause unexpectedly rapid potassium loss. However, the special form of licorice known as DGL (deglycyrrhizinated licorice) should not affect potassium levels.

Dong Quai, St. John's Wort

Possible Harmful Interaction

Loop diuretics have been reported to cause increased sensitivity to the sun, amplifying the risk of sunburn or skin rash. Because **St. John's wort** and **dong quai** may also cause this problem, taking these herbal supplements during treatment with loop diuretics might add to this risk.

It may be a good idea to wear a sunscreen or protective clothing during sun exposure if you take one of these herbs while using a loop diuretic.

Methotrexate

ALTERNATE NAMES: *Amethopterin, MTX*
TRADE NAMES: *Immunex, Folex PFS, Rheumatrex*
Potassium Citrate—Possible Harmful Interaction
St. John's Wort, Dong Quai—Possible Harmful Interaction
White Willow—Possible Harmful Interaction
Ipriflavone—Possible Harmful Interaction
Citrate—Possible Harmful Interaction
Folate—Supplementation Possibly Helpful

Methotrexate is used in cancer chemotherapy as well as for treating inflammatory diseases, such as rheumatoid arthritis and psoriasis.

Potassium Citrate

Possible Harmful Interaction

Potassium citrate and other forms of citrate (for example, calcium citrate, magnesium citrate) may be used to prevent kidney stones. These agents work by making the urine less acidic.

This effect on the urine may lead to decreased blood levels and therapeutic effects of methotrexate.

It may be advisable to avoid these citrate compounds during methotrexate therapy except under medical supervision.

Dong Quai, St. John's Wort

Possible Harmful Interaction

St. John's wort (*Hypericum perforatum*) is primarily used to treat mild to moderate depression.

The herb **dong quai** (*Angelica sinensis*) is often recommended for menstrual disorders such as dysmenorrhea, PMS, and irregular menstruation.

Methotrexate has been reported to cause increased sensitivity to the sun, amplifying the risk of sunburn or skin rash. Because St. John's wort and dong quai may also cause this problem, taking these herbal supplements during methotrexate therapy might add to this risk.

It may be a good idea to wear a sunscreen or protective clothing during sun exposure if you take one of these herbs while using methotrexate.

White Willow

Possible Harmful Interaction

The herb **white willow** (*Salix alba*), also known as willow bark, is used to treat pain and fever. White willow contains a substance that is converted by the body into a salicylate similar to aspirin.

Case reports suggest that salicylates can increase methotrexate blood levels and toxicity. For this reason, you should avoid combining white willow with methotrexate.

Ipriflavone

Possible Harmful Interaction

The supplement **ipriflavone** is used to treat osteoporosis. A 3-year, double-blind trial of almost 500 women, as well as a small study, found worrisome evidence that ipriflavone can reduce white blood cell count in some people. For this reason, anyone taking medications that suppress the immune system should avoid taking ipriflavone.

Citrate

Possible Harmful Interaction

Potassium citrate, sodium citrate, and potassium-magnesium citrate are sometimes used to prevent kidney stones. These supplements reduce urinary acidity and can therefore lead to decreased blood levels and effectiveness of methotrexate.

Folate

Supplementation Possibly Helpful

Folate (also known as folic acid) is a B vitamin that plays an important role in many vital aspects of health, including preventing neural tube birth defects and possibly reducing the risk of heart disease. Because inadequate intake of folate is widespread, if you are taking any medication that depletes or impairs folate even slightly, you may need supplementation.

Methotrexate is called a "folate antagonist" because it prevents the body from converting folate to its active form. In fact, this inactivation of folate plays a role in methotrexate's therapeutic effects. This leads to an interesting Catch-22: methotrexate use can lead to folate deficiency, but taking extra folate could theoretically prevent methotrexate from working properly.

However, evidence suggests that individuals who take methotrexate for rheumatoid arthritis, juvenile rheumatoid arthritis, or psoriasis can safely use folate supplements. Not only does the methotrexate continue to work properly, but its usual side effects may decrease also.

For example, in a 48-week, double-blind, placebo-controlled trial of 434 individuals with active rheumatoid arthritis, use of folate helped prevent liver inflammation caused by methotrexate. Other side effects did not improve. A slightly higher dose of methotrexate was needed to reach the same level of benefit as taking methotrexate alone, but researchers felt this was worth it.

In the study just described, folate supplements did not help reduce the incidence of mouth sores and nausea. However, in other studies folate supplements did reduce these side effects, both in individuals receiving methotrexate for rheumatoid arthritis and in those with psoriasis.

In addition, two studies of individuals with rheumatoid arthritis found that use of folate supplements corrected the methotrexate-induced rise in homocysteine without affecting disease control.

Note: Folate supplements have only been found safe as supportive treatment in the specific conditions noted above. It is not known, for example, whether folate supplements are safe for use by individuals taking methotrexate for cancer treatment.

Methyldopa

TRADE NAMES: *Aldomet*

Coenzyme Q$_{10}$ (CoQ$_{10}$)—Supplementation Possibly Helpful
Iron—Take at a Different Time of Day

Methyldopa is a medication that is sometimes used to control hypertension; however, it is not a first-line treatment due to the various health risks associated with its use.

Coenzyme Q$_{10}$ (CoQ$_{10}$)

Supplementation Possibly Helpful

There is some evidence that methyldopa might impair the body's ability to manufacture the substance **coenzyme** Q$_{10}$ (CoQ$_{10}$). Taking CoQ$_{10}$ supplements might make sense as a general precaution, but no specific benefit has been established.

Iron

Take at a Different Time of Day

Iron supplements can interfere with the absorption of methyldopa, so make sure you do not take iron during the 2 hours before or after your methyldopa dose.

Monoamine Oxidase Inhibitors

Ephedra—Dangerous Interaction

Scotch Broom—Dangerous Interaction

Green Tea—Probable Dangerous Interaction

Ginseng—Possible Dangerous Interaction

St. John's Wort—Possible Dangerous Interaction

S-Adenosylmethionine (SAMe), 5-Hydroxytryptophan (5-HTP)—Possible Dangerous Interactions

Monoamine oxidase inhibitors (MAO inhibitors) were the first antidepressant drugs invented. While they are quite effective, they can be dangerous if combined with the wrong foods, drugs, or supplements. The substance tyramine, found in some cheeses, beer, fermented soy products, and other foods, is particularly dangerous to combine with these medications. Stimulant drugs such as pseudoephedrine can also cause problems.

Antidepressants in this family include

➤ furazolidone (Furoxone),
➤ isocarboxazid (Marplan),
➤ phenelzine sulfate (Nardil),
➤ and tranylcypromine sulfate (Parnate).

Ephedra

Dangerous Interaction

Because it contains the stimulant ephedrine, combining the herb **ephedra** with MAO inhibitors can rapidly produce a severe, dangerous interaction and must be avoided.

Scotch Broom

Dangerous Interaction

The herb scotch broom contains high levels of tyramine, so it should not be taken with MAO inhibitors.

Green Tea

Probable Dangerous Interaction

Because it contains caffeine, **green tea** should not be combined with MAO inhibitors.

Ginseng

Possible Dangerous Interaction

According to one report, the combination of **ginseng** and the MAO inhibitor phenelzine caused worrisome symptoms. While this may have been due to caffeine contamination of the ginseng, we would recommend that you avoid ginseng–MAO inhibitor combinations at this time.

St. John's Wort

Possible Dangerous Interaction

Current thinking suggests that **St. John's wort** functions somewhat similarly to SSRI (selective serotonin-reuptake inhibitor) antidepressants. Since SSRIs should not be combined with MAO inhibitors, this herb probably should not be combined either.

S-Adenosylmethionine (SAMe), 5-Hydroxytryptophan (5-HTP)

Possible Dangerous Interactions

Based on one case report and current thinking on how they work, **SAMe** and **5-HTP** should not be combined with MAO inhibitors.

Nitrofurantoin

TRADE NAMES: *Furadantin, Macrobid, Macrodantin*
Magnesium—Take at a Different Time of Day
See also *Antibiotics (General)*.

Nitrofurantoin is sometimes taken on an ongoing basis to prevent bladder infections.

Magnesium

Take at a Different Time of Day

Magnesium supplements might impair the absorption of nitrofurantoin, so do not take magnesium during the 2 hours before or after your nitrofurantoin dose.

Nitroglycerin

TRADE NAMES: *Deponit, Minitran, Nitrek, Nitro-Bid, Nitro-Derm, Nitro-Dur, Nitro-Time, Nitrocine,*
Nitrodisc, Nitrogard, Nitroglyn, Nitrol, Nitrolingual, Nitrong, NitroQuick, Nitrostat, Transderm-Nitro
N-Acetyl Cysteine (NAC)—Possible Benefits and Risks
Vitamin C—Supplementation Possibly Helpful
Arginine—Supplementation Possibly Helpful
Folate—Supplementation Possibly Helpful
Vitamin E—Supplementation Possibly Helpful

Nitroglycerin (NTG) is one of the most commonly used treatments for quick relief of anginal pain. Related drugs include isosorbide dinitrate and isosorbide mononitrate.

N-Acetyl Cysteine (NAC)

Possible Benefits and Risks

N-acetyl cysteine (NAC) is a specially modified form of the dietary amino acid cysteine that has various proposed uses.

Nitrates such as nitroglycerin lose some of their effectiveness over time. According to some studies, but not all, the supplement N-acetyl cysteine might help these drugs work better. However, there's a catch: the combination of NAC and nitroglycerin appears to cause severe headaches.

Taking NAC with nitroglycerin may be beneficial in some cases. However, unpleasant side effects probably limit the use of this combination.

Note: Angina is too serious a disease for self-treatment. If you have angina, do not take any supplement except on a physician's advice.

Vitamin C

Supplementation Possibly Helpful

Vitamin C may help prevent the development of tolerance to nitrate medications, such as nitroglycerin. According to a double-blind study of 48 individuals, use of vitamin C at a dose of 2,000 mg 3 times daily helped maintain the effectiveness of nitroglycerin. These findings are supported by other studies as well.

Note: Angina is too serious a disease for self-treatment. If you have angina, do not take any supplement except on a physician's advice.

Arginine

Supplementation Possibly Helpful

According to a small, double-blind, placebo-controlled crossover study, use of **arginine** (700 mg 4 times daily) may help prevent tolerance to nitrate medications.

Note: Angina is too serious a disease for self-treatment. If you have angina, do not take any supplement except on physician's advice.

Folate

Supplementation Possibly Helpful

A small, double-blind trial suggests that **folate** supplements (at the high dose of 10 mg daily) may help prevent tolerance to nitrate medications.

Note: Angina is too serious a disease for self-treatment. If you have angina, do not take any supplement except on a physician's advice.

Vitamin E

Supplementation Possibly Helpful

A small, double-blind trial suggests that **vitamin E** at a dose of 200 mg 3 times daily may help prevent tolerance to nitrate medications.

Note: Angina is too serious a disease for self-treatment. If you have angina, do not take any supplement except on a physician's advice.

Nitrous Oxide

Folate, Vitamin B_{12}—Supplementation Possibly Helpful

Nitrous oxide gas is used primarily as a local anesthetic in dentistry as well as in certain phases of cardiac bypass surgery.

Folate, Vitamin B_{12}

Supplementation Possibly Helpful

Nitrous oxide can occasionally cause significant **vitamin B_{12}** deficiency, especially in people who are already borderline deficient in the vitamin (total vegetarians, for example) or those who are frequently exposed to the gas, such as dentists and anesthesiologists.

The effect on B_{12} impacts **folate**, too.

Taking folate and B_{12} supplements at the U.S. Dietary Reference Intake (formerly known as the Recommended Dietary Allowance) levels should prevent any problems from developing.

Nonsteroidal Anti-Inflammatory Drugs

Arginine—Possible Harmful Interaction

Feverfew—Possible Harmful Interaction

Garlic, Ginkgo—Possible Harmful Interaction

Policosanol (sugarcane source)—Possible Harmful Interaction

PC-SPES—Possible Harmful Interaction

Potassium Citrate—Possible Harmful Interaction

Reishi—Possible Harmful Interaction

Dong Quai, St. John's Wort—Possible Harmful Interaction

Vinpocetine—Possible Harmful Interaction

Vitamin E—Possible Mixed Interaction

White Willow—Possible Harmful Interaction

Herbs and Supplements—Possible Harmful Interaction

Citrate—Possible Harmful Interaction

Cayenne—Supplementation Possibly Helpful

Colostrum—Supplementation Possibly Helpful

Folate—Supplementation Possibly Helpful

Licorice—Supplementation Possibly Helpful

Vitamin C—Supplementation Possibly Helpful

Policosanol (beeswax form)—Possible Helpful Interaction

Chondroitin—Possible Harmful Interaction

Nonsteroidal anti-inflammatory drugs (NSAIDs) are used to treat pain, fever, and inflammation. Traditional NSAIDs block COX-1 and COX-2 enzymes that the body uses to manufacture substances called prostaglandins. Since COX-1 prostaglandins are stomach-protective, blocking this enzyme is associated with gastrointestinal toxicity, a known side effect of these drugs. Newer NSAIDs (called COX-2 inhibitors) block primarily COX-2 prostaglandins associated with pain, fever, and inflammation, and might be are less risky to the stomach. However, this is not proven, and some COX-2s have been taken off the market due to excess risk of heart attacks attributable to their use. Drugs in this family include

➤ aspirin, alternatively called acetylsalicylic acid or ASA (Adprin-B, Anacin, Arthritis Foundation Aspirin, Ascriptin, Aspergum, Asprimox, Bayer, BC, Bufferin, Buffex, Cama, Cope, Easprin, Ecotrin, Empirin, Equagesic, Fiorinal, Fiorital, Halfprin, Heartline, Genprin, Lanorinal, Magnaprin, Measurin, Micrainin, Momentum, Norwich, St. Joseph, ZORprin),

➤ bromfenac sodium (Duract),

➤ celecoxib (Celebrex),

➤ choline salicylate (Arthropan),

➤ choline salicylate/magnesium salicylate (Tricosal, Trilisate),

➤ diclofenac potassium (Cataflam, Voltaren Rapide),

➤ diclofenac sodium (Arthrotec, Voltaren, Voltaren SR, Voltaren-XR),

➤ diclofenac sodium/misoprostol (Arthrotec),

➤ diflunisal (Dolobid),

➤ etodolac (Lodine, Lodine XL),

➤ fenoprofen calcium (Nalfon),

➤ flurbiprofen (Ansaid),

➤ ibuprofen (Advil, Arthritis Foundation Ibuprofen, Bayer Select Ibuprofen, Dynafed IB, Genpril, Haltran, IBU, Ibuprin, Ibuprohm, Menadol, Midol IB, Motrin, Nuprin, Saleto),

➤ indomethacin (Indochron E-R, Indocin, Indocin SR, Indomethacin, Indomethacin SR, Novo-Methacin),

➤ ketoprofen (Actron, Orudis, Orudis KT, Oruvail),

➤ ketorolac tromethamine (Toradol),

➤ magnesium salicylate (Doan's, Magan, Mobidin, Backache Maximum Strength Relief, Bayer Select Maximum Strength Backache, Momentum Muscular Backache Formula, Nuprin Backache, Mobigesic, Magsal),

➤ meclofenamate sodium (Mecolfen, Meclomen),

➤ mefenamic acid (Ponstan, Ponstel),

➤ nabumetone (Relafen),

➤ naproxen (EC-Naprosyn, Napron X, Naprosyn),

➤ naproxen sodium (Aleve, Anaprox, Anaprox DS, Naprelan),

➤ oxaprozin (Daypro),

➤ piroxicam (Feldene),

➤ salsalate or salicylic acid (Amigesic, Argesic-SA, Arthra-G, Disalcid, Marthritic, Mono-Gesic, Salflex, Salgesic, Salsitab),

➤ sodium salicylate (Pabalate),

➤ sodium thiosalicylate (Rexolate),

➤ sulfasalazine (Azulfidine EN-tabs, Salazopyrin, SAS-500),

➤ sulindac (Clinoril),

➤ tolmetin sodium (Tolectin, Tolectin DS),

➤ and others.

Note: Besides reducing pain and inflammation, aspirin (and to a lesser extent, other NSAIDs) interfere with cells in the blood called platelets which facilitate clotting.

Arginine

Possible Harmful Interaction

Arginine is an amino acid found in many foods, including dairy products, meat, poultry, and fish. Supplemental arginine has been proposed as a treatment for various conditions, including heart problems.

Arginine has been found to stimulate the body's production of gastrin, a hormone that increases stomach acid. Because excessive acid can irritate the stomach, there are concerns that arginine could be harmful for individuals taking drugs that are also hard on the stomach (such as NSAIDs).

It may be best not to mix arginine with NSAIDs unless approved by your doctor.

Feverfew

Possible Harmful Interaction

The herb **feverfew** (*Tanacetum parthenium*) is primarily used for the prevention and treatment of migraine headaches.

NSAIDs are also used for migraines, so there is a chance that some individuals might use both the herb and drug at once, a combination that may present risks.

The biggest concern with NSAIDs is that they can cause stomach ulcers, which may progress to bleeding or perforation without pain or other warning symptoms. This stomach damage is due to drug interference with the body's protective prostaglandins. Newer NSAIDs called COX-2 inhibitors may be less likely to produce this side effect.

Feverfew also affects prostaglandins. Thus, combining it with an NSAID might increase the risk of stomach problems.

Garlic, Ginkgo

Possible Harmful Interaction

The herb **garlic** (*Allium sativum*) is taken to lower cholesterol, among many other proposed uses.

One of the possible side effects of garlic is a decreased ability of the blood to clot, leading to an increased bleeding tendency. Therefore, you should not combine garlic and aspirin or other NSAIDs except under medical supervision.

The herb **ginkgo** is used to treat Alzheimer's disease and ordinary age-related memory loss, among many other uses.

Some evidence suggests that ginkgo might also decrease the ability of the blood to clot, probably through effects on platelets. However, one double-blind study found that ginkgo does *not* increase the anticoagulant effects of aspirin. While this is reassuring, prudence still suggests that one should not take ginkgo while using aspirin or other NSAIDs except under medical supervision.

Policosanol (sugarcane source)

Possible Harmful Interaction

A sugarcane-derived form of the supplement **policosanal** is used to reduce cholesterol levels. It also interferes with platelet clumping, creating potential benefit as well as a risk of interactions with blood-thinning drugs.

For example, a 30-day, double-blind, placebo-controlled trial of 27 individuals with high cholesterol levels found that policosanol at 10 mg daily markedly reduced the ability of blood platelets to clump together. Another double-blind, placebo-controlled study of 37 healthy volunteers found evidence that the blood-thinning effect of policosanol increased as the dose was increased—the larger the policosanol dose, the greater the effect. Yet another double-blind, placebo-controlled study of 43 healthy volunteers compared the effects of policosanol (20 mg daily), aspirin (100 mg daily), and policosanol and aspirin combined at these same doses. The results again showed that policosanol substantially reduced the ability of blood platelets to stick together, and that the combined therapy exhibited additive effects.

Based on these findings, it would be advisable to avoid combining aspirin or other NSAIDs with sugarcane policosanol except under medical supervision. **Note:** Beeswax policosanol is substantially different from sugarcane policosanol, and is described separately below.

PC-SPES

Possible Harmful Interaction

PC-SPES is an herbal combination that has shown promise for the treatment of prostate cancer. One case report suggests that PC-SPES might increase risk of bleeding complications if combined with blood-thinning medications. Subsequent evidence has indicated that PC-SPES contains the strong prescription blood thinner warfarin, making this interaction inevitable.

Potassium Citrate

Possible Harmful Interaction

Potassium citrate and other forms of citrate (for example, calcium citrate, magnesium citrate) may be used to prevent kidney stones. These agents work by making the urine less acidic.

This effect on the urine may lead to decreased blood levels and therapeutic effects of several drugs, including aspirin and other salicylates (choline salicylate, magnesium salicylate, salsalate, sodium salicylate, sodium thiosalicylate).

It may be advisable to avoid these citrate compounds during therapy with aspirin or salicylates except under medical supervision.

Reishi

Possible Harmful Interaction

One study suggests that **reishi** impairs platelet clumping. This creates the potential for an interaction with any blood-thinning medication.

Dong Quai, St. John's Wort

Possible Harmful Interaction

St. John's wort (*Hypericum perforatum*) is primarily used to treat mild to moderate depression.

The herb **dong quai** (*Angelica sinensis*) is often recommended for menstrual disorders such as dysmenorrhea, PMS, and irregular menstruation.

Certain NSAIDs, including most notably piroxicam, can cause increased sensitivity to the sun, amplifying the risk of sunburn or skin rash. Because St. John's wort and dong quai may also cause this problem, taking these herbal supplements during NSAID therapy might add to this risk.

It may be a good idea to wear a sunscreen or protective clothing during sun exposure if you take one of these herbs while using an NSAID.

Vinpocetine

Possible Harmful Interaction

The substance **vinpocetine** is sold as a dietary supplement for the treatment of age-related memory loss and impaired mental function.

Vinpocetine is thought to inhibit blood platelets from forming clots. For this reason, it should not be combined with medications or natural substances that impair the blood's ability to clot normally, as this may lead to excessive bleeding. One study found only a minimal interaction between the blood-thinning drug warfarin (Coumadin) and vinpocetine, but prudence dictates caution anyway.

Vitamin E

Possible Mixed Interaction

Vitamin E appears to add to aspirin's blood-thinning effects. One study suggests that the combination of aspirin and even relatively small amounts of vitamin E (50 mg daily) may lead to a significantly increased risk of bleeding. In another study of 28,519 men, vitamin E supplementation at a low dose of about 50 IU (international units) daily was associated with an increase in fatal hemorrhagic strokes, the kind of stroke caused by bleeding within the brain. However, there was a reduced risk of the more common ischemic stroke, caused by obstruction of a blood vessel in the brain, and the two effects were found essentially to cancel each other out.

Weak evidence from one animal study hints that vitamin E might reduce stomach inflammation caused by NSAIDs.

The bottom line: Seek medical advice before combining vitamin E and aspirin.

White Willow

Possible Harmful Interaction

The herb **white willow** (*Salix alba*), also known as willow bark, is used to treat pain and fever.

White willow contains a substance that is converted by the body into a salicylate similar to aspirin. It is therefore possible that taking NSAIDs and white willow could lead to increased risk of side effects, just as would occur if you combined NSAIDs with aspirin.

Herbs and Supplements

Possible Harmful Interaction

Based on their known effects or constituents, the herbs **dong quai** (*Angelica sinensis*), **garlic** (*Allium sativum*), **ginger** (*Zingiber officinale*), **horse chestnut** (*Aesculus hippocastanum*), and **red clover** (*Trifolium pratense*), and the substances **fish oil**, **mesoglycan**, and **OPCs** (oligomeric proanthocyanidins) might conceivably present an increased risk of bleeding if combined with aspirin.

Citrate

Possible Harmful Interaction

Potassium citrate, sodium citrate, and potassium-magnesium citrate are sometimes used to prevent kidney stones. These supplements reduce urinary acidity and can therefore lead to decreased blood levels and effectiveness of NSAIDs.

Cayenne

Supplementation Possibly Helpful

Cayenne (*Capsicum annuum* or *C. frutescens*) and other hot peppers used in chili and various dishes contain as their "hot" ingredient capsaicin, a substance that is thought to be stomach-protective.

For years, people have believed that spicy foods were a cause of stomach ulcers. However, preliminary evidence suggests that cayenne peppers might actually help protect the stomach against ulcers caused by aspirin and possibly other NSAIDs.

In a study involving 18 healthy human volunteers, one group received chili powder, water, and aspirin; the control group received only water and aspirin. Chili powder was found to significantly protect the stomach against damage from aspirin, a known stomach irritant.

It was suggested that this protective effect might result from capsaicin-induced stimulation of blood flow in the lining of the stomach.

Further support for this theory comes from a study in rats which found that capsaicin protected the stomach against damage caused by aspirin, ethanol (drinking alcohol), and acid. Increasing the dose of capsaicin brought even greater benefit, as did increasing the time between giving capsaicin and the other agents. An earlier study in rats found that capsaicin exerted similar protection against aspirin damage.

Some researchers have used this data to advocate chili or capsaicin as treatment for peptic ulcer disease, but check with your doctor before trying to self-treat this serious condition.

Colostrum

Supplementation Possibly Helpful

Colostrum is the fluid that new mothers' breasts produce during the first day or two after birth. It gives newborns a rich mixture of antibodies and growth factors that help them get a good start.

According to one study involving rats, taking colostrum from cows (bovine colostrum) as a supplement might help protect against the ulcers caused by NSAIDs.

Folate

Supplementation Possibly Helpful

Folate (also known as folic acid) is a B vitamin that plays an important role in many vital aspects of health, including preventing neural tube birth defects and possibly reducing the risk of heart disease. Because inadequate intake of folate is widespread, if you are taking any medication that depletes or impairs folate even slightly, you may need supplementation.

There is some evidence that NSAIDs might produce this effect. In test-tube studies, many NSAIDs have been found to interfere with folate activity. In addition, a study of 25 people with arthritis receiving the drug sulfasalazine found evidence of folate deficiency. In another report, a woman taking 650 mg of aspirin every 4 hours for 3 days experienced a significant fall in blood levels of folate.

Based on this preliminary evidence, folate supplementation may be warranted if you are taking drugs in the NSAID family.

Licorice

Supplementation Possibly Helpful

Licorice root (*Glycyrrhiza glabra* or *G. uralensis*), a member of the pea family, has been used since ancient times as both food and medicine.

Preliminary evidence suggests that a specific form of licorice called DGL (deglycyrrhizinated licorice) might help protect the stomach against damage caused by the use of aspirin and possibly other NSAIDs. (DGL is a modified version of licorice that is safer to use.)

In a double-blind study of 9 healthy human volunteers, participants were given aspirin alone (325 mg) or aspirin (325 mg) plus DGL (175 mg). Stomach damage (as measured by blood loss) was found to be about 20% less when DGL was given with aspirin. As part of the same study, DGL was also found to reduce stomach damage caused by aspirin in rats, though the benefit was small. It is possible that larger doses of DGL might provide greater protection.

Vitamin C

Supplementation Possibly Helpful

Test-tube studies suggest that aspirin promotes the loss of **vitamin C** through the urine, which could lead to tissue depletion of the vitamin. In addition, low vitamin C levels have been noted in individuals with rheumatoid arthritis, and this has been attributed to aspirin therapy taken for this condition.

If you take aspirin regularly, vitamin C supplementation may be advisable.

Policosanol (beeswax form)

Possible Helpful Interaction

The supplement **policosanol** is a mixture of numerous related substances, and its exact composition varies with its source. Policosanol made from sugar cane appears to reduce cholesterol levels. Policosanol from beeswax may help protect the stomach from damage caused by NSAIDs. However, it is not clear whether beeswax policosanol might amplify the "blood thinning" effect of anti-inflammatory drugs in the same mannger as sugar-cane policosanol, as described above.

Chondroitin

Possible Harmful Interaction

Based on **chondroitin's** chemical similarity to the anticoagulant drug heparin, it has been suggested that chondroitin might have anticoagulant effects as well. There are no case reports of any problems relating to this, and studies suggest that chondroitin has at most a mild anticoagulant effect. Nonetheless, prudence suggests that chondroitin should not be combined with NSAIDs except under physician supervision.

Oral Contraceptives

ALTERNATE NAMES: *Birth Control Pills, Contraceptives*
Folate—Supplementation Possibly Helpful
Other Nutrients—Supplementation Possibly Helpful
St. John's Wort—Decreased Effectiveness of Drug
Indole-3-Carbinol —Possible Reduced Effectiveness of Drug
Dong Quai, St. John's Wort—Possible Harmful Interaction
Rosemary—Possible Harmful Interaction
Grapefruit Juice—Possible Harmful Interaction
Resveratrol—Possible Harmful Interaction
Milk Thistle—Possible Decreased Action of Drug
Androstenedione—Theoretical Harmful Interaction
Soy—Probably No Interaction

Oral contraceptives (OCs), or birth control pills, are some of the most effective contraceptive drugs. These medications include

➤ Alesse,
➤ Brevicon,
➤ Demulen,
➤ Desogen,
➤ Estrostep,
➤ Genora,
➤ Jenest,
➤ Levlen,
➤ Levlite,
➤ Levora,
➤ Loestrin,
➤ Lo/Ovral,
➤ Micronor,
➤ Mircette,
➤ Modicon,
➤ Nelova,
➤ Nordette,
➤ Norethin,
➤ Norinyl,
➤ Nor-Q.D.,
➤ Ortho-Novum,
➤ Ovcon,
➤ Ovral,
➤ Ovrette,
➤ Tri-Levlen,
➤ Tri-Norinyl,
➤ Triphasil,
➤ Ortho-Cept,
➤ Ortho Cyclen,
➤ Ortho Tri-Cyclen,
➤ Zovia,
➤ and others.

Folate

Supplementation Possibly Helpful

Although the evidence is not consistent, women who are taking OCs may need extra **folate**.

Since folate deficiency is fairly common even among women who are not taking OCs, and it's not wise to be lacking in an essential nutrient, taking a folate supplement on general principle is probably a good idea.

Other Nutrients

Supplementation Possibly Helpful

Evidence from several studies suggests that OCs might interfere with the absorption or metabolism of **magnesium**, **vitamin B$_2$**, **vitamin C**, and **zinc**. With the exception of the trials involving magnesium, these studies used older, high-dose OCs. Modern, low-dose OCs may not affect nutrients to the same extent; still, you should probably make sure you get enough of these nutrients.

St. John's Wort

Decreased Effectiveness of Drug

Reliable case reports, as well as controlled clinical trials, indicate that **St. John's wort** interferes with the effectiveness of oral contraceptives and may have led to unwanted pregnancies.

Indole-3-Carbinol

Possible Reduced Effectiveness of Drug

Indole-3-carbinol (I3C) is a substance found in broccoli that is thought to have cancer preventive effects. One of its mechanisms of action is thought to involve facilitating the inactivation of estrogen, as well as blocking its effects on cells. The net result could be decreased effectiveness of oral contraceptives.

Dong Quai, St. John's Wort

Possible Harmful Interaction

OCs have been reported to cause increased sensitivity to the sun, amplifying the risk of sunburn or skin rash. Because **dong quai** and **St. John's wort** may also cause this problem, taking these herbal supplements while taking OCs might add to this risk.

It may be a good idea to wear a sunscreen or protective clothing during sun exposure if you take one of these herbs while using OCs.

Rosemary

Possible Harmful Interaction

Weak evidence hints that the herb **rosemary** may enhance the liver's ability to deactivate estrogen in the body. This could potentially interfere with the activity of medications that contain estrogen.

Grapefruit Juice

Possible Harmful Interaction

Grapefruit juice slows the body's normal breakdown of several drugs, including estrogen, allowing it to build up to potentially excessive levels in the blood. A recent study indicates this effect can last for 3 days or more following the last glass of juice.

If you take estrogen, the safest approach is to avoid grapefruit juice altogether.

Resveratrol

Possible Harmful Interaction

The supplement **resveratrol** has a chemical structure similar to that of the synthetic estrogen diethylstilbestrol and produces estrogenic-like effects. For this reason, it should not be combined with prescription estrogen products.

Milk Thistle

Possible Decreased Action of Drug

One report has noted that an ingredient of **milk thistle**, silibinin, can inhibit a bacterial enzyme called beta-glucuronidase. This enzyme helps oral contraceptives work. Taking milk thistle could therefore reduce the effectiveness of OCs.

Androstenedione

Theoretical Harmful Interaction

Androstenedione has become popular as a sports supplement, on the theory that it increases testosterone levels as well as sports performance. However, there is no evidence that it is effective. In addition, androstenedione appears more likely to elevate estrogen than testosterone levels. This could increase risks of developing estrogen-related diseases, including breast and uterine cancers. Women taking estrogen should not take androstenedione.

Soy

Probably No Interaction

Fears have been expressed by some experts that **soy** or soy isoflavones might interfere with the action of oral contraceptives. However, one study of 36 women suggests that such concerns are groundless.

Oral Hypoglycemics

Vitamin B$_{12}$—Supplementation Possibly Helpful

Coenzyme Q$_{10}$ (CoQ$_{10}$)—Possible Benefits and Risks

Ipriflavone—Might Require Reduction in Medication Dosage

Magnesium—Might Require Reduction in Medication Dosage

Herbs and Supplements—Might Require Reduction in Medication Dosage

Potassium Citrate—Possible Harmful Interaction

Gingko Biloba—Possible Harmful Interactions

Dong Quai, St. John's Wort—Possible Harmful Interaction

These medications are used for controlling blood sugar in adult-onset diabetes.

Drugs in this family include

➤ acarbose (Prandase, Precose),
➤ acetohexamide (Dymelor),
➤ chlorpropamide (Diabinese),
➤ glimepiride (Amaryl),
➤ glipizide (Glucotrol, Glucotrol XL),
➤ glyburide or glibenclamide (DiaBeta, Glynase, Micronase),
➤ metformin (Glucophage),
➤ miglitol (Glyset),
➤ phenformin,
➤ pioglitazone (Actos),
➤ rosiglitazone (Avandia),
➤ repaglinide (Prandin),
➤ tolazamide (Tolinase),
➤ tolbutamide (Orinase),
➤ troglitazone (Rezulin),
➤ and others.

Vitamin B$_{12}$

Supplementation Possibly Helpful

The so-called biguanide oral hypoglycemic drugs, metformin and phenformin, are thought to cause malabsorption of **vitamin B$_{12}$**. Taking extra vitamin B$_{12}$ should solve this problem.

Coenzyme Q$_{10}$ (CoQ$_{10}$)

Possible Benefits and Risks

Studies suggest that the oral hypoglycemic drugs glyburide, phenformin, and tolazamide may inhibit the normal production of the substance **coenzyme Q$_{10}$ (CoQ$_{10}$)**. While there is as yet no direct evidence that taking extra CoQ$_{10}$ will provide any specific benefit, supplementing with CoQ$_{10}$ on general principle might make sense.

In addition, there is some evidence that use of CoQ$_{10}$ could improve blood sugar control for people with diabetes. While this could be helpful, keep in mind that if it works, you might need to reduce your medication dosage.

Ipriflavone

Might Require Reduction in Medication Dosage

There is some evidence that the supplement **ipriflavone** might increase blood levels of oral hypoglycemic drugs. This could lead to a risk of blood sugar levels falling too low. If you are taking oral hypoglycemic medications, don't take ipriflavone without first consulting your physician.

Magnesium

Might Require Reduction in Medication Dosage

Magnesium supplements might increase the absorption of chlorpropamide (and, by inference, other oral hypoglycemics), possibly requiring you to reduce your dose.

Herbs and Supplements

Might Require Reduction in Medication Dosage

Meaningful preliminary evidence suggests that use of the following herbs and supplements could potentially improve blood sugar control and require you to reduce your daily dose of oral hypoglycemic medication: **aloe, chromium, fenugreek, ginseng, gymnema,** and **vanadium**.

Weaker evidence suggests that the following herbs and supplements could potentially have the same effect under certain circumstances: *Anemarrhena asphodeloides,* **arginine,** *Azadirachta indica* (**neem**), **bilberry leaf, biotin, bitter melon, carnitine,** *Catharanthus roseus, Coccinia indica,* **coenzyme Q**$_{10}$, **conjugated linoleic acid** (CLA), *Cucumis sativus, Cucurbita ficifolia, Cuminum cyminum* (cumin), *Euphorbia prostrata,* **garlic, glucomannan,** *Guaiacum coulteri, Guazuma ulmifolia,* **guggul,** holy basil, *Lepechinia caulescens,* **lipoic acid,** *Medicago sativa* (**alfalfa**), *Musa sapientum* L. (banana), **niacinamide,** nopal cactus, onion, *Phaseolus vulgaris, Psacalium peltatum,* pterocarpus, *Rhizophora mangle,* **salt bush,** *Spinacea oleracea, Tournefortia hirsutissima, Turnera diffusa,* and **vitamin E**.

Potassium Citrate

Possible Harmful Interaction

Potassium citrate and other forms of citrate (for example, calcium citrate and magnesium citrate) may be used to prevent kidney stones. These agents work by making the urine less acidic.

This effect on the urine may lead to decreased blood levels and therapeutic effects of chlorpropamide and possibly other oral hypoglycemic drugs.

For this reason, it may be advisable to avoid these citrate compounds during treatment with oral hypoglycemic drugs.

Gingko Biloba

Possible Harmful Interactions

It has been suggested that **ginkgo** might cause problems for people with type 2 diabetes both by altering blood levels of medications as well as by directly affecting the blood sugar–regulating system of the body. However, the most recent and best designed studies have failed to find any such actions. Nonetheless, until this situation is clarified, people with diabetes should use ginkgo only under physician supervision.

Dong Quai, St. John's Wort

Possible Harmful Interaction

Some oral hypoglycemic drugs have been reported to cause increased sensitivity to the sun, amplifying the risk of sunburn or skin rash. Because **St. John's wort** and **dong quai** may also cause this problem, taking these herbal supplements during treatment with oral hypoglycemic drugs might add to this risk.

It may be a good idea to wear a sunscreen or protective clothing during sun exposure if you take one of these herbs while using an oral hypoglycemic medication.

Oxytetracycline/Sulfamethizole

TRADE NAMES: *Urobiotic*

This medication is a combination of the following drugs:

➤ Tetracyclines
➤ Trimethoprim/Sulfamethoxazole

Please see the separate articles on each one to find out about potential drug interactions. The interactions for each may be different, so read both articles carefully to find out the whole story.

Penicillamine

TRADE NAMES: *Cuprimine, Depen*

Copper—Avoid in Cases of Wilson's Disease

Vitamin B$_6$—Possible Need for Supplementation

Zinc—Supplementation Possibly Helpful, but Take at a Different Time of Day

Iron—Take at a Different Time of Day

The drug penicillamine is primarily used to treat Wilson's disease (an inherited disorder affecting copper metabolism, causing cirrhosis, brain and eye problems), and rheumatoid arthritis.

Copper

Avoid in Cases of Wilson's Disease

When used to treat Wilson's disease, penicillamine works by removing **copper** from the body. Taking copper supplements while you are using penicillamine for this condition is not a good idea.

Vitamin B$_6$

Possible Need for Supplementation

Penicillamine might increase the need for **vitamin B$_6$**. Taking 25 to 50 mg of supplemental B$_6$ daily is often recommended.

Zinc

Supplementation Possibly Helpful, but Take at a Different Time of Day

Long-term use of penicillamine can cause **zinc** deficiency. However, zinc can impair penicillamine absorption, so do not take zinc supplements during the 2 hours before or after your penicillamine dose.

Iron

Take at a Different Time of Day

Penicillamine attaches to the mineral **iron**, which impairs the absorption of both substances. The solution: If you need iron supplements, do not take them during the 2 hours before or after your penicillamine dose.

Phenobarbital

TRADE NAMES: *Bellatal, Solfoton*

RELATED DRUGS: *Mephobarbital, Mebaral, Methylphenobarbital*

Folate—Supplementation Possibly Helpful

Vitamin D—Supplementation Possibly Helpful

Vitamin K—Supplementation Helpful for Pregnant Women

Biotin—Supplementation Possibly Helpful, but Take at a Different Time of Day

St. John's Wort, Dong Quai—Possible Harmful Interaction

Ginkgo—Possible Harmful Interaction

Kava, Valerian, Passionflower, Hops—Possible Harmful Interaction

Glutamine—Theoretical Harmful Interaction

Phenobarbital and its relative phenobarbitone are sometimes used to control seizures.

Folate

Supplementation Possibly Helpful

Phenobarbital can reduce **folate** levels, perhaps by increasing the rate of breakdown of the vitamin. Over time such a decrease can cause anemia. Taking folate supplements can correct this anemia. Anticonvulsant-induced folate deficiency might also cause birth defects. Women who plan to become pregnant while on phenobarbital should be sure to take a supplement to prevent deficiency.

Vitamin D

Supplementation Possibly Helpful

Phenobarbital appears to interfere with the normal absorption or metabolism of **vitamin D**. In turn, this can impair calcium absorption. Making sure to get enough vitamin D (and calcium) should help prevent any problems from developing.

Vitamin K

Supplementation Helpful for Pregnant Women

Children born to women taking phenobarbital while pregnant may be deficient in **vitamin K**. This might lead to bleeding disorders and facial bone abnormalities. Supplementing with vitamin K during pregnancy should help; however, physician supervision is recommended.

Biotin

Supplementation Possibly Helpful, but Take at a Different Time of Day

Many antiseizure medications, including phenobarbital, are believed to interfere with the absorption of **biotin**. For this reason, individuals taking phenobarbital may benefit from extra biotin. Biotin should be taken 2 to 3 hours apart from your antiseizure medication. Do not exceed the recommended daily intake, because it is possible that too much biotin might interfere with the effectiveness of the medication.

Dong Quai, St. John's Wort

Possible Harmful Interaction

Phenobarbital has been reported to cause increased sensitivity to the sun, amplifying the risk of sunburn or skin rash. Because **St. John's wort** and **dong quai** may also cause this problem, taking them during treatment with this drug might add to this risk.

It may be a good idea to wear a sunscreen or protective clothing during sun exposure if you take one of these herbs while using this anticonvulsant.

Ginkgo

Possible Harmful Interaction

The herb **ginkgo** (*Ginkgo biloba*) has been used to treat Alzheimer's disease and ordinary age-related memory loss, among many other conditions.

This interaction involves potential contaminants in ginkgo, not ginkgo itself.

A recent study found that a natural nerve toxin present in the seeds of *Ginkgo biloba* made its way into standardized ginkgo extracts prepared from the leaves. This toxin has been associated with convulsions and death in laboratory animals.

Fortunately, the detected amounts of this toxic substance are considered harmless. However, given the lack of satisfactory standardization of herbal formulations in the United States, it is possible that some batches of product might contain higher contents of the toxin depending on the season of harvest.

In light of these findings, taking a ginkgo product that happened to contain significant levels of the nerve toxin might theoretically prevent an anticonvulsant from working as well as expected.

Hops, Kava, Passionflower, Valerian

Possible Harmful Interaction

The herb **kava** (*Piper methysticum*) has a sedative effect and is used for anxiety and insomnia.

Combining kava with anticonvulsants, which possess similar depressant effects, could result in "add-on" or excessive physical depression, sedation, and impairment.

Because of the potentially serious consequences, you should avoid combining other herbs having a sedative effect, such as **hops**, **passionflower**, and **valerian**, with phenobarbital unless advised by your physician.

Glutamine

Theoretical Harmful Interaction

Because phenobarbital works (at least in part) by blocking glutamate pathways in the brain, high dosages of **glutamine** might possibly overwhelm the drug and increase the risk of seizures.

Phenothiazines

Coenzyme Q$_{10}$ (CoQ$_{10}$)—Supplementation Possibly Helpful

Milk Thistle—Possible Helpful Interaction

Ginkgo—Possible Helpful Interaction

Vitamin E—Possible Helpful Interaction

Vitamin B$_6$—Possible Helpful Interaction

DHEA (dehydroepiandrosterone)—Possible Helpful Interaction

Phenylalanine—Possible Increased Risk of Tardive Dyskinesia

Kava—Possible Increased Risk of Dystonic Reactions

St. John's Wort, Other Herbs—Potential Increased Risk of Photosensitivity

Yohimbe—Possible Dangerous Interaction

Phenothiazine drugs are primarily used for the treatment of schizophrenia and other forms of psychosis. Medications in this family include

- chlorpromazine hydrochloride (Thorazine),
- fluphenazine (Permitil, Prolixin),
- mesoridazine besylate (Serentil),
- perphenazine (Trilafon),
- prochlorperazine (Compazine),
- promazine hydrochloride (Sparine),
- promethazine hydrochloride (Anergan [injectable], Phenergan),
- thioridazine hydrochloride (Mellaril),
- trifluoperazine hydrochloride (Stelazine),
- triflupromazine hydrochloride (Vesprin [injectable]),
- and others.

Coenzyme Q$_{10}$ (CoQ$_{10}$)

Supplementation Possibly Helpful

Preliminary studies suggest that phenothiazine drugs might deplete the body of **coenzyme Q$_{10}$** (CoQ$_{10}$). While there is as yet no evidence that taking CoQ$_{10}$ supplements provides any specific benefit, supplementing with CoQ$_{10}$ on general principle might be a good idea if you are taking phenothiazine drugs.

Milk Thistle

Possible Helpful Interaction

Milk thistle might protect against the liver toxicity sometimes caused by phenothiazine drugs.

Ginkgo

Possible Helpful Interaction

Preliminary evidence suggests that **ginkgo** might reduce the side effects and increase the efficacy of various antipsychotic medications.

Vitamin E

Possible Helpful Interaction

One of the most feared side effects of phenothiazines is the development of a permanent side effect called tardive dyskinesia (TD). This late-developing (tardy, or tardive) complication consists of annoying uncontrollable movements (dyskinesias), particularly in the face.

There is some evidence that high doses of **vitamin E** might reduce symptoms of tardive dyskinesia.

Vitamin B$_6$

Possible Helpful Interaction

A pilot study suggests that **vitamin B$_6$** may be helpful for the treatment of TD. In this 4-week, double-blind, crossover trial of 15 individuals, treatment with vitamin B$_6$ significantly improved TD symptoms as compared to placebo. Benefits were seen after 1 week of treatment. However, the dosage of vitamin B$_6$ used in this study was quite high (400 mg daily). Toxicity has been reported with daily intake of vitamin B$_6$ at half this dose.

Vitamin B$_6$ might also reduce symptoms of akathesia, a type of restlessness associated with phenothiazine antipsychotics.

DHEA (dehydroepiandrosterone)

Possible Helpful Interaction

One small double-blind study found that use of **DHEA** reduced the Parkinson-like movement disorders that may occur in people taking phenothiazine drugs.

Phenylalanine

Possible Increased Risk of Tardive Dyskinesia

There are some indications that using the supplement **phenylalanine** while taking antipsychotic drugs might increase your risk of developing tardive dyskinesia.

Kava

Possible Increased Risk of Dystonic Reactions

Besides the late-developing complication of tardive dyskinesia, antipsychotic drugs can cause more immediately another movement disorder: dystonic reactions, sudden intense movements of the neck and eyes. There is some evidence that the herb **kava** can increase the risk or severity of this side effect.

St. John's Wort, Other Herbs

Potential Increased Risk of Photosensitivity

Phenothiazines can cause increased sensitivity to the sun. Various herbs, including **St. John's wort** and **dong quai**, can also cause this problem. Combined treatment with herb and drug might increase the risk further.

Yohimbe

Possible Dangerous Interaction

The herb **yohimbe** is relatively toxic and can cause problems if used incorrectly. Phenothiazine medications may increase the risk of toxicity.

Phenytoin

TRADE NAMES: *Dilantin*

Ginkgo—Possible Harmful Interaction

Glutamine—Possible Harmful Interaction

Ipriflavone—Possible Harmful Interaction

Hops, Kava, Passionflower, Valerian—Possible Harmful Interaction

White Willow—Possible Harmful Interaction

Biotin—Supplementation Possibly Helpful, but Take at a Different Time of Day

Folate—Possible Benefits and Risks

Calcium—Supplementation Probably Helpful, but Take at a Different Time of Day

Carnitine—Supplementation Possibly Helpful

Vitamin D—Supplementation Possibly Helpful

Vitamin K—Supplementation Possibly Helpful for Pregnant Women

Phenytoin is an anticonvulsant agent used primarily to prevent seizures in conditions such as epilepsy. Drugs similar to phenytoin are ethotoin (Peganone) and mephenytoin (Mesantoin).

Other anticonvulsant agents include **carbamazepine**, **phenobarbital**, **primidone**, and **valproic acid**. In some cases, combination therapy with two or more anticonvulsant drugs may be used.

Ginkgo

Possible Harmful Interaction

The herb **ginkgo** (*Ginkgo biloba*) has been used to treat Alzheimer's disease and ordinary age-related memory loss, among many other conditions. Seizures have been reported with the use of ginkgo leaf extract in people with previously well-controlled epilepsy; in one case, the seizures were fatal. One possible explanation is contamination of ginkgo leaf products with ginkgo seeds. It has also been suggested that ginkgo might interfere with the effectiveness of some antiseizure medications, including phenytoin. Finally, it has been noted that the drug tacrine (also used to improve memory) has been associated with seizures, and ginkgo may affect the brain in ways similar to tacrine.

Glutamine

Possible Harmful Interaction

The amino acid **glutamine** is converted to glutamate in the body. Glutamate is thought to act as a neurotransmitter (a chemical that enables nerve transmission). Because anticonvulsants work (at least in part) by blocking glutamate pathways in the brain, high dosages of the amino acid glutamine might theoretically diminish an anticonvulsant's effect and increase the risk of seizures.

Ipriflavone

Possible Harmful Interaction

Ipriflavone, a synthetic isoflavone that slows bone breakdown, is used to treat osteoporosis.

Test-tube studies indicate that ipriflavone might increase blood levels of the anticonvulsants phenytoin and carbamazepine when they are taken therapeutically. Ipriflavone was found to inhibit a liver enzyme involved in the body's normal breakdown of these drugs, thus allowing them to build up in the blood. Higher drug levels increase the risk of adverse effects.

Because anticonvulsants are known to contribute to the development of osteoporosis, a concern is that the use of ipriflavone for this drug-induced osteoporosis could result in higher blood levels of the drugs, with potentially serious consequences.

People taking either of these drugs should use ipriflavone only under medical supervision.

Hops, Kava, Passionflower, Valerian

Possible Harmful Interaction

The herb **kava** (*Piper methysticum*) has a sedative effect and is used for anxiety and insomnia.

Combining kava with anticonvulsants, which possess similar depressant effects, could result in "add-on" or excessive physical depression, sedation, and impairment. In one case report, a 54-year-old man was hospitalized for lethargy and disorientation, side effects attributed to his having taken the combination of kava and the antianxiety agent alprazolam (Xanax) for 3 days.

Other herbs having a sedative effect that might cause problems when combined with anticonvulsants include **ashwagandha** (*Withania somnifera*), **calendula** (*Calendula officinalis*), **catnip** (*Nepeta cataria*), **hops** (*Humulus lupulus*), **lady's slipper** (*Cypripedium* species), **lemon balm** (*Melissa officinalis*), **passionflower** (*Passiflora incarnata*), sassafras (*Sassafras officinale*), **skullcap** (*Scutellaria lateriflora*), **valerian** (*Valeriana officinalis*), and yerba mansa (*Anemopsis californica*).

Because of the potentially serious consequences, you should avoid combining these herbs with anticonvulsants or other drugs that also have sedative or depressant effects unless advised by your physician.

White Willow

Possible Harmful Interaction
The herb **white willow** (*Salix alba*), also known as willow bark, is used to treat pain and fever. White willow contains a substance that is converted by the body into a salicylate similar to aspirin.

Higher doses of aspirin may increase phenytoin levels and toxicity during long-term use of both drugs. This raises the concern that white willow might have similar effects on phenytoin, though this has not been proven.

Biotin

Supplementation Possibly Helpful, but Take at a Different Time of Day
Anticonvulsants may deplete **biotin**, an essential water-soluble B vitamin, possibly by competing with it for absorption in the intestine. It is not clear, however, whether this effect is great enough to be harmful.

Blood levels of biotin were found to be substantially lower in 404 people with epilepsy on long-term treatment with anticonvulsants compared to 112 untreated people with epilepsy. The effect occurred with phenytoin, carbamazepine, phenobarbital, and primidone. Valproic acid appears to affect biotin to a lesser extent than other anticonvulsants.

A test-tube study suggested that anticonvulsants might lower biotin levels by interfering with the way biotin is transported in the intestine.

Biotin supplementation may be beneficial if you are on long-term anticonvulsant therapy. To avoid a potential interaction, take the supplement 2 to 3 hours apart from the drug.

Note: It has been suggested that the action of anticonvulsant drugs may be at least partly related to their effect of reducing biotin levels. For this reason, it may be desirable to take enough biotin to prevent a deficiency, but not an excessive amount.

Folate

Possible Benefits and Risks
Folate (also known as folic acid) is a B vitamin that plays an important role in many vital aspects of health, including preventing neural-tube birth defects and possibly reducing the risk of heart disease. Because inadequate intake of folate is widespread, if you are taking any medication that depletes or impairs folate even slightly, you may need supplementation.

Most drugs used for preventing seizures can reduce levels of folate in the body. Phenytoin in particular appears to decrease folate levels by interfering with its absorption in the small intestine as well as by accelerating its normal breakdown by the body.

The low blood levels of folate caused by anticonvulsants can raise **homocysteine** levels, a condition believed to increase the risk of heart disease.

Adequate folate intake is also necessary to prevent neural tube birth defects such as spina bifida and anencephaly (absence of a brain). Because anticonvulsant drugs deplete folate, babies born to women taking anticonvulsants are at increased risk for such birth defects. Anticonvulsants may also play a more direct role in the development of birth defects.

However, there can be problems with using folate supplements. High folate levels may speed up the normal breakdown of phenytoin. This can lead to breakthrough seizures.

For this reason, folate supplementation during phenytoin therapy should be supervised by a physician.

Calcium

Supplementation Probably Helpful, but Take at a Different Time of Day
Anticonvulsant drugs may impair **calcium** absorption and in this way increase the risk of osteoporosis and other bone disorders.

Calcium absorption was compared in 12 people on

anticonvulsant therapy (all taking phenytoin and some also taking phenobarbital, primidone, and/or carbamazepine) and 12 people receiving no treatment. Calcium absorption was found to be 27% lower in the treated participants.

An observational study found low calcium blood levels in 48% of 109 people taking anticonvulsants. Other findings in this study suggested that anticonvulsants might also reduce calcium levels by directly interfering with parathyroid hormone, a substance that helps keep calcium levels in proper balance.

A low blood level of calcium can itself trigger seizures and this might reduce the effectiveness of anticonvulsants.

Calcium supplementation may be beneficial for people taking anticonvulsant drugs. However, some studies indicate that antacids containing calcium carbonate may interfere with the absorption of phenytoin and perhaps other anticonvulsants. For this reason, take calcium supplements and anticonvulsant drugs several hours apart if possible.

Carnitine

Supplementation Possibly Helpful

Carnitine is an amino acid that has been used for heart conditions, Alzheimer's disease, and intermittent claudication (a possible complication of atherosclerosis in which impaired blood circulation causes severe pain in calf muscles during walking or exercising).

Long-term therapy with anticonvulsant agents, particularly valproic acid, is associated with low levels of carnitine. However, it isn't clear whether the anticonvulsants cause the carnitine deficiency or whether it occurs for other reasons. It has been hypothesized that low carnitine levels may contribute to valproic acid's damaging effects on the liver. The risk of this liver damage increases in children younger than 24 months and carnitine supplementation does seem to be protective. However, in one double-blind, crossover study, carnitine supplementation produced no real improvement in "well-being" as assessed by parents of children receiving either valproic acid or carbamazepine.

L-carnitine supplementation may be advisable in certain cases, such as in infants and young children (especially those younger than 2 years) who have neurologic disorders and are receiving valproic acid and multiple anticonvulsants.

Vitamin D

Supplementation Possibly Helpful

Anticonvulsant drugs may interfere with the activity of **vitamin D**. As proper handling of calcium by the body depends on vitamin D, this may be another way that these drugs increase the risk of osteoporosis and related bone disorders (see the above **Calcium** topic).

Anticonvulsants appear to speed up the body's normal breakdown of vitamin D, decreasing the amount of the vitamin in the blood. A survey of 48 people taking both phenytoin and phenobarbital found significantly lower levels of calcium and vitamin D in many of them as compared to 38 untreated people. Similar but lesser changes were seen in 13 people taking phenytoin or phenobarbital alone. This effect may be apparent only after several weeks of treatment.

Another study found decreased blood levels of one form of vitamin D but normal levels of another. Because there are two primary forms of vitamin D circulating in the blood, the body might be able to adjust in some cases to keep vitamin D in balance, at least for a time, despite the influence of anticonvulsants.

Adequate sunlight exposure may help overcome the effects of anticonvulsants on vitamin D by stimulating the skin to manufacture the vitamin. Of 450 people on anticonvulsants residing in a Florida facility, none were found to have low blood levels of vitamin D or evidence of bone disease. This suggests that environments providing regular sun exposure may be protective.

People regularly taking anticonvulsants, especially those taking combination therapy and those with limited exposure to sunlight, may benefit from vitamin D supplementation.

Vitamin K

Supplementation Possibly Helpful for Pregnant Women

Phenytoin, carbamazepine, phenobarbital, and primidone speed up the normal breakdown of **vitamin K** into inactive byproducts, thus depriving the body of active vitamin K. This can lead to bone problems such as osteoporosis. Also, use of these anticonvulsants can lead to a vitamin K deficiency in babies born to pregnant mothers taking the drugs, resulting in bleeding disorders or facial bone abnormalities in the newborns.

Mothers who take these anticonvulsants may need vitamin K supplementation during pregnancy to prevent these conditions in their newborns.

Potassium-Sparing Diuretics

Potassium—Likely Harmful Interaction

Arginine—Possible Harmful Interaction

Magnesium—Possible Harmful Interaction

White Willow—Possible Negative Interaction

Zinc—Possible Harmful Interaction

This family of diuretics was invented to avoid the potassium loss common with loop and thiazide diuretics.

Potassium-sparing diuretics include drugs such as amiloride hydrochloride (Midamor), spironolactone (Aldactone), and triamterene (Dyrenium) among others.

Potassium

Likely Harmful Interaction

Potassium-sparing diuretics cause the kidneys to hold **potassium** in the body. When you are taking these medications you generally should not take potassium supplements, because your potassium levels might rise too high.

Treatments that combine thiazide diuretics (which cause potassium loss) and potassium-sparing diuretics can affect potassium levels unpredictably. If you are taking such a combination medication, do not take potassium except on the advice of your physician.

Magnesium

Possible Harmful Interaction

Preliminary evidence from animal studies suggests that the potassium-sparing diuretic amiloride might cause the body to retain **magnesium** also, along with potassium. Therefore, taking magnesium supplements might conceivably present the risk of excessive magnesium levels.

Arginine

Possible Harmful Interaction

Based on experience with intravenous **arginine**, it is possible that the use of high-dose oral arginine might alter potassium levels in the body, especially in people with severe liver disease. This is a potential concern for individuals who take potassium-sparing diuretics.

White Willow

Possible Negative Interaction

The herb **white willow** contains substances very similar to aspirin. On this basis, it might not be advisable to combine white willow with potassium-sparing diuretics.

Zinc

Possible Harmful Interaction

The potassium-sparing diuretic amiloride was found to significantly reduce **zinc** excretion from the body. This means that if you take zinc supplements at the same time as amiloride, zinc accumulation could occur. This could lead to toxic side effects.

However, the potassium-sparing diuretic triamterene does not seem to cause this problem.

Primidone

TRADE NAMES: *Mysoline*

Folate—Supplementation Possibly Helpful

Vitamin D—Supplementation Possibly Helpful

Vitamin K—Supplementation Possibly Helpful for Pregnant Women

Biotin—Supplementation Possibly Helpful, but Take at a Different Time of Day

Glutamine—Theoretical Harmful Interaction

Vitamin B₃—Potentially Dangerous Interaction

St. John's Wort, Dong Quai—Possible Harmful Interaction

Ginkgo—Possible Harmful Interaction

Kava, Valerian, Passionflower, Hops—Possible Harmful Interaction

Like phenobarbital, to which it is closely related, primidone is used to control epileptic seizures.

Folate

Supplementation Possibly Helpful

Primidone can reduce **folate** levels perhaps by increasing the rate of breakdown of the vitamin. Over time, such a decrease can cause anemia. Taking folate supplements will correct this anemia. Anticonvulsant-induced folate deficiency might also cause birth defects. Women who plan to become pregnant while on primidone should be sure to take a supplement to prevent deficiency.

Vitamin D

Supplementation Possibly Helpful

Primidone appears to interfere with the normal absorption or metabolism of **vitamin D**. This in turn impairs calcium absorption, with many potential complications. To help avoid this problem, you should make sure that you get enough vitamin D.

Vitamin K

Supplementation Possibly Helpful for Pregnant Women

Children born to women taking primidone while pregnant may be deficient in **vitamin K**. This might lead to bleeding disorders and facial bone abnormalities. Supplementing with vitamin K during pregnancy should help; however, physician supervision is recommended.

Biotin

Supplementation Possibly Helpful, but Take at a Different Time of Day

Many antiseizure medications including primidone are believed to interfere with the absorption of **biotin**. For this reason, individuals taking primidone may benefit from extra biotin. Biotin should be taken 2 to 3 hours apart from your antiseizure medication. Do not exceed the recommended daily intake, because it is possible that too much biotin might interfere with the effectiveness of the medication.

Glutamine

Theoretical Harmful Interaction

Because many anti-epilepsy drugs, including primidone, work by blocking glutamate stimulation in the brain, high dosages of **glutamine** might counteract the drugs' effects, and pose a risk of increased seizures.

Vitamin B₃

Potentially Dangerous Interaction

Niacinamide (a form of **vitamin B₃**) might increase blood levels of primidone, possibly requiring reduction in drug dosage.

Dong Quai, St. John's Wort

Possible Harmful Interaction

Primidone has been reported to cause increased sensitivity to the sun, amplifying the risk of sunburn or skin rash. Because **St. John's wort** and **dong quai** may also cause this problem, taking them during treatment with this drug might add to this risk.

It may be a good idea to wear a sunscreen or protective clothing during sun exposure if you take one of these herbs while using this anticonvulsant.

Ginkgo

Possible Harmful Interaction

The herb **ginkgo** (*Ginkgo biloba*) has been used to treat Alzheimer's disease and ordinary age-related memory loss, among many other conditions.

This interaction involves potential contaminants in ginkgo, not ginkgo itself.

A recent study found that a natural nerve toxin present in the seeds of *Ginkgo biloba* made its way into standardized ginkgo extracts prepared from the leaves. This toxin has been associated with convulsions and death in laboratory animals.

Fortunately, the detected amounts of this toxic substance are considered harmless. However, given the lack of satisfactory standardization of herbal formulations in the United States, it is possible that some batches of product might contain higher contents of the toxin depending on the season of harvest.

In light of these findings, taking a ginkgo product that happened to contain significant levels of the nerve toxin might theoretically prevent an anticonvulsant from working as well as expected.

Hops, Kava, Passionflower, Valerian

Possible Harmful Interaction

The herb **kava** (*Piper methysticum*) has a sedative effect and is used for anxiety and insomnia.

Combining kava with anticonvulsants, which possess similar depressant effects, could result in "add-on" or excessive physical depression, sedation, and impairment.

Because of the potentially serious consequences, you should avoid combining other herbs having a sedative effect, such as **hops**, **passionflower**, and **valerian**, with primidone unless advised by your physician.

Protease Inhibitors

Glutamine—Possible Helpful Interaction

St. John's Wort—Dangerous Interaction

Grapefruit Juice—Possible Harmful Interaction

Vitamin C—Possible Harmful Interaction

Garlic—Possible Harmful Interaction

Milk Thistle—Possible Helpful Interaction

Protease inhibitors include

➤ amprenavir (Agenerase),
➤ indinavir (Crixivan),
➤ nelfinavir (Viracept),
➤ ritonavir (Norvir),
➤ and saquinavir (Fortovase, Invirase).

Glutamine

Possible Helpful Interaction

The amino acid glutamine is thought to have protective effects on the digestive tract. One small double-blind study found that use of glycine at 30 g daily reduced diarrhea caused by nelfinavir.

St. John's Wort

Dangerous Interaction

St. John's wort has been found to decrease blood levels of the HIV drug indinavir by an average of 57%. The reduction is substantial, and could lead to failure of the drug to keep the HIV virus in check. Similar effects are expected to occur with other protease inhibitors. To make matters worse, St. John's wort also appears to interact with another category of drugs used for HIV, **reverse transcriptase inhibitors**.

The bottom line: If you have HIV, don't take St. John's wort! Furthermore, if you have been stabilized on HIV medications while taking St. John's wort, don't stop taking the herb without consulting your physician. Discontinuing the herb might cause your blood levels of the drugs to rise, potentially leading to increased side effects.

Grapefruit Juice

Possible Harmful Interaction

Grapefruit juice impairs the body's normal breakdown of several drugs, allowing them to build up to potentially excessive levels in the blood. Saquinavir mesylate as well as other protease inhibitors may be affected. A recent study indicates that this effect can last for 3 days or more following the last glass of juice.

Because this could increase the risk of drug side effects, if you take protease inhibitors, the safest approach is to avoid grapefruit juice altogether.

Vitamin C

Possible Harmful Interaction

One study found that use of **vitamin C** at a dose of 1 g daily significantly reduced levels of indinavir. This was the first report of such an interaction with vitamin C, but the study was well designed and deserves to be taken seriously. People taking any protease inhibitor should either avoid taking vitamin C, or have their protease inhibitor levels checked whenever they start (or stop) taking vitamin C.

Garlic

Possible Harmful Interaction

The herb **garlic** is widely used in the belief that it can help prevent heart disease. However, it may not be safe to combine garlic supplements with protease inhibitors.

Two people with HIV experienced severe gastrointestinal toxicity from the drug ritonavir after taking garlic supplements. Garlic might also reduce the effectiveness of some drugs used for HIV.

Milk Thistle

Possible Helpful Interaction

The herb **milk thistle** is thought to have liver-protective properties, and some people with HIV may take milk thistle in hopes of minimizing liver-related side effects of HIV medications. While there is no evidence that milk thistle provides any benefit in this regard, one study did find that at least it does *not* interfere with levels of indinavir.

Proton Pump Inhibitors

St. John's Wort—Possible Harmful Interactions
Vitamin B$_{12}$—Supplementation Likely Helpful
Folate—Supplementation Possibly Helpful
Minerals—Supplementation Possibly Helpful

These drugs are the most powerful medications for reducing stomach acid levels; in fact, they almost completely shut down the stomach's ability to produce acid. (Their science fiction–sounding name comes from the last stage of the acid-secreting process, called the "proton pump.") Proton pump inhibitors are used for ulcers as well as for the treatment of moderate to severe esophageal reflux, commonly known as heartburn.

Drugs in this family include

➤ lansoprazole (Prevacid),
➤ omeprazole (Prilosec),
➤ and others.

St. John's Wort

Possible Harmful Interactions

The herb **St. John's wort** is known to interact with numerous drugs. There are two potential harmful interactions between St. John's wort and proton pump inhibitors.

One study found that use of St. John's wort greatly decreases levels of omeprazole in the body. This would be expected to lead to markedly reduced efficacy.

The other potential risk is more theoretical. When taken to excess, the herb St. John's wort can cause an increased risk of sunburn. Some evidence hints that proton pump inhibitors might increase this risk.

Vitamin B$_{12}$

Supplementation Likely Helpful

Vitamin B$_{12}$ deficiency is a concern with the use of all drugs that reduce stomach acidity.

In food, vitamin B$_{12}$ is always accompanied by proteins, and it must be separated from them before it can begin to be absorbed. Following separation, B$_{12}$ is then attached to a substance called intrinsic factor, which allows B$_{12}$ to be absorbed in the intestines.

Stomach acid plays a role in this separation. If you don't have enough stomach acid, the process of freeing vitamin B$_{12}$ from protein so that it can be bound to intrinsic factor may be impaired.

Studies suggest that treatment with proton pump inhibitors might significantly reduce the absorption of vitamin B$_{12}$.

Interestingly, there is some evidence that cranberry juice might increase B$_{12}$ absorption in individuals taking proton pump inhibitors, possibly because the juice is somewhat acidic.

Folate

Supplementation Possibly Helpful

Research on related medications suggests that proton pump inhibitors may slightly reduce the body's absorption of **folate**. The decrease in folate absorption should be quite small, but since folate deficiency is quite common and potentially harmful, taking extra folate might make sense as insurance.

Minerals

Supplementation Possibly Helpful

By reducing stomach acid levels, proton pump inhibitors might interfere with the absorption of **iron, zinc**, and perhaps other minerals. Taking mineral supplements to meet the U.S. Dietary Reference Intake (formerly known as the Recommended Dietary Allowance) levels for these nutrients should help.

Reverse Transcriptase Inhibitors

Coenzyme Q$_{10}$—Possible Benefits and Risks
St. John's Wort—Dangerous Interaction

The human immunodeficiency virus (HIV) contains genetic information in the form of RNA. When HIV infects a human T cell, it must convert this RNA to DNA. It does so by using an enzyme called reverse transcriptase. Reverse transcriptase inhibitors interfere with this process.

There are two major categories of reverse transcriptase inhibitors: *nucleoside/nucleotide reverse transcriptase inhibitors* (NRTIs) and *non-nucleoside reverse transcriptase inhibitors* (NNRTIs).

Reverse transcriptase inhibitors include

➤ Combivir (lamivudine and zidovudine),
➤ Emtriva (emtricitabine),
➤ Epivir (lamivudine),
➤ Epzicom (abacavir and lamivudine),
➤ Hivid (zalcitabine),
➤ Rescriptor (delaviridine),
➤ Retrovir (AZT, zidovudine),
➤ Trizivir (abacavir-lamivudine-zidovudine),
➤ Truvada (emtricitabine-tenofovir),
➤ Videx (didanosine),
➤ Viramune (nevirapine),
➤ Viread (tenofovir),
➤ Zerit (stavudine),
➤ and Ziagen (abacavir).

Coenzyme Q$_{10}$

Possible Benefits and Risks

The reverse transcriptase inhibitors lamivudine and zidovudine can cause damage to the mitochondria, the energy-producing subunits of cells. This may lead to symptoms such as lactic acidosis (a dangerous metabolic derangement), **peripheral neuropathy** (injury to nerves in the extremities), and lipodystrophy (cosmetically undesirable rearrangement of fat in the body). The supplement **CoenzymeQ$_{10}$** has been tried for minimizing these side effects. In one double-blind, placebo-controlled study, use of CoQ$_{10}$ improved general sense of well-being in people with HIV infection using reverse transcriptase inhibitors; however, for reasons that are unclear, it actually worsened symptoms of peripheral neuropathy. For this reason, people with HIV who have peripheral neuropathy symptoms should use CoQ$_{10}$ only with caution.

St. John's Wort

Dangerous Interaction

Use of the herb St. John's wort can lower blood levels of numerous medications, including **protease inhibitors** used for HIV. Case reports indicate St. John's wort also lowers blood levels of the non-nucleoside reverse transcriptase inhibitor nevirapine. **The bottom line:** If you have HIV, don't take St. John's wort! Furthermore, if you have been stabilized on HIV medications while taking St. John's wort and if you stop taking the herb, your blood levels of the drugs could rise, potentially leading to increased side effects.

Rifampin

TRADE NAMES: *Rifadin, Rimactane*
Vitamin D—Supplementation Possibly Helpful
See also *Antibiotics (General).*

R ifampin is often used along with isoniazid for the treatment of tuberculosis.

Vitamin D

Supplementation Possibly Helpful

Rifampin might interfere with the metabolism of **vitamin D**. Although it is not clear whether this interaction actually causes vitamin D deficiency, making sure that you get enough vitamin D on general principle is probably a good idea.

Selective Serotonin-Reuptake Inhibitors

5-Hydroxytryptophan (5-HTP), S-Adenosylmethionine (SAMe)—Possible Harmful Interaction

St. John's Wort—Possible Harmful Interaction

Folate—Supplementation Possibly Helpful

Ginkgo—Supplementation Probably Not Helpful

Ephedra—Supplementation probably not helpful

Since the development of Prozac, the first of the selective serotonin-reuptake inhibitors (SSRIs), this family of drugs has been expanding. The SSRIs are used for both severe and mild to moderate depression as well as for a variety of other conditions. These drugs work primarily by altering the action of the neurotransmitter (chemical messenger) serotonin in the brain. SSRI antidepressants include

➤ citalopram (Celexa),
➤ fluoxetine (Prozac),
➤ fluvoxamine (Luvox),
➤ paroxetine (Paxil),
➤ sertraline (Zoloft),
➤ and others.

Other antidepressants that increase serotonin activity include

➤ nefazodone (Serzone),
➤ trazodone (Desyrel),
➤ and venlafaxine (Effexor).

5-Hydroxytryptophan (5-HTP), S-Adenosylmethionine (SAMe)

Possible Harmful Interaction

The body uses the natural substance **5-hydroxytryptophan** (5-HTP) to manufacture serotonin and supplemental forms have been used for treating depression and migraine headaches.

S-adenosylmethionine (SAMe) is a naturally occurring compound derived from the amino acid methionine and the energy molecule adenosine triphosphate (ATP). SAMe is widely used as a supplement for treating osteoarthritis and depression.

Based on one case report and current thinking about how they work, SAMe and 5-HTP should not be taken with SSRIs, as they might increase the risk of serotonin syndrome.

This syndrome is a toxic reaction brought on by too much serotonin activity. The condition requires immediate medical attention, with symptoms including anxiety, restlessness, confusion, weakness, tremor, muscle twitching or spasm, high fever, profuse sweating, and rapid heartbeat.

The report describes a case of apparent serotonin syndrome in an individual taking SAMe with clomipramine, a **tricyclic antidepressant** that increases serotonin activity.

Although SAMe is not currently known to affect serotonin, it does appear to have antidepressant effects and may in some way increase serotonin activity.

Because SSRIs increase serotonin activity even more than clomipramine, a similar problem might occur if you combine SAMe with an SSRI.

The supplement 5-HTP is used by the body to manufacture serotonin, so it could also increase the risk of serotonin syndrome when combined with an SSRI.

St. John's Wort

Possible Harmful Interaction

The herb **St. John's wort** (*Hypericum perforatum*) is primarily used to treat mild to moderate depression. One of its actions appears to be increasing the activity of serotonin in the brain.

If you are taking an SSRI medication, do not take the herb St. John's wort at the same time. It is possible that your serotonin levels might be raised too high, causing a dangerous condition called serotonin syndrome (please see previous topic).

Several case reports appear to bear this out. Serotonin syndrome was reported in five elderly individuals who began using St. John's wort while taking sertraline (four reports) or nefazodone (one report). One individual had symptoms resembling serotonin syndrome after combining paroxetine (50 mg daily) and St. John's wort (600 mg daily). Another person taking St. John's wort with two other serotonin-enhancing drugs was reported to experience serotonin syndrome.

Furthermore, if you wish to switch from an SSRI to St. John's wort, you may need to wait a few weeks for the SSRI to wash out of your system before it is safe to start taking the herb. The waiting time required depends on which SSRI you are taking. Ask your physician or pharmacist for advice.

Folate

Supplementation Possibly Helpful

Folate is a B vitamin that offers many important health benefits. Not only does it help prevent birth defects and possibly reduce the risk of heart disease, a recent study suggests that folate can also help SSRI antidepressants work better.

In this double-blind, placebo-controlled trial, 127 individuals with severe depression were given either Prozac plus folate (500 mcg daily) or Prozac alone. Researchers wanted to see whether the vitamin would increase the medication's effectiveness.

The results were different for men and women. Female participants definitely benefited from receiving folate along with the medication. While just under 50% of the women taking Prozac alone fully recovered from their depression, combination treatment produced a recovery rate of nearly 75%. This is a very marked difference and one that makes a strong case for combining folate with antidepressant therapy.

Men, however, did not do any better on combination treatment than on Prozac alone. Researchers found evidence that a higher dose would have been necessary for male participants, perhaps 800 to 1,000 mcg daily. However, for dosages this high, medical supervision is necessary.

Ginkgo

Supplementation Probably Not Helpful

SSRIs can cause many sexual side effects, including inability to achieve orgasm (in women) and impotence (in men). Case reports and open studies raised hopes that the herb **ginkgo** could help reverse these problems. However, only double-blind, placebo-controlled studies can truly establish efficacy of a treatment, and when studies of this type were finally performed to evaluate ginkgo's potential effectiveness for this purpose, no benefits were seen.

Ephedra

Supplementation probably not helpful

As with ginkgo, ephedrine (extracted from the herb **ephedra**) does not appear any more effective than placebo for treatment of female sexual dysfunction caused by SSRIs.

Spironolactone/Hydrochlorothiazide

TRADE NAMES: *Aldactazide*

This medication is a combination of the following drugs:

➤ Potassium-Sparing Diuretics
➤ Thiazide Diuretics

Please see the separate articles on each one to find out about potential drug interactions. The interactions for each may be different, so read both articles carefully to find out the whole story.

Statin Drugs

Chaparral, Comfrey, and Coltsfoot—Possible Harmful Interaction

St. John's Wort—Possible Harmful Interaction

Grapefruit Juice—Possible Harmful Interaction

Vitamin B$_3$—Possible Benefits and Risks

Red Yeast Rice—Possible Harmful Interaction

Coenzyme Q$_{10}$ (CoQ$_{10}$)—Supplementation Probably Helpful

Fish Oil—Supplementation Probably Helpful

The statin drugs, also known as HMG-CoA reductase inhibitors, are the most popular and powerful medications for lowering cholesterol. They work by interfering with HMG-CoA reductase, an enzyme necessary for the body's manufacture of cholesterol. Drugs in this family include

- ➤ atorvastatin calcium (Lipitor),
- ➤ fluvastatin (Lescol),
- ➤ lovastatin (Mevacor),
- ➤ pravastatin (Pravachol),
- ➤ simvastatin (Zocor),
- ➤ and others.

Chaparral, Comfrey, and Coltsfoot

Possible Harmful Interaction

The herb chaparral (*Larrea tridentate* or *L. mexicana*) has been promoted for use in arthritis, cancer, and various other conditions, but there is insufficient evidence supporting its effectiveness. There are, however, concerns about its apparent liver toxicity.

Several cases of chaparral-induced liver damage have been reported, some of them severe enough to require liver transplantation.

Based on these reports, combining chaparral with other agents that are hard on the liver, such as statin drugs, may amplify the risk of potential liver problems. Other herbs that are toxic to the liver include comfrey (*Symphytum officinale*) and coltsfoot (*Tussilago farfara*).

St. John's Wort

Possible Harmful Interaction

The herb **St. John's wort**, used to treat depression, may decrease blood levels of various drugs in the statin family, including simvastatin, lovastatin, and atorvastatin (but not pravastatin).

Grapefruit Juice

Possible Harmful Interaction

Grapefruit juice impairs the body's normal breakdown of several drugs, including statins, allowing them to build up to potentially excessive levels in the blood. A recent study indicates that this effect can last for 3 days or more following the last glass of juice.

Because this could increase the risk of serious drug side effects, if you take interacting statins, the safest approach is to avoid grapefruit juice altogether. Grapefruit juice may not affect fluvastatin or pravastatin because these drugs are broken down differently than other statins.

Vitamin B$_3$

Possible Benefits and Risks

Niacin (nicotinic acid) is **vitamin B$_3$**. In high doses (often 1,500 mg daily or more), niacin is effective in lowering cholesterol levels. Its other form, niacinamide (nicotinamide), does not affect cholesterol.

Combining high-dose niacin with statin drugs further improves cholesterol profile by raising HDL ("good") cholesterol. Unfortunately, there are real concerns that this combination therapy could cause a potentially fatal condition called rhabdomyolysis.

A growing body of evidence, however, suggests that the risk is relatively slight in individuals with healthy kidneys. Furthermore, even much lower doses of niacin than the usual dose given to improve cholesterol levels (100 mg versus 1,000 mg or more) may provide a similar benefit. At this dose, the risk of rhabdomyolysis should be decreased. Nonetheless, it is not safe to try this combination except under close physician supervision.

Red Yeast Rice

Possible Harmful Interaction

Red yeast rice is an herbal cholesterol-lowering therapy. It contains a mixture of statins; its primary statin ingredient is lovastatin, making it most closely resemble the prescription drug Mevacor.

Based on the similarity of red yeast rice to statin drugs, the two should not be combined without medical supervision.

Coenzyme Q_{10} (CoQ_{10})

Supplementation Probably Helpful

Coenzyme Q_{10} (CoQ_{10}) is a vitamin-like substance that plays a fundamental role in the body's energy production and appears to be important for normal heart function.

Statin drugs inhibit the enzyme necessary for the body's synthesis of both cho-lesterol and CoQ_{10}. Several studies (including two double-blind trials) have found that these drugs reduce CoQ_{10} levels in the body. Because statin drugs are used to protect the heart by lowering cholesterol levels, their effect of inhibiting CoQ_{10} production might be counterproductive.

Taking CoQ_{10} supplements prevents the lowering of CoQ_{10} levels caused by statin drugs and does so without interfering with their therapeutic effects. However, as yet there is only minimal evidence that supplementation provides any benefit.

One study found that statin-induced lowering of tissue CoQ_{10} levels may worsen heart function in people with cardiomyopathy, a disease of the heart muscle. Individuals most vulnerable to this effect appear to be those with low CoQ_{10} levels and impaired heart function to begin with. When the study participants were given oral CoQ_{10} supplementation (100 to 200 mg/day), their CoQ_{10} blood levels increased and their deteriorating heart function improved.

Another study in a broader population failed to find any correlation between levels of CoQ_{10} and rate of adverse events. This was an observational study, however, and therefore not very reliable.

Fish Oil

Supplementation Probably Helpful

Fish oil is thought to help prevent heart disease. A 1-year, double-blind, placebo-controlled trial found that use of fish oil enhanced the benefits of simvastatin, further reducing triglyceride levels.

Sulfonamide Drugs

See *Trimethoprim/Sulfamethoxazole.*

Tamoxifen

TRADE NAME: *Nolvadex*

Tangeretin—Possible Harmful Interaction

Soy Isoflavones—Mixed Interaction

Tamoxifen is a drug related to estrogen. It is called an agonist/antagonist because it blocks the actions of estrogen and at the same time produces some estrogen-like actions. Tamoxifen is primarily used for the prevention and treatment of breast cancer.

Tangeretin

Possible Harmful Interaction

Tangeretin is a bioflavonoid found in citrus fruit and some **citrus bioflavonoid** supplements. Animal studies suggest that high intake of tangeretin reduces the effectiveness of tamoxifen. For this reason, people using tamoxifen should avoid supplements containing tangeretin and should also probably avoid excessive intake of citrus fruit.

Soy Isoflavones

Mixed Interaction

Like tamoxifen, **soy isoflavones** have both estrogen-like and anti-estrogen actions. Test-tube and animal studies suggest that relatively low doses of soy isoflavones interfere with the ability of tamoxifen to inhibit breast cancer growth, but high doses of isoflavones augment the effectiveness of tamoxifen.

Tetracyclines

Minerals—Take at a Different Time of Day
St. John's Wort, Dong Quai—Possible Harmful Interaction
Citrate—Possible Harmful Interaction
See also *Antibiotics (General).*

Tetracycline antibiotics are used to treat certain infections, such as chlamydia, as well as for the long-term treatment of acne. Drugs in this family include

➤ demeclocycline hydrochloride (Declomycin),
➤ doxycycline (Bio-Tab, Doryx, Doxy-Caps, Doxychel, Monodox, Periostat, Vibramycin, Vibra-Tabs),
➤ minocycline hydrochloride (Dynacin, Minocin, Vectrin),
➤ oxytetracycline hydrochloride (Terramycin, Uri-Tet),
➤ tetracycline hydrochloride (Achromycin V, Panmycin, Robitet, Sumycin, Teline, Tetracap, Tetracyn, Tetralan),
➤ and others.

Minerals

Take at a Different Time of Day

Numerous minerals, including aluminum (found in many antacids), bismuth (in Pepto-Bismol), **calcium**, **iron**, **magnesium**, and **zinc**, interfere with the absorption of medications in the tetracycline family (and vice versa).

The reason is that the minerals and the drugs attach to each other and form insoluble chemicals that simply pass out of the digestive tract. The best solution is to avoid taking supplements that contain these minerals within the 2 hours before or after your dose of tetracycline medication.

Dong Quai, St. John's Wort

Possible Harmful Interaction

Tetracycline antibiotics have been reported to cause increased sensitivity to the sun, amplifying the risk of sunburn or skin rash. Because St. John's wort and dong quai may also cause this problem, taking these herbal supplements during tetracycline treatment might add to this risk.

It may be a good idea to wear a sunscreen or protective clothing during sun exposure if you take one of these herbs with a tetracycline antibiotic.

Citrate

Possible Harmful Interaction

Potassium citrate, sodium citrate, and potassium-magnesium citrate are sometimes used to prevent kidney stones. These supplements reduce urinary acidity, and can therefore lead to decreased blood levels and effectiveness of tetracycline antibiotics.

Theophylline

TRADE NAMES: *Accurbron, Aerolate, Aquaphyllin, Asmalix, Elixomin, Elixophyllin, Lanophyllin, Quibron-T, Quibron-T-SR, Slo-bid, Slo-Phyllin, T-Phyl, Theo-24, Theo-Dur, Theo-Sav, Theo-X, Theobid, Theochron, Theoclear L.A., Theoclear-80, Theolair, Theolair-SR, Theospan-SR, Theostat 80, Theovent, Uni-Dur, Uniphyl*

RELATED DRUGS:
Aminophylline
    Phyllocontin, Somophyllin, Somophyllin-DF, Truphylline
Dyphylline
    Dilor, Lufyllin
Oxtriphylline
    Choledyl, Choledyl-SA
Vitamin B$_6$—Supplementation Possibly Helpful
St. John's Wort—Possible Interference with Action of Drug
Cayenne—Possible Increased Risk of Toxicity
Ipriflavone—Possible Increased Risk of Toxicity

Once among the most common treatments for asthma, theophylline is no longer widely used, having been replaced by drugs that cause fewer side effects.

Vitamin B$_6$

Supplementation Possibly Helpful

Theophylline appears to impair the normal conversion of **vitamin B$_6$** into the more active substance pyridoxal 5'-phosphate (PLP). These findings have led some researchers to suspect that some of the many side effects of theophylline could be caused, at least in part, by interference with B$_6$ activity. Indeed, one study found that B$_6$ supplements might help reduce theophylline-induced tremors.

St. John's Wort

Possible Interference with Action of Drug

Evidence suggests the herb **St. John's wort** can lower blood levels of theophylline, making it less effective.

Cayenne

Possible Increased Risk of Toxicity

Oral **cayenne** might increase the absorption of theophylline, which could lead to an increased risk of theophylline toxicity.

Ipriflavone

Possible Increased Risk of Toxicity

Like cayenne, the supplement **ipriflavone** may increase levels of theophylline in the body, possibly increasing the risk of toxicity.

Thiazide Diuretics

Potassium—Probable Need for Supplementation
Magnesium—Supplementation Possibly Helpful
Calcium—Possible Dangerous Interaction
Coenzyme Q_{10} (CoQ_{10})—Supplementation Possibly Helpful
Zinc—Supplementation Possibly Helpful
Licorice—Possible Dangerous Interaction

Thiazide diuretics are commonly used to treat hypertension. Drugs in this family include

➤ bendroflumethiazide (Naturetin),
➤ benzthiazide (Exna),
➤ chlorothiazide (Diurigen, Diuril),
➤ chlorthalidone (Hygroton, Thalitone),
➤ hydrochlorothiazide (Esidrix, Ezide, HydroDIURIL, Hydro-Par, Microzide, Oretic),
➤ hydroflumethiazide (Diucardin, Saluron),
➤ indapamide (Lozol),
➤ methyclothiazide (Aquatensen, Enduron),
➤ metolazone (Mykrox, Zaroxolyn),
➤ polythiazide (Renese),
➤ quinethazone (Hydromox),
➤ trichlormethiazide (Diurese, Metahydrin, Naqua),
➤ and others.

Potassium

Probable Need for Supplementation

Thiazide diuretics cause a constant and significant loss of potassium. The classic treatment for this is to eat bananas and drink orange juice. Potassium supplements are also frequently prescribed.

Medications that combine thiazides and potassium-sparing diuretics might produce an unpredictable effect on potassium levels in the body. If you are taking such medications, do not increase your potassium intake except on the advice of your physician.

Magnesium

Supplementation Possibly Helpful

Long-term use (more than 6 months) of thiazide diuretics might lead to **magnesium** deficiency. In turn, this loss of magnesium can increase the depletion of potassium.

Since magnesium deficiency is common anyway, if you take thiazide diuretics it would certainly make sense to take magnesium supplements at the U.S. Dietary Reference Intake (formerly known as the Recommended Dietary Allowance) dosage.

Calcium

Possible Dangerous Interaction

When taken over the long term, thiazide diuretics tend to increase levels of **calcium** by decreasing the amount excreted by the body and, indirectly, by affecting vitamin D. It's not likely that this will cause a problem. However, since greatly increased calcium levels in the body can cause side effects such as calcium deposits, if you are using thiazide diuretics you should consult with your physician on the proper dose of calcium and vitamin D for you.

Coenzyme Q_{10} (CoQ_{10})

Supplementation Possibly Helpful

Preliminary evidence suggests that thiazide diuretics might impair the body's ability to synthesize **coenzyme Q_{10}** (CoQ_{10}), a substance important for normal heart function. Although we don't know for sure that taking CoQ_{10} supplements will provide any specific benefit, supplementing with CoQ_{10} on general principle might be a good idea.

Zinc

Supplementation Possibly Helpful

Reportedly, thiazide diuretics can cause loss of **zinc** in the urine. Since zinc deficiency is relatively common, you should probably make sure that you get enough zinc when using these drugs.

Licorice

Possible Dangerous Interaction

If you are using thiazide diuretics, do not take **licorice** root. Licorice root could exacerbate the potassium depletion caused by thiazides. However, the special form of licorice known as DGL (deglycyrrhizinated licorice) should not cause this problem.

Thyroid Hormone

Calcium—Take at a Different Time of Day
Iron—Take at a Different Time of Day
Soy—Possible Harmful Interaction
Carnitine—Supplementation Possibly Helpful

Thyroid hormone supplements are primarily used to treat hypothyroidism, a condition caused by deficient secretion of thyroid hormone by the thyroid gland. Forms of thyroid hormone include

- dextrothyroxine (Choloxin),
- levothyroxine (Levoid, Levothroid, Levoxine, Levoxyl, Synthroid),
- liothyronine (Cytomel, Triostat),
- liotrix (Euthroid, Thyrolar),
- thyroglobulin (Proloid),
- and thyroid (Armour Thyroid).

Calcium

Take at a Different Time of Day

Two case reports suggest that calcium carbonate interferes with the body's absorption of thyroid hormone when both were taken at the same time.

A prospective cohort study has validated these case reports. Twenty individuals with hypothyroidism stabilized on long-term levothyroxine therapy were included in the trial. Participants were given calcium carbonate (1,200 mg daily of elemental calcium) for 3 months. During the period the calcium supplement was taken, thyroid hormone blood levels declined. But after calcium supplementation was stopped, thyroid levels climbed back up, slightly surpassing the levels measured at the beginning of the study.

It is thought that calcium chelates (combines) with thyroid hormone, thus reducing its absorption.

To prevent this interaction, take thyroid hormone and calcium supplements as far apart as possible.

Iron

Take at a Different Time of Day

Iron salts (including ferrous fumarate, ferrous gluconate, ferrous sulfate, and iron polysaccharide) may impair the effect of the thyroid hormone levothyroxine, probably by forming a complex with it and decreasing its absorption.

To prevent a problem, take iron supplements and thyroid hormones as far apart as possible.

Soy

Possible Harmful Interaction

Soy formula may interfere with the absorption of thyroid medication in infants. In addition, soy may directly interfere with thyroid function. The result may be a need to increase the infant's dosage of thyroid medication. However, if you stop giving an infant soy formula, the thyroid dosage may need to be decreased. Of course, all changes relating to thyroid treatment should be managed by a physician.

Based on these findings, individuals with impaired thyroid function should use soy (such as soybeans, soy milk, tofu) with caution.

Carnitine

Supplementation Possibly Helpful

Individuals with an enlarged thyroid gland are some-times given high doses of thyroid medication to shrink it. However, this treatment can cause unpleasant side effects, including bone loss, heart palpitations, and a feeling of malaise. A double-blind trial suggests that the supplement **L-carnitine** may safely reduce the adverse effects of this treatment.

Ticlopidine

TRADE NAMES: *Ticlid*

Ticlopidine is a drug that makes the blood clot less easily. It is used to reduce the risk of strokes, heart attacks, and other conditions caused by blood clots.

Numerous herbs and natural supplements might in-terfere with the ability of the blood to clot as well. If they are taken with clopidogrel, excess bleeding might occur. For a discussion of all these natural products, see the **Warfarin** article.

Tramadol

TRADE NAMES: *Ultram*

St. John's Wort, 5-Hydroxytryptophan (5-HTP), S-Adenosylmethionine (SAMe)—Possible Dangerous
   Interactions

Tramadol is a unique non-narcotic and non-anti-inflammatory analgesic medication used for the treat-ment of moderate pain. It has many effects in the body, including some that relate to endorphins and others that involve serotonin.

St. John's Wort, 5-Hydroxytryptophan (5-HTP), S-Adenosylmethionine (SAMe)

Possible Dangerous Interactions

There are two case reports that possibly implicate trama-dol in serotonin syndrome. This syndrome is caused by excessive levels of serotonin, which bring about various dangerous side effects.

Since **St. John's wort** and **5-Hydroxytryptophan (5-HTP)** might increase serotonin levels, and **S-adenosyl-methionine (SAMe)** has reportedly caused serotonin syn-drome, combining any of them with tramadol could be risky.

Triamterene/Hydrochlorothiazide

TRADE NAMES: *Dyazide, Maxzide*

This medication is a combination of the following drugs:

➤ Potassium-Sparing Diuretics
➤ Thiazide Diuretics

Please see the separate articles on each one to find out about potential drug interactions. The interactions for each may be different, so read both articles carefully to find out the whole story.

Tricyclic Antidepressants

Coenzyme Q_{10} (CoQ_{10})—Supplementation Possibly Helpful

St. John's Wort, Yohimbe, 5-Hydroxytryptophan (5-HTP), S-Adenosylmethionine (SAMe)—Possible Dangerous Interactions

St. John's Wort—Possible Harmful Interaction

For many years, the tricyclics were the most popular antidepressants. Although superseded today by the less side-effect prone SSRI drugs (Prozac family), they are still used in certain cases.

Antidepressants in this family include

➤ amitriptyline hydrochloride (Elavil),
➤ amoxapine (Asendin),
➤ clomipramine hydrochloride (Anafranil),
➤ desipramine hydrochloride (Norpramin),
➤ doxepin hydrochloride (Sinequan),
➤ imipramine (Tofranil),
➤ nortriptyline hydrochloride (Aventyl, Pamelor),
➤ protriptyline hydrochloride (Vivactil),
➤ trimipramine maleate (Surmontil),
➤ and others.

Coenzyme Q_{10} (CoQ_{10})

Supplementation Possibly Helpful

Preliminary evidence suggests that tricyclic antidepressants might deplete the body of coenzyme Q_{10} (CoQ_{10}), a substance that appears to be important for normal heart function. Based on this observation, it has been suggested (but not proved) that CoQ_{10} supplementation might help prevent the heart-related side effects that can occur with the use of tricyclic antidepressants.

St. John's Wort, Yohimbe, 5-Hydroxytryptophan (5-HTP), S-Adenosylmethionine (SAMe)

Possible Dangerous Interactions

Based on one case report and our general knowledge about the actions of **St. John's Wort, yohimbe, 5-HTP, SAMe**, taking any of these in combination with some tricyclic antidepressants could conceivably present a risk of elevating serotonin levels too high.

St. John's Wort

Possible Harmful Interaction

St. John's wort might decrease the effectiveness of tricyclic antidepressants by reducing blood levels of the drug. Conversely, if you are taking St. John's wort already and your physician adjusts your dose of medication, suddenly stopping the herb could cause blood levels of the drug to rise dangerously high.

Trimethoprim/Sulfamethoxazole

ALTERNATE NAMES: *TMP-SMZ*

TRADE NAMES: *Bactrim, Cotrim, Septra, Sulfatrim*

Folate—Supplementation Likely Helpful

Para-Aminobenzoic Acid (PABA)—Interference with Action of Drug

Potassium—Possible Harmful Interaction

White Willow—Possible Negative Interaction

St. John's Wort, Other Herbs—Potential Increased Risk of Photosensitivity

See also *Antibiotics (General)*.

Trimethoprim (Proloprim, Trimpex) is commonly combined with sulfamethoxazole (Gantanol) for an antibiotic combination that gives a one-two punch against bacteria.

Folate

Supplementation Likely Helpful

Both trimethoprim and sulfamethoxazole interfere with **folate**: The sulfamethoxazole makes it hard for invading bacteria to manufacture folate and the trimethoprim makes it hard for bacteria to use the folate. The net effect is to starve the bacteria of this necessary vitamin.

Humans and other mammals are much less affected by these antibiotics than are bacteria, due to the different way we process folate. However, trimethoprim can still interfere to some extent in your body's ability to utilize this essential nutrient. Folate supplementation may be helpful if you take this antibiotic for a long period of time (to prevent urinary tract infections, for example).

Para-Aminobenzoic Acid (PABA)

Interference with Action of Drug

The supplement **PABA** may make trimethoprim/sulfamethoxazole less effective. If you are being treated with this drug, do not take PABA except on medical advice.

Potassium

Possible Harmful Interaction

Trimethoprim/sulfamethoxazole might increase levels of **potassium** in the body. Therefore, if you are on long-term treatment with this antibiotic, you should not take potassium supplements except on the advice of a physician.

White Willow

Possible Negative Interaction

The herb **white willow** contains substances very similar to aspirin. On this basis, it might not be advisable to combine white willow with trimethoprim or sulfamethoxazole.

St. John's Wort, Other Herbs

Potential Increased Risk of Photosensitivity

Sulfa drugs can cause increased sensitivity to the sun. Various herbs, including **St. John's wort** and **dong quai**, can also cause this problem. Combined treatment with herb and drug might increase the risk further.

Valproic Acid

TRADE NAMES: *Depakene*

Carnitine—Supplementation Possibly Helpful

Vitamin D—Supplementation Possibly Helpful

Folate—Supplementation Possibly Helpful

Melatonin—Supplementation Possibly Helpful

Biotin—Supplementation Possibly Helpful, but Take at a Different Time of Day

Vitamin A—Possible Increased Risk of Birth Defects

Glutamine—Theoretical Harmful Interaction

White Willow—Possible Negative Interaction

Ginkgo—Possible Harmful Interaction

Dong Quai, St. John's Wort—Possible Harmful Interaction

Valproic acid is a commonly used anticonvulsant treatment. Drugs in this family include

➤ Divalproex Sodium,
➤ Depakote,
➤ Depakote Sprinkle,
➤ Sodium Valproate,
➤ and Depakene Syrup.

Carnitine

Supplementation Possibly Helpful

Carnitine is an amino acid that has been used for heart conditions, Alzheimer's disease, and intermittent claudication (a possible complication of atherosclerosis in which impaired blood circulation causes severe pain in calf muscles during walking or exercising).

Long-term therapy with anticonvulsant agents, particularly valproic acid, is associated with low levels of carnitine. However, it isn't clear whether the anticonvulsants cause the carnitine deficiency or whether it occurs for other reasons. It has been hypothesized that low carnitine levels may contribute to valproic acid's damaging effects on the liver. The risk of this liver damage increases in children younger than 24 months and carnitine supplementation does seem to be protective. However, in one double-blind, crossover study, carnitine supplementation produced no real improvement in "well-being" as assessed by parents of children receiving either valproic acid or carbamazepine.

L-carnitine supplementation may be advisable in certain cases, such as in infants and young children (especially those younger than 2 years) who have neurologic disorders and are receiving valproic acid and multiple anticonvulsants.

Vitamin D

Supplementation Possibly Helpful

Valproic acid slows down the liver's conversion of **vitamin D** into the active form of the vitamin that can be used by the body. This effect might lead to reduced calcium absorption, since the body needs active vitamin D to absorb calcium properly. Therefore, it might be advisable to take vitamin D supplements at the U.S. Adequate Intake (AI) dosage.

Folate

Supplementation Possibly Helpful

Folate (also known as folic acid) is a B vitamin that plays an important role in many vital aspects of health, including preventing neural tube birth defects and possibly reducing the risk of heart disease. Because inadequate intake of folate is widespread, if you are taking any medication that depletes or impairs folate even slightly, you may need supplementation.

Valproic acid appears to decrease the body's absorption of folate, and other antiseizure drugs can also reduce levels of folate in the body.

The low serum folate caused by anticonvulsants can

raise homocysteine levels, a condition believed to increase the risk of heart disease.

Adequate folate intake is also necessary to prevent neural tube birth defects, such as spina bifida and anencephaly. Because anticonvulsant drugs deplete folate, babies born to women taking anticonvulsants are at increased risk for such birth defects. Anticonvulsants may also play a more direct role in the development of birth defects.

However, the case for taking extra folate during anticonvulsant therapy is not as simple as it might seem. It is possible that folate supplementation might itself impair the effectiveness of anticonvulsant drugs, and physician supervision is necessary.

Melatonin

Supplementation Possibly Helpful

One double-blind study in children found that use of **melatonin** improved general quality of life in children on valproic acid. The most obvious way melatonin might help would involve improvements in sleep, as melatonin is a widely used treatment for insomnia. Another rather theoretical study by the same author suggests it might help in other, more subtle ways that involve the body's biochemistry.

Biotin

Supplementation Possibly Helpful, but Take at a Different Time of Day

Many antiseizure medications, including valproic acid, are believed to interfere with the absorption of **biotin**. For this reason, individuals taking valproic acid may benefit from extra biotin. Biotin should be taken 2 to 3 hours apart from your antiseizure medication. Do not exceed the recommended daily intake, because it is possible that too much biotin might interfere with the effectiveness of the medication.

Vitamin A

Possible Increased Risk of Birth Defects

Both valproic acid and **vitamin A** can increase the risk of birth defects. The effect might be additive, indicating that pregnant women should avoid such combination treatment.

Glutamine

Theoretical Harmful Interaction

Because valproic acid works (at least in part) by blocking glutamate pathways in the brain, high dosages of **glutamine** might possibly overwhelm the drug and increase the risk of seizures.

White Willow

Possible Negative Interaction

The herb **white willow** contains substances very similar to aspirin. On this basis, it might not be advisable to combine white willow with valproic acid.

Ginkgo

Possible Harmful Interaction

The herb **ginkgo** is widely used for improving memory and mental function. Seizures have also been reported with the use of ginkgo leaf extract in people with previously well-controlled epilepsy; in one case, the seizures were fatal. One possible explanation is contamination of ginkgo leaf products with ginkgo seeds. It has also been suggested that ginkgo might interfere with the effectiveness of some antiseizure medications, including phenytoin. Finally, it has been noted that the drug tacrine (also used to improve memory) has been associated with seizures and ginkgo may affect the brain in ways similar to tacrine.

Dong Quai, St. John's Wort

Possible Harmful Interaction

Valproic acid has been reported to cause increased sensitivity to the sun, amplifying the risk of sunburn or skin rash. Because **St. John's wort** and **dong quai** may also cause this problem, taking them during treatment with this drug might add to this risk.

Warfarin

TRADE NAMES: *Coumadin*

Alfalfa—Possible Harmful Interaction

Chamomile—Possible Harmful Interaction

Chondroitin—Possible Harmful Interaction

Coenzyme Q_{10} (CoQ_{10})—Possible Harmful Interaction

Cranberry—Possible Harmful interaction

Danshen—Possible Harmful Interaction

Devil's Claw—Possible Harmful Interaction

Dong Quai—Possible Harmful Interaction

Feverfew—Possible Harmful Interaction

Garlic—Possible Harmful Interaction

Ginger—Possible Harmful Interaction

Ginkgo—Possible Harmful Interaction

Ginseng—Possible Harmful Interaction

Low Carb, High Protein Diet—Possible Harmful Interaction

Green Tea—Possible Harmful Interaction

Ipriflavone—Possible Harmful Interaction

Papain, Bromelain—Possible Harmful Interaction

Vinpocetine—Possible Harmful Interaction

PC-SPES—Possible Harmful Interaction

Policosanol—Possible Harmful Interaction

Reishi—Possible Harmful Interaction

Soy—Possible Harmful Interaction

St. John's Wort—Possible Harmful Interaction

Vitamin A—Possible Harmful Interaction

Vitamin C—Possible Harmful Interaction

Vitamin E—Possible Harmful Interaction

Vitamin K—Possible Harmful Interaction

White Willow—Possible Harmful Interaction

Other Herbs and Supplements—Possible Harmful Interaction

Warfarin (Coumadin) is an anticoagulant used to thin the blood and prevent it from clotting. It is a somewhat dangerous drug that can be affected by many substances, including foods. **Note:** If you are taking warfarin, we don't recommend taking any herb or supplement except on a physician's advice.

Similar blood-thinning drugs are anisindione (Miradon) and dicumarol.

Alfalfa

Possible Harmful Interaction

The herb **alfalfa** (*Medicago sativa*) is promoted for a variety of conditions. The relatively high vitamin K content in alfalfa could reduce the effectiveness of warfarin. Vitamin K directly counteracts warfarin's blood-thinning effects. Since the amount of vitamin K in alfalfa varies widely, it's difficult to give an exact safe upper dose.

As a precaution, avoid alfalfa supplements during warfarin therapy except under medical supervision.

Chamomile

Possible Harmful Interaction

The herb **chamomile** contains substances in the coumarin family. Some coumarins have blood thinning actions that could interact with warfarin. One case report exists of a person in which it appears that combined use of chamomile and warfarin led to internal bleeding.

Chondroitin

Possible Harmful Interaction

Based on **chondroitin's** chemical similarity to the anticoagulant drug heparin, it has been suggested that chondroitin might have anticoagulant effects as well. There are no case reports of any problems relating to this, and studies suggest that chondroitin has, at most, a mild anticoagulant effect. Nonetheless, prudence suggests that chondroitin should not be combined with warfarin except under physician supervision.

Coenzyme Q_{10} (CoQ_{10})

Possible Harmful Interaction

Coenzyme Q_{10} (CoQ_{10}) is a vitamin-like substance that plays a fundamental role in the body's energy production.

CoQ_{10} is somewhat similar in structure to vitamin K and, reportedly, it too can reduce the therapeutic effects of warfarin. In three case reports, CoQ_{10} was found to interfere with warfarin's blood-thinning effects. A double-blind study found no interaction between CoQ_{10} and warfarin. However, in view of warfarin's low margin of safety, prudence indicates physician supervision before combining CoQ_{10} with warfarin.

Cranberry

Possible Harmful interaction

Five case reports indicate that **cranberry** juice can increase warfarin's action, causing dangerous and potentially fatal bleeding problems. However, a formal study failed to find evidence of such an interaction. This study was somewhat indirect, however, in that it did not evaluate the effects of cranberry on warfarin action, but rather on another drug that is metabolized similarly in the body. Prudence would therefore suggest continued caution at this time.

Danshen

Possible Harmful Interaction

The herb **danshen**, the root of *Salvia miltorrhiza*, is used in traditional Chinese medicine for treating heart disease.

Preliminary evidence, including several case reports, suggests that danshen can dangerously increase the effects of warfarin and cause significant bleeding problems.

Therefore, if you take warfarin, you should avoid danshen except under a physician's supervision.

Devil's Claw

Possible Harmful Interaction

The herb **devil's claw** (*Harpogophytum procumbens*) is used for various types of arthritis and digestive problems.

According to one case report, devil's claw might increase the risk of abnormal bleeding when taken with warfarin.

As a precaution, you should probably not combine devil's claw and warfarin except under a physician's supervision.

Dong Quai

Possible Harmful Interaction

The herb **dong quai** (*Angelica sinensis*) is used for menstrual disorders.

According to one case report, dong quai may add to the blood-thinning effects of warfarin, thus increasing the risk of abnormal bleeding.

You should probably avoid combining dong quai and warfarin without medical supervision.

Feverfew

Possible Harmful Interaction

The herb **feverfew** (*Tanacetum parthenium*) is primarily used for the prevention and treatment of migraine headaches.

In vitro studies suggest that feverfew thins the blood

by interfering with the ability of blood platelets to clump together. This raises the concern that feverfew might increase the risk of abnormal bleeding when combined with warfarin. However, there is as yet no evidence that the blood-thinning effect of feverfew is significant in humans.

Though an additive effect of feverfew and warfarin appears to be theoretical at this time, it may be best to avoid this combination except under medical supervision.

Garlic

Possible Harmful Interaction

The herb **garlic** (*Allium sativum*) is taken to lower cholesterol, among many other proposed uses.

One of the possible side effects of garlic is an increased tendency to bleed. This blood-thinning effect has been demonstrated in a double-blind trial of garlic in 60 volunteers, as well as in other studies and one case report.

According to two other case reports, the blood-thinning effects of warfarin were greatly enhanced in individuals taking garlic. This could amplify the risk of bleeding problems.

Based on these findings, you should avoid combining garlic and warfarin except under a physician's supervision.

Ginger

Possible Harmful Interaction

The herb **ginger** (*Zingiber officianale*) is used for nausea associated with motion sickness, morning sickness in pregnancy, and the postsurgical period.

Ginger appears to thin the blood by interfering with the ability of blood platelets to clump together. As with feverfew, this raises the concern that ginger might increase the risk of abnormal bleeding when taken with warfarin. However, there is no evidence at present that the blood-thinning effect of ginger is significant in humans.

Though an additive effect of ginger and warfarin appears to be theoretical based on current evidence, it may be best to avoid this combination except under medical supervision. Ginger flavored drinks should not present a problem, but candies containing whole dried ginger are potentially of concern.

Ginkgo

Possible Harmful Interaction

The herb **ginkgo** (*Ginkgo biloba*) has been used to treat Alzheimer's disease and ordinary age-related memory loss, among many other uses.

Inconsistent evidence suggests that ginkgo might reduce the ability of platelets (blood-clotting cells) to stick together. In addition, several case reports suggest that use of ginkgo may be associated with an increased risk of serious abnormal bleeding episodes in individuals taking the herb. These findings raise concern that ginkgo might add to the blood-thinning effects of warfarin and there is one report of abnormal bleeding in an individual who had been taking the herb and drug together. However, two double-blind studies found no interaction between ginkgo and warfarin. These findings are reassuring. Nonetheless, in view of warfarin's low margin of safety, prudence indicates physician supervision before combining ginkgo with warfarin.

Ginseng

Possible Harmful Interaction

The herb **ginseng** (*Panax ginseng*) is promoted as an adaptogen, a treatment that is said to help the body adapt to stress of all types.

A case report suggest that *Panax ginseng* can reduce the anticoagulant effects of warfarin; however, two double-blind studies failed to find any interaction. In general, double-blind studies are far more reliable than case reports and, therefore, it would appear that there is not too much reason for concern regarding this potential interaction. However, another double-blind trial that evaluated the closely related American ginseng species (*Panax quinquefolius*) found that use of the herb reduced the anticoagulant effects of warfarin, similarly to what was seen in the case report. At this point, therefore, it is reasonable to suggest that caution should be exercised when combining ginseng and warfarin.

Low Carb, High Protein Diet

Possible Harmful Interaction

Low carbohydrate, high-protein diets have been advocated for weight loss. According to two case reports, adoption of such diets may decrease the effectiveness of warfarin, possibly by increasing blood levels of a substance called albumin that might tend to bind and inactivate warfarin in the body.

Green Tea

Possible Harmful Interaction

Green tea (*Camellia sinensis*) contains strong antioxidant substances and may have cancer-preventive effects.

Because green tea contains vitamin K, which directly interferes with warfarin's blood-thinning action, drinking large amounts of it might reduce the therapeutic effects of the drug.

I|priflavone

Possible Harmful Interaction

Ipriflavone, a synthetic isoflavone that slows bone breakdown, is used to treat osteoporosis.

Warfarin use increases the risk of osteoporosis. Because ipriflavone has been found to help prevent osteoporosis in certain circumstances, you might be tempted to consider taking this supplement while you use warfarin. However, some evidence indicates that ipriflavone might interfere with the body's normal breakdown of warfarin. This could raise the levels of warfarin in your body and increase the risk of abnormal bleeding.

If you try this combination, you need to do so under physician supervision.

Papain, Bromelain

Possible Harmful Interaction

One case report suggests that **papain**, a digestive enzyme found in papaya extract (*Carica papaya*), might add to warfarin's blood-thinning effect.

Vinpocetine

Possible Harmful Interaction

The substance **vinpocetine** is sold as a dietary supplement for the treatment of age-related memory loss and impaired mental function. Vinpocetine is thought to inhibit blood platelets from forming clots. For this reason, it should not be combined with medications or natural substances that impair the blood's ability to clot normally, as this may lead to excessive bleeding. One study found only a minimal interaction between the blood-thinning drug warfarin and vinpocetine (and it actually involved an *increased* tendency for blood clotting), but prudence dictates caution anyway.

PC-SPES

Possible Harmful Interaction

PC-SPES is an herbal combination that has shown promise for the treatment of prostate cancer. One case report suggests that PC-SPES might increase risk of bleeding complications if combined with blood-thinning medications. Subsequent evidence has indicated that PC-SPES actually contains warfarin, making this interaction inevitable.

Policosanol

Possible Harmful Interaction

Policosanol, derived from sugarcane, is used to reduce cholesterol levels. It also interferes with platelet clumping, creating a risk of interactions with blood-thinning drugs.

For example, a 30-day, double-blind, placebo-controlled trial of 27 individuals with high cholesterol levels found that policosanol at 10 mg daily markedly reduced the ability of blood platelets to clump together. Another double-blind, placebo-controlled study of 37 healthy volunteers found evidence that the blood-thinning effect of policosanol increased as the dose was increased—the larger the policosanol dose, the greater the effect. Yet another double-blind, placebo-controlled study of 43 healthy volunteers compared the effects of policosanol (20 mg daily), the blood-thinner aspirin (100 mg daily), and policosanol and aspirin combined at these same doses. The results again showed that policosanol substantially reduced the ability of blood platelets to stick together, and that the combined therapy exhibited additive effects.

Based on these findings, you should not combine warfarin and policosanol except under medical supervision.

Reishi

Possible Harmful Interaction

One study suggests that **reishi** impairs platelet clumping. This creates the potential for an interaction with any blood-thinning medication.

Soy

Possible Harmful Interaction

One case report indicates that **soy** milk might decrease warfarin's effectiveness.

St. John's Wort

Possible Harmful Interaction

The herb **St. John's wort** (*Hypericum perforatum*) is primarily used to treat mild to moderate depression.

Evidence suggests that St. John's wort may interfere with warfarin, possibly requiring an increased dosage of the drug to maintain the proper therapeutic effect. Seven cases have been reported in which the blood-thinning effects of warfarin have been impaired in individuals taking St. John's wort.

A "hidden" risk lies in this type of interaction. Suppose your physician has raised the warfarin dose to take into account the effect of St. John's wort in holding down drug levels. If you then stop taking the herbal product, it would be like releasing the brakes and your warfarin levels could surge dangerously high.

For these reasons, if you take warfarin, avoid St. John's wort except under a physician's supervision.

Vitamin A

Possible Harmful Interaction

Supplemental **vitamin A** might increase the blood-thinning effects of warfarin and this could potentially lead to an increased risk of abnormal bleeding.

For this reason, it may be best to avoid combining vitamin A with warfarin unless supervised by a physician.

Vitamin C

Possible Harmful Interaction

Vitamin C taken in high dosages (more than 1,000 mg daily) has been reported to *reduce* the blood-thinning effect of warfarin. In one case, the person was taking 1,000 mg of vitamin C daily; another involved huge megadoses (about 16,000 mg daily).

As a precaution, if you take warfarin, consult with your physician before taking high-dose vitamin C supplements.

Vitamin E

Possible Harmful Interaction

On the basis that **vitamin E** "thins" the blood, it has been suggested not to combine vitamin E with warfarin. However, a 4-week, double-blind study of 25 individuals taking warfarin found no additive effect. None of the participants taking vitamin E at a daily dose of 800 or 1,200 international units (IU) showed an increased risk for abnormal bleeding.

In contrast, a case report indicated that vitamin E (800 IU daily) added to the effects of warfarin and resulted in abnormal bleeding. Because this effect did not become apparent until the fourth week, it is possible that problems might take longer to develop than the 4-week period covered by the double-blind study or that certain individuals might be more prone to an interaction. An unpublished 30-day study of three volunteers taking a warfarin-like drug also found an additive effect with only 42 IU of vitamin E daily.

Though the evidence supporting a possible interaction is scanty, it is best not to risk serious bleeding problems. Avoid combining vitamin E with warfarin except under the supervision of a physician.

Vitamin K

Possible Harmful Interaction

Vitamin K is an antidote to warfarin—it directly counteracts warfarin's blood-thinning effects. This is true for both supplemental vitamin K and foods high in vitamin K. For this reason, eating more vitamin K–rich vegetables can decrease warfarin's therapeutic effect and eating less of these foods can increase the drug's effect. Either situation can lead to potential life-threatening complications.

Therefore, once you are established on a certain dose of warfarin, you should not change your usual intake of vitamin K without medical supervision.

White Willow

Possible Harmful Interaction

The herb **white willow** (*Salix alba*), also known as willow bark, is used to treat pain and fever. White willow contains a substance that is converted by the body into a salicylate similar to the blood-thinner aspirin.

Because white willow, like aspirin, may enhance the blood-thinning effects of warfarin, this combination should be avoided unless medically supervised.

Other Herbs and Supplements

Possible Harmful Interaction

One case report suggests that a combination of the herbs **boldo** and **fenugreek** increased the effects of warfarin. Another isolated case report suggests that the same can happen when fish oil is combined with warfarin.

Based on their known effects or the effects of their constituents, the following herbs and supplements might not be safe to combine with warfarin, though this has not been proven: **chamomile** (*Matricaria recutita*), ***Coleus forskohlii*, ginger** (*Zingiber officinale*), **horse chestnut** (*Aesculus hippocastanum*), papaya (*Carica papaya*), **red clover** (*Trifolium pratense*), and **reishi** (*Ganoderma lucidum*), **mesoglycan, fish oil, OPCs** (oligomeric proanthocyanidins), and **phosphatidylserine.**

INDEX